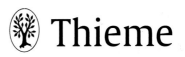

Gastroenterological Endoscopy

Meinhard Classen, MD
Professor Emeritus and former Chairman
Department of Internal Medicine
Technical University of Munich
Munich, Germany

Guido N. J. Tytgat, MD, PhD
Professor Emeritus of Gastroenterology
University of Amsterdam
Former Chief of Department of Gastroenterology
Academic Medical Center
Amsterdam, the Netherlands

Charles J. Lightdale, MD
Professor of Clinical Medicine and
Director of Clinical Research
Division of Digestive and Liver Diseases
New York Presbyterian Hospital/Columbia University
Medical Center
New York, USA

Associate Editors
Jacques J. G. J. M. Bergman, Alexander Meining,
D. Nageshwar Reddy, Hisao Tajiri, Michael B. Wallace

Second edition

With contributions by

Douglas G. Adler, Furqaan Ahmed, Hans-Dieter Allescher, Anthony T. R. Axon, Rami J. Badreddine, John Baillie, Juergen Barnert, Todd H. Baron, Hugh Barr, J. F. W. M. Bartelsman, Witold Bartnik, Vikram Bhatia, David Bjorkman, Wojciech Blonski, Lawrence J. Brandt, Marco J. Bruno, Andrew K. Burroughs, David Cave, Jean-Pierre Charton, Evangelos Cholongitas, Meinhard Classen, Guido Costamagna, Stefan von Delius, Michel Delvaux, James A. DiSario, Steven A. Edmundowicz, Axel Eickhoff, Shungo Endo, Pietro Familiari, Paul Feuerstadt, Hubertus Feußner, David E. Fleischer, Evan L. Fogel, Victor L. Fox, Gérard Gay, Karel Geboes, Joseph E. Geenen, Nalini M. Guda, Neil Gupta, Gregory B. Haber, Robert H. Hawes, Juergen Hochberger, Keiichi Ikeda, John M. Inadomi, Sreeni Jonnalagadda, Michael Jung, Abdel M. Kassem, Ralf Kiesslich, Kiyonori Kobayashi, David Kotlyar, Richard A. Kozarek, Shin-ei Kudo, Spiros D. Ladas, James Y. W. Lau, Glen A. Lehman, Blair S. Lewis, Gary R. Lichtenstein, Jenifer R. Lightdale, Juergen Maiss, Elisabeth M. H. Mathus-Vliegen, Koji Matsuda, Kai Matthes, Helmut Messmann, Hideyuki Miyachi, Faris M. Murad, Horst Neuhaus, H. Juergen Nord, Hiroyuki Ono, Jacek Pachlewski, Sandy H. Y. Pang, Shabana F. Pasha, Andrew T. Pellecchia, Jan-Werner Poley, Thierry Ponchon, Jeffrey L. Ponsky, Benjamin K. Poulose, Christian Prinz, D. Nageshwar Reddy, Jaroslaw Regula, Juergen F. Riemann, Thomas Roesch, Gurpal S. Sandha, Yasushi Sano, Shiv K. Sarin, Brian Saunders, Stefan Seewald, Marco Senzolo, Prateek Sharma, Stuart Sherman, Chan-Sup Shim, Nathan J. Shores, Nib Soehendra, Ma Somsouk, Joseph J. Y. Sung, Paul Swain, Hisao Tajiri, Shinji Tanaka, George Triadafilopoulos, Andrea Tringali, Kristien M. A. J. Tytgat, Guido N. J. Tytgat, Kenneth K. Wang, Jerome D. Waye, Justin C.Y. Wu, Byung Moo Yoo

1820 illustrations

Thieme
Stuttgart · New York

Library of Congress Cataloging-in-Publication Data is available from the publisher.

Important note: Medicine is an ever-changing science undergoing continual development. Research and clinical experience are continually expanding our knowledge, in particular our knowledge of proper treatment and drug therapy. Insofar as this book mentions any dosage or application, readers may rest assured that the authors, editors, and publishers have made every effort to ensure that such references are in accordance with **the state of knowledge at the time of production of the book.** Nevertheless, this does not involve, imply, or express any guarantee or responsibility on the part of the publishers in respect to any dosage instructions and forms of applications stated in the book. **Every user is requested to examine carefully** the manufacturers' leaflets accompanying each drug and to check, if necessary in consultation with a physician or specialist, whether the dosage schedules mentioned therein or the contraindications stated by the manufacturers differ from the statements made in the present book. Such examination is particularly important with drugs that are either rarely used or have been newly released on the market. Every dosage schedule or every form of application used is entirely at the user's own risk and responsibility. The authors and publishers request every user to report to the publishers any discrepancies or inaccuracies noticed. If errors in this work are found after publication, errata will be posted at www.thieme.com on the product description page.

© 2010 Georg Thieme Verlag,
Rüdigerstrasse 14, 70 469 Stuttgart, Germany
http://www.thieme.de
Thieme New York, 333 Seventh Avenue,
New York, NY 10 001, USA
http://www.thieme.com

Cover design: Thieme Publishing Group
Typesetting by primustype Hurler, Notzingen, Germany
Printed in China by Leo Paper Ltd, Hongkong
ISBN 978-3-13-125852-6   1 2 3 4 5 6

Preface

Seven years after the initial publication of our book we now present the second edition. This new edition employs the same proven concept as before. However, its content fully reflects the rapid advances that have characterized the development of gastroenterological endoscopy in recent years. This development is not solely the result of technical progress but has also been driven by an increasing interest in endoscopy of the gastrointestinal tract. It is evident that the number of endoscopic centers has continuously increased in recent years. We note with some satisfaction that this development has embraced every continent. The major endoscopic journals report both increasing subscriptions and increasing submissions of scientific papers. The major emerging economic powers in Asia, such as China and India, have apparently decisively influenced this development. We also note that scientific papers in the field of endoscopy no longer come exclusively from university hospitals, but increasingly from municipal hospitals and private practices as well.

This newly acquired knowledge extends to all aspects of gastroenterological endoscopy that are relevant to the patient: patient preparation prior to examination, premedication, screening of premalignant and malignant lesions, endoscopic diagnosis, and therapy.

Completely new technology and methods have been introduced. Not only has the endoscopist's field of endeavor expanded continuously as a result of this development, it has also undergone significant change.

The magic acronym NOTES has evoked fascination. It refers to transluminal invasive procedures in which the endoscope is advanced through the wall of the organ of approach (stomach, vagina, etc.) to reach the target organ in the abdominal or retroperitoneal space in order to remove the appendix, gallbladder, kidney, etc. Surgical teams that include gastroenterologists now see a completely new field of endeavor unfolding for the intrepid gastroenterological endoscopist.

Colorectal carcinoma is by far the most impressive example of the impact of health care policies on the field of endoscopy. Where colonoscopy is the established method of screening for colon cancer, as in the United States and many European countries, endoscopists are veritably flooded with screenees. Might this not mean that other equally important tasks of the physician are being neglected as a result? Obviously new biomarkers for colon cancer with high sensitivity and specificity are needed to filter out unsuitable candidates so that only those cases where a genuine suspicion exists are sent to colonoscopy.

Naturally, colonoscopy and the removal of adenomas are indispensable established methods of colon cancer screening. However, not every intervention detects precancerous lesions or small malignancies, permitting timely endoscopic or surgical removal. Obviously improvements to endoscopic methodology or completely new methods are required to reduce the number of interval carcinomas to near zero.

Recent findings that flat and dimpled adenomas and certain serrated polyps in the colon entail a higher risk of malignant degeneration are important. Here there is some good news. Clear improvements in the detection of changes in the epithelial surface of the gastrointestinal tract have resulted from enlarging the endoscopic image, using dyes, autofluorescence, high-definition endoscopy, and also by manipulating the wavelength of the applied light by means of narrow-band imaging (NBI) and Fujinon intelligent color enhancement (FICE). More precise evaluation of the substrate also permits endoscopic classification of changes as premalignant or malignant lesions; the Paris–Japan and Kudo classifications are convincing examples of such a system. But this is not all. With the aid of confocal laser microscopy it is possible to obtain images of the deeper layer of the intestinal mucosa beneath the epithelial surface. This modality can visualize high-grade dysplasia in ulcerative colitis that might go undetected with white light microscopy. Have we not come very close to many older endoscopists' dream of practicable "endoscopic histology"?

The endoscopic submucosal dissection (ESD) developed by our Japanese friends represents a great advance in both diagnosis and therapy. In contrast to endoscopic mucosal resection (EMR), ESD allows better en bloc resection of the tumor-bearing area of the wall, more precise histopathological diagnostic studies, and a deeper resection. In the first edition of our book we had described endoscopic mucosal resection as a revolutionary advance. Now this elegant method risks being supplanted by endoscopic submucosal dissection. This will hold true especially if the modification suggested by the American Apollo group, namely first marking the affected area of the wall laterally with electrocautery and lifting the wall by inflating a balloon in the submucosa, does indeed increase safety and reduce the time required for surgery.

New imaging modalities such as high-resolution–high-magnification endoscopy, autofluorescence, spectra modulation, etc., and new therapeutic technology were applied in the colon. This novel technology was also applied in other fields such as esophagus, stomach, and bilio-pancreatic area. Particularly Barrett's esophagus was favored to apply and evaluate all novel technology but progress in diagnostic and therapeutic possibilities was also made in the bilio-pancreatic field.

A true novelty in this second edition of the atlas is the in depth description of investigational possibilities for small intestinal diseases with capsule endoscopy and mono- and double balloon endoscopy. The last endoscopic frontier has now been tackled, allowing investigation of the entire intestinal tract, whenever clinically indicated.

In parallel with the amazing endoscopic evolution was the further development of diagnostic and particularly therapeutic endosonography. Something which was unthinkable in the past is now entering the arena of routine procedures in an optimally equipped and skilled endoscopic unit.

The key contributions of the gastroenterologal endoscopist to digestive oncology are hardly at risk of being usurped by other disciplines. The situation is different in the case of classic chemotherapy or the application of biologicals by gastroenterologists in advanced gastrointestinal tumors. This is common practice in certain European countries. Indeed, the use of biologicals is hardly new to gastroenterologists used to treating patients with chronic inflammatory bowel disease.

This book addresses all endoscopists throughout the world as well as colleagues from related fields. It is especially intended for our fellows, for gastroenterologists in private practice and those practicing in tertiary referral centers, who work closely with surgeons, pathologists, radiologists, and oncologists, as well as for all those who are involved in research and participate in clinical studies wherever possible. We are well aware of the great economic differences between the various regions and countries of the world, and we explicitly encourage our colleagues in the developing countries. Our express thanks go to those manufacturers of endoscopes and add-on devices who help to establish gastroenterological and endoscopic training centers for training physicians and assistants in the developing countries.

This edition has seen a change in the group of editors. Jacques Bergman, Alexander Meining, D Nageshwar Reddy, Michael Wallace, and Hisao Tajiri have been brought on board as associate editors in an effort to involve younger endoscopists with solid scientific and clinical reputations, who have already acquired experience and demonstrated sound critical judgment in both research and practice. These colleagues have also played a crucial role in designing the book and will be responsible for the coming editions. We felt it important that they already become familiar with the responsibilities of editors. It is essential for a textbook to keep abreast of the latest developments. New aspects and changing emphasis make it important to enlist younger authors as well. This approach has paid off. However, the majority of our authors had already contributed to the first edition. We know of few gastroenterological book projects with such a broad international group of contributing authors. The editors would like to thank all the authors for their understanding for our urgent wishes and for their outstanding cooperation.

The high quality of text and image material the editors strived for was nearly invariably achieved. We thank the enthusiastic donors (especially from Japan) for their excellent image material.

We present readers throughout the world with a book that does justice to the advances in medical science and to the development and importance of gastroenterological endoscopy. Gastroenterologists throughout the world will receive the information they require for planning an endoscopy department, for their endoscopic work in both private practice and the hospital, and for detecting and treating even rare pathology in the gastrointestinal tract and major digestive glands.

Our special thanks go to the staff of Thieme Publishers, especially Dr. Wachinger and Dr. Bergman. Ms. Rachel Swift not only did justice to her name, but won the editors' boundless admiration for her knowledge, patience, and kindness. Dr. Hauff was a generous publisher who agreed to give the book an excellent layout.

The editors

List of Contributors

Associate Editors

Jacques J. G. J. M. Bergman, MD
Professor
Academic Medical Center
Department of Gastroenterology
Amsterdam, the Netherlands

Alexander Meining, MD
Department of Gastroenterology
Technical University of Munich
Klinikum rechts der Isar
Munich, Germany

D. Nageshwar Reddy, MD
Chairman
Asian Institute of Gastroenterology
Hyderabad, India

Hisao Tajiri, MD
Chairman and Professor
Division of Gastroenterology
and Hepatology
Department of Internal Medicine
The Jikei University School of Medicine
Tokyo, Japan

Michael B. Wallace, MD
Associate Professor of Gastroenterology
Mayo Clinic
Jacksonville, FL, USA

Contributors

Douglas G. Adler MD, FACG, FASGE
Assistant Professor of Medicine
Director of Therapeutic Endoscopy
Gastroenterology and Hepatology
Huntsman Cancer Center
University of Utah
Salt Lake City, UT, USA

Furqaan Ahmed
Fellow, Division of Gastroenterology
and Hepatology
Department of Medicine
Indiana University Medical Center
Indianapolis, IN, USA

Hans-Dieter Allescher, MD
Professor
Klinikum Garmisch-Partenkirchen GmbH
Center for Internal Medicine
Garmisch-Partenkirchen, Germany

Anthony T. R. Axon, MD
Professor of Gastroenterology
The General Infirmary at Leeds
Leeds, United Kingdom

Rami J. Badreddine, MD
Division of Gastroenterology
and Hepatology
Mayo Clinic
Rochester, MN, USA

John Baillie, MB, ChB, FRCP, FACG
Professor, Internal Medicine
(Gastroenterology)
Director, Hepatobiliary and
Pancreatic Disorders Services
Wake Forest University Baptist
Medical Center
Medical Center Boulevard
Winston-Salem, NC, USA

Juergen Barnert, MD
Supervising Physician
3 rd Medical Department
Klinikum Augsburg
Augsburg, Germany

Todd H. Baron, MD, FASGE
Division of Gastroenterology
and Hepatology
Mayo Clinic
Rochester, MN, USA

Hugh Barr, MD, ChM, FRCS, FRCSE, FHEA
Professor
Cranfield Health
Gloucestershire Royal Hospital
Gloucester, UK

J. F. W. M. Bartelsman
Professor
Department of Gastroenterology
and Hepatology
Academic Medical Center
Amsterdam, the Netherlands

Witold Bartnik, MD
Professor
Department of Gastroenterology
and Hepatology
Medical Center for Postgraduate
Education and
the Maria Sklodowska-Curie
Memorial Cancer Center and Institute
of Oncology
Warsaw, Poland

Vikram Bhatia, MD, DM
Assistant Professor (Medical Hepatology)
Institute of Liver and Biliary Sciences
New Delhi, India

David Bjorkman, MD, MSPH
Dean, University of Utah School of Medicine
Executive Medical Director
Division of Gastroenterology
and Hepatology
Salt Lake City, UT, USA

Wojciech Blonski, MD, PhD
Division of Gastroenterology
University of Pennsylvania
Philadelphia, PA, USA
Department of Gastroenterology
and Hepatology
Medical University
Wroclaw, Poland

Lawrence J. Brandt, MD
Chief, Department of Gastroenterology
Montefiore Medical Center
Albert Einstein College of Medicine
Bronx, NY, USA

Marco J. Bruno, MD, PhD
Erasmus Medical Centre
University Medical Center Rotterdam
Depaertment of Gastroenterology
and Hepatology
Rotterdam, the Netherlands

Andrew K. Burroughs
Consultant Physician and Hepatologist
Liver Transplantation and
Hepatobiliary Medicine
Royal Free Hospital
London, UK

David Cave, MD, PhD
Professor of Medicine
Director of Clinical
Gastroenterology Research
UMass Memorial Medical Center
Worcester, MA, USA

Jean-Pierre Charton, MD
Consultant, Gastroenterology
Evangelisches Krankenhaus
Düsseldorf, Germany

Evangelos Cholongitas, MD
Liver Transplantation and
Hepatobiliary Medicine
Royal Free Hospital
London, UK

Meinhard Classen, MD
Professor Emeritus and former Chairman
Department of Internal Medicine
Technical University of Munich
Munich, Gerrmany

Guido Costamagna, MD, FACG
Università Cattolica del Sacro Cuore
A. Gemelli University Hospital
Digestive Endoscopy Unit
Rome, Italy

Stefan von Delius
Assistant Physician
2nd Medical Clinic
Klinikum rechts der Isar
Technical University of Munich
Munich, Germany

Michel Delvaux, MD, PhD
Department of Internal Medicine
and Digestive Pathology
Hopitaux de Brabois
University Hospital of Nancy
Nancy, France

James A. DiSario, MD
Adjunct Professor of Medicine
University of Utah Health Sciences Center
Utah, USA

Steven A. Edmundowicz, MD
FASGE Professor of Medicine
Chief of Endoscopy
Division of Gastroenterology
Washington University School of Medicine
St. Louis, MO, USA

Axel Eickhoff, MD
Medical Department C
Klinikum Ludwigshafen
Academic Hospital of the
University of Mainz
Ludwigshafen, Germany

Shungo Endo, MD
Digestive Disease Center
Showa University Northern
Yokohama Hospital
Yokohama, Japan

Pietro Familiari, MD, PhD
Università Cattolica del Sacro Cuore
A. Gemelli University Hospital
Digestive Endoscopy Unit
Rome, Italy

Paul Feuerstadt, MD
Fellow, Department of Gastroenterology
Montefiore Medical Center
Albert Einstein College of Medicine
Bronx, NY, USA

Hubertus Feußner, MD
Professor
Department of Surgery
Klinikum Rechts der Isar
Technical University of Munich
Munich, Germany

David E. Fleischer, MD
Professor of Medicine
Mayo Clinic College of Medicine
Division of Gastroenterology
and Hepatology
Scottsdale, AZ, USA

Evan L. Fogel
Professor of Clinical Medicine
Indiana University School of Medicine
Division of Gastroenterology
and Hepatology
Department of Medicine, Indiana University
Medical Center
Indianapolis, IN, USA

Victor L. Fox, MD, FAAP
Director, Gastroenterology Procedure Unit
Assistant Professor of Pediatrics
Harvard Medical School
Children's Hospital Boston
Boston, MA, USA

Gérard Gay, MD
Department of Internal Medicine
and Digestive Pathology
Hopitaux de Brabois
University Hospital of Nancy
Nancy, France

Karel Geboes, MD
Professor
Department of Pathology
University Hospital KULeuven
Leuven, Belgium

Joseph E. Geenen, MD
Clinical Professor of Medicine
Medical College of Wisconsin
Director, Pancreatobiliary Services
St.Luke's Medical Center
Milwaukee, WI, USA

Nalini M. Guda, MD
Clinical Associate Professor of Medicine
University of Wisconsin School of Medicine
and Public Health
Pancreatobiliary Services
St.Luke's Medical Center
Milwaukee, WI, USA

Neil Gupta, MD, MPH
Fellow, Division of
Gastroenterology/Hepatology
University of Kansas Medical Center
Kansas City Veterans Administration
Kansas City, MO, USA

Gregory B. Haber, MD
Director of Gastroenterology
Lenox Hill Hospital
New York, NY, USA

Robert H. Hawes, MD
Professor of Medicine
Peter Cotton Chair for
Endoscopic Innovation
Division of Gastroenterology
and Hepatology
Digestive Disease Center
Medical University of South Carolina
Charleston, SC, USA

Juergen Hochberger, MD, PhD
Professor of Medicine and Chairman
Department of Medicine III –
Gastroenterology, Interventional Endoscopy
St. Bernward Academic Teaching Hospital
Hildesheim, Germany

Keiichi Ikeda, MD
Department of Endoscopy
The Jikei University School of Medicine
Tokyo, Japan

John M. Inadomi, MD
GI Health Outcomes
Policy and Economics (HOPE)
Research Program
Department of Medicine
University of California
San Francisco, USA

Sreeni Jonnalagadda, MD
Associate Professor of Medicine
Director of Biliary and Pancreatic Endoscopy
Interventional Endoscopy Section
Washington University School of Medicine
St. Louis, MO, USA

Michael Jung, MD, FRCP
Professor and Chief Physician
Department of Gastroenterology
St. Hildegardis-Krankenhaus
Katholisches Klinikum Mainz
Mainz, Germany

Abdel Meguid Kassem, MD
Associate Professor
Department of Tropical Medicine
and GI-Endoscopy
Faculty of Medicine, Cairo University
Cairo, Egypt

Ralf Kiesslich
Professor and Chief
Endoscopy Unit
1st Medical Department
Johannes Gutenberg University
Mainz, Germany

Kiyonori Kobayashi, MD
Department of Gastroenterology
Kitasato University East Hospital
Sagamihara, Japan

David Kotlyar, MD
University of Pennsylvania
School of Medicine
Philadelphia
Pennsylvania, USA

Richard A. Kozarek, MD
FASGE Division of Gastroenterology
Virginia Mason Medical Center
Seattle, WA, USA

Shin-ei Kudo, MD
Digestive Disease Center
Showa University Northern
Yokohama Hospital
Yokohama, Japan

Spiros D. Ladas, MD
Professor of Medicine and Gastroenterology
Chairman, 1st Department of
Internal Medicine
Laiko General Hospital of Athens
Medical School, University of Athens
Athens, Greece

James Y. W. Lau, MD
Department of Surgery
Prince of Wales Hospital
Shatin
Hong Kong, China

Glen A. Lehman, M. D.
Indiana University Medical Center
Department of Medicine
Division of Gastroenterology
and Hepatology
Indianapolis, IN, USA

Blair S. Lewis, MD
The Mount Sinai School of Medicine
New York, NY, USA

Gary R. Lichtenstein, MD
Professor of Medicine
University of Pennsylvania
School of Medicine
Director, Center for
Inflammatory Bowel Disease
University of Pennsylvania Health System
Division of Gastroenterology
Philadelphia, PA, USA

Jenifer R. Lightdale, MD, MPH
Attending Physician
Gastroenterology and Nutrition
Children's Hospital Boston
Boston, MA, USA

Juergen Maiss, MD, PhD
Kerzel & Maiss
Gastroenterology Associates
Forchheim, Germany

Elisabeth M. H. Mathus-Vliegen, MD
Professor
Department of Gastroenterology
and Hepatology
Academic Medical Centre
Amsterdam, the Netherlands

Koji Matsuda, MD, PhD
Department of Endoscopy
The Jikei Unversity Aoto Hospital
Tokyo, Japan

Kai Matthes, MD, PhD
Division of Gastroenterology
Beth Israel Deaconess Medical Center
Harvard Medical School
Boston, MA, USA

Helmut Messmann, MD
Professor and Director
3 rd Medical Department
Klinikum Augsburg
Augsburg, Germany

Hideyuki Miyachi, MD
Digestive Disease Center
Showa University Northern
Yokohama Hospital
Yokohama, Japan

Faris M. Murad, MD
Advanced Fellow
Gastroenterology,
Advanced Therapeutic Endoscopy
Mayo Clinic
Rochester, MN, USA

Horst Neuhaus, MD
Professor and Chief Physician
Department of Gastroenterology
Evangelisches Krankenhaus
Düsseldorf, Germany

H. Juergen Nord,
MD, MACG, FACP, FASGE, AGAF
Professor of Medicine
University of South Florida
College of Medicine
Tampa, FL, USA

Hiroyuki Ono, MD
Chief of Endoscopy
Shizuoka Cancer Center
Shizuoka, Japan

Jacek Pachlewski, MD
Department of Gastroenterology
and Hepatology
Medical Center for Postgraduate Education
Maria Sklodowska-Curie Memorial
Cancer Center and Institute of Oncology
Warsaw, Poland

Sandy H. Y. Pang, MD
Department of Medicine and Therapeutics
Prince of Wales Hospital
Shatin
Hong Kong, China

Shabana F. Pasha, MD
Assistant Professor of Medicine
Division of Gastroenterology
and Hepatology
Mayo Clinic College of Medicine
Scottsdale, AZ, USA

Andrew T. Pellecchia, MD
Attending Physician
Department of Gastroenterology
Jacobi Medical Center /
Albert Einstein College of Medicine
Bronx, NY, USA

Jan-Werner Poley, MD
Erasmus Medical Centre
University Medical Center Rotterdam
Department of Gastroenterology
and Hepatology
Rotterdam, the Netherlands

Thierry Ponchon, MD
Professor
Department of Gastroenterology
and Hepatology
Hôpital Eduard Herriot
Lyon, France

Jeffrey L. Ponsky
Oliver H. Payne Professor and Chairman
Department of Surgery
Case Western Reserve University
School of Medicine
Case Medical Center
Cleveland, OH, USA

Benjamin K. Poulose, MD, MPH
Assistant Professor of Surgery
Vanderbilt University Medical Center
Nashville, TN, USA

Christian Prinz, MD
2nd Medical Department
Klinikum Rechts der Isar
Technical University of Munich
Munich, Germany

D. Nageshwar Reddy, MD
Chairman
Asian Institute of Gastroenterology
Hyderabad, India

Jaroslaw Regula, MD
Professor
Department of Gastroenterology
and Hepatology
Medical Center for Postgraduate Education
Maria Sklodowska-Curie Memorial
Cancer Center and Institute of Oncology
Warsaw, Poland

Jürgen F. Riemann, MD
Chairman and Professor
Medical Department C
Klinikum Ludwigshafen
Ludwigshafen, Germany

Thomas Rösch, MD
Chief of Endoscopy
Klinik rechts der Isar
Technical University of Munich
Munich, Germany

Gurpal S. Sandha
Assistant Professor
Division of Gastroenterology
University of Alberta
Edmonton, AB, Canada

Yasushi Sano, MD, PhD
Director and Chief
Gastrointestinal Center
Sano Hospital
Kobe, Japan

Shiv Kumar Sarin, MD, DM
Professor
Institute of Liver and Biliary Sciences
New Delhi, India

Brian Saunders, MD, FRCP
Consultant Gastroenterologist
and Specialist GI Endoscopist
Director, Wolfson Unit for Endoscopy
St. Mark's Hospital
Harrow, United Kingdom

Stefan Seewald, MD
Center of Gastroenterology
Klinik Hirslanden
Zurich, Switzerland

Marco Senzolo, MD
Liver Transplantation and
Hepatobiliary Medicine
Royal Free Hospital
London, United Kingdom

Prateek Sharma, MD
Professor
Division of Gastroenterology/Hepatology
University of Kansas Medical Center
Kansas City Veterans Administration
Kansas City, MO, USA

Stuart Sherman, MD
Professor of Medicine
Glen Lehman Professor in Gastroenterology
Division of Gastroenterology
and Hepatology
Department of Medicine
Indiana University Medical Center
Indianapolis, IN, USA.

Chan-Sup Shim, MD, PhD
Director of Digestive Disease Center
KonKuk University Medical Center
Seoul, Korea

Nathan J. Shores, MD
Fellow
Section on Gastroenterology
Department of Internal Medicine
Wake Forest University Health System
Winston-Salem, NC, USA

Nib Soehendra, MD
Professor Emeritus
Senior Advisor
Universitätsklinikum Hamburg-Eppendorf
Hamburg, Germany

Ma Somsouk, MD, MAS
GI Health Outcomes, Policy
and Economics (HOPE) Research Program
Department of Medicine
University of California, San Francisco
Division of Gastroenterology
and Hepatology
San Francisco General Hospital
San Francisco, CA, USA

Joseph J. Y. Sung, MBBS, MD, PhD, FRCP
Chairman and Professor of Medicine
Department of Medicine and Therapeutics
Director, Institute of Digestive Disease
The Chinese University of Hong Kong
Hong Kong, China

Paul Swain, MD
Professor of Gastrointestinal Endoscopy
Department of Surgical Oncology
and Technology
Imperial College of Science,
Technology and Medicine
London, United Kingdom

Hisao Tajiri, MD, PhD
Chairman and Professor
Division of Gastroenterology
and Hepatology
Professor
Department of Endoscopy
The Jikei University School of Medicine
Tokyo, Japan

Shinji Tanaka, MD, PhD
Professor and Director
Department of Endoscopy
Hiroshima University Hospital
Hiroshima, Japan

George Triadafilopoulos, MD
Department of Medicine
Division of Gastroenterology
and Hepatology
Stanford University
Stanford, CA, USA

Andrea Tringali, MD, PhD
Università Cattolica del Sacro Cuore
A. Gemelli University Hospital
Digestive Endoscopy Unit
Rome, Italy

K. M. A. J. Tytgat, MD, PhD
Department of Gastroenterology
Academic Medical Center
Amsterdam, the Netherlands

Guido N. J. Tytgat, MD, PhD
Professor Emeritus of Gastroenterology
University of Amsterdam
Former Chief of Department
of Gastroenterology
Academic Medical Center
Amsterdam, the Netherlands

Kenneth K. Wang, MD, PhD
Director
Advanced Endoscopy Group
Division of Gastroenterology
and Hepatology
Mayo Clinic
Rochester, MN, USA

Jerome D. Waye, MD
Department of Gastroenterology
Mount Sinai Medical Center
New York, NY, USA

Justin C.Y. Wu, MBChB, MD, FRCP
Associate Professor
Department of Medicine and Therapeutics
The Chinese University of Hong Kong
Hong Kong, China

Byung Moo Yoo, MD
Indiana University Medical Center
Department of Medicine
Division of Gastroenterology
and Hepatology
Indianapolis, IN, USA

Contents

Contents

Contents

V Therapeutic Procedures

Section editors: Guido N.J. Tytgat, Meinhard Classen, and Charles J. Lightdale

Contents

Contents

VI Upper Gastrointestinal Tract Disease

Section editors: Charles J. Lightdale, Hisao Tajiri, Jaques J.G.J.M. Bergman

VII Lower Gastrointestinal Tract Diseases

Section editors: Charles J. Lightdale, Guido N.J. Tytgat, Alexander Meining

Contents

VIII Biliopancreatic, Hepatic, and Peritoneal Diseases

Section editors: Charles J. Lightdale, Meinhard Classen, D. Nageshwar Reddy

IX Infectious Diseases of the Gastrointestinal Tract

Section editors: Guido N.J. Tytgat, Charles J. Lightdale, Michael B. Wallace

Contents

X Pediatric Endoscopy

Section editors: Guido N.J. Tytgat, Charles J. Lightdale, Meinhard Classen

Abbreviations

airway breathing and circulation	ABC
blood transfusion requirement index	ABRI
American Cystoscope Makers Inc.	ACMI
acute colonic pseudo-obstruction	ACPO
autofluorescence imaging	AFI
American Gastroenterological Association	AGA
acute gallstone pancreatitis	AGP
American Heart Association	AHA
acquired immune deficiency syndrome	AIDS
autoimmune pancreatitis	AIP
aminolevulinic acid	ALA
alanine aminotransferase .	ALT
American Medical Association	AMA
analysis of variance	ANOVA
Asia–Pacific Association for the Study of the Liver	APASL
adenomatous polyposis coli gene	APC
Argon plasma coagulation	APC
antireflux device	ARD
American Society of Anesthesiologists	ASA
adjustable silicone gastric banding	ASGB
American Society of Gastrointestinal Endoscopy	ASGE
aspartate aminotransferase	AST
arteriovenous malformation	AVM
BioEnterics Intragastric Balloon	BIB
bipolar electrocoagulation	BICAP
body mass index	BMI
biliopancreatic diversion	BPD
biliopancreatic diversion with duodenal switch	BPD-DS
balloon-occluded retrograde transvenous obliteration	BRTO
bovine spongiform encephalopathy	BSE
British Society of Gastroenterology	BSG
chronic antral gastritis	CAG
computer-assisted personalized sedation	CAPS
computer-based colonoscopy simulator	CBCS
common bile duct	CBD
charge-coupled device	CCD
colitis cystica profunda	CCP
Crohn disease	CD
Crohn Disease Activity Index	CDAI
Crohn Disease Endoscopic Index of Severity	CDEIS
carcinoembryonic antigen	CEA
capsule endoscopy Crohn disease activity index	CECDAI
cylindrical insertion	CI
cytokeratins	CKs
columnar-lined lower esophagus	CLE
confocal laser endomicroscopy	CLE
Cytomegalovirus	CMV
carbon dioxide	CO_2
Cyclooxygenase-2	COX-2
celiac plexus neurolysis	CPN
complete portal tracts	CPTs
colorectal cancer	CRC
controlled radial expansion	CRE
calcinosis Raynaud phenomenon sclerodactyly and telangiectasia	CRST
cylindrical surface	CS
clinically significant portal hypertension	CSPH
centimeter	cm
computed tomography	CT
computed-tomographic angiography .	CTA
diffuse antral gastritis	DAG
dysplasia-associated lymphoid mass	DALM
double-balloon endoscopy	DBE
dilated intercellular spaces	DIS
diisopropyl iminodiacetic acid	DISIDA
dimethyl sulfoxide	DMSO
desoxyribonucleic acid	DNA
direct percutaneous endoscopic jejunostomy	DPEJ
deep venous thrombosis	DVT
Erlangen Active Simulator for Interventional Endoscopy	EASIE
endoscopic band ligation	EBL
electrocardiography	ECG
enterochromaffin-like	ECL
early gastric cancer	EGC
esophagogastroduodenoscopy	EGD
epidermal growth factor receptor	EGFR
esophagogastric junction	EGJ
enterohemorrhagic E. coli	EHEC
electrohydrolic lithotripsy	EHL
electrohydraulic lithotripsy	EHL
electrohydrothermal [probes]	EHT
enteroinvasive E. coli	EIEC
endoscopic injection sclerotherapy	EIS
enzyme-linked immunosorbent assay	ELISA
endoscopic laser therapy	ELT
endoscopic mucosal resection	EMR
cap-assisted endoscopic mucosal resection	EMR-C
ligation-assisted EMR	EMR-L
endoscopic polypectomy	EP
European Panel on Appropriateness of Gastrointestinal Endoscopy	EPAGE
endoscopic papillary balloon dilation	EPBD
endoscopic papillotomy	EPT
endoscopic retrograde cholangiography	ERC
endoscopic retrograde cholangiopancreatography	ERCP
endoscopic resection using a hypertonic saline–epinephrine	ERHSE
endoscopic submucosal dissection	ESD
European Society of Gastrointestinal Endoscopy	ESGE
European Society of Gastroenterology and Endoscopy Nurses and Associates	ESGENA
endoscopic sphincterotomy	EST
extracorporeal shock-wave lithotripsy	ESWL
endoscopic transanal resection	ETAR
enteropathy-type T-cell lymphoma	ETL
endoscopic trimodality imaging	ETMI
European Board of Anesthesiology of the European Union of Medical Specialists	EUMS/UEMS
endoscopic ultrasonography	EUS
gastrointestinal endosonography	EUS

endoscopic variceal ligation	EVL	ileal pouch–anal anastomosis	IPAA
ethylene-vinyl alcohol	EVOH	immunoproliferative small-intestinal disease	IPSID
familial adenomatous polyposis	FAP	isosorbide dinitrate	ISDN
Food and Drug Administration	FDA	insulated-tip	IT
fresh frozen plasma	FFP	IT knife-2	IT-2
free hepatic venous pressure	FHVP	internal vena cava	IVC
Fujinon intelligent chromoendoscopy	FICE	Joule	J
fluorescent in-situ hybridization	FISH	jejunoileal bypass	JIB
fine-needle aspiration	FNA	jejunostomy through a PEG	JPEG
fine-needle aspiration biopsy	FNAB	juvenile polyposis syndrome	JPS
fine-needle injection	FNI	potassium titanyl phosphate	KTP
fine-needle puncture	FNP	liter	l
French size	Fr	laparoscopic adjustable silicone gastric banding	LASGB
front surface .	FS	laparoscopic cholecystotomy	LCT
gauge	G	laparoscopic–endoscopic procedure	LEP
gastric antral vascular ectasia	GAVE	lower esophageal sphincter	LES
gastric bypass	GBP	liver function tests	LFTs
gastroesophageal flap valve	GEFV	low-grade dysplasia	LGD
Garren–Edwards Gastric Bubble	GEGB	lower gastrointestinal bleeding	LGIB
gastroesophageal junction	GEJ	low-grade intraepithelial neoplasia	LGIN
gastroesophageal reflux disease	GERD	lymphogranuloma venereum	LGV
GERD health-related quality of life	GERD-HRQL	laser lithotripsy	LL
Groupe d'Etudes Thérapeutiques des Affections		low-molecular-weight heparin	LMWH
Inflammatoires du Tube Digestif	GETAID	low-osmolality nonionic contrast media	LOCM
gastroesophageal varices	GEV	laterally spreading tumor	LST
gastroesophageal varices	GEVs	*Mycobacterium avium* complex	MAC
gamma glutamyltransferase	gGT	mucosa-associated lymphoid tissue	MALT
gastrointestinal	GI	minilaparoscopy-assisted natural orifice surgery	MANOS
gastrointestinal stromal tumor	GIST	*MUTYH* gene–associated polyposis	MAP
Global Rating Scale .	GRS	magnetic endoscope imaging	MEI
glyceryl trinitrate	GTN	multiple endocrine neoplasia	MEN
graft-versus-host disease	GVHD	myocardial infarction	MI
gastric variceal obturation	GVO	milliliter	ml
highly active antiretroviral therapy	HAART	mechanical lithotripsy	ML
hepatitis B virus	HBV	millimeter	mm
hepatocellular carcinoma	HCC	mitochondrial neurogastrointestinal	
hepatitis C virus	HCV	encephalomyopathy	MNGIE
hernia diaphragmatica	HD	main pancreatic duct	MPD
high-grade dysplasia	HGD	magnetic resonance cholangiography	MRC
high-grade intraepithelial neoplasia	HGIN	magnetic resonance cholangiopancreatography	MRCP
hereditary hemorrhagic telangiectasia	HHT	magnetic resonance imaging	MRI
hepatoiminodiacetic acid	HIDA	microsatellite instability	MS
human immunodeficiency virus	HIV	microsatellite instability	MSI
hereditary nonpolyposis colorectal cancer	HNPCC	Men who have sex with men	MSM
hereditary nonpolyposis colorectal cancer	HNPCC	methyl *tert*-butyl ether	MTBE
holmium:yttrium–aluminum–garnet	Ho:YAG	temoporfin	mTHPC
human papillomavirus	HPV	metaplasia ulceration stricture and esophagitis	MUSE
herpes simplex virus	HSV	nucleic acid amplification tests	NAATs
hemolytic uremic syndrome	HUS	nurse-administered propofol sedation	NAPS
hepatic venous pressure gradient	HVPG	narrow-band imaging	NBI
hepatic venous pressure gradient	HVPG	neodymium:yttrium–aluminum–garnet	Nd:YAG
The Hygiene in Gastroenterology—Endoscope		North Italian Endoscopic Club	NIEC
Reprocessing study [*Hygiene in der*		National Institutes of Health	NIH
Gastroenterologie – Endoskop-Aufbereitung]	HYGEA	nanometer	nm
herz	Hz	number needed to treat	NNT
internal anal sphincter	IAS	Natural Orifice Surgery Consortium for	
inflammatory bowel disease	IBD	Assessment and Research	NOSCAR
International Conference on Capsule Endoscopy	ICCE	natural orifice transluminal endoscopic surgery	NOTES
intravenous indocyanine green	ICG	nonsteroidal anti-inflammatory drugs	NSAIDs
intraductal ultrasonography	IDUS	nonselective beta-blockers	NSBBs
idiopathic esophageal ulceration	IEU	New York Society for Gastrointestinal Endoscopy	NSYGE
immunoglobulin G	IgG	One-Action Stent Introduction System	OASIS
immunoglobulin G4	IgG4	optical coherence tomography	OCT
immunoglobulin M	IgM	World Organization of Digestive Endoscopy	
isolated gastric varices	IGVs	[Organisation Mondiale d'Endoscopie Digestive]	OMED
international normalized ratio	INR	ortho-phthalaldehyde	OPA

over-the-wire	OTW	squamous cell carcinoma	SCC
picture archiving and communication system	PACS	specialized columnar epithelium	SCE
analogue broadcasting systems	PAL and NTSC	squamocolumnar junction	SCJ
		submucosal endoscopy with mucosal flap	SEMF
periodic acid–Schiff	PAS	self-expanding metal stent	SEMS
patient-controlled analgesia–sedation	PCAS	self-expanding plastic stent	SEPS
polymerase chain reaction	PCR	Simple Endoscopic Score for Crohn Disease	SES-CD
photodynamic therapy	PDT	sphincter of Oddi dysfunction	SOD
percutaneous endoscopic cecostomy	PEC	stigmata of recent hemorrhage	SRH
percutaneous endoscopic colostomy	PEC	solitary rectal ulcer syndrome	SRUS
percutaneous endoscopic gastrostomy	PEG	secretin stimulation MRCP	ss-MRCP
polyethylene glycol–electrolyte solution	PEG-ELS	sodium tetradecyl sulfate	STD
percutaneous endoscopic jejunostomy	PEJ	stone–tissue discrimination system	STDS
positron-emission tomography	PET	sexually transmitted proctitis	STP
porfimer sodium	Photofrin	Tissue Apposition System	TAS
percutaneous liver biopsy	PLB	target-controlled infusion	TCI
pseudomembranous colitis	PMC	transendoscopic microsurgery	TEMS
peroral cholangioscopy	POC	transforming growth factor-β	TGF-β
pulsatile organ perfusion	POP	transoral incisionless fundoplication	TIF
proton-pump inhibitors	PPI	transjugular intrahepatic portosystemic shunt	TIPS
protoporphyrin IX	PpIX	transjugular liver biopsy	TJLB
positive predictive value	PPV	transient LES relaxations	tLESRs
packed red blood cells.	PRBC	tumor necrosis factor-α	TNF-α
primary sclerosing cholangitis	PSC	tumor node metastasis	TNM
percutaneous transhepatic biliary drainage	PTBD	transoral gastroplasty	TOGA
percutaneous transhepatic cholangiography	PTC	total pancreatectomy with islet cell	
percutaneous transhepatic cholangiographic drainage	PTCD	autotransplantation	TP-IAT
percutaneous transhepatic cholangioscopy	PTCS	through-the-scope	TTS
polytetrafluoroethylene	PTFE	ulcerative colitis	UC
percutaneous transhepatic papillary balloon dilation	PTPBD	ursodeoxycholic acid	UDCA
percutaneous ultrasound guidance	PUG	ultrasonography	US
Quality Assurance of Hygiene in Endoscopy		vertical banded gastroplasty	VBG
		video capsule endoscopy	VCE
[Qualitätssicherung der Hygiene in der Endoskopie]	QSHE	variant Creutzfeldt–Jakob disease	vCJD
randomized controlled trial	RCT	vascular endothelial growth factor	VGEF
radiofrequency	RF	Watt	W
Robotics Interactive Endoscopy Simulation	RIES	automated washer-disinfectors	WDs
relative risk	RR	wedged hepatic venous pressure	WHVP
Roux-en-Y gastric bypass	RYGB	walled-off pancreatic necroses	WOPNs
Society of American Gastrointestinal Endoscopic Surgeons	SAGES		
small bowel endoscopy	SBE		

I

Development of Endoscopy

Section editors:
Meinhard Classen, Guido N.J. Tytgat, Charles J. Lightdale

1 Two Centuries of Digestive Tract Endoscopy: a Concise Report

Meinhard Classen

Introduction

This report on the fascinating recent history of digestive tract endoscopy, its pioneers, and the sometimes revolutionary discoveries and developments that have been seen in the field makes no claim either to completeness or to absolute accuracy. In his excellent book on the history of endoscopy, Francisco Vilardell draws attention to the uncertainties involved in identifying the real originator of any method—whenever this author fails, it should always be regarded as a matter of *nescientia* rather than *ignorantia*. Important and first-rate histories of the field have been written by Irvin M. Modlin (*A Brief History of Endoscopy*) and Francisco Vilardell (*Digestive Endoscopy in the Second Millennium*)—books that can be strongly recommended to every endoscopist [1,2].

Nineteenth-Century Pioneers

Philipp Bozzini (1773–1809), a physician responsible for public health in Frankfurt am Main in Germany, is recognized as the founding father of endoscopy. The light-conducting system which he developed in 1806 and used to inspect the orifices featured a candle and a system of prisms (**Fig. 1.1**) [3]. A better light source was provided in 1853 by the alcohol–turpentine lamp used for cystoscopy by Antonin Desormeaux (1815–1894). The same light source was used in 1868 by Adolph Kussmaul (1822–1902, **Fig. 1.2**) [4], for the first examination of the esophagus, in a sword-swallower—with a rigid endoscope, of course.

The year 1879 is celebrated as heralding the birth of modern endoscopy, when Max Nitze (1848–1906) presented his *Blasenspiegel,* a cystoscope. The device included a distal platinum lamp and a magnifying optical system and was also capable of being used in the rectum. The surgeon Johannes von Mikulicz-Radecki (1850–1905, **Fig. 1.3**), is regarded as the pioneer of gastroscopy [5]. He was able to identify the pylorus and visualize carcinomas in the stomach.

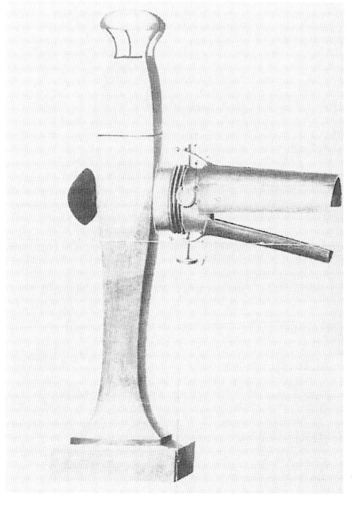

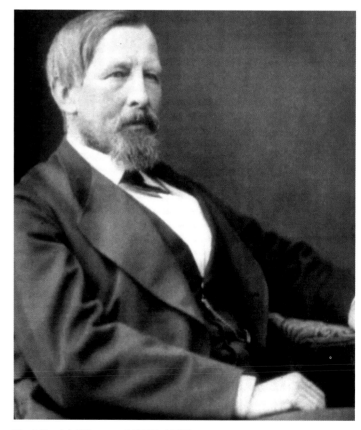

Fig. 1.2 Adolf Kussmaul (1822–1902).

◁ **Fig. 1.1** The original sketch of the light conductor, drawn by Philipp Bozzini himself.

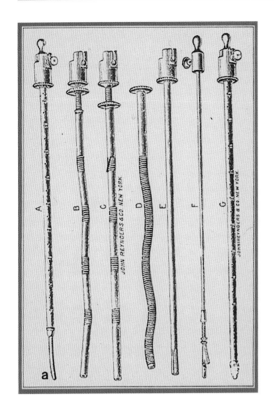

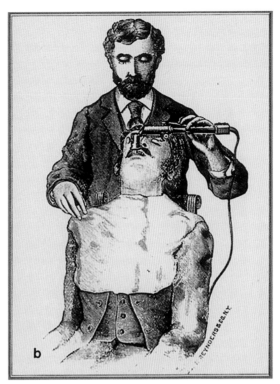

Fig. 1.3 Johannes von Mikulicz's esophagoscope, 1881.

The light bulb invented by Thomas Edison in 1870 was quickly incorporated into endoscopes. The next generation of endoscopes, from the workshop of instrument-maker Josef Leiter (1830–1892) in Vienna, was used for many generations for esophagoscopy, bronchoscopy, and thoracoscopy. With the technology available at the time, numerous further attempts to reduce the rigidity of the instruments, improve illumination conditions, and overcome the limited visualization in the organs being inspected remained unsuccessful.

Rudolf Schindler and the "Semiflexible" Endoscope

In 1932, Rudolf Schindler (1888–1968, **Fig. 1.6**), together with the instrument-maker Georg Wolf (1873–1938), developed a gastroscope in which the proximal end was still rigid but the distal end was capable of being angled up to 34°, so that it was slightly easier to introduce it into the stomach (**Fig. 1.5**) [6]. When using a successor model to this device, I personally found that passage of the instrument was not very easy—particularly in older patients with a short neck, limited cervical spine mobility, large teeth, and a small mouth. In addition, it was not possible to visualize the esophagus and duodenum at all, and only limited inspection of the stomach was possible. Later developments, such as the modification described by Norbert Henning (1896–1985), included a biopsy channel and a facility for photographic documentation [7]. The watercolor illustrations that had been used to record pathological findings before this are evidence of the artistic skills of Schindler and of Henning, as well as those of an endoscopy nurse working with the French gastroscopist François Moutier (1881–1961, **Fig. 1.7**). Schindler suffered the tragic fate of many refugees from Nazi Germany, after being imprisoned in the concentration camp in Dachau for 6 months in 1934. He left Germany and made a new home in the United States. Even today he is still honored as a missionary in the cause of endoscopy, and as the founder of the American Society for Gastrointestinal Endoscopy—thanks in particular to his charismatic qualities as a teacher. He died in Munich in 1968.

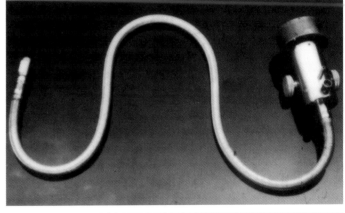

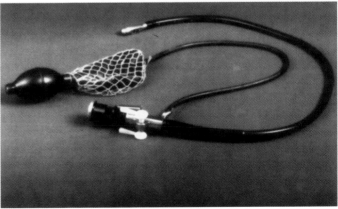

Fig. 1.4 Two gastroscopes.
a The prototype for the fiber gastroscope (1957).
b The first commercial Hirschowitz fiber gastroscope (1961).

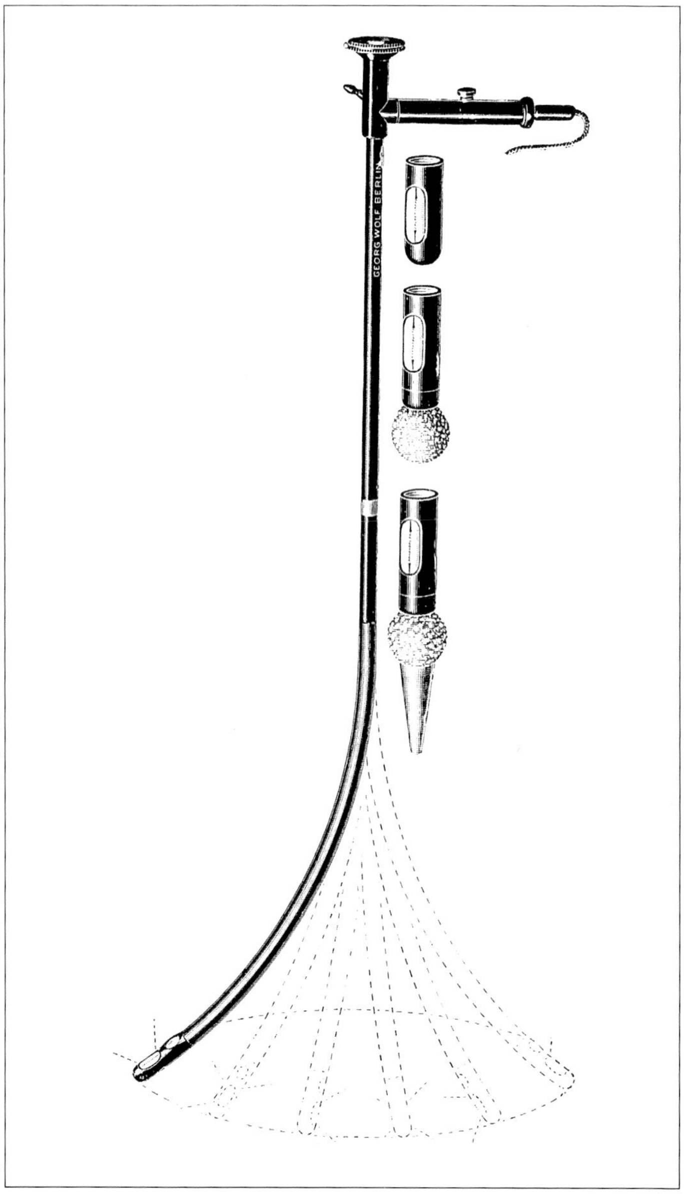

Fig. 1.5 The semiflexible Wolf–Schindler gastroscope (1932).

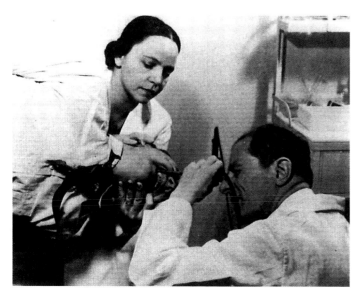

Fig. 1.6 Rudolf Schindler performing a gastroscopy, with his wife Gabriele holding the patient's head.

Fiberglass Endoscopy and Electronic Endoscopy

The watershed in endoscopy was the development of the fully flexible fiber endoscope by Basil Hirschowitz and colleagues [8]. Heinrich Lamm, a student in Munich, had already developed a model for transmitting light through glass fibers as early as 1927, which he showed to Rudolf Schindler [9]. In 1954, Hopkins and Kapany reported in the journal *Nature* on light transmission through a bundle of parallel glass fibers [10]. The decisive advances that followed involved the use of high-quality clear fiberglass and the isolation of each fiber to prevent light from crossing into neighboring fibers. The problems involved were overcome by Basil Hirschowitz's associates, and by Lawrence E. Curtiss in particular [11,12], and in 1957 the first laboratory prototype of a fiber gastroscope was able to produce a recognizable image of President Lincoln on an American stamp (**Fig. 1.4a**; **Fig. 1.8**).

Several years then passed before American Cystoscope Makers, Inc. (ACMI) developed an industrial product based on the prototype. A few years later, an instrument channel and Bowden cables for controlling the tip of the instrument were incorporated into it. In 1963, an esophagoscope with a second fiberglass bundle for transmitting light (cold light) was developed, followed by a "panendoscope" with prograde viewing that also made it possible to inspect the duodenum. It should also be mentioned that Rudolf Ottenjann, Rita Hohner, and H. Petzel in 1966 attached Bowden cables to the fiber gastroscope available at the time, which was flexible but had not hitherto been controllable, to allow regular visualization of the cardia by inverting the tip of the instrument [13].

Fiberglass endoscopes were quickly developed for inspection of the colon as well. Initial attempts to advance a fiberglass endoscope as far as the cecum were made by Provenzale and Revignas [14]. They used a plastic thread for the purpose; following peroral passage of the thread through the stomach and bowel, the colonoscope was pulled up on it into the right colon. In 1963, Overholt in the USA had already inspected the rectum and sigmoid using a fiberglass endoscope [15].

In electronic or video endoscopy, the coherent fiberglass bundle for image transmission is replaced with a tiny chip camera at the tip of the instrument. The American company Welch Allyn manufactured the first usable device of this type in 1983 [16–18]. The new types of device made by Japanese manufacturers took the world of endoscopy by storm. These instruments made the endoscopist's work easier by providing binocular vision and allowed many types of image processing and image alteration. The final domains reserved for fiberglass endoscopy—the narrow lumina in the bronchi and intrahepatic bile ducts, as well as in the pancreatic ductal system—have now also been conquered by chip endoscopes with a diameter of 1 mm.

Japanese Contributions to Digestive Tract Endoscopy

An early gastrocamera that had been developed by F. Lange and N. Meltzing in 1893 was unsuccessful, as it only provided monochrome images [19] (**Fig. 1.9**). By contrast, the gastrocamera produced by Tatsuro Uji together with the Olympus Optical Co. in Tokyo in 1952 provided the technology that allowed mass screening examinations to be carried out for early recognition of gastric cancer in Japan [20]. Keiichi Kawai and colleagues developed an endoscopic classification of early gastric carcinomas and were also able to show that these lesions develop further to become advanced carcinomas. Mass screening appears to have significantly reduced the mortality due to gastric cancer in Japan. Pioneering advocates of the gastrocamera

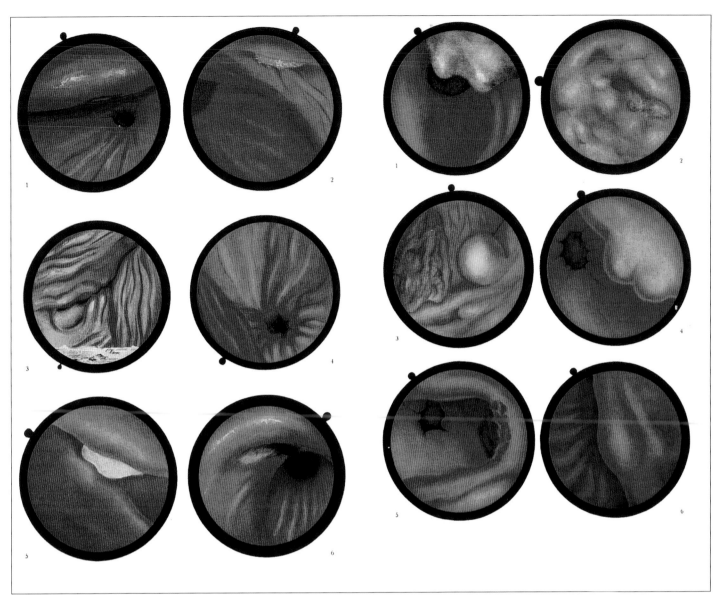

Fig. 1.7 Watercolors of pathological gastric findings made by endoscopy nurse Claire Escoube with François Moutier after a glimpse through the gastroscope (1925).

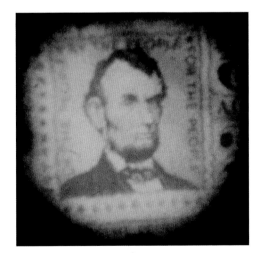

Fig. 1.8 The first photo taken through the new prototype instrument in 1975—a stamp showing President Lincoln.

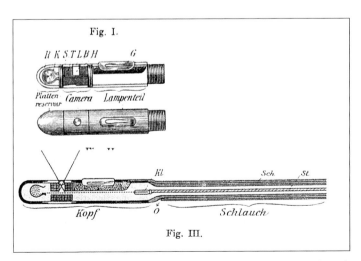

Fig. 1.9 Design drawing for the Meltzing and Langer gastrocamera (1898).

in Germany included K. Heinkel, A. Oshima, and U. von Gaisberg, but in contrast to endoscopy a breakthrough with this type of device was not achieved in Germany [21].

The history of endoscopy in Japan began with the purchase of a Hirschowitz gastroscope by Professor Kondo of Tokyo Women's Medical College in 1960. Kondo had to purchase the device personally, as no academic or other institutions were willing to accept the cost. But things then started to move very quickly. The powerful optical industry in Japan was able to offer a fiberglass gastroscope as early as 1963, and in 1966 the device became available with an angling mechanism and a biopsy channel (the GIF-D model by Olympus Optical Co., **Fig. 1.10**). The achievements of Japanese gastroenterologists and instrument manufacturers are evident throughout the present volume.

Colonoscopy

Initial efforts to construct a colonoscope were made as early as 1964 by Hirohumi Niwa, together with the Olympus Optical Co. [22]. Niwa's device was intended for the left colon, but Matsunaga was already planning an endoscope that would allow examination of the whole colon—although it was only able to reach the right colon in 8% of cases. Via numerous stages of development, a colonoscope approaching today's standard was ultimately developed, with an angle of vision of 140°, 160–80° angulation, and a diameter of 13.8 mm; the shaft had varying degrees of flexibility [23].

Numerous auxiliary instruments to make it easier to advance the device through the entire colon, such as stiffening wires and "sliding tubes," were proposed, but none of these was able to replace fluoroscopic guidance. The guidance method available today, using a magnetic localization system (the Olympus ScopeGuide three-dimensional control system), works without X-ray exposure and is particularly useful in helping beginners to reach the cecum or terminal ileum more quickly, and for recognizing and eliminating loops and loop formation. The localization system also makes it possible to precisely locate findings for subsequent surgical interventions [24].

As a completely new method, colonoscopy immediately attracted a great deal of attention. The major diseases of the large bowel and terminal ileum, such as polyps, carcinoma, chronic inflammatory bowel diseases, infectious and ischemic colitis, were redefined and reevaluated. The advantages of direct inspection of the bowel lumen and the use of auxiliary devices and methods—such as biopsy forceps, electrical snares, coagulation probes, injection needles, chromoscopy, mucosectomy, and balloon dilation—have become evident during the last few decades. In addition to the diseases mentioned above, diverticulitis, collagenous colitis, microscopic colitis, localization and treatment of occult bleeding sources such as vascular malformations, etc., were also redefined. Removal of colonic adenomas was identified as a method of pre-

venting colorectal carcinoma [25,26], and monitoring of chronic inflammatory bowel diseases was recognized as important for recognizing dysplasias and carcinomas as early as possible. Identifying the causes of unclear diarrhea and bleeding sources are also important indications for colonoscopy today.

In addition to Christopher Williams in England [23], the pioneers of colonoscopy include Hirohumi Niwa (Japan) [22], Bergein Overholt [15], Hiromi Shinya [27] and Jerome Waye [26] in the USA, and the innovative figures of Peter Deyhle [25] and Peter Frühmorgen in Ludwig Demling's research group in Erlangen, Germany [28]. The clinical and scientific work of V.P. Strekalovskiĭ (Moscow) is little known in Western countries.

Endoscopic Retrograde Cholangiopancreatography

The Americans McCune, Shorb, and Moscovitz [29] published the first report of successful exploration of the papilla of Vater (the major duodenal papilla) and retrograde demonstration of the ductal system opening there. However, the quality of the radiographs obtained with an Eder fiberoptic duodenoscope was so poor that Ludwig Demling and I felt unable to definitely identify a cholangiopancreatography on them. Using a fiber endoscope made by the Wolf Knittlingen company, we were also only able to probe the papilla of Vater in one patient in April 1970, and instillation of contrast medium into the pancreatic duct was incomplete. It was only when the Machida and Olympus companies in 1970 offered duodenoscopes with good optical characteristics and a mechanism for omnidirectional angulation that reliable introduction of the device into the duodenum, location and intubation of the papilla of Vater, and selective intubation of the ducts became routine. The papers presented by Itaru Oi on endoscopic retrograde cholangiopancreatography (ERCP) at the World Congress for Gastroenterology and Endoscopy held in Copenhagen in 1970 were *the* sensation of the conference [30] (**Fig. 1.11a–c**; **Fig. 1.13**). For the first time, gastroenterologists were now able to reliably diagnose morphological changes caused by diseases of the hepatobiliary and pancreatic ductal systems. Our own group received a JFB-1 instrument from Olympus in November 1970, and by the end of that year we had been able to demonstrate one or both ductal systems in 16 of 20 attempts [31]. Numerous research groups all over the world did pioneering work in identifying the potentialities and risks of ERCP. Pioneers alongside Kawai and Kawajima included Ogoshi et al. [32] and Fujita et al. [33] in Japan; N. Soehendra and E. Seifert in Germany; P.B. Cotton and P. Salmon in the United Kingdom; C. Liguory in France [34]; M. Cremer in Belgium [35]; L. Safrany in Hungary; J. E. Geenen, J. Vennes, and D. Zimmon in the USA; and G.C. Caletti in Italy (see references in the relevant chapters).

In 1976, an endoscopic piggyback system (the mother-and-baby scope) for cholangioscopy was presented by Olympus Optical Co. [36]. The mother device was introduced into the duodenum, and the thin baby scope (with an outer diameter of 2 mm) was then introduced through the papilla of Vater into the bile duct for direct inspection.

Percutaneous Transhepatic Cholangiography

In 1921, Hans Burkhardt and Walter Müller (surgeons in Marburg, Germany) for the first time injected a fluid contrast medium percutaneously into the gallbladder and bile ducts [37]. In 1937, the French surgeon Pierre Husard in Hanoi and his Vietnamese colleague Do-Xuan Hop were also able to inject Lipiodol into the bile ducts via a percutaneous transhepatic route [38]. An important pioneer in this field was Kunio Okuda, who was the first to combine

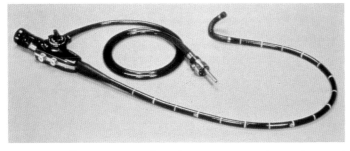

Fig. 1.10   A fiber gastroscope from the early 1970s, with omnidirectional angulation (Olympus GIF-D).

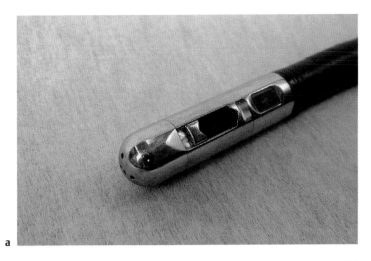

a

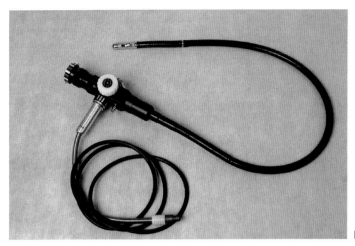

b

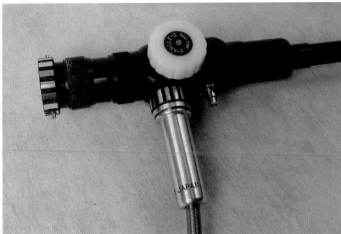

c

Fig. 1.11 The Machida duodenoscope with which Itaru Oi worked—an elegant but difficult device.

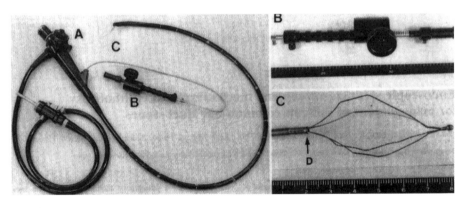

Fig. 1.12 An Olympus duodenoscope with a mechanical lithotriptor (B, C & D).

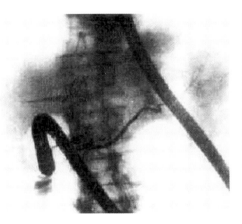

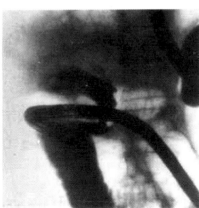

Fig. 1.13 The first images showing endoscopic retrograde cholangiopancreatography, which Itaru Oi presented at the Fourth World Congress of Gastroenterology in Copenhagen, 12–18 July 1970.

1

percutaneous cholangiography with external biliary drainage [39]. The Swedish surgeon Karl Ludvik Wiechel was the first to introduce percutaneous transhepatic cholangiography into more or less routine practice in Europe [40], succeeding against strong resistance.

ERCP, which entered clinical practice in 1970, did not make the percutaneous access route superfluous, as ERCP examinations (or at least complete examinations) were not possible in quite a few patients with biliary strictures, as well as in patients in whom access to the papilla of Vater was difficult. In 1975, Yamakawa et al. [41] first described the technique of percutaneous transhepatic cholangioscopy, which is still in use today. Stabilization of the puncture channel using mandrins, and subsequent enlargement of it up to 10–12 Fr in two or three steps over a period of 8–10 days, made it possible to introduce flexible cholangioscopes, which were initially equipped with fiberglass but now have charge-coupled device (CCD) chips for image transmission. This approach made it possible to carry out all of the therapeutic manipulations in the intrahepatic and extrahepatic biliary system that were difficult using the route through the papilla of Vater. These include lithotripsy (mechanical, electrohydraulic, and laser), stricture dilation, and tumor ablation.

However, the visual facilities provided by cholangioscopy were limited, illumination was poor, and breaks in the glass fibers led to reduced visibility, as did the yellow discoloring of the glass fibers caused by X-rays. By contrast, the new 1-mm thin chip endoscopes that have been available since 2003 for the same target area provide a clear view into the thin lumina.

Enteroscopy

For a long period, the small bowel stubbornly resisted every effort that was made to achieve complete inspection of it with flexible instruments. Initial attempts were made in 1972, when we managed to guide a 2-m long fiber endoscope through the entire gastrointestinal tract over a swallowed nylon thread [42]. Our efforts to inspect the small bowel remained incomplete, as there were a few regions that "raced past" the lens, and due to the nylon thread it was not always possible to distinguish definitively between superficial mucosal lesions and relevant changes. Complete visualization of the small bowel was still not possible later on, with push enteroscopy and probe enteroscopy. For intraoperative enteroscopy, it was necessary to know in advance at least the segment of the bowel in which a lesion was suspected.

Capsule endoscopy, developed by the ingenious Paul Swain and Given Imaging, Ltd., has now solved diagnostic problems in small-bowel diseases such as occult bleeding sources, tumors, and Crohn's disease lesions that cannot be identified with other methods. It can be usefully supplemented with enteroscopy using one or two balloons, and the latter method also allows biopsies and therapeutic interventions to be carried out [43,44].

Therapeutic Endoscopy

Endoscopy only played a very minor role, if any, in gastrointestinal diagnosis before 1960, but the diagnosis and treatment of numerous digestive tract diseases would be inconceivable without it today. It would be unthinkable nowadays for a gastroenterologist not to have good endoscopic skills, including skills in therapeutic endoscopy.

Foreign-body removal from the digestive tract viscera is the oldest method in therapeutic endoscopy. As early as 1906, Hugo Starck reported on 73 cases of foreign-body extraction from the esophagus [45]. He and Jean Guisez [46] were the pioneers of the method (**Fig. 1.14**). Today, it is primarily children and prisoners who swallow foreign bodies, and as long as these remain in the upper gastrointestinal tract, including the duodenum, they can be extracted

endoscopically using special auxiliary devices. Foreign bodies introduced into the rectum can also be mobilized and extracted by the endoscopist. General anesthesia and laparotomy are now only rarely needed for treatment of foreign bodies.

Esophageal dilation can now also be regarded as a method of only historical interest. The Starck dilator—a construction resembling an umbrella—was used right up to the 1970s for achalasia, as was the Gottstein balloon. Starck also popularized the method of bougienage of long esophageal strictures—e. g., strictures due to caustic injuries. Hard cicatricial strictures in the esophagus used to be incised using an endoscopically controlled esophagotome. All of these procedures were guided using a rigid esophagoscope, and this continued to be quite customary in some otorhinolaryngology departments even up to the 1990s. Gastroenterologists, by contrast, were already using fiber endoscopy for foreign-body extraction and controlled balloon dilation at the end of the 1960s [47]. The balloons that are in use today have a ring-shaped mark to allow precise endoscopic and/or fluoroscopic positioning within the stricture. Modern treatment of achalasia using botulinum toxin (Botox) is based on the principle of reducing the pressure in the lower esophagus [48].

Palliative treatment of malignant stenoses is another of the older methods in therapeutic endoscopy. Endoscopic stent treatment for stenotic esophageal tumors was developed to clinical maturity by Atkinson and Ferguson [49] and by Guido Tytgat's group in Amsterdam [50]. The earlier plastic stents have now been replaced with self-expanding metal stents. The first description of the use of a spiral metal stent was published in 1982 by Eckart Frimberger, who was then still a member of Rudolf Ottenjann's research group [51]. Covered metal stents with small hooks at each end are usually able to hold the metal stent in the desired position and are often also used to close esophagobronchial fistulas.

The procedure of hemostasis with palliative ablation of stenotic tumor tissue using neodymium:yttrium–aluminum–garnet (Nd:YAG) laser coagulation was originally developed by Kiefhaber et al. [52]. This method is now only rarely used, in stenoses that are barely passable.

Photodynamic diagnosis and treatment. Initial experimental treatments with fluorescent dyes were carried out as long ago as 1903 [53]. In premalignant and malignant epithelial structures, porfimer sodium (Photofrin) and Δ-aminolevulinic acid (ALA) enhance more strongly than in the normal neighboring epithelium. This characteristic can be helpful for diagnosis and targeted treatment in patients with chronic inflammatory bowel diseases, and particularly in ulcerative colitis and Barrett's epithelium with circumscribed high-grade dysplasia/carcinomas that are difficult to recognize endoscopically. Marianne Ortner was the first to use photodynamic diagnosis and therapy in patients with biliary malignancies [54].

Endoscopic polypectomy. The origins of endoscopic polyp removal using rigid esophagoscopes and rectoscopes are difficult to trace, but certainly go back a long time. Following the introduction of fiber colonoscopy, Hirohumi Niwa in Tokyo was able in 1968 to remove colonic polyps using an isolated biopsy forceps (hot biopsy), and later using a coagulation probe. In 1969, he reported at a conference of Japanese endoscopists on the first snare polypectomies in the colon, although these were apparently unsuccessful [55]. His research was obstructed for several years when protesting students barricaded his laboratory door. The first fiber-endoscopic polypectomies in the colon were carried out by Peter Deyhle and colleagues [56] in 1970, and procedures in the stomach were reported in 1971 by our own group and Ottenjann's group in Germany simultaneously [57,58] and by William Wolff and Hiromi Shinya in New York [59]. The importance of polypectomy in the colon as a means of preventing cancer was impressively demonstrated by Sidney Winawer and colleagues in the National Polyp Study in the USA [60].

Polypectomy significantly reduces not only the mortality from colorectal carcinomas, but also the incidence of the lesions.

Modern techniques for enlarging the endoscopic image and enhancing structures by applying stains (chromoendoscopy) are nowadays able to improve image perception and allow better classification in differentiating between surface structures that are suspicious for malignancy [61], particularly in small depressed and malignant lesions, which infiltrate the submucosa in 50% of cases. They also differ from polypoid carcinomas with regard to pathogenesis and tumor biology. The basic research carried out by Shin'ei Kudo is therefore of immense interest here [62].

Endoscopic mucosal resection (EMR) and endoscopic submucosal dissection (ESD). Endoscopists are nowadays undaunted by superficial and broad-based tumors, even when the lesions have already infiltrated the submucosa. Inoue and Endo [63] in Japan, as well as Soehendra's group [64] in Hamburg, can claim the merit of being the first authors to report on mucosectomy (see Chapter 30). The techniques differ, but the results are comparable. Younger endoscopists—particularly Japanese colleagues such as Yahagi—are ablating wall areas with a diameter of 10 cm or more in the esophagus, stomach, and colon using endoscopic submucosal dissection in operations lasting several hours [65]. Perforations that occasionally occur are closed by the endoscopist from inside the lumen using Endoclips, and by the laparoscopist from the serosal side. As an alternative to extensive submucosal dissection, combined laparoscopic full-thickness wall resection with endoscopic guidance is possible (see Chapter 30).

Christian Ell and his research group have recently presented a report—including what is probably the largest group of patients in the world to have received this form of treatment—impressively describing the potential of endoscopic therapy in premalignant and malignant lesions in Barrett's esophagus [66].

Drainage and endoprostheses in the bile duct. Endoscopic placement of drains in the bile duct was perfected by my former associate, Dietmar Wurbs, with an ingeniously pre-shaped probe construction [67]. Shortly afterward, Soehendra and Reynders-Frederix reported the first common bile duct stent made of plastic material [68]. These two approaches—both developed in Hamburg—for drainage of the biliary tract and pancreas have not only made ERCP, endoscopic papillotomy, and other interventions in this area safer, but have also added new indications for the treatment of biliary and pancreatic diseases to the list of indications for endoscopy. Septic cholangitis has lost its seriousness if it is treated early enough, and post-ERCP pancreatitis can be avoided more often through stenting of the pancreatic duct with a thin stent (3 Fr) made of plastic. The relevant chapters of this book describe numerous other indications for stenting through the papilla of Vater.

As in the esophagus, self-expanding metal stents are now commonplace in the palliative treatment of malignant tumors in the bile duct. Frimberger et al. can take credit for being the first to report this technique [69]. Laser therapy and radiotherapy (with the afterloading technique) for malignant stenoses [70,71] currently only have a negligible role.

Hemostasis. Massive acute hemorrhage from the upper gastrointestinal tract has presented physicians with almost insurmountable problems in every period of history [72–74]. Esophageal varices were first treated in 1939 by Crafoord and Frenkner, using sclerosing agents [75]. Sclerotherapy for esophageal varices was particularly advocated by Loren Pitcher [76], but has now been largely replaced by rubber-band ligation ("banding") [77], a form of treatment that has long been used in the treatment of hemorrhoids. The ulcers resulting after esophageal banding are smaller and heal more quickly than the ulcers produced when sclerosants are injected. In accordance with a method originally suggested by Soehendra et al., bleeding from fundic varices can be arrested by injecting an acrylic resin [78].

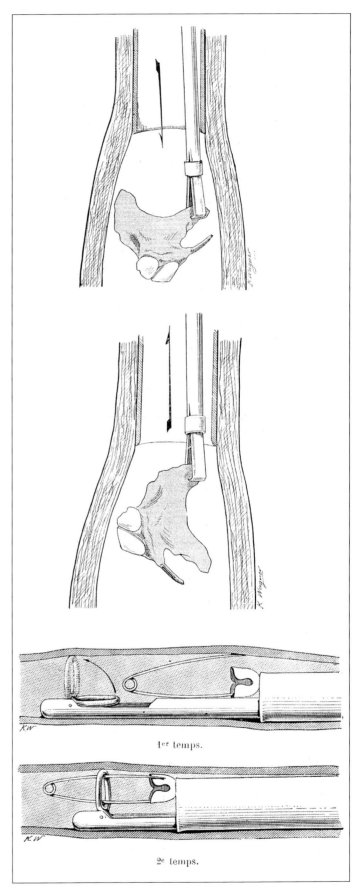

Fig. 1.14 Instructions on how to extract foreign bodies, from Jean Guisez's *Traité des maladies de l'oesophage*, 1911 [46].

The debate between the proponents of argon and Nd:YAG laser treatment for hemostasis [52,79] has long since been settled. Today, the modern argon beamer has proved its value, particularly in patients with mild bleeding and in cases of seeping hemorrhage, as well as for tissue ablation. Safe prevention or treatment of bleeding can be achieved with mechanical methods such as the Endoloop and hemoclip. The latter was already developed in the 1970s, but due to a technical problem did not gain acceptance. Experiments with endoscopic suturing machines (Heinzl, Buess) by several groups have now been resolved by Paul Swain [80,81]. The Swain model has been used to treat hiatus hernia in the context of reflux disease, and also for hemostasis.

Percutaneous endoscopic gastrostomy (PEG) was introduced by Gauderer et al. in the USA in 1980 [82]. PEG is certainly the most important method of overcoming transit disturbances for food and saliva in parts of the upper gastrointestinal tract closer to the mouth—whether the disturbances are neurogenic or caused by malignancies. If gastric dilation needs to be treated, a nutritional probe can be advanced through the gastric stoma into the jejunum. Information regarding ethical problems with PEG nutrition in patients with senile dementia and those in the terminal stages of disease is provided in Chapter 40.

Endoscopic papillotomy (EPT) and endoscopic sphincterotomy (ES, EST). Immediately after the introduction of diagnostic ERCP, the search began for a treatment approach to solve the "new diseases" for which only palliative treatment variants were available using endoscopic drainage or stenting. Even in their first approaches to the problem, Ludwig Demling and his research group started by modifying the polypectomy snare developed in Erlangen, which could be introduced without difficulty into the papilla and the ductal systems that emerge there. Electrical incision with the snare did not appear to be fully controllable endoscopically; in particular, there were concerns regarding potential trauma to the opening of the pancreatic duct, and a variant method was therefore sought. This was found in 1973 in discussions held by Ludwig Demling, particularly with Peter Frühmorgen, Hermann Bünte, and myself. Initial experiments in animals and at autopsies confirmed that the resulting instrument—known as the "Erlangen papillotome"—was practicable. It was first used in June 1973, and the procedure was successful [83]. Kawai's research group in Kyoto pursued a different technical principle, in which an electrical knife (known as the push papillotome) is advanced into the papilla and the bile duct. Keiichi Kawai used this device in a patient for the first time in August 1973 [84]. It was subsequently found that the Erlangen papillotome was superior in terms of controllability and safety, and it is still being used throughout the world today. A miniature version of the Erlangen papillotome—which was also used for the first time by our group—may be helpful when there are anatomic variants in the ampullary orifice or in cases of stricture. The needle-knife is an important additional aid, and debate continued for several years over the indications for its use and on whether only experienced practitioners should use it or whether all endoscopists were able to do so (see Chapter 34).

Balloon dilation is an alternative to incision into the papilla of Vater, and this was first described by Staritz et al. [85]. It is now clear that anyone who carries out a dilation procedure also needs to be able to do a papillotomy.

When the length of the incision is sufficient, endoscopic papillotomy leaves a gaping common bile duct orifice and an easily recognizable pancreatic duct orifice. Endoscopists soon began to consider endoscopic treatment options for stones, parasites, inflammations, strictures, and tumors in the biliary and pancreatic ducts. Examples include mechanical lithotripsy with a reinforced Dormia basket (**Fig. 1.12**), electrohydraulic lithotripsy [86–89], laser lithotripsy [90,91], pancreatic duct stenting in chronic pancreatitis (M. Cremer), and sphincter of Oddi dyskinesia (J.E. Geenen, G. Lehman),

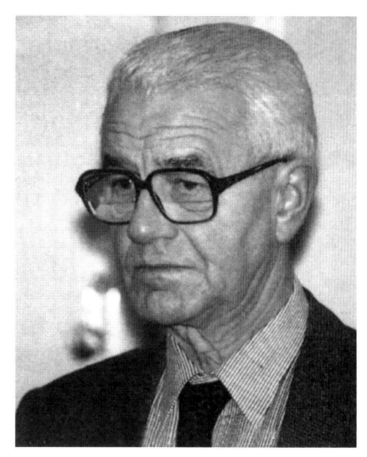

Fig. 1.15 Ludwig Demling.

treatment for recurrent pancreatitis in patients with pancreas divisum (P.B. Cotton), drainage [65], and bile duct stenting in patients with septic cholangitis or acute pancreatitis. As endoscopic papillotomy is a prerequisite for most endoscopic treatment methods in the bile ducts and pancreatic ductal system, it is often described as the "pattern for pancreaticobiliary procedures."

Endoscopic Ultrasonography

The method of endoscopic ultrasonography (EUS) is undoubtedly one of the greatest advances that has been made in the field of digestive tract endoscopy, as it provides the endoscopist with unrivaled visualization of the wall of the bowel with its typical layers, as well as a glimpse of the neighboring structures. Initial experiments were conducted by Wild and Reid, who introduced a mechanically rotating scanner into the rectum in 1957 [92]. The difficulties involved in introducing a scanner into the esophagus and stomach were only solved many years later. Initial clinical experience was gained in 1980 [93–95]. The "marriage" of endoscopy and ultrasound was particularly fruitful for the staging of tumors in the upper gastrointestinal tract and pancreas. EUS using a probe in the narrow lumina of the pancreas and biliary tract is known as intraductal ultrasonography (IDUS). It provides remarkably clear images. Procedures conducted using EUS guidance—such as choledochoduodenostomy, neurolysis (e.g., of the celiac plexus) and in particular cystogastrostomy and cystoenterostomy—show the growing potential of this method [96].

Laparoscopy

In 1902, Georg Kelling (1866–1945), one of the most important personalities among the pioneers of endoscopy (including esophagoscopy and gastroscopy) inspected the abdominal cavity of a dog using a cystoscope [97,98] (**Fig. 1.16**). By 1910, he had reported a few "celioscopies" using a pneumoperitoneum and port placement. In the same year, Hans-Christen Jacobaeus in Stockholm—without knowing anything of Kelling's work—described a procedure he called "laparoscopy" [99]. For decades, laparoscopy then played an important role, primarily in central Europe, in the morphological diagnosis of liver diseases and other conditions in the peritoneal cavity. Particular achievements in this area were made by Kalk et al. [100], Harald Lindner, and others. An outstanding atlas and textbook of laparoscopy by Henning et al. was produced by Thieme, the present publishers, in 1994 [101]. Minilaparoscopy for the diagnosis of abdominal emergencies and unclear findings in the liver and peritoneum is unfortunately nowadays only used in a few centers [102]. Ultrasound-guided biopsy of hepatic lesions appears to be replacing laparoscopy in internal medicine departments. Abdominal surgeons have relabeled laparoscopy-assisted treatment procedures as "minimally invasive surgery." Keyhole surgery has now progressed well beyond the areas of its initial success in appendectomy and cholecystectomy [103–107], and surgery for benign gastric and intestinal diseases has now also entered the range of indications for minimally invasive procedures. Earlier warnings against carrying out oncological procedures using the laparoscope are now no longer heeded. The present volume has for the first time grouped new types of procedure under the heading of natural orifice transluminal endoscopic surgery (NOTES). Access to the abdominal organs is achieved via the body's natural orifices (peroral, transgastric, transrectal, and transvaginal). The role of the gastroenterologist is thoughtfully outlined by Robert Hawes in Chapter 23.

Summary and Prospects

Forty years ago, endoscopy of the digestive tract only had a negligible role in the diagnosis and treatment of digestive diseases, with the exception of rectoscopy and laparoscopy. I would estimate that some 200 completely new diseases have since been discovered and correctly understood with regard to their etiology and pathogenesis, or have since become amenable to causal treatment. In most cases, this has been achieved with the help of endoscopy, biopsy, histology, radiology, microbiology, molecular biology, genetics, and other endoscopy-supported methods. The most outstanding example of this is the discovery of *Helicobacter pylori* and the diseases caused by the bacterium. Further examples of the tremendous importance of endoscopy include early recognition of gastrointestinal tumors and prevention of carcinoma in the colon using polypectomy. In comparison with other imaging methods, endoscopy is the diagnostic standard for most diseases of the digestive tract and bile ducts.

Not only has the professional profile of the gastroenterologist been fundamentally transformed, with a gastroenterologist nowadays having to be an endoscopist as well—the work of other specialists, such as radiologists, surgeons, pathologists, microbiologists, etc., has also changed drastically. Endoscopy of the upper and lower digestive tract has led to pathologists moving from the autopsy table to the sickbed. The diagnosis of endoscopic biopsies, including the latest molecular-genetic methods, is now the pathologist's major concern, instead of the dissection of cadavers. Early advocates of this transformation included Basil Morson, Konrad Elster, Manfred Stolte, and Cyrus Rubin. Procedures that used to be surgical ones,

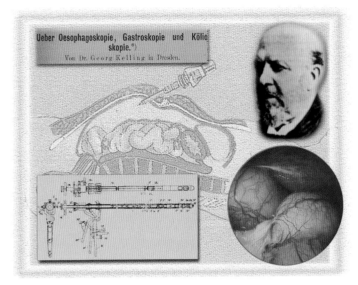

Fig. 1.16 George Kelling of Dresden and his 1902 publication.

such as choledochotomy, polypectomy, and many other interventions, have joined the range of indications for the less traumatic field of endoscopy. The most important aspect of this reallocation of territory is the outcome for the patient, which has been substantially improved. In the future, the science of endoscopy will show even more clearly than before, and in a multitude of ways, that it can produce practical and economic advantages both for patients and for health-care funding in the management of digestive and metabolic diseases. In polypectomy, stent therapy in the biliary and pancreatic ducts, drainage and endoprostheses, stricture dilation, PEG, hemostasis, and laparoscopy-assisted treatment procedures, the advantages of endoscopy are clear—even though strict scientific proof in the form of well-planned controlled clinical studies is not always available. Another example of the immense importance of endoscopy lies in early recognition of gastrointestinal tumors and carcinoma prevention in the colon using polypectomy. In the past, diseases of the bile ducts and pancreas belonged to the field of surgery, which was associated with considerable morbidity and mortality rates. ERCP, EPT, treatment for stones, dilation, stenting and drainage were the appropriate responses provided by endoscopy. These advances were of course only possible thanks to ingenious partners among the manufacturers of endoscopes and devices, such as Dr. Karl Storz, Dr. Herbert Schubert, Dr. I. Kawahara, A. Fukami, the Machida brothers, Reinhold Wappler, Don Wilson, and many others.

Developments are sure to continue at a breathtaking pace. Even now, there is nothing prophetic in suggesting that the endoscopy capsule, which has already proved its value for small-bowel diagnosis, will also become capable of retrograde movement and will be externally controllable and able to carry out therapeutic interventions. It is already possible to use biosensors on flexible endoscopes, and optical coherence tomography (OCT) is an example of this. Molecular imaging, bioendoscopy, and optical biopsy are the key words for the new endoscopic era. The next step will be to combine various types of spectroscopy with endoscopy in order to solve the problem of how to recognize neoplasia in flat areas of inflammation—as in Barrett's esophagus or ulcerative colitis, for example. Using ingenious "beacons," it is already possible today to use fluorescence spectroscopy to depict colonic adenomas with a diameter of 50 μm in the mouse. The future is already here. I am convinced it will be at least as exciting, fascinating, and dazzling as the last 50 years.

References

1. Modlin IM. A brief history of endoscopy. Milan: MultiMed; 2000.
2. Vilardell F. Digestive endoscopy in the second millennium: from the *Lichtleiter* to echoendoscopy. Madrid: Aula Medica Ediciones/Stuttgart: Thieme; 2006.
3. Bozzini P. Der Lichtleiter, oder Beschreibung einer einfachen Vorrichtung und ihrer Anwendung zur Erleuchtung innerer Höhlen und Zwischenräume des lebenden animalischen Körpers. Stuttgart: Max-Nitze-Museum; 1988 [reprint of ed. Weimar: Verlage des Landes-Industrie-Comptoirs; 1807].
4. Kluge F. Adolf Kussmaul, 1822–1902. Arzt und Forscher—Lehrer der Heilkunst. Freiburg im Breisgau, Germany: Rombach; 2002.
5. Mikulicz J. Über Gastroskopie und Ösophagoskopie. Wien Med Press 1881; 22: 1629–31.
6. Schindler R. Gastroscopy: the endoscopic study of gastric pathology. 2nd ed. Chicago: University of Chicago Press; 1950.
7. Henning N, Keilhack H. Die gezielte Farbenphotographie in der Magenhöhle. Dtsch Med Wochenschr 1938; 64: 1392–3.
8. Hirschowitz BI. A fibre optic flexible oesophagoscope. Lancet 1963; ii (7304): 388.
9. Lamm H. Biegsame optische Geräte. Z Instrumentenkd 1930; 50: 579–81.
10. Hopkins HH, Kapany NS. A flexible fiberscope using static scanning. Nature 1954; 173: 39–41.
11. Hirschowitz BI, Curtiss LE, Peters CW. A flexible light transmitting tube. U. S. patent no. 3,010,357. Washington, DC: US Patent Office; 1961.
12. Hirschowitz BI, Curtiss LE, Peters CW, Pollard HM. Demonstration of a new gastroscope, the fiberscope. Gastroenterology 1958; 35: 50–3.
13. Ottenjann R, Petzel H. [Endogastric inversion of the fiber gastroscope for the endoscopy of the stomach fornix]. Med Klin 1966; 61: 1543–4. German.
14. Provenzale L, Revignas A. Transanale Kolonoskopie mittels Fiberoptik. Bericht einer neuen Methode zur Untersuchung des gesamten Dickdarms. In: Fortschritte der Endoskopie (2nd Conference of the Deutsche Gesellschaft für Endoskopie, Erlangen, February 1968), vol. 1. Stuttgart: Schattauer; 1969: 167.
15. Overholt BF. The history of colonoscopy. In: Hunt RH, Waye JD, editors. Colonoscopy: techniques, clinical practice, and colour atlas. London: Chapman-Hall, 1981; 1–7.
16. Classen M, Phillip J. Electronic endoscopy of the gastrointestinal tract: initial experience with a new-type endoscope that has no fiberoptic bundle for imaging. Endoscopy 1984; 16: 16–9.
17. Haubrich WS. History of endoscopy. In: Sivak MV Jr, editor. Gastroenterologic endoscopy. Philadelphia: Saunders; 1987; 2–19.
18. Sivak MV Jr, Fleischer DE. Colonoscopy with a video endoscope: preliminary experience. Gastrointest Endosc 1984; 30: 1–5.
19. Lange F, Meltzing CA. Die Photographie des Mageninneren. Münch Med Wochenschr 1898; 50: 1585–8.
20. Uji T. The gastrocamera. Tokyo Med J 1952; 61: 135–8.
21. Von Gaisberg U. Bedeutung der Gastrocamera. Stuttgart: Edition Medi-Text; 2005.
22. Niwa H, Fujino M, Yoshitoshi Y. Colonic fiberscopy for routine practice. In: Advances in gastrointestinal endoscopy: proceedings of the Second Congress of the International Society of Gastrointestinal Endoscopy, Rome, July 1972). Padua, Italy: Piccin Medical, 1972; 549–55.
23. Williams C, Muto T. Examination of the whole colon with fibreoptic colonoscope. Br Med J 1972; 3: 278–81.
24. Olympus Europe Medical Systems and Endoscopy [Internet]. Hamburg, Germany: Olympus Europa, Ltd.; 2009. ScopeGuide: new imaging technique for colonoscopy. Available from: http://www.olympus-europa.com/endoscopy/431_ScopeGuide.htm. Accessed 12 March 2009.
25. Deyhle P, Demling L. Coloscopy: technique, results, indication. Endoscopy 1971; 3: 143–51.
26. Waye J. Colonoscopy. Surg Clin North Am 1972; 52: 1013–24.
27. Wolff WI, Shinya H. Colonofiberoscopy. JAMA 1971; 217: 1509–12.
28. Demling L, Classen M, Frühmorgen P, editors. Atlas of enteroscopy: endoscopy of the small and large bowel, retrograde cholangio-pancreatography. Berlin: Springer; 1974.
29. McCune WS, Shorb PE, Moscovitz H. Endoscopic cannulation of the ampulla of Vater: a preliminary report. Ann Surg 1968; 167: 752–6.
30. Oi I, Kobayashi S, Kondo T. Endoscopic pancreatocholangiography. Endoscopy 1970; 2: 103.
31. Demling L, Classen M. Duodenojejunoscopy. Endoscopy 1970; 2: 115–7.
32. Ogoshi K, Tobita Y, Hara Y. Endoscopic observation of the duodenum and endoscopic pancreatocholangiography. Gastroenterol Endosc 1970; 12: 83–94.
33. Fujita R, Sohma S, Kidokoro T. Endoscopy of the duodenum (experience using Olympus JF-2). Gastroenterol Endosc 1970; 12: 97–106.
34. Liguory C, Meduri B, Coelho F, Ahl-Kampf C, Leger L. Traitement endoscopique d'un faux kyste sur pancréas divisum. Chirurgie 1982; 108: 273–8.
35. Cremer M, Devière J, Delhaye M, Baize M, Vandermeeren A. Stenting in severe chronic pancreatitis: results of medium-term follow-up in 76 patients. Endoscopy 1991; 23: 171–6.
36. Nakajima M, Akasaka Y, Fukumoto K, Misuyoshi Y, Kawai K. Peroral cholangiopancreatoscopy (PCPS) under duodenoscopic guidance. Am J Gastroenterol 1976; 66: 241–7.
37. Burckhardt H, Müller W. Versuche über die Punktion der Gallenblase und ihre Röntgendarstellung. Dtsch Z Chir 1921; 162: 168–97.
38. Huard P, Do XH. La ponction transhépatique des canaux biliaires. Bull Soc Méd Chir Indoch 1937; 28: 1090–100.
39. Okuda K, Tanikawa K, Emura S, et al. Nonsurgical percutaneous transhepatic cholangiography diagnostic significance in medical problems of the liver. Dig Dis 1974; 19: 21–7.
40. Sandberg AA. Karl Ludwig Wiechel. Profiler svensk kirurgi. Sven Kir 2008; 66: 6.
41. Yamakawa T, Komaki F, Shikata JI. Biliary tract endoscopy with an improved choledochofiberscope. Gastrointest Endosc 1978; 24: 110–3.
42. Classen M, Frühmorgen P, Koch H, Demling L. Peroral enteroscopy of the small and large intestine. Endoscopy 1972; 4: 157–62.
43. Iddan G, Meron G, Glukhovsky A, Swain P. Wireless capsule endoscopy. Nature 2000; 405: 417.
44. May A, Nachbar L, Wardak A, Yamamoto H, Ell C. Double-balloon enteroscopy: preliminary experience in patients with obscure gastrointestinal bleeding or chronic abdominal pain. Endoscopy 2003; 35: 985–91.
45. Starck H. Lehrbuch der Ösophagoskopie, 2nd ed. Würzburg, Germany: Kabitsch; 1914.
46. Guisez J. Traité des maladies de l'oesophage. Paris: Baillière, 1911.
47. Witzel L. Treatment of achalasia with a pneumatic dilator attached to a gastroscope. Endoscopy 1981; 13: 176–7.
48. Storr M, Born P, Frimberger E, Weigert N, Rösch T, Meining A, et al. Treatment of achalasia: the short-term response to botulinum toxin injection seems to be independent of any kind of pretreatment. BMC Gastroenterol 2002; 2: 19.
49. Atkinson M, Ferguson R. Fibreoptic endoscopic palliative intubation of inoperable oesophagogastric neoplasms. Br Med J 1977; 1: 266–7.
50. Tytgat GNJ, den Hartog Jäger FCA, Haverkamp HJ. Positioning of a plastic prosthesis under fiberendoscopic control in the palliative treatment of cardio-esophageal cancer. Endoscopy 1976; 8: 180–5.
51. Frimberger E. Expanding spiral—a new type of prosthesis for the palliative treatment of malignant esophageal stenoses. Endoscopy 1983; 15 (Suppl 1): 213–4.
52. Kiefhaber P, Nath G, Moritz K. Endoscopical control of massive gastrointestinal hemorrhage by irradiation with a high-power Neodymium-Yag laser. Prog Surg 1977; 15: 140–55.
53. Tappeiner HV, Jesionck A. Therapeutische Versuche mit fluoreszierenden Farbstoffen. Münch Med Wochenschr 1903; 1: 2042.
54. Ortner ME, Caca K, Berr F, Liebetruth J, Mansmann U, Huster D, et al. Successful photodynamic therapy for nonresectable cholangiocarcinoma: a randomized prospective study. Gastroenterology 2003; 125: 1355–63.
55. Niwa H. Endoscopic polypectomy using high-frequency current. [Paper presented at the Eighth Kanto Branch Meeting of the Japanese Gastroenterological Endoscopy Society.]
56. Deyhle P, Seibarth K, Jenny S, Demling L. Endoscopic polypectomy in the proximal colon. Endoscopy 1971; 3: 103–5.
57. Classen M, Demling L. Operative Gastroskopie: Fiberendoskopische Polypenabtragung im Magen. Dtsch Med Wochenschr 1971; 37: 1466–7.
58. Rösch W, Elster K, Ottenjann R. [Endoscopic and biopsy diagnosis of stomach polyps]. Dtsch Med Wochenschr 1971; 96: 39–40. German.
59. Wolff WI, Shinya H. Polypectomy via the fiberoptic colonoscope. Removal of neoplasms beyond reach of the sigmoidoscope. N Engl J Med 1973; 288: 329–32.
60. Winawer SJ, Zauber AG, Ho MN, O'Brien MJ, Gottlieb LS, Sternberg SS, et al. Prevention of colorectal cancer by colonoscopic polypectomy. The National Polyp Study Workgroup. N Engl J Med 1993; 329: 1977–81.
61. Niwa H. The history of digestive endoscopy. In: Niwa H, Tajiri H, Nakajima M, Yasuda K, editors. New challenges in gastrointestinal endoscopy. Tokyo: Springer, 2008; 3–28.
62. Kudo S. Early colorectal cancer: detection of depressed types colorectal carcinomas. Tokyo/New York: Igaku Shoin; 1996.
63. Inoue H, Endo M. Endoscopic esophageal mucosal resection using a transparent tube. Surg Endosc 1990; 4: 198–201.

64. Soehendra N, Binmoeller KF, Bohnacker S, et al. Endoscopic snare mucosectomy in the esophagus without any additional equipment: a simple technique for resection of flat early cancer. Endoscopy 1997; 29: 380–3.

65. Yahagi N. Is esophageal endoscopic submucosal dissection an extreme treatment modality, or can it be a standard treatment modality? Gastrointest Endosc 2008; 68: 1073–5.

66. Manner H, May A, Pech O, et al. Early Barrett's carcinoma with "low-risk" submucosal invasion: long-term results of endoscopic resection with a curative intent. Am J Gastroenterol 2008; 103: 2589–97.

67. Wurbs D, Dammermann R, Classen M. [Palliative non-surgical bile duct drainage]. Dtsch Med Wochenschr 1979; 104: 1831–2. German.

68. Soehendra N, Reynders-Frederix V. [Palliative biliary duct drainage. A new method for endoscopic introduction of a new drain]. Dtsch Med Wochenschr 1979; 104: 206–7. German.

69. Frimberger E, Kühner W, Ottenjann R. [Spiral prosthesis for the common bile duct]. Dtsch Med Wochenschr 1982; 107: 1985–6. German.

70. Phillip J, Hagenmüller F, Manegold K, Szepesi S, Classen M. [Endoscopic intraductal radiotherapy of high bile-duct carcinoma]. Dtsch Med Wochenschr 1984; 109: 422–6. German.

71. Hagenmüller F, Sander C, Sander R, Ries G, Classen M. Laser and endoluminal 192-iridium radiation. Endoscopy 1987; 19 (Suppl 1): 16–8.

72. Pitcher JL. Therapeutic endoscopy and bleeding ulcers: historical overview. Gastrointest Endosc 1990; 36 (Suppl 5): S 2–7.

73. Desneux JJ. [Emergency endoscopy in acute digestive hemorrhages]. Arch Mal Appar Dig Mal Nutr 1958; 47: 1163–8. French.

74. Palmer ED. The vigorous diagnostic approach to upper-gastrointestinal tract hemorrhage. A 23-year prospective study of 1,400 patients. JAMA 1969; 207: 1477–80.

75. Crafoord C, Frenckner P. New surgical treatment of varicous veins of the oesophagus. Acta Otolaryngol 1939; 27: 422–9.

76. Pitcher JL. Medical management of bleeding esophagogastric varices. In: Bárány FR, Torsoli A, editors. Gastrointestinal emergencies: proceedings of the First International Symposium held at the Wenner-Gren Center, Stockholm, September 1975. Oxford: Pergamon Press, 1977; 261–8.

77. Van Stiegmann G, Cambre T, Sun JH. A new endoscopic elastic band ligating device. Gastrointest Endosc 1986; 32: 230–3.

78. Soehendra N, Nam VC, Grimm H, Kempeneers J. Endoscopic obliteration of large esophagogastric varices with bucrylate. Endoscopy 1986; 18: 25–6.

79. Frühmorgen P, Bodem F, Reidenbach HD, Kaduk B, Demling L. Endoscopic laser coagulation of bleeding gastrointestinal lesions with report of the first therapeutic application in man. Gastrointest Endosc 1976; 23: 73–5.

80. Gong F, Swain P, Kadirkamanathan S, et al. Cutting thread at flexible endoscopy. Gastrointest Endosc 1996; 44: 667–74.

81. Swain CP. New technology for diagnostic and therapeutic endoscopy. In: Classen M, Tytgat GNJ, Lightdale CJ, editors. Gastroenterological endoscopy. Stuttgart: Thieme; 2002: p.62–70.

82. Gauderer MW, Ponsky JL, Izant RJ Jr. Gastrostomy without laparotomy: a percutaneous endoscopic technique. J Pediatr Surg 1980; 15: 872–5.

83. Classen M, Demling L. [Endoscopic sphincterotomy of the papilla of Vater and extraction of stones from the choledochal duct]. Dtsch Med Wochenschr 1974; 99: 496–7. German.

84. Kawai K, Akasaka Y, Murakami K, Tada M, Koli Y. Endoscopic sphincterotomy of the ampulla of Vater. Gastrointest Endosc 1974; 20: 148–51.

85. Staritz M, Ewe K, Meyer zum Büschenfelde KH. Endoscopic papillary dilation (EPD) for the treatment of common bile duct stones and papillary stenosis. Endoscopy 1983; 15: 197–8.

86. Riemann JF, Demling L. Lithotripsy of bile duct stones. Endoscopy 1983; 15 (Suppl 1): 191–6.

87. Nakajima M, Yasuda K, Cho E. Endoscopic sphincterotomy and mechanical basket lithotripsy for management of difficult common bile duct stones. J Hepatobiliary Pancreat Surg 1997; 4: 5–10.

88. Frimberger E, Kühner W, Weingart J, Ottenjann R. [A new method of electrohydraulic cholelithotripsy (lithoklasia)]. Dtsch Med Wochenschr 1982; 107: 213–5. German.

89. Koch H, Rösch W, Walz V. Endoscopic lithotripsy in the common bile duct. Gastrointest Endosc 1980; 26: 16–8.

90. Lux G, Ell C, Hochberger J, Müller D, Demling L. The first successful endoscopic retrograde laser lithotripsy of common bile duct stones in man using a pulsed neodymium-YAG laser. Endoscopy 1986; 18: 144–5.

91. Neuhaus H, Hoffmann W, Gottlieb K, Classen M. Endoscopic lithotripsy of bile duct stones using a new laser with automatic stone recognition. Gastrointest Endosc 1994; 40: 708–15.

92. Wild JJ, Reid JM. Diagnostic use of ultrasound. Br J Phys Med 1956; 19: 248–57.

93. Strohm WD, Phillip J, Hagenmüller F, Classen M. Ultrasonic tomography by means of an ultrasonic fiberendoscope. Endoscopy 1980; 12: 241–4.

94. DiMagno EP, Buxton JL, Regan PT, et al. Ultrasonic endoscope. Lancet 1980; 1: 629–31.

95. Hisanaga K, Hisanaga A, Nagata K, Ichie Y. High speed rotating scanner for transgastric sonography. AJR Am J Roentgenol 1980; 135: 627–9.

96. Hawes RH, van Dam J, Varadarajulu S, editors. Diagnostic and interventional endoscopic ultrasound: 16th International Symposium on Endoscopic Ultrasonography, September 12–13, 2008, San Francisco, California. Gastrointest Endosc 2009; 69 (2 Suppl): S 1–S 266 [special issue].

97. Kelling G. Über Oesophagoskopie, Gastroskopie und Kölioskopie. Münch Med Wochenschr 1902; 49: 21.

98. Kelling G. Endoskopie für Speiseröhre und Magen. Münch Med Wochenschr 1898; 50: 1591–5.

99. Jacobaeus HC. Über Laparo- und Thorakoskopie bei Untersuchung seröser Höhlungen anzuwenden. Münch Med Wochenschr 1910; 58: 2090–2.

100. Kalk H, Wildhirt E, Burgmann W. Lehrbuch und Atlas der Laparoskopie und Leberpunktion. Stuttgart: Thieme; 1962.

101. Henning HI, Lightdale CJ, Look D. Color atlas of diagnostic laparoscopy. New York: Thieme Medical; 1994.

102. Helmreich-Becker I, Meyer zum Büschenfelde KH, Lohse AW. Safety and feasibility of new minimally invasive diagnostic laparoscopy technique. Endoscopy 1998; 30: 756–62.

103. Semm K. Endoscopic appendectomy. Endoscopy 1983; 15: 59–64.

104. Mühe E. Die erste Cholezystektomie durch das Laparoskop. Langenbecks Arch Chir 1986; 369: 804–6.

105. Mouret PH. From the first laparoscopic cholecystectomy to the frontiers of laparoscopic surgery: the future perspectives. Dig Surg 1991; 8: 124–5.

106. Dubois F, Berthelot G, Levard H. [Cholecystectomy by coelioscopy]. Presse Méd 1989; 18: 980–2. French.

107. Perissat J, Collet D, Belliard R. Gallstones: laparoscopic treatment—cholecystectomy, cholecystostomy, and lithotripsy. Our own technique. Surg Endosc 1990; 4: 1–5.

1

2 Quality Assurance

Anthony T. R. Axon

Introduction

In recent years, quality assurance has become an integral part of health-care provision. This has arisen in response to demands from health-care purchasers, providers and staff, and more particularly as a result of increasing patient expectations.

Patients undergoing digestive endoscopy have a right to understand why the procedure is necessary, what it will entail, and what alternatives there are. They must be aware of the risks they will be taking and must be assured that the examination will be performed in an efficient and well-run department by qualified personnel with experience and a good track record. Patients expect to be treated politely and with consideration shown both to themselves and to the relatives and friends who accompany them. After the procedure, they expect the findings to be discussed with them without delay, their follow-up to be organized efficiently, and to return home safely with advice on how to seek emergency assistance if required.

Quality assurance in endoscopy is designed to ensure that examinations are carried out to the accepted current standard. If applied properly with regular auditing, this leads to continued improvement in the quality of the service provided. This is to the advantage not only of the patient, whose experience is by far the most important aspect, but also of health-care purchasers, providers, and health-care workers as well.

History of Quality Assurance

The Emperor Augustus (63 BC–14 AD) said, "I found Rome built of bricks; I leave her clothed in marble" [1]. Quality was an important concept in the ancient world. The skills employed by the Roman builders in the construction of public buildings and civil engineering can still be seen today in monuments that testify to the quality of their workmanship. Throughout the history of civilization, governments have employed inspectors to ensure that major projects were carried out to specification. In the Middle Ages, trade guilds were set up to protect both craftsmen and the public by ensuring that only those who had served an apprenticeship could become master tradesmen and charge at the appropriate rate. Nevertheless, for most articles purchased or services received, there was no guarantee and it was a case of "buyer beware."

The Industrial Revolution led to the employment of less skilled workers in factories. In order to maintain quality standards, they worked under the supervision of a foreman. During the First World War, governments employed inspectors in the munitions factories to encourage better-quality products.

Modern quality assurance began in the USA in the 1930s, when "statistical quality control" was established on production lines. Following the Second World War, quality control was introduced into Japan by the Americans in order to help rebuild the country's industrial base. It was this that led to quality assurance—a concept based not just on following specifications laid down by an employer, but also on taking customer feedback into account. As a result, Japanese industry flourished during the 1970s. Quality assurance expanded to encompass employee education and working conditions, when it became recognized that employee satisfaction was essential for producing high-quality products.

Quality assurance in medicine has taken longer to develop. In England, the Royal College of Physicians was established in 1517, but practitioners belonging to the College largely practiced in the upper echelons of society. The Society of Apothecaries (founded as an offshoot from the Society of Grocers in 1617) provided the medical care available to most of the population. The Company of Barber-Surgeons formed in 1540 from the union of the Fellowship of Surgeons and the Company of Barbers. This partnership remained uneasy until in 1745, the surgeons broke away and formed a separate Company of Surgeons. In 1800, the Company of Surgeons was granted a Royal Charter and became The Royal College of Surgeons in London, later of England. These organizations restricted membership of the guild or college on the basis of an individual's educational training. During the 18th century, a visit to the "quack doctor" was also a social event (**Fig. 2.1**).

During the 19th and 20th centuries, medicine became scientific. Medical practitioners were obliged to obtain a license to practice, but having done so they had a free hand to practice as they wished (although their licence could be withdrawn if they practiced unethically). Specialist registration was not introduced in the United Kingdom until the 1970s. Since then, with the rapid advances in new and specialized medical, diagnostic, and therapeutic techniques, there have been radical changes in health care. Its costs have increased exponentially, medicine has become politicized, litigation has increased, and most of all patients' expectations have soared.

In the 1970s and early 1980s, the concept of medical auditing was introduced. Medical audits were aimed at assessing outcomes such as mortality, drug expenditure, and complications of surgery. Identifying the reasons why mortality or complications occurred, or why drug expenditure was high, made it possible to establish guidelines to rectify problems. The auditing loop was closed by repeating the audit at a later date and if necessary modifying the guidelines in the light of the new audit.

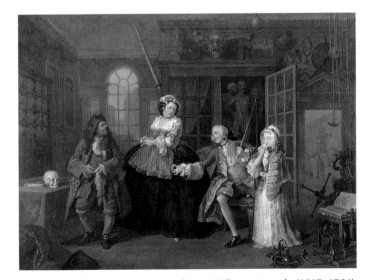

Fig. 2.1 Quality assurance in medicine. William Hogarth (1697–1764), *Marriage à la Mode, 3: The Inspection,* also known as *The Visit to the Quack Doctor* (ca. 1743; © The National Gallery, London).

Auditing drew attention to the variability of medical practice between one institution and another. A highly publicized investigation into excessive mortality in children undergoing heart surgery at Bristol Royal Infirmary in England during the years 1983–1995 revealed that no mechanisms were in place to identify problems automatically. These concerns, allied with the rapidly increasing cost of health care, led health contractors and patients to demand reassurance about the effectiveness of interventions and the standard of care. It became apparent that the only way to prevent inadequate practice was to introduce some form of quality assurance.

Quality Assurance in Endoscopy

Quality assurance involves setting a standard of care and ensuring that it is maintained. Health care can be divided into the elements of structure, process, and outcome [2]. In the case of endoscopy, examples of structure would include the endoscopy unit, equipment, and staff; the process would be the actual endoscopic procedure; and the outcome would be the change in health status resulting from the endoscopic procedure. Quality assurance therefore needs to address all three aspects; good structure will increase the likelihood of a good process, and a good process the likelihood of a good outcome. It is essential to place the patient at the center of quality assurance. This involves assessment and quantification of the clinical quality of the procedure provided for the patient, and also the quality of the patient's experience itself.

The next step is to consider what to measure when assessing quality. "Indicators" known to reflect the quality of care are required. Once these have been identified, a minimum standard can be set and performance can be measured against it. Failure to reach such a standard would demonstrate a poor quality of care and would result in action being taken to improve practice [3].

▥ Quality Indicators

The measurement of quality in endoscopy has been addressed in detail by a working party of the American Society of Gastrointestinal Endoscopy (ASGE) and the American College of Gastroenterology [4]. The resulting recommendations are available free of charge on the ASGE web site (www.asge.org). The task force produced a comprehensive and practical approach to quality indicators. The report includes a general introduction applicable to all gastrointestinal endoscopic procedures and then deals individually with esophago-gastroduodenoscopy, colonoscopy, endoscopic retrograde cholangiopancreatography (ERCP), and endoscopic ultrasonography. Recommendations are graded according to the quality of evidence in the literature that supports the various recommendations—ranging at best from grade 1A, where there is a clear benefit supported by randomized trials without important limitations and leading to a strong recommendation that can be applied to most clinical settings; down to grade 3, where the clarity of benefit is unclear, the evidence is based on expert opinion only, and the implication of the recommendation is weak and likely to change as further data become available.

Table 2.1 Preprocedural quality indicators

- Patient demographics
- Indication
- Timeliness
- Consent
- Clinical status and risk assessment
- Special precautions
- Sedation plan
- Team pause ("time out")

▥ Preprocedural Quality Indicators

Quality indicators in digestive endoscopy can be broadly divided into three aspects: preprocedural, intraprocedural, and postprocedural. Table 2.1 sets out the general preprocedural quality indicators based on the recommendations made by the American working party. Most of these indicators form part of the written endoscopy report.

Indication for Endoscopy

The indication for the procedure must be stated. An endoscopic examination will generally be undertaken only if the potential findings are likely to influence the management of the patient. Endoscopy is contraindicated when the risks of the procedure outweigh its potential benefit, or when the patient, having been fully informed of the advantages and disadvantages of the procedure, decides against having it done. There is a gray area in which the benefits of endoscopy are marginal, or when the cost or inconvenience of the procedure may outweigh the benefit. A number of authorities have made recommendations regarding which clinical situations merit endoscopy and which do not [5,6], but it is not unusual for significant pathology to be identified in a proportion of patients who would fall into the "inappropriate" group [7–9]. National guidelines on indications cannot necessarily be applied in other countries, as the epidemiology of diseases, the facilities available, and prosperity vary from country to country.

Timeliness

The timeliness of the procedure is of importance; patients usually expect a diagnosis without delay. Timeliness must be judged in relation to the indication—for example, a patient presenting with melena will require a more urgent endoscopy than one with dyspeptic pain.

Informed Consent

The issue of informed consent has assumed considerable importance in recent years [10]. Patients in most developed countries today expect to receive a full explanation as to why they require an endoscopy, what it will involve, how much it will cost, the risks it will entail, and how complications would be managed. They should also be aware of what alternative investigations could be used and when the procedure can be carried out. Each patient should receive an easily understood information sheet to take home. Ideally, unless it is an emergency procedure, the patient should sign the consent form at a later date, after they have had time to reflect and if necessary discuss it with friends, relations, or other professionals. The form should not be signed in the endoscopy suite just before the procedure takes place.

Preliminary Assessment

Before the endoscopy procedure, the patient's health status should be assessed, the American Society of Anesthesiology (ASA) score should be recorded (Table 2.2), and any potential risks should be noted—for example, whether antibiotic prophylaxis is needed or whether advice should be given to the examiner regarding the patient's anticoagulation treatment or diabetes. Special precautions may be needed, such as avoidance of latex rubber gloves. The patient may have drug allergies, or in those with sleep apnea it may be necessary to have an anesthetist in attendance. A sedation plan should be drawn up and discussed with the patient so that he or she is aware of what will take place.

Team Pause

The American guidelines suggest that before sedation is administered or the endoscope is inserted, a pause should be observed and documented, during which the team are clear that they have the correct patient and that the appropriate procedure will be done, and to reassess any other data that might influence the endoscopy procedure.

Intraprocedural Quality Indicators

Table 2.3 shows the intraprocedural quality indicators for EGD. Quality indicators vary according to which procedure is being performed.

Monitoring

All patients require monitoring of some kind. For those receiving sedation, intravenous access is essential, pulse oximetry and oxygen saturation is now standard, and most units monitor blood pressure. Electrocardiography may be necessary in certain patients.

Drugs and Sedation

Any medication given must be documented. It is helpful for the nursing staff to record the degree of sedation and any discomfort experienced by the patient or lack of cooperation. These data can be linked to the amount of sedation given to the patient and may lead to the conclusion that an endoscopist is either using too much or too little sedation, or possibly the endoscopic technique requires improvement.

Recordings

A photographic record of the procedure should be made. In some units, a video of the examination is retained. The timing of the procedure is valuable, particularly in colonoscopy, where the time taken to reach the cecum may provide some assessment of the examiner's endoscopic skill, whilst—perhaps more importantly—the time to extubation, if not long enough, may lead to a smaller harvest of polyps.

Postprocedural Quality Indicators

Table 2.4 sets out the quality indicators for the postprocedural period.

Discharge Criteria

An in-house protocol should be in place setting out the discharge criteria for patients. These should be documented at discharge, and the patient should be provided with written instructions as to what to do in the immediate post-discharge period. The patient must be

Table 2.2 American Society of Anesthesiology (ASA) score

Class	Findings
I	Healthy patients
II	Mild systemic disease, no functional limitations, no acute problems (e. g., controlled hypertension, mild diabetes)
III	Severe systemic disease, definite functional limitation (e. g., brittle diabetic, frequent angina, myocardial infarction)
IV	Severe systemic disease with acute, unstable symptoms (e. g., myocardial infarction within last 3 months, congestive heart failure, acute renal failure, uncontrolled active asthma)
V	Severe systemic disease with imminent risk of death

Table 2.3 Intraprocedural quality indicators recorded for esophagogastro-duodenoscopy

- Instruments
- Monitoring
- Medication
- Completeness of examination
- Location of Z line
- Findings
- Photographic record
- Procedure time
- Patient discomfort
- Endoscopic therapy given
- Outcome
- Biopsies taken
- Complications

Table 2.4 Postprocedural quality indicators

- Predetermined discharge criteria
- Written instructions for patient
- Pathology results
- Follow-up
- Report
- Complications
- Patient satisfaction
- Communication with referring clinician
- Postprocedural drug treatment

informed about the follow-up arrangements and when pathology results will become available.

The Report

The endoscopy report is the most important part of the quality assurance exercise, as it contains most of the information that will be required for analysis. It should include the patient's name and demographic details, the name of the referring clinician, and the indication for the procedure. The patient's ASA grade should be recorded, together with the nature and amount of sedation given and the instrument used for the examination. Any peculiarities or difficulties experienced in the procedure should be noted. In the case of colonoscopy, the quality of bowel preparation should be indicated. Then the extent of the procedure should be described—for example, whether the cecum was reached or the ileum. Any abnormalities identified should be described, along with the procedures undertaken—specifically, whether biopsies were taken and if so, from where and what number. Complications are recorded, as well as the use of any additional sedation or reversal agents.

Specific quality indicators collected by the nursing staff, such as the degree of sedation, discomfort, and pre-assessment and post-

Table 2.5 Intraprocedural quality indicators for endoscopic retrograde cholangiopancreatography (ERCP; in addition to those given in Table 2.2)

- Assessment of procedural difficulty
- Cannulation success
- Use of precut
- Size and number of biliary stones
- Stone clearance success
- Extraction technique used
- Stent placement
- Clinical success rate

Table 2.6 Intraprocedural quality indicators in colonoscopy (in addition to those given in Table 2.2)

- Quality of bowel preparation
- Cecal intubation
- Small-bowel intubation
- Number of polyps detected
- Number of polyps retrieved
- Size of polyps
- Time to cecum
- Withdrawal time

assessment details should be recorded separately by nursing staff and included in the computerized report.

Discharge

A letter should be despatched to the referring clinician indicating the findings of the endoscopy. The staff responsible for discharging the patient must be certain that the patient is fully appraised of any change in medication that is to take place after the endoscopy, such as restarting anticoagulant treatment. Patients should be provided with an emergency phone number, so that if there are any problems they can access medical advice after leaving the endoscopy unit.

Patient Satisfaction

Information should be gathered about patient satisfaction. This is usually done by encouraging patients to complete a questionnaire. The number of patients who respond is limited, and it is difficult to know how much confidence can be attached to these results. There are similar issues with late complications. Prospective studies identify more complications than those obtained retrospectively or by questionnaire. Inability to record accurately patients' views and any complications that occur is a serious drawback in assessing patient satisfaction.

It is beyond the scope of this chapter to discuss in detail all of the quality indicators for each type of procedure, but suggested intraprocedural indicators for ERCP and colonoscopy are listed in **Tables 2.5** and **2.6**, and the American guidelines mentioned above can be consulted.

Nursing Involvement in Quality Assurance

Quality assurance is a team activity. It involves the director of the endoscopy unit, the nurse in charge, the nursing staff, the hospital administration, secretarial and reception staff, and those responsible for cleaning and maintenance of the department. However, documentation of the quality indicators rests mainly with the medical and nursing staff, who are largely responsible for the prelimi-

nary assessment, intraprocedural monitoring, and postprocedural assessment.

Other areas besides the procedure itself require quality control. These include tracking of the equipment used, cleaning and disinfection of endoscopic equipment, and auditing of these processes. Ordering of equipment and inventory maintenance are necessary for the smooth and efficient running of an endoscopy unit.

Staff Safety and Satisfaction

Staff safety, efficient and personalized rostering, the provision of changing facilities, showers, and access to refreshment all encourage a happy working environment. Nursing staff often regard the quality of their working time and in particular their hours of work and scheduling as more important than the level of their salary, so it is incumbent upon those in charge of endoscopy units to ensure that working conditions are as good as they possibly can be in order to retain experienced staff and thereby provide a better-quality service.

How Should Quality Indicators Be Recorded?

Most of the quality indicators discussed above will be recorded routinely in the endoscopy report. For the purposes of quality assurance, however, it is essential that all relevant quality indicators for a particular procedure should be included.

In colonoscopy, the quality of the bowel preparation, the amount of sedation given, the colonoscopist's expertise, the time spent reaching the cecum and during withdrawal, the number of polyps identified, and instruments used are all interrelated. If these comprehensive data are not available and cannot be analyzed, the cause of a poor outcome by an endoscopist or by an endoscopy unit cannot be identified.

The incidence of bleeding, perforation, and pancreatitis in ERCP may be related to the skill of the operator, the time taken to do the procedure, the patient's age, gender, and indication, and the use of the needle precut technique. Unless all of these indicators can be analyzed, the reason why an individual examiner has a higher incidence of postprocedural pancreatitis may not be apparent. The purpose of continued quality improvement is to identify areas in which individual endoscopists or units can improve their outcomes, so complete data collection is necessary and the ability to analyze the data is critical.

Quality Assurance and Information Technology

Many endoscopists still complete their examination reports by dictation or freehand rather than using a computerized reporting system. This means that quality indicators are often not fully recorded and manual retrospective analysis is required for quality assurance.

The advantage of a computerized system is that software can be created that insists on quality indicators being entered. Further development of the software enables comparisons to be made between oxygen desaturation, the amount of sedation, and successful cecal intubation, for example. At present, the major drawback with quality assurance is the absence of commercially available software systems that are able to record and analyze the relevant data in the way indicated above. Some argue that the use of computerized endoscopic reporting seriously prolongs the time taken to complete the report. This is certainly true of a number of software systems that have been developed. However, the better-designed ones can be used with considerable speed once the endoscopist has completed the learning curve.

There is a need for better and more readily available systems using generally accepted terminology, such as the Minimal Standard Terminology published by the World Organization of Digestive Endoscopy/*Organisation Mondiale d'Endoscopie Digestive* (OMED) [11]. A further advantage of a computerized system is that it provides a typed (and therefore legible) report that is immediately available for despatch to referring clinicians or the patients themselves. A computer-generated report saves secretarial time and storage space and allows immediate access to previous endoscopy reports.

For individuals and departments without access to computerized reporting, quality assurance is limited to retrospective analysis of written or typed reports, or specific prospective audits undertaken as a separate exercise, which is often incomplete and subjective.

A simple example of the colonoscopy success rate obtained from eight colonoscopists working in a department in England over a 3-month period is shown in **Fig. 2.2**. Similar data can be extrapolated in graphic form showing the ASA grades of the patients examined, the number of polyps identified, and the average dose of sedation used [12].

How Should Quality Assurance Data Be Used?

Quality Standards

The aim of quality assurance is to ensure that patients receive a high standard of care within the endoscopy unit. For this to be possible, it is necessary to set certain quality standards. For example, a department, a health-care provider, or a national endoscopy society might recommend that endoscopists should be able to perform total colonoscopy 90 % of the time and that they should be able to retrieve at least one tubular adenoma from at least 15 % of the examinations that they undertake. By monitoring the endoscopists in a unit using the techniques outlined above, it would become apparent which endoscopists were not reaching the prescribed quality level. This would lead to an analysis of that endoscopist's data to see whether, for example, he or she was not spending sufficient time trying to reach the cecum, whether the patient mix was different or the patients were less well prepared, older, or less healthy, or whether insufficient sedation was being used. Remedial action could then be taken, which might involve the endoscopist concerned having a period of performing endoscopy under supervision.

Quality assurance should not be threatening. The data in **Fig. 2.2** are anonymized and were sent to all eight colonoscopists, each of whom knew his or her own number but was not able to identify the others. All of the numbers were known to the quality assurance supervisor, an experienced colonoscopist who was able to take individual action if it became necessary. The availability of these data, circulated by e-mail, enabled those who were less successful to identify where their examinations were falling short.

Trainees

Routine prospective collection of data is helpful in assessing the progress of trainees. The use of this technology allows more objective assessment of the trainees' success, which is a better method of determining competence than assessing it on the basis of the number of procedures performed or one or two endoscopies carried out under supervision.

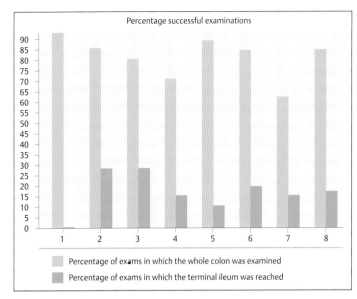

Fig. 2.2 Success for total colonoscopy (%).

Continuous Quality Improvement

Quality assurance should not be used to provide only a minimum quality of treatment. When applied correctly, it should engender continuous improvement in quality, and this can be done only by frequent monitoring of quality indicators, with regular assessment as to how the quality can be improved. This should be applied across the whole range of the service being provided and include waiting times, scheduling, cost management, efficiency in the endoscopy unit, and staff satisfaction, in addition to improving technical success rates and clinical outcomes. In the United Kingdom, this approach has been introduced into the National Health Service using the endoscopy Global Rating Scale (GRS).

The Endoscopy Global Rating Scale

Total control of medicine by the government ("socialized medicine") enables government to introduce quality regulations and insist that they be followed. In the United Kingdom, the Department of Health has introduced a web-based questionnaire that all National Health Service endoscopy units are expected to complete [13]. It is divided into two separate dimensions: clinical quality and quality of patient experience. Each of these two dimensions includes 12 patient-centered items (**Table 2.7**). Each of the 24 items in turn has a series of statements to which the endoscopy director has to answer "yes" or "no" online. On the basis of these replies, the Department of Health is able to derive a global rating score, the lowest level being D and the highest A. Since its inception, the percentage of units scoring A or B has increased. To achieve a high rating means that there has to be continuous monitoring of a variety

Table 2.7 The twelve patient–centered standards used in the United Kingdom Global Rating Scale for endoscopy

Clinical quality	Quality of patient experience
• Appropriateness	• Equality
• Information/consent	• Timeliness
• Safety	• Choice
• Comfort	• Privacy and dignity
• Quality	• Aftercare
• Timely results	• Ability to provide feedback

Source: www.grs.nhs.uk.

of quality indicators, with an achievement of a colonoscopy completion rate of over 90 %, and an adenoma detection rate of over 10 %, with a polyp recovery rate of more than 90 %. Sedation and analgesia, comfort levels, good-quality bowel preparation, and continuous monitoring for complications have to be performed. Further details, together with a list of quality and safety indications for endoscopy, are available on the GRS web site (www.grs.nhs.uk).

Impact of Quality Assurance on Endoscopic Practice

The introduction of quality assurance undoubtedly increases the workload not just for the endoscopist, but for most of the team working in the endoscopy unit and in particular the chief nurse and endoscopy director. Continuous monitoring and regular auditing increases the cost of running the endoscopy unit, and in addition will identify defective equipment requiring replacement. Examinations take longer if the endoscopist adheres to recommended standards—for example, it takes longer to obtain informed consent, and the extubation time at endoscopy may have to be increased to maximize the number of polyps identified.

Quality assurance also covers efficiency in the endoscopy unit and should lead to more appropriate scheduling, a reduction in the numbers of unnecessary endoscopies performed, and more efficient methods of reducing turnaround time. Improved patient satisfaction should lead to fewer complaints and a reduction in litigation. The most important outcome should be an improvement in the clinical effectiveness of endoscopy [14,15], fewer complications, more satisfied patients, and improved conditions for staff, leading to a higher rate of staff retention, better morale, and pride in the service being provided.

What Are the Next Steps?

The principles underlying quality assurance in endoscopy are now firmly established. There is general agreement on which quality indicators should be recorded. To date, however, there is no universal consensus regarding the level of quality that should be achieved. National and international organizations are beginning to appreciate that it is necessary to set certain standards that will have to be reached if an individual endoscopist is to remain in practice or if a department is to continue to provide a service. We can expect to see the introduction of specific parameters within the next few years.

Standards will be set on the basis of what is considered to be good practice. Provided that individual endoscopists are competently trained and that they continue to perform a sufficient number of procedures on a regular basis and attend courses in professional development, there should be little difficulty in maintaining an acceptable endoscopic standard. No doctor enjoys practicing suboptimally. Among those who practice within accepted guidelines, the risk of litigation will fall. Refresher courses will be required for those who would benefit from them.

Managing the Endoscopy Unit

It is becoming recognized that specific skills and training are required for individuals who manage endoscopic services. OMED initiated a series of Endoscopy Directors' Workshops in 2005 in order to improve the standard of endoscopy worldwide. Many aspects of the workshops are concerned with quality in one way or another, but an important section is specifically designed to discuss quality assurance in the endoscopy unit. A group within the ASGE is also hoping to set up a section within the society to address issues relating to endoscopy unit management [16]. These workshops and meetings have identified important areas of management not previously addressed by health-care providers or by national societies. A major deficiency is the inadequate provision of information technology in endoscopy. Although some organizations have attempted to stimulate industry to take an interest in this area, the products created have not fulfilled requirements. Considerable work is needed in this area.

References

1. Suetonius. The twelve Caesars, trans. Robert Graves, rev. ed. James Rives. London: Penguin; 2007; p. 59.
2. Donabedian A. Evaluating the quality of medical care. Milbank Mem Fund Q 1966; 44: 166–206.
3. Brown RD, Goldstein JL. Quality assurance in the endoscopy unit: an emphasis on outcomes. Gastrointest Endosc Clin N Am 1999; 9: 595–607.
4. Bjorkman DJ. Measuring the quality of endoscopy. Gastrointest Endosc 2006; 63: S 1–2.
5. American Society for Gastrointestinal Endoscopy. Appropriate use of gastrointestinal endoscopy. Gastrointest Endosc 2000; 52: 831–7.
6. Vader JP, Burnand B, Froehlich F, Dubois RW, Bochud M, Gonvers JJ. The European Panel on Appropriateness of Gastrointestinal Endoscopy (EPAGE): project and methods. Endoscopy 1999; 31: 575–8.
7. Adler A, Roll S, Marowski B, Drossel R, Rehs HU, Willich SN, et al. Appropriateness of colonoscopy in the era of colorectal cancer screening: a prospective, multicenter study in a private-practice setting (Berlin Colonoscopy Projecct I, BECOP). Dis Colon Rectum 2007; 50: 1628–38.
8. Hassan C, Bersani G, Buri L, Zullo A, Anti M, Bianco MA, et al. Appropriateness of upper-GI endoscopy: an Italian survey on behalf of the Italian Society of Digestive Endoscopy. Gastrointest Endosc 2007; 65: 767–74.
9. Chan TH, Goh KL. Appropriateness of colonoscopy using the ASGE guidelines: experience in a large Asian hospital. Chin J Dig Dis 2006; 7: 24–32.
10. Shepherd H, Hewett D. Guidance for obtaining a valid consent for elective endoscopic procedures. A report of the Working Party of the British Society of Gastroenterology. London: British Society of Gastroenterology; 2008. Available from: http://www.bsg.org.uk/images/stories/docs/clinical/guidelines/endoscopy/consent08.pdf.
11. World Organization of Digestive Endoscopy. Minimal Standard Terminology MST 3.0. Munich, Germany: OMED Committee of Documentation and Standardization, 2008. Available from: http://www.omed.org/index.php/resources/re_mst/.
12. Naylor G, Gatta L, Butler A, Duffet S, Wilcox M, Axon AT, et al. Setting up a quality assurance program in endoscopy. Endoscopy 2003; 35: 701–7.
13. GRS Global Rating Scale [Internet]. Available from: www.grs.nhs.uk.
14. Ball JE, Osbourne J, Jowett S, Pellen M, Welfare MR. Quality improvement programme to achieve acceptable colonoscopy completion rates: prospective before and after study. BMJ 2004; 329: 665–7.
15. Imperiali G, Minoli G, Meucci GM, Spinzi G, Strocchi E, Terruzzi V, et al. Effectiveness of a continuous quality improvement program on colonoscopy practice. Endoscopy 2007; 39: 314–8.
16. Al-Kawas FH. Proposed endoscopy directors SIG. ASGE News 2008; 15: 26.

3 Advanced Imaging in Endoscopy

Ralf Kiesslich and Hisao Tajiri

Introduction

The prognosis for patients with gastrointestinal tract malignancies is strictly dependent on early detection of premalignant and malignant lesions. However, small, flat, or depressed neoplastic lesions are still difficult to detect with conventional techniques, which are therefore of limited value for polyp and cancer screening. What would the ideal advanced imaging method be capable of? Three steps are important: recognition, characterization, and confirmation (**Fig. 3.1**).

- *Recognition* of lesions in the gut can be improved using better scopes that provide better imaging quality, such as high-resolution or high-definition imaging. Autofluorescence may also be helpful in allowing better recognition of lesions.
- *Characterization* of the lesion type and surface architecture is important for predicting the histology, and chromoendoscopy or digital chromoendoscopy can make this easier. New software modalities are emerging here. A proposal for a consensus terminology for new imaging modalities is available and should be used [1].
- Histological *confirmation* is needed in order to establish whether or not cancer is present. It can be provided by conventional histology, or most recently also with in vivo histology (confocal laser endomicroscopy). Molecular imaging may be able to open up new prospects for tailored and individualized diagnosis.

New diagnostic tools are being developed in order to allow targeted therapy. New endoscopic techniques such as endoscopic submucosal dissection (ESD) and natural orifice transluminal endoscopic surgery (NOTES) are now available, and these will broaden the therapeutic options available in gastrointestinal endoscopy in the near future.

High-Resolution and Magnifying Endoscopy

High-resolution and magnification endoscopes provide an imaging quality that is significantly better than that of the first-generation video endoscopes and the older fiberoptic systems. The *resolution* of an endoscopic image is a different quality from its *magnification* and is defined as the ability to distinguish between two points that are located close together. High-resolution imaging improves the ability to discriminate details, while magnification enlarges the image. In digital video imaging, resolution is a function of pixel density. As they use charged-coupled devices (CCDs) that have a high pixel density, high-resolution endoscopes can provide slightly magnified views of the gastrointestinal tract with greater mucosal detail. Magnification endoscopy uses a movable lens controlled by the endoscopist to vary the degree of magnification, which ranges from 1.5× to 150×. Newly designed magnification endoscopes include high-resolution and magnification features.

High-definition endoscopes have recently become available. CCDs convert light information into electronic signals, which are processed into an image by the video processor. The standard analogue broadcasting systems (PAL and NTSC) generate approximately 480–576 scanning lines on a screen. The new high-definition endo-scopes can generate up to 1080 scanning lines on a screen, which further increases the resolution. Surface analysis of distinct lesions can be done even before magnification (**Fig. 3.2**). For screening colonoscopy, convincing data are available to show that high-definition endoscopy leads to increased detection rates in patients who have at least one adenoma [2].

Chromoendoscopy

Chromoendoscopy, or tissue staining, is a comparatively old endoscopic technique that has been in use for decades. It involves the topical application of stains or pigments in order to improve the localization, characterization, or diagnosis of lesions [3]. It is a useful adjunct to endoscopy, with the contrast between normally stained and abnormally stained epithelium enabling the endoscopist to make a diagnosis and/or to target biopsies on the basis of a specific reaction or enhancement of the surface morphology (**Fig. 3.2**).

The staining technique is simple and easy to learn. Chromoendoscopy can be done in an untargeted fashion, including a whole segment (panchromoendoscopy), or can be directed towards a specific lesion (targeted staining). During untargeted spraying of dye in the colon, the endoscopist has to direct the endoscope and catheter tip toward the colorectal mucosa and use a combination of clockwise/counterclockwise rotation with simultaneous withdrawal of the endoscope tip.

During the 1990s, surface analysis of stained colorectal lesions provided new visual impressions for endoscopists. Kudo et al. [4] first reported that there are regular staining patterns that are often seen in hyperplastic polyps or normal mucosa, whereas an unstructured surface architecture is associated with malignancy. The type of adenoma (tubular vs. villous) can also be identified by detailed

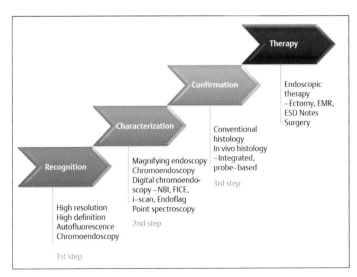

Fig. 3.1 Three diagnostic steps to targeted therapy: new options. EMR, endoscopic mucosal resection; ESD, endoscopic submucosal dissection; FICE, Fujinon Intelligent Chromoendoscopy; NBI, narrow-band imaging; NOTES, natural orifice transluminal endoscopic surgery.

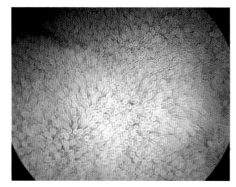

a

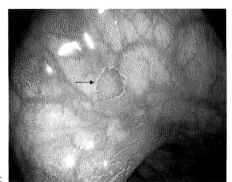

b

Fig. 3.2   High definition and chromoendoscopy. **a** High-definition image of the terminal ileum. **b** Individual villi can be differentiated on closer observation even without further magnification, due to the high-resolution charge-coupled device (CCD) and high-definition imaging. **c** Chromoendoscopy—e. g., with methylene blue staining—can be used to unmask flat lesions (arrow). **d** An aberrant crypt focus is clearly visible after magnification. The blue bands and lines represent the epithelial cell layer.

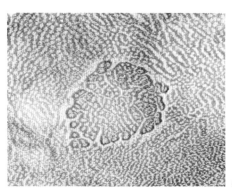

c

d

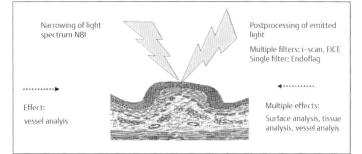

Fig. 3.3   Digital chromoendoscopy is available simply by pressing a button on the endoscope. Narrow-band imaging (NBI) focuses on the vessel architecture by narrowing the spectrum of the light emitted to the mucosa. Fujinon Intelligent Chromoendoscopy (FICE), i-scan, and Endoflag are technologies that use the reflected light for postprocessing filtering, which is used to produce different effects (such as surface, tissue, and vessel enhancement).

inspection. This led to a categorization of the different staining patterns seen in the colon. Known as the pit-pattern classification [4], this system distinguishes between five types, with several subtypes. Types 1 and 2 are staining patterns that predict nonneoplastic lesions, whereas types 3 to 5 predict neoplastic lesions. With the help of this classification, the endoscopist is able to predict the histology with a good level of accuracy. The pit-pattern classification was developed with the help of magnifying endoscopes, and the question arises of whether endoscopic differentiation of different staining patterns is also possible using the more widely available high-resolution endoscopes.

Chromoendoscopy has been shown to have significant advantages for detecting flat colorectal neoplasia and colitis-associated neoplasia [5], but its value in the upper gastrointestinal tract is still a matter of controversy, and no clear recommendations about its use can be made. However, the success of chromoendoscopy in the lower gastrointestinal tract has stimulated instrument manufacturers to develop new light filters that can mimic chromoendoscopy. The systems available are known as narrow-band imaging

(NBI), Fujinon Intelligent Chromoendoscopy (FICE; Fujinon Europe, Ltd., Willich, Germany), and i-scan (Pentax Europe Ltd., Hamburg, Germany). New systems are also being developed and may offer new computer-assisted diagnostic algorithms.

Digital Chromoendoscopy

Conventional white-light endoscopy uses the full range of visible wavelengths to produce a red–green–blue image. In contrast, narrow-band imaging, in combination with magnification endoscopy, illuminates the tissue surface using special filters that narrow the respective red, green, and blue bands. This enhances the tissue microvasculature, mainly due to the differential optical absorption of light by hemoglobin in the mucosa, associated with the initiation and progression of dysplasia, particularly in the blue range. The resulting images produce an appearance that could be described as chromoendoscopy without the need for dye (**Figs. 3.3, 3.4**).

Alternatively, the light reflected from the mucosa can be modified using postprocessing computer algorithms (e. g., FICE and i-scan). These can be modulated to produce different types of enhancement, leading to accentuation of the vasculature, surface architecture, or pattern visualization (**Figs. 3.2, 3.5**).

Narrow-band imaging is not useful for recognizing lesions in the colon (see **Fig. 3.1**). However, it can be used to characterize previously identified lesions on the basis of their vascular architecture [6–8]. Narrow-band imaging is becoming very widely used in the upper gastrointestinal tract, as it can help unmask high-grade intraepithelial neoplasia and early cancers in patients with Barrett's esophagus and squamous-cell cancer [9].

New filtering techniques are also available that use adaptive image-processing algorithms (filtering and logic) for segmentation and extraction of image irregularities. This can be achieved irrespective of the size, shape, contrast, and color of the irregularities. Endoflag (Endopix Ltd., Tel Aviv, Israel), for example, is a single-filter, single-pass system that processes standard or high-definition video sequences (**Fig. 3.6**) [10].

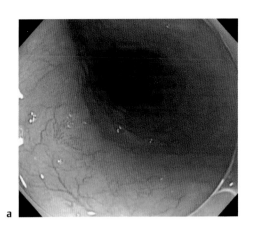
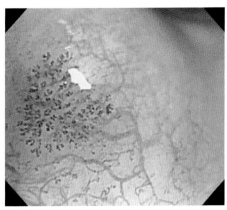

Fig. 3.4 Squamous cell cancer of the upper esophagus.
a White light imaging within the upper esophagus identifies irregularities of the superficial vasculature.
b NBI clarifies the angiogenesis and delineate the borders of the early cancer (2 mm). The lesion was removed subsequently with EMR.

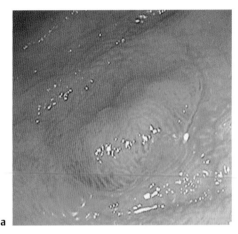
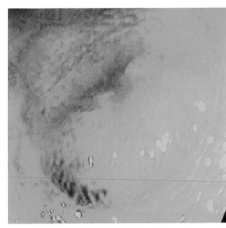

Fig. 3.5 Digital chromoendoscopy (i-scan) and chromoendoscopy of a flat adenoma.
a High-definition white-light imaging. **b** i-scan V: increased vasculature is displayed with an intense blue. **c** i-scan P: pattern analysis is possible, and the villous architecture can be identified. **d** Chromoendoscopy with indigo carmine leads to better visualization of tissue details.

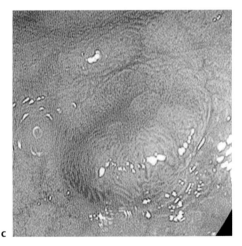
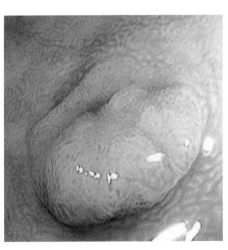

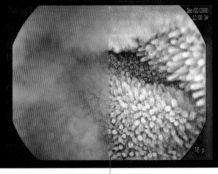
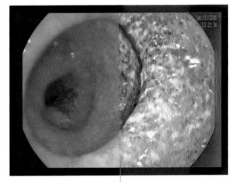

Fig. 3.6 Postprocessing with an adaptive intelligent filter system. Images are postprocessed during the ongoing procedure, with the enhanced image being displayed on one half of the monitor. Multiple displays (with two monitors and the region of interest) are possible to assist the endoscopist.
a Normal terminal ileum: single villi can be differentiated after postprocessing. **b** In a patient with ulcerative colitis, the inflammation is better visualized after postprocessing.

Standard view | Online postprocessing

Standard view | Online postprocessing

Functional Imaging

In standard endoscopy, reflection and absorption are the two interactions between light and tissue that are used to generate an image. When incident light hits the mucosa, several other tissue interactions such as autofluorescence, elastic scattering, and Raman scattering also occur. The optical signals resulting from these light–tissue interactions depend on the molecular and structural composition of the tissue. As neoplastic progression in tissue leads to changes in its composition, information from these interactions can be used for tissue diagnosis (i. e., functional imaging).

Point Spectroscopy

Light–tissue interactions can also be investigated using point spectroscopy. This is a probe-based technique in which a fiberoptic probe is passed through the accessory channel of an endoscope and placed in close contact with the mucosa. Depending on the optical signal to be investigated, a specific light source generates excitation light, which is transported to the mucosa via efferent optic fibers in the probe. Afferent optic fibers then collect the light signals that return to the probe from the tissue and transport these back to an optical analyzer (spectrograph) outside the endoscope. The signals emitted can be displayed as light spectra on a computer and subsequently analyzed for tissue diagnosis.

Fluorescence Spectroscopy

When tissue is exposed to light that has a short wavelength (e. g., ultraviolet light or blue light), excitation of certain endogenous substances occurs, leading to the emission of light with a longer wavelength (i. e., autofluorescence). Normal tissue may have different autofluorescence spectra in comparison with neoplastic tissue, due to changes in the molecular distribution and architecture of neoplastic tissue.

Autofluorescence spectroscopy has been shown to allow identification of early neoplastic lesions in patients with Barrett's esophagus, with a high level of sensitivity (86–100%) and specificity (76–97%) [11–13]. In addition, exogenous fluorescing substances can be used to induce fluorescence in tissues of interest (i. e., drug-induced fluorescence) [14,15].

Elastic Scattering Spectroscopy

During light–tissue interactions, incident photons can be deflected without alterations in wavelength (a phenomenon known as elastic scattering). Elastic scattering spectroscopy measures the behavior of white light when it leaves the tissue after multiple scattering events. The scattering spectra depend on the size and density of nuclei in the uppermost epithelial cells [16]. In early neoplastic tissue, the size and density of nuclei (i. e., the nucleus–cytoplasm ratio) is increased in comparison with normal tissue. On the basis of this phenomenon, it is possible to distinguish between low-grade and high-grade intraepithelial neoplasia with acceptable sensitivity and specificity rates [17].

Raman Spectroscopy

This technique detects scattered light that has undergone small shifts in wavelength (inelastic scattering) after single-wavelength excitation. The wavelength shifts correspond to specific vibrations of common molecular bonds in tissue. Raman spectroscopy is a very promising technology that may be able to generate very specific spectra, potentially providing a high degree of accuracy in differentiating early neoplastic tissue from normal tissue. However, the weak signals produced by Raman spectroscopy require sophisticated instruments and complex statistical techniques for detecting and analyzing the spectral differences between different tissues [18].

Multimodal Spectroscopy

Different spectroscopy techniques measure different optical properties of tissue and may be able to provide complementary diagnostic information when used together. This may result in more accurate spectroscopic diagnosis. Georgakoudi et al. showed that a combination of autofluorescence, reflectance, and elastic scattering spectroscopy resulted in better sensitivity and specificity in comparison with the diagnostic performance of each of the modalities alone [12]. An important drawback with point spectroscopy, however, is that it samples only small areas of tissue ($1–2\,mm^3$). The future success of all types of spectroscopy will therefore be strictly dependent on whether they can be incorporated into real-time full-viewing endoscopy systems that can screen large surface areas.

Autofluorescence Imaging

A new autofluorescence imaging system has recently been developed that uses a video endoscope with two CCDs—one for high-resolution white-light endoscopy and one for autofluorescence imaging (AFI). The autofluorescence image is a pseudocolored image composed from three integrated images: total autofluorescence after blue light excitation (395–475 nm), green reflectance (540–560 nm), and red reflectance (600–620 nm). The additional value of AFI was investigated by Kara et al. in a feasibility study including 60 patients with Barrett's esophagus [19]. Early neoplasia was detected in 21 patients; 14 patients had lesions detected with high-resolution white-light endoscopy (which were also positive on AFI), whereas seven patients were diagnosed solely with AFI. In addition, in six patients in whom lesions were visible with white light, AFI detected 11 additional neoplastic lesions. This uncontrolled study suggests that this video AFI system may be able to improve the detection of early neoplasia in patients with Barrett's esophagus. However, the drawback in the study was a high false-positive rate of approximately 50% with AFI.

In a proof-of-principle study, Kara et al. also later combined video AFI endoscopy with NBI to try to reduce the high false-positive rate [20]. In this study, high-resolution endoscopy and AFI were used for primary detection of suspicious lesions, with NBI then being used for detailed inspection of the suspicious lesions. Twenty-eight lesions with early neoplasia were detected; 17 were identified using high-resolution endoscopy (61%) and 28 using AFI (100%). AFI detected a total of 47 suspicious lesions; 28 contained early neoplasia and 19 were false-positive findings (40%). With NBI, suspicious patterns were found in all lesions with early neoplasia.

Another new system has recently become available that incorporates high-resolution endoscopy, AFI, and NBI into a single system—endoscopic trimodality imaging (ETMI). This system uses a new autofluorescence algorithm in which the fluorescence image is composed of two integrated images instead of three: total autofluorescence after blue light excitation (395–475 nm) and green reflectance (**Figs. 3.7**, **3.8**). The results of an international multicenter feasibility study using this system showed that AFI increased the sensitivity for detecting early neoplasia from 53% for high-resolution white-light endoscopy to 90%. In addition, NBI reduced the

, b

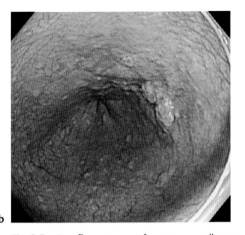
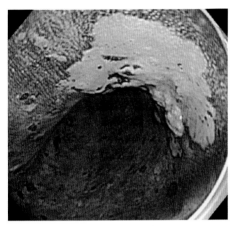
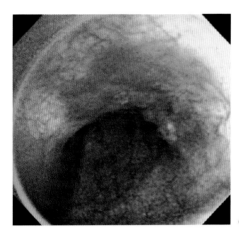

c

Fig. 3.7 Autofluorescence of squamous cell cancer in the esophagus.
a Discrete nodularities are visible in the mid portion of the esophagus.
b Autofluorescence shows the malignant spread in a pinkish coloration.

c The tumour extend could be confirmed using Lugol's solution. The malignant changes remain unstained.

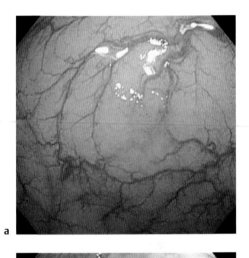
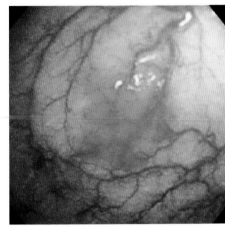

a

b

Fig. 3.8 Autofluorescence in the colon.
a A reddish area can be identified using white light imaging.
b Autofluorescence indicate a flat adenoma.
c The extend and surface pattern can be identified after chromoendoscopy.
d The flat adenoma was resected endoscopically and a tubular adenoma with low-grade intraepithelial neoplasia could be confirmed.

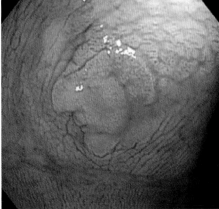
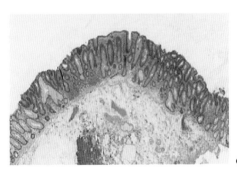

c

d

high false-positive rate of AFI from 81% to 26% [21]. The main advantage of this new prototype is that it incorporates multiple imaging modalities, including high-resolution white-light endoscopy, into one system. However, the true additional value of these imaging modalities (AFI and NBI) has yet to be established in high-quality randomized cross-over studies.

Optical Coherence Tomography

Optical coherence tomography (OCT) is a high-resolution cross-sectional imaging technique. It is analogous to B-mode high-resolution endosonography, but uses light waves instead of acoustic waves. As a result, OCT has high resolution (up to 10 times higher than high-frequency ultrasound), allowing microstructural features of tissue to be identified, although it has a limited sampling depth of 1–2 mm [22]. OCT measures the intensity of back-scattered light from tissue at various depths using low-coherence interferometry (**Figs. 3.9, 3.10**).

Interferometry measures the interference produced by two light beams derived from a single source. One beam is directed at the tissue sample and the other at a reference mirror, the location of which is precisely known. The light reflected from the sample and the reference beam is recombined at a detector, and the interference between the two beams is measured. Using a light source with a short coherence length allows the distance traveled by the sample

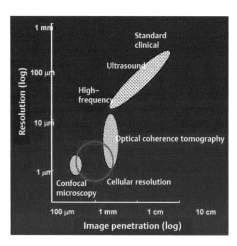

Fig. 3.9 The resolution and image penetration available with different imaging modalities.

raphy, OCT can be performed without a coupling medium (e.g., water). The OCT catheter has to be positioned adjacent to the mucosa within the system's focal distance (1–5 mm), which may be difficult due to movements of the esophagus caused by peristalsis and heartbeat. In addition, compression artifacts may be seen when the probe comes into contact with the mucosa.

The use of OCT was first described in ophthalmology and dermatology in the early 1990s. The first report describing endoscopic in vivo OCT was published by Sergeev et al. in 1997 [23]. The five-layered structure of the normal esophageal wall (i.e., squamous epithelium, lamina propria, muscularis mucosae, submucosa, and muscularis propria) was clearly identified using OCT and correlated well with the histopathological findings.

OCT can easily differentiate normal epithelium from abnormal tissue with a high degree of accuracy. However, detecting and grading high-grade dysplasia and early cancer continue to be challenging. Future developments in OCT, such as ultrahigh-resolution OCT, spectroscopic OCT, Doppler OCT, and optical frequency-domain imaging, may enhance the accuracy of OCT in detecting dysplasia and give rise to further applications.

beam to be determined, as interference only occurs when the path lengths of both light beams are matched to within the coherence length of the light source. The axial resolution of OCT is thus determined by the coherence length of the light source. By recording the location of the reference mirror, the magnitude of the back-reflected light signal from the sample can be determined as a function of depth. This measurement is referred to as an "axial scan." To create a two-dimensional image, axial scans are performed rapidly while the interrogating beam is swept across the sample. Images are usually displayed as gray-scale images, which can represent high back-reflection signals as either dark or light.

OCT is a probe-based technique in which the probe is passed through the accessory channel of an endoscope. Unlike endosonog-

Endocytoscopy

Endocytoscopy is based on the principle of light contact microscopy. The initial studies using this system were conducted in the field of otolaryngology. After application of methylene blue, the tip of a rigid endoscope was placed in direct contact with the tissue surface. The method makes it possible to visualize cytological details directly, allowing direct observation of living cells [24]. However, the rigid instrument used in the first endocytoscopy system was not practical

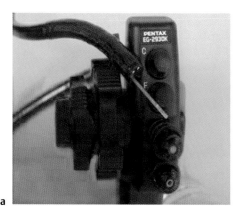

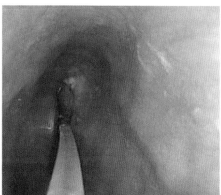

a

b

Fig. 3.10 Optical coherence tomography (OCT). **a** The probe is passed over the working channel. **b** The OCT probe is placed on the region of interest (in this case the distal esophagus). **c** An OCT image showing the different layers of the esophagus. **d** The corresponding histological findings.

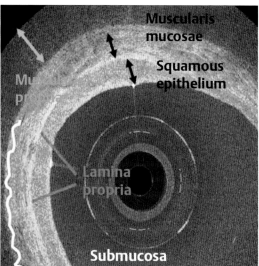

c

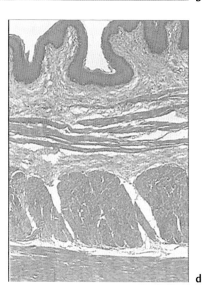

d

for use in the gastrointestinal tract. A novel endocytoscope system has therefore been developed, known as the endocytoscope. This consists of two flexible endoscopes with a diameter of 3.2 mm, which can easily pass through an accessory channel with a diameter of 3.7 mm—a low-magnification endocytoscope with a maximum magnification of 450× and a high-magnification endocytoscope with a maximum magnification of 1100×. The endocytoscope has also recently been integrated into an otherwise conventional endoscope.

Endocytoscopy is used to identify the cellular and nuclear architecture of the surface layer of the epithelium. Residual mucin and motion artifacts can alter its accuracy. The combination of macroscopy (white-light endoscopy) and microscopy (endocytoscopy) has led to a better understanding of the surface microarchitecture. The current system is not capable of visualizing the deeper layers of the epithelium and is therefore not yet suitable for evaluating the depth of invasion in early neoplasia. In addition, the system requires the use of 1 % methylene blue, which significantly reduces the brightness of the white-light image and may increase DNA damage in the tissue after illumination [25].

Confocal Laser Endomicroscopy

Confocal laser endomicroscopy is a new imaging modality for gastrointestinal endoscopy. It allows in vivo imaging of the mucosal layer at cellular and even subcellular resolution, making in vivo histology possible during ongoing endoscopy. This new imaging modality provides more information than conventional histology, as cellular interactions can be observed over time (physiological processes) and distinct changes can be identified (pathophysiological processes).

▨ Principle of Confocal Microscopy

Confocal microscopy provides better spatial resolution in comparison with conventional fluorescence microscopy, as the images are not contaminated by light scattering from other focal planes. A low-powered laser is focused to a single point within a defined microscopic field of view, and the same lens is used as both condenser and objective folding optical path. The point of illumination thus coincides with the point of detection within the specimen. Light emanating from that point is focused through a pinhole to a detector, and light emanating from outside the illuminated spot is excluded from detection. The illumination and detection system are on the same focal plane, and the process is therefore termed "confocal." All of the signals detected from the illuminated spot are captured and measured. The gray-scale image created is an optical section representing one focal plane within the specimen being examined. The image of a scanned region can then be constructed and digitized by measuring the light returning to the detector from successive points.

Series of confocal images in successive planes can be used to observe fine cellular or subcellular structures, and in addition three-dimensional structures of specimens can be created. Confocal microscopy has become a standard method for molecular imaging in basic research, in conjunction with fluorescence labeling techniques, making it possible to localize specific proteins at distinct cellular locations. However, the method has so far mainly been used experimentally, rather than at the bedside [26].

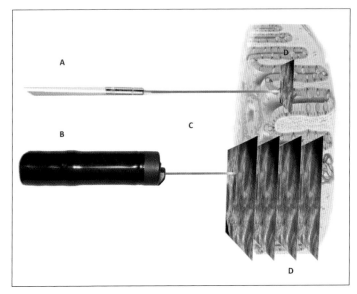

Fig. 3.11 Types of confocal endomicroscopy. Two different confocal endomicroscopic systems are currently available. The miniprobe (**A**) can be passed over the working channel of standard endoscopes (Cellvizio, Mauna Kea Technologies, Paris, France). The endomicroscope (**B**) is embedded in an otherwise standard endoscope (Pentax, Japan). The blue laser light is applied onto and into the mucosa (**C**). The fluorescence and reflected light is measured, and gray-scale images of the mucosal microarchitecture are displayed on an additional monitor. The miniprobe has a fixed imaging plane depth (**D**), whereas the confocal endoscope can vary the imaging plane depth during imaging, from the surface down to the deepest parts of the mucosal layer.

▨ Endoscopic Confocal Microscopy

Endoscopic confocal microscopy is an outgrowth of conventional laboratory confocal microscopy. Currently, two confocal imaging systems are available for in vivo detection of gastrointestinal diseases: confocal imaging that relies on tissue reflectance, and confocal imaging based on tissue fluorescence. Reflectance endomicroscopy was first described by Sakashita et al. [27] in 2003. The method suffers from poor resolution and poor contrast.

Fluorescence confocal imaging has overcome these limitations. The first publication on integrating a confocal fluorescence microscope into the distal tip of a conventional colonoscope (Pentax EC-3830FK; Pentax, Tokyo, Japan) appeared in 2004 [28] and showed that in vivo microscopy at a subcellular resolution (0.7 μm), simultaneously displayed with white-light endoscopy, was possible and provided a high degree of accuracy. This approach, known as confocal laser endomicroscopy (CLE), allowed immediate diagnosis of colorectal intraepithelial neoplasias using fluorescein or acriflavine as contrast agents.

A probe-based confocal endomicroscope has recently been developed that can be passed through the working channel of standard endoscopes. This further miniaturization using fiber-bundle technology provides a lateral resolution of 3.5 μm, axial resolution of 15 μm, and a field of view of 600 × 500 μm, with a fixed imaging plane depth [29] (**Fig. 3.11**).

▨ Contrast Agents

Fluorescence confocal imaging is only possible using exogenous fluorescence contrast agents. Potentially suitable agents are fluorescein, acriflavine, and cresyl violet [26].

The most common contrast agents are acriflavine hydrochloride (0.05 % in saline; topical use only) or fluorescein sodium (5–10 mL of

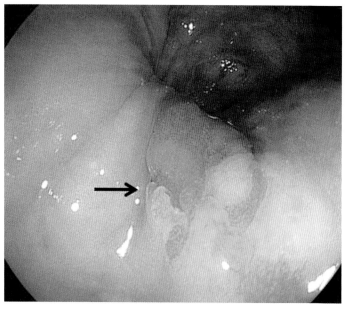

a

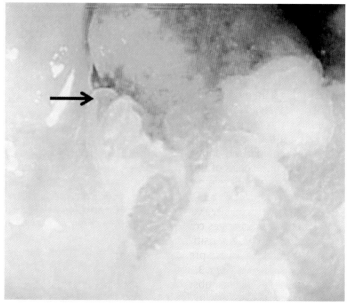

b

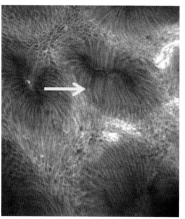

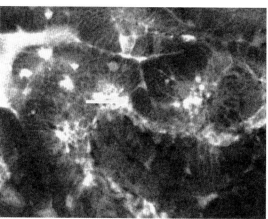

c, d

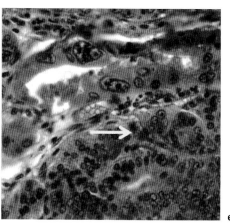

e

Fig. 3.12 Confocal endomicroscopy of early Barrett's cancer.
a Short-segment Barrett's esophagus is visible with white-light endoscopy. A subtle depression can be identified (arrow). **b** The i-scan function (postprocessing light filter) helps highlight the subtle changes (arrow). **c** Normal, nonneoplastic Barrett's glands are characterized by their roundish appearance and the presence of goblet cells (arrow). **d** Malignant cellular architecture is characterized by dark irregular cells with different shapes and sizes (arrow). Infiltration of malignant cells into the lamina propria can be observed, indicating at least mucosal cancer. **e** Endomicroscopy-guided mucosal resection revealed early Barrett's cancer (m2, well-differentiated).

a 10 % solution; intravenous administration). Confocal imaging following staining with acriflavine hydrochloride and fluorescein sodium reveals a characteristic morphology in mucosal tissue. Whereas topically administered acriflavine hydrochloride strongly labels the superficial epithelial cells, including nuclei, intravenously applied fluorescein sodium distributes throughout the entire mucosa, with strong contrast in connective tissue and the capillary network. Fluorescein binds to serum albumin, and unbound dye molecules that remain pass across systemic capillaries and enter the tissue, highlighting the extracellular matrix. Confocal images can be generated simultaneously with endoscopic images, making it possible to identify typical histologic structures in the upper and lower gastrointestinal tract.

Clinical Data in Endomicroscopy

Endomicroscopy can be used to observe living cells during ongoing endoscopy, enabling the examiner to identify a plethora of changes. Thorough familiarity with mucosal pathology is mandatory to allow reliable diagnosis.

Barrett's Esophagus

Barrett's esophagus is a recognized premalignant condition in patients with gastroesophageal reflux disease, and most adenocarcinomas of the distal esophagus have been shown to arise in Barrett's tissue. Barrett's esophagus is defined histologically as the presence of specialized columnar epithelium (SCE) with goblet cells. The columnar-lined lower esophagus (CLE) can be identified during standard upper endoscopy. SCE is often present in a patchy mosaic distribution within CLE and may be overlooked when random biopsies are taken, resulting in biopsies of the cardia or gastric type of mucosa without goblet cells. However, it has been suggested that four-quadrant step biopsies within CLE can serve as the gold standard for diagnosing Barrett's epithelium and Barrett's-associated neoplastic changes (**Fig. 3.12**).

Endomicroscopy makes it possible to identify CLE macroscopically and identify goblet cells microscopically in the distal esophagus, allowing immediate and reliable diagnosis of Barrett's esophagus. In the first endomicroscopic study of Barrett's esophagus, including 63 patients, different types of epithelial cell could be distinguished and cellular and vascular changes were detected using fluorescein-guided endomicroscopy [30]. A classification of confocal images for the diagnosis of Barrett's epithelium and Barrett's-associated neoplasias was developed on the basis of a comparison of the in vivo and conventional ex vivo histology. The classification distinguishes between three types of epithelium: gastric epithelium; Barrett's epithelium without neoplastic changes; and Barrett's epithelium with neoplastic changes.

In the first study dealing with endomicroscopy in patients with Barrett's esophagus [30], 156 areas and 3012 images were reassessed in accordance with the newly developed confocal Barrett classification and compared with the targeted biopsies (411 biopsies). The comparison showed that Barrett's esophagus could be predicted on the basis of the identification of goblet cells with the help of confocal endomicroscopy with a sensitivity of 98.1 % and a specificity of 94.1 % (accuracy 96.8 %; positive predictive value 97.2 %; negative predictive value 96.0 %). In addition, Barrett's-associated neoplastic changes could be predicted on the basis of irregular black cells with a sensitivity of 92.9 % and a specificity of 98.4 % (accuracy 97.4 %; positive predictive value 92.9 %; negative predictive value 98.4 %) (see **Fig. 3.2**).

This initial study was subsequently confirmed prospectively with a cross-over design [6]. In this study, confocal guided biopsies improved the yield for detecting neoplasia from 17 % to 33 % in a group of patients with suspected nonlocalized endoscopically invisible high-grade dysplasia (n = 16). In patients undergoing routine surveillance of Barrett's esophagus (n = 23), it was possible to avoid mucosal biopsies in almost two-thirds of the cases, as no neoplasia was found to be present during endomicroscopic imaging.

Confocal endomicroscopy (with the Pentax system) with targeted biopsies can thus allow the endoscopist to obtain biopsies in a better-targeted way and could potentially reduce the delay arising before definitive therapy can be offered to patients with Barrett's-associated neoplasia [31]. Endomicroscopy is also able to guide mucosal resection [32]. Data have also recently become available for miniprobe-based endomicroscopy [33]. A total of 296 biopsy sites in 38 consecutive patients with Barrett's esophagus were examined using standard high-resolution endoscopy and miniprobe endomicroscopy. Endomicroscopically examined areas were matched with biopsies using argon beamer marking of the tissue examined. Criteria for Barrett's and associated neoplasia were established on the basis of 15 patients, and these criteria were prospectively investigated in 23 patients using video recording of the endomicroscopic examination. In a per-biopsy analysis, the sensitivity and specificity for two independent investigators were 75.0 % and 88.8 %, and 75.0 % and 91.0 %, respectively—translating at best into a positive predictive value of 44.4 % and a negative predictive value of 98.8 %. Interobserver agreement was good ($\kappa = 0.6$).

The diagnostic yield of miniprobe-based endomicroscopy appears to be lower than that of the integrated type of endomicroscopy, possibly due to the lower resolution and fixed imaging plane depth of the miniprobe.

Gastritis and Gastric Cancer

Gastritis is defined histologically by various stages of inflammatory changes. These include infiltration of inflammatory cells into the lamina propria, often combined with alterations and defects in the mucosal surface, such as erosions.

Helicobacter pylori and nonsteroidal anti-inflammatory drugs can induce gastritis, which can lead to atrophic gastritis and intestinal metaplasia, increasing the risk for gastric cancer. *H. pylori* and intestinal metaplasia are easily identified using confocal laser endomicroscopy [34–36]. *H. pylori* can be found on the surface of the gastric mucosa, and acriflavine can be used as a topical contrast agent to identify it. Intestinal metaplasia is best visualized using fluorescein contrast. The tissue has a much brighter appearance in

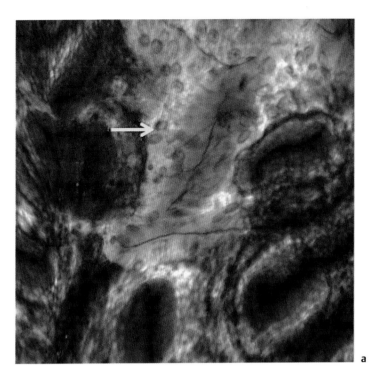

a

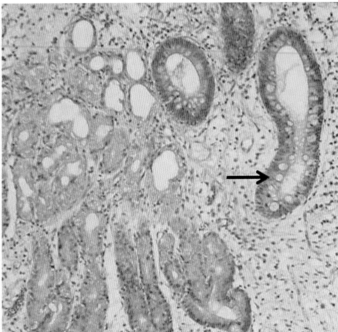

b

Fig. 3.13 Atrophic gastritis and intestinal metaplasia in the stomach. **a** The different tissue components (normal gastric mucosa and intestinal metaplasia) are readily identified due to their distinct staining patterns. Intestinal metaplasia is characterized by a brighter appearance, with the presence of goblet cells (arrow). **b** Endomicroscopy-guided biopsies confirmed the presence of intestinal metaplasia (arrow) and atrophic gastritis.

comparison with the surrounding normal mucosa, and goblet cells can be identified due to their characteristic target sign (**Fig. 3.13**).

Zhang et al. [35] investigated the pattern and in vivo architecture of gastritis and gastric cancer in 132 consecutive patients. Confocal images obtained from the 132 patients were compared with the histopathologic findings in biopsy specimens from the corresponding confocal imaging sites in a prospective and blinded fashion. The gastric pit-pattern cellular architecture was classified into seven types (**Fig. 3.14**).

Category	The appearance of pit patterns by confocal endomicroscopy	Distribution area	Diagram
Type A	Round pits with round opening	Normal mucosa with fundic gland	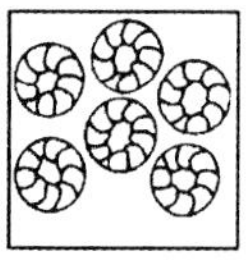
Type B	Non-continuous short rod-like pits with short thread-like opening	Corporal mucosa with chronic inflammation	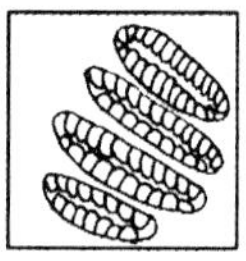
Type C	Continuous short rod-like pits with slit-like opening	Normal mucosa with pyloric gland	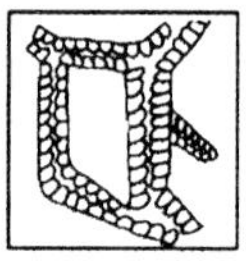
Type D	Elongated and tortuous branch-like pits	Antral mucosa with chronic inflammation	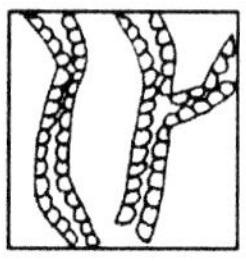
Type E	The number of pits decreasing and pits prominently dilating	Chronic atrophy gastritis	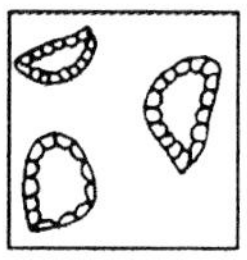
Type F	Villus-like appearance, interstitium in the centre and goblet cells appearing	Intestinal metaplastic mucosa	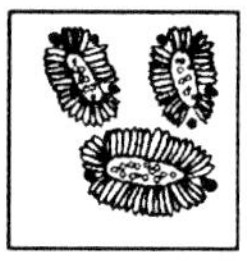
Type G			
Type G_1	Normal pits disappearing, with the appearance of diffusely atypical cells	Signet-ring cell carcinoma and poorly differentiated tubular adenocarcinoma	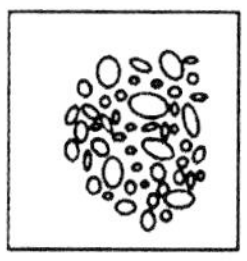
Type G_2	Normal pits disappearing, with the appearance of atypical glands	Differentiated tubular adenocarcinoma	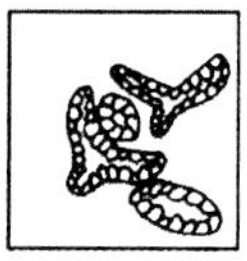

Fig. 3.14 The classification of gastric pit patterns by confocal endomicroscopy. Reprinted from Gastrointestinal Endoscopy Vol. 67, No. 6, Zhang et al. Classification of gastric pit patterns by confocal endomicroscopy, 843–853: 2008, with permission from Elsevier.

Fluorescein-guided endomicroscopy displays the vessel architecture, which can be used to differentiate between nonneoplastic and neoplastic lesions. Vascular function can be observed, and leakage of fluorescein into the lamina propria is characteristic of inflammation or neo-angiogenesis [35].

Endoscopic detection of early gastric cancer is challenging, as most of the lesions are usually nonpolypoid. Endomicroscopy allows immediate microscopic analysis of the gastric mucosa during ongoing endoscopy. Intra-individual comparison of regular and altered gastric mucosa facilitates the interpretation of the confocal images.

Changes in tissue and microvascular architecture, as well as changes in cell morphology, are valuable endomicroscopic criteria for defining neoplasia. Nuclear changes are best observed using acriflavine as a topical contrast agent, as shown by Kakeji et al. [37]. Kitabatake et al. were able to demonstrate differences in the mucosal vasculature depending on the grade of tumor differentiation using endomicroscopy. The accuracy of endomicroscopy for diagnosing gastric cancer was over 90 % if good imaging quality was available [38].

Endomicroscopy is ideally suited to diagnosing intestinal metaplasia in patients with atrophic gastritis. H. pylori can be identified in vivo, and distinct cellular and vascular changes can be used to target biopsies to areas of neoplastic change.

▓ Celiac Disease

Celiac disease is very common in Western countries. It is associated with a risk of malignant transformation and severe illness due to malabsorption. Current endoscopic techniques are unable to diagnose celiac disease as accurately as histopathological assessment. The value of confocal endomicroscopy in patients with celiac disease was recently evaluated, with very promising results [39].

Patients with celiac disease and control individuals prospectively underwent endomicroscopy using fluorescein as a contrast agent.

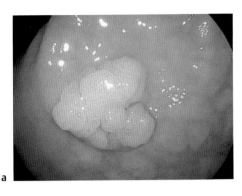
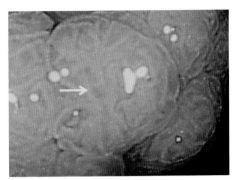

a

b

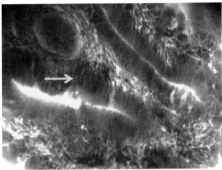
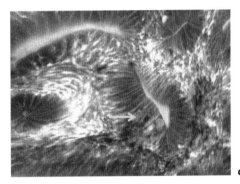

c

d

Fig. 3.15 Tubulovillous adenoma in the rectum. **a** A flat adenoma is present in the sigmoid. **b** Close observation using magnifying endoscopy unmasks the surface staining pattern (Kudo classification III L). Epithelial cell bands can be identified (arrow). **c** Endomicroscopy confirms the presence of tubular adenoma. The tubular architecture, as well as single cells, can be identified (arrow). **d** Depletion of goblet cells indicates the presence of intraepithelial neoplasia (arrow).

Features of villous atrophy and crypt hypertrophy were defined endomicroscopically. A scoring system for measuring the severity of celiac disease in vivo was devised and validated against the diagnosis of celiac disease and blinded histopathology. Receiver operating characteristics, sensitivity to change after treatment, and reliability of findings were assessed. In 31 patients (six with untreated celiac disease, 11 with treated celiac disease, and 14 controls), 7019 confocal endomicroscopy images paired with 326 biopsy specimens were obtained. The accuracy of confocal endomicroscopy for diagnosing celiac disease was excellent (receiver operating characteristics area under the curve 0.946; sensitivity 94%, specificity 92%) and the findings correlated well with the Marsh grading (R^2 0.756). Confocal endmicroscopy differentiated patients with celiac disease from controls ($P < 0.0001$) and was sensitive to changes after treatment with a gluten-free diet (1787 optical biopsies; $P = 0.012$). The intraclass correlation of reliability was high (0.759–0.916). Of the 17 patients with diagnosed celiac disease, 16 (94%) were diagnosed correctly using endomicroscopy, but only 13 of them (76%) had detectable histopathological changes. The procedure was safe and well tolerated. Endomicroscopy thus has great potential for improving the efficiency of endoscopy and the clinical algorithm in patients with celiac disease [39].

Colorectal Cancer

Colorectal cancer is still one of the leading causes of cancer-related death in the world. Screening colonoscopy is widely accepted as the gold standard for early diagnosis of cancer. The prognosis for patients with colonic neoplasia is strictly dependent on the depth of infiltration, and therefore depends on early detection of preinvasive and neoplastic changes. Early detection makes it possible to cure the patient with immediate endoscopic resection.

In 2003, Inoue et al. reported initial experience with real-time confocal endoscopy in ex vivo specimens [40]. The prototype endomicroscope that was used (Olympus Optical Ltd., Tokyo, Japan) was passed through the working channel of an endoscope. The aim of the study was to establish new criteria for distinguishing between benign lesions and high-grade dysplasia or cancer. The authors

examined 100 endoscopically or surgically visualized lesions in normal colonic mucosa or hyperplastic polyps; neoplastic lesions were visible more often. Conversely, goblet cells were visible less often in malignant or premalignant lesions. However, it should be noted that it was not individual nuclei, but rather dark areas within irregular cells that were visible. The study found a statistically significant difference between nonneoplastic and neoplastic lesions in relation to the detection rate of nuclei (dark areas) in laser-scanning confocal microscopy images.

On the basis of these results, the authors recommended preliminary criteria for a confocal imaging classification of high-grade intraepithelial neoplasia and cancer. Neoplasia was characterized by the presence of any structural abnormality and clear visualization of nuclei. However, the sensitivity of this method for predicting colorectal neoplasms was only 60%, reflecting the limited resolution of the system that was used.

In the first study using the newly developed endomicroscopic system, 42 patients with indications for screening or surveillance colonoscopy after previous polypectomy underwent in vivo endomicroscopy with the confocal laser endoscope [28]. The aim of the study was to assess the histology in vivo during ongoing colonoscopy in order to diagnose intraepithelial neoplasias or colon cancer. Fluorescein-guided endomicroscopy of intraepithelial neoplasias and colon cancers showed a tubular, villous, or irregular architecture, with a reduced number of goblet cells. In addition, neovascularization in neoplasms was characterized by irregular vessel architecture with fluorescein leakage.

A simple classification of the confocal pattern, based on initial experience with confocal endomicroscopy, was developed to allow differentiation between neoplastic and nonneoplastic tissue. Macroscopic and microscopic images were taken together to allow an immediate prediction of the histopathology. It was possible to predict the presence of neoplastic changes using the newly developed confocal pattern classification with a sensitivity of 97.4%, a specificity of 99.4%, and an accuracy of 99.2% [28] (**Fig. 3.15**).

3

Ulcerative Colitis

It is not possible to examine the whole surface of the colon in the endomicroscopic mode. In patients with ulcerative colitis, it is therefore important to combine endomicroscopy with chromoendoscopy. Panchromoendoscopy with either methylene blue or indigo carmine is a valid diagnostic tool for improving the diagnostic yield of intraepithelial neoplasia using the SURFACE recommendations (strict patient selection; unmask surface; reduce peristaltic waves; full-length staining; augmented detection with dyes; crypt architecture analysis; endoscopic targeted biopsies) [41]. Chromoendoscopy can reveal circumscribed lesions, and chromoendoscopy-guided confocal laser endomicroscopy can be used to predict intraepithelial neoplasias with a high degree of accuracy [42]. This allows targeted biopsies of relevant lesions to be taken, and rapid confirmation of neoplastic changes using confocal laser endoscopy during colonoscopy may lead to significant improvements in the clinical management in comparison with the histological results.

In the first randomized trial of endomicroscopy in ulcerative colitis, 153 patients with long-term ulcerative colitis who were in clinical remission were randomly assigned at a ratio of 1:1 to undergo either conventional colonoscopy or panchromoendoscopy using 0.1% methylene blue in conjunction with endomicroscopy to detect intraepithelial neoplasia or colorectal cancer [42]. Circumscribed lesions in the colonic mucosa detected by chromoendoscopy were evaluated with endomicroscopy for cellular and vascular changes in accordance with the confocal pattern classification for predicting neoplasia. Targeted biopsies from the areas examined were taken and histologically graded according to the new Vienna classification.

In the standard colonoscopy group, randomized biopsies were taken every 10 cm between the anus and cecum, as well as targeted biopsies of visible mucosal changes. The primary outcome analysis was a histological diagnosis of neoplasia. Using chromoendoscopy in conjunction with endomicroscopy (80 patients, average examination time 42 min), significantly more intraepithelial neoplasia was detected (19 versus four cases; $P = 0.007$) than with standard colonoscopy (73 patients, average examination time 31 min). Endomicroscopy revealed different cellular structures (epithelial and blood cells), capillaries, and connective tissue limited to the mucosal layer. A total of 5580 confocal images from 134 circumscribed lesions were compared with the histological results from 311 biopsies. The presence of neoplastic changes was predicted with a high degree of accuracy (sensitivity 94.7%, specificity 98.3%, accuracy 97.8%) [42].

In summary, chromoendoscopy is able to reveal circumscribed lesions, and confocal laser microscopy can be used to confirm intraepithelial neoplasias with a high degree of accuracy. Biopsies can therefore be limited to targeted sampling of relevant lesions. In vivo histology with endomicroscopy may lead to significant improvements in the clinical management of patients with ulcerative colitis, with reduced numbers of biopsies being needed for confirmation of the condition and time being gained for immediate therapeutic intervention.

Microscopic Colitis

The term "microscopic colitis" is used for clinicopathological entities characterized by chronic watery diarrhea, normal radiographic and endoscopic appearances, and microscopic abnormalities. Specific histopathological appearances can be used to further classify collagenous colitis, lymphocytic colitis, and other conditions. Collagenous colitis differs from lymphocytic colitis through the presence of a subepithelial collagen band ($\geq 10\,\mu m$) adjacent to the basal membrane. Both diseases cause inflammatory changes in the lamina propria and superficial epithelial damage. Microscopic colitis is considered a rare condition, but increasing awareness of these entities among pathologists and clinicians has resulted in more frequent diagnosis. The incidence of the diseases is unclear, but the incidence of lymphocytic colitis is about three times higher than that of collagenous colitis, and microscopic colitis should be considered as a major possibility in the work-up of chronic diarrhea in older women.

Endomicroscopy makes it possible to locate and measure the distribution and thickness of collagenous bands underneath the epithelial layer, thus allowing targeted biopsies—a new approach in collagenous colitis, particularly in patients with disrupted subepithelial collagen deposits. At present, randomized biopsies are recommended, preferably from the right colon. The distribution of the collagenous bands can be patchy and segmental in the colon. Confocal endomicroscopy helps differentiate between affected and normal sites and can guide biopsies [43,44].

Future of Endomicroscopy

Endomicroscopy can be used for other purposes as well as histological assessment. The great potential of the method lies in displaying and observing physiologic and pathophysiologic changes during ongoing endoscopy. It also makes molecular imaging possible.

Cell shedding is a physiologic process. After cell shedding, epithelial gaps occur that are sealed within seconds. Patients with inflammatory bowel disease have defective gap closure, which can lead to bacterial invasion of the lamina propria (**Fig. 3.16**). These changes can be observed with endomicroscopy, and the findings may lead to new options becoming available in the treatment of inflammatory bowel diseases [45]. Endomicroscopy can display not only the tissue, but also bacterial interaction with the mucosal layer [46].

Molecular imaging has already been achieved [47] (**Fig. 3.17**). Dysplastic colonic crypts were selectively stained with heptapeptides linked with fluorescein. This approach will open the door to new clinical algorithms based on the endomicroscopic findings (e.g., for predicting the efficacy of chemotherapy). The diagnostic range of endomicroscopy is constantly expanding, and the boundaries of the gastrointestinal tract have already been crossed. Endomicroscopy can be used to investigate the bile duct, liver, and cervix [48–50].

Endomicroscopy is thus a revolutionary technique that has significantly broadened the diagnostic range of gastrointestinal endoscopy. It allows in vivo histological assessment, which is currently mainly being used to guide biopsy. In the future, however, endomicroscopy will also be used to develop a better understanding of physiology and pathophysiology, leading to new diagnostic algorithms based on newly discovered microscopic alterations in the mucosal layer. The method has tremendous potential, which is only beginning to be explored. It will be a crucial tool in the endoscopist's armamentarium in the future.

Conclusions

New imaging modalities are rapidly evolving in gastrointestinal endoscopy that will have a substantial influence on everyday work in the very near future. These advances in endoscopic technology follow substantial innovations in the fields of IT (information technology) and multimedia. This will be the beginning of a new era in which computer-assisted solutions and technical innovations will greatly influence diagnostic strategies. The main goal is to achieve

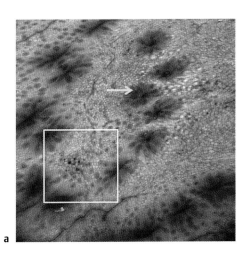
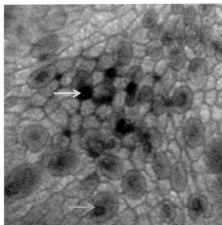

Fig. 3.16 Differentiation of goblet cells and epithelial gaps.
a Healthy colonic mucosa is visible on endomicroscopy with acriflavine contrast. Single round crypts are present (arrow). Epithelial gaps are present after cell shedding (square). **b** Further magnification shows the difference between gaps (yellow arrow) and goblet cells (blue arrow). Goblet cells have a distinct target sign, whereas gaps are displayed as completely black roundish areas.

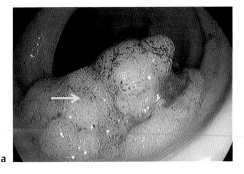
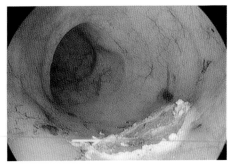

Fig. 3.17 Molecular imaging.
a A villous adenoma in the sigmoid. **b** The resection area after mucosal resection. **c** The resected specimen was incubated in antibody solution (against epidermal growth factor receptor). Antibodies were linked with fluorescein. Active receptors at the cell membrane can be visualized 3 min after resection. **d** Further magnification. In vivo molecular imaging is to become available soon.

3

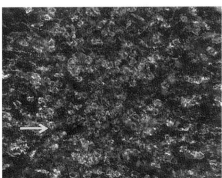
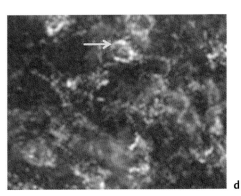

early detection of gastrointestinal cancer in order to save lives and reduce costs.

Evolving technologies are helping to improve diagnosis—advancing from the ability to merely recognize lesions to characterizing them. These steps are essential for targeted endoscopic therapy and making new resection techniques possible. Endoscopic mucosal resection is an already established method, and endoscopic submucosal dissection is following in its footsteps.

References

1. Tajiri H, Niwa H. Proposal for a consensus terminology in endoscopy: how should different endoscopic imaging techniques be grouped and defined? Endoscopy 2008; 40:775–8.
2. Rex DK, Helbig CC. High yields of small and flat adenomas with high-definition colonoscopes using either white light or narrow band imaging. Gastroenterology 2007; 133: 42–7.
3. Canto MI. Staining in gastrointestinal endoscopy: the basics. Endoscopy 1999; 31: 479–86.
4. Kudo S, Tamura S, Nakajima T, Yamano H, Kusaka H, Watanabe H. Diagnosis of colorectal tumorous lesions by magnifying endoscopy. Gastrointest Endosc 1996; 44: 8–14.
5. Kiesslich R, Fritsch J, Holtmann M, Koehler HH, Stolte M, Kanzler S, et al. Methylene blue-aided chromoendoscopy for the detection of intraepithelial neoplasia and colon cancer in ulcerative colitis. Gastroenterology 2003; 124: 880–8.
6. Machida H, Sano Y, Hamamoto Y, Muto M, Kozu T, Tajiri H, et al. Narrow-band imaging in the diagnosis of colorectal mucosal lesions: a pilot study. Endoscopy 2004; 36: 1094–8.
7. Kaltenbach T, Friedland S, Soetikno R. A randomised tandem colonoscopy trial of narrow band imaging versus white light examination to compare neoplasia miss rates. Gut 2008; 57: 1406–12.
8. Adler A, Aschenbeck J, Yenerim T, Mayr M, Aminalai A, Drossel R, et al. Narrow-band versus white-light high definition television endoscopic imaging for screening colonoscopy: a prospective randomized trial. Gastroenterology 2009; 136: 410–6.
9. Curvers WL, Bohmer CJ, Mallant-Hent RC, Naber AH, Ponsioen CI, Ragunath K, et al. Mucosal morphology in Barrett's esophagus: interobserver agreement and role of narrow band imaging. Endoscopy 2008; 40: 799–805.
10. Kiesslich R, Goetz M, Schumacher B, Santo EM, Neurath MF, Guissin R, et al. Endoflag—a new video processing technology greatly enhancing recognition and characterization of gastrointestinal lesions seen with standard or high definition endoscopes [abstract]. Gastrointest Endosc 2008; 67: AB135.
11. Panjehpour M, Overholt BF, Vo-Dinh T, Haggitt RC, Edwards DH, Buckley FP 3rd. Endoscopic fluorescence detection of high-grade dysplasia in Barrett's esophagus. Gastroenterology 1996; 111: 93–101.
12. Georgakoudi I, Jacobson BC, Van Dam J, Backman V, Wallace MB, Müller MG, et al. Fluorescence, reflectance, and light-scattering spectroscopy for evaluating dysplasia in patients with Barrett's esophagus. Gastroenterology 2001; 120: 1620–9.
13. Bourg-Heckly G, Blais J, Padilla JJ, Bourdon O, Etienne J, Guillemin F, et al. Endoscopic ultraviolet-induced autofluorescence spectroscopy of the esophagus: tissue characterization and potential for early cancer diagnosis. Endoscopy 2000; 32: 756–65.
14. von Holstein CS, Nilsson AM, Andersson-Engels S, Willén R, Walther B, Svanberg K. Detection of adenocarcinoma in Barrett's oesophagus by means of laser induced fluorescence. Gut 1996; 39: 711–6.
15. Brand S, Wang TD, Schomacker KT, Poneros JM, Lauwers GY, Compton CC, et al. Detection of high-grade dysplasia in Barrett's esophagus by spectroscopy measurement of 5-aminolevulinic acid-induced protoporphyrin IX fluorescence. Gastrointest Endosc 2002; 56: 479–87.
16. Backman V, Wallace MB, Perelman LT, Arendt JT, Gurjar R, Müller MG, et al. Detection of preinvasive cancer cells. Nature 2000; 406: 35–6.
17. Wallace MB, Perelman LT, Backman V, Crawford JM, Fitzmaurice M, Seiler M, et al. Endoscopic detection of dysplasia in patients with Barrett's esophagus using light-scattering spectroscopy. Gastroenterology 2000; 119: 677–82.
18. Wong Kee Song LM, Wilson BC. Endoscopic detection of early upper GI cancers. Best Pract Res Clin Gastroenterol 2005; 19: 833–56.
19. Kara MA, Peters FP, Ten Kate FJ, Van Deventer SJ, Fockens P, Bergman JJ. Endoscopic video autofluorescence imaging may improve the detection of early neoplasia in patients with Barrett's esophagus. Gastrointest Endosc 2005; 61: 679–85.
20. Kara MA, Peters FP, Fockens P, ten Kate FJ, Bergman JJ. Endoscopic video-autofluorescence imaging followed by narrow band imaging for detecting early neoplasia in Barrett's esophagus. Gastrointest Endosc 2006; 64: 176–85.
21. Curvers WL, Singh R, Song LM, Wolfsen HC, Ragunath K, Wang K, et al. Endoscopic tri-modal imaging for detection of early neoplasia in Barrett's oesophagus; a multi-centre feasibility study using high-resolution endoscopy, autofluorescence imaging and narrow band imaging incorporated in one endoscopy system. Gut 2008; 57: 167–72.
22. Das A, Sivak MV Jr, Chak A, Wong RC, Westphal V, Rollins AM, et al. High-resolution endoscopic imaging of the GI tract: a comparative study of optical coherence tomography versus high-frequency catheter probe EUS. Gastrointest Endosc 2001; 54: 219–24.
23. Sergeev AM, Gelikonov VM, Gelikonov GV, Feldchtein FI, Kuranov RV, Gladkova ND, et al. In vivo endoscopic OCT imaging of precancer and cancer states of human mucosa. Opt Express 1997; 1: 432–40.
24. Inoue H, Sasajima K, Kaga M, Sugaya S, Sato Y, Wada Y, et al. Endoscopic in vivo evaluation of tissue atypia in the esophagus using a newly designed integrated endocytoscope: a pilot trial. Endoscopy 2006; 38: 891–5.
25. Curvers WL, Kiesslich R, Bergman JJ. Novel imaging modalities in the detection of oesophageal neoplasia. Best Pract Res Clin Gastroenterol 2008; 22: 687–720.
26. Kiesslich R, Galle PR, Neurath MF, editors. Atlas of endomicroscopy. Heidelberg: Springer, 2008.
27. Sakashita M, Inoue H, Kashida H, Tanaka J, Cho JY, Satodate H, et al. Virtual histology of colorectal lesions using laser-scanning confocal microscopy. Endoscopy 2003; 35: 1033–8.
28. Kiesslich R, Burg J, Vieth M, Gnaendiger J, Enders M, Delaney P, et al. Confocal laser endoscopy for diagnosing intraepithelial neoplasias and colorectal cancer in vivo. Gastroenterology 2004; 127: 706–13.
29. Meining A, Saur D, Bajbouj M, Becker V, Peltier E, Höfler H, et al. In vivo histopathology for detection of gastrointestinal neoplasia with a portable, confocal miniprobe: an examiner blinded analysis. Clin Gastroenterol Hepatol 2007; 5: 1261–7.
30. Kiesslich R, Gossner L, Goetz M, Dahlmann A, Vieth M, Stolte M, et al. In vivo histology of Barrett's esophagus and associated neoplasia by confocal laser endomicroscopy. Clin Gastroenterol Hepatol 2006; 4: 979–87.
31. Dunbar K, Okolo P, Montgomery E, Canto MI. Confocal endomicroscopy in Barrett's esophagus and endoscopically inapparent Barrett's neoplasia: a prospective randomized double-blind controlled crossover trial. Gastrointest Endosc 2009; 69 [in press].
32. Leung KK, Maru D, Abraham S, Hofstetter WL, Mehran R, Anandasabapathy S. Optical EMR: confocal endomicroscopy-targeted EMR of focal high-grade dysplasia in Barrett's esophagus. Gastrointest Endosc 2009; 69: 170–2.
33. Pohl H, Rösch T, Vieth M, Koch M, Becker V, Anders M, et al. Miniprobe confocal laser microscopy for the detection of invisible neoplasia in patients with Barrett's oesophagus. Gut 2008; 57: 1648–53.
34. Guo YT, Li YQ, Yu T, Zhang TG, Zhang JN, Liu H, et al. Diagnosis of gastric intestinal metaplasia with confocal laser endomicroscopy in vivo: a prospective study. Endoscopy 2008; 40: 547–53.
35. Zhang JN, Li YQ, Zhao YA, Yu T, Zhang JP, Guo YT, et al. Classification of gastric pit patterns by confocal endomicroscopy. Gastrointest Endosc 2008; 67: 843–53.
36. Kiesslich R, Goetz M, Burg J, Stolte M, Siegel E, Maeurer MJ, et al. Diagnosing *Helicobacter pylori* in vivo by confocal laser endoscopy. Gastroenterology 2005; 128: 2119–23.
37. Kakeji Y, Yamaguchi S, Yoshida D, Tanoue K, Ueda M, Masunari A, et al. Development and assessment of morphologic criteria for diagnosing gastric cancer using confocal endomicroscopy: an ex vivo and in vivo study. Endoscopy 2006; 38: 886–90.
38. Kitabatake S, Niwa Y, Miyahara R, Ohashi A, Matsuura T, Iguchi Y, et al. Confocal endomicroscopy for the diagnosis of gastric cancer in vivo. Endoscopy 2006; 38: 1110–4.
39. Leong RW, Nguyen NQ, Meredith CG, Al-Sohaily S, Kukic D, Delaney PM, et al. In vivo confocal endomicroscopy in the diagnosis and evaluation of celiac disease. Gastroenterology 2008; 135: 1870–6.
40. Inoue H, Cho JY, Satodate H, Sakashita M, Hidaka E, Fukami S, et al. Development of virtual histology and virtual biopsy using laser-scanning confocal microscopy. Scand J Gastroenterol Suppl 2003; (237): 37–9.
41. Kiesslich R, Neurath MF. Surveillance colonoscopy in ulcerative colitis: magnifying chromoendoscopy in the spotlight. Gut 2004; 53: 165–7.
42. Kiesslich R, Goetz M, Lammersdorf K, Schneider C, Burg J, Stolte M, et al. Chromoscopy-guided endomicroscopy increases the diagnostic yield of intraepithelial neoplasia in ulcerative colitis. Gastroenterology 2007; 132: 874–82.
43. Kiesslich R, Hoffman A, Goetz M, Biesterfeld S, Vieth M, Galle PR, et al. In vivo diagnosis of collagenous colitis by confocal endomicroscopy. Gut 2006; 55: 591–2.
44. Zambelli A, Villanacci V, Buscarini E, Bassotti G, Albarello L. Collagenous colitis: a case series with confocal laser microscopy and histology correlation. Endoscopy 2008; 40: 606–8.
45. Kiesslich R, Goetz M, Angus EM, Hu Q, Guan Y, Potten C, et al. Identification of epithelial gaps in human small and large intestine by confocal endomicroscopy. Gastroenterology 2007; 133: 1769–78.

46. Günther U, Epple HJ, Heller F, Loddenkemper C, Grünbaum M, Schneider T, et al. In vivo diagnosis of intestinal spirochaetosis by confocal endomicroscopy. Gut 2008; 57: 1331–3.

47. Hsiung PL, Hardy J, Friedland S, Soetikno R, Du CB, Wu AP, et al. Detection of colonic dysplasia in vivo using a targeted heptapeptide and confocal microendoscopy. Nat Med 2008; 14: 454–8.

48. Meining A, Frimberger E, Becker V, Von Delius S, Von Weyhern CH, Schmid RM, et al. Detection of cholangiocarcinoma in vivo using miniprobe-based confocal fluorescence microscopy. Clin Gastroenterol Hepatol 2008; 6: 1057–60.

49. Goetz M, Kiesslich R, Dienes HP, Drebber U, Murr E, Hoffman A, et al. In vivo confocal laser endomicroscopy of the human liver: a novel method for assessing liver microarchitecture in real time. Endoscopy 2008; 40: 554–62.

50. Tan J, Delaney P, McLaren WJ. Confocal endomicroscopy: a novel imaging technique for in vivo histology of cervical intraepithelial neoplasia. Expert Rev Med Devices 2007; 4: 863–71.

3

4 Evidence-Based Endoscopy

John M. Inadomi and Ma Somsouk

Background

Evidence-based medicine provides a framework for using the medical literature to solve clinical problems and provide better patient care [1]. While many practitioners are skeptical about the value of this approach, which they perceive as being "cookbook" and dismissive of clinical judgment, the value of practicing evidence-based medicine is as much about understanding how little evidence is available to support our daily decision-making as it is about guiding practice based on results of quality clinical studies. "EBM" stands for evidence-based medicine—but it is meant to complement experience-based medical practice, not replace it.

This chapter will provide the foundation for understanding the principles of evidence-based medicine, using practical examples from endoscopy to illustrate the application of EBM. We will identify the critical components necessary to validate studies of therapy, diagnosis, harm, and prognosis. Armed with these tools, it is hoped that the reader will understand which aspects of his or her practice are based on firm evidence, which are based on guidelines or standards that may not be derived from solid evidence, and which are simply dogma based on experience. As my mentor Dr. Marvin Sleisenger is fond of saying, "It's not what we don't know that will kill us but rather what we think we know that is wrong."

Each of the following sections will focus on a different type of clinical problem, opening with a clinical scenario to frame the question, followed by the accepted components of a study that would provide valid evidence, and closing with recommendations about how to incorporate study results into clinical practice. The basis of these concepts has been presented previously by the Evidence-Based Medicine Working Group and published in a series of articles in *JAMA* entitled "Users' Guides to the Medical Literature." These comprehensive resources are listed as references, and interested readers can peruse details of the concepts of evidence-based medicine through these publications [1–7].

The template for discussing evidence-based methods includes three universal questions, each of which has subtopics, that ask: firstly, are the results of the study valid? Secondly, what are the results? And thirdly, will the results help me in caring for my patients? Since the second and third questions are irrelevant if the first question is not answered affirmatively, emphasis is placed on determining whether the study methods are valid. The whole essence of a valid study design boils down to a simple goal: reduce bias. What is bias? In technical terms, it is "the consistent, repeated divergence of the sample statistic from the population parameter in the same direction." In plain English, it is the presence of something that causes the study to provide an answer that is not correct. Most often, it results from the presence of confounders, which are measured or unmeasured factors that are associated with both the predictor or exposure under scrutiny and the outcome. Instead of going through the mathematical or statistical derivations of bias, we will explore these ideas through various examples in this chapter.

Studies of Therapy

Clinical Scenario

You are consulted by your hospitalist to evaluate a patient with coffee-ground emesis and melena. Upper endoscopy revealed a large duodenal ulcer with a visible vessel that was not actively bleeding. Initial treatment was complicated by active bleeding, but you achieved hemostasis with epinephrine injection, thermocoagulation, and continuous infusion of a proton-pump inhibitor. Unfortunately, rebleeding occurred within 24 h. You feel that you have given it your best shot and feel wary about repeating an endoscopy. You question whether or not repeated endoscopy is warranted after initial endoscopy, or whether you should refer the patient for surgery.

Are the Results Valid?

The issues that need to be addressed in order to determine whether a study of therapy is valid are shown in **Table 4.1** and consist of: 1, randomization; 2, blinding; 3, concealed allocation; 4, complete follow-up; 5, intention-to-treat analysis; and 6, co-interventions [5].

Randomization refers to the process of randomly assigning patients to one group versus another. If this were done by deliberate assignment, it could result in unequal distribution of patients, with confounders in the study groups based on investigator bias. For example, assignment of patients with peptic ulcer hemorrhage could be biased if the investigators preferentially assigned patients without stigmata of recent hemorrhage to a new endoscopic therapy while assigning patients with stigmata to medical therapy. In this case, the confounder would be stigmata of hemorrhage, which could drive the outcome of recurrent hemorrhage more heavily than the intervention. While it would be possible to manually assign patients in equal numbers to each arm of a trial and thus reduce bias, the advantage of randomization is that it can adjust for unknown

Table 4.1 Studies of therapy

Are the results of the study valid?
1. Randomization
2. Blinding
3. Concealed allocation
4. Complete follow-up
5. Intention-to-treat analysis
6. Co-interventions

What were the results?
1. Magnitude of the treatment effect
2. Precision of the treatment effect

Will the results help me in caring for my patients?
1. Application of the study to my patients
2. Clinically important outcomes
3. Treatment benefits versus harms and costs

confounders as easily as known confounders, while manual assign-ment can only adjust for the latter. A nice example of this occurred with studies of ulcer hemorrhage, where prior to our knowledge of *Helicobacter pylori* we could not have specified enrollment based on this important etiologic factor; however, randomization would have ensured equal distribution of patients with and without *H. pylori* into competing arms of any trial.

Blinding. Study investigators may treat patients or assess them differently if they know that they are on a new medication versus a standard medication or placebo. Patients themselves may report different outcomes if they know whether they are on an active therapy or placebo. For these reasons, it is essential to blind the patients and investigators or study observers responsible for assess-ing outcomes.

Concealed allocation and baseline differences. Despite random-ization, it is possible that study groups may differ in important prognostic factors at baseline. This tends to occur more commonly in small trials, where there is an increased risk of imbalance be-tween study groups in the number of patients with different poten-tial confounders. More importantly, group differences may occur at the time of enrollment prior to randomization, in the absence of concealed allocation. This term refers to the blinding of the person responsible for enrolling patients to the sequence of group assign-ment. If an investigator is enrolling patients into a study comparing a new intervention versus standard therapy, there may be conscious or subconscious efforts to enroll healthier patients if it is known that the strategy to which they would be randomized is the new inter-vention, while excluding other potentially "sicker" candidates from enrollment on the basis of subjective exclusion criteria. Typically, the first table in a study of therapy will list baseline characteristics and identify significant differences between study groups to ensure that baseline differences are minimized. If significant differences remain, it is still possible to adjust for the differences statistically, but the power to detect significant outcomes may be reduced.

Complete follow-up. If a substantial proportion of patients en-rolled in a trial are not followed to its conclusion, the possibility of biased ascertainment of end points may occur. Patients whose out-come is unknown could have dropped out because they were doing so well they did not feel the need to return; conversely, they might have been unable to attend for follow-up because they were too ill or had in the meantime died. A general rule of thumb is that if the dropout rate is less than 10%, the conclusions are not likely to change with complete ascertainment of end points from the lost patients. If dropout is greater, a sensitivity analysis can be per-formed in which a "bad" outcome is assigned to all patients ran-domly assigned to the intervention or strategy being tested who do not have complete follow-up, while a "good" outcome is assigned to all patients randomly assigned to the comparator or placebo arm who do not have complete follow-up. If the conclusions of the study do not change, the lack of complete follow-up is unlikely to interfere with the study's conclusions; however, if the conclusions do change, an iterative analysis can be performed to find the threshold propor-tion of dropouts in each group who must have a "bad" or "good" outcome in order for the conclusions to change. In this way, the reader can be provided with a confidence interval depicting the range of potential outcomes.

Intention to treat. Patients should be analyzed by the intervention or strategy to which they were initially randomized, regardless of whether they were managed by that strategy. While this may ap-pear overly harsh, the reasons for this requirement should be appa-rent from the following example. The studies that compared endo-scopic treatment to surgical therapy for the management of bleed-ing esophageal varices examined endoscopic sclerotherapy and portocaval shunting [8]. Most patients randomly assigned to endo-scopic therapy received this within hours of enrollment; however, many patients randomly assigned to surgical therapy never re-ceived the shunt, because they either exsanguinated before surgery or became too unstable to undergo the procedure. For this reason, the patients who actually received shunt surgery were "healthier" than those who were randomized to endoscopic therapy, since the sickest patients in the surgical arm had died or could not undergo surgery. Thus, despite randomization, the patients who actually received the therapy to which they were randomized were different with regard to the overall morbidity and risk of mortality. If the data from this study were subjected to a per-protocol analysis, the con-clusions would be biased to find better outcomes in the surgical arm.

Per-protocol analysis, in which patients are analyzed by the actual management received, may be considered the "best-case scenario" for that strategy. It may be useful to report a per-protocol analysis, as it provides an estimate of what could be achieved, but due to the bias illustrated above it should not be considered the primary outcome.

Co-interventions. It is important to reduce differences in manage-ment between study groups so that any difference in outcome can be ascribed to the intervention under investigation, not differences in other factors (termed "co-interventions"). Double-blinding as-sists in this process, but it is possible that certain interventions, such as surgical procedures, do not allow complete blinding. Careful adherence to study protocols to reduce co-interventions will there-fore be necessary.

If the study methods are deemed valid after each of the steps mentioned above has been confirmed, then it is appropriate to assess the results and determine the potential impact on the clinical care of patients [2].

What Are the Results?

Magnitude of treatment effect. To assess the results of a study of therapy, one needs to determine the magnitude and precision of the treatment effect. In general, the results of a study of therapy report the proportion of patients who achieve the primary end point in the intervention group in comparison with the control or standard therapy group. In this case, there will be a comparison of propor-tions between these groups and some determination of the statis-tical and clinical importance of the differences. The differences can be described as the absolute risk reduction, which is simply the difference between rates. Alternatively, one may report the relative risk reduction, which is the percentage reduction in risk between strategies [(baseline risk – intervention risk) / baseline risk]. The rel-ative risk reduction can be somewhat misleading, as it may appear to magnify the actual reduction in risk. For example, assume a baseline risk of pancreatitis after endoscopic retrograde cholangio-pancreatography (ERCP) of 2%. A new therapy that results in a 1% risk of post-ERCP pancreatitis nets an absolute risk reduction of 1%; however, the results can also be stated as a 50% relative risk reduc-tion [(2% – 1%) / 2%].

Precision of treatment effect. One must remember that a study can only identify a "point estimate" of the treatment effect, since only a sample of the entire population at risk for the outcome has been assessed in a clinical trial. If the study were to be repeated multiple times, the results might differ, and this variation in results reflects the precision. The confidence interval is used to describe the varia-tion in study results that could be expected with repeated studies. By convention, a 95% confidence interval is used to report the range of values within which the risk reduction is expected to fall 95% of the time if such a study is repeated over and over again. In general, the larger the sample size of the study, the narrower the range of the confidence interval. Thus, when assessing the "power" of a study, which is the ability to detect a significant difference in treatment outcomes between competing strategies, the confidence interval is useful to determine whether the study is large enough to provide a definitive answer. Small studies may report a point estimate of relative risk reduction representing a positive treatment effect; however, the confidence interval may include 1 (no benefit) or even indicate potential harm with the intervention. Using the example above, an intervention to reduce post-ERCP pancreatitis may have a point estimate of a relative risk equal to 0.5 (50% relative risk reduction) but a confidence interval of 0.2 to 1.1, which means that the benefit could be as large as an 80% reduction in pancreatitis but potentially a 10% increase in pancreatitis. The P value of results is linked to the confidence interval. If $P < 0.05$, this implies that the 95% confidence interval does not cross "1" and that significant differences are present, meaning that the confidence interval for relative risk in treatment benefit lies entirely above (or entirely below) 1 and the probability that the difference was observed purely by chance is less than 5%.

Will the Results Help Me in Caring for My Patients?

In this section, the key issues are to determine whether the results of the study could be applied to one's own patients, whether all clinically relevant outcomes are considered, and whether the treatment benefits outweigh the potential harms and costs of therapy. The results of a trial can be directly applicable to patients if they fit the inclusion criteria required for entry into the study and do not possess any of the exclusion criteria. More than likely, however, there are various factors that would not have allowed your particular patient to have enrolled in the trial. In this case, some judgment needs to be applied to assess whether there is reason to suspect that the study results would not apply to your patient [2].

While study design makes it possible to report statistically significant differences, it is more important to determine whether clinically significant differences can be expected with new therapies or interventions. This refers not only to the magnitude of the treatment effect, but also the quality of effect. For example, trials assessing the efficacy of endoscopic therapy for Barrett's esophagus generally use elimination of dysplasia or intestinal metaplasia; however, the clinically relevant end point for practitioners is whether the therapy reduces the development of esophageal adenocarcinoma. Since few studies provide data regarding the latter, it may be difficult to support the adoption of a new endoscopic therapy that is based solely on the reduction of esophageal dysplasia or metaplasia. Similarly, it may be possible for a new therapy to reduce the incidence of esophageal adenocarcinoma but increase the risk of morbidity or mortality due to periprocedural factors. These adverse events must be factored into the assessment of the effectiveness of new therapy. Finally, we are often provided with results that illustrate a statistically significant reduction in the risk of an outcome we wish to avoid; however, the magnitude of that risk reduction is not clinically important, in which case one should compare the expected treatment benefits in contrast to the potential harm and costs associated with therapy.

One method of assessing the clinical relevance of a treatment benefit is to calculate the number of patients one would need to treat (number needed to treat, NNT) with the experimental therapy in comparison with the standard therapy in order to observe one episode of improved outcome as defined by the study. This incorporates not only the relative risk reduction, but also the baseline risk of the outcome in question. The NNT is defined as the inverse of the absolute risk reduction. For example, a hypothetical endoscopic therapy reduces the lifetime risk of esophageal adenocarcinoma by half, a relative risk reduction of 50%. The baseline risk of cancer in your patient is 2%, thus the absolute risk reduction is 1%. The NNT is $1/0.01 = 100$, meaning that applying this endoscopic therapy in 100 patients will yield one less case of esophageal adenocarcinoma over the lifetime of this cohort of patients.

This treatment benefit should be viewed in conjunction with the treatment costs and potential harms, either implicitly or explicitly (as in formal cost-effectiveness or cost–benefit analysis). There are no solid guidelines regarding the threshold NNT to support the use of an intervention. Instead, this decision should be made on the basis of the impact of disease on mortality and quality of life and the magnitude of the treatment effect, balanced by the costs and potential adverse events.

Resolution of the Clinical Scenario

You find an article that supported upper endoscopy after a first episode of rebleeding. The study randomly assigned 92 patients with rebleeding to immediate surgery versus endoscopy for hemostasis. It suggested a 73% probability of hemostasis with repeated endoscopic therapy, without any significant difference in the death rate at 30 days (five of 48 who received a second endoscopy and eight of 42 with immediate surgery; $P = 0.37$). More complications occurred in the surgical arm. Your repeat endoscopy reveals an adherent clot that you can easily remove. The lesion is again a visible vessel; you treat it this time with Endoclips, and the patient has no recurrent hemorrhage [9].

Studies of Diagnosis

Clinical Scenario

You are seeing a patient in clinic who has just turned 50 years old. He has no family history of colorectal polyps or cancer. He has heard of virtual colonoscopy and asks whether this test is good enough to exclude the risk of cancer developing if the results are normal.

Are the Results Valid?

The criteria for assessing the validity of a study of a diagnostic test are presented in **Table 4.2** [4]. A new diagnostic test should be assessed through blinded, independent comparison with an established reference, or with an acceptable alternative if there is no established standard. All patients should undergo the reference test, regardless of the result of the new diagnostic test. Methods of conducting the test should be provided in sufficient detail for the results to be to replicated, and the study should assess patients who are representative of the population in which the test would be clinically applied.

Independent blind comparison with a reference standard. It is not possible to assess the characteristics of a new diagnostic test unless

Table 4.2 Studies of diagnosis

Are the results of the study valid?
1. Independent, blind comparison with reference standard
2. Reference standard performed regardless of test result
3. Test examined in population similar to that intended for clinical use
4. Methods for test performance described with sufficient detail to reproduce
What were the results?
1. Likelihood ratios
Will the results help me in caring for my patients?
1. Test reproducible in clinical setting
2. Results applicable to patients
3. Results change management
4. Patients' health care improved by test results

4

there is a definition of the presence or absence of disease based on a reference or "gold standard." This reference test should be associated with greater risk, greater costs, or more inconvenience than the new test, otherwise there would be no reason to consider the new test. In some instances, however, there is no acknowledged gold standard. In these cases, an appropriate surrogate must be employed that may require multiple tests or clinical follow-up. In the case of computed tomographic (CT) colonography, the usual reference standard, colonoscopy, is known—on the basis of tandem colonoscopy studies and interval lesion development—to be incompletely sensitive for detecting polyps. Several multicenter trials used colonoscopy with sequential unblinding of CT colonography as the gold standard. This surrogate gold standard has been shown to be superior to either method alone, although it is unfeasible for use in clinical practice [10–12]. In this case, the test characteristics of colonoscopy are based on the initial examination during scope withdrawal, which is blinded to the results of the CT colonography, but the gold standard includes sequential unblinding of CT results, with colonoscopic reexamination if there is a lesion noted on CT that was not detected during the initial colonoscopic withdrawal. While the absolute sensitivity of either test may be overestimated, as there are lesions that could be missed by both modalities, blinded independent examinations can be conducted to compare the test characteristics relative to each other.

When assessing a new diagnostic test, the results should be determined independently without knowledge of the results of the reference test (blinding) [4]. This is important, as knowledge of the results of one test may influence the reading of subsequent tests. Certainly, if endoscopists had knowledge of abnormal lesions on CT colonography, they could inspect the suspicious regions more closely and use multiple passes or other maneuvers that would not ordinarily be performed in clinical practice to enhance detection, thereby biasing the results in favor of colonoscopy.

Reference standard performed regardless of test result. Verification bias or "work-up bias" is possible if the results of a diagnostic test influence the decision to perform or not perform the reference test. While this is not a problem in clinical trials of CT colonography, since all of the patients included underwent colonoscopy, other endoscopic studies of diagnosis face this issue. For example, when evaluating endoscopic ultrasonography with fine-needle aspiration for the diagnosis of pancreatic cancer, only those patients who are diagnosed with cancer undergo pancreatectomy. The true sensitivity of fine-needle aspiration for detecting cancer is unknown, since not all patients receive the gold standard, total pancreatic histopathology. Verification bias invariably increases test sensitivity, because the analysis is limited to the individuals who finally undergo pancreatectomy. Extreme efforts are needed to decrease the impact of verification bias—such as using long-term follow-up to establish the absence of cancer in individuals who do not undergo pancreatectomy.

Test examined in a population similar to that in which it is intended for clinical use. The characteristics of a new diagnostic test cannot be adequately assessed unless the research setting uses patients in whom the test is intended for use in clinical practice. Many studies, however, evaluate a new test in an enriched population with a high risk of disease or with severe disease. This example of spectrum bias will favor the diagnostic test, as it is fairly simple to distinguish healthy from severely diseased individuals, yet most diagnostic tests are used to separate patients with similar presentations caused by different etiologies. An example of this problem was seen in the evaluation of fecal DNA testing for colorectal cancer. One of the initial studies in which DNA exfoliated into stool was assayed for the presence of various markers associated with colorectal cancer (K-*ras*, p53, APC, Bat-26, highly amplifiable DNA) reported a sensitivity of 91 % for cancer and 82 % for adenomas ≥ 1 cm [13]. The study examined 22 patients with colorectal cancer, 11 with adenomas, and

28 individuals without colonic polyps, for a cancer prevalence of 36 % and an adenoma prevalence of 18 %. A subsequent study in which fecal DNA was tested in an average-risk, asymptomatic population with a cancer prevalence of 0.7 %, however, revealed that the sensitivity for invasive cancer dropped to 51.6 %, and while fecal DNA detected 32.5 % of adenomas with high-grade dysplasia, only 10.7 % of tubular adenomas ≥ 1 cm were identified [14]. This example highlights the necessity of evaluating a new diagnostic test in the target population in which the test is intended for clinical use. A test's sensitivity and specificity should not depend on the prevalence of disease; however, several studies have illustrated the way in which spectrum bias can overestimate the power, or relative diagnostic odds ratio, through selective enrollment of disease-positive and disease-negative patients from separate populations, or through nonconsecutive patient sampling [15–17].

Method for test performance described with sufficient detail to reproduce. Finally, the method by which the test is performed should be explained in sufficient detail to allow replication of the test in settings outside of research. This may include not only testing methods, but also patient preparations, analysis, and interpretation. If all the prerequisites cited above and in **Table 4.2** are met, the methods of a study evaluating a new diagnostic test are likely to be valid, and further exploration of what the results mean and how they may affect clinical care is warranted [3].

■ What Are the Results?

Most clinical studies of diagnostic tests report the sensitivity and specificity of the test for the presence of disease. The sensitivity represents the proportion of patients with the disease who have a positive test, while the specificity refers to the proportion of patients without the disease who have a negative test. In the example provided in **Table 4.3**, these can be calculated as: sensitivity = $a/(a+c)$ = $90/(90+10)$ = 90%; specificity = $d/(d+b)$ = $810/(810+90)$ = 90%. As stated above, these characteristics are independent of the prevalence of disease in the population; however, the positive or negative predictive values, which reflect the proportion of patients with a positive test who have the disease $[a/(a+b) = 90/(90+90) = 50\%]$ or the proportion of patients with a negative test who do not have the disease $[d/(d+c) = 810/(810+10) = 98.8\%]$ depends on the disease prevalence (in this example, 10 %).

Despite reliance on these traditional measures of test characteristics, results from studies examining diagnostic tests are best presented through likelihood ratios [3]. This concept highlights the ability of a test to change the likelihood that a patient has a particular condition from the probability before testing, known as the pretest probability, to the probability of disease after application of the test, or the post-test probability. The direction and magnitude of this change in likelihood is expressed through likelihood ratios that are not conveyed through traditional parameters. In the example provided in **Table 4.3**, the likelihood ratio of a positive test is the

Table 4.3 Diagnostic tests

		Disease		Totals
		Present	**Absent**	
Diagnostic test result	Positive	90	90	180
		a	b	
	Negative	c	d	
		10	810	820
Totals		100	900	1000

sensitivity/(1-specificity) or 90%/10% = 9, which means that a positive result is nine times more likely to be seen in someone with the disease than in someone without disease. Conversely, the likelihood ratio of a negative test is (1-sensitivity)/specificity = 10%/90% = 0.11, which means that a negative test is one-ninth less likely to be seen in someone with disease than in someone without disease. In general, likelihood ratios greater than 10 or less than 0.1 are associated with conclusive changes between pretest and post-test probability, while ratios from 5 to 10 or 0.1 to 0.2 represent moderate shifts in probability. Ratios from 2 to 5 or 0.2 to 0.5 generate small changes in probability, and ratios from 1 to 2 or 0.5 to 1 alter probability only modestly and are unlikely to change clinical decision-making. The statistical method used to calculate the change from pretest to post-test probability is based on the Bayes theorem. Mathematically, one can convert the pretest probability to odds, multiply the result by the likelihood ratio, and convert the post-test odds to probabilities. A much easier method is to use a nomogram that incorporates these calculations to convert pretest to post-test probability [18]. **Figure 4.1** depicts this nomogram, which is used by drawing a line from the pretest probability through the likelihood ratio and noting where the line intersects the post-test probability scale. That point represents the probability of disease after the result of the test is known. In the example provided in **Fig. 4.1**, if the pretest probability is 20% and the likelihood ratio is 25, the resulting probability of disease with a positive test is 86%. The nomogram also illustrates the advantage of likelihood ratios, in that they provide a numerical range of the probability of disease presence as opposed to the simple dichotomy of sensitivity and specificity for disease detection. One final comment concerns the estimation of the pretest probability. In the absence of other empirical data, the pretest probability can be estimated as the prevalence of disease in the population. If more accurate estimates of prevalence are available for specific subgroups of the population, these are preferred.

▦ Will the Results Help Me in Caring for My Patients?

Test reproducible in the clinical setting. In order for a test to gain acceptance in clinical practice, it must be reproducible with regard to performance and interpretation. If variation in test performance occurs in the clinical practice setting, or if interpretation requires subjective analysis, this may have a negative impact on accuracy. It should be noted that even if reproducibility is poor, the test may still be usable if it discriminates between patients with and without disease. Conversely, even if reproducibility is high, the test may not gain clinical acceptance if it requires highly skilled interpretation that may not be available in clinical practice [3]. A weighted kappa statistic (κ) can be used to identify the agreement in interpretation between or within observers. Values of 1.0 and 0.0 represent perfect agreement and disagreement, while 0.6–0.8 indicate good agreement, 0.4–0.6 fair agreement, and values <0.4 poor agreement [3].

Results applicable to patients. The study must be generalizable to patients in one's own practice in order to support the use of a new diagnostic test. This specifically relates to the variation in disease severity within the study versus the clinical population. If the study population was enriched with patients who had severe disease, the characteristics of the test, including the likelihood ratios, will exaggerate the discriminatory value of the test; in contrast, if the clinical population has a greater proportion of patients with mild disease, the ability of the test to distinguish between disease and health will be reduced.

Results change management and improve patient health care. Finally, it is imperative to ensure that any testing is performed with the intent to change management on the basis of the test

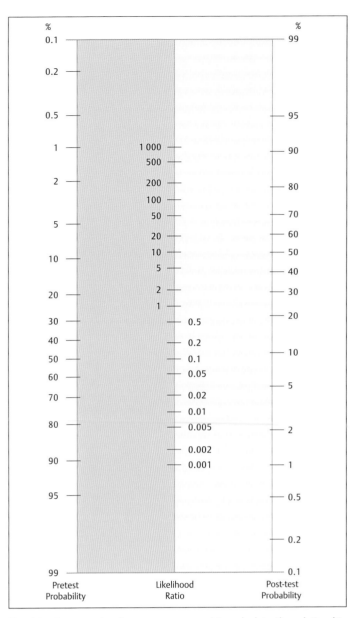

Fig. 4.1 An example of a nomogram, used to calculate the relationship between pretest probability and post-test probability.

results, and that patients will be better off as a result of the test. Screening to detect Barrett's esophagus in elderly patients may be an example. The competing risk of mortality from other disease may be so great in certain patients that even complete elimination of the risk for developing esophageal adenocarcinoma will not increase life expectancy. In this case, detection of Barrett's esophagus and dysplasia during surveillance may not lead to surgical or endoscopic therapy.

▦ Resolution of the Clinical Scenario

You review the literature and find a study comparing virtual colonoscopy and traditional colonoscopy. The per-patient sensitivity was 90% for adenomas or cancers ≥ 10 mm; however, the sensitivity drops significantly for smaller polyps, with a sensitivity of 65% if the cut-off is ≥ 5 mm. You explain to the patient that each test has its advantages and disadvantages, and after learning that the preparation is similar and positive results on virtual colonoscopy require evaluation with traditional colonoscopy, he opts to undergo the latter [19].

Studies of Harm

■ Clinical Scenario

You are seeing a 60-year-old woman in clinic who has had long-standing gastroesophageal reflux disease. Her endoscopy was unremarkable and her symptoms are well controlled while taking a proton-pump inhibitor twice daily. She is concerned about news related to hip fracture and its association with acid suppression. She also adds that her mother had a hip fracture. She wants to know whether she should continue taking the proton-pump inhibitor.

■ Are the Results Valid?

Criteria for assessing studies investigating potential harm from exposure to various agents have been previously published [7]. **Table 4.4** describes the steps necessary to determine whether a study of harm is valid and should be used to influence clinical practice.

Clearly identified comparison groups that are similar with respect to important determinants of outcome other than the one of interest. A *randomized controlled trial* (RCT) will provide solid evidence regarding the presence and magnitude of harm resulting from exposure. The strength of randomization is that potential confounders, either known or unknown, are allocated in equal proportions between study groups, thereby reducing biased results. The major barriers to RCTs examining potentially harmful exposure are ethical and feasibility issues. *Cohort studies,* in which individuals exposed and not exposed to the agent of interest are followed to determine the incidence of outcome events, may overcome the ethical issues. Cohort studies may be prospective or retrospective with regard to data collection. However, selection bias due to the baseline differences in other factors that may be important in determining the outcome between exposed and unexposed individuals may overwhelm the ability of the analysis to adjust for these effects. *Case–control studies* are retrospective studies and are especially advantageous when examining rare outcomes. This design first identifies patients with documented disease, as well as patients documented not to have disease, and looks backward in time to determine the odds that members of either group were exposed to the factor being investigated. As in cohort studies, case–control studies attempt to adjust for the presence of confounders that may be linked to both the exposure and the outcome; however, confounders that are either unmeasured or unknown may still bias the results.

Table 4.4 Studies of harm

Are the results of the study valid?

1. Clearly identified comparison groups that are similar with respect to important determinants of outcome, other than the one of interest
2. Outcomes and exposures measured in the same way in the groups being compared
3. Follow-up is sufficiently long and complete
4. Correct temporal relationship
5. Dose–response gradient

What are the results?

1. Strength of association between exposure and outcome
2. Precision of the risk estimate

Will the results help me in caring for my patients?

1. Results applicable to practice
2. Magnitude of risk
3. Elimination of exposure

The exposures and outcomes are measured in the same way in the groups being considered. Depending on the study design, one or both of these elements are crucial for validation. In case–control studies, verification of the exposure is critical—if based on patient query, *recall bias* may induce patients (cases) to respond positively to questions about the exposure that may not be reported as frequently among control individuals who do not have disease. Concurrently, researchers querying patients may probe more deeply among cases to elicit exposure than among controls (*interviewer bias*), which may result in a higher proportion of cases with positive exposure [7]. Validation of the controls is also important—it is possible for a patient classified as a control to have the disease in question, although it has been missed because the diagnosis has not been pursued.

In cohort studies and RCTs, validation of the outcome is critical. Once a patient is known to have an exposure, it is possible that he or she will receive greater scrutiny and investigation to seek evidence of the outcome than patients not known to have been exposed. This apparent enhanced risk is termed *surveillance bias* and requires strict enforcement of the protocol for detecting outcomes among unexposed and exposed patients [7].

Follow-up is sufficiently long and complete. Expanding on the theme of outcome assessment, incomplete follow-up threatens the validity of cohort studies or RCTs examining harmful exposure in a similar manner as in studies of therapy. A sensitivity analysis that assumes exposed patients do not suffer detrimental outcomes and that unexposed patients do experience the outcome may illustrate whether the proportion lost to follow-up affects the conclusions of the study.

The temporal relationship is correct. Retrospective studies may only illustrate association. To increase the strength of association to support causation, one must first verify that the exposure occurred prior to the outcome. A converse finding could indicate that the factor considered the "exposure" was in fact a result of, rather than the cause of, the disease.

Dose–response gradient. To further support the hypothesis of causation, one seeks to identify a dose–response relationship in which increasing amounts of exposure result in an increased risk of disease. A large case–control study examining the influence of heartburn on the risk of esophageal adenocarcinoma found strong dose responses with the frequency, severity, and duration of heartburn, which bolstered the investigators' hypothesis that there existed a causal relationship between gastroesophageal reflux disease and esophageal adenocarcinoma [20].

■ What Are the Results?

The strength of the association between exposure and outcome. The most straightforward manner in which to describe the association between an exposure and an outcome is the relative risk, which is the incidence of outcome among patients in the exposed group compared with (divided by) the incidence of outcome in the unexposed group. Harmful exposures are associated with a relative risk greater than 1, while protective exposures will result in a relative risk less than 1. Calculation of the relative risk requires knowledge of the true incidence of outcome—only possible in RCTs and cohort studies. Since the prevalence of disease is set by the ratio of cases to controls in a case–control study, the incidence of disease is not known. Due to this limitation, a case–control study reports the odds ratio, which compares the odds of a case versus a control having been exposed to the factor under scrutiny. Patients, however, are much more interested in their risk of disease after exposure, which is represented by the relative risk. Case–control studies are generally limited to examining outcomes that are rare and require long follow-up; otherwise, prospective cohort studies would be a more powerful study design. Fortunately, as the incidence of outcomes decreases, the odds ratio more closely approximates the relative risk. Table 4.5 illustrates this point by example. It should be recalled that risk is represented by the number of outcomes per number of chances, while odds depict the number of outcomes compared to the number of non-outcomes. As can be seen in the table when events are common, the odds ratio and relative risk greatly differ; however, the smaller the risk, the closer the odds ratio approximates the relative risk, especially when the risk of outcomes drops below 1 %.

Precision of the risk estimate. As in the case of studies assessing therapy, confidence intervals can be calculated to illustrate the magnitude of uncertainty surrounding the point estimate of risk. It should be recalled that confidence intervals that span 1 illustrate the lack of statistical significance of the findings, assuming $P < 0.05$ and 95 % confidence intervals.

Will the Results Help Me in Caring for My Patients?

Results applicable to practice. As with the other types of study discussed above, it is important to determine whether the patients examined in the study are similar enough to those seen in clinical practice for comparable outcomes to be expected. For example, there are reports illustrating an association between a radiation dose equivalent to that received during an abdominal CT scan and subsequent development of cancer. The implications for radiation are important, in the light of recent proposals to use CT colonography to detect cancer and adenomatous polyps among average-risk patients. The exposure in these studies, however, was based on radiation exposure among survivors of the atomic bomb explosions in Japan [21,22]. Single time-point whole-body exposure may cause a different biological outcome from multiple focal dose exposures, despite a similar cumulative dose; other differences in the type of radiation and a high organ-specific dose despite a low whole-body effective dose may be important in estimating the cancer risk from screening CT colonography.

Magnitude of risk. The relative risk or odds ratio compares outcomes among exposed versus unexposed patients. The absolute risk of an adverse outcome is not provided in these numbers, and thus the clinically relevant estimation of the absolute magnitude of risk is missing. We can calculate the number of patients exposed to a potentially harmful factor that would be necessary to observe one excess adverse event using a method that is similar to the "number needed to treat" presented in the section on studies of therapy. The inverse of the absolute increase in risk [1 / (risk in exposed – risk in unexposed)] yields the "number needed to harm" that provides the estimation of risk magnitude. For example, if two out of 2000 patients not receiving nonsteroidal anti-inflammatory drugs (NSAIDs) suffer upper gastrointestinal hemorrhage and three out of 2000 patients taking NSAIDs have hemorrhage, the absolute increase in risk is one in 2000, and the number needed to harm is 2000 [7].

Elimination of exposure. The issues that should be considered when approaching this question include the strength of the evidence supporting harm, the magnitude of harm associated with the exposure, and the potential adverse consequences of reducing exposure [7]. If the study results are valid and the magnitude of the effect is deemed sufficiently high (in comparison with the risk of adverse events), the decision to avoid exposure should be relatively straightforward. Reductions in validity or magnitude, or adverse consequences of reducing exposure, will temper this argument.

Table 4.5 Odds ratio versus relative risk. Odds ratio depicts the proportion of patients in whom the outcome event occurred, in comparison with patients in whom the outcome event did not occur. Relative risk depicts the proportion of patients in whom the outcome event occurred, in comparison with the total number of patients. Each of the rows depicts the odds ratio and relative risk associated with the same number of outcomes and patients

Odds ratio		Relative risk	
1 : 1	100 %	1/2	50 %
1 : 2	50 %	1/3	33 %
1 : 4	25 %	1/5	20 %
1 : 10	10 %	1/11	9 %
1 : 100	1 %	1/101	1 %

Resolution of the Clinical Scenario

You review the literature and find the biological basis for acid secretion and absorption of divalent cations such as calcium. You also find a positive association between proton-pump inhibitor use and hip fractures in a study using a large case–control design. The adjusted odds ratio was 1.44 (95 % CI, 1.30 to 1.59), with a causal inference supported by a positive dose-dependent and duration-dependent relationship with hip fractures. However, the absolute risk of hip fracture among users of proton-pump inhibitors was 0.4 % annually [23]. You advise that although the absolute risk of hip fracture is small, the risk should be minimized by using the lowest possible PPI dose, while discussing alternative options with the patient's primary care provider such as increasing dietary calcium and vitamin D, doing weight-bearing exercises, and taking bisphosphonates.

How to Use an Article about Prognosis

The criteria for assessing the validity of a study about prognosis are shown in **Table 4.6**. In general, a study of prognosis answers questions about the risk factors associated with the development of disease as a function of time [6].

Clinical Scenario

You are seeing a patient with Barrett's esophagus who, on surveillance endoscopy and random biopsies of flat mucosa, is found to have high-grade dysplasia. You discuss with him the various management options, including endoscopic treatment, surgical resection, and continued surveillance. During the discussion, he asks whether there are additional factors that can help him understand his personal risk of cancer. You turn to the literature to determine whether there are prognostic factors that may provide better information about his risk of cancer.

Are the Results Valid?

Representative and well-defined cohort at a similar point in the course of the disease. The first part of this statement influences the generalizability of the study to other populations. In many instances, a cohort assembled at an academic institution consists of tertiary or quaternary referral patients who have a more severe or advanced disease process. This "referral bias" can result in an exaggerated rate of poor outcomes, which may not reflect the average population of patients with the condition being studied. An example of referral bias can be seen in the initial reports concerning the incidence of

4

Table 4.6 Studies of prognosis

Are the results valid?

1. Representative and well-defined cohort at a similar point in the course of disease
2. Follow-up sufficiently long and complete
3. Objective and unbiased outcome criteria
4. Adjustment for important prognostic variables

What are the results?

1. Magnitude of risk of outcome events
2. Precision of estimates

Will the results help me in caring for my patients?

1. Study cohort similar to patients
2. Results prompt management change
3. Results useful for counseling or reassuring patients

esophageal adenocarcinoma reported among patients diagnosed with Barrett's esophagus. The observations published from academic medical centers included annual cancer rates of 2–5%; subsequent reports showed a more modest cancer risk of approximately 0.5% per year [24]. In addition to focusing on a representative cohort, it is important to ensure that all patients are at a similar, well-defined point in the course of their disease. A good example illustrating the importance of this requirement is seen in the recommendations for surveillance among patients with ulcerative colitis. Clear epidemiological evidence supports the view that the duration (as well as the extent) of the disease influences the development of colorectal cancer in patients with ulcerative colitis [25]. If an investigator reported a cancer incidence from a group of patients with pancolitis, the results would be much more informative if the cohort consisted of patients who had been followed since the onset of symptoms than if the follow-up was initiated at the time they were first seen at a tertiary care referral center. The latter would include a heterogeneous group of patients with varying durations of disease, and the observed cancer incidence would be difficult to apply to other populations.

Follow-up sufficiently long and complete. The adequacy of the follow-up period depends on the disease being studied. Follow-up to determine recurrent bleeding after peptic ulcer hemorrhage is likely to be adequate after 6–8 weeks [26]. The development of esophageal adenocarcinoma among a cohort of patients with Barrett's esophagus, on the other hand, requires years for the outcome to be adequately assessed [27]. It is self-evident that if the follow-up of the cohort is shorter than the time expected for the outcome to be observed, then the results may be invalid. As in the case with studies of therapy, losses to follow-up compromise the validity of results of prognosis studies. Cases in which the follow-up data are incomplete may be due to both good outcomes (with the patient doing so well that no medical contact is necessary) or bad outcomes (the patient is too ill to report his or her condition, or has died). The significance of incomplete follow-up can be assessed by assuming the extremes of possibility, where all patients lost to follow-up are assumed to have sustained the outcome, while all patients with complete data are assumed to have avoided the outcome. On this basis of this "confidence interval," one can determine whether a threshold for management change has been crossed and the study provides incomplete resolution of a clinical question.

Objective and unbiased outcome criteria. Some outcomes, such as death, are objective and fairly easy to assess. Others, including quality of life and symptom severity, are more qualitative and potentially influenced by either the patient or by the individual assessing the outcomes—especially if they know whether factors influencing the development of the outcome are present. Blinding the assessor to the status of the prognostic factors is important, as is use of a standardized data abstraction process that minimizes the potential for observer bias.

Adjustment for important prognostic variables. This criterion complements the requirement for defining a cohort at a similar stage in the disease course. If it is not possible or not desirable to limit the cohort to one disease stratum, it is essential to adjust or stratify the results by known prognostic factors that influence disease outcomes. For example, in the case of colorectal cancer development in ulcerative colitis, one may choose to initiate follow-up of patients at the time of symptom onset; however, the extent of disease among these patients may not be identical. Instead of eliminating patients in whom pancolitis is not present, an investigator may choose to follow all patients but plan to stratify them by disease extent—in this case perhaps by proctitis alone, left-sided disease, and pancolitis. In this manner, the relative risk of outcomes can be compared between various subgroups of the cohort, adding knowledge about the magnitude of the effect of these prognostic factors on outcomes. Similarly, differences in treatment can be used to stratify patients so that outcomes can be adjusted for these differences.

What Are the Results?

Magnitude of risk of outcome events. The results of a study of prognosis may report outcomes as binary events, such as the proportion of patients alive or dead after a specified duration of follow-up. While this may be informative, greater information may be revealed by using survival curves, in which the numbers of outcome events are plotted as a function of time. This allows a more accurate description of outcomes whose likelihood of occurrence changes over time. The reader is then able to determine whether outcome events are more likely early in the course of the disease or whether they are more likely to occur with a longer duration of disease.

Precision of estimates. As is the case with all studies, the measured result reflects the interaction between the prognostic factor and outcome in the specific sample of patients being studied. Even if the results are valid, they should be expressed in the larger context of the entire population at risk for the outcome through the use of confidence intervals. Reporting 95% confidence intervals provides estimates of the high and low range of results, and it should be expected that survival curves will have greater precision (narrower confidence intervals) early in the course of disease, but that as follow-up losses accrue over time, there will be a reduction in the precision and the confidence intervals will widen.

Will the Results Help Me in Caring for My Patients?

Study cohort similar to patients. A study will provide information pertinent to the patients studied. It follows that if one's own patients are very similar to the patients in the trial, the results are likely to be similar to expected outcomes in one's own practice. However, if the study patients differ with regard to prognostic features including age, severity of disease, comorbid factors, etc., it may be that one's own patients will experience different outcomes.

Results prompt management change. Ideally, the results of a study of prognosis will assist the provider in determining whether a particular intervention is warranted, and if so at what point in the disease course it is best carried out. For example, early studies of Barrett's esophagus showed relatively high rates of cancer incidence among patients with high-grade dysplasia, leading to recommendations for esophagectomy in this group [28]. Later reports illustrated a much lower rate of malignancy, leading to modification of the guidelines and allowing endoscopic therapy to be used in patients with Barrett's esophagus and high-grade dysplasia [29,30].

Results useful for counseling or reassuring patients. In some cases, the information provided by a study of prognosis does not lead to a management change. In these cases, it is expected that the data will provide a means for counseling patients and their families, to inform them of the risk of outcomes that may require mental or emotional preparation. Alternatively, the data may allow a provider to reassure a patient that the risk of an adverse outcome is low, in an effort to reduce anxiety.

▪ Resolution of the Clinical Scenario

You find an article that examined the cancer risk among patients with high-grade dysplasia. The authors reported 12 cancers that developed among a cohort of 75 patients with Barrett's esophagus and high-grade dysplasia during a mean follow-up period of 7.3 years [27]. Only one patient who developed cancer died of this disease; the remainder of deaths were due to unrelated causes. On the basis of this information, the patient states a preference for less invasive treatment and opts for endoscopic instead of surgical therapy.

Conclusions

Evidence-based medicine provides a framework for identifying, critically evaluating, and implementing relevant research findings in clinical practice. It is designed to complement, rather than replace, clinical experience and judgment. In fact, as one uses the methods of EBM more and more, it becomes clear that the vast majority of clinical questions have not been explicitly answered with the rigor necessary to deem the majority of practice "evidence-based." In this case, the impact of experience and clinical judgment become even more critical in allowing one to translate what has been discovered in research to related, but not identical, clinical scenarios. It is hoped that by using the tools provided in this chapter, readers will be better able to critique studies published in journals, understand their strengths and limitations, and use the information constructively to help improve outcomes for patients in their care.

References

1. Oxman AD, Sackett DL, Guyatt GH. Users' guides to the medical literature. I. How to get started. The Evidence-Based Medicine Working Group. JAMA 1993; 270: 2093–5.
2. Guyatt GH, Sackett DL, Cook DJ. Users' guides to the medical literature. II. How to use an article about therapy or prevention. B. What were the results and will they help me in caring for my patients? Evidence-Based Medicine Working Group. JAMA 1994; 271: 59–63.
3. Jaeschke R, Guyatt GH, Sackett DL. Users' guides to the medical literature. III. How to use an article about a diagnostic test. B. What are the results and will they help me in caring for my patients? The Evidence-Based Medicine Working Group. JAMA 1994; 271: 703–7.
4. Jaeschke R, Guyatt G, Sackett DL. Users' guides to the medical literature. III. How to use an article about a diagnostic test. A. Are the results of the study valid? Evidence-Based Medicine Working Group. JAMA 1994; 271: 389–91.
5. Guyatt GH, Sackett DL, Cook DJ. Users' guides to the medical literature. II. How to use an article about therapy or prevention. A. Are the results of the study valid? Evidence-Based Medicine Working Group. JAMA 1993; 270: 2598–601.
6. Laupacis A, Wells G, Richardson WS, Tugwell P. Users' guides to the medical literature. V. How to use an article about prognosis. Evidence-Based Medicine Working Group. JAMA 1994; 272: 234–7.
7. Levine M, Walter S, Lee H, Haines T, Holbrook A, Moyer V. Users' guides to the medical literature. IV. How to use an article about harm. Evidence-Based Medicine Working Group. JAMA 1994; 271: 1615–9.
8. Cello JP, Grendell JH, Crass RA, Weber TE, Trunkey DD. Endoscopic sclerotherapy versus portacaval shunt in patient with severe cirrhosis and acute variceal hemorrhage. Long-term follow-up. N Engl J Med 1987; 316: 11–5.
9. Lau JY, Sung JJ, Lam YH, Chan AC, Ng EK, Lee DW, et al. Endoscopic retreatment compared with surgery in patients with recurrent bleeding after initial endoscopic control of bleeding ulcers. N Engl J Med 1999; 340: 751–6.
10. Pickhardt PJ, Choi JR, Hwang I, Butler JA, Puckett ML, Hildebrandt HA, et al. Computed tomographic virtual colonoscopy to screen for colorectal neoplasia in asymptomatic adults. N Engl J Med 2003; 349: 2191–200.
11. Cotton PB, Durkalski VL, Pineau BC, Palesch YY, Mauldin PD, Hoffman B, et al. Computed tomographic colonography (virtual colonoscopy): a multicenter comparison with standard colonoscopy for detection of colorectal neoplasia. JAMA 2004; 291: 1713–9.
12. Rockey DC, Paulson E, Niedzwiecki D, Davis W, Bosworth HB, Sanders L, et al. Analysis of air contrast barium enema, computed tomographic colonography, and colonoscopy: prospective comparison. Lancet 2005; 365: 305–11.
13. Ahlquist DA, Skoletsky JE, Boynton KA, Harrington JJ, Mahoney DW, Pierceall WE, et al. Colorectal cancer screening by detection of altered human DNA in stool: feasibility of a multitarget assay panel. Gastroenterology 2000; 119: 1219–27.
14. Imperiale TF, Ransohoff DF, Itzkowitz SH, Turnbull BA, Ross ME. Fecal DNA versus fecal occult blood for colorectal-cancer screening in an average-risk population. N Engl J Med 2004; 351: 2704–14.
15. Lijmer JG, Mol BW, Heisterkamp S, Bonsel GJ, Prins MH, van der Meulen JH, et al. Empirical evidence of design-related bias in studies of diagnostic tests. JAMA 1999; 282: 1061–6.
16. Rutjes AW, Reitsma JB, Di Nisio M, Smidt N, van Rijn JC, Bossuyt PM. Evidence of bias and variation in diagnostic accuracy studies. CMAJ 2006; 174: 469–76.
17. Whiting P, Rutjes AW, Reitsma JB, Glas AS, Bossuyt PM, Kleijnen J. Sources of variation and bias in studies of diagnostic accuracy: a systematic review. Ann Intern Med 2004; 140: 189–202.
18. Fagan TJ. Letter: Nomogram for Bayes theorem. N Engl J Med 1975; 293: 257.
19. Johnson CD, Chen MH, Toledano AY, Heiken JP, Dachman A, Kuo MD, et al. Accuracy of CT colonography for detection of large adenomas and cancers. N Engl J Med 2008; 359: 1207–17.
20. Lagergren J, Bergstrom R, Lindgren A, Nyren O. Symptomatic gastroesophageal reflux as a risk factor for esophageal adenocarcinoma. N Engl J Med 1999; 340: 825–31.
21. Preston DL, Cullings H, Suyama A, Funamoto S, Nishi N, Soda M, et al. Solid cancer incidence in atomic bomb survivors exposed in utero or as young children. J Natl Cancer Inst 2008; 100: 428–36.
22. Pierce DA, Preston DL. Radiation-related cancer risks at low doses among atomic bomb survivors. Radiat Res 2000; 154: 178–86.
23. Yang YX, Lewis JD, Epstein S, Metz DC. Long-term proton pump inhibitor therapy and risk of hip fracture. JAMA 2006; 296: 2947–53.
24. Shaheen NJ, Crosby MA, Bozymski EM, Sandler RS. Is there publication bias in the reporting of cancer risk in Barrett's esophagus? Gastroenterology 2000; 119: 333–8.
25. Jess T, Loftus EV Jr, Velayos FS, Harmsen WS, Zinsmeister AR, Smyrk TC, et al. Risk of intestinal cancer in inflammatory bowel disease: a population-based study from Olmsted county, Minnesota. Gastroenterology 2006; 130: 1039–46.
26. Stedman CA, Barclay ML. Review article: comparison of the pharmacokinetics, acid suppression and efficacy of proton pump inhibitors. Aliment Pharmacol Ther 2000; 14: 963–78.
27. Schnell TG, Sontag SJ, Chejfec G, Aranha G, Metz A, O'Connell S, et al. Long-term nonsurgical management of Barrett's esophagus with high-grade dysplasia. Gastroenterology 2001; 120: 1607–19.
28. Sampliner RE. Practice guidelines on the diagnosis, surveillance, and therapy of Barrett's esophagus. The Practice Parameters Committee of the American College of Gastroenterology. Am J Gastroenterol 1998; 93: 1028–32.
29. Wang KK, Wongkeesong M, Buttar NS. American Gastroenterological Association technical review on the role of the gastroenterologist in the management of esophageal carcinoma. Gastroenterology 2005; 128: 1471–505.
30. Wang KK, Sampliner RE. Updated guidelines 2008 for the diagnosis, surveillance and therapy of Barrett's esophagus. Am J Gastroenterol 2008; 103: 788–97.

4

II

The Patient and Endoscopy

Section editors:
Guido N.J. Tytgat, Meinhard Classen, Charles J. Lightdale

5 Informed Consent for Gastrointestinal Endoscopy

Spiros D. Ladas

Historical Perspectives

Medical ethics originated on the Greek island of Kos with the "father of medicine," Hippocrates (ca. 460–377 BC; **Fig. 5.1**). A fundamental axiom in Hippocratic ethics is that "The physician must ... have two special objects in view with regard to disease, namely, to do good or to do no harm" [1]—a maxim that is familiar in its modern Latin version, *primum non nocere*. For many ages, physicians provided their patients with treatment "in accordance with their ability and judgment." The doctor's knowledge and expertise placed him in a position of authority over the patient. In this paternalistic model of medicine, the doctor determines what is in the patient's best interests, including how much the patient should know and whether the patient should be told the truth about the disease and its prognosis. The patient's role is to follow the doctor's orders. During the last 50 years, however, this paternalistic approach has been replaced by partnership—i.e., an approach based on sharing of information, decision-making, and responsibilities between physicians and patients [2].

Patients' rights are an aspect of human rights, which became internationally established on 10 December 1948, when the United Nations General Assembly adopted the Universal Declaration of Human Rights. Article 25 states: "Everyone has the right to a standard of living adequate for the health and well-being of himself and of his family, including ... medical care and necessary social services ... " [3]. Important declarations relevant here include the World Health Organization's 1994 European Consultation on the Rights of Patients [4], the Consumer Bill of Rights introduced in the USA in 1997 [5], and the American Medical Association (AMA) Code of Medical Ethics [6].

The Concept of Informed Consent

Informed consent derives from the principle of respecting patients' self-determination and autonomy—i.e., the patient has the right to decide about a proposed treatment or procedure. Physicians therefore have to give full and unbiased information to patients and encourage them to participate in the process of decision-making. Informed consent is not merely getting a patient to sign on a standardized form listing the complications of a procedure. It is a dynamic process of physician–patient communication, during which the physician discloses all relevant information about a suggested diagnostic procedure or therapy or intervention and provides the patient with adequate time to ask questions. This information should be explained in simple, understandable terms, adapted to the patient's educational level and intelligence. During the patient–physician communication, the patient has the chance to ask questions and have them answered to his or her satisfaction, so that he or she can make an informed decision to proceed with or to decline the suggested therapy.

Several major national and international gastroenterological societies have published guidelines for informed consent in order to help physicians in communicating with their patients. These include the British Society of Gastroenterology (BSG; 1999) [7], the European Society of Gastrointestinal Endoscopy (ESGE; 2003) [8], and

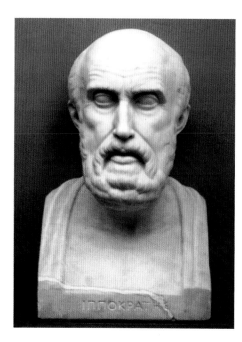

Fig. 5.1 Hippocrates of Kos, ca. 460–377 BC.

the American Society for Gastrointestinal Endoscopy (ASGE; 2007) [9]. In addition, the Council of Europe in 1997 published a declaration on the "Convention for the protection of human rights and dignity of the human being with regard to the application of biology and medicine: convention on human rights and biomedicine" [10]. In the same year, a similar declaration on the "Consumer Bill of Rights" was adopted in the USA [5]. It is distributed by the American Hospital Association to patients and is written in clear and understandable language, providing adequate information on patients' rights.

This chapter includes important extracts from these documents, which should also be studied in the original full versions.

Declarations Protecting Patients' Rights

In the "Convention for the Protection of Human Rights," Chapter 2—Consent, Article 5, states [10]: "An intervention in the health field may only be carried out after the person concerned has given free and informed consent to it. This person shall beforehand be given appropriate information as to the purpose and nature of the intervention as well as on its consequences and risks. The person concerned may freely withdraw consent at any time."

The American "Consumer Bill of Rights", Chapter VI—Participation in Treatment Decisions, states [5]: "Consumers have the right and responsibility to fully participate in all decisions related to their health care. Consumers who are unable to fully participate in treatment decisions have the right to be represented by parents, guardians, family members, or other conservators." In order to ensure consumers' rights and their ability to participate in treatment decisions, health-care professionals should provide patients with easily understood information and an opportunity to decide among treat-

ment options consistent with the informed consent process. Specifically, health-care professionals should:
- Discuss all treatment options with a patient in a culturally competent manner, including the option of no treatment at all.
- Ensure that persons with disabilities have effective communication with members of the health-care system in making such decisions.
- Discuss all current treatments a consumer may be undergoing, including alternative treatments that are self-administered.
- Discuss all risks, benefits, and consequences of treatment or nontreatment.
- Give patients the opportunity to refuse treatment and to express preferences about future treatment decisions.

Informed Consent for Gastrointestinal Endoscopy

Consent is the voluntary agreement of the patient to allow a diagnostic examination, therapy, or intervention proposed by a physician. Consent is valid provided that the patient has the functional capacity to take decisions and that the physician has disclosed to (and discussed with) the patient all the relevant information about the proposed intervention. The competence of patients to understand this information should be assessed by the endoscopist. All information given should be evidence-based and updated to the current state of scientific knowledge from published studies [8,11].

A crucial unresolved issue is the amount of information that the endoscopist should provide to the patient about the complication and mortality rates of the suggested procedure. Too much information about risks may frighten patients and deter them from undergoing the suggested endoscopic procedure, while too little information may leave the endoscopist open to claims of invalid consent. A published survey concluded that most patients wish to be informed about risks greater than one in 1000 [12]. By contrast, another survey showed that 14–19% of gastroscopy and colonoscopy patients wanted to know all possible complications, no matter how inconsequential or rare they were [13], and a third survey reported that 16% of solicitors specializing in clinical negligence in the United Kingdom expected that patients should be told of risks of one in 1 000 000 [14]. The endoscopist needs to consider and discuss with the patient the nature of the risks, how serious they could be, the probability that they may occur, and the imminence of the risk—i. e., immediate or late complications. The more serious and the higher the probability of the risk, the more its disclosure is warranted [15]. The current practice is to disclose only those risks and complications that occur "with significant frequency" and those "of a serious nature" [9]. This information is regarded as sufficient for a "reasonable patient" to make an informed decision. In addition, the hospital and the physician's personal outcome data on each endoscopic procedure, if different from national standards [12,15–17], should be available if the patient requests them. Hospital administrators and directors of endoscopy units may expose themselves to liability (known as "vicarious liability") for granting privileges to poorly trained or inexperienced endoscopists [18].

Obtaining informed consent is not only an ethical requirement for the physician, but also a legal one in most parts of the world. Written consent should be obtained for any procedure or treatment carrying any substantial risk or substantial side effect, and informed consent to undergo gastrointestinal endoscopy should therefore be provided in written form [8,19]. According to the ESGE and ASGE guidelines, the essential elements to be disclosed to patients undergoing gastrointestinal endoscopy include [8,19]:
- What the patient's disease is and its prognosis
- The nature of the proposed procedure

- The reason why the procedure is necessary and its benefits for the patient
- The complications of the procedure, including their relative incidence and severity
- Reasonable alternatives to the proposed procedure, including their risks for the patient
- The patient's prognosis if endoscopy is declined

Additional information should include:
- Who is in overall charge of the case and who will perform the procedure
- If it is a therapeutic endoscopy, its relative success rate
- Details of the procedure—i. e., use of conscious sedation, taking biopsies, use of radiation and videotaping of the procedure

▥ Exceptions to Informed Consent

There are certain exceptions to the informed consent process. These exceptions are recognized by law and include: emergency situations, waiver, therapeutic privilege, and legal mandate.

Emergency situations. When there is a real threat to a patient's life and there is insufficient time to inform the patient and involve him or her in the decision-making process—e. g., in cases of bleeding from esophageal varices—the treating endoscopist may forgo obtaining informed consent from the patient. The definition of an emergency situation lies in the judgment of the endoscopist, who has to do his or her best in providing endoscopic treatment to save the patient's life through the construct of "implied consent." The rationale underlying this is that any mentally competent patient would consent to treatment in an emergency. The endoscopist must declare the patient's condition an emergency and document clearly in the medical record the reasons for this, using established guidelines wherever possible.

Waiver. Waiver of informed consent is an intentional relinquishment of a known right. This is a legally recognized exception to informed consent and is referred to as a waiver. When a patient expresses a desire not to participate in the informed consent process, the endoscopist is not required to obtain informed consent. However, the endoscopist should be certain that the patient has full knowledge and understanding of his or her right to informed consent and that he or she is voluntarily relinquishing it. Appropriate documentation, including a written acknowledgment of the waiver signed by the patient, is essential.

Therapeutic privilege. The exception of therapeutic privilege recognizes that certain patients may have an adverse reaction to the information disclosed to them. For endoscopic procedures, the likely incidence of this exception is small, but an endoscopist may invoke it in selected clinical situations. In case of therapeutic privilege, obtaining consent from the patient's legal guardian is mandatory.

Legal mandate. A judge's order supersedes the process of informed consent. In these cases, the patient's and/or the public's welfare and interest overshadow the patient's right to informed consent. Typical examples are endoscopic examination of prisoners for removal of evidence such as a foreign body, or treatment of sexually transmitted diseases.

▥ Additional Issues on Informed Consent

Mentally Impaired Adults

The judgment as to whether a patient lacks decision-making capacity is made by the attending physician or the endoscopist. The law protects incapacitated patients' rights. It is strongly advisable for the endoscopist to be aware of locally applicable laws regarding patient capacity, guardianship, and surrogate regulations.

Various laws apply in each country regarding the protection of mentally impaired patients. In the USA, the endoscopist has a duty to obtain informed consent from a parent, legal guardian, or surrogate [9]. In England and Wales, the Mental Capacity Act 2005 not only provides an ethical approach but also sets out clear legal requirements for assessing competence and for treating incompetent patients. The act requires that the views of family members on what is in the patient's best interests should be taken into account, but they have no legal power to consent on behalf of their incompetent relative [20]. The situation is not the same in several countries in continental Europe and the Middle East countries. There is a requirement for a legally nominated family member or a justice of the peace to give consent on behalf of the incompetent patient in Israel, while in countries such as Greece, Poland, and Slovenia, it is common practice for relatives to give written approval before any medical procedure. During the Second European Symposium on Ethics in Gastroenterology and Digestive Endoscopy, held on the island of Kos in Greece in 2006, the following consensus statement was accepted: when mentally impaired or elderly patients require endoscopy, discussion with the closest available relative is strongly advised, but it is not advisable to have them sign an agreement, the overall responsibility resting with the physician [21].

Incompetent Patients

Incompetence is not actually an exception to informed consent. Gastroenterologists should be able to perform cognition tests [22], as cognitive impairment is rare in patients younger than 60, but it may exceed 40 % in patients older than 85. Special care therefore needs to be taken in obtaining informed consent from patients who have a reduced ability to communicate, such as elderly patients, those with less formal education, and patients with a below-average IQ. Obtaining unbiased informed consent from geriatric patients is not a simple matter, as they often have a reduced ability to communicate due to visual and or hearing impairment. Information should be given to these patients in understandable language, adapted to their intelligence and needs. Written information should also be provided on the basis of local outcome data for their age group, and should be given early to allow patients to discuss the issue with their relatives [23].

Children

In children, both parents have parental responsibility in the United Kingdom [7]. An unmarried mother has sole responsibility, and the parents or guardians provide consent on behalf of a child up to the age of 16 years. If the parents appear not to be acting in the child's best interests, or if there is conflict between the parents, the endoscopist has to act to protect the patient's best interests within the locally applicable law [8]. It may then be necessary to ask the courts for permission to perform the endoscopic procedure.

Jehovah's Witnesses

In Jehovah's Witnesses, the need for informed consent applies in the same way as for any other patient. However, these patients should specifically state in advance that they refuse to receive transfusions of blood or blood products in case of procedure-related complications such as postpolypectomy or post-sphincterotomy bleeding, as their will cannot be overridden even in life-threatening situations [7,8].

Withdrawal of Consent (Halfway through an Endoscopy)

A fundamental issue is that the patient has the right to withdraw informed consent at any time during an examination or therapy [15]. But what about a struggling patient under the influence of conscious sedation, who asks for a colonoscopy or ERCP to be stopped? This is an unsettled area of consent withdrawal, which the endoscopist should be aware of. In published guidelines on informed consent, the British Society of Gastroenterology [7] suggests that if the endoscopic procedure is near the end, some extra sedation is the best course of action. However, if the procedure is likely to take more than an extra few minutes, then it is better to stop the procedure, allow the patient time to recover, and then to discuss with him or her whether to repeat endoscopy under propofol or general anesthesia.

Informed Refusal

An issue related to informed consent is informed refusal. The essence of this doctrine is that the patient who refuses a procedure or any medical treatment must have an opportunity to decline in a knowing way. One example of informed refusal is that of a 55-year-old patient who refuses screening colonoscopy for colorectal cancer despite being informed that he or she belongs to a high-risk group, as both parents died of colorectal cancer. In the event that the patient declines the procedure, the gastroenterologist should document the patient's response on an "informed refusal" form. This form follows the informed consent format, but at the end, instead of electing to undergo the suggested endoscopic examination, the patient states that he or she will forego it. If a patient refuses to sign the refusal form, it is important to document this in the patient's medical records.

Medicolegal Issues

Informed consent is the cornerstone of good medical practice. In addition, it protects doctors against complaints from patients and claims of malpractice. Although gastroenterology ranked 23rd among 28 specialty groups with regard to the number of claims reported in the USA (1985–1999), there is a concern that the severity of paid claims has been increasing over the last 4 years [19]. However, this should not lead to a form of "defensive medicine," in which the doctor's actions are focused on avoiding liability rather than on treating the patient. Endoscopists should be aware of a number of legal issues when practicing endoscopy [24].

▦ Breach of Duty

Breach of duty is defined as a failure to satisfy ethical, legal, or moral obligations. For endoscopists, these obligations are judged against the national standards—i. e., the physicians should be well trained, in good professional standing, and practicing with reasonable diligence. The typical question at a negligence lawsuit is: would a reasonable endoscopist in a similar situation have done the same thing as the person being sued?

▦ Malpractice in Gastrointestinal Endoscopy

Endoscopies are invasive procedures. Although the complication rate is low, complications are unavoidable when practicing endoscopy [25] and there is a real threat of malpractice claims. Successful risk management strategies reduce the frequency of preventable endoscopic injuries [18]. The endoscopists are liable only for adverse effects due to negligence. A perforation resulting from a properly indicated colonoscopy for which informed consent was correctly obtained, which was performed with technical proficiency, and which was properly diagnosed and treated should not be regarded as malpractice and is defensible.

Causes of Malpractice Claims in Endoscopy

Suboptimal performance. Performance errors have been the most frequent allegations for any type of endoscopic procedure.

Iatrogenic injuries. Significant iatrogenic injuries are those related to perforation and/or direct injuries to the gastrointestinal tract. Standards of practice therefore require the endoscopist to disclose all significant risks to the patient during the informed consent process, including the rare risk of perforation at colonoscopy or ERCP [16,26].

Diagnostic error. Missing polyps or colon cancer at colonoscopy is not an uncommon diagnostic error. Endoscopists evaluating the colon must therefore consider the adequacy of their evaluation carefully [27]. A recently published study from Canada concluded that "Complete colonoscopy was strongly associated with fewer deaths from left-sided colorectal cancer (33% reduction), but not from right-sided colorectal cancer (1% reduction)." The authors commented that this might be due to false-negative colonoscopies and delay in diagnosis after a false-negative result leading to poorer outcomes [28]. The study attracted a great deal of media attention, including from the *New York Times,* questioning colonoscopy's effectiveness in preventing right-sided colon cancer. This worrisome publicity prompted a public reply by the American Society for Gastrointestinal Endoscopy presenting the following points [29]:

- Colonoscopies in this study were performed primarily by non-gastroenterologists (family practice, primary-care doctors and surgeons) who are not trained to the same extent as gastro-enterologists. Studies have shown that missed lesion rates are higher among internists and family-practice physicians.
- This was a retrospective study and may not reflect current practices; currently, bowel preparation is better, examination techniques are slower, and there is increased recognition of right-sided lesions.
- The way in which data were collected in this study does not provide any assurance that the right colon was fully evaluated, as there is no documentation that a full colonoscopy was actually performed when a full examination is listed.
- Colonoscopy is not a perfect test, but it is the best test for preventing colorectal cancer. Patients must find an expertly trained gastrointestinal endoscopist and ask the physician about their qualifications before undergoing a colonoscopy.

Medication error. Errors in the administration of conscious sedation are not a common allegation in malpractice claims directly linked to endoscopy [25].

Informed consent–associated issues. Informed consent is the most common issue leading to malpractice claims following an endoscopic procedure [16,30]. All endoscopic examinations, no matter whether they involve ERCP or diagnostic endoscopy, have similar legal risks. The informed consent process should therefore be used before any endoscopic procedure.

Issues relating to conscious sedation. As stated above, patients should be informed about possible risks and consent to administration of sedation and analgesia. The information given should include benefits, risks, and alternatives. The benefits of sedation are a painless procedure and amnesia relating to the endoscopic examination. The risks associated with sedation have a very low incidence, but should be reported. An ASGE and FDA survey found that in about 20 000 cases in which midazolam or diazepam was used, serious cardiopulmonary complications occurred in 5.4 out of 1000 cases and death in three out of 10 000 cases [31]. Recently, propofol has come to be widely used because of its rapid onset and offset of action. However, it has a narrow therapeutic window and there is no reversing agent available for it. Propofol administered by a gastroenterologist or nurse appears to be safe, but the occurrence of severe respiratory depression and the lack of a rescue agent continue to be concerns. As sedation may account for up to 40% of complications resulting from endoscopy [32,33], patients should be informed, but reassured that all measures have been taken to prevent complications. These measures include administration of supplementary oxygen and continuous monitoring with pulse oximetry, electrocardiography (ECG), blood pressure, and capnography, and should be used in all cases to prevent cardiopulmonary complications of sedation. In addition, at least one person in the endoscopy team should have experience in advanced life-support measures and resuscitation medication [33]. Endoscopists must remember that informed consent is an independent cause of legal action; "Had I known about these risks, I would never have agreed to sedation by a nonanesthesiologist" [34].

In recent years, drug delivery methods have been developed that are aimed at reducing the total amount of the sedative drug administered. These include patient-controlled analgesia–sedation (PCAS), target-controlled infusion (TCI), and computer-assisted personalized sedation (CAPS) [35]. PCAS uses a computerized pump controlled by the patient, delivering predetermined programmed doses of medications intravenously. The TCI drug-delivery system provides the drug intravenously at a rate calculated by a computer system to maintain a target concentration of the sedative. In the CAPS system, the computer uses feedback data from patient monitoring devices (pulse oximetry, capnometry, ECG, blood pressure) combined with patient responses to audible and tactile stimuli and delivers intravenous sedative as needed. The latter two systems have been used for propofol administration, with promising results [35].

The alternative to sedated endoscopy is nonsedated endoscopy. There are countries in which sedation is used for any diagnostic endoscopic examination [33], while in others most examinations are performed without any sedation [36]. The truth lies in between these policies. It is ethically and legally justified that we, the endoscopists, should not cause pain to our patients, but when possible we should not to expose them to the risks of sedation. For example, many elderly patients may tolerate upper gastrointestinal endoscopy without any sedation, as it is an unpleasant but not a painful procedure. In addition, once an intravenous line has been inserted, sedation and analgesia may be given on patient demand during colonoscopy, although certain patients may tolerate the procedure without any sedation or analgesia.

How and When Informed Consent Should be Obtained

The ASGE recommends that informed consent must be obtained within a reasonable time before the endoscopic procedure, in outpatient or in-patient settings [7]. The BSG recommends that it is desirable for each endoscopy unit to develop a code of practice suitable to its mode of operation—but never arranging for a patient to sign a consent form immediately before the procedure, because this does not constitute a valid informed consent. The patient should be fully informed by the endoscopist, ideally at least 24 h before the procedure, and should then be asked to sign a consent form [9]. This is not always possible for busy units. The referring clinician or practitioner should therefore be involved in the process of providing information.

5

The attending clinician proposing an endoscopic procedure should explain why it needs to be performed and should describe its essential elements. The patient should receive an appropriately written pamphlet along with the appointment. This pamphlet should describe the procedure in detail, including the administration of conscious sedation, as well as the benefits, risks, and complications of the procedure. It should also describe what will happen before and after endoscopy. If the patient is given an appointment for an endoscopy session during which trainees will be present, this should be mentioned.

The information sheet should also contain a checklist covering important aspects of general health, current drug therapy, and other questions to indicate that the patient has read the pamphlet and has been given the opportunity to ask questions. On arrival at the endoscopy unit, the patient should be welcomed and interviewed by a physician trainee in endoscopy or a qualified endoscopy nurse, who should check the level of understanding, provide further explanation and reassurance, deal with any residual concerns, and convey such concerns to the endoscopist. The endoscopist should then deal with any last-minute questions. If the consent form has not been signed yet, the endoscopist should ask the patient to sign it.

It is advisable to have a separate patient information sheet describing what endoscopy is and what patients should know about it for each type of endoscopic procedure, because of the different indications, types of preparation, and type and rate of immediate and late complications. Examples can easily be found with a Google search using appropriate key words. They are published by gastroenterological societies or hospitals and can be adapted and translated if needed.

Despite the recommendations and guidelines published by endoscopy societies in several countries [7–9], there is growing evidence that there are many deficiencies in the process of obtaining a valid informed consent. A recent publication in the United Kingdom investigated the completeness of the consent process in outpatients undergoing gastroscopy. It showed that about 10 % of the patients did not understand why they were having a gastroscopy [37]. Another survey conducted by the ESGE in its member societies showed that patients do not sign a consent form before gastroscopy in more than half of the responders' endoscopy units [38]. All of this shows that there are numerous deficiencies in the process of obtaining informed consent for gastrointestinal endoscopic procedures in many European countries and that informed consent issues should be included in the training curriculum for endoscopists.

Additional Issues on Obtaining Informed Consent

▦ Personnel Responsible for Obtaining Informed Consent

There is considerable variation from country to country in the personnel obtaining informed consent. In a survey of ASGE members, 30 % of physicians stated that they left the task of obtaining consent to other hospital or office personnel. Twenty-one percent of the respondents had been sued, and in 42 % of these instances, the informed consent process was an issue [30]. In a survey of ESGE members, information was given by the endoscopist in 23 % of the countries and by the endoscopy team—i. e., the endoscopy assistant or nurse—in 62 % [38].

It should be emphasized that the responsibility for obtaining informed consent lies with the endoscopist who is to perform the procedure. The ASGE guidelines include the recommendation: "The endoscopist is best advised to obtain the patient's informed consent personally. In general, this duty should not be delegated to health-care providers not directly involved with the procedure" [9]. In Germany, detailed information regarding complications and risks reported in the medical literature, as well as in the endoscopic unit in which the procedure is to be performed, should be given by the endoscopist or an associate who is familiar with these facts, but not by a nurse.

▦ Open-Access Gastrointestinal Endoscopy

Open-access gastrointestinal endoscopy is a rapidly evolving system in which the aim is to reduce the costs associated with endoscopy. Patients are referred directly for endoscopy by primary-care physicians—i. e., without any previous consultation with a gastroenterologist, implying that the patient has not had any contact with the endoscopist before the examination. To improve the information the patient has about the endoscopic procedure, an informed consent package including educational material [39], such as a booklet including a consent form, diagrams, or videos is sent to the patients by post at the time when their appointment for endoscopy is arranged. This "postal consent" should be mailed to patients well in advance of the procedure. It is a useful decision-making aid for the patient, but it is not a substitute for the physician–patient interaction [9].

Studies that addressed the effect of open-access endoscopy on the adequacy of informed consent found that patients reported being less adequately informed about their endoscopic procedure than patients who were referred by a gastroenterology department or specialist [40]. In a recently published study evaluating the informed consent process in an open-access gastroscopy service in Britain, it was shown that almost half of the patients were not told about the risks of the procedure and were not given an opportunity to decline, either before or on the day of the procedure. In addition, 39 % did not read the consent form before signing it [37]. The use of postal leaflets to obtain informed consent also does not address the problem of providing information about the choice between available options, as the procedure has already been chosen by the open-access endoscopy service. The consent obtained for such procedures needs to be associated with the best information possible within the practical constraints surrounding the provision of this kind of service.

▦ Obtaining Informed Consent for Teaching and Learning Endoscopy

The goal of ethical teaching is to train endoscopists in a way that does not harm patients and exposes them to training in a fair way, respecting their right to self-determination. This part of the chapter draws on an important workshop on ethics in teaching and learning endoscopy [41], which should be studied in detail by those interested on this topic.

Both trainers and patients know that endoscopies done by trainees are in several respects inferior to those done by trained endoscopists [42]. It is therefore clearly unethical to allow trainees with insufficient competence to practice endoscopy unsupervised. A trainer should be in charge of the procedure, deciding what procedures the trainee is competent in performing and when to take over [24,43].

The general information that patients receive on notification of an appointment should include the fact that training is integrated into the department's endoscopic activities. This will allow the individual patient a real choice with regard to finding another hospital, should the issue of training be a problem. However, if patients decline to undergo procedures performed by trainees, the entire process of teaching endoscopy may be jeopardized [41].

The issue of obtaining a patient's acceptance of a trainee being involved in the endoscopic procedure can in most cases be resolved by discussion in an atmosphere of reassurance and confidence, stressing the fact that the procedure is a team effort in which the supervisor is in charge of everything that is done. The following are essential elements of the informed consent process to be followed by teaching endoscopy units:

- The needs of the patient must always be weighed up against those of the trainee.
- Patients should be informed about the department's training activities.
- They should be reassured that the supervisor is responsible for the endoscopic procedure.
- Written consent should be obtained, stating that the patient accepts that a trainee may be involved in the procedure.
- The individual patient must have an opportunity to decline a trainee procedure.

Obtaining Informed Consent for Endoscopy-Based Research

Informed consent for endoscopy-based investigational procedures in which a new treatment is compared to the current standard treatment usually requires more information than the consent for any routine clinical investigation or standard therapy. Any new therapeutic procedure—e. g., endoscopic repair of a hiatus hernia—should first be successfully tested in animals and then balanced against an established treatment in patients [44]. The new technique must be evaluated in randomized, controlled trials and performed by expert endoscopists in accordance with high safety standards.

An institutional review board should approve the detailed protocol. This should clearly define the aims of the study, consider any potential procedure-related risks and benefits, disclose conflicts of interest, and be valid as long as the patient does not change his or her mind in the light of continuous information presented during the progress of the study. Participants should know whether there is any randomization to treatment versus no treatment or an established therapy and must be assured that withdrawal of consent does not imply any current or future disadvantages [45]. They should also be informed that this is a new endoscopic method that is being evaluated and that long-term results are not available. Informed consent for taking blood or tissue samples should always be obtained. This should explain the reason for taking biopsies and the method of doing so, the side effects, expected results, and potential future implications. Researchers must always ask patients if they want feedback about results.

The informed consent process should be properly designed to help patients weigh all of the pros and cons, so that they can make an informed decision for themselves and choose freely whether to enrol in the study or not to participate. Researchers must evaluate the patients' ability to understand the information about the study protocol before they sign the consent form.

Obtaining Informed Consent for Live Endoscopy Demonstrations

"Patients agreeing to be endoscoped during a live course do so because they have confidence in the specialists … They believe they will receive not only the best possible care … but also be treated by one of the best" [46]. However, there are ethical concerns about endoscopy demonstrations, mainly because the invited experts are not working in their "home" facilities and are under pressure to succeed. Concerns are frequently raised with regard to a higher rate of procedure-related complications. An important issue is that the treatment of the patient must not be delayed while the live endoscopy course is awaited. A couple of weeks' delay for a mucosectomy of a flat rectal adenoma is not clinically important, but this period is crucial for endoscopic therapy in a jaundiced patient with either common bile duct stones or malignant obstruction, who should be treated within 2–3 days. The patient's safety should be the first concern and should take priority over all other considerations.

The creation of a genuine physician–patient relationship is difficult with invited experts. Informed consent should be obtained from the patient by the local organizer, and should include information about the procedure and information about the live endoscopy course, presenting its advantages and potential risks, and explaining that the endoscopy might be delayed [47]. There should be an additional informed consent process between the expert and the patient. Appropriate translation should be provided if necessary. The informed consent procedure should include information about what will be done, who will perform the examination, and when the examination will be performed.

Informed Consent and Endoscopy by Nonphysicians

Due to the increasing demand for diagnostic gastrointestinal endoscopy, the shortage of trained physician endoscopists in several countries, and the availability of low-cost training of nonphysician medical personnel, nonphysician endoscopists have been trained to carry out screening sigmoidoscopy examinations, and in some cases upper gastrointestinal endoscopy and colonoscopy in certain countries [48]. Most of the comments below are based on extracts from the ASGE guidelines on endoscopy by nonphysicians [49] and a more recent ASGE report on ensuring competence in endoscopy [50].

Technical skills can be taught to nonphysicians to allow them to perform an endoscopic procedure such as sigmoidoscopy. Competent endoscopic practice requires thorough training in both the technical and cognitive aspects of endoscopy. However, cognitive skills include knowledge of procedural indications and contraindications, risks, benefits, and alternatives, as well as accurate identification and interpretation of gross pathology [49]. There are several ethical and even legal issues relating to endoscopy being practiced by nonphysicians, mostly arising from the informed consent possess [29,49].

- Nonphysicians do not have the knowledge to assess the implications of information regarding the patient's condition and the capability to integrate endoscopic findings into clinical practice [49]. Nonphysician sigmoidoscopy for the evaluation of patients' symptoms is therefore not currently recommended [50].
- Nonphysicians do not achieve the cognitive expertise necessary for optimum patient care as is expected of a physician.
- Obtaining informed consent for gastrointestinal endoscopy is an ethical and legal duty of physicians, because it assumes a thorough medical knowledge of gastrointestinal diseases. This duty cannot be transferred to nonphysician personnel.
- Patients wish to know who will perform the procedure, and they have the right to choose the best-trained endoscopist [29,50].
- Following training, a nonphysician should not carry out endoscopy unsupervised and should never perform a therapeutic procedure—e. g., removal of a polyp [50].
- What are the legal implications for the hospital and endoscopy unit director in case of a serious complication, such as esophageal or bowel perforation?

The ASGE recommendations on this debatable subject are as follows [49,50]: "The medical literature supports the utilization of nonphysician endoscopists for screening flexible sigmoidoscopy only … It is recommended that a trained physician endoscopist be available for immediate assistance and confirmation of findings."

References

1. Hippocrates. The genuine works of Hippocrates, trans. Francis Adams. London: Sydenham Society, 1849; I.II.5.
2. Coulter A. Paternalism or partnership? BMJ 1999;319:719–20.
3. United Nations. UN Web Services Section, Department of Public Information. The universal declaration of human rights. Available from: http://www.un.org/Overview/rights.html.
4. World Health Organization, WHO Regional Office for Europe. Declaration on the promotion of patients' rights in Europe: European consultation on the rights of patients, Amsterdam 28–30 March 1994. Copenhagen: WHO Regional Office for Europe, 1994. Available from: www.who.int/entity/genomics/public/eu_declaration1994.pdf.
5. President's Advisory Commission on Consumer Protection and Quality in the Health Care Industry. Appendix A: consumer bill of rights and responsibilities. Report to the President of the United States. November 1997. Available from: http://www.hcqualitycommission.gov/final/append_a.html.
6. American Medical Association. Code of Medical Ethics. Opinion 8.08, informed consent. [Report: Issued March 1981. Updated November 2006.] Available from: http://www.ama-assn.org/ama1/pub/upload/mm/Code_of_Med_Eth/opinion/opinion808.html.
7. British Society of Gastroenterology. Guidelines for informed consent for endoscopic procedures. London: British Society of Gastroenterology, 1999. Available from: http://www.bsg.org.uk/images/stories/docs/clinical/guidelines/endoscopy/consent.pdf.
8. Stanciu C, Novis B, Ladas S, Sommerville A, Zabowowski P, Isaacs P, et al. Recommendations of the ESGE workshop on informed consent for digestive endoscopy. First European Symposium on Ethics in Gastroenterology and Digestive Endoscopy, Kos, Greece, June 2003. Endoscopy 2003;35:772–4.
9. American Society for Gastrointestinal Endoscopy Standards of Practice Committee, Zuckerman MJ, Shen B, Harrison ME 3 rd, Baron TH, Adler DG, et al. Informed consent for GI endoscopy. Gastrointest Endosc 2007;66:213–8.
10. Council of Europe. Convention for the Protection of Human Rights and Dignity of the Human Being with regard to the Application of Biology and Medicine: Convention on Human Rights and Biomedicine. Oviedo, 4 April 1997. Available from: http://conventions.coe.int/Treaty/en/Treaties/Html/164.htm.
11. Clancy CM, Cronin K. Evidence-based decision making: global evidence, local decisions. Health Aff (Millwood) 2005;24:151–62.
12. Newton-Howes PA, Bedford ND, Dobbs BR, Frizelle FA. Informed consent: what do patients want to know? N Z Med J 1998;111:340–2.
13. Brooks AJ, Hurlstone DP, Fotheringham J, Gane J, Sanders DS, McAlindon ME. Information required to provide informed consent for endoscopy: an observational study of patients' expectations. Endoscopy 2005;37:1136–9.
14. Mayberry MK, Mayberry JF. Towards better informed consent in endoscopy: a study of information and consent processes in gastroscopy and flexible sigmoidoscopy. Eur J Gastroenterol Hepatol 2001;13:1467–76.
15. Feld AD. Informed consent: not just for procedures anymore. Am J Gastroenterol 2004;99:977–80.
16. Cotton PB. Analysis of 59 ERCP lawsuits: mainly about indications. Gastrointest Endosc 2006;63:378–82.
17. Kirsch M. The myth of informed consent. Am J Gastroenterol 2000;95:588–9.
18. Frakes JT. The ERCP-related lawsuit: "best avoid it!" Gastrointest Endosc 2006;63:385–8.
19. American Society for Gastrointestinal Endoscopy. Medical malpractice claims and risk management in gastroenterology and gastrointestinal endoscopy. Oak Brook, IL: American Society for Gastrointestinal Endoscopy, 2007. Available from: http://www.asge.org/MembersOnlyindex.aspx?id=52.
20. Corfield L, Granne I. Treating non-competent patients. BMJ 2005;331:1353–4.
21. Ladas SD, Novis B, Triantafyllou K, Schoefl R, Rokkas T, Stanciu C, et al. Ethical issues in endoscopy: patient satisfaction, safety in elderly patients, palliation, and relations with industry. Second European Symposium on Ethics in Gastroenterology and Digestive Endoscopy, Kos, Greece, July 2006. Endoscopy 2007;39:556–65.
22. Hall KE, Proctor DD, Fisher L, Rose S. American Gastroenterological Association Future Trends Committee report: effects of aging of the population on gastroenterology practice, education, and research. Gastroenterology 2005;129:1305–38.
23. Ladas SD. Ethical issues in the management of elderly patients in gastroenterology and digestive endoscopy. Expert Rev Gastroenterol Hepatol 2007;1:257–63.
24. Ahuja V, Tandon R. Ethics in diagnostic and therapeutic endoscopy. In: Stanciu C, Ladas S, editors. Medical ethics: focus on gastroenterology and digestive endoscopy. Athens: Beta Medical Publishers; 2002. p. 97–108.
25. Thompson AM, Wright DJ, Murray W, Ritchie GL, Burton HD, Stonebridge PA. Analysis of 153 deaths after upper gastrointestinal endoscopy: room for improvement? Surg Endosc 2004;18:22–5..
26. Neale G. Reducing risks in gastroenterological practice. Gut 1998;42:139–42.
27. Rex DK, Bond JH, Feld AD. Medical-legal risks of incident cancers after clearing colonoscopy. Am J Gastroenterol 2001;96:952–7.
28. Baxter NN, Goldwasser MA, Paszat LF, Saskin R, Urbach DR, Rabeneck L. Association of colonoscopy and death from colorectal cancer. Ann Intern Med 2009;150:1–8.
29. American Society for Gastrointestinal Endoscopy. ASGE urges patients to seek a qualified endoscopist before undergoing a colonoscopy for colorectal cancer [press release, 16 December 2008]. Oak Brook, IL: American Society for Gastrointestinal Endoscopy. Available from: http://www.asge.org/PressroomIndex.aspx?id=6024.
30. Levine EG, Brandt LJ, Plumeri PA. Informed consent: a survey of physician outcomes and practices. Gastrointest Endosc 1995;41:448–52.
31. Arrowsmith JB, Gerstman BB, Fleischer DE, Benjamin SB. Results from the American Society for Gastrointestinal Endoscopy/U.S. Food and Drug Administration collaborative study on complication rates and drug use during gastrointestinal endoscopy. Gastrointest Endosc 1991;37:421–7.
32. Cohen LB, Delegge MH, Aisenberg J, Brill JV, Inadomi JM, Kochman ML, et al. AGA Institute review of endoscopic sedation. Gastroenterology 2007;133:675–701.
33. Standards of Practice Committee of the American Society for Gastrointestinal Endoscopy, Lichtenstein DR, Jagannath S, Baron TH, Anderson MA, Banerjee S, et al. Sedation and anesthesia in GI endoscopy. Gastrointest Endosc 2008;68:815–26.
34. Feld AD. Endoscopic sedation with propofol: legal risks and risk management. Gastroenterol Hepatol Ann Rev 2006;1:103–5. Available from: http://www.gastro.org/user-assets/Documents/08_Publications/06_GI-Hep_Annual_Review/Articles/Feld.pdf.
35. Pambianco DJ. Future directions in endoscopic sedation. Gastrointest Endosc Clin N Am 2008;18:789–99.
36. Ladas SD, Aabakken L, Rey JF, Nowak A, Zakaria S, Adamonis K, et al. Use of sedation for routine diagnostic upper gastrointestinal endoscopy: a European Society of Gastrointestinal Endoscopy survey of national endoscopy society members. Digestion 2006;74:69–77.
37. Woodrow SR, Jenkins AP. How thorough is the process of informed consent prior to outpatient gastroscopy? A study of practice in a United Kingdom district hospital. Digestion 2006;73:189–97.
38. Triantafyllou K, Stanciu C, Kruse A, Malfertheiner P, Axon A, Ladas SD; European Society of Gastrointestinal Endoscopy. Informed consent for gastrointestinal endoscopy: a 2002 ESGE survey. Dig Dis 2002;20:280–3.
39. Shepherd HA, Bowman D, Hancock B, Anglin J, Hewett D. Postal consent for upper gastrointestinal endoscopy. Gut 2000;46:37–9.
40. Bassi A, Brown E, Kapoor N, Bodger K. Dissatisfaction with consent for diagnostic gastrointestinal endoscopy. Dig Dis 2002;20:275–9.
41. Axon AT, Aabakken L, Malfertheiner P, Danielides I, Ladas S, Hochberger J, et al. Recommendations of the ESGE workshop on ethics in teaching and learning endoscopy. First European Symposium on Ethics in Gastroenterology and Digestive Endoscopy, Kos, Greece, June 2003. Endoscopy 2003;35:761–4.
42. Tassios PS, Ladas SD, Grammenos I, Demertzis K, Raptis SA. Acquisition of competence in colonoscopy: the learning curve of trainees. Endoscopy 1999;31:702–6.
43. Plumeri PA. Endoscopic training directors: a few legal and ethical considerations. Gastrointest Endosc Clin N Am 1995;5:447–55.
44. Devière J, Hochberger J, Neuhaus H, Ponchon T, Eugenidis N, Neumann C, et al. Recommendations of the ESGE workshop on ethical, clinical, and economic dilemmas arising from the implementation of new techniques. First European Symposium on Ethics in Gastroenterology and Digestive Endoscopy, Kos, Greece, June 2003. Endoscopy 2003;35:768–71.
45. Malfertheiner P, Mantzaris GJ, Farthing M, Niv Y, Escourrou J, Treiber G, et al. Recommendations of the ESGE workshop on ethics in gastrointestinal endoscopy-based research. First European Symposium on Ethics in Gas-

troenterology and Digestive Endoscopy, Kos, Greece, June 2003. Endoscopy 2003;35:775–7.

46. Carr-Locke DL, Gostout CJ, Van Dam JA. A guideline for live endoscopy courses: an ASGE White Paper. Gastrointest Endosc 2001;53:685–8.

47. Devière J, Ponchon T, Beilenhoff U, Neuhaus H, Costamagna G, Schmit A, et al. Recommendations of the ESGE workshop on ethical-legal issues concerning live demonstrations in digestive endoscopy. First European Symposium on Ethics in Gastroenterology and Digestive Endoscopy, Kos, Greece, June 2003. Endoscopy 2003;35:765–7.

48. Meaden C, Joshi M, Hollis S, Higham A, Lynch D. A randomized controlled trial comparing the accuracy of general diagnostic upper gastrointestinal endoscopy performed by nurse or medical endoscopists. Endoscopy 2006;38:553–60.

49. American Society for Gastrointestinal Endoscopy. Endoscopy by non-physicians: guidelines for clinical application. Gastrointest Endosc. 1999;49:826–8.

50. ASGE Taskforce on Ensuring Competence in Endoscopy/American College of Gastroenterology Executive and Practice Management Committees. Ensuring competence in endoscopy. Oak Brook, IL/Bethesda, MD: American Society for Gastrointestinal Endoscopy/American College of Gastroenterology [n.d.]. Available from: http://www.asge.org/WorkArea/showcontent.aspx?id=3384.

5

6 Patient Preparation and Sedation for Endoscopy

Jenifer R. Lightdale

Preparing and sedating patients are fundamental components of gastrointestinal endoscopy, despite persistent and wide differences in practices at the local and global levels. In many countries, patients are increasingly presenting on the day of their procedure, without previously encountering a gastroenterologist. Adding complexity to the preparation of patients, endoscopists around the world vary greatly in determining which procedures warrant sedation, who should administer it, and which drugs should be used, in what doses, and to what effect. These variations appear to be based in part on cultural norms and endoscopic training, but also increasingly reflect diverse policies on the part of institutions, third-party payers, and government. While patient safety remains paramount, cost has clearly emerged as a central consideration for health-care systems worldwide.

Sedation is defined as a drug-induced depression in the level of the patient's consciousness that can range from minimal anxiolysis to general anesthesia. The primary goals of sedation for patients undergoing gastrointestinal endoscopy are to ensure their safety, comfort, and cooperation throughout procedures. Secondary goals of providing sedation for gastrointestinal endoscopy may include ensuring patient amnesia for the procedure, immobility, and willingness to undergo repeat procedures. For clinicians, sedation may provide an ideal environment for performing gastrointestinal endoscopy, while enhancing cost-effectiveness and procedural efficiency.

In recent years, there has been an increased emphasis on understanding how sedation choices may heavily impact not only the safety and quality of gastrointestinal procedures, but also the efficiency of procedural units. Propofol, in particular, has emerged as a pharmaceutical agent particularly suited to endoscopy, as it allows for rapid induction and recovery, as well as a wide range of sedation levels. Although in the United States and other countries there are local legislative differences that may dictate whether propofol can be administered by nonanesthesiologists, administration of propofol by gastroenterologists and nurses has increased dramatically worldwide, with reports including large numbers of patients who have received nonanesthesiologist-administered propofol for endoscopic procedures without complications. Nevertheless, many questions remain regarding which clinicians should be allowed to administer propofol and how they should be best trained to do so. There has also been ongoing discussion regarding medicolegal and political issues that may affect the use of propofol for endoscopy.

In an effort to standardize the practice of sedation at national levels, a number of medical societies have released new guidelines for gastrointestinal procedures. In particular, the European Board of Anesthesiology of the European Union of Medical Specialists (EUMS/UEMS), the American Gastroenterological Association (AGA), the American Society of Gastrointestinal Endoscopy (ASGE), and the American Society of Anesthesiologists (ASA) Committee for Sedation and Analgesia by Nonanesthesiologists have released statements and recommendations based on a growing body of literature and primary clinical research. Nevertheless, more randomized and controlled trials regarding many de facto sedation practices are needed in order to provide an evidence basis for sedation decisions around the world.

Levels of Sedation

Sedation guidelines have universally defined levels of sedation as stretching along a continuum without clear boundaries from "light" to "deep" [1–4]. The consensus also dictates that levels of sedation are directly related to patient risks.

- *Light sedation* implies the retention of a patient's ability to respond voluntarily to vocal commands and to maintain a patent airway with protective reflexes.
- *Deep sedation* implies a medically controlled state of depressed consciousness from which the patient is not easily aroused.
- *General anesthesia* describes the deepest level of sedation, in which the patient is unarousable with painful stimuli and has inadequate spontaneous ventilation, requiring airway management.

Depth of sedation is directly related to cardiovascular stability; the deeper the level of sedation, the more at risk a patient is for cardiopulmonary events (**Fig. 6.1**).

It is imperative that endoscopists target a level of sedation before starting the procedure. On the other hand, one of the most difficult assessments for endoscopists to make during a procedure is often the level of sedation that has been achieved. Many patients slip into deeper levels of sedation than anticipated. In some procedures of a more prolonged, painful nature, or when patients are unable to tolerate endoscopic stresses at a lighter level, deep sedation may be deliberately achieved.

Viewed from the perspective of a continuum of sedation, targeting light levels of sedation by definition creates the potential for patients to become deeply sedated. Regardless of the sedative or regimens employed, as doses increase, a patient may lose consciousness and protective reflexes. Other patient or procedural factors may also be relevant and affect the level of sedation. For instance,

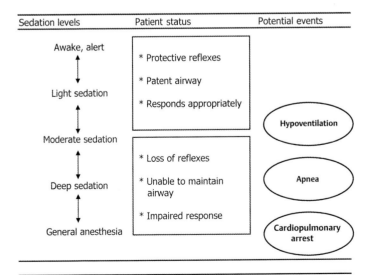

Fig. 6.1 Terms commonly used to describe sedation and their relationship to the continuum of sedation levels.

deep sedation may develop in lightly sedated patients because of delayed drug absorption, or because the stimulus of the procedure lessens (e. g., after successful navigation of the hepatic flexure during colonoscopy). Accordingly, it has been recommended that all providers be prepared to rescue patients from deeper levels of sedation than targeted.

Gastrointestinal societies have increasingly also acknowledged that most endoscopic procedures are performed with moderate sedation, as opposed to the previously used term "conscious sedation." The latter term has in fact been declared inaccurate, as it describes patients who can respond to simple commands such as "take a deep breath" or "turn on your back" [1,5]. The term "moderate sedation" provides a better description of the sedated state in which patients are able to tolerate unpleasant procedures while maintaining adequate cardiorespiratory function, protective reflexes, and the ability to react to verbal or tactile stimulation [5]. This type of sedation may also be known as "procedural sedation."

Of course, optimal levels of sedation may be different for upper endoscopy and colonoscopy. In upper endoscopy, a major goal of sedation may be to avoid gagging and to increase patient cooperation; in colonoscopy, the goal of sedation is often to avoid visceral pain associated with looping. Patient anxiety levels may also be different for different procedures. Generally speaking, endoscopy appears to be better tolerated by older than by younger individuals, by men than women, and by patients who have had a previous endoscopy [6]. The ability to tolerate procedures without sedation may be enhanced by older age and decreased pharyngeal sensitivity [7], while a history of poor tolerance of prior examinations may be predictive of patients who require deep sedation [8].

Patient Preparation and Assessment for Sedation

All patients undergoing sedation for gastrointestinal procedures should be informed of and agree to the level of sedation that will be targeted during their procedure [3,9]. In particular, patients should understand the benefits, risks, and limitations of the sedation that will be administered, including the possibility that they will experience lighter or deeper levels than anticipated. Targeted levels of sedation should match the patient's expectations as closely as possible. Patients should also be told about alternative regimens, including the option of forgoing sedation for their procedure.

■ Fasting Instructions

It is generally accepted that patients undergoing sedated upper and lower endoscopy should cease to eat and drink at some point prior to the administration of sedation, to minimize the potentially life-threatening risk of aspiration. While aspiration during colonoscopy has been described [10], upper endoscopy is perceived to be more strongly associated with aspiration of gastric contents during gastrointestinal procedures. Nonetheless, there is an absence of supporting data for this supposition, and there are accordingly no absolute guidelines as to the timing of fasting before gastrointestinal procedures [2,11]. The American Society of Anesthesiology recommends that patients fast a minimum of 2 h after consuming clear liquids and 6 h after consuming light meals [4]. With regard to emergency situations or in situations of delayed gastric emptying, the ASGE recommends that fasting status be considered in the light of three factors: 1, the level of sedation to be targeted; 2, risks of delaying the procedure; and 3, plans for endotracheal intubation [3].

■ Patient Medical History and Examination

A careful medical history must be obtained from all patients before sedation is administered, as there are a number of known risk factors for complications during sedated gastrointestinal procedures (**Table 6.1**). Inquiries must include a history of all current medications, untoward or allergic reactions, alcohol or other substance abuse, chronic use of sedatives or analgesics, and past endoscopic experiences. Risk assessments should also include patient age, comorbid illnesses or organ dysfunction, pregnancy, and obesity. A history of cardiopulmonary disease, a cardiac pacemaker, surgical history, radiation therapy, cirrhosis, and other conditions that might affect access to a patient's airway should also be obtained. Finally, it is increasingly recommended that patients should be asked if they suffer from stridor, snoring, or sleep apnea [2,3].

The patient's medical history may affect the choice of sedatives, as well as other intraprocedural medications. Depending on the underlying conditions in the patient and the planned procedure, periprocedural antibiotic prophylaxis may be indicated (**Table 6.2**) [12]. A major departure in recent years from previous guidelines concerns the recommendation against administering antibiotic prophylaxis for patients with underlying cardiac disease solely in order to prevent infective endocarditis [12]. According to the American Heart Association and numerous gastroenterological societies, there are no data demonstrating a link between endoscopy and endocarditis, nor are there any data demonstrating that antibiotic prophylaxis prevents endocarditis [12,13].

Table 6.1 Potential patient risk factors for complications during endoscopy with sedation

Systemic conditions

Sepsis
Shock
Dehydration
History of drug allergy
Pregnancy
Obesity
History of radiation therapy

Cardiovascular conditions

Arrhythmias
Cardiac pacemaker
Coronary artery disease
History of myocardial ischemia
Congestive heart failure

Neurologic conditions

Seizure disorders
History of stroke

Gastrointestinal/hepatic conditions

Active gastrointestinal bleeding
Liver dysfunction
Cirrhosis

Genitourinary conditions

Renal dysfunction
Urinary retention

Social conditions

Elderly or young age
Chronic use of prescribed sedatives
Substance abuse

Psychiatric conditions

Uncooperative attitude
Mental disorders

Table 6.2 Antibiotic prophylaxis in endoscopy

Patient condition	Procedure contemplated	Antibiotic prophylaxis	Goal of prophylaxis
All cardiac conditions	Any endoscopic procedure	Not indicated	Prevention of infective endocarditis
Bile duct obstruction in the absence of cholangitis	ERCP with complete drainage	Not recommended	Prevention of cholangitis
Bile duct obstruction in absence of cholangitis	ERCP with anticipated incomplete drainage (e. g., PSC, hilar strictures)	Recommended; continue antibiotics after procedure	Prevention of cholangitis
Sterile pancreatic fluid collection (e. g., pseudocyst, necrosis), which communicates with pancreatic duct	ERCP	Recommended	Prevention of cyst infection
Sterile pancreatic fluid collection	Transmural drainage	Recommended	Prevention of cyst infection
Solid lesion along upper GI tract	EUS-FNA	Not recommended	Prevention of local infection
Solid lesion along lower GI tract	EUS-FNA	Insufficient data to make firm recommendation	Prevention of local infection
Cystic lesions along GI tract (including mediastinum)	EUS-FNA	Recommended	Prevention of cyst infection
All patients	Percutaneous endoscopic feeding tube placement	Recommended	Prevention of peristomal infection
Cirrhosis with acute GI bleeding	Required for all patients, regardless of endoscopic procedures	On admission	Prevention of infectious complications and reduction of mortality
Synthetic vascular graft and other nonvalvular cardiovascular devices	Any endoscopic procedure	Not recommended	Prevention of graft and device infection
Prosthetic joints	Any endoscopic procedure	Not recommended	Prevention of septic arthritis

ERCP, endoscopic retrograde cholangiopancreatography; EUS-FNA, endoscopic ultrasound–guided fine-needle aspiration; GI, gastrointestinal; PSC, primary sclerosing cholangitis.

All patients should be asked if they are taking anticoagulants or antiplatelet agents, including daily aspirin, as this common situation may be associated with an increased intraprocedural risk of bleeding. According to a number of international societies (including the British Society of Gastroenterology, the British Committee for Standards in Haematology, the American Society of Gastrointestinal Endoscopy, the American College of Gastroenterology, the American Heart Association, and the Japanese Gastroenterological Endoscopy Society), the cardiovascular risks involved in stopping therapy before the procedure may outweigh the risks of bleeding during the procedure [14–17]. However, for high-risk endoscopic procedures in patients at low risk for coagulopathies, warfarin should be temporarily discontinued as much as 5 days before endoscopy and clopidogrel should be stopped 7 days prior to the procedure [14]. There is currently no mandate to discontinue aspirin or nonsteroidal anti-inflammatory agents for most endoscopic procedures [15,17].

A physical examination should also be performed before administering sedation. The examination can be focused, but must include: 1, vital signs and patient weight; 2, auscultation of heart and lungs; and 3, an assessment of a patient's baseline level of consciousness. In addition, it may be appropriate for endoscopists to perform a standardized, detailed airway evaluation. The goal of an airway evaluation is to identify patient risk factors or oropharyngeal anatomic variations that may complicate airway management. For example, obese patients or patients with a short, thick neck, cervical spine disease, decreased hyoid–mental distance, or structural abnormalities of the mouth, jaw, and oral cavity may require special provisions for safe sedation. At a minimum, patients with these risk factors may be difficult to intubate in an unlikely emergency, and this should be taken into account when administering sedation.

Airway Evaluation

The Mallampati score has been proposed as a standardized way of identifying patients who may be at risk for difficult planned or unanticipated endotracheal intubation (**Fig. 6.2**) [18]. To assess the airway using this score, the patient is asked to sit straight, extend the head forward, open the mouth and stick out the tongue. In general, in grades I and II, in which the soft palate and uvula are visible, intubation can be performed without difficulty if necessary. Patients who are scored as having either grade III or IV, in whom the soft palate and uvula are less visible, may prove to be at risk for difficult endotracheal intubation. If deep sedation for endoscopic procedures is planned, anesthesiologist assistance should be considered for patients who have Mallampati scores of III or IV. There are known relationships between obesity, neck circumference, and higher Mallampati scores [19]. The relationship between obesity and sedation risks during gastrointestinal procedures has not been well elucidated [20].

It is also well accepted that endoscopists may always choose to work with a dedicated anesthesiologist for the duration of a gastrointestinal procedure. In this connection, the American Society of Anesthesiologists has devised a physical status classification system that may be of use in helping endoscopists determine which patients would be best served by anesthesiologists (**Table 6.3**). The ASA patient classification system was not specifically developed to estimate anesthesia risk, but rather to provide relative guidelines for identifying patients in whom moderate sedation is safe and which patients should be considered for general anesthesia. Generally, patients with status 1 and 2 are considered good candidates for moderate sedation. Status 3 patients should be evaluated carefully, while status 4 and 5 patients are likely to require general anesthesia. ASA classes represent crude categories and may not be useful for capturing complex clinical scenarios. Disagreement regarding patient status between nurses, endoscopists, and anesthesiologists may also be common.

6

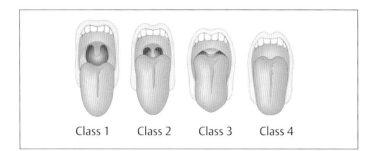

Class 1   Class 2   Class 3   Class 4

Fig. 6.2 Mallampati classification of variations in airway views [18].

Table 6.3 American Society of Anesthesiologists (ASA) classification of patients' physical status

ASA class	Physical status
1	Normal healthy patient
2	Patient with mild systemic disease
3	Patient with severe systemic disease
4	Patient with severe systemic disease that is a constant threat to life
5	Moribund patient not expected to survive without the operation

As a final consideration before entering the procedure room, patients must be carefully assessed as to their level of cooperation for endoscopy. Uncooperative patients present a special situation in which general anesthesia is often required. Of course, patients vary considerably in how they react to sedative medications in both the rapidity and the depth of sedation achieved. A careful discussion of what to expect during the procedure, delivered in a relaxed and reassuring manner—the so-called "vocal local"—may decrease the anxiety level in some patients, allowing reduced medication doses to achieve the desired effect. In addition, a recent meta-analysis suggests that using music to create an ambience in the endoscopy suite may help soothe patients [21].

Special Patient Considerations

As part of the general assessment of patients, all women of child-bearing age should be asked whether or not they might be pregnant, as common sedatives are teratogenic, especially early in the first trimester. History and physical examination may be insufficient to identify early pregnancy, and an endoscopy facility should develop a standardized protocol for pregnancy testing. One study found that the incidence of unrecognized true positive pregnancies on the day of a surgical procedure was four of 2588, or 0.15 % [22].

If endoscopic procedures have to be performed during pregnancy, consultation with an obstetrician or an anesthesiologist, or both, regarding medication use during pregnancy should be considered [23,24]. No pregnancy category A drugs are used for endoscopy sedation. Instead, pethidine, a category B drug, alone is preferred. If necessary, pethidine can be followed by small doses of midazolam (category D), although midazolam should be avoided if possible during the first trimester [24].

The bottom line is that endoscopists need to be flexible in choosing sedation agents and in administering them, largely basing sedation choices on patient assessment. For instance, sedation with midazolam may exacerbate subclinical hepatic encephalopathy in patients with cirrhosis [25]. As another example, elderly patients, who are often highly sensitive to narcotic–benzodiazepine combinations, might have these agents given in half the usual doses and at twice the incremental intervals, or the narcotic agent may be omitted altogether. In an era of open-access endoscopy in which prior outpatient consultation with a gastroenterologist may not occur, it may be even more essential for the endoscopist to carefully evaluate each patient in a systematic manner in order to best develop a sedation plan [11].

Procedures without Sedation

Most upper gastrointestinal procedures in Western populations are carried out with sedation, while Asian endoscopists more frequently carry out the same procedures in unsedated patients. A recent survey of members of the European Society of Gastrointestinal Endoscopy suggests that in 47 % of member countries, fewer than a quarter of patients receive sedation for routine upper endoscopy [26]. A survey of members of the American Society of Gastrointestinal Endoscopy suggests that only half of members perform any unsedated upper endoscopies, with those who do so performing less than 25 such procedures a year [27]. Worldwide, there is growing interest in performing upper endoscopy with thin instruments (< 6 mm) using only topical pharyngeal anesthesia or even a transnasal approach [28,29].

Sedation practice during colonoscopy is particularly variable, running the gamut from no sedation to general anesthesia [30–32]. Some procedures, such as flexible sigmoidoscopy, are almost never performed with sedation in any setting. Methods reported to minimize patient discomfort or enhance cecal intubation during unsedated colonoscopy include hypnosis, music, distraction, use of a pediatric colonoscope, use of a gastroscope, as well as inhalation of nitrous oxide or insufflation of carbon dioxide [32].

The main advantage of not sedating patients for procedures lies in minimizing complication risks and costs [33]. In fact, many studies have indicated that complications from sedation are the most frequent adverse events associated with gastrointestinal procedures and are much more common than procedural complications themselves, such as perforation or bleeding [34–36]. The cost reductions associated with not using sedation can be attributed to reduced costs for medication, elimination of the cost of oxygen administration, and shorter recovery times.

Conversely, by not sedating patients, endoscopists incur the risk of not completing procedures in a satisfactory way for both the doctor and the patient. For the most part, the decision to use sedation during endoscopy is based on clinical perception of the discomfort associated with a given procedure. Patients are often unwilling to undergo unsedated procedures, due to cultural expectations [27]. On the other hand, performing procedures in the absence of sedation allows the patient an almost immediate return to normal functioning, including the ability to drive an automobile and resume employment. Some patients may expect or request no sedation for these reasons.

Pharmacological Options for Endoscopy

The choice of which medications to use for procedural sedation during endoscopy should be tailored to the procedure and the patient. A well-reasoned risk–benefit approach always suggests the least sedation possible—better for the patient, as the lowest risk associated with sedation will be incurred. However, thorough knowledge of all the options for sedation and analgesia improves the chances of a procedure being completed successfully without undue risk of complications or of unpleasantness for the patient. **Table 6.4** lists different sedation agents and their potential risks and side effects.

Table 6.4 Common agents for procedural sedation in endoscopy and their side effects

Class, name	Potential adverse events and complications
Topical	
Benzocaine	Methemoglobinemia
Lidocaine	Potential for systemic absorption and toxicity
Benzodiazepines	
Diazepam	Respiratory depression; apnea; thrombophlebitis
Midazolam	Respiratory depression; apnea
Opioids	
Pethidine	Respiratory and central nervous system depression; seizures, nausea; vomiting
Fentanyl	Apnea, bradycardia; chest wall and glottic rigidity
Antagonists	
Flumazenil	Short duration of action; resedation
Naloxone	Catecholamine release, tachyarrhythmias, sudden death
Propofol	Rapid progression to general anesthesia; impaired gastrointestinal contractility
Adjuvant	
Anticholinergics	Vasoconstriction; dry mouth; headache; glaucoma
Droperidol	Dissociative state, unpleasant procedural experience; nightmares

Topical Agents

In patients undergoing upper endoscopy, there may be some benefit derived from applying a topical anesthetic such as Cetacaine (benzocaine, butyl aminobenzoate, and amethocaine) or lidocaine to the posterior pharynx. Spray preparations may be more effective than gargles or lozenges.

While it is not clear that the routine use of topical anesthetics affects the degree of sedation required for gastrointestinal procedures in most patients [37], a recent systematic review of five randomized controlled trials suggests that it is beneficial [38]. In this meta-analysis, pharyngeal anesthesia before upper endoscopy was found to be related to improved ease of endoscopy as rated by the endoscopists and improved patient tolerance as reported by patients.

Studies have shown that topical application is only effective when the anesthetic is delivered to the posterior pharynx, rather than to the tongue and mouth. Topical drug delivery therefore often requires depression of the tongue and elicitation of a gag reflex with a tongue blade during spraying, which may be highly unpleasant for the patient but maximizes the effectiveness of the drug.

The practice of administering pharyngeal topical agents is not without risk. In particular, several case reports have documented methemoglobinemia related to topical benzocaine administration before upper endoscopy [39–41]. However, these complications remain extremely rare and as yet should not dissuade endoscopists from routinely using topical anesthesia before endoscopy.

Benzodiazepines

Benzodiazepines are the most commonly used sedatives during endoscopic procedures. In particular, diazepam and midazolam are considered to be comparable in terms of efficacy and safety. Although both have high therapeutic indices, midazolam may be preferable to diazepam for its faster onset of action, shorter duration of action, and strong anamnestic effects [3,42].

The same characteristics that make benzodiazepines attractive for endoscopy also mandate their administration in small serial increments with close monitoring to clinically determine sedation levels. Yet, incremental administration of benzodiazepines until a goal depth of sedation has been achieved may heighten the risk of accidentally progressing from light to deep sedation. Patients often initially appear to require more doses, only to quickly become deeply sedated as unanticipated delayed pharmacokinetics effectively leads to unintended overdosage.

Diazepam

Diazepam is generally used alone or in combination with opioids for sedation in patients undergoing gastrointestinal procedures. As the metabolism of diazepam is primarily hepatic, this drug should be used with caution in patients with liver disease. Respiratory depression with diazepam, as with all benzodiazepines, is particularly likely when it is combined with narcotics. Its main disadvantages are a long duration of action, pain associated with intravenous administration, and thrombophlebitis. To avoid these, emulsified versions of diazepam have been developed that are associated with less pain on injection, less thrombophlebitis, and significantly lower cost [43].

Midazolam

Midazolam is three to six times more potent than diazepam and has become the mainstay benzodiazepine for gastrointestinal procedural sedation, due to its significant clinical advantages over diazepam for the endoscopist. Midazolam is water-soluble, which greatly diminishes the pain associated with intravenous or even intramuscular administration. Also, its beta elimination half-life is significantly shorter than that of diazepam, which is particularly advantageous for brief procedures.

One of midazolam's most desirable side effects is its retrograde and anterograde amnesia for procedures. According to the Versed brand package insert (Roche Laboratories), 71 % of patients sedated with midazolam were shown to have no recall of introduction of the endoscope, and 82 % had no recall of withdrawal of the endoscope. In a systematic review and meta-analysis of randomized controlled trials of moderate sedation for routine endoscopic procedures, midazolam provided superior patient satisfaction in comparison with diazepam, and far less frequent memory of the procedure [44].

Midazolam generally produces a calm, compliant patient who is receptive to nonthreatening procedures. Its main disadvantage is that it appears to have much greater potential for causing respiratory depression in elderly patients, and generally it is given in smaller doses to this population. In fact, well-controlled studies continue to suggest that even octogenarians can safely undergo sedation with midazolam for upper gastrointestinal endoscopy without undue risks of desaturation or hypotension [45,46].

6

Opioids

Opioids are primarily analgesic agents, but they do have a mild sedative effect that is especially notable when used in combination with benzodiazepines. Opioids have been demonstrated to improve patient tolerance for endoscopy when used alone. Alternatively, it is in combination with benzodiazepines that opioids have been shown to maximally enhance tolerance and amnesia. Of course, the same combination of opioids and benzodiazepines has also been shown to significantly depress the central nervous system's ventilatory response to carbon dioxide, thereby causing CO_2 retention and hypoxemia.

Pethidine (Meperidine)

One of the opioids most commonly used by endoscopists in both the United States and the United Kingdom is pethidine (U.S. Adopted Name meperidine). Pethidine has a serum half-life of 3–4 h and should therefore be used primarily for procedures lasting longer than 30 min. For similar reasons, pethidine should only be used when there are adequate facilities for monitoring the patient during recovery. In terms of drawbacks, pethidine has been shown to cause apnea and insensitivity to painful stimuli in doses that may not be adequate to induce sleep.

Fentanyl

The opioid fentanyl has a more rapid onset of action and is associated with a lower incidence of nausea compared with pethidine. Fentanyl is approximately 100 times more potent than morphine, due to a high degree of fat solubility that allows rapid penetration of the blood–brain barrier. The resulting onset of opioid effect is therefore much faster for fentanyl than for pethidine (the onset of action is 30 s–5 min, versus 5–10 min). Nonetheless, comparisons of fentanyl with pethidine do not necessarily suggest that it is superior for effecting patient comfort [47].

The termination of action of fentanyl when administered in successive doses is primarily determined by redistribution from the plasma, rather than metabolism. This property of fentanyl puts the patient at risk for dissociation between analgesia and respiratory depression. The opioid effects of fentanyl may last for 30–45 min, but the respiratory depression may last far longer. Fentanyl has also been reported to cause chest wall and glottic rigidity, especially when rapidly administered. Therefore, although the kinetics and dynamics of fentanyl make it desirable for most gastrointestinal procedures, these inherent properties increase the risks of untoward complications. Most suggested guidelines for safe administration involve slow titration, allowing several minutes between doses.

Adjuvant Agents

A number of medications have been postulated to enhance sedation with benzodiazepine and opioid regimens. In particular, the American Society of Gastrointestinal Endoscopy has listed diphenhydramine, promethazine, and droperidol as medications that may potentiate a sedation regimen. To date, none of these has been accepted in general practice, but they continue to garner interest as alternatives in special situations, including patients in whom sedation is difficult.

Diphenhydramine hydrochloride is a histamine H1-receptor antagonist with anticholinergic and sedative properties. Its onset of action is fairly quick, within several minutes, but its duration of effect may be up to 4–6 h. One placebo-controlled randomized trial of diphenhydramine as an adjunct to pethidine and midazolam for colonoscopy suggested lower pain scores and lower doses of sedatives in the diphenhydramine group, without affecting recovery times [48]. However, the adverse effects of diphenhydramine may preclude its routine use and include hypotension, dizziness, blurred vision, dry mouth, wheezing, and urinary retention.

Promethazine is a phenothiazine with antihistamine, sedative, antiemetic and anticholinergic effects. It is best known as a treatment for postoperative nausea and vomiting, and has not been well studied as an adjunctive agent for endoscopy. While it may enhance sedation, promethazine is associated with a number of unpleasant side effects, including oculogyric crisis.

Droperidol is another antiemetic that may be useful as an adjuvant agent for endoscopic sedation, at the risk of causing hypotension and extrapyramidal signs. In addition, droperidol has been given a black box warning by the American Food and Drug Administration that it should be used only when first-line sedative agents fail, as it is associated with prolongation of the QT interval. Use of droperidol should be avoided in patients with cardiovascular risk factors including congestive heart failure, bradycardia, diuretic use, hypokalemia, hypomagnesemia, and use of other drugs that prolong the QT interval.

The mechanism of action of droperidol is to interfere with central neurotransmission by α-adrenergic blockade and produce a dissociative state. Its onset of action is 3–10 min after intravenous administration, and its duration of action is typically 3–6 h, although it can continue for up to 12 h.

It has been postulated that droperidol might be useful in patients in whom sedation is difficult, such as alcoholics and other substance abusers [49]. Then again, its long duration of action can also extend to side effects, including muscle rigidity, visual disturbances, hallucinations, oculogyric crises, and dysphoria, which may last up to 24 h from administration. In addition, patients who receive droperidol may require less restraint, but have less favorable impressions of the procedure, possibly because droperidol does not impart any amnestic effects and leaves patients highly aware of their surroundings [50]. Administration of a narcotic can help ameliorate these effects, but again risks may outweigh benefits for routine use.

Propofol

Propofol (2,6-diisopropylphenol) is a very short-acting hypnotic agent that features a rapid onset of action and a short recovery time. The time from intravenous administration to the onset of sedation is typically 30–60 s, with a duration of effect of 4–8 min. Propofol can be used to induce and maintain a spectrum of sedation levels, ranging from moderate to deep anesthesia. It also confers excellent amnesia, with no analgesia.

Propofol has a high first-pass hepatic degradation profile that limits its administration to intravenous routes only and accounts for its rapid termination of effects and the patient's quick return to consciousness. The level of sedation achieved by propofol is dose-dependent and it is highly lipophilic, rapidly crossing the blood–brain barrier. The most common preparation of propofol is an oil–water emulsion consisting of 1 % propofol, 10 % soybean oil, 2.25 % glycerol, and 1.2 % egg lecithin. Propofol is therefore generally contraindicated in patients with hypersensitivity to eggs or soybean. (A less common preparation uses bisulfites and should be avoided if a patient has a bisulfite allergy.) Propofol is a pregnancy category B drug and should be used with caution during lactation.

The use of propofol for endoscopic sedation in both adults and children worldwide has increased dramatically over the past decade. In particular, physicians have been more satisfied with its efficacy as a sedative and with its recovery profile [2,44]. Propofol is used currently for routine upper and lower endoscopy, as well as therapeutic procedures such as endoscopic retrograde cholangio-pancreatography (ERCP), which may require patient immobility [51,52]. On the other hand, because propofol can swiftly produce a state of general anesthesia, there is consensus that it should not be used by individuals unqualified in airway management. Debate still continues on whether administration should be limited to anesthesiologists.

"Gastroenterologist-administered propofol" refers to either the practice of endoscopists themselves providing direct delivery of propofol, or providing supervision of propofol administration by registered nurses. "Nurse-administered propofol sedation" (NAPS) was originally used to refer to a single-agent regimen of propofol delivered in a bolus [53]. More recently, it has been recognized that propofol is more effectively administered as part of combination therapy with low doses of opioids or benzodiazepines [54]. What has been termed "balanced propofol sedation" [54], or combination gastroenterologist-directed propofol, has become the preferred sedation regimen for nonanesthesiologists working with propofol and has been found to be safe in large series reporting on half a million patients throughout the world [55].

A review of the published literature suggests that administration of propofol by endoscopists or endoscopy nurses has been readily adopted in many countries, including Switzerland, Japan, Australia, Spain, China, Thailand, and Germany [54,56]. While a national survey of U.S. endoscopists found that more than 25% were using propofol, only 7% were administering it themselves. The results of this survey also suggested that the majority of American endoscopists would like to administer propofol but are reluctant to do so because of a widespread perception of increased risks [51].

Propofol may impair gastrointestinal contractile activity [57], although the clinical relevance of this pharmaceutical characteristic following short-term administration for procedural sedation is not known. A more clinically relevant drawback of propofol is a high incidence of pain, which occurs in 30% of patients with intravenous administration. Such pain can be reduced by prior administration of lidocaine intravenously before propofol administration, or by administering propofol through a large vein (e.g., the antecubital vein). Finally, propofol may have a less reliable amnestic effect than midazolam. Investigations into combination sedation with propofol and midazolam suggest that the two drugs together are effective in improving patient comfort and providing amnesia for the procedure. It is less clear whether combination sedation prolongs postprocedural recovery times [44,58].

Antagonists

Antagonists for both benzodiazepines and opioids are available and should be stocked in endoscopy facilities. Antagonists to benzodiazepines and opioids allow near-immediate reversal of adverse side effects or overdosage of these medications, but are unlikely to prevent major complications of oversedation. As another caveat, it is essential to recognize that reversal effects are nearly always shorter than the effects of the drugs being reversed. It is therefore imperative for patients to be carefully observed for an extended period following reversal of sedation, as they are at high risk for recurrent deep sedation.

▨ Flumazenil

Flumazenil is a specific benzodiazepine receptor antagonist that is available in Europe and North America. It produces rapid awakening from benzodiazepine-related respiratory depression and coma, and

may serve as a key means of treatment as well as diagnosis in patients with possible overdose. In patients who have been sedated with a benzodiazepine–opioid combination, flumazenil may be useful at reversing the benzodiazepine's component of central nervous system depression. A history of seizures or use of tricyclic medications are contraindications to the use of flumazenil. The duration of flumazenil's effect is shorter than that of many of the benzodiazepines, and resedation may occur and require repeated doses. A minimum of 2 h of observation is therefore currently recommended following flumazenil treatment for benzodiazepine overdose.

▨ Naloxone

Naloxone is a competitive antagonist to opioids, and should be given intravenously to improve ventilation, reverse coma, and correct hypotension. Although there are no direct contraindications to its use, naloxone's very effectiveness can lead a patient to experience sudden severe pain and catecholamine release, and can increase the risk of tachyarrhythmias and sudden death, especially in patients with underlying cardiac disease. Also, patients habituated to narcotics may experience severe withdrawal reactions to naloxone. Naloxone should therefore not be used routinely to reverse opioid analgesia, but rather reserved for circulatory decompensation or respiratory arrest secondary to opioid administration during endoscopy. The effect of naloxone is dose-dependent. The use of small doses titrated to clinical response is preferable; in a true emergency, a full ampule (0.4 mg) can be administered.

Care and Monitoring of the Patient during Endoscopy

Safe sedation of all patients undergoing endoscopy requires a systematically applied, protective net of skilled staff members, caution, monitoring devices, common sense in patient and drug selection, emergency response equipment, and the availability of drugs to sustain life. Consensus dictates that a well-trained assistant who can closely monitor the patient represents the principal factor in effective patient monitoring during gastrointestinal procedures. Endoscopy personnel should be trained in advanced cardiopulmonary life support and airway management, and—perhaps even more critically—should understand the difference between ventilation and oxygenation.

▨ Electronic Monitoring and Intervention

Intraprocedural monitoring using a combination of a dedicated staff member and electronic monitors can detect changes in the patient's vital signs before clinically significant events occur. Most cardiopulmonary events during gastrointestinal endoscopy stem from hypoventilation cascading into hypoxia and cardiac decompensation. Accordingly, endoscopy staff should be comfortable with basic airway management maneuvers, including jaw-thrusts, chin-lifts, and bag-mask ventilation (**Fig. 6.3**). During moderate and deep sedation, a patient's level of consciousness needs to be continually assessed, and documented at the least before the procedure begins, at initial sedation administration, at regular intervals during the procedure, at the beginning of the recovery period, and before discharge [3].

As a basic component of monitoring, pulse oximetry has become a standard of care in endoscopy units around the world. However, pulse oximeters may not adequately reflect impending hemodynamic instability or vasoconstrictive shock. In particular, patients may be well saturated with oxygen and still be suffering from

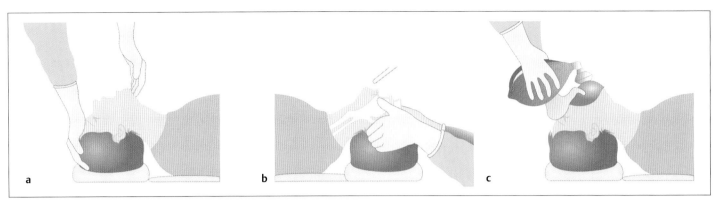

Fig. 6.3   Basic airway management skills.
a   Chin lift.

b   Jaw thrust.
c   Correct positioning for bag-mask ventilation.

significant carbon dioxide retention. This type of discrepancy between oxygenation and ventilation (gas exchange) may be present particularly when supplemental oxygen is used.

Recently, technological advances have enabled the measurement of real-time end-tidal carbon dioxide in nonintubated patients. Capnography has in this way emerged as a noninvasive method of measuring the patient's ventilation. While there is currently insufficient evidence to support its use during routine sedation in upper and lower endoscopy, a number of studies have suggested that intervention based on capnographic detection of hypoventilation will decrease hypoxemia in patients undergoing gastrointestinal procedures [59,60]. These studies have suggested that monitoring for a lack of respiratory activity is adequate for detecting hypoventilation, which is often not recognized by clinical staff dedicated to visually monitoring the patient.

Finally, several gastrointestinal societies have joined with the American Society of Anesthesiologists in recommending that a patient's blood pressure be assessed at the least before, during, and after endoscopic procedures. For high-risk patients with a history of underlying cardiopulmonary disease, blood pressure measurements every 5–10 min and continuous electrocardiography monitoring are recommended [4].

References

1. Knape JT, Adriaensen H, van Aken H, Blunnie WP, Carlsson C, Dupont M, et al. Guidelines for sedation and/or analgesia by non-anaesthesiology doctors. Eur J Anaesthesiol 2007;24:563–7.
2. Cohen LB, Delegge MH, Aisenberg J, Brill JV, Inadomi JM, Kochman ML, et al. AGA Institute review of endoscopic sedation. Gastroenterology 2007;133:675–701.
3. Standards of Practice Committee, Lichtenstein DR, Jagannath S, Baron TH, Anderson MA, Banerjee S, et al. Sedation and anesthesia in GI endoscopy. Gastrointest Endosc 2008;68:205–16.
4. American Society of Anesthesiologists Task Force on Sedation and Analgesia by Non-Anesthesiologists. Practice guidelines for sedation and analgesia by non-anesthesiologists. Anesthesiology. 2002;96:1004–17.
5. American Society of Anesthesiology, Economics Committee. Distinguishing monitored anesthesia care ("MAC") from moderate sedation/analgesia (conscious sedation). (Approved by the ASA House of Delegates on October 27, 2004 and last updated on September 2, 2008). Available at: www.asahq.org/publicationsAndServices/standards/35.pdf.
6. Bell GD. Preparation, premedication, and surveillance. Endoscopy 2004; 36:23–31.
7. Abraham N, Barkun A, Larocque M, Fallone C, Mayrand S, Baffis V, et al. Predicting which patients can undergo upper endoscopy comfortably without conscious sedation. Gastrointest Endosc 2002;56:180–9.
8. Campo R, Brullet E, Montserrat A, Calvet X, Moix J, Rué M, et al. Identification of factors that influence tolerance of upper gastrointestinal endoscopy. Eur J Gastroenterol Hepatol 1999;11:201–4.
9. Standards of Practice Committee, Zuckerman MJ, Shen B, Harrison ME 3 rd, Baron TH, Adler DG, et al. Informed consent for GI endoscopy. Gastrointest Endosc 2007;66:213–8.
10. Gabel A, Muller S. Aspiration: a possible severe complication in colonoscopy preparation of elderly people by orthograde intestine lavage. Digestion 1999;60:284–5.
11. Mitty RD, Wild DM. The pre- and postprocedure assessment of patients undergoing sedation for gastrointestinal endoscopy. Gastrointest Endosc Clin N Am 2008;18:627–40.
12. ASGE Standards of Practice Committee, Banerjee S, Shen B, Baron TH, Nelson DB, Anderson MA, et al. Antibiotic prophylaxis for GI endoscopy. Gastrointest Endosc 2008;67:791–8.
13. Wilson W, Taubert KA, Gewitz M, Lockhart PB, Baddour LM, Levison M, et al. Prevention of infective endocarditis: guidelines from the American Heart Association: a guideline from the American Heart Association Rheumatic Fever, Endocarditis, and Kawasaki Disease Committee, Council on Cardiovascular Disease in the Young, and the Council on Clinical Cardiology, Council on Cardiovascular Surgery and Anesthesia, and the Quality of Care and Outcomes Research Interdisciplinary Working Group. Circulation 2007;116:1736–54.
14. Veitch AM, Baglin TP, Gershlick AH, Harnden SM, Tighe R, Cairns S. Guidelines for the management of anticoagulant and antiplatelet therapy in patients undergoing endoscopic procedures. Gut 2008;57:1322–9.
15. Bhatt DL, Scheiman J, Abraham NS, Antman EM, Chan FK, Furberg CD, et al. ACCF/ACG/AHA 2008 expert consensus document on reducing the gastrointestinal risks of antiplatelet therapy and NSAID use: a report of the American College of Cardiology Foundation Task Force on Clinical Expert Consensus Documents. J Am Coll Cardiol 2008;52:1502–17.
16. Fujishiro M, Oda I, Yamamoto Y, Akiyama J, Ishii N, Kakushima N, et al. Multi-center survey regarding the management of anticoagulation and antiplatelet therapy for endoscopic procedures in Japan. J Gastroenterol Hepatol 2009;24:214–8.
17. Eisen GM, Baron TH, Dominitz JA, Faigel DO, Goldstein JL, Johanson JF, et al. Guideline on the management of anticoagulation and antiplatelet therapy for endoscopic procedures. Gastrointest Endosc 2002;55:775–9.
18. Mallampati SR, Gatt SP, Gugino LD, Desai SP, Waraksa B, Freiberger D, et al. A clinical sign to predict difficult tracheal intubation: a prospective study. Can Anaesth Soc J 1985;32:429–34.
19. Gonzalez H, Minville V, Delanoue K, Mazerolles M, Concina D, Fourcade O. The importance of increased neck circumference to intubation difficulties in obese patients. Anesth Analg 2008;106:1132–6.
20. Moos DD. Obstructive sleep apnea and sedation in the endoscopy suite. Gastroenterol Nurs 2006;29:456–63.
21. Rudin D, Kiss A, Wetz RV, Sottile VM. Music in the endoscopy suite: a meta-analysis of randomized controlled studies. Endoscopy 2007;39:507–10.
22. Kahn RL, Stanton MA, Tong-Ngork S, Liguori GA, Edmonds CR, Levine DS. One-year experience with day-of-surgery pregnancy testing before elective orthopedic procedures. Anesth Analg 2008;106:1127–31.
23. Gilinsky NH, Muthunayagam N. Gastrointestinal endoscopy in pregnant and lactating women: emerging standard of care to guide decision-making. Obstet Gynecol Surv 2006;61:791–9.
24. Qureshi WA, Rajan E, Adler DG, Davila RE, Hirota WK, Jacobson BC, et al. ASGE guideline: guidelines for endoscopy in pregnant and lactating women. Gastrointest Endosc 2005;61:357–62.

25. Assy N, Rosser BG, Grahame GR, Minuk GY. Risk of sedation for upper GI endoscopy exacerbating subclinical hepatic encephalopathy in patients with cirrhosis. Gastrointest Endosc 1999;49:690–4.

26. Ladas SD, Aabakken L, Rey JF, Nowak A, Zakaria S, Adamonis K, et al. Use of sedation for routine diagnostic upper gastrointestinal endoscopy: a European Society of Gastrointestinal Endoscopy Survey of national endoscopy society members. Digestion 2006;74:69–77.

27. Faulx AL, Vela S, Das A, Cooper G, Sivak MV, Isenberg G, et al. The changing landscape of practice patterns regarding unsedated endoscopy and propofol use: a national Web survey. Gastrointest Endosc 2005;62:9–15.

28. Horiuchi A, Nakayama Y. Unsedated ultrathin EGD by using a 5.2-mm-diameter videoscope: evaluation of acceptability and diagnostic accuracy. Gastrointest Endosc 2006;64:868–73.

29. Cheung J, Bailey R, Veldhuyzen van Zanten S, McLean R, Fedorak RN, Morse J, et al. Early experience with unsedated ultrathin 4.9 mm transnasal gastroscopy: a pilot study. Can J Gastroenterol 2008;22:917–22.

30. Knox L, Hahn RG, Lane C. A comparison of unsedated colonoscopy and flexible sigmoidoscopy in the family medicine setting: an LA Net study. J Am Board Fam Med 2007;20:444–50.

31. Chen PJ, Shih YL, Chu HC, Chang WK, Hsieh TY, Chao YC. A prospective trial of variable stiffness colonoscopes with different tip diameters in unsedated patients. Am J Gastroenterol 2008;103:1365–71.

32. Leung FW. Methods of reducing discomfort during colonoscopy. Dig Dis Sci 2008;53:1462–7.

33. Abraham NS, Fallone CA, Mayrand S, Huang J, Wieczorek P, Barkun AN. Sedation versus no sedation in the performance of diagnostic upper gastrointestinal endoscopy: a Canadian randomized controlled cost-outcome study. Am J Gastroenterol 2004;99:1692–9.

34. Sharma VK, Nguyen CC, Crowell MD, Lieberman DA, de Garmo P, Fleischer DE. A national study of cardiopulmonary unplanned events after GI endoscopy. Gastrointest Endosc 2007;66:27–34.

35. Rudner R, Jalowiecki P, Kawecki P, Gonciarz M, Mularczyk A, Petelenz M. Conscious analgesia/sedation with remifentanil and propofol versus total intravenous anesthesia with fentanyl, midazolam, and propofol for outpatient colonoscopy. Gastrointest Endosc 2003;57:657–63.

36. Thakkar K, El-Serag HB, Mattek N, Gilger MA. Complications of pediatric EGD: a 4-year experience in PEDS-CORI. Gastrointest Endosc 2007;65:213–21.

37. Ristikankare M, Hartikainen J, Heikkinen M, Julkunen R. Is routine sedation or topical pharyngeal anesthesia beneficial during upper endoscopy? Gastrointest Endosc 2004;60:686–94.

38. Evans LT, Saberi S, Kim HM, Elta GH, Schoenfeld P. Pharyngeal anesthesia during sedated EGDs: is "the spray" beneficial? A meta-analysis and systematic review. Gastrointest Endosc 2006;63:761–6.

39. Byrne MF, Mitchell RM, Gerke H, Goller S, Stiffler HL, Golioto M, et al. The need for caution with topical anesthesia during endoscopic procedures, as liberal use may result in methemoglobinemia. J Clin Gastroenterol 2004;38:225–9.

40. Dahshan A, Donovan GK. Severe methemoglobinemia complicating topical benzocaine use during endoscopy in a toddler: a case report and review of the literature. Pediatrics 2006;117:e806–9.

41. Moos DD, Cuddeford JD. Methemoglobinemia and benzocaine. Gastroenterol Nurs 2007;30:342–5.

42. Waring JP, Baron TH, Hirota WK, Goldstein JL, Jacobson BC, Leighton JA, et al. Guidelines for conscious sedation and monitoring during gastrointestinal endoscopy. Gastrointest Endosc 2003;58:317–22.

43. Van Houten JS, Crane SA, Janardan SK, Wells K. A randomized, prospective, double-blind comparison of midazolam (Versed) and emulsified diazepam (Dizac) for opioid-based, conscious sedation in endoscopic procedures. Am J Gastroenterol 1998;93:170–4.

44. McQuaid KR, Laine L. A systematic review and meta-analysis of randomized, controlled trials of moderate sedation for routine endoscopic procedures. Gastrointest Endosc 2008;67:910–23.

45. Ma WT, Mahadeva S, Kunanayagam S, Poi PJ, Goh KL. Colonoscopy in elderly Asians: a prospective evaluation in routine clinical practice. J Dig Dis 2007;8:77–81.

46. Arora A, Singh P. Colonoscopy in patients 80 years of age and older is safe, with high success rate and diagnostic yield. Gastrointest Endosc 2004;60:408–13.

47. Agency for Healthcare Research and Quality (AHRQ). Medical errors: the scope of the problem. Rockville, MD: Agency for Healthcare Research and Quality, 2000 (fact sheet, publication no. AHRQ 00-P037). Available at: http://www.ahrq.gov/qual/errback.htm.

48. Tu RH, Grewall P, Leung JW, Suryaprasad AG, Sheykhzadeh PI, Doan C, et al. Diphenhydramine as an adjunct to sedation for colonoscopy: a double-blind randomized, placebo-controlled study. Gastrointest Endosc 2006;63:87–94.

49. Cohen J, Haber GB, Dorais JA, Scheider DM, Kandel GP, Kortan PP, et al. A randomized, double-blind study of the use of droperidol for conscious sedation during therapeutic endoscopy in difficult to sedate patients. Gastrointest Endosc 2000;51:546–51.

50. Rizzo J, Bernstein D, Gress F. A randomized double-blind placebo-controlled trial evaluating the cost-effectiveness of droperidol as a sedative premedication for EUS. Gastrointest Endosc 1999;50:178–82.

51. Cohen LB, Wecsler JS, Gaetano JN, Benson AA, Miller KM, Durkalski V, et al. Endoscopic sedation in the United States: results from a nationwide survey. Am J Gastroenterol 2006;101:967–74.

52. Lightdale JR, Mahoney LB, Schwarz SM, Liacouras CA. Methods of sedation in pediatric endoscopy: a survey of NASPGHAN members. J Pediatr Gastroenterol Nutr 2007;45:500–2.

53. Rex DK, Overley CA, Walker J. Registered nurse-administered propofol sedation for upper endoscopy and colonoscopy: Why? When? How? Rev Gastroenterol Disord 2003;3:70–80.

54. Rex DK, Deenadayalu V, Eid E. Gastroenterologist-directed propofol: an update. Gastrointest Endosc Clin N Am 2008;18:717–25.

55. Deenadayalu V, Eid E, Goff JS, et al. Non-anesthesiologist administered propofol sedation for endoscopic procedures: a worldwide safety review [abstract]. Gastrointestinal Endoscopy 2008;67:AB107.

56. Heuss LT, Peter S. Propofol use by gastroenterologists—the European experience. Gastrointest Endosc Clin N Am 2008;18:727–38.

57. Lee TL, Ang SB, Dambisya YM, Adaikan GP, Lau LC. The effect of propofol on human gastric and colonic muscle contractions. Anesth Analg 1999;89:1246–9.

58. Wurz SM, Bernstein B. Propofol or process: what really affects efficiency? Gastroenterol Nurs 2004;27:69–73.

59. Lightdale JR, Goldmann DA, Feldman HA, Newburg AR, Dinardo JA, Fox VL. Microstream capnography improves patient monitoring during moderate sedation: a randomized, controlled trial. Pediatrics 2006;117:1170–8.

60. Qadeer MA, Rocio Lopez A, Dumot JA, Vargo JJ. Risk factors for hypoxemia during ambulatory gastrointestinal endoscopy in ASA I–II Patients. Dig Dis Sci 2009;54:1035–40.

6

7 Endoscopy in Special Clinical Situations

Douglas G. Adler and David Bjorkman

Introduction

While most endoscopic procedures are performed in patients in whom there are no special requirements or relative contraindications, there are several special clinical situations in which additional precautions before, during, or after the procedure are warranted in an effort to maximize patient safety and minimize complications and poor outcomes. This chapter focuses on three of the most commonly encountered special situations: gastrointestinal endoscopy in pregnant and lactating women; in the elderly; and in patients who require anticoagulant therapy.

Endoscopy in Pregnant and Lactating Women

Although endoscopy in pregnant and lactating women has been performed extensively, there are relatively few studies involving these patient populations. This situation is probably due to the fact that women in these groups are often specifically excluded from enrollment in prospective trials, and institutional approval to perform procedures in pregnant patients is extremely difficult to obtain even in the context of a research study.

▪ Endoscopy in Pregnant Patients

In general, most practitioners would prefer to avoid performing any endoscopic procedures in pregnant women, owing to very real concerns about causing harm to either the mother or the fetus, either as a result of the endoscopy itself, the use of sedation, and/or possible fetal exposure to radiation. There are consequently relatively few indications for endoscopy in pregnant women. Endoscopy in pregnant patients is often performed to identify and treat relatively serious conditions that could endanger the life of the mother or the fetus. While no strict criteria exist, the American Society of Gastrointestinal Endoscopy has produced a list of generally accepted indications, a modified version of which is presented in **Table 7.1** [1].

In most pregnant patients, gastrointestinal endoscopy can be safely performed. Some special precautions are generally required to ensure that the procedure involves the minimal acceptable risk. Patients should have the procedure performed, when possible, by the most experienced endoscopist available—preferably someone with experience in performing procedures in pregnancy—in an effort to minimize the duration of the procedure. Maternal and fetal monitoring equipment should be used appropriately, and fetal heart tones should be assessed before, during, and after the endoscopy. Consultation with the patient's obstetrician is often very helpful when planning endoscopy in pregnant patients, and if the patient is in the advanced stages of pregnancy it is often helpful to have a representative of the obstetric team present or available on short notice in the event of any obstetric complications or the development of any evidence of fetal distress. Patients should be placed in the left pelvic tilt or left lateral decubitus position in an effort to avoid compression of the gravid uterus, aorta, or internal vena cava (IVC). If fluoroscopy is to be used, appropriate shielding of the fetus

Table 7.1 Indications for considering endoscopy in pregnant patients

- Known or suspected gastrointestinal bleeding
- Severe abdominal pain
- Severe and/or refractory nausea and vomiting
- Dysphagia
- Odynophagia
- Strong suspicion of gastrointestinal malignancy
- Severe diarrhea of unclear etiology
- Biliary pancreatitis
- Choledocholithiasis
- Cholangitis
- Known or suspected biliary or pancreatic ductal injury

Adapted from Qureshi et al. [1].

is warranted and an effort to expose the patient to as little radiation as possible should be made. If possible, only category A or B medications should be used for sedation and anesthesia, and consideration should be given to having an anesthesiologist administer medications and assist in monitoring the patient. Lastly, if possible, endoscopy should be deferred until the second trimester, by which time the majority of fetal development has already occurred.

Upper endoscopy, flexible sigmoidoscopy, and colonoscopy have been evaluated in a limited number of studies in pregnant patients with proper indications, and have been generally been found to be safe and have not been associated with poor fetal outcome or spontaneous abortion [2–5].

Endoscopic retrograde cholangiopancreatography (ERCP) in pregnant patients (**Fig. 7.1**) has been an area of special interest. This is likely due to the high-risk nature of the procedure, which typically involves exposing the patient and the fetus to radiation via fluoroscopy, and the fact that the indications for performing ERCP in pregnancy (e. g., cholangitis) tend to be quite serious and may be potentially life-threatening.

ERCP in pregnancy has been reported, collectively, in fewer than 100 patients, although it has doubtlessly been performed on a much larger scale [6–10]. Almost all reported patients had choledocholithiasis with or without cholangitis, although a small number of patients underwent ERCP for the treatment of other diagnoses (i. e., chronic pancreatitis). Biliary sphincterotomy, stone extraction, and biliary stenting all appear to be safe in pregnancy. In general, complications (e. g., post-ERCP pancreatitis, post-sphincterotomy bleeding, etc.) did not result in fetal or maternal death, although preterm labor has been reported in these settings. In studies that included follow-up, the health of the children after delivery also usually did not appear to be affected by the procedure. In studies that reported fetal complications (birth defects, etc.) these could not be decisively linked to the ERCP [8].

Fluoroscopy exposure should be minimized and, if available, dosimeters should be placed on the patient to record the level of radiation exposure. Most ERCPs in pregnant patients have been accomplished with an extremely low fluoroscopy time (60 s or less) [9,10]. Actual radiation doses have not been universally reported, but tended to be low and well below the presumed safe threshold for pregnant or potentially pregnant patients [9,11]. If access to the biliary tree can be confirmed without fluoroscopy

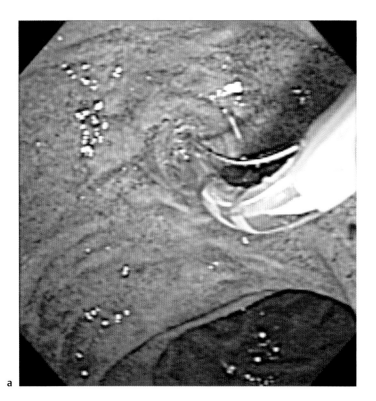

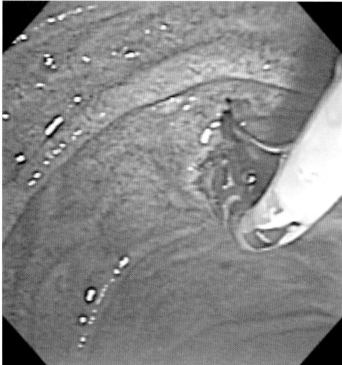

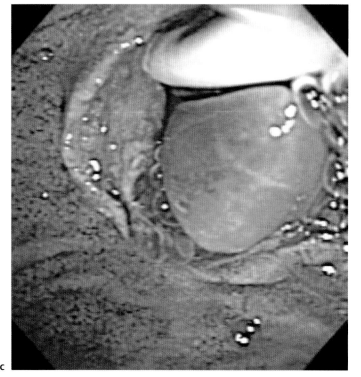

Fig. 7.1 Endoscopic retrograde cholangiopancreatography in the pregnant patient.
a The native papilla in a 19-year-old woman who developed jaundice and cholelithiasis during the second trimester of pregnancy.
b Biliary sphincterotomy was performed after deep cannulation had been achieved.
c Stone extraction using standard occlusion/extraction balloons.

(via the aspiration of pure bile), ERCP with therapeutic maneuvers can be safely performed without the use of any fluoroscopy [8].

With regard to endoscopic technique, some physicians prefer simply to place a stent in patients with obstructive jaundice, choledocholithiasis and/or cholangitis, avoiding the risks of biliary sphincterotomy and the increased procedure time required to extract stones or perform other therapeutic maneuvers. In these patients, the stent is simply left in place to provide biliary drainage until after delivery, at which time a second ERCP can be performed in a more standard fashion without any additional precautions being required. Others have approached these patients with the intention of performing all of the required maneuvers in a single

session, thus minimizing the chance of a repeat procedure being required before delivery. No general consensus on this point exists, and treatment should be individualized.

Endoscopy in Lactating Patients

Endoscopy in patients who are lactating can be performed in almost all clinical situations. Patients can safely undergo upper and lower endoscopy, endoscopic ultrasonography, and can undergo procedures requiring fluoroscopy such as ERCP. The chief modification with regard to endoscopic practice in these patients involves the avoidance, when possible, of certain medications that can be potentially transmitted to a child via breast milk.

Fentanyl, meperidine, midazolam, and propofol are the agents most commonly used for sedation during gastrointestinal endoscopy. These are all, to some extent, excreted in breast milk [12–16]. In general, these agents reach undetectable levels in human breast milk within 4–24 h, with meperidine being detectable in breast milk the longest after administration [1]. There is limited evidence to suggest that at least meperidine, transmitted via breast milk, can affect infant behavior [13,14,17]. The safety of the reversal agents naltrexone and naloxone in lactating women has currently not been described, but these medications should be used clinically if a patient is manifesting signs or symptoms of oversedation during or after endoscopy.

In general, if a lactating patient is to undergo endoscopy with these medications as sedation, breast milk should be stored in advance to be used in the postprocedure period. If this is not an option, or a means of storing breast milk in advance is not available, the patient should switch to formula in the postprocedure period and discard any breast milk obtained during this period—a process referred to as "pump and dump."

Endoscopy in the Elderly

As the population ages, endoscopy in older persons will continue to become more commonplace. Endoscopy in the elderly, who are generally (although not universally) defined as patients over 65 years of age, has been evaluated in a variety of contexts, and the role of specific procedures in these patients varies considerably. As a general rule of thumb, the same indications (and contraindications) for any form of endoscopy should apply to elderly patients.

Preparation for endoscopy in the elderly is generally similar to that performed in younger patients. Upper endoscopy requires the same period of preprocedure fasting, unless the patient has known or suspected gastroparesis, in which case this period can be extended or preceded by a period of dietary restriction (i.e., liquids only) to facilitate gastric emptying [18]. For colonoscopy, either polyethylene glycol or sodium phosphate preparations can be used, although the latter carries an increased risk of electrolyte abnormalities (Na, K, PO_4) and renal dysfunction and should be used with some degree of caution, especially in patients with pre-existing cardiac or renal compromise.

Elderly patients are more likely to have implantable pacemakers and/or cardiac defibrillators, and appropriate care should be exercised when using electrocautery (consultation with cardiologists, proper placement of grounding pads, use of magnets to deactivate implanted devices, etc). It should be noted that there are limited data suggesting that capsule endoscopy does not appear to interfere with implanted cardiac defibrillators [19,20].

Sedation in the elderly should be performed with additional care. Elderly patients tend to have a more impressive and profound response to drugs commonly used for conscious sedation and have an increased risk of cardiovascular depression and aspiration [21,22]. In general, drugs with a shorter half-life, such as fentanyl or propofol, should be used in the elderly when possible, and at reduced doses with a longer titration time between doses [23,24]. If possible, consideration should be given to unsedated endoscopy using ultrathin instruments in patients who are likely to have poor tolerance for sedation.

Esophagogastroduodenoscopy (EGD) is frequently performed in the elderly to investigate symptoms ranging from dyspepsia to melena. Alarm symptoms such as dysphagia, weight loss, or upper gastrointestinal bleeding are more likely to be associated with malignancy in older patients [25,26].

Colonoscopy, performed for a variety of indications, has largely been found to be safe and effective in elderly patients, with a few caveats. Procedure times may be somewhat longer in comparison with younger patients; the rate of terminal ileal intubation may be lower; and a higher incidence of poor bowel preparation has been reported. In addition, there may be a higher rate of incomplete examinations, possibly due to decreased patient tolerance or poor preparation [27–31].

Colonoscopy performed specifically as a screening modality is a powerful tool for detecting adenomatous polyps and reducing the risk of death from colorectal cancer [32]. Most screening colonoscopy guidelines do not address the issue of an upper age limit. However, the role of screening colonoscopy in elderly patients is somewhat complicated, and the issue has been addressed by several authors [33–35]. There are no firm guidelines for deciding at what age individuals should cease to undergo screening colonoscopy. On the one hand, robust seniors with at least 5 years of anticipated future lifespan seem to be reasonable candidates for colorectal cancer screening by colonoscopy. Similarly, frail elderly patients with multiple or significant comorbid conditions are unlikely to be referred for screening colonoscopy, given the difficulties of bowel preparation and the inherent risks of the procedure.

Issues that should be taken into consideration for performing screening colonoscopy in the elderly include consideration of the lead time between the screening examination and any potential benefit, the patient's comorbid medical illnesses (if any), and the presumed life expectancy.

Elderly patients are more likely to experience cerebrovascular accidents or strokes and are thus more likely to be considered for interventional procedures to provide enteral access when swallowing becomes impossible or unsafe, such as percutaneous endoscopic gastrostomy (PEG) or percutaneous endoscopic jejunostomy (PEJ) tubes. These procedures are more often considered and subsequently performed in elderly patients [36,37]. PEG tubes appear to be safe to place in elderly patients, and their placement can be viewed as a relatively low-risk procedure [38]. Gastrostomy tubes may be more frequently associated with upper gastrointestinal bleeding due to severe esophagitis in the elderly, but otherwise appear to have a similar risk–benefit profile in comparison with their use in younger patients [39]. The short-term mortality in these patients tends to be high and related to the underlying disease and overall performance status. It should be emphasized that PEG tubes do not appear to prolong life in most cases. In addition, the placement of a PEG or PEJ tube in an elderly patient comes with a significant burden to their caregivers, who will be called upon to manage the daily operation of the tube and attend to any tube-related problems. The decision on whether or not to place a PEG tube in an elderly patient who has suffered a severe illness or who is not expected to regain significant function remains controversial [40,41].

ERCP has been specifically evaluated, given the increased risk associated with the procedure and its almost exclusively therapeutic nature, combined with the tendency for elderly patients to have more baseline comorbid conditions that could complicate or increase the risk of such procedures. Preprocedure risk assessment in these patients needs to focus not just on the risks of the endoscopy itself, but also on the risk of anesthesia (especially if deep sedation with propofol or general anesthesia is being considered). Consideration should therefore be given to evaluation by an anesthesiologist or cardiologist before an elective procedure is scheduled, to evaluate and maximize the patient's cardiac function.

Köklü et al. evaluated ERCP outcomes in patients aged 70 or over in a prospective trial of 299 patients, 97 of whom were deemed elderly and the remainder of whom were in the control group [42]. The authors reported a decrease in the incidence of benign biliary findings (benign strictures, etc.) and a higher overall incidence of

7

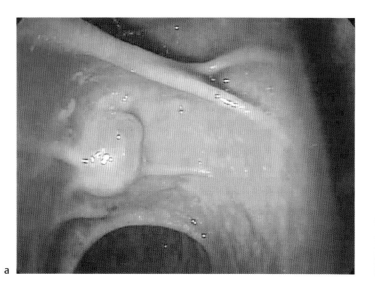

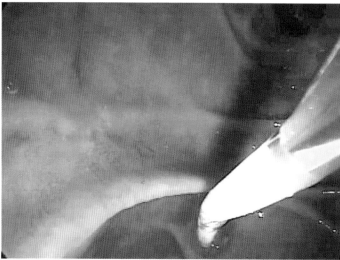

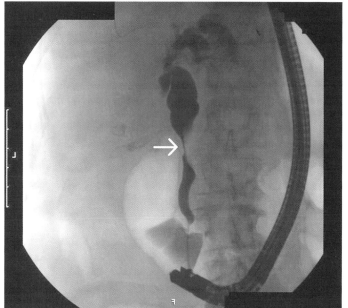

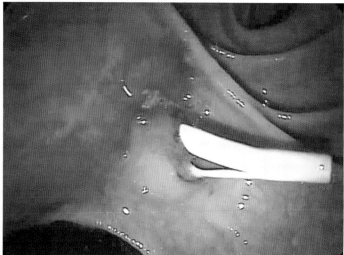

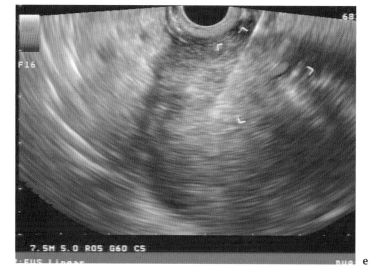

Fig. 7.2 Endoscopic retrograde cholangiopancreatography and endoscopic ultrasonography (EUS) in an elderly patient.

a A 93-year-old woman with a Billroth II gastrectomy was suffering from painless jaundice. The typical Billroth II configuration of the native papilla in the afferent limb should be noted.

b Cannulation with an inverted sphincterotome.

c Cholangiogram, showing a malignant-appearing stricture (arrow).

d After brushings had been obtained from the stricture, a plastic biliary stent was placed for ductal decompression.

e A 7.5-MHz linear EUS examination in the same patient. The echoendoscope has been advanced up the afferent limb to the ampulla, and a large solid pancreatic head mass was seen. Fine-needle aspiration was performed with a 22-gauge needle and revealed a pancreatic adenocarcinoma.

malignancy in patients deemed elderly. There were more complications in the group of patients over the age of 70, although the authors performed precut papillotomy in approximately half of the cases, which could have contributed to this finding.

Several authors have investigated ERCP in patients over the age of 80 [43–45]. Collectively, these studies include 407 patients who underwent ERCP at least once, although several underwent multiple procedures. Complications tended to be more common in elderly patients in comparison with controls, although the difference did not always reach statistical significance. Patients who had a complication were more likely to die from it in comparison with younger patients, especially in the event of perforation or postprocedure cholangitis. Still, the authors considered that ERCP was safe and effective in octogenarians.

With regard to the very elderly (**Fig. 7.2**), two studies have been published regarding ERCP in patients over the age of 90 [46,47].

Collectively including 79 patients, who were mainly women, these studies reported similar outcomes in comparison with control patients with regard to procedure success and complication rates. However, the studies were somewhat less detailed in their reporting and were both retrospective in nature.

In all studies of ERCP elderly patients, the survival period after the procedure was shorter overall, but this may be an artifact of the higher incidence of malignancy in these patients, who were more likely to undergo ERCP for palliation.

Endoscopy in Patients Requiring Anticoagulation or Antiplatelet Medications

Given the widespread use of antiplatelet and anticoagulant medications, endoscopists are frequently called upon to perform a variety of procedures on patients who have an increased risk for bleeding. The risk frequently extends beyond the actual procedure itself and into the postprocedure period, and the timing not only of stopping the medications but also of restarting them needs to be considered.

Not all procedures require modification of anticoagulant or antiplatelet medications. Low-risk procedures that do not include therapeutic or invasive maneuvers can often be performed without any adjustment to the patient's medication regimen. Mucosal biopsies from any location can generally be performed safely using standard biopsy forceps without risk of severe hemorrhage. Procedures such as EGD, colonoscopy, push enteroscopy, endoscopic ultrasonography (EUS) without fine-needle aspiration (FNA), and ERCP without sphincterotomy therefore do not require modification of antiplatelet or anticoagulant regimens. Conversely, procedures of a more invasive nature with an inherent potential for bleeding, such as ERCP with sphincterotomy, EUS with FNA, PEG or PEJ tube placement, or pneumatic/bougie dilation of strictures, etc., do require appropriate cessation of antiplatelet and anticoagulation agents [48].

◼ Management of Antiplatelet Agents

In general and if possible, aspirin and other over-the-counter non-steroidal anti-inflammatory drugs (NSAIDs) should be discontinued 7–10 days before planned endoscopic procedures. The data on the use of aspirin and NSAIDs in certain high-risk procedures are conflicting, and the question of whether or not to stop these agents has yet to be definitively resolved. For example, some have suggested that aspirin increases the risk of post-sphincterotomy bleeding during ERCP, while others have not seen this effect or have noted only clinically insignificant bleeding [49,50]. Many hospitals have created institutional guidelines or policies regarding the use and/or discontinuation of aspirin and NSAIDs before endoscopic procedures. If such guidelines exist, physicians should defer to their institutional policies whenever possible.

Modern antiplatelet agents, such as ticlopidine, clopidogrel, dipyridamole, and the glycoprotein IIb/IIIa inhibiting agents are generally prescribed in patients with more significant or serious underlying cardiovascular conditions. Clopidogrel is routinely used in patients with recent myocardial infarction (MI), stroke, or severe peripheral vascular disease. Dipyridamole is used for the secondary prevention of stroke, and the glycoprotein IIb/IIIa platelet inhibitor agents are often used in acutely ill patients with active angina or MIs.

Patients taking any of these medications who are undergoing low-risk procedures can generally proceed to endoscopy without discontinuing them, although patients on clopidogrel and aspirin should consider taking one agent, preferably aspirin, before endoscopy [48].

Patients with active gastrointestinal bleeding may need to have their medication stopped if the presumed risk of bleeding is greater than the risk of thrombosis. Patients taking antiplatelet agents who experience bleeding while hospitalized for an acute MI are commonly encountered, and modifications to antiplatelet therapy have to be individualized in this group.

Patients receiving ticlopidine and clopidogrel who need to undergo higher-risk endoscopic procedures should discontinue these agents 7–10 days in advance if possible. Data on dipyridamole are largely lacking. Patients requiring glycoprotein IIb/IIIa agents should have these stopped between 4 and 24 h before the procedure, depending on the specific agent, as these are short-acting drugs [48].

◼ Management of Warfarin and Heparins

Warfarin inhibits vitamin K–dependent clotting factors and is routinely used to treat patients with known deep venous thrombosis (DVT) and pulmonary emboli, and in patients at risk for these conditions. In addition, warfarin is frequently used to treat patients with thromboembolic disorders (atrial fibrillation, indwelling mechanical heart valves, etc.) and as prophylaxis in patients with inherited hypercoagulable states and low flow states (peripheral vascular disease), among other conditions. It should be noted that some of these conditions carry a relatively low risk of thromboembolic events (the risk of a thrombosis in a patient with atrial fibrillation is only 5–7 % per year, while the risk in a patient with a mechanical heart valve may be substantially higher) [51,52].

Patients receiving warfarin who plan to undergo low-risk procedures can generally continue to take the medication without interruption. If patients are supratherapeutic with regard to their international normalized ratio (INR), they should be brought into the therapeutic range before the procedure [53].

Patients receiving warfarin who need to undergo high-risk procedures or therapeutic interventions should be evaluated in relation to the inherent risk of their underlying conditions. Patients with low-risk conditions (such as atrial fibrillation) can often simply stop warfarin use 3–7 days before the procedure without the use of intravenous unfractionated heparin or low-molecular-weight heparin (LMWH) and restart the anticoagulation 3–7 days after the procedure, depending on the nature of the therapeutic maneuvers performed.

Patients receiving warfarin who have high-risk conditions (known DVT, ball-cage mechanical heart valve, etc.) who need to undergo high-risk procedures will likely require some form of bridging therapy to provide anticoagulation as close to the time of the procedure as possible. Bridge therapy is most commonly delivered in the form of intravenous unfractionated heparin or LMWH, which is typically administered via subcutaneous injections once or twice a day. Patients can start to receive a heparin agent when they discontinue their warfarin, to provide adequate anticoagulation. Unfractionated heparin should be discontinued approximately 6 h before the procedure, and LMWH should be discontinued approximately 12 h before the procedure [53,54].

With regard to restarting anticoagulation after endoscopic procedures that have included therapeutic maneuvers in which the patients are at increased risk for bleeding (sphincterotomy, endoscopic mucosal resection, etc.), there are no firm guidelines, and treatment must be individualized. The risk of bleeding has to be weighed against the risk of a thromboembolic event on the basis of the patient's personal history and underlying medical conditions. It should be emphasized that in these situations there is often no "right" or "wrong" decision and that the risks of any treatment plan should be discussed with the patient before therapy is instituted. In general, most patients can resume anticoagulation approximately 7 days after high-risk endoscopic interventions, with a relatively low risk for hemorrhage.

Endoscopy in Patients with Hemophilia

Patients with hemophilia represent a small subgroup of patients who may require gastrointestinal endoscopy on either an elective or emergency basis. These patients require appropriate age-related colorectal cancer screening and have an increased risk of developing pigment gallstones and thus choledocholithiasis. They may therefore require ERCP at some time during their lives. The published literature on these patients is scant, although most reports focus on the value of treatment with appropriate clotting factors before and after endoscopy. Biliary sphincterotomy for stone extraction, treatment of bleeding solitary rectal ulcer syndrome, and the treatment of gastrointestinal bleeds using standard devices in combination with clotting factors, have all been reported with good outcomes [55–59].

Restarting Anticoagulation

There are no firm guidelines regarding when to restart anticoagulation after endoscopy. Care needs to be taken to individualize therapy—for example, patients undergoing colonoscopy involving a simple biopsy and/or small polypectomy with cold forceps or cold snares are likely to be able to restart anticoagulation sooner than a patient who has undergone a biliary sphincterotomy with stone extraction. The underlying cardiopulmonary risk of withholding anticoagulation must also be balanced against the risk of gastrointestinal bleeding. For example, a patient with a history of thromboembolic central nervous system events who requires warfarin or a heparin would probably be allowed to restart anticoagulation sooner than a patient with atrial fibrillation after undergoing a biliary sphincterotomy. Consultation with the patient's referring providers is often helpful in deciding when to restart anticoagulants.

Conclusion

Endoscopy in pregnant and lactating women, the elderly, and patients receiving antiplatelet or anticoagulant medications can usually be safely performed. For many of these situations, there are no specific guidelines, or guidelines are based on limited data. Proper preprocedural preparation and consultation is often critical in minimizing complications and adverse outcomes.

References

1. Qureshi WA, Rajan E, Adler DG, Davila RE, Hirota WK, Jacobson BC, et al. ASGE guideline: guidelines for endoscopy in pregnant and lactating women Gastrointest Endosc 2005;61:357–62.
2. Cappell MS, Colon V, Sidhom OA. A study of eight medical centers of the safety and clinical efficacy of esophagogastroduodenoscopy in 83 pregnant females with follow-up of fetal outcome and with comparison to control groups. Am J Gastroenterol 1996;91:348–54.
3. Capell MS, Sidhom O. A multicenter, multiyear study of the safety and clinical utility of esophagogastroduodenoscopy in 20 consecutive pregnant females with follow-up of fetal outcome. Am J Gastroenterol 1993;88:1900–5.
4. Capell MS, Sidhom O. Multicenter, multiyear study of safety and efficacy of flexible sigmoidoscopy during pregnancy in 24 females with follow-up of fetal outcome. Dig Dis Sci 1995;40:472–9.
5. Siddiqui U, Proctor D. Flexible sigmoidoscopy and colonoscopy during pregnancy. Gastrointest Endosc Clin N Am 2006;16:59–69.
6. Tham TC, Vandervoort J, Wong RC, Montes H, Roston AD, Slivka A, et al. Safety of ERCP during pregnancy. Am J Gastroenterol 2003;98:308–11.
7. Tarnasky PR, Simmons DC, Schwartz AG, Macurak RB, Edman CD. Safe delivery of bile duct stones during pregnancy. Am J Gastroenterol 2003;98:2100–1.
8. Simmons DC, Tarnasky PR, Rivera-Alsina ME, Lopez JF, Edman CD. Endoscopic retrograde cholangiopancreatography (ERCP) in pregnancy without the use of radiation. Am J Obstet Gynecol 2004;190:1467–9.
9. Kahaleh M, Hartwell GD, Arseneau KO, Pajewski TN, Mullick T, Isin G, et al. Safety and efficacy of ERCP in pregnancy. Gastrointest Endosc 2004;60:287–92.
10. Gupta R, Tandan M, Lakhtakia S, Santosh D, Rao GV, Reddy DN. Safety of therapeutic ERCP in pregnancy—an Indian experience. Indian J Gastroenterol 2005;24:161–3.
11. Medical radiation exposure of pregnant and potentially pregnant women. NCRP Report no. 54. Washington, DC: National Council on Radiation Protection and Measurements; 1977.
12. Matheson I, Lunde PK, Bredesen JE. Midazolam and nitrazepam in the maternity ward: milk concentrations and clinical effects. Br J Clin Pharmacol 1990;30:787–93.
13. Freeborn SF, Calvert RT, Black P, Macfarlane T, D'Souza SW. Saliva and blood pethidine concentrations in the mother and the newborn baby. Br J Obstet Gynaecol 1980;87:966–9.
14. Wittels B, Scott DT, Sinatra RS. Exogenous opioids in human breast milk and acute neonatal neurobehavior: a preliminary study. Anesthesiology 1990;73:864–9.
15. Steer PL, Biddle CJ, Marley WS, Lantz RK, Sulik PL. Concentration of fentanyl in colostrum after an analgesic dose. Can J Anaesth 1992;39:231–5.
16. Dailland P, Cockshott ID, Lirzin JD, Jacquinot P, Jorrot JC, Devery J, et al. Intravenous propofol during cesarean section: placental transfer, concentrations in breast milk, and neonatal effects. A preliminary study. Anesthesiology 1989;71:827–34.
17. Ito S. Drug therapy for breast-feeding women. N Engl J Med 2000;343:118–26.
18. Faigel DO, Eisen GM, Baron TH, Dominitz JA, Goldstein JL, Hirota WK, et al. Preparation of patients for GI endoscopy. Gastrointest Endosc 2003;57:446–50.
19. Leighton JA, Sharma VK, Srivathsan K, Heigh RI, McWane TL, Post JK, et al. Safety of capsule endoscopy in patients with pacemakers. Gastrointest Endosc 2004;59:567–9.
20. Leighton JA, Srivathsan K, Carey EJ, Sharma VK, Heigh RI, Post JK, et al. Safety of wireless capsule endoscopy in patients with implantable cardiac defibrillators. Am J Gastroenterol 2005;100:1728–31.
21. Shaker R, Ren J, Bardan E, Easterling C, Dua K, Xie P, et al. Pharyngoglottal closure reflex: characterization in healthy young, elderly and dysphagic patients with predeglutitive aspiration. Gerontology 2003;49:12–20.
22. Muravchick S. Anesthesia for the geriatric patient. In: Barash PG, Cullen BF, Stoelting RK, editors. Clinical anesthesia. 4th ed. Philadelphia: Lippincott Williams and Wilkins; 2001; p. 1205–16.
23. Heuss LT, Schnieper P, Drewe J, Pflimlin E, Beglinger C. Conscious sedation with propofol in elderly patients: a prospective evaluation. Aliment Pharmacol Ther 2003;17:1493–501.
24. Darling E. Practical considerations in sedating the elderly. Crit Care Nurs Clin N Am 1997;9:371–80.
25. Salo M, Collin P, Kyrönpalo S, Rasmussen M, Huhtala H, Kaukinen K. Age, symptoms and upper gastrointestinal malignancy in primary care endoscopy. Scand J Gastroenterol 2008;43:122–7.
26. Liou JM, Lin JT, Wang HP, Huang SP, Lee YC, Shun CT, et al. The optimal age threshold for screening upper endoscopy for uninvestigated dyspepsia in Taiwan, an area with a higher prevalence of gastric cancer in young adults. Gastrointest Endosc 2005;61:819–25.
27. Sardinha TC, Nogueras JJ, Ehrenpreis ED, Zeitman D, Estevez V, Weiss EG, et al. Colonoscopy in octogenarians: a review of 428 cases. Int J Colorectal Dis 1999;14:172–6.
28. Arora A, Singh P. Colonoscopy in patients 80 years of age and older is safe, with high success rate and diagnostic yield. Gastrointest Endosc 2004;60:408–13.
29. Chatrenet P, Friocourt P, Ramain JP, Cherrier M, Maillard JB. Colonoscopy in the elderly: a study of 200 cases. Eur J Med 1993;2:411–3.
30. Ure T, Dehghan K, Vernava AM 3rd, Longo WE, Andrus CA, Daniel GL. Colonoscopy in the elderly. Low risk, high yield. Surg Endosc 1995;9:505–8.
31. Duncan JE, Sweeney WB, Trudel JL, Madoff RD, Mellgren AF. Colonoscopy in the elderly: low risk, low yield in asymptomatic patients. Dis Colon Rectum 2006;49:646–51.

32. Lieberman DA, Weiss DG, Bond JH, Ahnen DJ, Garewal H, Chejfec G. Use of colonoscopy to screen asymptomatic adults for colorectal cancer. Veterans Affairs Cooperative Study Group 380. N Engl J Med 2000;343:162–8.

33. Kahi CJ, Azzouz F, Juliar BE, Imperiale TF. Survival of elderly persons undergoing colonoscopy: implications for colorectal cancer screening and surveillance. Gastrointest Endosc 2007;66:544–50.

34. Ko CW, Sonnenberg A. Comparing risks and benefits of colorectal cancer screening in elderly patients. Gastroenterology 2005;129:1163–70.

35. Miller K, Waye JD. Colorectal polyps in the elderly: what should be done? Drugs Aging 2002;19:393–404.

36. Piccinni G, Angrisano A, Testini M, Merlicco D, Nacchiero M. Venting direct percutaneous jejunostomy (DPEJ) for drainage of malignant bowel obstruction in patients operated on for gastric cancer. Support Care Cancer 2005;13:535–9.

37. Phillips TE, Cornejo CJ, Hoffer EK, McCormick WC. Gastrostomy and jejunostomy placement: the urban hospital perspective pertinent to nursing home care. J Am Med Dir Assoc 2005;6:390–5.

38. Callahan CM, Haag KM, Weinberger M, Tierney WM, Buchanan NN, Stump TE, et al. Outcomes of percutaneous endoscopic gastrostomy among older adults in a community setting. J Am Geriatr Soc 2000;48:1048–54.

39. Dharmarajan TS, Yadav D, Adiga GU, Kokkat A, Pitchumoni CS. Gastrostomy, esophagitis, and gastrointestinal bleeding in older adults. J Am Med Dir Assoc 2004;5:228–32.

40. Cervo FA, Bryan L, Farber S. To PEG or not to PEG: a review of evidence for placing feeding tubes in advanced dementia and the decision-making process. Geriatrics 2006;61:30–5.

41. Arvanitakis M, Ballarin A, Van Gossum A. Ethical aspects of percutaneous endoscopic gastrostomy placement for artificial nutrition and hydration. Acta Gastroenterol Belg 2006;69:317–20.

42. Köklü S, Parlak E, Yüksel O, Sahin B. Endoscopic retrograde cholangiopancreatography in the elderly: a prospective and comparative study. Age Ageing 2005;34:572–7.

43. Ashton CE, McNabb WR, Wilkinson ML, Lewis RR. Endoscopic retrograde cholangiopancreatography in elderly patients. Age Ageing 1998;27:683–8.

44. Fritz E, Kirchgatterer A, Hubner D, Aschl G, Hinterreiter M, Stadler B, et al. ERCP is safe and effective in patients 80 years of age and older compared with younger patients. Gastrointest Endosc 2006;64:899–905.

45. Thomopoulos KC, Vagenas K, Assimakopoulos SF, Giannikoulis C, Arvaniti V, Pagoni N, et al. Endoscopic retrograde cholangiopancreatography is safe and effective method for diagnosis and treatment of biliary and pancreatic disorders in octogenarians. Acta Gastroenterol Belg 2007;70:199–202.

46. Mitchell RM, O'Connor F, Dickey W. Endoscopic retrograde cholangiopancreatography is safe and effective in patients 90 years of age and older. J Clin Gastroenterol 2003;36:72–4.

47. Katsinelos P, Paroutoglou G, Kountouras J, Zavos C, Beltsis A, Tzovaras G. Efficacy and safety of therapeutic ERCP in patients 90 years of age and older. Gastrointest Endosc 2006;63:417–23.

48. Zuckerman MJ, Hirota WK, Adler DG, Davila RE, Jacobson BC, Leighton JA, et al. DOASGE guideline: the management of low-molecular-weight heparin and nonaspirin antiplatelet agents for endoscopic procedures. Gastrointest Endosc 2005;61:189–94.

49. Hui CK, Lai KC, Yuen MF, Wong WM, Lam SK, Lai CL. Does withholding aspirin for one week reduce the risk of post-sphincterotomy bleeding? Aliment Pharmacol Ther 2002;16:929–36.

50. Hussain N, Alsulaiman R, Burtin P, Toubouti Y, Rahme E, Boivin JF, et al. The safety of endoscopic sphincterotomy in patients receiving antiplatelet agents: a case–control study. Aliment Pharmacol Ther 2007;25:579–84.

51. Laupacis A, Albers G, Dunn M, Feinberg W. Antithrombotic therapy in atrial fibrillation. Chest 1992;102(4 Suppl):426S–433 S.

52. Cannegieter SC, Rosendaal FR, Wintzen AR, van der Meer FJ, Vandenbroucke JP, Briet E. Optimal oral anticoagulant therapy in patients with mechanical heart valves. N Engl J Med 1994;333:11–7.

53. Eisen GM, Baron TH, Dominitz JA, Faigel DO, Goldstein JL, Johanson JF, et al. Guidelines on the management of anticoagulation and antiplatelet therapy for endoscopic procedures. Gastrointest Endosc 2002;55:775–9.

54. Constans M, Santamaria A, Mateo J, Pujol N, Souto JC, Fontcuberta J. Low-molecular-weight heparin as bridging therapy during interruption of oral anticoagulation in patients undergoing colonoscopy or gastroscopy. Int J Clin Pract 2007;61:212–7.

55. Katsinelos P, Pilpilidis I, Paroutoglou G, Tsolkas P, Galanis I, Giouleme O, et al. Endoscopic sphincterotomy in adult hemophiliac patients with choledocholithiasis. Gastrointest Endosc 2003;58:788–91.

56. Bishop PR, Nowicki MJ, Subramony C, Parker PH. Solitary rectal ulcer: a rare cause of gastrointestinal bleeding in an adolescent with hemophilia A. J Clin Gastroenterol 2001;33:72–6.

57. Yamada M, Fukuda Y, Koyama Y, Nakano I, Urano F, Katano Y, et al. Prophylactic endoscopic ligation of high-risk oesophageal varices in a cirrhotic patient with severe haemophilia A. Eur J Gastroenterol Hepatol 1998;10:151–3.

58. Kadayifci A, Simsek H. Epinephrine injection therapy for peptic ulcer bleeding in hemophilia patients. Eur J Haematol 1996;56:321–2.

59. Mittal R, Spero JA, Lewis JH, Taylor F, Ragni MV, Bontempo FA, et al. Patterns of gastrointestinal hemorrhage in hemophilia. Gastroenterology 1985;88:515–22.

7

8 The Endoscopy Suite

Hans-Dieter Allescher

Endoscopic techniques are developing rapidly, and new techniques and combinations with other diagnostic modalities are becoming more and more important and clinically relevant. These changing demands in relation to technical equipment and combination with information technology need to be taken into account when planning and designing a new endoscopy suite. Earlier guidelines can only partly be adapted to these changes, and new demands on imaging flexibility and connectivity need to be met. In general, the space and facilities required in endoscopy units depend on the range and numbers of procedures carried out. In addition, it is important to establish beforehand which endoscopic techniques may be performed or introduced in the future. If necessary, the facilities should be sufficiently versatile and flexible to allow emergency cases to be handled without disrupting routine procedures.

There are a few general questions and considerations that should be answered on a check-list before the planning and building of an endoscopy suite is started.

General Questions and Considerations

- What purpose is the endoscopy suite used for?
  - Only elective/planned procedures?
  - Only outpatients, or also bedridden patients?
  - Estimated number of procedures and procedure types per day?
  - Number and frequency of complex procedures (e.g., endoscopic submucosal dissection, double-balloon endoscopy)
  - What types of therapeutic and invasive procedure are performed?
- How is sedation performed in the endoscopic suite?
  - Percentage of procedures with sedation?
  - What type of sedation is used, and how are the patients monitored during and after the procedure?
  - Need for and frequency of general anesthesia?
  - How is general anesthesia performed?
- What types of complex procedure are performed?
  - Frequency of radiography and radiological requirements?
  - Need for navigated work or procedures?
  - Need for combined imaging (e.g., endoscopic ultrasonography plus radiology)?
  - Are there plans for natural orifice transluminal endoscopic surgery (NOTES) procedures?
  - Are other procedures and tests (manometry, capsule endoscopy, function tests) performed in the unit?
- What type of hygiene approach is planned?
  - Processing of endoscopes within the unit or in central facility?
  - Reuse of materials or single use?
  - What type of room plan (ceiling supplies or trolleys) is envisaged?
- What are the flow routes for materials, patients, doctors, and nurses?
  - What is the most effective route for patients from admission to the end of recovery?
  - Which pathway is most effective for nurses and endoscopes?
  - How can the time and movement of the doctors be optimized?
  - How and when is the endoscopic report generated and given/explained to the patient?

Guidelines for Planning an Endoscopy Suite

The room plan for an endoscopic suite is influenced by many factors [1–8]. If the endoscopy suite is being planned from scratch or established in a new building, an ideal room plan can be achieved. However, if the unit is being incorporated into an existing building, a compromise between requirements and technical feasibility has to be reached. The number of endoscopy suites depends on several factors, such as the estimated number of endoscopic procedures and their breakdown by type, complexity, and the need for fluoroscopy or radiography. Exact updated numbers and a development plan for future years should be made available for planning, as these statistics are often outdated [1].

In addition, transport and waiting times, as well as the management of patients outside of the procedure rooms is relevant. Particularly when patients are receiving sedation, clearly defined and structured monitoring of the patients is mandatory and sufficient space, monitors, and staff have to be considered. Some units have individual rooms for each patient in which the patients are assessed, undress, recover, dress, and are reviewed before discharge. In some countries, the requirements for postprocedural recovery are clearly regulated and should be taken into account during planning [9]. If space for the recovery rooms is limited, or if several patients share a room, there should be one or two interview rooms available for consultation after the procedure (**Figs. 8.1, 8.2**).

Pathways for Patients, Staff and Materials

When a new unit is being planned, it is advisable first of all to plan the routes that will be taken by individual patients (inpatients and outpatients), materials and endoscopes, and doctors and nursing staff first. Where does the patient (outpatient or bedridden) enter the endoscopy unit? Where do preparation, changing, and interview take place? How and where does the patient leave the unit? If possible, preparation and recovery should take place separately from the procedure rooms, as this increases the unit's flexibility and productivity. On the other hand, separate recovery areas require more staff and space. In addition, it is advisable to separate patients who are waiting for procedures from those who are recovering. The numbers and timing of outpatient procedures without sedation also have to be estimated, as these patients require less infrastructure and nearby changing rooms, possibly with direct access to the procedure room.

For endoscopy physicians, it is important to define the endoscopic workflow beforehand. Who will be performing sedation (specialized staff, an anesthetist, or a second doctor)? When and how is report-writing carried out? Will a report be given to the patient immediately before he or she leaves the unit, or will it be finalized in a second step? Routes (location for computer-based generation, printout, and signing of the report) have to be developed depending on the answers to these questions. Similar path-

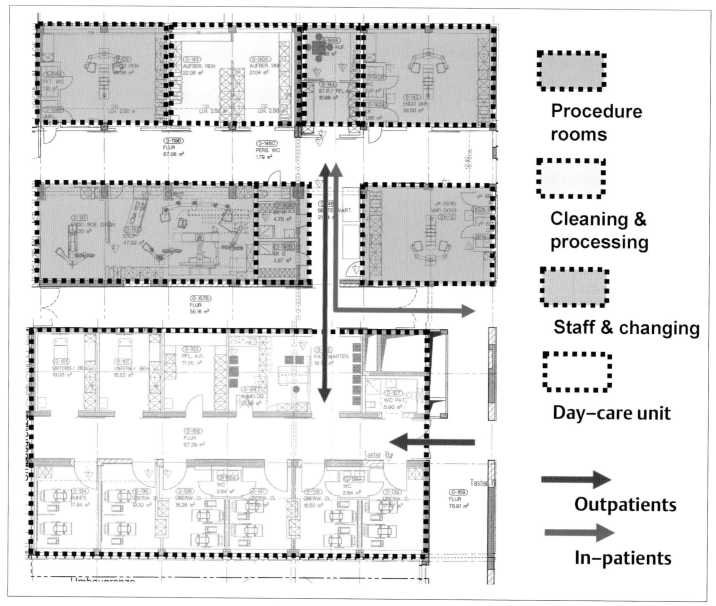

Fig. 8.1 A possible general plan for an endoscopy unit with an adjacent day-care unit. It is important to visualize routes for patients, doctors, and staff in order to optimize the workflow.

ways should be defined for materials, including endoscopes, and endoscopic staff. Close proximity between the procedure rooms and the cleaning and disinfection area is desirable. In this context, it is important to define how used endoscopes are to be transported back to the unclean area of the cleaning facilities and how clean endoscopes are to be transported back to the procedure room. In many modern endoscopy units, a special closed trolley system with cleaning solution is used for this purpose.

Location of the Unit

The strategic location of the unit is crucial and should be based on the number of in-patient and/or outpatient procedures. If the majority of endoscopic examinations are outpatient procedures, a location next to the outpatient department or day-care unit is desirable (**Figs. 8.1, 8.2**), unless day-care facilities are fully provided for within the unit itself [1,10]. The majority of patients will walk into the unit, but a significant minority will arrive in wheelchairs or trolleys, or even on beds. A suitable reception area is therefore desirable, as well as an area for patients to await endoscopy on

trolleys, on which they will be transported into the endoscopy room. Changing facilities in or near this waiting area must be provided. The waiting area can also serve as the recovery area to which patients are wheeled after endoscopy, although it is advisable to have separate waiting and recovery areas. Waiting and recovery areas must also be provided with toilet facilities. After full recovery, ambulant patients should await discharge in the reception area, which can also be used by waiting relatives and friends. Waiting-room space can be calculated on the basis of eight chairs for each endoscopy procedure room. This is based on two or three seats for the waiting patient and family members, and two each for family members of the two patients in recovery and the patient undergoing the procedure.

If outpatients and in-patients are to be treated simultaneously, separate patient flow pathways for ambulant patients and those confined to bed should be aimed for, and these should certainly be available if pediatric gastrointestinal care is given (**Fig. 8.1**). There should be an interview room in which the details of the procedure can be discussed in privacy with the patients and/or their relatives, as appropriate, before the endoscopy and where the results of the

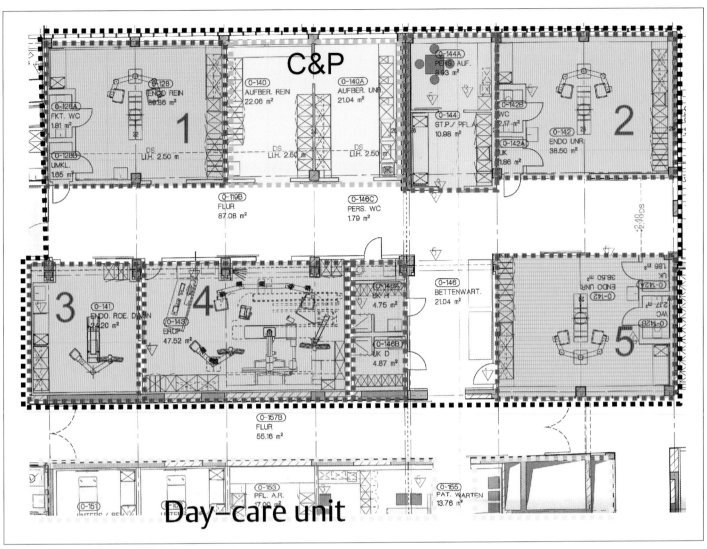

Fig. 8.2 Plan of the endoscopic suite in more detail, showing the procedure rooms (pink), the area for endoscope cleaning and processing (green), and the staff areas (blue).

examination and further arrangements can be discussed afterwards.

Number of Rooms

In general, upper and lower gastrointestinal tract endoscopy are separated, so that a minimum of two endoscopy rooms is required even for a small unit. For larger units, approximately one endoscopy room per 1000 examinations (diagnostic and low-level therapeutic) annually is a rough estimate for capacity planning. The British Society of Gastroenterology recommends a minimum of two plus one endoscopy rooms for 3000 endoscopies per year [10,11].

In larger units, the concept should also include a radiography unit and a multipurpose room for various procedures such as laser therapy, endoscopic ultrasonography, and emergencies [2]. The handling of emergencies has to be standardized and separated into cases suitable for the endoscopy unit and cases in which the patients should be treated in the intensive-care unit. If many emergency patients are seen, it is important to have at least one additional room for flexibility in dealing with emergencies and extra work without interrupting the routine list [10].

With the further development of additional tests such as capsule endoscopy, a further additional room for nonendoscopic gastrointestinal tests and function tests and for reviewing capsule endo-

scopy should be planned. In larger units or specialized centers performing 6000 procedures (the "four plus two" room model), a dedicated room for endoscopic ultrasonography, laser therapy, and photodynamic therapy should also be present.

Therapeutic endoscopic procedures are increasingly time-consuming and result in lower productivity per room. Newer techniques such as endoscopic submucosal dissection (ESD) and double-balloon endoscopy in particular have long procedure times and learning curves, which should be taken into account.

The amount of teaching taking place in the endoscopy unit has also a considerable impact on procedure performance time and can amount to as much as an additional 30% of time per procedure.

In addition, the plan for report generation has to be taken into account (see below). If the report is generated immediately after the procedure using a computer-based documentation system, the time can be used for switching patients and cleaning of the room. This would allow a single endoscopist to work continuously in one room. However, a system in which the endoscopist switches rooms between procedures is often used. This increases the individual endoscopist's productivity, but report writing and documentation may be less accurate. Capacity planning is important, and all calculations for procedure-room capacity have to incorporate a realistic period (e.g., 10–15 min) for cleaning and setting up the room for the next procedure [12,13]. However, capacity and productivity planning are often substantially affected by waiting times, in-house transportation, and recovery facilities. Room productivity is greatly reduced if patients have to remain in the procedure room for any length of time because of a lack of recovery facilities. An easy accessible recovery area thus increases the productivity of the endoscopy suite. The productivity of a procedure room is also influenced be the availability of instruments (endoscopes) and the cleaning preparation cycles.

Radiographic Requirements

Several therapeutic endoscopic interventions in addition to endoscopic retrograde cholangiopancreatography (ERCP) and percutaneous transhepatic cholangiographic drainage (PTCD), such as dilation, placement of stents and probes, and double-balloon endoscopy require radiographic control or guidance. If a unit requires more than 200–500 radiographic examinations per year, then its own radiography room is desirable. In this case, either the third room in the "two plus one" model should have such facilities, or they should be available in a separate room. If the radiography facilities are shared with other departments, there is a considerable loss of effective procedure time for setting up the room with the endoscopic equipment. In addition, the sensitive equipment has to be moved constantly, which reduces its lifespan and also has a negative effect on the safety and reliability of endoscope installation.

In most modern hospitals, a picture archiving and communication system (PACS) with central storage is available that allows digital archiving and distribution of radiographs. If this is not available, a film-processing area must be provided near the procedure room. As PACS provides digital radiographs, high-quality monitors for displaying the digital images have to be included in the plans for the various procedure rooms.

The Endoscopic Examination Room

Size of the Rooms

A central problem and point of discussion is the minimum size of an endoscopy room. A general or multipurpose endoscopy room, primarily intended for gastrointestinal endoscopy, should have a floor surface area of not less than 35 m² (Fig. 8.3). There should be at least two entrances, preferably one with double swinging doors to allow for the movement of trolleys and beds, and the other(s) connecting with the preparation, cleaning, and storage facilities, etc. The width of the entrance and corridors should be sufficient to allow for the transportation of beds, stretchers, and wheelchairs. It must be possible to turn beds round in the corridor. The standard door width should be 1.28 m, and the opening should have sliding doors. An "engaged" or "in use" sign as well as signs for "laser" or "x-ray" should be present on the entrance doors to endoscopy rooms, where appropriate.

Requirements for adequate working space have also been described by the British Society of Gastroenterology [11]. A room measuring 25–30 m² is considered adequate if there is sufficient storage space outside the room for endoscopes and ultrasound and laser equipment. A two-monitor television system is important in order to provide an unobstructed view of the screen for the endoscopist, gastrointestinal assistants, and fellows. The endoscopy room based on these requirements would be approximately 6.25 × 4.75 m or 30 m² in size [4]. Space must also be available to accommodate the expansion of endoscopy procedures and changes in technology. For emergency therapeutic endoscopy, the third room in the "two plus one" model should be calculated to include space for resuscitation equipment (30–35 m²).

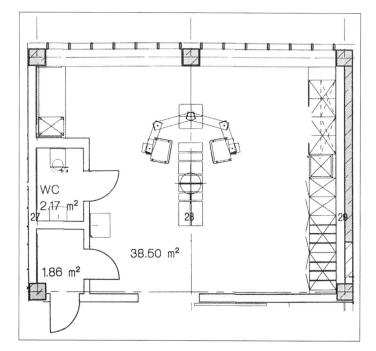

Fig. 8.3 Plan of a procedure room in more detail. The area of the room is 38.5 m². Facilities include a ceiling supply unit with a two-monitor system, fitted cupboards (right side), a computer documentation area (upper left corner), changing room, and toilet (WC).

Equipment

The endoscopy room should contain a mobile examination table with adjustable height and positioning (e. g., for placing the patient in the reverse Trendelenburg or Trendelenburg position), a desk and chair, a radiograph viewing facility, a work surface with a double sink and cupboards, a slop sink, and two television monitors, optionally with a closed-circuit connection to other endoscopy rooms. Storage space for accessories should be available in the endoscopy room or in an adjacent storage area. The accessories include instruments for polypectomy, coagulation, and photography, and video, laser, and ultrasound equipment [14].

There should be fitted cupboards for endoscopes and ancillary equipment and washing facilities for staff and equipment. The procedure rooms should be equipped with wall-mounted radiography viewing screens and/or with high-quality video screens for viewing of digital images. The floor must be easy to clean and must conform to anesthetic and high-frequency electric requirements. In addition, there should be waste containers, wheeled chairs for endoscopists and assistants, and other miscellaneous equipment.

It is essential to have piped oxygen gas and suction facilities, as well as pressured air. As CO_2 endoscopy will be performed more frequently, especially in longer endoscopy procedures and during interventional procedures, piped CO_2 could also be considered, with sockets close to the endoscopic processor. The positioning of the terminals for piped oxygen and suction has to be well planned, as the lines to the patient or the endoscope should not cross the working area or the floor. Suction should thus be close to the endoscopic processor and oxygen could be close to the patient's head for pulse oximetry. There should be plenty of electric sockets, either wall-mounted or attached to the ceiling supply units. The electric sockets should be connected to various circuits, and one group of sockets—which should be used for the endoscopic light source and video processor, as well as the surveillance monitors—should have an uninterrupted emergency power supply.

Especially in the endoscopy room, ventilation and temperature control must be optimal. If there are outside windows, blinds or blackout facilities are needed. Ceiling lighting should be bright, but easily dimmed. There is a new trend to use colored lights such as blue or green light for procedure rooms, as blue light should increase the contrast and facilitates viewing of the monitor image while still providing enough surrounding light for handling and controlling the patient. There are new approaches in which the various functions of the endoscopic procedure room (room light, video recording, picture documentation, video switching and video streaming, video sources for the monitor, communications) can be handled using a touch screen–based device. There are several commercial systems available that offer this type of functionality as a complete room service package (e. g., Endo-Alpha by Olympus, OR1 by Storz). Other optional features such as writing surfaces and dictation facilities depend on the method of report generation selected (see below).

Monitor Systems and Anesthesia

Surveillance monitors should be present in each procedure room for supervision of patients during the procedure as well as during the recovery period. The monitor display should be positioned in such a way that it can be easily viewed and controlled. The monitor system should include noninvasive blood-pressure measurement, pulse oximetry, and electrocardiography. The monitor should also be positioned to take into account the fact that cables and lines connecting to the patients should not cross the endoscopist's working area. Positioning the monitor system opposite the endoscopist, near the video monitor, is a possible solution that avoids these problems (**Fig. 8.4**). The suction equipment can either be free-standing or placed on a trolley, or incorporated into a ceiling supply unit (**Fig. 8.4**).

In addition, resuscitation equipment should be available in the unit. A resuscitation trolley should be in the endoscopy room or easily available. In some units, it has been found convenient to place markers on the floor so that mobile equipment is placed correctly.

As general anesthesia has changed mostly to intravenous anesthesia, the installation requirements for general anesthesia have decreased. However, the anesthesiologist's needs should be taken into account during initial planning. There should be anesthesiology trolleys or equipment and infrastructure—pressure air and oxygen sockets, as well as information technology (IT) connections—to accommodate the anesthetist's needs. Preferably, the radiography room should be equipped with such facilities.

Video Integration and Computer-Based Documentation

Endoscopy almost exclusively consists of video endoscopy. In most units, closed-circuit color televisions are used, and video recording is mostly carried out with analogue recording equipment (SVHS video recording, CD or DVD recorders). However, new imaging qualities are dependent on the high-definition video standard (Full HD), and digital techniques and video streaming are increasingly being used even in the procedure rooms. Video recording is mostly digital and is either computer-based or carried out centrally via a video streaming system. Alternatively, videos can be stored directly in endoscopic documentation systems.

Computer-based documentation of endoscopic procedures is becoming more and more important. A specialized area for computer documentation in the procedure room therefore has to be planned. This area should be located outside either the sterile or contaminated procedure areas, but should be close enough for checking or consultation of written or computer-documented in-

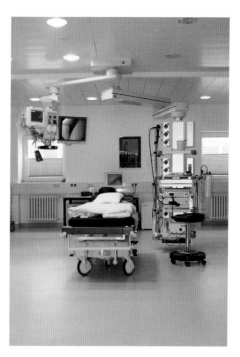

Fig. 8.4 An example of an endoscopic room for upper gastrointestinal endoscopy, with optimized positioning of video monitors and surveillance monitors.

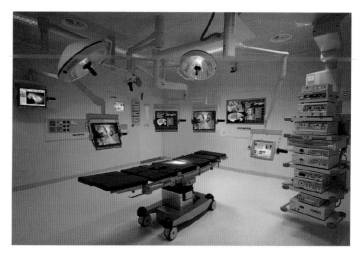

Fig. 8.5 A high-tech interventional endoscopic procedure room with an integrated platform solution (Olympus EndoAlpha). (Reproduced with permission of Olympus Europe, Germany.)

formation. In the radiographic procedure room, this documentation area must be located outside the radiation area.

Various commercial endoscopic documentation systems with integrated report generation are available. As endoscopic terminology has been widely standardized, standardized reports can be generated with these systems. Integrated systems will also allow video streaming and video switching (**Fig. 8.5**). To integrate additional equipment, additional video inputs and video lines have to be planned and installed. It is advisable to have a separate video planning concept for a new unit. In most larger units, it is advisable to centralize video information to a central video switchboard, which allows central video streaming or storage. Most integrated systems (EndoAlpha, OR1) are based on this type of approach (**Fig. 8.5**).

Endoscopes and Endoscopic Equipment

Sufficient endoscopes must be available for the endoscopist to continue with the next patient while the endoscope used in the previous patient is being disinfected. Sufficient power outlets are necessary to ensure flexible working conditions. Some power outlets should also be connected to the hospital's emergency energy supply. The compressed air supply, intravenous fluid hooks, suction lines, and connections for closed-circuit television should preferably be fixed to the ceiling to prevent cables from crossing the floor. Cubicles, or at least curtained-off partitions and washing facilities, should be available for patients who have undergone sigmoidoscopy or colonoscopy.

In addition to the equipment in the procedure room itself, a mobile endoscopy trolley carrying all essential instruments should always be on standby, as occasionally an endoscopy has to be carried out in other parts of the hospital, such as the intensive-care unit or the surgical or radiological department.

Endoscopic Ultrasound and Laser Treatment Room, Radiography Room

Large endoscopy units, from the so-called "four plus two" room model and upwards, should have a dedicated room for endoscopic ultrasonography, laser, or photodynamic therapy. As these procedures tend to be slower, they should not interfere with general routine endoscopic activities. Radiographic facilities should be available when required during ERCP, dilation procedures, insertion of stents, etc. Such facilities avoid the inconvenience and waste of time involved in transporting patients and fragile equipment to and from the radiography department. An alternative for smaller endoscopy units is to modify one of the rooms in the radiography department to accommodate endoscopy.

The choice of radiography system should take the endoscopist's special needs into account. In most modern units, a C-arm system with flexible x-ray planes is used. Digital radiography is strongly preferable in comparison with older analogue machines. A solid-phase x-ray detector is a new radiographic standard with fewer movement artifacts, which is helpful especially in ERCP and PTCD interventions.

The radiographic procedure room is often used with additional imaging modalities such as endosonography or cholangiography. The display capacity in this room therefore has to be planned for versatile and flexible working (see below). A "two and two" or "three and two" monitor system is recommended, with flexible inputs to the various monitors—e. g., using a special switching device. The radiography monitor and the video-endoscopic monitor should be mounted together and positioned in such a way that the endoscopist and assistant personnel have direct, unobstructed views. The main monitor system preferably consists of one radiographic and one endoscopic monitor, while the third monitor should be used for reference (radiography) or additional imaging modalities (endoscopic ultrasonography, cholangiography, mother–baby endoscopy). The second monitor system for the assistant staff should consist of one radiography and one endoscopy monitor.

The radiographic room should have enough space for an x-ray protection system and should be especially equipped for procedures performed with the patient under general anesthesia.

Preparation and Recovery Room

Preparation and recovery rooms should be located close to the endoscopy unit. In general, three beds per endoscopy room are required [4,5]. Seven square meters per bed is standard. The use of sedatives such as midazolam and/or propofol during upper or lower tract endoscopy requires recovery facilities (with nursing supervision), as it may be up two hours before these patients are able to leave the endoscopy unit. An insufficient number of recovery beds will invariably lead to stagnation. Oxygen and suction devices are essential in addition to pulse oximeters, electrocardiography monitoring, and resuscitation equipment.

Cleaning and Disinfection Area

A central cleaning and disinfection area must be provided adjacent to the endoscopy rooms. There are two different concepts for the cleaning area. In one, the cleaning area is accessible directly from the procedure room. This is only practicable in smaller units. In larger units, the cleaning area should be centrally located and separated into an unclean und clean area, preferably with a one-way system for endoscope transport and processing. This avoids possible contamination of the endoscope. The cleaning of the endoscopes should be carried out by fully automated washing and disinfection machines.

Basically, the area should contain stainless-steel work surfaces, with a double sink and an ultrasound bath for initial cleaning. There should be 1.5 m on either side of the sink to position the endoscopes. There should be enough room for brushing, ultrasonic cleaner, tightness control, and a compressed-air system for mechanical cleaning. The volume of disinfection equipment and washing machines required depends on the number of examinations, the time planned per examination, and the time needed to clean, disinfect, and dry the endoscope. Vapors from disinfectants need to be removed via a powerful ventilation system, to exclude the possibility of toxic or allergenic vapors being inhaled. There should be separate containers for waste, dirty linen, etc. There should be at least one slop sink.

Staffing

Assisting with gastrointestinal endoscopy is a task for fully trained professional nurses [15,16]. Nursing staff carry a major responsibility for patient safety. In some countries, nursing staff can be trained and specialized for administration of sedative and surveillance of the patient during the endoscopic procedure [9]. There must be one properly trained nurse assistant in each procedure room, and two for any complex procedures such as ERCP and sophisticated therapy. One head nurse should be in charge of the unit for the day, and at least one other handling the recovery area. Lower-level staff can be trained to perform cleaning and disinfection effectively and to assist with recovery duties. However, the procedure-related nurses should maintain their skills in handling these functions and may occasionally rotate through these areas. As emergency procedures performed out of hours are often the most difficult and dangerous ones, it is essential to have gastrointestinal nursing staff on 24-h call. This will also ensure a more consistent approach to cleaning and disinfection of endoscopic equipment for patient safety. The extent to which the nurse manager is involved in actual procedures will depend on the size of the unit. In a department with four or five procedure rooms, the nurse manager should allocate at least half of his or her time for office and managerial activities. The amount of secretarial assistance will depend on the methods used for scheduling and reporting. An appropriate technician must be available if radiography equipment is in use—not only to assist with the procedures, but also to help in maintaining and monitoring radiation safety standards.

References

1. Mulder CJJ. The endoscopy unit. In: Tytgat GNJ, Mulder CJJ, editors. Procedures in hepatogastroenterology. 2nd ed. Dordrecht: Kluwer Academic; 1997. p. 345–53.

2. Mulder CJJ, Tan AC, Huibregtse K. Guidelines for designing an endoscopy unit: report of the Dutch Society of Gastroenterologists. Endoscopy 1997;29:i–vi.

3. Phillip J, Allescher HD, Hohner R, editors. Endoskopie: Struktur und Ökonomie; Planung, Einrichtung und Organisation einer Endoskopieeinheit. Bad Homburg/Englewood, NJ: Normed-Verlag, 1998.

4. Waye JD, Rich ME. Planning an endoscopy suite for office and hospital. New York: Igaku-Shoin Medical, 1990.

5. Burton D, Ott BJ, Gostout CJ, DiMagno EP. Approach to designing a gastrointestinal endoscopy unit. Gastrointest Endosc Clin N Am 1993;3:525–40.

6. Sivak MV, Senick JM. The endoscopy unit. In: Sivak MV, editor. Gastroenterologic endoscopy. Philadelphia: Saunders; 1987. p. 42–66.

7. Marasco JA, Marasco RF. Designing the ambulatory endoscopy center. Gastrointest Endosc Clin N Am 2002;12:185–204.

8. Seifert E, Weismüller J. How to run an endoscopy unit? Experience in the Federal Republic of Germany. Results of a survey of 31 centers. Endoscopy 1986;18:20–4.

9. Riphaus A, Wehrmann T, Weber B, Arnold J, Beilenhoff U, Bitter H, et al. [S 3-guidelines—sedation in gastrointestinal endoscopy]. Z Gastroenterol 2008;46:1298–330. German.

10. [No authors listed.] Provision of gastrointestinal endoscopy and related services for a district general hospital: Working Party of the Clinical Services Committee of the British Society of Gastroenterology. Gut 1991;32:95–105.

11. Lennard-Jones JE, Williams CB, Axon A. Provision of gastrointestinal endoscopy and related services for a district general hospital: report of the British Society of Gastroenterology. London: British Society of Gastroenterology; 1990.

12. Staritz M, Alkier R, Krzoska B, Holzer R, Grosse A. Zeitbedarf für endoskopische Diagnostik und Therapie: Ergebnisse einer Multicenterstudie. Z Gastroenterol 1992;30:505–18.

13. Phillip J, Sahl RJ, Ruus P, Rösch T, Classen M. Zeitaufwand für endoskopische Untersuchungen. Z Gastroenterol 1990;28:1–9.

14. Marmarinou J. The autonomous endoscopy unit: designing it for maximum efficiency. AORN J 1990;51:764–73.

15. Axon ATR. Staffing of endoscopy units. Acta Endosc 1989;19:213–6.

16. Lennard-Jones JE, Slade GE. Report of a working party on the staffing of endoscopy units. Gut 1987;29:1682–5.

8

9 Cleaning and Disinfection in Endoscopy

Michael Jung and Thierry Ponchon

Flexible endoscopes are complex instruments with narrow channels partly connected to each other via branches (**Fig. 9.1**). Mechanical devices such as biopsy ports and Albaran levers, as well as valves and caps, are also sometimes critical components during reprocessing.

When they have been used for a prolonged period, the narrow-lumen channels of the endoscope develop irregular inner surfaces and grooves, caused by the introduction of accessories such as biopsy forceps. These grooves can be colonized by bacteria. There are no procedures that can provide definite information about the surface characteristics of the channels. Endoscopes are also heat-sensitive, so that reprocessing procedures need to take the integrity of the instruments into account. High standards therefore have to be met to allow reprocessing and reuse of endoscopes and endoscopic accessories (e. g., biopsy forceps, loops, and papillotomes) [1].

Spaulding Criteria

The principles of reprocessing are based on the Spaulding classification, in accordance with which it is obligatory for instruments that penetrate tissue or enter sterile hollow viscera to be sterile [2]. Instruments that come into contact with intact mucosa have to be disinfected. The Spaulding classification categorizes flexible endoscopes (gastroscopes, colonoscopes, and duodenoscopes) as "semicritical devices," for which high-level disinfection, but not necessarily sterilization, is recommended. All devices that come into contact with nonintact mucosa or are associated with opening of blood vessels (e. g., for mucosal biopsy) are regarded as critical instruments and have to be sterilized.

Sterilization is defined as the complete destruction of all microorganisms, including bacterial spores. *Disinfection*, by contrast, means irreversible inactivation or destruction of a substantial proportion of the microorganisms, in numbers that allow safe reuse of the instrument in other patients. Sterilization is defined by the Food and Drug Administration (FDA) in the United States as a reduction by a factor of 10^{12} of bacterial spores, which are regarded as being the most resistant microorganisms. High-level disinfection means destruction of 10^6 resistant, non–spore-forming microorganisms, including *Mycobacterium tuberculosis,* in defined conditions (in terms of temperature, contact time, and pH). High-level disinfection is not synonymous with sterilization and is recommended when sterilization is not absolutely necessary. Conversely, disinfection is a prerequisite for sterilization and should be carried out immediately after the cleaning process.

The standards and terminology used in the guidelines in North America and Europe show minor differences, but the degree of disinfection is consistently defined [1,3–6]. Reprocessing procedures in endoscopy have to be sufficiently effective to exclude contamination from the instruments.

Mechanisms of Infection in Endoscopy

Microorganisms can be transferred from one patient to the next by flexible endoscopes and endoscopic accessories. According to Spach, an exogenous infection can be caused in two ways—firstly from the patient undergoing endoscopy, and secondly via the materials and fluids used in the cleaning process [7] (**Fig. 9.2**). The patient undergoing endoscopy transfers his or her normal bacterial flora, partic-

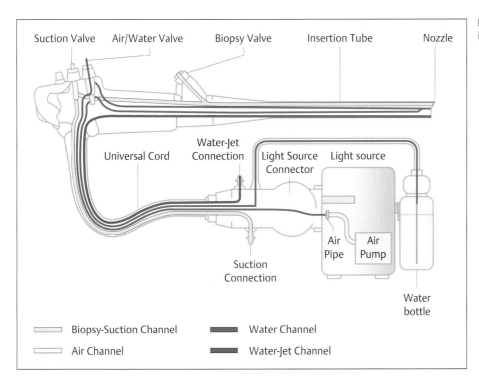

Fig. 9.1 The air, water, and suction system of a flexible endoscope.

Suction Valve   Air/Water Valve   Biopsy Valve   Insertion Tube   Nozzle

Water-Jet Connection

Universal Cord

Light Source Connector   Light source

Air Pipe   Air Pump

Suction Connection

Water bottle

▭ Biopsy-Suction Channel   ▬ Water Channel

▭ Air Channel   ▬ Water-Jet Channel

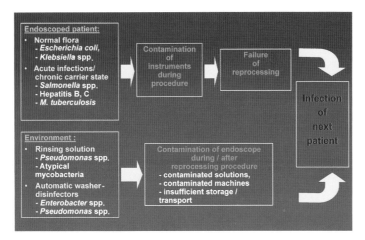

Fig. 9.2 Exogenous infections: nosocomial transmission of microorganisms via endoscopy [7].

Table 9.1 Indicator organisms for quality control

Organisms identified in microbiological tests	Indication of origin
Escherichia coli, enterococci, and Enterobacteriaceae	Insufficient cleaning and/or disinfection procedures, e.g.: ● No brushing ● Inadequate concentrations or exposure times of process chemicals Mechanical or electronic defects of washer-disinfector, e.g.: ● Incorrect amounts and/or concentration of processing chemicals ● Design flaws in washer-disinfector, with dead volumes
Pseudomonas aeruginosa and other Gram-negative nonfermenters	● Insufficient final rinsing ● Contamination of final rinsing water ● Contamination of washer-disinfector due to mechanical or electronic defects ● Contamination of filter systems ● Design flaws in washer-disinfector, with dead volumes ● Insufficient drying of endoscopes before storage
Staphylococcus aureus, *S. epidermidis*	Recontamination of endoscopes due to: ● Inadequate storage and transport ● Inadequate hand hygiene ● Contamination from sampling
Atypical mycobacteria, *Legionella* organisms	Contamination of washer-disinfector and water system

Adapted from Beilenhoff et al. [8].

ments. Pathogens are then passed on during the next examination and can cause an infectious chain reaction. Contaminated solutions and water, washer-disinfectors that are colonized with bacteria, and inadequate storage and transport conditions provide a breeding-ground for bacterial and viral transfer.

Indicator Bacteria

Inadequacies in the reprocessing procedure can be identified by demonstrating the presence of specific microorganisms that are typical for the individual processing steps (**Table 9.1**). The microorganisms concerned can thus be regarded as indicator bacteria [8]. For example, the presence of intestinal bacteria (*E. coli*, enterococci) indicates inadequacies in manual cleaning or disinfection or defects in the WD. What are known as "wet bacteria"—*Pseudomonas* and nonfermenter bacteria—are involved in transference when there is inadequate rinsing and drying, and they may be present as contaminating bacteria in the washer-disinfector's rinsing water. *Staphylococcus aureus* and *S. epidermis* indicate recontamination by staff members (due to inadequate handwashing) and inappropriate transport, storage, and drying conditions. Finally, atypical mycobacteria and also *Legionella* species may indicate contamination of the water system, with additional contamination of the washer-disinfector.

When the problem of prions emerged, debate over the correct reprocessing of endoscopes and endoscopic accessories revived [9]. As prions are resistant in principle to conventional disinfection and sterilization procedures (for example, they even resist autoclaving at 134 °C for 20 min), and as they are highly heat-stable, there were fears that it would be possible for them to be transferred via endoscopes [10,11]. In addition, disinfectants, particularly aldehydes, are capable of fixing protein particles (prions), so that clusters or biofilms can form in the narrow channels. Although there is practically no relationship with the digestive tract in sporadic Creutzfeldt–Jakob disease, the variant form (vCJD) has attracted considerable attention. Consumption of contaminated beef containing the bovine spongiform encephalopathy (BSE) agent is regarded as causing the disease. Since prions can be demonstrated in lymphatic tissue and in the intestines, tonsils, appendix, ileum, and rectum in vCJD, the condition is relevant in gastrointestinal endoscopy, with special consideration needing to be given to the handling of the endoscopes used.

Infections in Endoscopy

Serial infections associated with endoscopic procedures are rare. In a recent overview including 134 scientific articles, 140 events were identified over a period of 30 years [12]. In a critical analysis, 90 % of the infections described were classified as avoidable if correct reprocessing had been carried out. Severe events are evidently less frequent in gastrointestinal endoscopy than in bronchoscopic examinations. The largest infection chain reported involved 48 cases of bacterial infection in 414 patients who underwent bronchoscopy (11.5 %) [13]. The cause was inadequate disinfection of the biopsy channel port, with formation of a moist chamber. The wet bacteria *Pseudomonas aeruginosa* and *Serratia marcescens* led to three deaths [14].

By contrast, case reports of bacterial transfer in gastroenterological endoscopy are well documented. These show that viruses (hepatitis C virus), as well as all types of bacteria—*Helicobacter pylori*, *P. aeruginosa*, salmonella, and *S. marcescens*—can be transferred via the endoscope [15–18]. The common factor among these documented cases of infection and transference in endoscopy involved

ularly intestinal bacteria (*Escherichia coli, Klebsiella,* etc.), or infectious bacteria to the endoscope and instruments used in the examination. In addition, salmonella, hepatitis viruses and tuberculosis bacteria can contaminate the endoscope and endoscopic accessories (forceps, papillotomes, loops, etc.). If the reprocessing procedure is faulty, the pathogens can be transferred to the next patient and can then cause infections. As a patient's infectious status is not usually known, all patients have to be regarded as potentially contagious [1].

A similar transfer process can occur if the cleaning solutions, as well as the instruments and machines, automated washer-disinfectors (WDs), and ultrasound solutions used in the procedure are already contaminated and in turn transfer bacteria to the instru-

errors and inadequacies in reprocessing, which diverged from the relevant hygiene guidelines.

While bacterial transfer can be quickly recognized as infection after endoscopy, obtaining evidence of viral infections is more problematic. Hepatitis viruses are only associated with disease symptoms after several months, making it difficult to trace them back to endoscopy as the actual causal event. The first evidence confirming a hepatitis C virus (HCV) infection transferred from one patient to others was only obtained by genomic evidence of the same HCV virus 6 months after the colonoscopy procedure [15]. Although larger studies have in the meantime disproved the risk of transference of hepatitis C, an endoscopic examination is still regarded as being a risk factor among blood donors [19–21]. In France and Germany, an endoscopy during the previous 6 months is regarded as a reason for excluding an individual from donating blood.

As obtaining virological evidence is considered to be extremely expensive, only colony-forming bacteria are tested during hygiene checks. When these tests are positive, the bacteria are also regarded as indicators for possible viral contamination.

Guidelines

Numerous national and international guidelines on the reprocessing of endoscopes and endoscopic accessories have been published. The guidelines of the European Society for Gastroenterological Endoscopy (ESGE) and European Society of Gastroenterology and Endoscopy Nurses and Associates (ESGENA) are subject to constant review, and the latest version was published in 2008 [1]. The American "Multi-society Guideline for Reprocessing Flexible Gastrointestinal Endoscopes" dates from 2003 [3]. The guidelines are comparable, but differ in details. There is a consensus that the reprocessing of endoscopes—due to the complex structure and unstable covering of the devices—can only be carried out with high-level disinfection, but not with sterilization. Endoscopes can be reprocessed using machines, but manual reprocessing is also possible. Endoscopic accessories (e. g., forceps, loops, and papillotomes) have to undergo sterile reprocessing or should be single-use articles.

The reprocessing of endoscopic equipment must be carried out in rooms specially designed for the purpose (**Fig. 9.3**) [1,5]. This prevents cross-contamination of potentially infectious materials, protects staff and patients from chemical agents, and minimizes the risk of infection and contamination for staff and patients. In the reprocessing room, there should be separate areas for soiled materials and for cleaned equipment. Reprocessing rooms should be equipped with adequate ventilation to reduce the risk of exposure to chemical vapors. Ideally, hygiene staff should work separately from the endoscopic examinations.

The reprocessing of endoscopes involves four working steps:

- Preliminary cleaning and removal of macroscopically visible materials on the exterior surfaces and interior of the channels immediately after use
- Manual cleaning, including leak testing, external cleaning and internal brush cleaning, as well as rinsing
- Disinfection to inactivate all microorganisms up to a level at which no subsequent contamination is possible
- Rinsing, drying and storage

Preliminary cleaning and manual cleaning, including brushing of the channels, must be carried out manually. After this, the disinfection procedure can continue using the automated washer-disinfector or manually. Preliminary cleaning, with flushing and surface cleaning, as well as function checking, is done in the endoscopy room. Manual cleaning with brushing through the instrument and leak testing, including subsequent disinfection, takes place in the separate reprocessing room. Detergents with enzymatic and/or al-

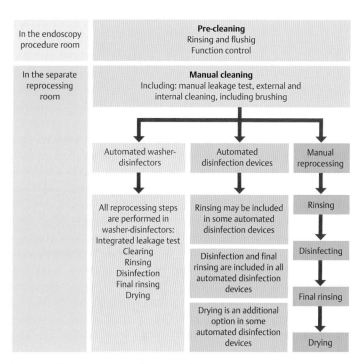

Fig. 9.3 Various methods of reprocessing endoscopes.

kaline boosters or detergents that contain antimicrobial agents are used for the cleaning process. Pre-cleaning and cleaning are essential components of the reprocessing procedure in order to achieve a bacterial reduction of three to four log steps [22,23]. Careful cleaning is regarded as being a prerequisite for disinfection [1,5,6]. In principle, the whole reprocessing procedure can be carried out manually. However, this method is open to several sources of (human) error, and for this reason automated reprocessing is nowadays universally recommended.

The agents used should not include aldehyde-containing detergents during the cleaning process, as these denature and coagulate proteins and can therefore fix them before the later disinfection process. As a disinfectant, 2 % glutaraldehyde is used as a reference product worldwide. Glutaraldehyde leads to the destruction of viruses such as human immunodeficiency virus (HIV), hepatitis B virus (HBV), and HCV within 5–20 min [23,24]. This achieves an additional bacterial reduction by six log steps [25]. The substance is effective and relatively inexpensive, and does not damage the endoscopes or endoscopic accessories. It is the agent most widely used throughout the world. However, glutaraldehyde has a number of adverse events due to toxic vapors, which can cause allergies, dermatitis, conjunctivitis, rhinitis, and asthma. In addition, the quantity of glutaraldehyde residues in flexible endoscopes is greater after manual reprocessing than after automated processing [26]. Due to protein fixation, the disinfectant can also allow the formation of biofilms, and thus bacterial and viral adhesion, as well as prion clusters, in endoscopy channels.

Automated reprocessing in washer-disinfectors provides a standardized, operator-independent reprocessing procedure that results in greater working safety and reduced health risks. As all of the subsequent working steps take place in the washer-disinfector, systematic reprocessing of the endoscopes, with validation, documentation, and traceability is possible. Evidence that the endoscope has been correctly reprocessed is provided by a print-out. Automated reprocessing is also economically advantageous, as staff no longer have to be committed full-time to the reprocessing procedure.

The 2007 European ESGE/ESGENA guideline describes in detail the procedure validation and routine testing applicable to reprocessed endoscopes in washer-disinfectors in accordance with the European standard (European Standard prEN ISO 15883) [27]. Automated reprocessing thus involves the steps of cleaning/disinfection, rinsing, and drying in a closed system. The critical part is the final rinsing of the reprocessed water, which is carried out by ultraviolet lamps or sterile filtration. This prevents recontamination of the endoscopes, internal rinsing/washing chamber, and subsequent pipe systems inside the machine.

Purely manual reprocessing carried out by staff consists of the working steps of rinsing, disinfection, final rinsing, and drying. It has to be ensured that the endoscopes are completely submerged in the disinfectant solution and that all channels and openings can be flushed with the disinfectant. In contrast to machine reprocessing, the manual process is not capable of being validated. As the advantages of automated reprocessing make it clearly superior to manual reprocessing, and the automated procedure also establishes a standardized and validated reprocessing cycle, the guidelines recommend automated reprocessing.

Complete drying of the endoscopes after the completion of reprocessing is absolutely necessary and prevents recontamination by wet bacteria [28]. Drying of the channels can be achieved by blowing compressed air through them. Additional rinsing with 70% isopropyl alcohol is recommended in the United States [3]. The European guidelines refer to responsibility for checking the drying quality and, where necessary, completing the drying process with medical compressed air [1]. Additional rinsing with alcohol is regarded critically in the European guidelines, as there is no clear evidence that alcohol actually supports drying and protects against proliferation of wet bacteria [29]. In some countries (e. g., Germany), alcohol rinsing is explicitly not recommended because of its fixing properties. If used, alcohol should only be introduced at the end of the examination, as alcohol residues can lead to problems with the use of high-frequency instruments.

Improved drying can also be achieved with special drying chambers [30,31]. The use of these chambers is well-established in the United Kingdom, Netherlands, and France in particular. With this in mind, the availability of a validated and verifiable protocol for the drying and storage phases is also desirable. Where drying and storage chambers are used, the European guidelines recommend regular maintenance and microbiological testing of the chambers, as they are another potential source of recontamination.

After 5–7 days of correct storage in the drying cabinet, reprocessed endoscopes are ready for immediate use. Studies in recent years have shown that there is no risk of recontamination during this period [32]. Reprocessing for safety reasons after 7 days' storage is therefore not necessary provided that complete and scrupulous drying was carried out. The quality of drying determines which storage options are possible.

Reprocessing of Endoscopic Accessories

Among endoscopic accessories, there is a distinction between single-use articles and reprocessable materials. All disposables are ready for use in their existing packaging and may only be used immediately after opening. However, single use does exclude reuse. According to the European guidelines, reprocessing of single-use materials is not permissible [1]. In the United States, this position is controversial for reasons of cost [33].

Reprocessed endoscopic materials, which also include forceps, have to be sterilized. Sterilization is carried out after the cleaning process, following a detailed reprocessing protocol. According to the European criteria, injection needles and extraction balloons for biliary and pancreatic endoscopy are not suitable for reprocessing [1]. As with endoscopes, accessories can be disinfected either automatically or manually (**Fig. 9.4**). A step consisting of preliminary

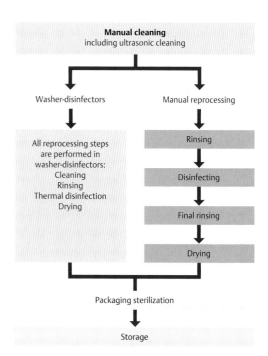

Fig. 9.4 Reprocessing of endoscopic accessories.

cleaning and ultrasound cleaning precedes washer-disinfector processing. For ultrasound cleaning, 30 min at a frequency of 38–47 kHz and an operating temperature of 45 °C are recommended. The subsequent disinfection step, including flushing and drying, can be carried out automatically or manually. Sterilization is defined as 134 °C for 20 min prevacuum. Subsequent storage must be in closed chambers/receptacles and protected from dust. Storage in an open space reduces the duration of storage.

Doubts have repeatedly been expressed as to whether auxiliary materials with complex and delicate mechanisms such as forceps and papillotomes are capable of being reprocessed, since liquids and sterilization steam are not able to penetrate into every component of a complex mechanism and complete dismantling into the individual components is not possible (**Figs. 9.5, 9.6**). However, studies on biopsy forceps, as well as on papillotomes, have also repeatedly shown that reprocessing following a strict protocol is successful and meets the criteria for sterilization [34–37]. However, the fashion has long since switched to single-use products, as their quality and pricing have become more favorable and they avoid the need for reprocessing. In the European Union, there are currently ten states that recommend single-use articles generally for the whole of endoscopy.

New Agents and Disinfectants

The use of glutaraldehyde as a disinfectant has been questioned in the wake of the prion problem. The health authorities in France have issued a general ban on it, as glutaraldehyde fixes protein, potentially leading to adhesion of prion particles [10]. When it is expected that an endoscope is going to be used in patients with sporadic Creutzfeldt–Jakob disease (e. g., for percutaneous endoscopic gastrostomy), a special endoscope is required in Germany that is subject to elaborate reprocessing. In a case of suspected vCJD disease, the instrument must be destroyed or has to undergo double cleaning with an alkaline detergent, plus disinfection with an oxidating agent. No cases of prions being transferred during endoscopy have ever been documented. In recent years, alternative agents and methods have been sought in order to avoid the disadvantages of glutaraldehyde.

13. Srinivasan A, Wolfenden LL, Song X, Mackie K, Hartsell TL, Jones HD, et al. An outbreak of *Pseudomonas aeruginosa* infections associated with flexible bronchoscopes. N Eng J Med 2003;348:221–7.

14. Kirschke DL, Jones TF, Craig AS, Chu PS, Mayernick GG, Patel JA, et al. *Pseudomonas aeruginosa* and *Serratia marcescens* contamination associated with a manufacturing defect in bronchoscopes. N Engl J Med 2003;348:214–20.

15. Bronowicki JP, Venard V, Botté C, Monhoven N, Gastin I, Choné L, et al. Patient-to-patient transmission of hepatitis C virus during colonoscopy. N Engl J Med 1997;337:237–40.

16. Langenberg W, Rauws EA, Oudbier JH, Tytgat GN. Patient-to-patient transmission of *Campylobacter pylori* by fiberoptic gastroduodenoscopy and biopsy. J Infect Dis 1990;161:507–11.

17. Tennenbaum R, Colardelle P, Chochon M, Maisonneuve P, Jean F, Andrieu J. [Hepatitis C after retrograde cholangiography.] Gastroenterol Clin Biol 1993;17:763–4. French.

18. Nelson DB, Muscarella LF. Current issues in endoscope reprocessing and infection control during gastrointestinal endoscopy. World J Gastroenterol 2006;12:3953–64.

19. Ponchon T. Transmission of hepatitis C and prion diseases through digestive endoscopy: evaluation of risk and recommended practices. Endoscopy 1997;29:199–201.

20. Ciancio A, Manzini P, Castagno F, D'Antico S, Reynaudo P, Coucourde L, et al. Digestive endoscopy is not a major risk factor for transmitting hepatitis C virus. Ann Intern Med 2005;142:903–9.

21. Andrieu J, Barny S, Colardelle P, Maisonneuve P, Giraud V, Robin E, et al. [Prevalence and risk factors of hepatitis C virus infection in a hospitalized population in a gastroenterology unit. Role of endoscopic biopsies.] Gastroenterol Clin Biol 1995;19:340–5. French.

22. Cronmiller JR, Nelson DK, Salman G, Jackson DK, Dean RS, Hsu JJ, et al. Antimicrobial efficacy of endoscopic disinfection procedures: a controlled, multifactorial investigation. Gastrointest Endosc 1999;50:152–8.

23. Chanzy B, Duc-Bin DL, Rousset B, Morand P, Morel-Baccard C, Marchetti B, et al. Effectiveness of a manual disinfection procedure in eliminating hepatitis C virus from experimentally contaminated endoscopes. Gastrointest Endosc 1999;50:147–51.

24. Hanson PJ, Gor D, Jeffries DJ, Collins JV. Elimination of high titre HIV from fiberoptic endoscopes. Gut 1990;31:657–9.

25. Kovacs BJ, Chen YK, Kettering JD, Aprecio RM, Roy I. High-level disinfection of gastrointestinal endoscopes: are current guidelines adequate? Am J Gastroenterol 1999;94:1546–50.

26. Farina A, Fievet MH, Plassart F, Menet MC, Thuillier A. Residual glutaraldehyde levels in fiberoptic endoscopes: measurement and implications for patient toxicity. J Hosp Infect 1999;43:293–7.

27. Beilenhoff U, Neumann CS, Biering H, Blum R, Schmidt V, Rey JF, et al. ESGE/ESGENA guideline for process validation and routine testing for reprocessing endoscopes in washer-disinfectors, according to the European Standard prEN ISO 15883 parts 1, 4, and 5. Endoscopy 2007;39:85–94.

28. Muscarella LF. Inconsistencies in endoscope-reprocessing and infection-control guidelines: importance of endoscope drying. Am J Gastroenterol 2006;101:2147–54.

29. Leiss O, Bader L, Mielke M, Exner M. [Five years of the Robert Koch Institute guidelines for reprocessing of flexible endoscopes. A look back and a look forward]. Bundesgesundheitsbl Gesundheitsforsch Gesundheitsschutz 2008;51:211–20. German.

30. Pineau L, Villard E, Duc DL, Marchetti B. Endoscope drying/storage cabinet: interest and efficacy. J Hosp Infect 2008;68:59–65.

31. Pietsch M. Safe storage of endoscopes: change in our guidelines? Endoscopy 2007;39:831–2.

32. Vergis AS, Thompson D, Pieroni P, Dhaila S. Reprocessing flexible gastrointestinal endoscopes after a period of disuse: is it necessary? Endoscopy 2007;39:737–9.

33. Fireman Z. Biopsy forceps: reusable or disposable? J Gastroenterol Hepatol 2006;21:1089–92.

34. Jung M, Beilenhoff U, Pietsch M, Kraft B, Rippin G. Standardized reprocessing of reusable colonoscopy biopsy forceps is effective: results of a German multicenter study. Endoscopy 2003;35:197–202.

35. Kozarek RA, Raltz SL, Ball TJ, Patterson DJ, Brandabur JJ. Reuse of disposable sphincterotomes for diagnostic and therapeutic ERCP: a one-year prospective study. Gastrointest Endosc 1999;49:39–42.

36. Prat F, Spieler JF, Paci S, Pallier C, Fritsch J, Choury AD, et al. Reliability, cost-effectiveness, and safety of reuse of ancillary devices for ERCP. Gastrointest Endosc 2004;60:246–52.

37. Sautereau D, Palazzo L. [Single-use biopsy forceps for digestive endoscopy: a wise decision or a caricature of precaution principles?]. Gastroenterol Clin Biol 2001;25:653–5. French.

38. Kampf G, Bloss R, Martiny H. Surface fixation of dried blood by glutaraldehyde and peracetic acid. J Hosp Infect 2004;57:139–43.

39. Napoléon B, Chapuis C. Le point sur le désinfecteur Cleantop. Acta Endosc 2004;34:390–4.

40. Tsuji S, Kawano S, Oshita M, Ohmae A, Shinomura Y, Miyazaki Y, et al. Endoscope disinfection using acidic electrolytic water. Endoscopy 1999;31:528–35.

41. Lee JH, Rhee PL, Kim JH, Kim JJ, Paik SW, Rhee JC, et al. Efficacy of electrolyzed acid water in reprocessing patient-used flexible upper endoscopes: Comparison with 2% alkaline glutaraldehyde. J Gastroenterol Hepatol 2004;19:897–903.

42. Pox C, Schmiegel W, Classen M. Current status of screening colonoscopy in Europe and in the United States. Endoscopy 2008;39:168–73.

43. Bader L, Blumenstock G, Birkner B, Leiss O, Heesemann J, Riemann JF, et al. [HYGEA (hygiene in gastroenterology—endoscope reprocessing): study on quality of reprocessing flexible endoscopes in hospitals and in the practice setting]. Z Gastroenterol 2002;40:157–70. German.

44. QSHE-Pilotprojekt (Qualitätssicherung der Hygiene in der Endoskopie) der Kassenärztlichen Vereinigung Bayerns. Gastro-Nachr 2003;37:6–7.

45. Heudorf U, Hofmann H, Kutzke G, Otto U, Exner M. [Hygiene in endoscopy in the clinic and practice, 2003: Results of infection hygiene survey on endoscopy services in Frankfurt am Main by the public health service]. Z Gastroenterol 2004;42:669–76. German.

9

Teaching and Learning

Section editors:
Meinhard Classen, Guido N.J. Tytgat, Charles J. Lightdale

10 Education and Training

Juergen Hochberger, Juergen Maiss, Kai Matthes, Guido Costamagna, and Robert H. Hawes

Introduction

Diagnostic and interventional endoscopy are in a state of continuous technological advancement, and interventional endoscopy has replaced surgery for many gastrointestinal disorders during the past few decades. Optimal patient care and quality management are playing an increasing role in clinical medicine. Public awareness and growing legal pressure to show and document competence have further contributed to the importance of training in interventional medicine. A debate over training standards aroused recent interest in connection with the effect of the learning curve on the complication rates observed with various procedures. While evidence-based medicine is rapidly becoming the "gold standard" for treatment modalities, the responsibility for obtaining education and further training—including the theoretical background, as well as acquiring and refining manual skills in gastrointestinal endoscopy—still lies in the hands of the individual physician. Practical skills are routinely acquired by practicing on patients, initially under the supervision of a senior endoscopist. Over the years, specialist medical societies have produced guidelines and recommendations for establishing minimum quality requirements for the unsupervised performance of the various endoscopic techniques (**Table 10.1**) [1–4]. However, in most of these guidelines, terms such as "self-reliance" and "under supervision" are not clearly defined, and the required procedures have been defined only in terms of number, rather than quality. In addition, educational considerations and the special demands of manual training have not yet been regarded as an important part of systematic curricula. Structured training programs and mandatory teaching curricula for gastrointestinal endoscopy are still not established. Recently, endoscopy simulators have rekindled debate on whether training in basic manual skills is better provided outside the patient. This chapter presents an overview of training issues and simulators.

Table 10.1 Recommendations regarding the minimum numbers of procedures required for competence

Organization	EGD	Colonoscopy	ERCP
American Society for Gastrointestinal Endoscopy [1]	100	100	100
British Society for Gastroenterology [2]	300	100	150
Conjoint Committee for Recognition of Training in Gastrointestinal Endoscopy (Australia) [3]	200	100	200
European Diploma of Gastroenterology [4]	300	100	150

EGD, esophagogastroduodenoscopy; ERCP, endoscopic retrograde cholangiopancreatography.

Clinical Education

Clinical Training in EGD and Colonoscopy: Studies and Guidelines

In surgery, there is a long tradition that surgeons keep a logbook of the procedures they carry out. Since the early 1980s, trainees have been formally required to keep a record of every gastrointestinal endoscopy procedure they carry out [5].

Medical societies then also started to address the issue of the numbers of procedures required. Information about clinical experience during the learning process was collected for training in esophagogastroduodenoscopy (EGD) and colonoscopy in particular. As it is necessary to examine the whole colon in order to be confident that lesions have not been missed, the ability to reach the cecum is the most common criterion by which colonoscopies have been judged. In nearly 50 % of cases, missed cancers are due to incomplete examinations [6]. Data from existing studies and minimal numbers of procedures required are outlined in **Tables 10.1** and **10.2** [1–26].

Table 10.2 Reported cecal intubation rates after performance of the stated number of procedures

First author, ref.	Year	Specialty	Trainees (n)	Procedures (n)	Cecal intubation (%)	Estimated 90 % success after n procedures
Parry [8]	1991	Surgery	1	305	91	261
Godreau [9]	1992	Family practice	1	157	83	
Rodney [10]	1993	Family practice	1	100	52	551
Cass [11])	1993	Gastroenterology and surgery	12	100	84	97
Cass [12]	1996	Gastroenterology	35	200	90	34
Church [13]	1993	Surgery	8	100	62	
Church [14]	1995	Surgery	10	125	72	376
Marshall [15]	1995	Gastroenterology	6	328	86	
Chak [16]	1996	Gastroenterology	7	123	64	
Hopper [17]	1996	Family practice	1	1048	75	
Tassios [18]	1999	Gastroenterology	8	180	77	188

Marshall followed nine gastroenterology fellows and measured their success in reaching the cecum during the last 7 months of the first and second years of study [15]. He found a success rate of only 86% for reaching the cecum after trainees had performed a mean of 328 procedures. Chak et al. followed five first-year and seven second-year gastroenterology fellows in a 2-year fellowship program over a 4-month period and observed their performance [16]. They found that after 123 colonoscopies, trainees reached the cecum in only 63.7% of the procedures. Church followed surgical residents and reported on their first 125 procedures [13]. By the last 25 procedures, the cecum was intubated only 72% of the time.

Tassios et al. followed eight trainees who were learning how to carry out colonoscopy during a 2-year gastroenterology fellowship [18]. Regression analysis was used to estimate cecal intubation success rates of only 67% after 100 procedures and 77% after 180 procedures. In an attempt to gather as much data as possible, Cass et al. again performed a 14-center study of 135 gastroenterology fellows throughout their 3-year fellowship. Preliminary data were presented in 1996. The authors concluded that at least 130 EGDs and 140 colonoscopies had to be completed to meet all criteria for competence consistently on over 90% of occasions [12]. With these data available, medical societies began to increase the number of procedures they recommended for acquiring competence [1–3,27].

It is quite evident that further data from medical practice, including outcomes after 30 days, for example, are needed in order to provide firm, evidence-based recommendations on the minimum numbers of supervised procedures required before endoscopy is carried out independently in patients.

However, when one examines some of the earlier data mentioned above, mainly obtained during the early period of colonoscopy screening, there is an important aspect that needs to be taken into consideration: the colonoscopes in use today are not comparable with the devices used 20 years ago. The facility for three-step rigidity or variable-stiffness adjustment of the instrument's shaft makes intubation much easier in comparison with older instruments, which were often very soft. Today, completion rates in colonoscopy would not be the only focus when evaluating competence; in addition, an individual physician's polyp and colon cancer detection rates over time would be taken into consideration.

Sarker and colleagues developed a self-appraisal tool for trainees in lower gastrointestinal endoscopy [28]. A total of 135 endoscopic procedures were performed by nine consultants and 12 registrars. The mean interrater reliability Cronbach α was 0.83 and 0.80 ($P \leq 0.05$) for generic and specific skills, respectively, for each procedure. The validity results using analysis of variance (ANOVA) for consultants and trainees were significant for each procedure ($P = 0.005$; $P = 0.003$ for generic and $P = 0.012$, $P = 0.004$ for specific technical skills). The authors concluded that this new assessment/self-appraisal tool for lower gastrointestinal endoscopy appears to have face, content, concurrent, and construct validity. The tool is also capable of being used for training and self-appraisal. The authors intend to modify and apply the tool to other endoscopic procedures in the future, such as endoscopic retrograde cholangiopancreatography (ERCP) and endoluminal and transluminal procedures.

Studies and Guidelines on Clinical Training in ERCP

Proficiency in all aspects of ERCP requires several years of practical training and continuous refinement of knowledge [29–33]. A standardized mandatory teaching program for ERCP has not yet been established.

Historically, endoscopic training in ERCP has consisted primarily of "learning by doing" under the supervision of an experienced endoscopist [34,35]. However, endoscopic therapy—e.g., for com-

mon bile duct stones—may nowadays include the whole range from sphincterotomy to complex laser lithotripsy [36–41]. With the advent of noninvasive tests such as magnetic resonance cholangiopancreatography (MRCP) and endoscopic ultrasonography (EUS), ERCP is moving from being a diagnostic procedure to an almost purely therapeutic one [42,43]. This is creating a new challenge in the training of young endoscopists, as ERCP procedures are becoming more concentrated in large-volume or mid-volume endoscopy centers, while the numbers of ERCPs performed in smaller hospitals are decreasing. Smaller hospitals are often located in rural areas and provide limited ERCP services such as sphincterotomy, stone extraction, and stent implantation. Threshold figures for numbers of ERCP procedures that have to be performed by trainees in order to receive credentials were published in the Gastroenterology Core Curriculum in 1996 [34]. The document indicated that fellows had to complete 100 ERCPs, including 25 therapeutic cases (20 sphincterotomies and five stent placement cases). Jowell et al. found that a minimum of 180–200 ERCPs needed to be performed before a trainee could be regarded as competent for unsupervised ERCP [44]. Approximately 80–100 ERCPs per endoscopist per year appear to be necessary to continue to maintain adequate competence for biliary procedures. More than 250 ERCPs per endoscopist per year are deemed mandatory for developing and maintaining expertise level in complex therapeutic procedures in the pancreas [45]. The ERCP volume plays a role in complication rates. In various studies, a minimum of 40–50 sphincterotomies (ESTs) per endoscopist per year was found to be associated with a lower complication rate in comparison with endoscopists with a lower EST frequency [46,47]. Rabenstein and Hahn showed that not only the number of ERCPs and ESTs performed in the past, but also the number of ERCPs currently being performed by an endoscopist, influence the success and complication rates [48]. Objective outcomes of an individual endoscopist and medicolegal concerns may play an increasing role in gastrointestinal practice in the future [29,49,50].

Practical Training in ERCP

Before acquiring the skills necessary for the performance of ERCP in a safe, effective, and comfortable manner, the endoscopist first has to understand the indications for the procedure and its risks and limitations. In addition to this, a competent endoscopist also needs training and proficiency in manual and technical skills. To achieve this, the American Society for Gastrointestinal Endoscopy (ASGE) published a new core curriculum for training in ERCP in March 2006 [51].

In most fellowship training programs, traditional ERCP training follows education in diagnostic gastroscopy and colonoscopy and is often begun when the trainee has been introduced to polypectomy, hemostasis, or EUS training as part of a "learning pyramid" (**Fig. 10.1**) [52]. Fellows begin their ERCP training by observing the procedure and/or assisting the primary endoscopist. In Europe, this initial experience may involve maneuvering the radiographic equipment during the procedure, or in some institutions the trainee may perform the duties of the assisting endoscopy nurse in order to learn how to properly handle catheters, guide wires, and other accessories. Accompanying learning aids include the review of video material, ERCP atlases, and interactive computer programs. In most cases, the first practical steps in learning ERCP involve understanding how to maneuver a side-viewing endoscope by passing the endoscope during the early stages of the procedure. This involves incrementally learning how to intubate the esophagus, maneuver along the lesser curvature of the stomach, appreciate the "setting-sun phenomenon" at the passage of the pylorus, and finally how to bring the endoscope into an appropriate "short" position in front of the papilla.

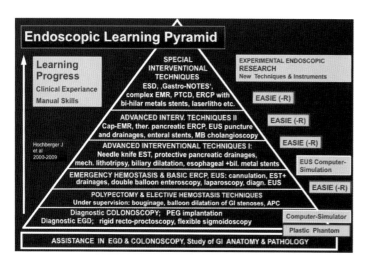

Fig. 10.1 The "learning pyramid" as an example of stepwise clinical training in interventional endoscopy.

Now that most ERCPs are performed for therapeutic purposes, it is a matter of controversy whether cannulation is the next technique for the trainee to learn after he or she is able to maneuver the duodenoscope to the papilla competently. For example, it is well known that for routine stent exchanges in the setting of a prior sphincterotomy, fewer procedures (n = 60) are needed to obtain competence than is the case with cannulation of a native papilla (n = 180–200), and it is also known that stent exchanges are associated with a lower risk profile [44,53]. Patients with benign biliary strictures, chronic obstructive pancreatitis, and recurrent bile duct stones in the setting of prior sphincterotomy may be good cases for the trainee to perform in the early stages of ERCP experience.

Schutz and Abbot developed an ERCP grading scale based on procedural difficulty. In a single-center study, they used benchmarks such as cannulation rates to gauge competence in attempted procedures. A modification of this score was adopted by the ASGE as part of their quality-assessment document [51,54]. Absolute numbers of procedures partially performed by a fellow may not realistically reflect competence. Where possible, trainee logbook records should specify particular skills completed by the fellow (cannulation, sphincterotomy, stent placement, tissue sampling), and should also indicate cases that the trainee completed without assistance.

The ASGE guidelines for advanced endoscopic training state that most fellows require at least 180 cases to achieve competence, with at least half of these cases being therapeutic. Although nearly all gastrointestinal training programs offer some exposure to ERCP, not all of the trainees may ultimately perform ERCP after the completion of their training. All fellows should at least develop an understanding of the diagnostic and therapeutic role of the procedure, including indications, contraindications, and possible complications. This is generally accomplished in the context of a 3-year gastroenterology fellowship training program [51].

In 2003, Kowalski et al. carried out a survey concerning ERCP training among U.S. gastroenterology fellows [55]. In a short questionnaire, they assessed the training program, personal ERCP experience, perceptions regarding training adequacy, and post-training practice plans. Graduating fellows performed a median of 140 ERCPs and 35 sphincterotomies during training, with an associated median comfort level for independently performing sphincterotomy of 7.5 on a scale of 1–10. The median estimated success rate for independent free cannulation was 75%. Based on nonparametric correlation and regression analysis, 180 ERCPs would be necessary to achieve a free cannulation rate of 80% and 69 sphincterotomies to achieve a comfort level of 8 on a scale of 1–10. Only 36% of the fellows achieved the relevant number of procedures and cannula-

tion success. Sixty-four percent of fellows did not achieve procedural competence, and 33% reported inadequate ERCP training. Nevertheless, 91% of the fellows said they expected to perform unsupervised ERCP after training. The authors concluded that the majority of graduating fellows did not achieve an acceptable success rate during training, yet still intended to perform ERCP after training.

The decision by a program director as to whether to train one or more fellows each year to achieve sufficient competence will depend in some measure on the volume of ERCPs performed at the institution and the availability of experts in ERCP to supervise the training of fellows. With data from Jowell et al. suggesting that well over 200 cases are required for most trainees to consistently cannulate the desired duct (**Fig. 10.2**) [44,56], programs with a limited case volume will have to weigh their training objectives with what is feasible. For example, with an annual volume of 400 cases and three fellows, it would be reasonable to have one fellow perform 300 or more cases and provide the other two with an exposure to ERCP, rather than have all three individuals equally share cases, with a low likelihood that any of the three would reach competence by the end of the fellowship.

Trainees who elect to pursue additional training in ERCP so as to attain procedural competence should have completed at least 18 months of a standard gastroenterology training program as per the Gastroenterology Core Curriculum. The minimum duration of training required to achieve advanced technical and cognitive skills is usually 12 months. This period of advanced training can be incorporated into the standard 3-year fellowship program, or may be completed during an additional year dedicated to advanced endoscopic procedures [51].

■ Complementary Video Courses

The initial introduction of video endoscopy to replace fiberoptic procedures was an important aid in everyday clinical teaching [57]. Live endoscopy courses, interactive teaching programs, and video materials can help trainees to recognize pathology better and to understand the appropriate application of therapeutic techniques. However, such passive activities cannot replace the performance of actual procedures with real-time personal feedback from an experienced tutor. This is especially true when new techniques are practiced for the first time [58,59].

Current Training Models

■ Plastic Phantoms and Other Static Models

The initial experimental models for endoscopy training were made of plastic. In 1974, Classen and Ruppin in Erlangen presented an anatomically shaped plastic phantom that allowed examination of the upper gastrointestinal tract using a flexible panendoscope [60]. Christopher Williams and his group in London have been working on the development of semirigid phantoms making it possible to acquire basic skills in flexible colonoscopy since the beginning of the 1970s [61].

A number of initiatives aimed at improving limitations in training have been launched in the past [51,62–65]. Courses using plastic dummies for gastroscopy and colonoscopy should be mentioned in this context. However, these models had the disadvantage of allowing virtually no interventions to be carried out and were never suitable for ERCP training.

Currently, by far the most advanced static simulator is the Interphant model developed by Lange and Grund in Tübingen, Germany [65]. These innovative artificial tissues have also been used for

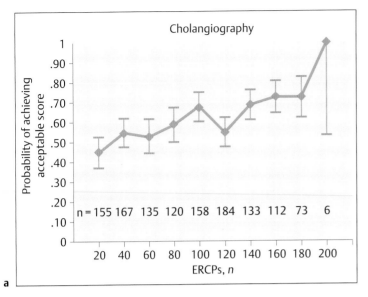

a

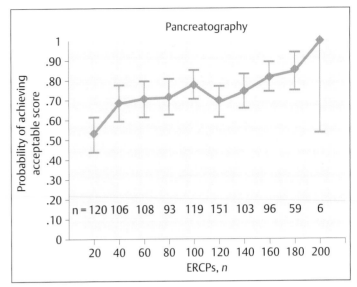

b

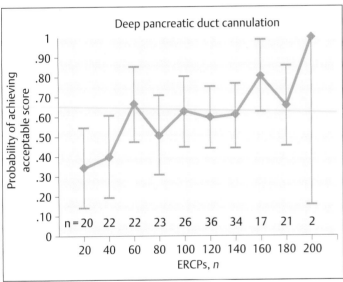

c

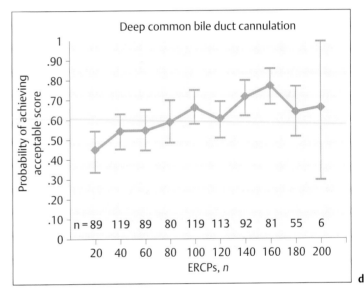

d

Fig. 10.2 The probability (with 95% confidence intervals) of achieving an acceptable score for cholangiography (**a**), pancreatography (**b**), deep pancreatic cannulation (**c**), and deep biliary cannulation (**d**) during training of fellows in endoscopic retrograde cholangiopancreatography (ERCP), as reported by Jowell et al. for 17 gastroenterology fellows during 1450 ERCP procedures [44,56].

specific ERCP techniques. The models employ a plastic bile duct and a papilla made from a chicken heart to allow training of sphincterotomy techniques. Unfortunately, so far as we are aware the model is not commercially available and there are no published data validating its use in training.

Computer Simulators

Apart from mechanical simulators, various computer simulation systems have been developed since 1982 [35,52,64,67]. In Baltimore, Maryland, Mark Noar began in the mid-1980s developing an interesting realistic, computer-assisted simulator—the Robotics Interactive Endoscopy Simulation (RIES) system for esophagogastroduodenoscopy (EGD) and ERCP [68–70]. His aim was to integrate a functioning endoscope into an interactive environment, thus creating a realistic visual appearance. The system reached a high level of technical sophistication, with functioning sphincters at the papilla of Vater and tactile feedback. Due to rapid developments in computer technology and electronics after 2000, a second generation of computer simulators emerged. The first of these models was

the Simbionix GI-Mentor, in the shape of a dummy ("Mr Silverman") [71]. The current GI-Mentor II model (Simbionix Corporation, Cleveland, Ohio), as well as the AccuTouch computer simulator (Immersion Medical Inc., Gaithersburg, Maryland) allow not only the simulation of different diagnostic and interventional procedures at different levels, but also include teaching modules—for example, with anatomy and pathology atlases (**Fig. 10.3**) [34,67]. Both systems create a relatively realistic virtual endoscopy environment. EUS and ERCP modules with parallel radiographic and endoscopic simulations, virtual sphincterotomy, stone extraction, etc., have been implemented (**Figs. 10.4–10.6**).

Various studies have demonstrated the benefits of additional computer simulator training in connection with colonoscopy [67]. Using the Immersion Medical device, Sedlack and Kolars developed a computer-based colonoscopy simulator (CBCS) course for first-year gastroenterology fellows [72,73]. Initially, performance on the simulator was tested in 10 faculty experts, five partially trained endoscopists, and two untrained gastroenterology assistants. Based on the performance standards for the three groups, the investigators concluded that the greatest benefit for trainees would be during the early stages of training. The curriculum developed included 1 h of

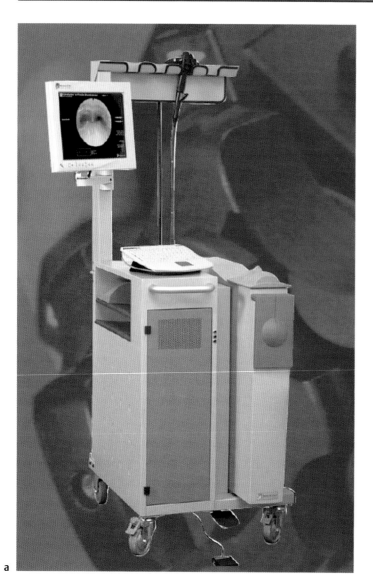

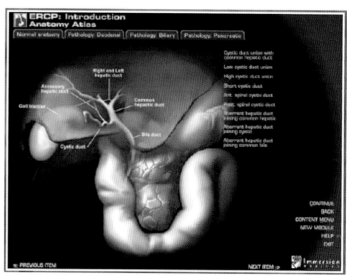

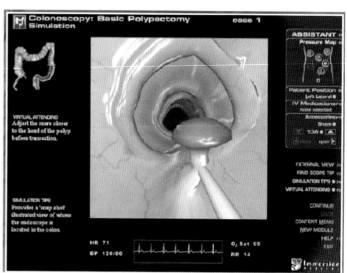

Fig. 10.3 A computer simulation model (Immersion Medical, Inc., Gaithersburg, Maryland, USA; **a**), with an anatomy tool (**b**) and simulation of an endoscopic polypectomy (**c**).

multimedia tutorial and 9 h of CBCS training, including completion of 25 colonoscopy cases. The investigators set standards for advancement to live colonoscopy, including an ability to view the entire colon in less than 15 min with minimal pain and no complications (evidence level B) [73].

In a subsequent validation study by Sedlack et al., performance in two virtual colonoscopies were assessed for 10 faculty experts, six gastroenterology fellows, and six medical residents [74]. There were significant differences with regard to total procedure time, insertion time, and readout time between the experts and the other test groups, but there were no other significant differences for the other test parameters. The faculty found the cases to be realistic, but also easier than actual colonoscopy (evidence level B).

In a prospective study using computer-based colonoscopy simulation, four novice fellows at the Mayo Clinic received 6 h of simulator-based training, compared with four novice fellows without training [75]. The simulator-trained fellows outperformed the traditionally trained fellows during their initial 15 colonoscopies in all performance aspects except for insertion time ($P < 0.05$). The simulator-trained fellows inserted the endoscope significantly further and reached the cecum independently nearly twice as often during this early training period. Three parameters (depth of insertion, independent completion, and ability to identify landmarks) demonstrated a continued advantage up to 30 colonoscopies. Be-

yond 30 procedures, there were no differences in performance between the two groups (evidence level B) [75]. The role of the colonoscopy simulator in training awaits further prospective studies. However, current evidence suggests that it is beneficial during the early learning period.

The easy accessibility and availability of new endoscopy simulators enhances the argument that the trainee should learn basic manual skills outside of patient care. Computer simulators may play an important role in the early phase of endoscopic training, especially in the early stages of colonoscopy [70,71,75–84]. However, for the most realistic training in complex therapeutic interventions, such as ERCP techniques, computer simulators still have problems, as they do not adequately simulate tissue elasticity. In addition, virtual endoscopes handle considerably differently from actual endoscopes [35,85,86].

Training Courses with Live Animals

Training courses using animal models offer a realistic and animate working environment for learning endoscopy. However, a substantial organizational, technical, and financial effort is required [85,87,88]. Since the early 1990s, anesthetized pigs and dogs have been used in systematic endoscopy training courses, especially for

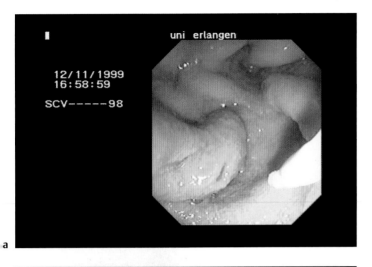

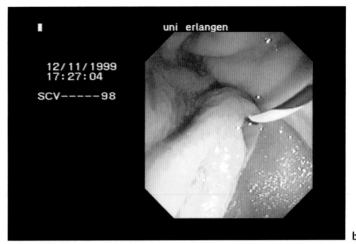

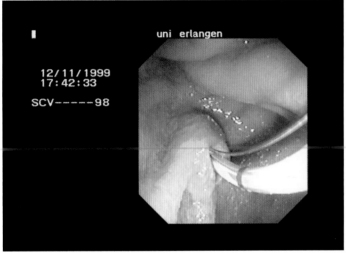

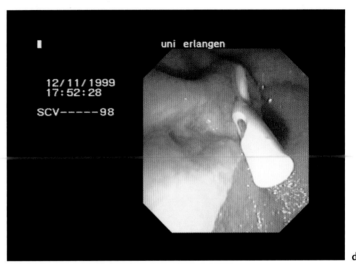

Fig. 10.4 Training in endoscopic retrograde cholangiopancreatography using a pig specimen. **a** Cannulation, **b** guide-wire insertion, **c** sphincterotomy, **d** stent implantation.

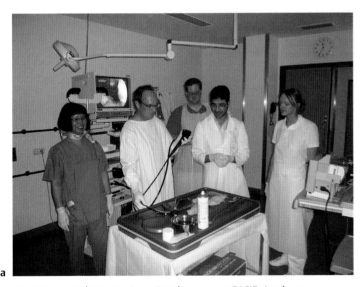

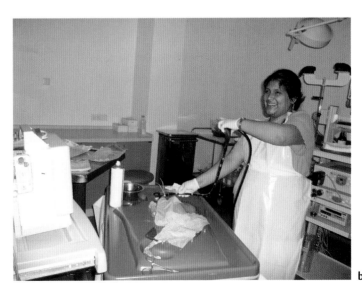

Fig. 10.5 Hands-on training using the compactEASIE simulator.
a Groups of three or four fellows per simulator and teacher receiving instructions.
b Individual practice—e. g., for basic gastroscopy.

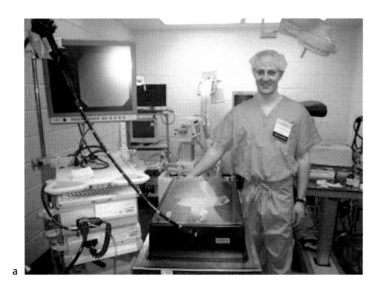

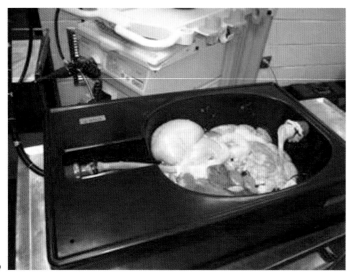

Fig. 10.6
a   The EASIE-R model designed by Kai Matthes and colleagues for providing training in interventions in the upper and lower gastrointestinal tract, as well as for training in natural orifice transluminal endoscopic surgery (NOTES). Embalmed pig specimens are used for repeated applications.
b   An endoscopic ultrasound (EUS) training setting with the EASIE-R simulator, with organs surrounded by gelatin and inclusion of an artificial cyst for EUS puncture and drainage techniques.

training. A polyp-like structure at the pylorus known as the torus pyloricus resembles a papilla with an impacted stone and can be used for practicing needle-knife techniques. Problems encountered during examination of the upper gastrointestinal tract in pigs include the often dilated stomach and the excessive distance to the pylorus due to the long snout. Perforation of the bile duct is not infrequent during ERCP training courses, necessitating sacrifice of the animal earlier than one would expect.

▣ Ex Vivo Porcine Tissue Models (EASIE, Erlanger Endo-Trainer, EASIE-R)

Pig stomachs have been used for training in diagnostic gastroscopy for many years. In 1997, Hochberger and Neumann presented the first generation of training models, which used specially prepared pig specimens for training in flexible interventional gastrointestinal endoscopy [90,91]. The Erlangen Active Simulator for Interventional Endoscopy (EASIE) was developed by integrating an endoscopic environment into the surgical Neumann Biosimulation Model, primarily designed for laparoscopy and open surgical interventions. The original 30-kg surgical simulator consisted of a rotatable plastic thorax–abdomen dummy. Upper gastrointestinal organ packages, obtained from normal slaughter processes in the meat industry, are thoroughly cleaned and placed in a special simulator mold. As in the pulsatile organ perfusion (POP) simulator described by Szinicz et al. [92], a roller pump can be used to drive artificial blood circulation with citrated and diluted blood through the arteries of previously heparinized organs for parenchymal resections. Hochberger et al. used this perfusion system to simulate spurting arterial bleeding in hollow gastrointestinal viscera for the first time [52]. This was achieved by suturing segments of porcine splenic arteries into the anterior wall of the stomach and connecting them to an artificial blood circuit. This made it possible to reproduce spurting arterial bleeding, to provide training in ulcer hemostasis for the first time.

The "compactEASIE" device is a simplified version of the original biosimulation model and was developed in 1998. CompactEASIE is a lightweight (15 kg) and shallow model (height 15 cm) that allows easy storage and shipping and is focused exclusively on interventional endoscopic applications (**Fig. 10.7 a**). The modified Neumann biosimulation model was then renamed as the Erlangen Endo-Trainer for endoscopic applications [93,94]. The two simulators have been described in greater detail elsewhere [35,52,93]. A study comparing the original Neumann model and the later compactEASIE did not identify any limitations with regard to training with the lightweight compactEASIE simulator [95].

Specially prepared porcine upper gastrointestinal organ packages (esophagus, stomach, and duodenum, and including the common bile duct, gallbladder, and liver) are used. After preparation from fresh meat, they are deep-frozen and then thawed for 6 h before use. The organ package can be varied depending on the workshop being planned—e. g., for hemostasis, EMR, or ERCP training. Thanks to the modular concept underlying the compactEASIE model for training in EGD, ERCP, and EMR, the roller pump (which is only needed to create pulsatile spurting bleeding in hemostasis training) can be left out (**Fig. 10.7 b, c**).

Training in more than 30 interventional endoscopic techniques can be provided. In addition to the compactEASIE model, a special lightweight colon model has been developed (coloEASIE), which can be used to practice stricture management, proctoscopic interventions, and EMR in the lower gastrointestinal tract, for example (see **Table 10.3**).

For ERCP interventions such as sphincterotomy and stent placement (**Fig. 10.4**), the hepatobiliary system with the liver, extrahepatic bile ducts, and gallbladder is dissected and added to the upper gastrointestinal tract. It is possible to perform conventional endo-

ERCP techniques [70,87–89]. The major advantages of using live animals for training are the natural tissue sensation, elasticity, and realistic tactile feedback resulting from organ structures similar to those found in humans. Ethical considerations, animal welfare, and problems of hygiene, along with the need for dedicated endoscopes for animal use and substantial staff and financial expenditure are major restrictions. In addition, the procedures have to be performed in special animal facilities, which may require separate permission for animal experiments, with the procedures needing veterinary support. An adequate fasting time in pigs is mandatory for training, as the stomach would otherwise be filled with food, impairing endoscopic visualization. The anatomy of the upper gastrointestinal tract in the swine is relatively similar to that in humans. However, there are differences, such as two separate papillae for the bile duct and pancreatic duct. The biliary papilla is located about 1.5–2 cm distal to the pylorus at the roof of the duodenal bulb. The pancreatic papilla is located more distally and is often difficult to find due to its small size and deep location in the duodenum. In contrast to the biliary papilla, the pancreatic papilla is usually not suitable for ERCP

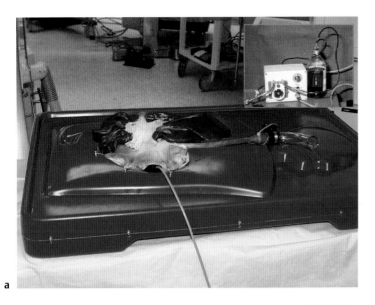

Fig. 10.7

a The compactEASIE model for hands-on training using specially prepared pig organs.

b A roller pump drives artificial blood into vessels that have been sutured into a pig stomach, to provide training in hemostasis procedures in realistic conditions.

c Practicing hemoclipping with the compactEASIE simulator.

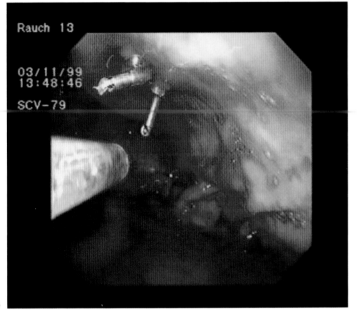

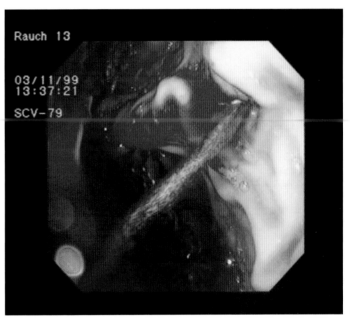

scopic sphincterotomy (EST), as well as needle-knife techniques. Techniques that can be practiced include selective cannulation of the left and right hepatic ducts or the cystic duct, in order to demonstrate guide-wire steering and catheter manipulation. Unihilar and bihilar stent placement can be performed using plastic and metal stents. Bile duct stones can be simulated by inserting pieces of 8.5-Fr or 10-Fr plastic stents with a length of 3–5 mm into the bile duct. Extraction techniques can then be demonstrated using baskets and balloons after EST.

Matthes and Cohen have reported an interesting model called the "neopapilla" [96]. As in the Grund Interphant or Susi simulators, a chicken heart is used to simulate the muscles of the sphincter apparatus. The authors were even able to simulate the human anatomical situation by incorporating a separate bile and pancreatic duct. In addition, it was possible to transfer the papilla deeper into the duodenum.

All organs used for these simulations are subject to veterinary inspection and comply with the relevant food hygiene regulations. The organ packages have to be specifically prepared and adapted to the subjects and objectives of the courses they are being used in. Organs from recently slaughtered animals can be stored for several months in sealed plastic bags at a temperature of about –18 °C. The organs are thawed on the night before the training session.

Since 2002, simple versions of the original compactEASIE and Endo-Trainer simulators have become available. The company Hammerhead Design (Mt. Pleasant, South Carolina) has developed a simple two-part plastic mold similar to the compactEASIE simulator. However, instead of screw pins, this simulator uses a flexible net suspended over the specimen to keep the stomach in position on the mold. The ASGE has also developed a simulator mold similar to the compactEASIE model, known as Endotrainer X, which also uses a plastic net that is fixed over the specimen.

The most recent further development of the compactEASIE simulator is known as EASIE-R (**Fig. 10.6**). The side walls of the EASIE-R model are considerably higher in comparison with compactEASIE, forming a central "bowl." The model allows implantation of organs from the upper as well as lower gastrointestinal tract and can also be used for training in natural orifice transluminal endoscopic surgery (NOTES) procedures. In combination with a special cover, it can be used for combination techniques involving laparoscopy and flexible endoscopy.

10

Table 10.3 Selection of endoscopic interventions for which training can be carried out using the compactEASIE simulator

Training goal	Technique
Ulcer hemostasis	Epinephrine injection Fibrin glue Hemoclipping Thermal probes Argon plasma coagulation
Variceal treatment	Esophageal sclerotherapy Multiple band ligation of esophageal and esophagogastric varices Miniloop application Cyanoacrylate (Histoacryl) Injection of esophageal and esophagogastric varices Experimental techniques (clipping, etc.)
Polypectomy, EMR, vital staining	Conventional polypectomy Polypectomy: stripping technique Polypectomy: Loop Indigo carmine staining (as well as training in the method of applying Lugol solution, ACC + methylene blue; educationally suitable, although there is no active absorption in dead tissue) EMR: stripping technique EMR: band-and-snare technique EMR: distal attachment (Olympus) EMR: experimental techniques—e. g., isolated tip (IT)-knife
ERCP	
Basic	Cannulation, standard Sphincterotomy Stone extraction (balloon, basket) Stenting, plastic Guide-wire exchange techniques (standard and rapid exchange, etc.)
Advanced	Steerable catheters (selective cannulation left/right) Cannulation of difficult papilla, sphincterotome and guide-wire cannulation Precut techniques (needle-knife, etc.) Stricture management (high-pressure balloon, bougienage) Stenting, metal New techniques (bihilar metal stenting, etc.) Cholangioscopy Laser lithotripsy, method of applying "smart lasers"
Tumor treatment and stricture management	Esophageal stenting Duodenal and enteral stenting Balloon dilation Argon plasma coagulation for ablation and diffuse bleeding Laser coagulation

Training Courses

Ways of integrating educational, demonstration, practice, feedback and evaluation into a comprehensive workshop. Regular training workshops on endoscopic hemostasis using the compactEASIE simulator have been available since 1997 in the Department of Medicine at the University of Erlangen-Nuremberg in Germany, and recently in Hildesheim, Germany, as well as in numerous international teaching centers and endoscopy courses provided by national societies throughout the world.

The EASIE group has promoted what is known as the EASIE team-training method for simultaneous training of doctors and nurses in different interventional endoscopic techniques using this type of simulator [35,97–99]. The EASIE team-training method was first

described in detail in 2001 [35]. It consists of a four-block sequence. The first block occurs before actual training; trainees are evaluated individually on the model to assess baseline endoscopy skills. This allows identification of deficiencies in both theoretical knowledge and practical skills. The workshop can then be adjusted in accordance with the pretraining performance evaluation. This evaluation is conducted using supervisors' and fellows' self-assessment forms.

Brain–hand coordination is an essential skill for interventional endoscopy. An important aspect is the ability to convert a thought or intention in the cerebral motor cortex into coordinated three-dimensional movement of the endoscope and associated devices. The position of the device can potentially be influenced by four different sets of controls, each moving in two opposite directions: by turning the vertical (up/down) wheel or horizontal (left/right) wheel of the endoscope, by body movement to the left or right, and by advancing or retracting the device. To be able to perform well-controlled three-dimensional movement of the device, the brain has to integrate all four controls or eight different maneuvering options into a single coordinated direction. The aim is to convert the intention generated in the cerebral hemisphere into a coordinated subhemispheric action that does not require conscious reflection about how to change the position of the device. With repetitive training and developing expertise, the four control mechanisms come to be used in an automated fashion without the need for abstract thinking about how to steer the device in a certain direction. Proficiency in this skill distinguishes the novice from the expert endoscopist.

Basic skills. To assess an individual's capacity for brain–hand coordination, we developed a practical simulator test for manual skills. For this hand–eye dexterity test performed before the training course, four 2–3-mm dots are created on the anterior wall of the ex vivo porcine simulator using a thermal device. The dots are arranged in the form of a square standing on one corner, with a diagonal length of 2 cm. Precision in the brain–hand coordination test can be evaluated by asking the trainee to touch each mark with the probe in a clockwise fashion. The trainees are instructed to "draw" a circle through the four points on the gastric wall with the probe while in an oblique position at close range. Performance is assessed using an ordinal scale from 1 to 10 points (with 1 representing the poorest performance and 10 representing the best). Mistakes are noted when generating the overall score. The time needed to complete the task is also measured. In this exercise, precision is weighted more heavily than speed.

Studies on training using ex vivo simulators (e. g., compactEASIE) for fellows and the EASIE team-training method. In 1997, we initiated the EASIE team-training method for physicians and gastroenterology assistants. Small groups of usually three doctors and their nurses are trained as teams by one skilled endoscopist and one nurse during a 1-day training course [91]. In addition to hemostasis, polypectomy, EMR/ESD, and ERCP courses, training in stricture management and ways of handling complications can be provided. The EASIE model has recently been successfully adapted for providing training in double-balloon enteroscopy, including ERCP in patients who have undergone Roux-en-Y surgery [100].

Since the introduction of the EASIE simulator, considerable efforts have been made to assess the value of additional simulator training using the EASIE model in endoscopic hemostasis. Despite ample and highly positive feedback from participants in the EASIE courses, the data obtained initially represented only the participants' subjective impressions [101]. Several prospective trials have been conducted in recent years to provide objective evidence that participants benefit from simulator training [35,102]. A prospective randomized study conducted by our group in Erlangen in collaboration with the New York Society for Gastrointestinal Endoscopy (NSYGE) was undertaken. The results provided the first evidence of benefit from simulator training in the treatment of upper gastro-

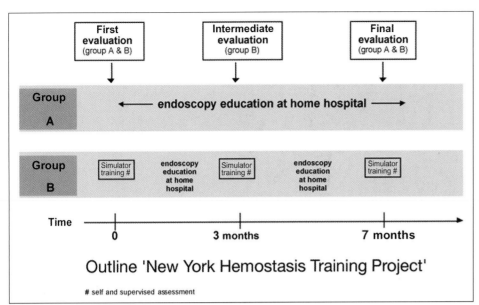

Fig. 10.8 Outline of a prospective and randomized study of training conducted in New York City, comparing conventional clinical education in endoscopic hemostasis provided for14 gastroenterology fellows with 14 fellows who received additional hands-on training in simulators in three 1-day workshops. After a period of 7 months, the intensive training group had significantly improved in all disciplines, while the conventional clinical group had only improved in variceal band ligation [102].

intestinal bleeding [103,104]. In this prospective training project, 37 gastroenterology fellows from nine hospitals in New York were first evaluated in five endoscopic techniques using the compactEASIE simulator [103]. These included manual skills, ulcer hemostasis using injection, a coagulation probe and hemoclipping, as well as variceal band ligation. Technical skills were evaluated and the time needed to complete individuals tasks was recorded. Twenty-eight fellows with comparable skills were then randomly assigned either to an intensive training group attending three 1-day simulator hands-on workshops over a period of 7 months or to a control group only receiving traditional clinical training in endoscopy in their home hospitals (**Fig. 10.8**) [103].

During the 7-month study period, it was demonstrated that the additional simulator training in four endoscopic hemostasis techniques significantly enhanced the participants' skills in comparison with fellows who only received a clinical training. In particular, the evaluation of clinical cases following the training period showed a higher initial hemostasis rate and a lower complication rate among simulator-trained fellows, although the difference in the complication rate was not significant [103]. These results were confirmed in a national training project conducted in France on training in endoscopic hemostasis which started 1 year later, with a similar study design [104,105]. The efficacy of the EASIE simulator was also confirmed in another project including novice endoscopists, in which remarkable levels of skill in hemostatic techniques were achieved using intensified simulator training every second week [106].

A recent study was designed to evaluate the best strategy for education in diagnostic gastroscopy [107]. A three-armed prospective randomized trial was conducted comparing clinical training alone with simulator training alone (computer simulators, plastic phantoms, and partly animal simulators), as well as a combined strategy (with clinical and simulator training) over a 6-month period. A final blinded evaluation was performed in clinical cases as well as in the simulator. In summary, clinical education accompanied by structured simulator training was found to be the best strategy for training in diagnostic gastroscopy. Simulator training alone does not appear to be sufficient for acquiring skills in diagnostic upper gastrointestinal endoscopy [107].

In addition, the value of the EASIE simulator as a tool for testing the efficacy of endoscopic hemostasis devices has been established, opening the way to preclinical testing of new devices in realistic and reliable conditions [108].

Neumann et al. have also published a pilot study using the Erlangen Endo-Trainer for ERCP. An experienced endoscopist and

nurse used the simulator to demonstrate positioning of the duodenoscope, cannulation, guide-wire insertion, sphincterotomy, stone extraction, and plastic stent placement [93]. In 2007, Maiss et al. presented their experience with interventional ERCP training using the compactEASIE biological simulator [106]. They analyzed nine structured training courses from March 1999 to July 2001 designed for team-training groups of three doctors and three nurses per simulator. A total of 188 participants received training. The workshops included three 30-min theoretical lectures and video demonstrations with an introduction to ERCP, sphincterotomy techniques, pathological findings at ERCP, treatment of biliary stones and strictures, as well as pitfalls, tips, and tricks. The course included three blocks of 90 min, 90 min, and 1 h of hands-on training. After demonstration by the tutor, the trainees were supervised in performing papillary cannulation, sphincterotomy techniques, guidewire exchange techniques, stone extraction and stenting. Only advanced trainees received simulator experience in needle-knife techniques and metal stent placement. Each group was instructed by an experienced endoscopist and gastroenterology assistant. At the end of the course, a standardized questionnaire was used to evaluate the course. A total of 132 trainees (78 doctors and 53 nurses, one unspecified) among the 188 trainees (70%) completed the questionnaire. Nearly all of the trainees (97%) rated the training as excellent or good. The participants' evaluation of the single techniques in which training was provided are listed in Table 1 in the article by Maiss et al. Evaluations of the realism of the anatomical environment, optical impression, and tactile feedback are listed in Table 2 [106]. Since then, workshops with different levels of difficulty for beginners, advanced endoscopists, and experts have been developed in Erlangen and Hildesheim, Germany (**Table 10.3**).

Comparison of Teaching Models for Training Courses

Sedlack et al. compared three different ERCP training methods used at an ASGE advanced ERCP training course in February 2002 [85]. A live anesthetized pig model was compared with the compactEASIE ex vivo simulator and the Simbionix GI Mentor ERCP module. Ten course participants and 10 experienced faculty practiced biliary cannulation and other interventional maneuvers for 20–30 min per model and then evaluated the model parameters using a seven-point Likert scale. The compactEASIE porcine model scored highest for realism and usefulness in teaching basic and advanced

10

ERCP skills. The scores for the computer model were significantly lower ($P < 0.05$) than those for the live and compactEASIE porcine models in nearly all areas except for papillary anatomy. The course faculty favored the Erlangen model, whereas the course participants favored the live pig model. Further validation and clinical studies are awaited with ERCP simulation models.

Acquiring Teaching Skills as a Tutor

The benefit of hands-on workshops for the trainee probably lies in a combination of the amount of unsupervised time using the model, expert instruction, high faculty-to-student ratios, and formal skill evaluations with an opportunity for feedback. To make simulator training accessible to more physicians, an expanded number of experts need to receive training on how to use these models to teach others. Potential instructors need to know how to set up the equipment, how to conduct the workshops, and how to evaluate the trainees using the model. The training of tutors who are available over a wide geographic area should make it possible for more simulators to be used locally. This is the only way in which simulator-based workshops can be integrated into standard endoscopy training. An additional benefit of focusing efforts to develop the educational skills of endoscopy instructors that it promotes uniformity in endoscopy training.

For hemostasis training, we conducted a pilot study that examined the feasibility of short "train-the-trainer" sessions to achieve these goals. Seven senior endoscopists without prior EASIE simulator experience were enrolled in the study to serve as a new tutors group. Five expert endoscopists with EASIE team-training experience instructed the new tutors in a 1-day train-the-trainers session. The next day, eight additional gastroenterology fellows attended a 1-day hemostasis workshop conducted by the new tutors group and underwent pretraining and post-training evaluations on the simulator by their instructors. In nearly all of the parameters assessed, fellows under the direction of newly trained trainers made significant progress in just 1 day. Tutors trained in this manner were able to provide an educational experience similar to that provided by experts who had conducted many hands-on workshops.

Open Questions and Future Prospects

Maintaining Skills in Complex Procedures

Simulator training in interventional endoscopy provides an effective opportunity for endoscopy trainees to gain considerable experience in ERCP techniques without time limitations and patient risk. In the New York study on EASIE simulator training in hemostasis, the trainees achieved significant improvement in the performance of multiple skills on the simulator after only three workshops [103]. It appears that a structured educational program with access to simulator training, in addition to supervised real cases in the hospital, would also increase the effectiveness of ERCP education. Such efforts should benefit patients by improving trainees' skill levels before they perform real cases and could result in lower complication rates when trainees are involved with actual cases, leading to better patient outcomes. The results of the real hemostasis cases performed in the New York study highlight this potential [103].

However, there is little doubt that the knowledge and skills gained in hands-on courses decline over time. Little is known about the volume of ERCP cases, for example, needed to maintain skills acquired during these sessions in order to continue to achieve good outcomes. While simulator training has the potential to facilitate the maintenance of ERCP skills as well as to teach individuals how to use new devices in practice, there are no data confirming this. In addition, there are no data regarding the frequency with which refresher courses of this type may be needed [53].

Incorporating Simulator Training into Educational Programs

Simulator training in interventional endoscopy provides an effective opportunity for learning. Modern simulators are able to assess the percentage of the colon surface visualized by the endoscopist. National cancer screening programs could follow up patients with adenomas or colon cancer and include data on individual endoscopists' performance skills. However, it will probably take 10 years for this to be implemented.

The easy accessibility and availability of new endoscopy simulators provides further support for the argument that the trainee should learn basic manual skills outside of patient care. Computer simulators may play an important role during the early phase of endoscopic training, especially in the early stages of colonoscopy [70,71,75–84]. However, for realistic training in complex therapeutic interventions such as ERCP techniques, there are still problems with computer simulators, as they do not simulate tissue elasticity adequately.

Prospects for the future include training interventional endoscopists in special institutions with periods of intensive hands-on training, theoretical lectures, and tests, combined with periods of training in their home institutions as well as in certified teaching hospitals. The training program could finish with a board-certified theoretical examination and hands-on inspection using ex vivo simulator models. This could be accompanied by long-term supervision of the trainee over the first 5 years, including clinical evaluations with visits by auditors.

Training in NOTES and the Future Endoscopic Interventionalist

Minimally invasive laparoscopic surgery and interventional gastrointestinal endoscopy currently appear to be merging, particularly since the development of natural orifice transluminal endoscopic surgery (NOTES) [109]. This new field uses natural orifices to access the abdominal cavity—e. g., by actively opening the anterior gastric wall and introducing a sterile overtube plus a sterile endoscope into the abdomen. Pioneers in this field include Anthony Kalloo at the Johns Hopkins University School of Medicine in Baltimore and the Apollo Group, which he founded with both American and international experts in endoscopy [110,111].

Surgeons are therefore preparing themselves to carry out flexible endoscopy and NOTES and are trying to increase their experience in flexible endoscopy [112]. Simulator training, especially using the EASIE-R simulator, may play an important role in a systematic training curriculum for NOTES interventionalists and for the endoscopic interventionalist of the future.

References

1. Methods of granting hospital privileges to perform gastrointestinal endoscopy. American Society for Gastrointestinal Endoscopy Standards of Training and Practice Committee. Gastrointest Endosc 1992;38:765–7.
2. Farthing M, Walt RP, Allan RN, Swan CH, Gilmore I, Mallinson CN. A national training programme for gastroenterology and hepatology. Gut 1996;38:459–70.
3. Conjoint Committee for Recognition of Training in Gastrointestinal Endoscopy. Information for supervisors: changes to endoscopic training. Sydney: Conjoint Committee for Recognition of Training in Gastrointestinal Endoscopy, 1997.

4. Beattie AD, Greff M, Lamy V, Mallinson CN. The European Diploma of Gastroenterology: progress towards harmonization of standards. Eur J Gastroenterol Hepatol 1996;8:403–6.

5. American Society for Gastrointestinal Endoscopy. Trainee evaluation form. Manchester, Massachusetts: American Society for Gastrointestinal Endoscopy; 1982.

6. Haseman JH, Lemmel GT, Rahmani EY, Rex DK. Failure of colonoscopy to detect colorectal cancer: evaluation of 47 cases in 20 hospitals. Gastrointest Endosc 1997;45:451–5.

7. Federation of Digestive Disease Societies. Guidelines for training in endoscopy. Manchester, Massachusetts: Federation of Digestive Disease Societies; 1981.

8. Parry BR, Williams SM. Competency and the colonoscopist: a learning curve. Aust N Z J Surg 1991;61:419–22.

9. Godreau CJ. Office-based colonoscopy in a family practice. Fam Pract Res J 2001;12:313–20.

10. Rodney WM, Dabov G, Cronin C. Evolving colonoscopy skills in a rural family practice: the first 293 cases. Fam Pract Res J 1993;13:43–52.

11. Cass OW, Freeman ML, Peine CJ, Zera RT, Onstad GR. Objective evaluation of endoscopy skills during training. Ann Intern Med 1993;118:40–4.

12. Cass OW. Acquisition of competency in endoscopic skills during training: a multicenter study [abstract]. Gastrointest Endosc 1996;43:308A.

13. Church J. Learning colonoscopy: the need for patience (patients). Am J Gastroenterol 1993;88:1569.

14. Church J. Training. In: Church J, ed. Endoscopy of the colon, rectum and anus. New York: Igaku-Shoin; 1995. p. 214–25.

15. Marshall JB. Technical proficiency of trainees performing colonoscopy: a learning curve. Gastrointest Endosc 1995;42:287–91.

16. Chak A, Cooper GS, Blades EW, Canto M, Sivak MV Jr. Prospective assessment of colonoscopic intubation skills in trainees. Gastrointest Endosc 1996;44:54–7.

17. Hopper W, Kyker KA, Rodney WM. Colonoscopy by a family physician: a 9-year experience of 1048 procedures. J Fam Pract 1996;43:561–6.

18. Tassios PS, Ladas SD, Grammenos I, Demertzis K, Raptis SA. Acquisition of competence in colonoscopy: the learning curve of trainees. Endoscopy 1999;31:702–6.

19. Wigton RS. Measuring procedural skills. Ann Intern Med 1996;125:1003–4.

20. Wigton RS, Blank LL, Monsour H, Nicolas JA. Procedural skills of practicing gastroenterologists. A national survey of 700 members of the American College of Physicians. Ann Intern Med 1990;113:540–6.

21. Wigton RS, Nicolas JA, Blank LL. Procedural skills of the general internist: a survey of 25 000 physicians. Ann Intern Med 1989;111:1023–34.

22. Wigton RS, Steinmann WC. Procedural skills training in the internal medicine residency. J Med Educ 1984;59:392–400.

23. American Board of Internal Medicine. Results of procedure survey of gastroenterology program directors. Am Board Intern Med Newsl Spring/Summer 1990:4–5.

24. Cass OW. Objective evaluation of competence: technical skills in gastrointestinal endoscopy. Endoscopy 1995;27:86–9.

25. Church JM. Complete colonoscopy: how often? And if not, why not? Am J Gastroenterol 1994;89:556–60.

26. Church J, Oakley J, Milsom J, Strong S, Hull T. Colonoscopy training: the need for patience (patients). ANZ J Surg 2002;72:89–91.

27. American Association for the Study of Liver Diseases; American College of Gastroenterology; American Gastroenterological Association (AGA) Institute; American Society for Gastrointestinal Endoscopy. The Gastroenterology Core Curriculum, third edition. Gastroenterology 2007;132:2012–8.

28. Sarker SK, Albrani T, Zaman A, Patel B. Procedural performance in gastrointestinal endoscopy: an assessment and self-appraisal tool. Am J Surg 2008;196:450–5.

29. Baron TH, Petersen BT, Mergener K, Chak A, Cohen J, Deal SE, et al. Quality indicators for endoscopic retrograde cholangiopancreatography. Am J Gastroenterol 2006;101:892–7.

30. Renewal of endoscopic privileges: guidelines for clinical application. From the ASGE. American Society for Gastrointestinal Endoscopy. Gastrointest Endosc 1999;49:823–5.

31. Principles of training in gastrointestinal endoscopy. From the ASGE. American Society for Gastrointestinal Endoscopy. Gastrointest Endosc 1999;49:845–53.

32. Guidelines for credentialing and granting privileges for gastrointestinal endoscopy. American Society for Gastrointestinal Endoscopy. Gastrointest Endosc 1998;48:679–82.

33. Position statement. Maintaining competency in endoscopic skills. American Society for Gastrointestinal Endoscopy. Gastrointest Endosc 1995;42:620–1.

34. Gastroenterology Leadership Council. Training the gastroenterologist of the future: the gastroenterology core curriculum. Gastroenterology 1996;110:1266–300.

35. Hochberger J, Maiss J, Magdeburg B, Cohen J, Hahn EG. Training simulators and education in gastrointestinal endoscopy: current status and perspectives in 2001. Endoscopy 2001;33:541–9.

36. Hochberger J, Tex S, Maiss J, Hahn EG. Management of difficult common bile duct stones. Gastrointest Endosc Clin N Am 2003;13:623–34.

37. Carr-Locke DL. Cholelithiasis plus choledocholithiasis: ERCP first, what next? Gastroenterology 2006;130:270–2.

38. NIH state-of-the-science statement on endoscopic retrograde cholangiopancreatography (ERCP) for diagnosis and therapy. NIH Consens State Sci Statements 2002;19:1–26.

39. Hochberger J, Bayer J, May A, Muhldorfer S, Maiss J, Hahn EG, et al. Laser lithotripsy of difficult bile duct stones: results in 60 patients using a rhodamine 6G dye laser with optical stone tissue detection system. Gut 1998;43:823–9.

40. Hochberger J, Bayer J, Maiss J, Tex S, Hahn EG. [Clinical results with a new frequency-doubled, double pulse Nd:YAG laser (FREDDY) for lithotripsy in complicated choledocholithiasis]. Biomed Tech (Berl) 1998;43(Suppl):172.

41. Kozarek R. Role of ERCP in acute pancreatitis. Gastrointest Endosc 2002;56:S 231–6.

42. Carr-Locke DL, Conn MI, Faigel DO, Laing K, Leung JW, Mills MR, et al. Technology status evaluation: magnetic resonance cholangiopancreatography: November 1998. From the ASGE. American Society for Gastrointestinal Endoscopy. Gastrointest Endosc 1999;49:858–61.

43. Mergener K, Kozarek RA. Therapeutic pancreatic endoscopy. Endoscopy 2005;37:201–7.

44. Jowell PS, Baillie J, Branch MS, Affronti J, Browning CL, Bute BP. Quantitative assessment of procedural competence. A prospective study of training in endoscopic retrograde cholangiopancreatography. Ann Intern Med 1996;125:983–9.

45. Freeman ML. Adverse outcomes of endoscopic retrograde cholangiopancreatography: avoidance and management. Gastrointest Endosc Clin N Am 2003;13:775–98, xi.

46. Freeman ML, Nelson DB, Sherman S, Haber GB, Herman ME, Dorsher PJ, et al. Complications of endoscopic biliary sphincterotomy. N Engl J Med 1996;335:909–18.

47. Huibregtse K. Complications of endoscopic sphincterotomy and their prevention. N Engl J Med 1996;335:961–3.

48. Rabenstein T, Hahn EG. Post-ERCP pancreatitis: is the endoscopist's experience the major risk factor? JOP 2002;3:177–87.

49. Cotton PB. Analysis of 59 ERCP lawsuits: mainly about indications. Gastrointest Endosc 2006;63:378–82.

50. Cotton PB. Evaluating ERCP is important but difficult. Gut 2002;51:287–9.

51. Chutkan RK, Ahmad AS, Cohen J, Cruz-Correa MR, Desilets DJ, Dominitz JA, et al. ERCP core curriculum. Gastrointest Endosc 2006;63:361–76.

52. Hochberger J, Maiss J, Hahn EG. The use of simulators for training in GI endoscopy. Endoscopy 2002;34:727–9.

53. Jowell PS. Endoscopic retrograde cholangiopancreatography: toward a better understanding of competence. Endoscopy 1999;31:755–7.

54. Schutz SM, Abbott RM. Grading ERCPs by degree of difficulty: a new concept to produce more meaningful outcome data. Gastrointest Endosc 2000;51:535–9.

55. Kowalski T, Kanchana T, Pungpapong S. Perceptions of gastroenterology fellows regarding ERCP competency and training. Gastrointest Endosc 2003;58:345–9.

56. Hochberger J, Menke D, Maiss J. ERCP training. In: Baron TH, Kozarek R, Carr-Locke DL, editors. ERCP. Philadelphia: Saunders/Elsevier; 2008. p. 61–72.

57. Carr-Locke DL. Videoendoscopy in clinical application. Impact on teaching. Endoscopy 1990;22(Suppl 1):19–21.

58. Carr-Locke DL, Gostout CJ, Van Dam J. A guideline for live endoscopy courses: an ASGE White Paper. Gastrointest Endosc 2001;53:685–8.

59. Devière J, Hochberger J, Neuhaus H, Ponchon T, Eugenidis N, Neumann C, et al. Recommendations of the ESGE workshop on ethical, clinical, and economic dilemmas arising from the implementation of new techniques. First European Symposium on Ethics in Gastroenterology and Digestive Endoscopy, Kos, Greece, June 2003. Endoscopy 2003;35:768–71.

60. Classen M. [Endoscopy of the digestive tract in the continuing education of internists and gastroenterologist]. Internist (Berl) 1982;23:243–4.

61. Williams CB. Fiberoptic colonoscopy: teaching. Dis Colon Rectum 1976;19:395–9.

10

62. Axon AT, Aabakken L, Malfertheiner P, Danielides I, Ladas S, Hochberger J, et al. Recommendations of the ESGE workshop on ethics in teaching and learning endoscopy. First European Symposium on Ethics in Gastroenterology and Digestive Endoscopy, Kos, Greece, June 2003. Endoscopy 2003;35:761–4.

63. Waye JD. Teaching basic endoscopy. Gastrointest Endosc 2000;51:375–7.

64. Williams CB, Baillie J, Gillies DF, Borislow D, Cotton PB. Teaching gastrointestinal endoscopy by computer simulation: a prototype for colonoscopy and ERCP. Gastrointest Endosc 1990;36:49–54.

65. Frakes JT. An evaluation of performance after informal training in endoscopic retrograde sphincterotomy. Am J Gastroenterol 1986;81:512–5.

66. Lange V, Grund KE. [Education in intraluminal endoscopy—experiences up to now]. Chirurg 2001;72(Suppl):164–5.

67. Gerson LB, Van Dam J. Technology review: the use of simulators for training in GI endoscopy. Gastrointest Endosc 2004;60:992–1001.

68. Noar MD. Endoscopy simulation: a brave new world? Endoscopy 1991;23:147–9.

69. Noar MD. Robotics interactive endoscopy simulation of ERCP/sphincterotomy and EGD. Endoscopy 1992;24(Suppl 2):S39–41.

70. Noar MD, Soehendra N. Endoscopy simulation training devices. Endoscopy 1992;24:159–66.

71. Bar-Meir S. A new endoscopic simulator. Endoscopy 2000;32:898–900.

72. Sedlack RE, Kolars JC. Colonoscopy curriculum development and performance-based assessment criteria on a computer-based endoscopy simulator. Acad Med 2002;77:750–1.

73. Sedlack RE, Kolars JC. Validation of a computer-based colonoscopy simulator. Gastrointest Endosc 2003;57:214–8.

74. Sedlack RE, Baron TH, Downing SM, Schwartz AJ. Validation of a colonoscopy simulation model for skills assessment. Am J Gastroenterol 2007;102:64–74.

75. Sedlack RE, Kolars JC. Computer simulator training enhances the competency of gastroenterology fellows at colonoscopy: results of a pilot study. Am J Gastroenterol 2004;99:33–7.

76. Dunkin BJ. Flexible endoscopy simulators. Semin Laparosc Surg 2003;10:29–35.

77. MacDonald J, Ketchum J, Williams RG, Rogers LQ. A lay person versus a trained endoscopist: can the preop endoscopy simulator detect a difference? Surg Endosc 2003;17:896–8.

78. Ladas SD, Malfertheiner P, Axon A. An introductory course for training in endoscopy. Dig Dis 2002;20:242–5.

79. Aabakken L, Adamsen S, Kruse A. Performance of a colonoscopy simulator: experience from a hands-on endoscopy course. Endoscopy 2000;32:911–3.

80. Ferlitsch A, Glauninger P, Gupper A, Schillinger M, Haefner M, Gangl A, et al. Evaluation of a virtual endoscopy simulator for training in gastrointestinal endoscopy. Endoscopy 2002;34:698–702.

81. Datta V, Mandalia M, Mackay S, Darzi A. The PreOp flexible sigmoidoscopy trainer. Validation and early evaluation of a virtual reality based system. Surg Endosc 2002;16:1459–63.

82. Gerson LB, Van Dam J. The future of simulators in GI endoscopy: an unlikely possibility or a virtual reality? Gastrointest Endosc 2002;55:608–11.

83. Williams CB, Saunders BP, Bladen JS. Development of colonoscopy teaching simulation. Endoscopy 2000;32:901–5.

84. Baillie J, Jowell P, Evangelou H, Bickel W, Cotton P. Teaching by endoscopy simulation. Endoscopy 1991;23:239–40.

85. Sedlack R, Petersen B, Binmoeller K, Kolars J. A direct comparison of ERCP teaching models. Gastrointest Endosc 2003;57:886–90.

86. Sedlack RE, Petersen BT, Kolars JC. The impact of a hands-on ERCP workshop on clinical practice. Gastrointest Endosc 2005;61:67–71.

87. Noar MD. An established porcine model for animate training in diagnostic and therapeutic ERCP. Endoscopy 1995;27:77–80.

88. Gholson CF, Provenza JM, Silver RC, Bacon BR. Endoscopic retrograde cholangiography in the swine: a new model for endoscopic training and hepatobiliary research. Gastrointest Endosc 1990;36:600–3.

89. Gholson CF, Provenza JM, Doyle JT, Bacon BR. Endoscopic retrograde sphincterotomy in swine. Dig Dis Sci 1991;36:1406–9.

90. Hochberger J, Neumann M, Hohenberger W, Hahn EG. Neuer Endoskopie-Trainer für die therapeutische flexible Endoskopie [abstract]. Z Gastroenterol 1997;35:722–3.

91. Hochberger J, Neumann M, Maiss J, Hohenberger W, Hahn EG. EASIE—Erlangen Active Simulator for Interventional Endoscopy—a new bio-simulation model—first experiences gained in training workshops [abstract]. Gastrointest Endosc 1998;47(Suppl):AB116.

92. Szinicz G, Beller S, Bodner W, Zerz A, Glaser K. Simulated operations by pulsatile organ-perfusion in minimally invasive surgery. Surg Laparosc Endosc 1993;3:315–7.

93. Neumann M, Hochberger J, Felzmann T, Ell C, Hohenberger W. Part 1. The Erlanger endo-trainer. Endoscopy 2001;33:887–90.

94. Neumann M, Mayer G, Ell C, Felzmann T, Reingruber B, Horbach T, et al. The Erlangen Endo-Trainer: life-like simulation for diagnostic and interventional endoscopic retrograde cholangiography. Endoscopy 2000;32:906–10.

95. Hochberger J, Euler K, Naegel A, Hahn EG, Maiss J. The compact Erlangen Active Simulator for Interventional Endoscopy: a prospective comparison in structured team-training courses on "endoscopic hemostasis" for doctors and nurses to the "Endo-Trainer" model. Scand J Gastroenterol 2004;39:895–902.

96. Matthes K, Cohen J. The Neo-Papilla: a new modification of porcine ex vivo simulators for ERCP training (with videos). Gastrointest Endosc 2006;64:570–6.

97. Hochberger J, Maiss J, Neumann M, Hildebrand V, Bayer J, Hahn EG. EASIE-team-training in endoscopic hemostasis—acceptance of a systematic training in interventional endoscopy by 134 trainees [abstract]. Gastrointest Endosc 1999;49:AB143.

98. Maiss J, Nägel A, Tex S, Hahn EG, Hochberger J. EASIE-team-training ERCP—experiences with a new training concept for interventional ERCP. Endoscopy 2000;32:E65.

99. Hochberger J, Maiss J, Nägel A, Tex S, Hahn EG. Polypectomy, endoscopic staining techniques, mucosectomy—a new structured team training course in a close to reality endoscopy simulator (EASIE). Endoscopy 2000;32:E23.

100. Maiss J, Diebel H, Naegel A, Muller B, Hochberger J, Hahn EG, et al. A novel model for training in ERCP with double-balloon enteroscopy after abdominal surgery. Endoscopy 2007;39:1072–5.

101. Maiss J, Hahn EG, Hochberger J. A prospective evaluation of 14 EASIE Team-Trainings-Workshops on endoscopic hemostasis. Endoscopy 2000;32:E23.

102. Hochberger J, Maiss J. Currently available simulators: ex vivo models. Gastrointest Endosc Clin N Am 2006;16:435–49.

103. Hochberger J, Matthes K, Maiss J, Koebnick C, Hahn EG, Cohen J. Training with the compactEASIE biologic endoscopy simulator significantly improves hemostatic technical skill of gastroenterology fellows: a randomized controlled comparison with clinical endoscopy training alone. Gastrointest Endosc 2005;61:204–15.

104. Maiss J, Wiesnet J, Proeschel A, Matthes K, Prat F, Cohen J, et al. Objective benefit of a 1-day training course in endoscopic hemostasis using the "compactEASIE" endoscopy simulator. Endoscopy 2005;37:552–8.

105. Maiss J, Prat F, Wiesnet J, Proeschel A, Matthes K, Peters A, et al. The complementary Erlangen active simulator for interventional endoscopy training is superior to solely clinical education in endoscopic hemostasis—the French training project: a prospective trial. Eur J Gastroenterol Hepatol 2006;18:1217–25.

106. Maiss J, Millermann L, Heinemann K, Naegel A, Peters A, Matthes K, et al. The compactEASIE is a feasible training model for endoscopic novices: a prospective randomised trial. Dig Liver Dis 2007;39:70–80.

107. Ende A, Zopf Y, Naegel A, Heide R, Hahn EG, Maiss J. Strategies for training in diagnostic upper GI-endoscopy. Gut 2007;56(Suppl III):A2.

108. Maiss J, Baumbach C, Zopf Y, Naegel A, Wehler M, Bernatik T, et al. Hemodynamic efficacy of the new resolution clip device in comparison with high-volume injection therapy in spurting bleeding: a prospective experimental trial using the compactEASIE simulator. Endoscopy 2006;38:808–12.

109. Rattner D, Kalloo A. ASGE/SAGES Working Group on Natural Orifice Transluminal Endoscopic Surgery. October 2005. Surg Endosc 2006;20:329–33.

110. Kalloo AN, Singh VK, Jagannath SB, Niiyama H, Hill SL, Vaughn CA, et al. Flexible transgastric peritoneoscopy: a novel approach to diagnostic and therapeutic interventions in the peritoneal cavity. Gastrointest Endosc 2004;60:114–7.

111. Kantsevoy SV, Jagannath SB, Niiyama H, Chung SS, Cotton PB, Gostout CJ, et al. Endoscopic gastrojejunostomy with survival in a porcine model. Gastrointest Endosc 2005;62:287–92.

112. Morales MP, Mancini GJ, Miedema BW, Rangnekar NJ, Koivunen DG, Ramshaw BJ, et al. Integrated flexible endoscopy training during surgical residency. Surg Endosc 2008;22:2013–7.

IV Diagnostic Procedures and Techniques

Section editors:
Meinhard Classen, Guido N.J. Tytgat, Michael B. Wallace

Upper Gastrointestinal Endoscopy

Michel Delvaux and Gérard Gay

Esophagogastroduodenoscopy (EGD), also often called "gastroscopy" or "fibroscopy," has become the gold standard for endoscopic examination of the upper gastrointestinal tract down to the second part of the duodenum. It allows the complete examination of the mucosa of the esophagus, stomach, and proximal duodenum.

During the historical development of EGD, various attempts were made to visualize the gastric mucosa using semirigid endoscopes, which were poorly tolerated by patients and were difficult to use, with a high risk of perforation [1,2]. The era of modern EGD started in 1957, with the first report by Hirschowitz et al. of the use of a flexible endoscope equipped with bundles of optical fibers [3]. EGD then rapidly expanded, benefiting from the introduction of electronic endoscopes during the 1980s. The technique for the procedure has been standardized for routine examinations, and in the meantime EGD has also made it possible to develop numerous additional procedures, increasing its diagnostic yield in many pathological conditions and allowing them to be treated endoscopically.

This chapter describes the technical characteristics of the current endoscopes used to perform EGD, the additional procedures available through EGD, the normal anatomy of the upper gastrointestinal tract as observed during an EGD, the indications and contraindications for the procedure, and the complications.

Technical Description of the Gastroscope

The standard fiber and video gastroscopes in use nowadays have direct forward viewing and a four-directional banding facility at the tip, controlled by two wheels. They are equipped with an air/water injection channel, allowing insufflation of the digestive tract and cleaning of the optical lens during the procedure, and an operating channel linked to a suction device, which makes it possible to remove liquid or excessive air during the procedure and to insert instruments for additional procedures (**Fig. 11.1**). Most procedures are currently carried out using electronic video endoscopes, with which the image is captured by an electronic chip (charge-coupled device, CCD) at the tip of the endoscope and is displayed on an external monitor in real time. The latest endoscopes have a wide angle of view (usually 140–150°) and high-definition imaging with over 1.4 million pixels. Fiberscopes are still helpful in emergency situations, as they can be transported to the bedside in intensive-care units. Video gastroscopes used in everyday practice are less than 10 mm in diameter at the level of the shaft and have a 2.8-mm working channel, allowing the insertion of standard instruments such as biopsy forceps, polypectomy snares, and injection needles.

Modified endoscopes have been developed for specific situations in therapeutic endoscopy and to provide new diagnostic features. Therapeutic gastroscopes are equipped with larger operating channels (3.8–4.2 mm). Double-channel gastroscopes allow two devices to be inserted simultaneously and have at least one large operating channel. More recently, an interesting prototype has been released for endoscopic submucosal dissection, with two operating channels each equipped with a perpendicular elevator (Olympus XGIF-2TQ240R). Endoscopes with large working channels are needed for the insertion of through-the-scope prostheses for palliative treatment of malignant stenoses [4].

Diagnostic tools have also been incorporated into the latest endoscopes, increasing the quality of mucosal examination of the mucosa. High-definition endoscopes have a larger number of pixels and provide a larger and more detailed image on the monitor [5]. Some endoscope series are equipped with powerful zoom capabilities [6]. The magnifying examination of the mucosa, combined with chromoendoscopy either with natural dyes or using electronic image processing [7,8] increases the diagnostic yield for small flat malignant lesions [9].

Pediatric endoscopes have been developed for procedures in infants and children under the age of 7. These endoscopes are thinner than the usual gastroscopes, with an external shaft diameter from 5.8 to 8.5 mm [10]. Some of these thin endoscopes have an operating channel of 2.2 mm, so that it is only possible to insert specially designed accessories for therapeutic endoscopy.

Transnasal gastroscopy has been developed to improve the tolerance of the procedure by unsedated patients, avoiding the nausea induced by stimulation of the uvula [11]. However, a controlled study showed that patients experienced more pain and discomfort during transnasal endoscope insertion than during transoral insertion [12], and in another study, the use of local anesthesia did not show any significant benefit [13]. In a large multicenter trial in France, nasogastroscopy appeared to be feasible in 93 % of patients, but the results were still better with the standard peroral gastroscopy [14]. The place of transnasal gastroscopy in everyday practice remains to be defined; some thin endoscopes have a banding mechanism limited to one plane. On the other hand, the need to buy a new endoscope needs to be taken into account, as well recent developments in capsule endoscopy that could be of interest in connection with screening for esophageal diseases [15].

Table 11.1 summarizes the main technical characteristics of currently available gastroscopes.

Description of the Procedure

▪ Sedation

EGD is usually performed without general anesthesia and with or without conscious sedation, depending on local resources and usual practices, as well as on the extent of the patient's compliance and the purpose of the examination. Deep sedation or general anesthesia is preferred for therapeutic procedures that may require a long examination time, or when chromoendoscopy is used. The presence of liquids or food residues in the esophagus represents a risk of reflux and aspiration into the trachea—e. g., during EGD with chromoendoscopy, or in patients with active bleeding and a large quantity of blood in the stomach. In patients with active bleeding, it is usually recommended either not to use any sedation or to perform the examination with the patient under general anesthesia with tracheal intubation [16].

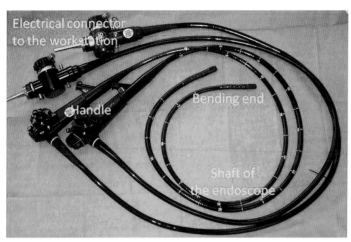

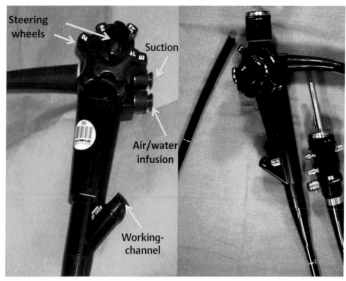

a

b

c

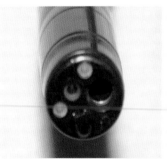

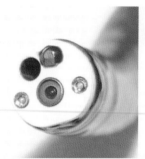

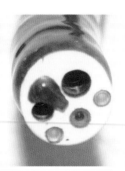

Fig. 11.1 Endoscopes commonly used for upper gastrointestinal endoscopy.
a Video endoscopes currently used in video gastroscopy.
b Close-up view of the handle, showing the control wheels.
c A fiberscope.
d The distal ends of various types of endoscope used for diagnostic and therapeutic upper gastrointestinal endoscopy. 1, Common video endoscope 2, zoom video endoscope; 3, Two-channel therapeutic video endoscope; 4, duodenoscope (side-viewing); 5, prototype endoscope for endoscopic dissection.

11

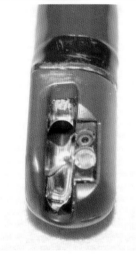

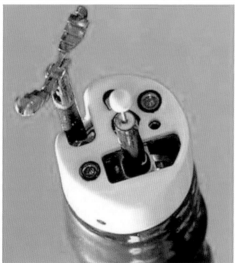

d

Preparation of the Patient

The patient should fast from midnight and avoid smoking. Loose clothing is recommended and the belt should be left open. The patient must be informed of the nature of the procedure and the associated risks, and consent should be obtained before the procedure. The clinical interview and physical examinations should identify any contraindications. Clothing tests must be checked, especially when a therapeutic procedure is scheduled.

Local anesthesia in the throat may help prevent a gag reflex during the insertion of the endoscope into the hypopharynx. The patient is placed in the left lateral position with a cushion under the head and is asked to bend the head forward so that the chin is near the chest wall. This position allows wider opening of the hypopharynx and easier insertion of the endoscope. A mouthpiece is then placed between the teeth to protect the endoscope during the examination.

Insertion of the Endoscope

The endoscope is usually inserted under direct visual control, down to the upper esophageal sphincter. The patient is then asked to swallow, and the endoscope is pushed gently into the esophagus. Infusing a small amount of water with the endoscope's wash pump may help the patient trigger the swallow. Insertion under visual control is preferable as it is safer, especially in elderly patients, who have a higher incidence of Zenker diverticulum.

Alternatively, the endoscope can be inserted blindly, directed by the index and middle fingers of the examiner's left hand, which are

Table 11.1 Technical characteristics of the various types of endoscope used in upper gastrointestinal endoscopy

	Viewing angle	Optical characteristics	Shaft outer diameter (mm)	Working length (cm)	Operating channel (mm)	Use
Ordinary gastroscopes (forward-viewing)						
Fiberscope	105–120°	Image provided by a bundle of optical fibers	9–11	100–105	2.8	Emergency endoscopy
Video gastroscope	140°		8.8–9.8	105–110	2.8	Routine EGD
Zoom video gastroscope	140°	Magnification, zoom	11.5	105–110	2.8	Routine EGD, chromoendo-scopy
HD gastroscope	140°	Zoom, high-definition image with 1080 scanning lines	9.8	105–110	2.8	Electronic chromoendoscopy (NBI, FICE)
Nasogastroscope	120°		5.8	110	2.0	Transnasal insertion, pediatric patients, patients with tight stenoses
Pediatric gastroscope	140°		5.8–8.8	100–110	2.2	Pediatric patients, patients with tight stenoses
Duodenoscopes (Lateral view)						
Video endoscope	100°		11.5–13.1	125–140	2.8–4.2	Examination of the duodenum and papilla area; ERCP
Therapeutic gastroscopes						
One large channel	140°		10.8	105–110	3.2–4.2	Therapeutic endoscopy
Two channels	140°		12.6	105–110	2.8/3.7–4.2	EMR, ESD
ESD prototype Olympus XGIF-2TQ 240R	140°	Zoom, magnification, HD		105–110		ESD

EGD, esophagogastroduodenoscopy; EMR, endoscopic mucosal resection; ERCP, endoscopic retrograde cholangiopancreatography; ESD, endoscopic submucosal dissection; FICE, Fujinon Intelligent Chromoendoscopy; HG, high definition; NBI, narrow-band imaging.

introduced into the mouth to depress the tongue. When the tip of the endoscope encounters some resistance, the patient is then instructed to swallow, while gentle pressure is applied until the cricopharyngeal sphincter has been passed. Blind intubation may be more difficult with thin endoscopes, as they may coil in the lateral sinus. On the other hand, a Zenker diverticulum may be overlooked, increasing the risk of pharyngeal perforation.

After intubation, the endoscope is pushed along the esophagus and the stomach down to the second part of the duodenum. Excessive air insufflation, which can make the access to the pylorus more difficult, should be avoided. Careful inspection of the mucosal surface has to be carried out both during scope insertion and during slow withdrawal of the instrument (see below).

▦ Advancement of the Endoscope and Maneuvering for a Complete Examination

The various maneuvers used to achieve complete visualization of the esophagus, stomach, and duodenum are illustrated in **Fig. 11.2**. The procedure starts with an examination of the esophageal mucosa. When the endoscope has entered the esophageal lumen, it is slowly pushed down to the lower third of the esophagus—i.e., approximately 30 cm from the incisors. Careful examination of the distal esophagus and esophagogastric junction is carried out before the scope is passed through the cardia into the stomach. Examination of the upper third of the esophagus—i.e., the segment between the upper esophageal sphincter and 20 cm from the incisors—is usually better carried out at the end of the procedure, during withdrawal of the endoscope.

Examination of the stomach requires a systematic sequence of maneuvers that allow visualization of all segments of it, particularly of areas that cannot be examined during advancement of the endoscope. It is preferable to examine the stomach after examining the duodenum, in order to avoid excessive air insufflation. The anatomical axes of the esophageal and gastric lumina are almost perpendicular. Advancement into the duodenum is therefore achieved by pushing the endoscope along the lesser curvature by means of 60–80° clockwise rotation, avoiding rubbing of the tip of the endoscope on the anterior wall. Advancement continues with a gentle downward flexion of the tip of the endoscope, bringing it in front of the pylorus. When the endoscope is pulled back in the stomach after examination of the duodenum, the instrument is rotated along its axis to allow examination of the whole circumference of the antral mucosa and gastric body mucosa. The fundus can be observed only during the retroflexion of the endoscope. To achieve this maneuver, the tip of the endoscope is placed almost in the middle of the antrum and a complete upward flexion is performed; at the same time, the endoscope is pushed down in the direction of the pylorus. This allows visualization of the angular incisure and then the lesser curvature. Finally, the endoscope is pulled back with 180° counterclockwise rotation to enter the fundus in a retrograde fashion and examine the gastric side of the cardia and fundus. At this point, the endoscope can be seen emerging from the esophagus.

The duodenal bulb is intubated by advancing the tip of the scope as closely as possible to the pyloric ring and then applying gentle pressure; usually, however, the tip of the endoscope comes close to the mucosa of the anterior wall of the bulb. After sufficient air has been used to inflate the bulb, the mucosa is examined during a few forward–backward movements with the endoscope. To enter the second part of the duodenum, the tip of the scope placed at the end of the bulb is flexed rightward and rotated 90° clockwise. During the passage through the genu superius, where the endoscope is often blindly pushed forward and the tip is bent upward. Once it has reached the second part of the duodenum, the endoscope can be inserted deeper by pulling it back and rotating it 120–180° clockwise.

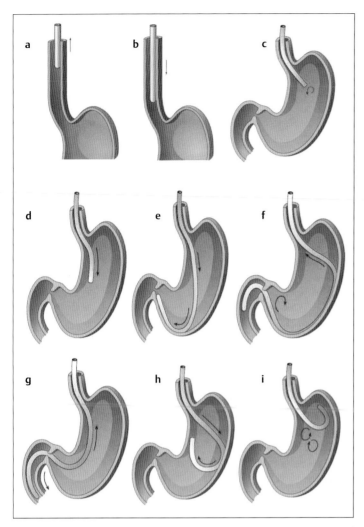

Fig. 11.2 Advancement of the endoscope in the upper gastrointestinal tract, showing the different phases of a complete examination of the upper tract.
a Examination of the proximal esophagus.
b Examination of the distal esophagus and esophageal side of the cardia.
c The endoscope advances into the stomach. The upper part is examined without insufflation, with gentle rotation to enter the distal part.
d Advancement along the lesser curvature.
e Advancing in the antrum down to the pylorus. The endoscope follows the greater curvature and leans on it to reach the pylorus.
f The endoscope is passed through the pylorus to examine the duodenal bulb and is then pushed gently forward through the genu superius to the vertical part of the duodenum.
g By pulling the endoscope back and rotating it counterclockwise, the endoscope enters deeper into the second part of the duodenum.
h During withdrawal, the endoscope is flexed in a retrograde fashion for examination of the fundus and lesser curvature, from the angular incisure.
i Continuing to pull back the endoscope during retroflexion results in a closer view of the gastric side of the cardia.

After the Procedure

Before the endoscope is withdrawn from the patient, air and fluids should be aspirated from the stomach as completely as possible to prevent postprocedural bloating and the risk of false passage into the airways, especially in patients who have received local anesthesia in the throat. For the same reason, the patients should be instructed not to drink or eat for at least 90–120 min after the end of the procedure. Patients who have undergone sedation or general anesthesia will require appropriate postprocedural surveillance.

Normal Endoscopic Anatomy of the Upper Gastrointestinal Tract

This section discusses the normal anatomy of the upper gastrointestinal tract, with the anatomical landmarks used in the procedure and for locating any findings. The various endoscopic patterns are shown in **Fig. 11.3**, where the images are arranged in the same sequence as in the various phases of advancement of the endoscope shown in **Fig. 11.2**.

Esophagus

The esophagus is anatomically divided into three parts:
- The cervical esophagus, from the upper esophageal sphincter or cricopharyngeal sphincter, located at approximately 16 cm from the incisors, to the entry of the esophagus into the chest, 2 or 3 cm down. This lower boundary is not visible at endoscopy.
- The intrathoracic part, which is almost 20 cm long and ends when the esophagus enters the abdominal cavity through the diaphragm, at approximately 38–40 cm from the incisors.
- The intra-abdominal part is short and can be seen during endoscopy. It ends at the esophagogastric junction on the mucosal side and the lower esophageal sphincter.

At 25 cm, the aorta crosses the esophagus and appears as an external compression on the left side of the lumen. The location of findings in the esophagus is usually defined by their distance from the incisors. The upper and lower limits of the lesion and its circumferential extent are given. The normal esophageal mucosa appears flat, with a pink color, and corresponds to the squamous epithelium. The transition to gastric mucosa, which often appears orange, is described as the Z line, as it looks like a broken line.

Various terms are used in everyday practice to describe the area of the esophagogastric junction; they are usually regarded as synonyms, and confusion has occurred as a result. An attempt was made to clarify the situation in the Minimal Standard Terminology for Digestive Endoscopy [17] and more recently by the Consensus Conference on Barrett's Esophagus [18]. The term "lower esophageal sphincter" is difficult to identify endoscopically, as it is a functional entity and cannot be used as a fixed point for locating an individual lesion. The term "esophagogastric junction" implies a transition from the esophagus to the stomach, and it is usually characterized by the level of the mucosal junction (Z line). The word "hiatus" refers to the orifice in the diaphragm, which can be difficult to identify, and this tends to cause difficulties when defining a hiatus hernia. Finally, the term "cardia" characterizes the part of the gastric cavity that surrounds the entrance of the lower end of the esophagus. In patients with normal anatomy, these entities are located almost at the same level, but difficulties occur in patients with a hiatus hernia or Barrett's esophagus. Following initial testing of the terminology, it became apparent that it led to problems in descriptions of a hiatus hernia or the length of a Barrett's esophagus segment. The following landmarks have been suggested (**Fig. 11.4**):
- The position of the Z line (given in centimeters from the incisors), characterizing the change of the mucosal pattern from squamous to columnar epithelium.
- The hiatal narrowing is used, with a distance measured from the incisors, to characterize the lower limit of a hiatus hernia. This anatomical reference point, when combined with the distance measured for the Z line, should define the length of a hiatus hernia more precisely.
- The upper end of gastric folds is used as a measure of distance for Barrett's esophagus. When combined with the distance meas-

11

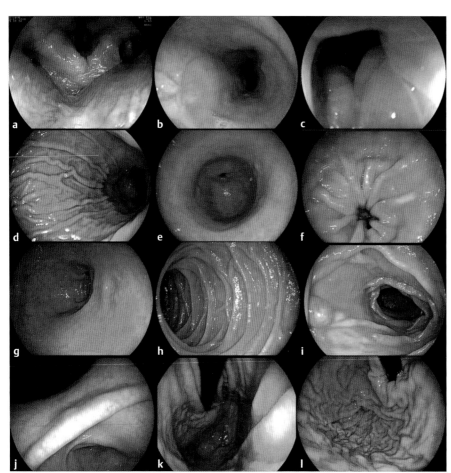

Fig. 11.3 Normal endoscopic anatomy in the upper gastrointestinal tract.
a The hypopharynx, with the origin of the trachea.
b The middle esophagus, with the aortic impression.
c The esophagogastric junction, with the esophageal mucosa appearing pale pink and the gastric mucosa orange.
d Upper view of the gastric body: the lesser curvature is on the right; the greater curvature is on the lower left (mucosal folds); the anterior wall is on the upper left; and the posterior wall is on the lower right.
e Forward view of the antrum, with the pylorus in the middle of the image.
f Antral contraction, with concentric mucosal folds.
g The duodenal bulb as seen from the pylorus.
h The second part of the duodenum.
i The second part of the duodenum, with the papilla visible on the left side of the image.
j The angular incisure as seen at the beginning of the retroflexion maneuver. The antrum and pylorus are partly visible in the lower part of the image; the gastric body is starting to appear in the retroflexed view in the upper part.
k Retroflex view of the gastric body.
l Retroflex view of the cardia and fundus.

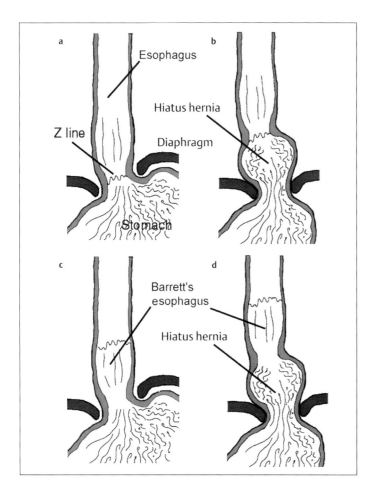

Fig. 11.4 a–d Anatomical landmarks used to define the cardia and the esophagogastric junction.

ured for the Z line, this location should define the length of a Barrett's esophagus segment more precisely.

Stomach

The stomach is divided into two main parts: the fundus and the antrum (**Fig. 11.5**). The cardia is the short segment of the stomach that surrounds the esophagogastric junction. It continues into the fundus, which constitutes the main part of the gastric body, extending from the cardia down to the angular incisure. The fornix is the upper part of the stomach that lies at the left side of the cardia, just under the diaphragm, and it is only visible during a retroflex maneuver. The lower boundary of the fundus is defined by the angular incisure and the end of the mucosal folds, which are characteristic of the fundus on the greater curvature. When the endoscope is straight in the proximal stomach, the anterior wall corresponds to the left part of the image, the posterior wall to the right side; the lesser curvature appears at the top of the image and the greater curvature at the bottom. The antrum is characterized by an absence of mucosal folds. It ends with the pylorus, which appears as a rounded short channel giving access to the duodenal bulb. Peristaltic contractions are often observed at this level. The contractions may temporarily close the pyloric channel, and it then appears as a protrusion in front of the endoscope in the antrum, with regular radial folds. The normal gastric mucosa has an orange to light red color. Some small submucosal veins are visible in the fornix and the gastric body. The gastric folds usually disappear completely when the stomach is inflated with air. Persistent folds should be regarded as pathological and require biopsies.

Duodenum

The duodenum starts with the duodenal bulb, an enlarged segment with an almost triangular shape, layered with pale, flat mucosa. The duodenal bulb ends at the genu superius, where the folds characteristic of the intestinal mucosa develop. These folds are circular and smooth, and high-resolution endoscopes allow visualization of the mucosal villi. As the axis of the bulb is almost perpendicular to that of the antrum, the anterior wall corresponds to the upper left quadrant of the image obtained with a forward-viewing endoscope and the posterior wall to the lower right quadrant, the upper edge being located between them on the right and the lower edge on the left. The duodenal papilla, where the biliary and pancreatic ducts open into the duodenum, is located on the internal face of the second part of the duodenum, usually recognizable by the presence of a vertical fold. In some patients, the papilla is difficult to recognize with a forward-viewing endoscope, and a duodenoscope with lateral viewing is needed to examine it properly. The minor papilla is often located 1.5 cm above the main papilla, usually on the anterior wall of the genu superius. In routine EGD, the duodenum is explored down to the second part and the genu inferius. The mucosa has an orange color, usually paler than the gastric mucosa.

Anatomical Variants

Some abnormal patterns may be found during an EGD that should not be regarded as pathological. Small islets of gastric mucosa may be recognized in the upper part of the esophagus, right down to the upper esophageal sphincter (**Fig. 11.6 a**). These islets do not have any pathological significance and should not be confused with Barrett's esophagus. Similarly, small venous ectasias are often recognized in the upper third of the esophagus (**Fig. 11.6 b**) and should not be confused with esophageal varices.

In the stomach, the left part of the liver may cause external compression, without pathological significance. An external compression of the gastric cavity should be interpreted cautiously and should persist when the stomach is completely distended with air.

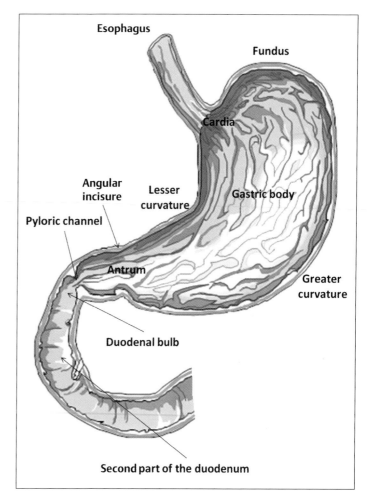

Fig. 11.5 Anatomical landmarks in the upper gastrointestinal tract that are used to describe the location of lesions and other findings.

In the duodenal bulb, the mucosa may appear nodular, without any change in color (**Fig. 11.7**). This nodular pattern is due to a hypertrophy of Brunner glands, the pathological significance of which is not known. In the second part of the duodenum, the mucosa may appear diffusely whitish, corresponding to lymphatic stasis, which may be secondary to other findings or may nonspecifically suggest a metabolic disorder.

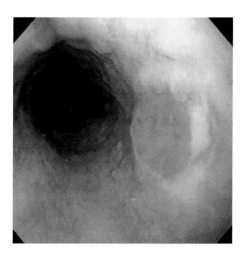 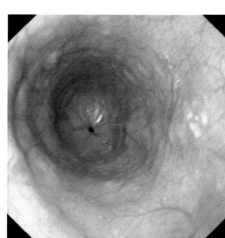

Fig. 11.6 Nonpathological alterations in the upper esophagus.
a Mucosal inlets, characterized by the presence of small areas of gastric mucosa located immediately beyond the upper esophageal sphincter.
b Enlarged submucosal veins characterizing venous ectasias, not to be confused with esophageal varices.

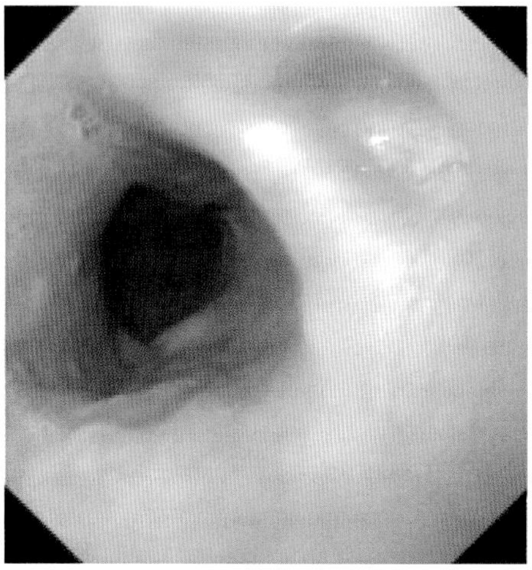

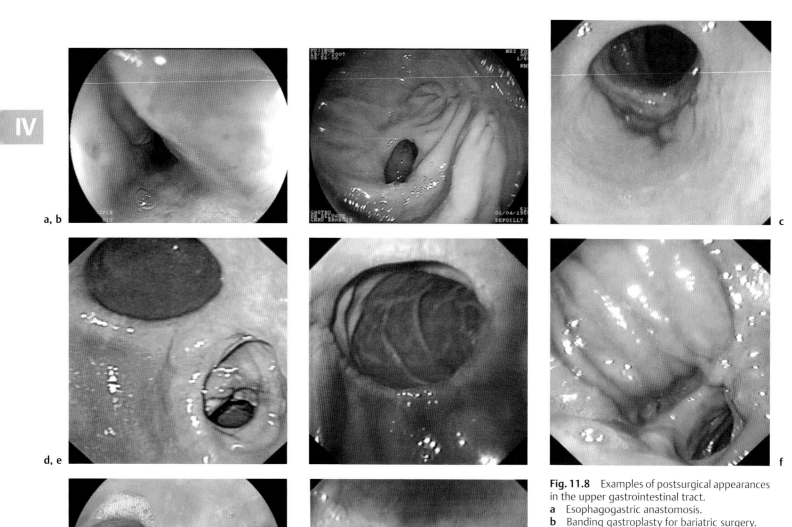

Fig. 11.7 An example of Brunner gland hyperplasia in the duodenal bulb, appearing as a nodular pattern in the mucosa.

Surgically Modified Anatomy

Most surgical interventions cause permanent changes in the anatomy. Postsurgical status must be described by indicating the extent of the resection—i.e., the missing segments of the digestive tract, the type and location of the anastomosis, and the accessibility of the major anatomical landmarks that usually define a complete examination through the existing pathway.

Anastomoses are often seen as a narrowed ring in the lumen, with a sharp transition between two types of mucosa. Suture material (surgical wire, staples) may be found at this level. Some anastomoses have a narrowed appearance, but allow easy passage of the endoscope and should not be regarded as pathological stenoses requiring dilation. **Table 11.2** and **Fig. 11.8** show the various types of surgical anastomosis in the upper gastrointestinal tract.

a, b

c

d, e

f

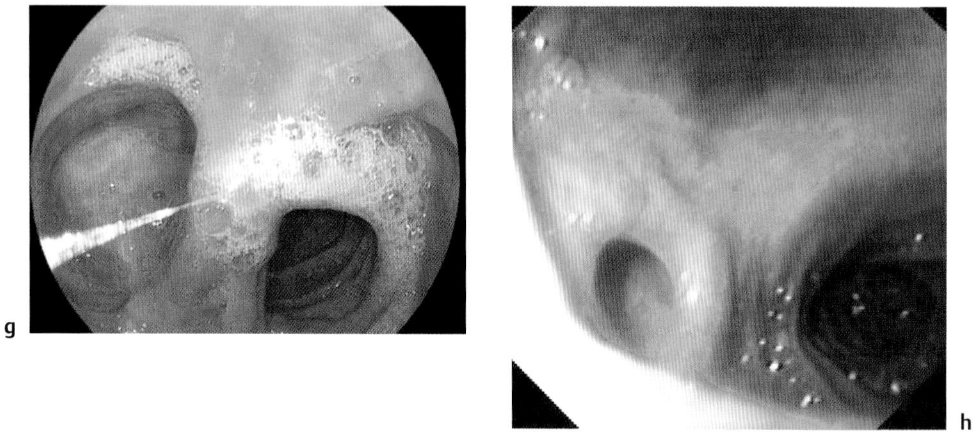

g

h

Fig. 11.8 Examples of postsurgical appearances in the upper gastrointestinal tract.
a Esophagogastric anastomosis.
b Banding gastroplasty for bariatric surgery.
c Esophagocolonic anastomosis.
d Gastrojejunal anastomosis without gastric resection: the anastomosis is seen in the lower right part of the image, the antrum at the upper left.
e Gastroduodenal anastomosis after antrectomy (Billroth I).
f Gastrojejunal anastomosis after partial gastrectomy (Billroth II).
g Esophagojejunal anastomosis after total gastrectomy.
h Choledochoduodenal anastomosis.

Table 11.2 Various types of surgical anastomosis and postsurgical status often encountered during upper gastrointestinal endoscopy

Original organ	Type of intervention	Type of anastomosis	Location of the anastomosis	Endoscopic pattern
Esophagus				
	Partial esophagectomy	Esophagogastric	Middle part of the esophagus	One ostium
		Esophagocolonic	Middle part of the esophagus, area of the cardia	Upper anastomosis between the esophageal remnant and the colonic segment. Lower anastomosis between the colonic transplant and the stomach body
	Total esophagectomy	Esophagogastric	Upper third of the esophagus, usually 1–2 cm down the upper esophageal sphincter	One ostium
		Esophagocolonic	Upper third of the esophagus, usually 1–2 cm down the upper esophageal sphincter, area of the cardia	Upper anastomosis between the esophageal remnant and the colonic segment. Lower anastomosis between the colonic transplant and the stomach body
Stomach				
	Antireflux surgery	–	Cardia in retroflexion	Mucosal folds tightened around the endoscope coming out of the esophagus and corresponding to the antireflux valve
	Pyloroplasty	–	Pylorus	Asymmetric pattern of the pyloric channel
	Antrectomy	Gastroduodenal (Billroth I)	Duodenal bulb/genu superius	One ostium, papilla visible down from the anastomosis
	Partial gastrectomy	Gastrojejunal (Billroth II)	Middle part of the gastric body	Two jejunal loops, one efferent in front of the endoscope, one afferent, usually posterior and more difficult to intubate (retroflexion)
	Total gastrectomy	Esophagojejunal	Diaphragmatic ostium	Two jejunal loops: one efferent, one afferent
		Roux-en-Y	One anastomosis (esophagojejunal) at the level of the diaphragmatic ostium; a lower jejunojejunal anastomosis between the afferent loop coming from the liver and pancreatic anastomoses and the efferent loop, arriving from the esophagus	One short blind loop and one efferent loop; two ostia visible in front of the endoscope. The ostium of the afferent loop is usually right-sided
	Gastroentero-anastomosis	Gastrojejunal	Posterior wall of the gastric body	Two jejunal loops, one efferent in front of the endoscope, one afferent usually posterior and more difficult to intubate; no resection is performed and the duodenum remains accessible through the pylorus
	Bariatric surgery	Adjustable silicone ring	Upper part of the gastric body	External compression, looking like a ring with a narrowed passage to the distal stomach. The ring may ulcerate the gastric wall and become visible in some patients.
		Vertical banded gastroplasty	Upper part of the gastric body	The stapling is performed on the greater curvature, appearing as a linear pattern in the mucosal folds, with a narrowed ostium giving access to the distal stomach
		Gastric bypass	Upper part of the gastric body	The small neocavity is anastomosed to the distal jejunum and separated by a suture from the distal stomach. The main part of the stomach becomes accessible only through the Roux-en-Y loop, requiring the use of a double balloon technique
Duodenum				
	Choledochoduodenal anastomosis	Choledochoduodenal	Genu superius	Small lateral orifice with bile flowing out

Changes in the anatomy are more difficult to identify after certain procedures, particularly if resection has not been performed. Antireflux surgery is often recognized by a narrowed cardia, sometimes passed with smooth rubbing of the endoscope. In retroflexion, the mucosa shows folds converging at the cardia, which are characteristic of the antireflux valve (**Fig. 11.9 a**). After complete bilateral vagotomy, gastric emptying is impaired and there is an associated pyloroplasty characterized by an enlarged and often asymmetric pyloric channel (**Fig. 11.9 b**).

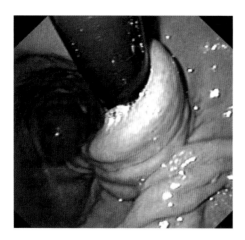
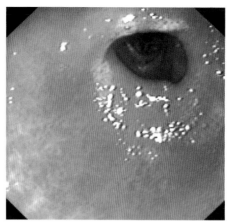

Fig. 11.9   Additional examples of postsurgical appearances in the upper gastrointestinal tract.
a   Nissen fundoplication.
b   Pyloroplasty.

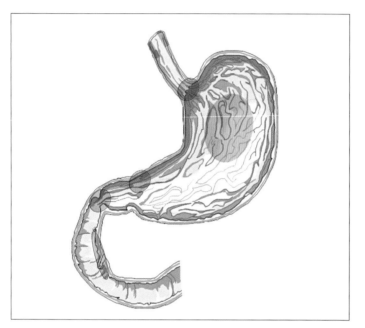

Fig. 11.10   Areas that may be difficult to examine during an upper gastrointestinal endoscopy, requiring slight rotation or twisting of the endoscope so that the tip of the instrument can be placed in front of the mucosal surface.

Difficult-to-Examine Anatomical Locations

Despite careful examination, some areas of the mucosa may not be properly examined during an EGD, as special maneuvers are required to place the endoscope in front of them, or because it is difficult to stabilize the endoscope, especially in unsedated patients. **Figure 11.10** shows these areas in which the examination requires more careful positioning of the endoscope during retroflexion or slower advancement, with circular movements and more air insufflation, to unfold the lumen adequately.

Indications and Contraindications

Indications

A detailed description of the indications for performing an EGD is beyond the scope of this chapter. Some are discussed in other chapters, and several endoscopic societies have published guidelines on indications for EGD in standard practice [19,20]. Generally, any disease or condition that involves the upper digestive tract may

constitute an indication for EGD. **Table 11.3** summarizes the most common indications, which fall into three categories:

- *Diagnostic EGD,* for diseases that are diagnosed by the presence of specific alterations in the mucosa or tumor growth in the upper gastrointestinal tract. Diagnostic EGD may also be indicated for further investigation of abnormal patterns found on radiography.
- *Mucosal biopsies* or samples of biological fluids may be required in some instances—e. g., patients with chronic diarrhea in whom duodenal biopsies are indicated in order to search for or rule out villous atrophy suggesting celiac disease.
- *Therapeutic EGD* is indicated to treat lesions or conditions that have been recognized at a previous endoscopy or with a different imaging modality. It is also primarily indicated in patients with upper gastrointestinal bleeding revealed by hematemesis or melena.

Contraindications

There are very few contraindications to EGD. Absolute contraindications include known or suspected perforation of a hollow organ, massive upper gastrointestinal bleeding leading to a suspicion of aortoduodenal fistula, and patients with acute unstabilized cardiorespiratory failure. Other contraindications should be regarded as relative and do not prevent an experienced endoscopist from performing an EGD, provided that all safety issues are managed. High-risk conditions include Zenker diverticulum, proximal esophageal or pharyngeal obstruction, excessive deformity of the cervical spine, aortic aneurysm with compression of the esophagus, gastric volvulus, and massive gastrointestinal bleeding. In most cases, these conditions are uncommon, and their presence does not prevent an experienced operator from performing the endoscopy.

In infants and children, as well as patients expected to have poor compliance during the procedure and patients with massive bleeding, general anesthesia may be considered in order to facilitate a complete and relevant procedure.

Appropriateness of Indications

The appropriateness of the indications for an upper gastrointestinal endoscopy is usually evaluated in relation to the guidelines published by endoscopic societies [19,20]. In the late 1990s, the European Panel on Appropriateness of Gastrointestinal Endoscopy (EPAGE) issued guidelines for the appropriateness of digestive endoscopies and opened an interactive web site allowing practitioners to test the indications they use personally [21]. As a result, it was shown that appropriate endoscopies had a higher diagnostic yield than inappropriate ones and that no significant lesions were dis-

Table 11.3 Indications for upper gastrointestinal endoscopy

Symptoms

Upper abdominal pain with associated alarm symptoms (weight loss, fever)

Upper abdominal pain that persists despite an adequate trial of therapy

Dysphagia, odynophagia

Persistent nausea/vomiting

Hematemesis, melena

Heartburn, regurgitation suggesting gastroesophageal reflux

Incidental or voluntary ingestion of caustic substances

Diseases and conditions

Gastroesophageal reflux
- Diagnosis
- Assessment of therapeutic efficacy in case of discrepancy with symptoms
- Screening/surveillance of Barrett's esophagus

Gastroduodenal ulcer
- Diagnosis
- Assessment of mucosal healing (+ biopsies) for gastric ulcers only

Liver cirrhosis
- Assessment of portal hypertension
- Screening of esophageal varices
- Treatment of esophageal varices

Obscure digestive bleeding, chronic iron-deficiency anemia

Malignancies of the upper gastrointestinal tract
- Diagnosis
- Treatment
  - Curative: ESD, EMR
  - Palliative: stenting
- Post-therapeutic surveillance

Premalignant conditions in the upper gastrointestinal tract: screening and diagnosis
- Familial adenomatous polyposis
- Peutz–Jeghers syndrome
- Gastric atrophy (Biermer disease)
- Patients with known ENT or epidermoid lung cancers
- Barrett's esophagus
- Ménétrier disease
- Achalasia
  Removal of foreign bodies

Assessment and sampling

Gastric biopsies
- Folate/vitamin B_{12} deficiency
- Iron deficiency
- Chronic diarrhea

Duodenal biopsies
- Suspicion of celiac disease
- Chronic diarrhea
- Iron deficiency

Assessment of any abnormal pattern observed during previous investigations (e. g., radiography, capsule endoscopy)

Assessment of the upper gastrointestinal tract before other therapies
- Pretransplantation check-up
- Prebariatric surgery

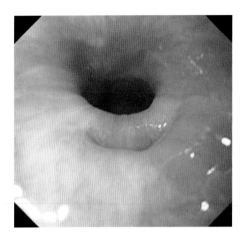

Fig. 11.11 Example of a Zenker diverticulum.

outcome of first-diagnosis EGD in a consecutive series of 2900 patients [24]. When indications were regarded as appropriate when associated with clinically relevant endoscopic findings, the diagnostic yield ranged from 42 % in patients with gastrointestinal bleeding to 20 % in patients with dyspeptic symptoms.

On the other hand, it must be emphasized that an endoscopy with negative findings is not necessarily devoid of clinical relevance. The clinical relevance of an endoscopic examination is generally defined by the effect of the procedure on the management of the patient—i. e., initiation of effective therapy. The tendency to regard an endoscopy with negative findings as useless does not take account of the positive impact of this in reassuring the patient, or in influencing the further diagnostic work-up by ruling out a diagnostic hypothesis on the basis of pathological biopsy results.

Complications

Complication rates as low as 0.1–0.2 % in diagnostic upper gastrointestinal endoscopy were reported in early studies [25,26]. More recent studies have shown that the procedure is well tolerated, with an overall complication rate of 0.07 % [27]. The complication rate in diagnostic EGD has declined due to the use of thinner endoscopes with a wider viewing angle, reducing the rate of blind advancement of the scope during esophageal insertion and intubation of the second part of the duodenum.

Life-threatening complications occur in only 0.03 % of the procedures and mainly involve perforations [28]. Perforations occur mainly when the endoscope is pushed blindly, especially during esophageal intubation, when the tip of the endoscope may be pushed laterally into the piriform fossa or when a Zenker diverticulum is overlooked (**Fig. 11.11**).

Nowadays, complications mainly occur during therapeutic endoscopies and are related to the type of therapeutic intervention. In a prospective 2-year study, 75 % of complications were found to be related to therapeutic procedures [27].

Documentation of an EGD Procedure

Every endoscopic procedure requires an accurate description of the examination, findings, and additional maneuvers undertaken during it. These data constitute the material included in the endoscopic report that is generated by the endoscopist at the end of the procedure. The ASGE guideline on the content of an endoscopic report provides a detailed example of a complete and accurate report [29]. Recent advances in information technology have supported the widespread use of computerized endoscopic reports generated by endoscopic information systems that are linked to the hospital

covered during inappropriate examinations [22]. In a multicenter prospective evaluation, Minoli et al. assessed the appropriateness of upper gastrointestinal endoscopy in an open-access system, using the American Society for Gastrointestinal Endoscopy (ASGE) guidelines [23]. The results of an analysis of 3414 EGDs showed that 23 % of the procedures would have been inappropriate. Inappropriate endoscopic examinations occurred mainly during the follow-up of healed benign disease and were more frequent when the examination was prescribed by the family doctor. Another study assessed the

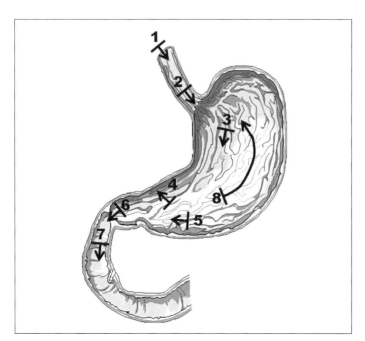

Fig. 11.12 Standardized points at which endoscopic images should be obtained for accurate documentation of an upper gastrointestinal endoscopy. A total of 8 images should be taken.

IV

information system [30]. Several systems and software programs are currently available for editing computerized reports in endoscopy. Ideally, they should use a standard terminology in order to promote readability and data exchange [31]. In addition, when used in combination with electronic endoscopes, they make it possible to include good-quality images to document the procedure. Standardization of the number and content of the images captured during an EGD has been advocated in an ESGE guideline [32]. The guidelines recommend capturing at least eight images at standardized points during the withdrawal of the endoscope (**Fig. 11.12**).

Conclusion

Esophagogastroduodenoscopy is nowadays regarded as the gold standard for the investigation of diseases and conditions involving the upper gastrointestinal tract. In most instances, it is the first-line examination. Advances in endoscope design and the development of various therapeutic and diagnostic instruments for use during EGD have dramatically increased diagnostic and therapeutic options. The indications are better defined and guidelines are available to help any practitioner in everyday practice to accurately identify patients who can be expected to benefit from the procedure. Complications have also become rarer, and in most instances a primary EGD is cost-effective and saves further investigations.

References

1. Moutier F. Traité de gastroscopie et de pathologie endoscopique de l'estomac. Paris: Masson, 1935.
2. Schindler R. Ein völlig ungefährliches, flexibles Gastroskop. Münch Med Wochenschr 1932;32:1268–9.
3. Hirschowitz BI, Curtiss LE, Peters CW, Pollard HM. Demonstration of a new gastroscope, the "fiberscope." Gastroenterology 1958;35:50–3.
4. Dormann A, Meisner S, Verin N, Wenk Lang A. Self-expanding metal stents for gastroduodenal malignancies: systematic review of their clinical effectiveness. Endoscopy 2004;36:543–50.
5. Curvers WL, Kiesslich R, Bergman JJ. Novel imaging modalities in the detection of oesophageal neoplasia. Best Pract Res Clin Gastroenterol 2008;22:687–720.
6. Yao K, Iwashita A, Tanabe H, Nagahama T, Matsui T, Ueki T, et al. Novel zoom endoscopy technique for diagnosis of small flat gastric cancer: a prospective, blind study. Clin Gastroenterol Hepatol 2007;5: 869–78.
7. Nakayoshi T, Tajiri H, Matsuda K, Kaise M, Ikegami M, Sasaki H. Magnifying endoscopy combined with narrow band imaging system for early gastric cancer: correlation of vascular pattern with histopathology (including video). Endoscopy 2004;36:1080–4.
8. Coriat R, Chryssostalis A, Zeitoun JD, Deyra J, Gaudric M, Prat F, et al. Computed virtual chromoendoscopy system (FICE): a new tool for upper endoscopy? Gastroenterol Clin Biol 2008;32:363–9.
9. Lambert R, Saito H, Saito Y. High-resolution endoscopy and early gastrointestinal cancer: dawn in the East. Endoscopy 2007;39:232–7.
10. Ament ME, Berquist WE, Vargas J, Perisic V. Fiberoptic upper intestinal endoscopy in infants and children. Pediatr Clin North Am 1988;35: 141–55.
11. Dean R, Dua K, Massey B, Berger W, Hogan WJ, Shaker R. A comparative study of unsedated transnasal esophagogastroduodenoscopy and conventional EGD. Gastrointest Endosc 1996;44:422–4.
12. Zaman A, Hahn M, Hapke R, Knigge K, Fennerty MB, Katon RM. A randomized trial of peroral versus transnasal unsedated endoscopy using an ultrathin videoendoscope. Gastrointest Endosc 1999;49:279–84.
13. Leder SB, Ross DA, Briskin KB, Sasaki CT. A prospective, double blind, randomized study on the use of a topical anesthetic, vasoconstrictor, and placebo during transnasal flexible fiberoptic endoscopy. J Speech Lang Hear Res 1997;40:1352–7.
14. Dumortier J, Napoleon B, Hedelius F, Pellissier PE, Leprince E, Pujol B, et al. Unsedated transnasal EGD in daily practice: results with 1100 consecutive patients. Gastrointest Endosc 2003;57:198–204.
15. Galmiche JP, Coron E, Sacher-Huvelin S. Recent developments in capsule endoscopy. Gut 2008;57:695–703.
16. Standards of Practice Committee, Lichtenstein DR, Jagannath S, Baron TH, Anderson MA, Banerjee S, et al. Sedation and anesthesia in GI endoscopy. Gastrointest Endosc 2008;68:205–16.
17. Korman LY, Delvaux M, Crespi M. The minimal standard terminology in digestive endoscopy: perspective on a standard endoscopic vocabulary. Gastrointest Endosc 2001;53:392–6.
18. Sharma P, Dent J, Armstrong D, Bergman JJ, Gossner L, Hoshihara Y, et al. The development and validation of an endoscopic grading system for Barrett's esophagus: the Prague C & M criteria. Gastroenterology 2006; 131:1392–9.
19. The American Society for Gastrointestinal Endoscopy. Appropriate use of gastrointestinal endoscopy: a consensus statement from the American Society for Gastrointestinal Endoscopy, revised Aug. 1992. Manchester, MA: American Society for Gastrointestinal Endoscopy; 1992.
20. Axon A, Bell G, Jones R, Quine M, McCloy R. Guidelines on appropriate indications for upper gastrointestinal endoscopy. Br Med J 1995;310: 853–6.
21. Vader JP, Burnand B, Froehlich F, Dubois RW, Bochud M, Gonvers JJ. The European Panel on Appropriateness of Gastrointestinal Endoscopy (EPAGE): project and methods. Endoscopy 1999;31:572–8.
22. Froehlich F, Repond C, Müllhaupt B, Vader JP, Burnand B, Schneider C, et al. Is the diagnostic yield of upper GI endoscopy improved by the use of explicit panel-based appropriateness criteria? Gastrointest Endosc 2000;52:333–41.
23. Minoli G, Prada A, Gambetta G, Formenti A, Schalling R, Lai L, et al. The ESGE guidelines for the appropriate use of upper gastrointestinal endoscopy in an open access system. Gastrointest Endosc 1995;42:387–9.
24. Adang RP, Vismans JF, Talmon JL, Hasman A, Ambergen AW, Stockbrugger RW. Appropriateness of indications for diagnostic upper gastrointestinal endoscopy: association with relevant endoscopic disease. Gastrointest Endosc 1995;42:390–7.
25. Meyers MA, Ghahremani GG. Complications of fiberoptic endoscopy. 1. Esophagoscopy and gastroscopy. Radiology 1975;115:293–300.
26. Mandelstrom P, Sugawa C, Silvis SE, Nebel OT, Rogers G. Complications associated with esophagogastroduodenoscopy and with esophageal dilatation. Gastrointest Endosc 1976;23:16–9.
27. Denis B, Ben Abdelghani M, Peter A, Weiss AM, Bottlaender J, Goineau J. Two years of mortality and morbidity conferences in a hospital gastrointestinal endoscopy unit. Gastroenterol Clin Biol 2003;27:1100–4.
28. Shamir M, Schuman BM. Complications of fiberoptic endoscopy. Gastrointest Endosc 1980;26:86–91.
29. ASGE Computers Committee. Standard format and content of endoscopic procedure report. Oak Brook, IL: ASGE; 1992.

30. Delvaux M, Crespi M, Armengol-Miro JR, Hagenmüller F, Teuffel W. The GASTER Project: building a computer network in digestive endoscopy. The experience of the European Society for Gastrointestinal Endoscopy. J Clin Gastroenterol 1999;29:118–26.

31. Delvaux M. Minimal Standard Terminology for data processing in digestive endoscopy: a trend towards standardization of endoscopic reports. Dig Endosc 1999;11:301–14.

32. Rey JF, Lambert R, ESGE Quality Assurance Committee. ESGE recommendations for quality control in gastrointestinal endoscopy: guidelines for image documentation in upper and lower GI endoscopy. Endoscopy 2001;33:901–3.

11

117

12 Enteroscopy Techniques

Blair S. Lewis and Kiyonori Kobayashi

Introduction

Endoscopic evaluation of the small bowel became possible with the advent of capsule endoscopy. The small bowel was previously regarded as a place where little happens, and endoscopic evaluation was limited to only a few centers. By 2008, however, more than 750 000 capsule endoscope ingestions had been carried out worldwide—leading to a corresponding need for a "therapeutic arm." Enteroscopy has become a companion to capsule endoscopy, allowing reexamination of areas considered abnormal at capsule endoscopy and allowing therapeutic interventions such as cauterization or removal of lesions identified at capsule endoscopy, as well as allowing tattooing of lesions so that they can be identified during subsequent surgery. Other indications include obscure gastrointestinal bleeding that continues following a negative capsule examination and examination of the duodenum or stomach in patients with altered anatomy following bariatric surgery. Enteroscopy may also be helpful in selected patients with unexplained chronic diarrhea, in patients with undefined radiographic abnormalities of the small bowel, and for following up patients with previously identified intestinal diseases [1].

Endoscopic evaluation of the small bowel has gone through extensive development. Initially, pediatric colonoscopes were used to advance an instrument through the stomach and into the duodenum and proximal jejunum. These initial instruments were 135 cm long and only allowed examination as far as the proximal jejunum. During instrument development, it became clear that although longer instruments could be manufactured, it was difficult to create an instrument that would be capable of being pushed through the multiple bends of the bowel in the free intraperitoneal space. The maximum length appeared to be approximately 2.5 m. This length extended enteroscopy only as far as the mid- to distal jejunum.

Other avenues of development included a thread-guided method of enteroscopy, known as rope-way enteroscopy, which was the first technique used to achieve complete intubation of the small bowel [2]. In this technique, the patient swallowed a guide string, which was allowed to pass through the whole gut until it emerged from the anus. The string was then exchanged for a stiffer Teflon tube, over which an endoscope was passed, either orally or transnasally. This method was quickly abandoned, as it was quite traumatic for the patient, time-consuming, and often required general anesthesia. Sonde enteroscopy involved a thin endoscope with a balloon on its tip that was dragged by peristalsis through the small bowel, much like a Cantor tube [3]. The endoscopic examination was performed during instrument withdrawal. This technique never gained widespread acceptance and has also been abandoned.

At present, two major forms of enteroscopy are practiced. One is termed balloon-assisted enteroscopy, and the other is intraoperative enteroscopy. Intraoperative enteroscopy was considered the gold standard for enteroscopy, but has largely been replaced by balloon-assisted enteroscopy, as the latter provides a more stable platform for viewing the small bowel and can be repeated should the need arise.

Balloon-Assisted Enteroscopy

Double-balloon enteroscopy (DBE), first described by Yamamoto in 2001, can allow total small-intestinal intubation using a 200-cm enteroscope coupled with a 140-cm overtube (Fujinon Inc., Saitama, Japan) [4]. Balloons are located at the tip of the enteroscope and at the tip of the overtube (**Fig. 12.1**). This assembly allows pleating or accordioning of the small bowel onto the overtube. The procedure is modeled on intraoperative enteroscopy, in which the small bowel is pleated onto the shaft of an endoscope by a surgeon who pushes the bowel onto the instrument and holds the pleats in place while the examination is performed. In double-balloon enteroscopy, the balloons act to hold the wall of the small bowel with friction, and withdrawal of the assembly pulls the pleats onto the overtube. The method has been described as resembling opening curtains over a curtain rod [5]. Double-balloon enteroscopy thus allows deeper intubation than push enteroscopy. The procedure can be performed not only from the standard peroral route; the instrument can also be advanced into the small bowel in a retrograde manner using a peranal approach (**Fig. 12.2**). The examination is not performed quickly, as each "reduction" involves several maneuvers: advancing the enteroscope, inflating the enteroscope balloon, then deflating the overtube balloon, advancing the overtube to the enteroscope's tip, inflating the overtube balloon, and then finally pulling the entire assembly backward to pleat the bowel onto the overtube. During an average examination, this series of maneuvers is performed 12 times, and the examination can thus easily last more than 1 h.

American experience with double-balloon enteroscopy has shown that the technique, even when performed from both the oral and transrectal approaches, does not allow viewing of the entire small bowel [6]. Despite this latest technology, total intubation of the small bowel cannot be achieved in every patient, and thus not every small-bowel lesion is amenable to nonsurgical therapy. Double-balloon enteroscopy appears to be limited in patients with a high body mass index, in whom fat in the mesentery restricts the ability to pleat the bowel, and in patients who have undergone previous surgery, in whom the bowel is tethered by adhesions and cannot be pleated.

Double-balloon enteroscopy presently has four major roles: 1, as a method for treating lesions identified by capsule endoscopy; 2, as a diagnostic tool if capsule endoscopy is negative and the patient has continuing bleeding; 3, as a removal tool in cases of capsule retention; and 4, to allow endoscopic retrograde cholangiopancreatography (ERCP) in patients with altered anatomy following bariatric surgery. It can also be used to clarify capsule findings that are not interpretable.

Double-balloon enteroscopy's major role is a therapeutic one, allowing endoscopic cautery of bleeding sites in the small bowel. Angiectasias represent the major cause of obscure gastrointestinal bleeding, accounting for approximately 80 % of cases. Endoscopic therapy has been shown to be effective in controlling bleeding from intestinal angiectasias, for which the depth of intubation was previously limited [7]. Before the development of double-balloon enteroscopy, the only option for a patient with a bleeding site in the mid- to distal small bowel was surgery guided by intraoperative

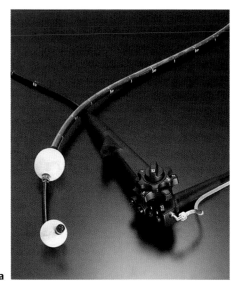

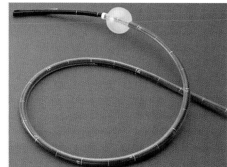

Fig. 12.1
a A double-balloon enteroscope.
b A single-balloon enteroscope.

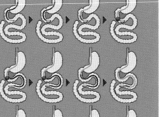

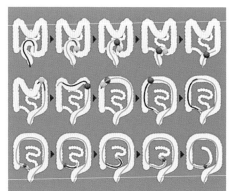

Fig. 12.2 The principles and methods of inserting a double-balloon enteroscope.
a Anterograde approach.
b Retrograde approach.

IV

enteroscopy. Double-balloon enteroscopy has now replaced intra-operative enteroscopy for re-identifying causes of bleeding seen on capsule endoscopy and providing therapy. Another therapeutic use for the double-balloon method is to tattoo mass lesions seen on capsule endoscopy that are considered to be too small to allow laparoscopic identification and resection. Double-balloon entero-scopy has numerous advantages over intraoperative enteroscopy, including reduced invasiveness, a shorter procedure time, improved visibility, and the ability to repeat the examination. Double-balloon enteroscopy can also be performed in patients in whom surgery is considered to be contraindicated due to severe medical conditions such as heart disease. Another advantage of this targeted approach is that it limits the time taken to perform the double-balloon exami-nation, a major factor that has limited the adoption of this new technology. Experience with double-balloon enteroscopy is encour-aging [8,9]. Obscure bleeding is the indication for DBE in 36–100% of examinations, and the overall diagnostic yield of the method ranges from 43% to 80%. Diagnostic or therapeutic success is achieved in 55–75% of examinations. In patients in whom obscure bleeding is the indication for DBE, the success rate is higher.

Proper localization of a lesion identified at capsule endoscopy remains a challenge, and this is important in choosing a procedure to allow re-identification and treatment of the finding. The physi-cian has to determine whether the finding is within reach of push enteroscopy, double-balloon enteroscopy with an oral approach, or double-balloon with a transrectal approach. Initial attempts to use the capsule passage time from the pylorus to the lesion proved inaccurate, as total small-bowel passage times vary between indi-viduals due to varying peristalsis rates. Mark Appleyard has advo-cated using the percentage of the passage time to determine where a finding is located (personal communication). The time of capsule passage from the pylorus to the lesion is divided by the total small-bowel passage time. He has suggested that passage percentages of less than 10% are within reach of a push enteroscope. Lesions within 70% can be reached from an oral approach, while those longer than 70% can only be reached by transrectal passage. This concept was applied by Gay et al., who used capsule endoscopy as a "filter" for double-balloon enteroscopy and were able select the appropriate examination route using this percentage method [10].

Although guidelines advocate capsule endoscopy in patients with obscure gastrointestinal bleeding after negative colonoscopy and upper endoscopy [11,12], the appropriate management of these patients if the capsule examination is negative is not clear. As stated previously, the yields of capsule endoscopy in patients with obscure bleeding average 70%. A pooled data analysis suggested that the overall miss rate for capsule endoscopy is 20%, with approximately 10% of patients having a bleeding site finally identified outside the small intestine [13]. The data suggest that most patients have no further bleeding if capsule endoscopy is negative [14]. However, some patients do continue to bleed, and the management is unclear in these cases. Two approaches have been suggested. One option is to repeat the capsule examination, while the other is to pursue double-balloon enteroscopy. Jones et al. repeated capsule studies for a variety of indications in 24 patients [15]. Repeat capsule endo-scopy revealed additional findings in 75% of the patients and led to a change in management in 62%. Limited data are available for the use

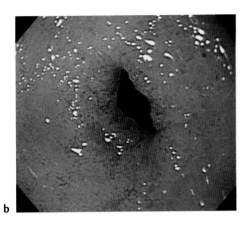
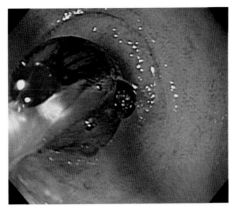
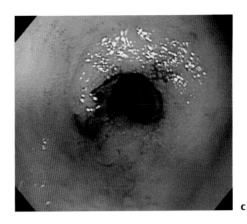

b   **c**

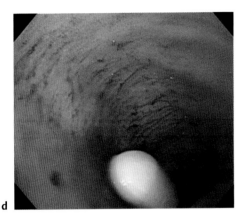
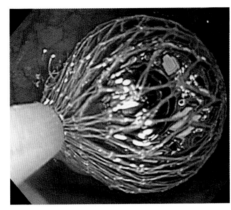

Fig. 12.3 A retained capsule in the small intestine, removed using a balloon enteroscope.
a Enteroscopic examination showed an intestinal stricture caused by radiation enteritis in the ileum.
b Endoscopic balloon dilation was performed.
c After treatment, the enteroscope was able to pass though the stricture.
d The retained capsule was found on the oral side of the stricture.
e The capsule was grasped with a net forceps.

d   **e**

of double-balloon enteroscopy in cases of negative capsule examinations. Chong et al. reported on four patients who underwent enteroscopy after negative capsule studies, in whom three diagnoses were made [16].

Another role for double-balloon enteroscopy is to remove a retained capsule (**Fig. 12.3**). Retention of the capsule in the small bowel continues to be a major concern for physicians performing capsule endoscopy, as it could potentially lead to a need for surgery in a patient who might otherwise have been treated medically for the same illness. This applies in particular to patients with Crohn's disease or nonsteroidal anti-inflammatory drug (NSAID) enteropathy. The International Conference on Capsule Endoscopy (ICCE) consensus statement on capsule retention reported a 1.5 % risk of retention when capsule endoscopy is performed in the setting of obscure bleeding [17]. The consensus statement defined capsule retention as having a capsule endoscope remain in the digestive tract for a minimum of 2 weeks. Retention was also defined as the capsule permanently remaining in the bowel lumen unless extracted by endoscopic or surgical methods, or if passed as a result of medical therapy. There are no data on the success of medical therapies for retention, such as initiating a course of steroids or infliximab, stopping NSAIDs, or using prokinetics or cathartics to aid in passage of the capsule. There is no time limit for instituting management for capsule removal, and the physician and patient together can decide on the best management choice. The choice of surgical or endoscopic management once capsule retention has been diagnosed depends on the cause of the retention and the indication for the examination in the first place. If retention occurs behind a tumor or mass, surgical intervention is typically pursued quickly. If retention occurs behind a Crohn's stricture or NSAID stricture and the patient has had pronounced bleeding, again surgical intervention may prove the most efficacious method, not only for removing the capsule but also for dealing with the cause of

hemorrhage. The same applies to retention in a patient with known Crohn's disease and recurrent symptoms but without documented disease by any other method and failure to respond to medical therapy before the capsule examination. Finally, for patients in whom bleeding is not pronounced or in whom prior disease was only suspected but not treated, capsule retention behind an NSAID or Crohn's stricture can be managed with double-balloon enteroscopy [18]. This technique allows capsule retrieval, and the patient can then be treated medically for the underlying illness.

Another form of balloon-assisted enteroscopy is single-balloon enteroscopy. This technique is similar to double-balloon enteroscopy, except that there is no balloon on the tip of the enteroscope, only a single balloon on the overtube tip [19] (**Fig. 12.1 b**). To achieve similar holding at the enteroscope tip, the enteroscope is deflected into a U-turn to hook on the small bowel during the withdrawal phase (**Fig. 12.4**). Although double-balloon enteroscopy was developed in 2001, the single-balloon method was only introduced in 2008, and only limited experience has therefore been reported in publications so far. Tsujikawa and colleagues first reported the single-balloon technique in 78 procedures performed in 41 patients [19]. As in double-balloon enteroscopy, the indications varied and included obscure bleeding, suspected Crohn's disease, unexplained abdominal pain, and a suspected small bowel tumor (**Figs. 12.5–12.8**). Kawamura and colleagues reported using the single-balloon method in 37 examinations in 27 patients [20]. Procedure times were similar to those with double-balloon enteroscopy, averaging 83–90 min, depending on whether the route was oral or transrectal. Although there have been no direct comparisons between the double-balloon and single-balloon techniques, both methods appear to allow total small-bowel intubation in a subset of individuals. The time required to set up the equipment is shorter with single-balloon enteroscopy, as a tip balloon is not affixed to the enteroscope.

IV

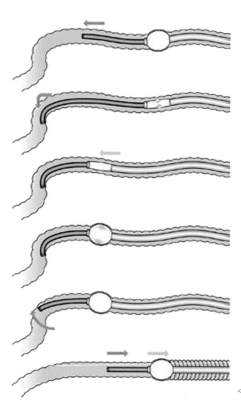

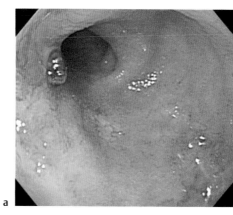

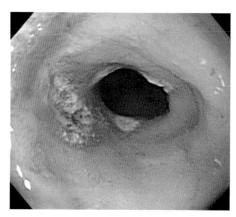

Fig. 12.5 Bleeding from a nonsteroidal anti-inflammatory drug (NSAID) ulcer in the small intestine.
a A small ulcer with a visible vessel in the ileum secondary to NSAID enteropathy.
b The appearance after argon plasma coagulation treatment.

◁ **Fig. 12.4** The principles and methods of inserting a single-balloon enteroscope. Orange arrow: motion of the scope; green arrow: motion of the sliding tube.

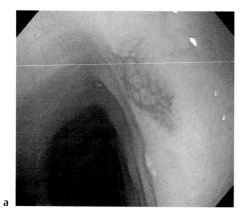

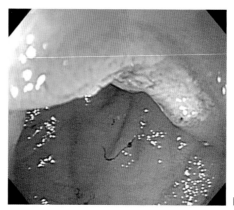

Fig. 12.6 Bleeding from an intestinal angiectasia.
a The enteroscopic examination showed typical angiectasia in the ileum.
b The appearance after argon plasma coagulation treatment.

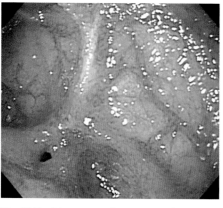

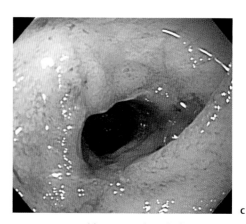

Fig. 12.7 Diagnosis and treatment of a Crohn's stricture.
a Enteroscopic examination, showing a tight stricture in the ileum.
b Endoscopic balloon dilation was carried out, allowing passage of the scope.

c After treatment, the enteroscope was able to pass though the stricture and the patient's abdominal symptoms improved.

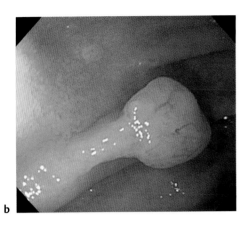

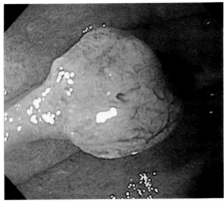

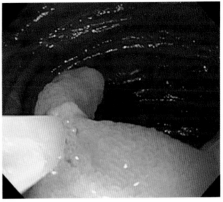

b

c

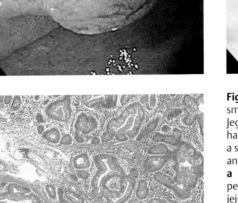

e

Fig. 12.8 Endoscopic ablation of a polyp in the small intestine in a 29-year-old man with Peutz–Jeghers syndrome. Small-intestinal radiography had revealed multiple polyps in the jejunum, and a single-balloon enteroscope was inserted via the anterograde approach.

a Enteroscopic examination showed a semi-pedunculated polyp in the middle part of the jejunum.

b Observation with narrow-band imaging allowed a clear evaluation of the vascular structures on the surface of the polyp.

c Three polyps were resected by endoscopic mucosal resection.

d For retrieval, the polyps were grasped with a tripod forceps. The enteroscope was then withdrawn, leaving the sliding tube in the small intestine.

e The histopathological findings showed that all of the polyps were hamartomatous.

Both balloon-assisted techniques have been used to perform ERCP in patients with altered anatomy [21,22] (**Fig. 12.9**). These are typically patients who have undergone gastric bypass procedures or Roux-en-Y operations, such as choledochojejunostomy or hepaticojejunostomy during liver transplantation. These examinations are lengthy and difficult, as the endoscopist first has to reach the Roux-en-Y anastomosis, which is located 1 m past the ligament of Treitz in gastric bypass patients. The afferent limb then has to be identified and intubated to the second portion of the duodenum. Since the instruments are forward-viewing, biliary tract cannulation rates are lower than in standard ERCP and have been reported as ranging from 60 % to 80 % [23].

Further innovations in the design and use of overtubes are likely to come. The idea of an active overtube that allows the endoscopist to reach and then treat areas not previously accessible is continuing to drive instrument design. A spiral overtube has been cleared by the Food and Drug Administration (FDA) for marketing. This overtube is spun over an enteroscope, pulling the small bowel up the overtube with its spiral design [24].

Intraoperative Enteroscopy

After capsule endoscopy, intraoperative enteroscopy remains the most common form of total small-bowel endoscopic examination. Colonoscopes are routinely employed for this examination, although a push enteroscope can also be used. The instrument does not need to be sterile, as the recommended technique involves peroral intubation of the small intestine. The proximal jejunum is intubated before the laparotomy is carried out, since once the abdomen is open it may be difficult to advance the instrument around

the ligament of Treitz due to excessive, and unopposed, bowing of the endoscope shaft along the greater curvature of the stomach. With oral intubation of an adult colonoscope, the endotracheal tube cuff may need to be deflated to allow passage of the wide-caliber endoscope. Once the colonoscope is placed within the proximal jejunum, laparotomy is performed. A noncrushing clamp is placed across the ileocecal valve to prevent distension of the colon with insufflated air. Colonic distension can lead to difficulties with subsequent abdominal closure. The endoscopic examination is performed by having the surgeon grasp the endoscope tip and hold a short segment of bowel straight to allow endoscopic inspection. The view is best when the overhead lights are dimmed, allowing the surgeon to examine the transilluminated bowel. Once it has been examined both internally and externally, the small bowel is pleated onto the shaft of the endoscope and the next section of bowel is examined. Active bleeding in the small bowel may limit the effectiveness of this method. Generally, the examination is performed only during intubation, since mucosal trauma occurs with the pleating, causing artifacts that may be confused with the appearance of angiectasia. Lesions identified with intraoperative enteroscopy are marked by the surgeon with a suture placed on the serosal surface of the small intestine. At the end of the examination, the endoscope is withdrawn, and resection sites are identified by the sutures.

Other intraoperative enteroscopy techniques are also available. An alternative is to create an enterotomy through which an enteroscope covered with a sterile plastic sheath is placed. The site of the enterotomy is generally determined by findings at capsule endoscopy. For example, a distal lesion seen on capsule endoscopy is approached through an enterotomy in the distal small bowel. An enterotomy performed in the mid-small bowel allows both proximal and distal intestinal intubation. Using an enterotomy allows

12

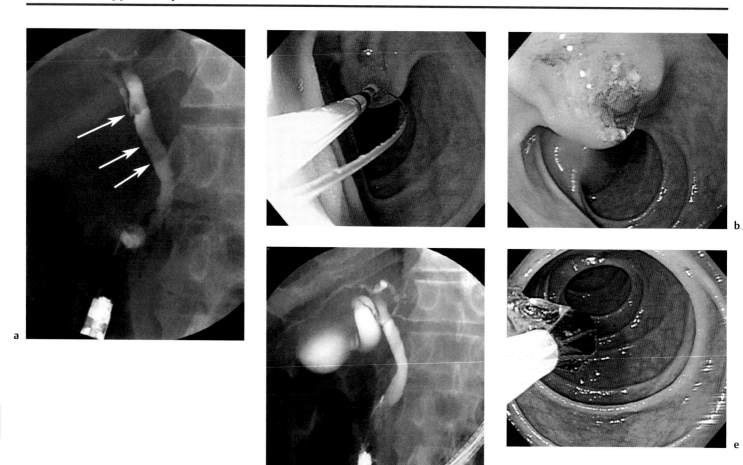

Fig. 12.9 Endoscopic retrograde cholangiopancreatography (ERCP) using the balloon enteroscope.
a The ERCP image obtained with a single-balloon enteroscope in a patient following Billroth II resection, in whom a pediatric colonoscope was not able to reach the ampulla. Multiple filling defects in the common bile duct (arrow) are seen.

b Endoscopic papillotomy was carried out using a prototype endoscopic sphincterotomy (EST) knife.
c The endoscopic findings, showing the duodenal papilla after EST.
d ERCP image showing the common bile duct stone, caught with the basket catheter inserted via the duodenal papilla.
e The stone was removed using the basket catheter.

the examination to be performed in a laparoscopically assisted manner with a much smaller incision [25].

Intraoperative endoscopy has been used for several reasons. It is presently the endoscopic method most widely used for identifying small intestinal sites of bleeding [26]. This most typically involves bleeding sites identified on capsule endoscopy that are not approachable endoscopically. Intraoperative enteroscopy is also used in cases in which surgical guidance is needed to limit small-bowel resection. This is especially the case in patients with hereditary hemorrhagic telangiectasia syndrome, in whom there are often diffuse lesions that are limited to the jejunum. The diffuse nature of the lesions limits enteroscopic management, and the surgeon needs to know where the lesions stop. Intraoperative enteroscopy is also used in patients with small-bowel polyposis such as Peutz–Jeghers syndrome. Multiple polypectomies can be performed and the specimens can be removed through the enterotomy, limiting resection. In patients with suspected multicentric carcinoid, intraoperative enteroscopy is able to identify small, nonpalpable lesions and thus guide complete resection of the tumor. Finally, intraoperative enteroscopy has been used to identify and guide resection procedures for diaphragm disease of the small bowel. These stenoses of the small bowel are not palpable, and endoscopic guidance is often necessary intraoperatively.

References

1. Upchurch Br, Vargo JJ. Small bowel enteroscopy. Rev Gastroenterol Disord 2008;8:169–77.
2. Classen M, Frühmorgen P, Koch H. Peroral enteroscopy of the small and large intestine. Endoscopy 1972;4:157–9.
3. Seensalu R. The sonde examination. Gastrointest Endosc Clin N Am 1999;9:37–59.
4. Yamamoto H, Sekine Y, Sato Y, Higashizawa T, Miyata T, Iino S, et al. Total enteroscopy with a nonsurgical steerable double-balloon method. Gastrointest Endosc 2001;53:216–20.
5. Gerson L, Flodin J, Miyabayashi K. Balloon-assisted enteroscopy: technology and troubleshooting. Gastrointest Endosc 2008;68:1158–67.
6. Mehdizadeh S, Ross A, Gerson L, Leighton J, Chen A, Schembre D, et al. What is the learning curve associated with double balloon enteroscopy? Technical details and early experience in 6 U.S. tertiary care centers. Gastrointest Endosc 2006;64:740–50.
7. Askin M, Lewis B. Push enteroscopic cauterization: long-term follow-up of 83 patients with bleeding small intestinal angiodysplasia. Gastrointest Endosc 1996;43:580–3.
8. Yamamoto H, Kita H, Sunada K, Hayashi Y, Sato H, Yano T, et al. Clinical outcomes of double-balloon endoscopy for the diagnosis and treatment of small-intestinal diseases. Clin Gastroenterol Hepatol 2004;2:1010–6.
9. Di Caro S, May A, Heine DG, Fini L, Landi B, Petruzziello L, et al. The European experience with double-balloon enteroscopy: indications,

IV

methodology, safety, and clinical impact. Gastrointest Endosc 2005;62: 545–50.

10. Gay G, Delvaux M, Fassler I. Outcome of capsule endoscopy in determining indication and route for push and pull enteroscopy. Endoscopy 2006;38:49–58.

11. Raju GS, Gerson L, Das A, Lewis B; American Gastroenterological Association. American Gastroenterological Association (AGA) Institute medical position statement on obscure gastrointestinal bleeding. Gastroenterology 2007;133:1694–6.

12. ASGE Technology Committee, DiSario JA, Petersen BT, Tierney WM, Adler DG, Chand B, et al. Enteroscopes. Gastrointest Endosc 2007;66:872–80.

13. Lewis B, Eisen G, Friedman S. A pooled analysis to evaluate results of capsule endoscopy trials. Endoscopy 2005;37:960–5.

14. Lai LH, Wong GL, Chow DK, Lau JY, Sung JJ, Leung WK. Long-term follow-up of patients with obscure gastrointestinal bleeding after negative capsule endoscopy. Am J Gastroenterol 2006;101:1224–8.

15. Jones BH, Fleischer DE, Sharma VK, Heigh RI, Shiff AD, Hernandez JL, et al. Yield of repeat wireless video capsule endoscopy in patients with obscure gastrointestinal bleeding. Am J Gastroenterol 2005;100:1058–64.

16. Chong AK, Chin BW, Meredith CG. Clinically significant small-bowel pathology identified by double-balloon enteroscopy but missed by capsule endoscopy. Gastrointest Endosc 2006;64:445–9.

17. Cave D, Legnani P, de Franchis R, Lewis B. ICCE consensus for capsule retention. Endoscopy 2005;37:1065–7.

18. Tanaka S, Mitsui K, Shirakawa K, Tatsuguchi A, Nakamura T, Hayashi Y, et al. Successful retrieval of video capsule endoscopy retained at ileal stenosis of Crohn's disease using double-balloon endoscopy. J Gastroenterol Hepatol 2006;21:922–3.

19. Tsujikawa T, Saitoh Y, Andoh A, Imaeda H, Hata K, Minematsu H, et al. Novel single-balloon enteroscopy for diagnosis and treatment of the small intestine: preliminary experience. Endoscopy 2008;40:11–5.

20. Kawamura T, Yasuda K, Tanaka K, Uno K, Ueda M, Sanada K, et al. Clinical evaluation of a newly developed single-balloon enteroscope. Gastrointest Endosc 2008;68:1112–6.

21. Dellon E, Kohn G, Morgan D, Grimm I. Endoscopic retrograde cholangio-pancreatography with single-balloon enteroscopy is feasible in patients with a prior Roux-en-Y anastomosis. Dig Dis Sci 2008 [Epub ahead of print].

22. Koornstra JJ. Double balloon enteroscopy for endoscopic retrograde cholangiopancreaticography after Roux-en-Y reconstruction: case series and review of the literature. Neth J Med 2008;66:275–9.

23. Chu Y, Yang C, Yeh Y, Chen C, Yueh S. Double-balloon enteroscopy application in biliary tract disease—its therapeutic and diagnostic functions. Gastrointest Endosc 2008;68:585–91.

24. Akerman PA, Agrawal D, Cantero D, Pangtay J. Spiral enteroscopy with the new DSB overtube: a novel technique for deep peroral small-bowel intubation. Endoscopy 2008;40:974–8.

25. Hotokezaka M, Jimi S, Hidaka H, Eto T, Chijiiwa K. Intraoperative enteroscopy in minimally invasive surgery. Surg Laparosc Endosc Percutan Tech 2007;17:492–2.

26. Raju GS, Gerson L, Das A, Lewis B; American Gastroenterological Association. American Gastroenterological Association (AGA) Institute technical review on obscure gastrointestinal bleeding. Gastroenterology 2007;133: 1697–717.

12

13 Wireless Video Capsule Endoscopy

David Cave

Introduction

Video capsule endoscopy (VCE) became a clinical reality in 2001, with Food and Drug Administration (FDA) approval of the M2A capsule (Given Imaging, Inc., Yoqneam, Israel) on the basis of a study comparing push enteroscopy with the capsule in patients with obscure gastrointestinal bleeding [1]. For clinicians interested in disorders of the small intestine, the arrival of capsule endoscopy was timely. Conventional endoscopic technology was severely limited; push enteroscopy allowed examination of up to 100 cm distal to the ligament of Treitz; ileoscopy allowed examination of the distal ileum; intraoperative enteroscopy was and still is the "gold standard" for small-bowel examination, but is far from perfect and is invasive [2]. The indications and limitations of VCE are now quite well understood around the world. In 2007, the FDA approved the EndoCapsule (Olympus America, Inc., Center Valley, Pennsylvania, USA) [3]. Capsules developed in China and the MiRo capsule from Korea have also been demonstrated [4], but are not yet clinically available in Western countries. With the concurrent development of other novel enteroscopic devices—double-balloon enteroscopes [5] (Fujinon Inc., Wayne, New Jersey, USA), single-balloon enteroscopes [6] (Olympus America), and spiral overtubes [7] (Endo-Ease Discovery SB; Spirus Medical, Inc., Stoughton, Massachusetts, USA) for diagnosis and/or therapy—interest in the small intestine has undergone a renaissance. This chapter reviews the technology of VCE, the indications for the procedure, and its complications and provides a perspective on it in relation to other enteroscopic techniques.

Technology

The PillCam SB, EndoCapsule, and MiRo capsule are similar in size, shape, weight, and imaging capabilities. The MiRo capsule uses electrical field propagation to transmit images (**Table 13.1**). Both the PillCam and EndoCapsule are single-ended imaging devices that are able to take two images per second for a total of about 55 000 images over the life of the silver oxide battery. The images created by the VCE are transmitted to a portable hard drive worn on the patient's belt, via eight sensor arrays adherent to the abdominal skin. After an 8-h period, the recorder is transferred from the patient to a workstation, and the images are processed into a video. The image quality of the two FDA-approved devices is excellent, but subjectively different. The slightly larger field of view of the PillCam SB has yet to be shown to be clinically useful. The images are magnified 1 : 8, allowing resolution of individual villi (**Fig. 13.1**). Since there is clear succus entericus in the lumen for much of the length of the small bowel, conditions are met for immersion endoscopy. The villi are often seen to be "floating," analogous to seaweed on a submerged rock. There is considerable variation in the normal characteristics of the villi. In at least 75 % of studies, the entire length of the intestine is visualized. In the remaining 25 %, transit of the capsule is incomplete after 8 h, but fewer than 1 % of capsules are retained for a long period. Transient retention usually occurs at the ileocecal valve.

Table 13.1 Comparison of video capsules

	EndoCapsule	PillCam SB	MiRo
Length	26	26	24
Diameter	11	11	10.8
Weight	3.8	3.45	3.3
Frame rate	2 fps	2 fps	2fps
Image sensor	CCD	CMOS	CMOS
Field of view	145	156	150
Illumination	6 white LEDs	6 white LEDs	6 white LEDs
Antennas	8 body leads	8 body leads	Electrical field propagation
Real-time viewing	VE-1 viewer	Yes	No
Documentation	DVD	CD	?

CCD, charge-coupled device; CD, compact disk; CMOS, complementary metal oxide semiconductor; DVD, digital video disk; fps, frames per second; LED, light-emitting diode.

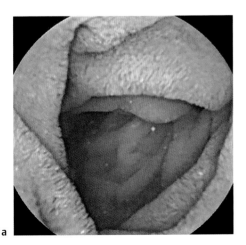
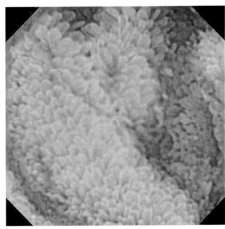

Fig. 13.1
a Normal villi.
b Edematous villi.

a

b

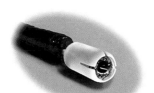

Fig. 13.2 Capsule placement device.

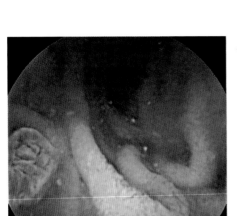

Fig. 13.3 Ampulla of Vater.

It consists of a plastic film encasing a lactose–barium mixture and a small transponder [14,15]. At each end of it there is a dissolvable plug, which starts to disintegrate after about 36 h of contact with digestive juice. The concept is that this type of device can be useful when there is a suspected stricture that cannot be demonstrated by other means. The capsule is swallowed, and 30 h later the abdomen is scanned with a device to detect the transponder, or using a plain abdominal film. If the capsule is not detected or is in the colon, there is sufficient lumen for the video capsule to pass. The video capsule may still not complete its passage through the small bowel before the battery runs out. This device is particularly useful in patients known to have Crohn's disease, in whom there is a capsule retention risk of up to 13%. In patients without Crohn's disease or those in whom it is only suspected, the retention rate is 1% or less. The device was originally designed with a single plug, which dissolved erratically and was associated with a few cases of obstruction.

Preparation of the patient remains controversial. Many small studies have been performed, but all have the fundamental problem of not being able to objectively measure what constitutes good preparation. Furthermore, it is not clear whether there is an increased diagnostic yield if the preparation is better; preparation may wash away small amounts of blood and thereby reduce the diagnostic value of the procedure [16].

The use of simethicone as a bubble-reducing agent is also controversial, as are prokinetics. There is some evidence that placing the bed-ridden patient in the right lateral decubitus position reduces gastric transit time, but this has not been confirmed in ambulatory patients. Clinically, the most commonly used preparations are nothing by mouth for 12 h before the procedure or 2 L of a polyethylene glycol solution the night before the procedure. The present author does not routinely use preparation, except in patients in whom there is evidence of reduced motility.

The PillCam SB is approved for use in children down to the age of 10, but anecdotally it has been used in children as young as 2 years of age without mishap. Children who are unable to swallow the capsule need to have the capsule placed endoscopically under general anesthesia (**Fig. 13.2**).

Relatively recently, the PillCam ESO (Given Imaging, Inc., Yoqneam, Israel) has been approved by the FDA [8,9] for screening patients for Barrett's esophagus and detecting esophageal varices. The device is the same size as the other capsules described above, but is double-ended and is used to take seven frames per second at each end. It has now been upgraded to take nine frames per second. Optimal imaging is obtained by placing the patient in the left lateral position. After rinsing out the mouth, the patient swallows the capsule with 15 mL of water, followed every 30 s by 15 mL of water ingested from a large-tipped syringe [10]. This position eliminates gravity and minimizes bubbles, and esophageal motility is such that that several minutes of imaging of the esophageal mucosa are possible. The battery life is only 30 min, but excellent views of the gastric mucosa and proximal small bowel can also be obtained. Images front the front and back are reviewed in parallel, and as the length of the capsule is known, it becomes possible to measure the length of abnormalities. However, at current pricing levels the device is not cost-effective and it has not caught on in the clinical arena. One study has reported sensitivity, specificity, and positive and negative predictive values for Barrett's esophagus in comparison with esophagogastroduodenoscopy (EGD) as 97%, 100%, 100%, and 98%, respectively. However, a second study including 96 patients only showed a sensitivity of 67% and a specificity of 84% [9,11].

This capsule has also been approved for detection of varices. In this context, it has potential value in very ill patients with decompensated liver disease who are reluctant to undergo endoscopy, to check whether they have esophageal varices [12].

A colon capsule has been developed and is undergoing trials in Europe [13]. This is larger, 30 mm long, and is again double-ended. Unfortunately, the withdrawal of the prokinetic agent tegaserod (Novartis), has put the trials in the USA on hold pending the availability of a new small-bowel prokinetic agent.

The Agile patency capsule (Given Imaging, Inc., Yoqneam, Israel) has undergone development to the point that it is now a useful tool.

Limitations

The technology is not perfect. In the majority of patients, 75% of the full length of the small bowel may be visualized, but the mucosal surface is incompletely seen. The duodenal sweep is usually poorly imaged, and the ampulla of Vater is seen about 5% of the time (**Fig. 13.3**). This is for two reasons—firstly, the lumen is not distended, so that it is not possible to see deeply between the plicae; and secondly, the capsule has been shown to tumble. This was demonstrated in the FDA trial for the Olympus capsule, in which a PillCam SB and EndoCapsule were swallowed by the same patient 40 min apart [3]. In some of the patients, the second capsule caught up with the first and imaged the leading capsule in a variety of postures, including tumbling and with the lens hood buried in the mucosa. This possibility was alluded to in an early paper in which beads were attached in a dog's intestinal mucosa. Subsequent study with VCE did not detect all the beads [17].

Interpretation is a major issue. The American Society for Gastrointestinal Endoscopy has recommended credentialing guidelines, which should be regarded as minimalist. There is the problem of the learning curve, particularly learning the range of normal variation. There is considerable confusion in interpreting abnormalities associated with intraluminal bubbles and what constitutes a submucosal mass. Thirdly, there is disagreement, even between experts, as to when a red spot becomes an angiectasia; the level of disagreement may be as high as 25% [3]. The capsule is also not the perfect tool for detecting small-bowel polyps or tumors, but is still better

IV

than other noninvasive techniques. Lastly, some abnormalities may require great concentration on the part of the reader—e.g., a single angiectasia on only one image.

Complications

VCE is remarkably safe. No deaths attributed to the device have been reported, despite more than 800,000 ingestions. One perforation has been attributed to a capsule, and there is rare anecdotal evidence of transient small-bowel obstruction, probably as the VCE is squeezed through a tight stricture over hours or days. There have been concerns about pacemakers and implanted cardiac defibrillators, and indeed there is an FDA warning regarding this on the label. However, several publications have examined the issue and have not found any problems either with the device interfering with the capsule or with the capsule interfering with the implanted device.

Occasional impaction of the capsule in the piriform fossa has been noted (**Fig. 13.4**). The capsule is best retrieved using an endoscope and a Roth retrieval net with the patient in the head-down position. Symptomatic dysphagia usually requires endoscopic placement, with or without dilation, depending on the reason for the dysphagia. Previous gastric surgery, such as a Billroth II procedure, is not usually a problem, but Roux-en-Y procedures for obesity management can be troublesome, as the gastrojejunal anastomosis may not allow passage of the capsule. Entrapment of the capsule in a duodenal or jejunal diverticulum is usually transient, but may lead to an incomplete study.

Indications and Contraindications

Obscure gastrointestinal bleeding. The indications for VCE are evolving (**Table 13.2**). The major indication is for obscure gastrointestinal bleeding, which may be overt or occult. This is defined as the absence of a bleeding site that is detectable using good upper endoscopy and colonoscopy examinations. The American Gastroenterological Association technical review suggests that about 5% of cases of gastrointestinal bleeding are in the obscure category [18]. The rate at which a source is identified has ranged from 50% to over 70%, and much depends on case selection [19,20]. The yield will be higher in patients who require transfusion than in those patients with a simple iron-deficiency anemia. Care needs to be taken to distinguish a capsule "finding"—an abnormality on the video—from the true diagnosis, or better still a final diagnosis based on pathology or a therapeutic intervention. This is because seeing an angiectasia on the video does not always mean that that is the source of the bleeding. In addition, when active bleeding without a clear source is seen, localizing its precise position longitudinally in the small bowel may be a real challenge (**Fig. 13.5**). The new deep enteroscopic techniques may be very helpful in this context. The author's preference is to maintain anticoagulation during VCE and enteroscopy in order to maximize the chance of finding a bleeding source. There is evidence that performing VCE as close as possible in time to the bleeding episode maximizes the diagnostic yield [19].

A meta-analysis of 14 studies including 396 patients with obscure bleeding demonstrated a 63% yield overall, with a clinically significant yield of 56% for VCE. This was significantly higher than for barium studies (8%) and for push enteroscopy (26%). The increased yield of VCE in comparison with push enteroscopy and small-bowel barium radiography for clinically significant findings was 30% or more, with a number needed to treat of three. In a study of 100 patients, Pennazio et al. demonstrated a very high yield of 92% in a subgroup of 26 patients with obscure overt bleeding. Previously, the yield for overt bleeding in 31 patients was 13% and 44% in patients with iron-deficiency anemia. In these patients, the

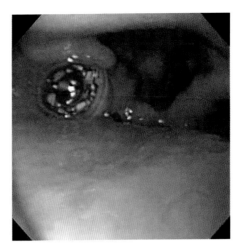

Fig. 13.4 Impaction of a capsule in a piriform fossa.

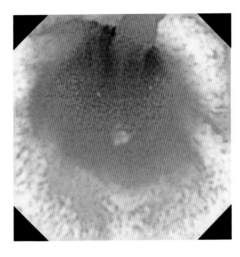

Fig. 13.5 Active small-bowel bleeding; the source is not seen.

Table 13.2 Indications and possible indications for video capsule endoscopy

Indications
Obscure gastrointestinal bleeding
Suspected Crohn's disease
Suspected small-intestinal tumor
Screening for Barrett's esophagus
Screening for varices
Possible indications
Chronic diarrhea
Abdominal pain
Diagnosis of celiac disease/malabsorptive states
Graft-versus-host reaction
Detection of the cause of partial small-bowel obstruction

most common finding was angiectasia (29%) [19] (**Fig. 13.6**). The sources of bleeding in this study and others are shown in **Table 13.3**. It is important to take a history of whether a patient is using or has used nonsteroidal anti-inflammatory drugs (NSAIDs). These drugs most frequently cause no more than breaks in the small-bowel mucosa. Much less frequently, they cause ulceration, and more rarely still the formation of very short (usually ulcerated) stenoses, which may present as obscure gastrointestinal bleeding, anemia, or abdominal pain. These probably idiosyncratic and rare lesions are a frequent cause of capsule retention (**Fig. 13.7**).

13

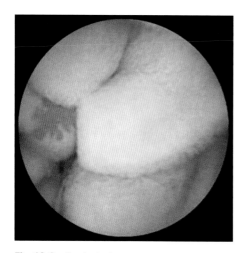

Fig. 13.6 Angiectasia.

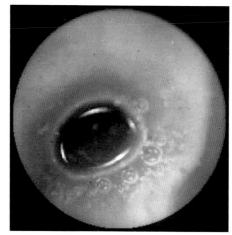

Fig. 13.7 Nonsteroidal anti-inflammatory drug (NSAID) ulcerated stricture.

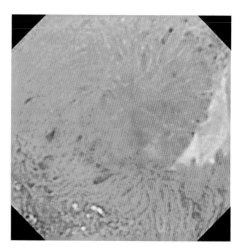

Fig. 13.8 Ileal Crohn's disease: ulcer and villous edema.

Table 13.3 Sources of obscure gastrointestinal bleeding

Origin of bleeding	
Normal	33 %
Angiectasia	15 %
Source not seen	14 %
Dieulafoy lesion	5 %
Crohn's disease	7 %
On specific ulcers	4 %
NSAID lesion	4 %
GAVE	4 %
Small-bowel varices	1 %
Tumors	2–8 %

NSAID, nonsteroidal anti-inflammatory drug; GAVE, gastric antral vascular ectasia.

Table 13.4 Differential diagnosis of small-bowel ulceration

Crohn's disease

NSAID ulcers/webs

Eosinophilic gastroenteritis

Jejunoileitis associated with celiac disease

Radiation enteritis

Behçet disease

Enteritis—systemic lupus erythematosus, Churg–Strauss syndrome, vasculitis

Chronic nonspecific stenosing ulceration (CNSU)

Graft-versus-host reaction

Suspected Crohn's disease. This indication is quite strongly supported in the literature, but the data are not uniform. The diagnostic utility of VCE also revolves around the question of how to define Crohn's disease using VCE, and to date there has been little discussion and no consensus on this. The recently described Lewis index is helpful for semiquantification of villous abnormalities, ulceration, and stenoses in the small intestine, but it is not specific to Crohn's disease [21]. The finding of a single aphthoid ulcer is clearly not diagnostic. However, multiple serpiginous ulcers with surrounding edema in an appropriate clinical context might be diagnostic (**Fig. 13.8**). In reality, the VCE findings may provide useful information that should be taken into consideration in the context of a good history, physical examination, and other tests, since there is no pathognomonic feature for the diagnosis of Crohn's disease. It

should be remembered that there is a significant differential diagnosis in small-bowel ulceration (**Table 13.4**; **Fig. 13.9**). The first report on the use of VCE in patients with suspected Crohn's disease detected abnormalities in 12 of 17 patients from all over Israel, selected due to diagnostic difficulty [22]. In a recent study that compared four different techniques for the investigation—computed-tomographic enterography, small-bowel series, colonoscopy, and ileoscopy—VCE was as sensitive as the other techniques, but was limited by the potential for retention by strictures that might have caused partial small-bowel obstruction [23]. A meta-analysis suggested that VCE is the most useful test in nonstricturing Crohn's disease, with a number needed to treat (NNT) of three relative to small-bowel radiography and an NNT of seven relative to colonoscopy and ileoscopy [24].

Established Crohn's disease. There are two possible uses in this context; one is to identify whether healing has occurred. The paradigm shift from symptomatic control to mucosal healing supports this use, but there are no systematic data on the topic. Secondly, in about 20–30 % of cases of small-bowel Crohn's disease, it can be very difficult to resolve whether there is a true flare of disease or whether there is concurrent exacerbation of an irritable bowel disorder [25]. Clarification of this diagnostic issue in these patients has major implications for cost containment and for avoiding risks of unnecessary and potentially hazardous medications.

VCE has rarely been used as a measure of therapeutic response in Crohn's disease trials [26]. This is partly because of concerns about capsule retention, and partly because of additional expense. However, in the study concerned, colonoscopy was the only test used to assess anastomotic recurrence. The possibility of more proximal recurrence was ignored, except in one patient in whom colonoscopy was not possible and who required capsule endoscopy.

Indeterminate colitis. In approximately 15 % of patients with colitis, it is difficult or impossible to categorize them as having either Crohn's disease or ulcerative colitis on the basis of current clinical histological and other available assessments. There are limited data on the use of VCE in this context. The data do suggest that the device may be useful, but a long-term prospective follow-up is needed [27].

Suspected small-bowel tumors. VCE clearly has a role to play in the detection of small-bowel tumors, whether benign, malignant, or metastatic (**Fig. 13.10**). It is not perfect, but when used in conjunction with radiographic imaging and/or deep enteroscopy it is valuable. The leading indication is obscure bleeding, as this is the most common early manifestation of most tumors. The overall incidence

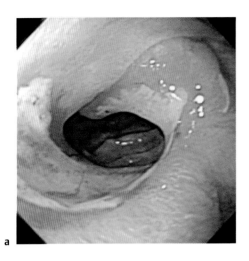

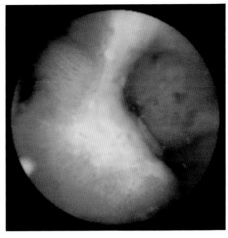

a

b

Fig. 13.9
a Duodenal Crohn's disease at upper endoscopy.
b The same lesion as seen by video capsule endoscopy.

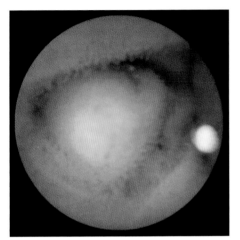

Fig. 13.10 Carcinoid.

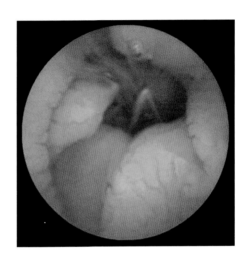

Fig. 13.11 Celiac disease with scalloping of the jejunal plicae.

13

of tumors in this diagnostic category is 6–8 % [28,29]. VCE has a role to play in the initial diagnosis and follow-up of the polyposis syndromes, particularly Peutz–Jeghers syndrome and familial adenomatous polyposis. Polyps may be missed, especially in the duodenum in the area of the papilla, due to rapid transit of the capsule though the duodenal sweep. The fact that the papilla is seen on only 5 % of studies is a reflection of this limitation.

Barrett's esophagus and esophageal varices. The PillCam ESO has been approved for detection of varices and for Barrett's esophagus, but due to the availability of preexisting technology (particularly EGD), the inability to take biopsies, and the expense of VCE, it is not use in widespread use [30].

▥ Potential Indications for VCE

There are a variety of indications for VCE that may be useful in the right clinical context (**Table 13.2**). Patients with unexplained chronic diarrhea may have a variety of inflammatory conditions that are sometimes not easily diagnosed, including Crohn's disease and eosinophilic gastroenteritis. Using VCE to diagnose the cause of abdominal pain is generally unrewarding [31], with a diagnostic yield of less than 20 %.

Several reports on the use of VCE in the diagnosis of celiac disease show that it is comparable to EGD in visual terms, but lacks the ability to obtain tissue—a critical issue in Marsh 1 patients who only have an increase in intraepithelial lymphocytes. VCE is a useful tool in patients who do not wish to undergo EGD [32]. A more important

role for it lies in the evaluation of refractory celiac disease, with or without ulcerative jejunitis (**Fig. 13.11**). VCE is able to detect possible enteropathy-associated T cell lymphoma, but biopsy at enteroscopy is still need to confirm monoclonality (type 2 refractory celiac disease).

Initial observations in patients with graft-versus-host disease after small-bowel transplantation or bone-marrow transplantation have been reported. The use of VCE appears promising in this very sick population, who are best studied when possible with noninvasive techniques [33].

Interplay between VCE and Deep Enteroscopy

The rapid and parallel development of deep enteroscopy and VCE has raised questions about their relative benefits and drawbacks. Obviously, VCE is limited to observation, while the enteroscopic technologies are both diagnostic and therapeutic. However, they are much more invasive and time-consuming. Until recently, there has been as scarcity of comparative data, as many centers only had one or other of the technologies. If both are available, VCE appears to have a slightly greater diagnostic capability than balloon enteroscopy [34]. The overall consensus appears to be that VCE should be the initial test for obscure gastrointestinal bleeding if both systems are available and that it can be used to guide the approach—antegrade or retrograde—in deep enteroscopy to avoid having to do both directions. In patients with massive bleeding, deep anterograde enteroscopy is probably the test of choice.

Summary

The small bowel is no longer a forgotten corner of endoscopic activity. VCE allows the investigation of the entire length of the intestine, including the esophagus, small bowel, and colon. The formally recognized indications are proving to be no bar to the investigation of other disorders of the small intestine. Obscure gastrointestinal bleeding is no longer the nightmare clinical challenge that it used to be. The combined use of VCE and deep enteroscopy is proving to be of great benefit to patients, by providing more accurate diagnoses more quickly and with a reduced need for intraoperative enteroscopy.

References

1. Lewis BS, Swain P. Capsule endoscopy in the evaluation of patients with suspected small intestinal bleeding: results of a pilot study. Gastrointest Endosc 2002;56:349–53.
2. Lewis BS, Waye JD. Small bowel enteroscopy in 1988: pros and cons. Am J Gastroenterol 1988;83:799–802.
3. Cave DR, Fleischer DE, Leighton JA, Faigel DO, Heigh RI, Sharma VK, et al. A multicenter randomized comparison of the EndoCapsule and the PillCam SB. Gastrointest Endosc 2008;68:487–94.
4. Bang S, Park JY, Jeong S, Kim YH, Shim HB, Kim TS, et al. First clinical trial of the "MiRo" capsule endoscope by using a novel transmission technology: electric-field propagation. Gastrointest Endosc 2009;69:253–9.
5. Yamamoto H, Sekine Y, Sato Y, Higashizawa T, Miyata T, Iino S, et al. Total enteroscopy with a nonsurgical steerable double-balloon method. Gastrointest Endosc 2001;53:216–20.
6. Kawamura T, Yasuda K, Tanaka K, Uno K, Ueda M, Sanada K, et al. Clinical evaluation of a newly developed single-balloon enteroscope. Gastrointest Endosc 2008;68:1112–6.
7. Akerman PA, Agrawal D, Cantero D, Pangtay J. Spiral enteroscopy with the new DSB overtube: a novel technique for deep peroral small-bowel intubation. Endoscopy 2008;40:974–8.
8. Lin OS, Schembre DB, Mergener K, Spaulding W, Lomah N, Ayub K, et al. Blinded comparison of esophageal capsule endoscopy versus conventional endoscopy for a diagnosis of Barrett's esophagus in patients with chronic gastroesophageal reflux. Gastrointest Endosc 2007;65:577–83.
9. Eisen GM, Eliakim R, Zaman A, Schwartz J, Faigel D, Rondonotti E, et al. The accuracy of PillCam ESO capsule endoscopy versus conventional upper endoscopy for the diagnosis of esophageal varices: a prospective three-center pilot study. Endoscopy 2006;38:31–5.
10. Gralnek IM, Rabinovitz R, Afik D, Eliakim R. A simplified ingestion procedure for esophageal capsule endoscopy: initial evaluation in healthy volunteers. Endoscopy 2006;38:913–8.
11. Galmiche JP, Sacher-Huvelin S, Coron E, Cholet F, Soussan EB, Sebille V, et al. Screening for esophagitis and Barrett's esophagus with wireless esophageal capsule endoscopy: a multicenter prospective trial in patients with reflux symptoms. Am J Gastroenterol 2008;103:538–45.
12. de Franchis R, Eisen GM, Laine L, Fernandez-Urien I, Herrerias JM, Brown RD, et al. Esophageal capsule endoscopy for screening and surveillance of esophageal varices in patients with portal hypertension. Hepatology 2008;47:1595–603.
13. Schoofs N, Devière J, Van GA. PillCam colon capsule endoscopy compared with colonoscopy for colorectal tumor diagnosis: a prospective pilot study. Endoscopy 2006;38:971–7.
14. Spada C, Shah SK, Riccioni ME, Spera G, Marchese M, Iacopini F, et al. Video capsule endoscopy in patients with known or suspected small bowel stricture previously tested with the dissolving patency capsule. J Clin Gastroenterol 2007;41:576–82.
15. Spada C, Riccioni ME, Costamagna G. Patients with known small bowel stricture or with symptoms of small bowel obstruction secondary to Crohn's disease should not perform video capsule endoscopy without being previously tested for small bowel patency. Am J Gastroenterol 2007;102:1542–3.
16. Rokkas T, Papaxoinis K, Triantafyllou K, Pistiolas D, Ladas SD. Does purgative preparation influence the diagnostic yield of small bowel video capsule endoscopy? A meta-analysis. Am J Gastroenterol 2009;104:219–27.
17. Appleyard M, Fireman Z, Glukhovsky A, Jacob H, Shreiver R, Kadirkamanathan S, et al. A randomized trial comparing wireless capsule endoscopy with push enteroscopy for the detection of small-bowel lesions. Gastroenterology 2000;119:1431–38.
18. Raju GS, Gerson L, Das A, Lewis B. American Gastroenterological Association (AGA) Institute technical review on obscure gastrointestinal bleeding. Gastroenterology 2007;133:1697–717.
19. Pennazio M, Santucci R, Rondonotti E, Abbiati C, Beccari G, Rossini FP, et al. Outcome of patients with obscure gastrointestinal bleeding after capsule endoscopy: report of 100 consecutive cases. Gastroenterology 2004;126:643–53.
20. Pennazio M, Eisen G, Goldfarb N. ICCE consensus for obscure gastrointestinal bleeding. Endoscopy 2005;37:1046–50.
21. Gralnek IM, Defranchis R, Seidman E, Leighton JA, Legnani P, Lewis BS. Development of a capsule endoscopy scoring index for small bowel mucosal inflammatory change. Aliment Pharmacol Ther 2008;27:146–54.
22. Eliakim R, Suissa A, Yassin K, Katz D, Fischer D. Wireless capsule video endoscopy compared to barium follow-through and computerised tomography in patients with suspected Crohn's disease—final report. Dig Liver Dis 2004;36:519–22.
23. Solem CA, Loftus EV Jr, Fletcher JG, Baron TH, Gostout CJ, Petersen BT, et al. Small-bowel imaging in Crohn's disease: a prospective, blinded, 4-way comparison trial. Gastrointest Endosc 2008;68:255–66.
24. Triester SL, Leighton JA, Leontiadis GI, Gurudu SR, Fleischer DE, Hara AK, et al. A meta-analysis of the yield of capsule endoscopy compared to other diagnostic modalities in patients with non-stricturing small bowel Crohn's disease. Am J Gastroenterol 2006;101:954–64.
25. Buchman AL, Miller FH, Wallin A, Chowdhry AA, Ahn C. Videocapsule endoscopy versus barium contrast studies for the diagnosis of Crohn's disease recurrence involving the small intestine. Am J Gastroenterol 2004;99:2171–7.
26. Regueiro M, Schraut W, Baidoo L, Kip KE, Sepulveda AR, Pesci M, et al. Infliximab prevents Crohn's disease recurrence after ileal resection. Gastroenterology 2009;136:441–50.
27. Mow WS, Lo SK, Targan SR, Dubinsky MC, Treyzon L, Abreu-Martin MT, et al. Initial experience with wireless capsule enteroscopy in the diagnosis and management of inflammatory bowel disease. Clin Gastroenterol Hepatol 2004;2:31–40.
28. Rondonotti E, Pennazio M, Toth E, Menchen P, Riccioni ME, De Palma GD, et al. Small-bowel neoplasms in patients undergoing video capsule endoscopy: a multicenter European study. Endoscopy 2008;40:488–95.
29. Urbain D, De Looze D, Demedts I, Louis E, Dewit O, Macken E, et al. Video capsule endoscopy in small-bowel malignancy: a multicenter Belgian study. Endoscopy 2006;38:408–11.
30. Rubenstein JH, Inadomi JM, Brill JV, Eisen GM. Cost utility of screening for Barrett's esophagus with esophageal capsule endoscopy versus conventional upper endoscopy. Clin Gastroenterol Hepatol 2007;5:312–8.
31. Keuchel M, Hagenmuller F. Video capsule endoscopy in the work-up of abdominal pain. Gastrointest Endosc Clin N Am 2004;14:195–205.
32. Rondonotti E, Spada C, Cave D, Pennazio M, Riccioni ME, De Vitis I, et al. Video capsule endoscopy in the diagnosis of celiac disease: a multicenter study. Am J Gastroenterol 2007;102:1624–31.
33. de Franchis R, Rondonotti E, Abbiati C, Beccari G, Merighi A, Pinna A, et al. Capsule enteroscopy in small bowel transplantation. Dig Liver Dis 2003;35:728–31.
34. Pohl J, Delvaux M, Ell C, Gay G, May A, Mulder CJ, et al. European Society of Gastrointestinal Endoscopy (ESGE) guidelines: flexible enteroscopy for diagnosis and treatment of small-bowel diseases. Endoscopy 2008;40:609–18.

IV

14 Colonoscopy: Basic Instrumentation and Technique

Brian Saunders

Introduction

In 1969, Shinya and Wolff described the first total colonoscopy, heralding a new era in the diagnosis and treatment of colonic disease [1]. Today, modern video colonoscopes provide breathtaking views of the colonic and terminal ileal mucosa revealing even the subtlest abnormalities of contour and color. Due to the biopsy and therapeutic capability of colonoscopy, it is the procedure of choice for investigation of colonic symptoms and is widely accepted as the "gold standard" procedure for the detection and prevention of colorectal neoplasia [2,3]. Despite the clear advantages of colonoscopy, insertion to the cecum is technically difficult in some patients and requires patience, manual dexterity, hand–eye coordination, and a good understanding of the anatomical basis for loop formation. The demand for colonoscopy is continuing to increase, and with this comes a duty for the endoscopist to ensure a safe, comfortable, and complete examination.

Indications

The European Society for Gastrointestinal Endoscopy (ESGE) has published comprehensive guidelines on the appropriateness of colonoscopy [4], and the American Society for Gastrointestinal Endoscopy (ASGE) recommendations are shown in **Tables 14.1–14.3**.

The detailed color image provided by colonoscopy and its biopsy and therapeutic potential make it the ideal examination for the detection of subtle inflammatory changes, vascular lesions, and neoplasia. It is therefore the procedure of choice for patients presenting with chronic diarrhea, anemia, and rectal bleeding, and as surveillance for those considered at high risk of developing colorectal cancer, in whom there may be a higher incidence of small, flat, advanced neoplastic lesions. Definitions of high-risk individuals and recommendations on surveillance intervals remain controversial and, in practical terms, are intimately linked to whether or not population screening is available nationally. Broadly speaking, there has been a trend toward extending surveillance for adenoma follow-up. In the U.S. National Polyp Study, there was no significant benefit in terms of advanced neoplasia detection (adenoma > 1 cm in size, severe dysplasia, or villous histology), comparing initial, 1-yearly plus 3-yearly, and 3-yearly colonoscopic surveillance [5]. Provided there is no family history of colorectal cancer (CRC), it appears that patients with one or two small, tubular adenomas can be left safely for 5 years or more [6] following a normal and complete examination. On the other hand, patients with "high-risk" adenomas (severe dysplasia, multiple adenomas, family history, and villous histology) may benefit from closer surveillance at 1–3-yearly intervals. Clearly, surveillance has to be tailored to the individual and not continued if biologically irrelevant—that is, if the risks of colonoscopy outweigh potential long-term benefits from CRC prevention. In the USA, colonoscopy screening at 10-yearly intervals from the age of 50 for average-risk individuals is a widely practiced and apparently successful cancer prevention strategy [6]. Other countries, such as Germany, Switzerland, and Poland have also used colonoscopy as the primary screening test, generally with high completion and low complication rates [7,8]. Aggressive colo-

Table 14.1 Colonoscopy is generally indicated in the following circumstances

- Evaluation of an abnormality on barium enema that is likely to be clinically significant, such as a filling defect or stricture
- Evaluation of unexplained gastrointestinal bleeding:
  - Hematochezia in the absence of a convincing anorectal source
  - Melena after an upper gastrointestinal source has been excluded
  - Presence of fecal occult blood
- Unexplained iron-deficiency anemia
- Surveillance for colonic neoplasia:
  - Examination to evaluate the entire colon for synchronous cancer or neoplastic polyps in a patient with treatable cancer or neoplastic polyp
  - Clearing colonoscopy at or around the time of curative resection of cancer, followed by colonoscopy at 3 years and 3–5 years thereafter to detect metachronous cancer
  - Following adequate clearance of neoplastic polyp(s), survey at 3–5-year intervals
  - Patients with significant family history:
    a. Hereditary nonpolyposis colorectal cancer (HNPCC): colonoscopy every 2 years beginning at the earlier of age 25, or 5 years younger than the earliest age of diagnosis of colorectal cancer. Annual colonoscopy should begin at age 40.
    b. Sporadic colorectal cancer before the age of 60: colonoscopy every 5 years beginning at age 10 years earlier than the affected relative, or every 3 years if adenoma is found
    In patients with ulcerative pancolitis of 8 or more years' duration or left-sided colitis of 15 or more years' duration, every 1–2 years with systematic biopsies to detect dysplasia
- Chronic inflammatory bowel disease of the colon if more precise diagnosis or determination of the extent of activity of disease will influence immediate management
- Clinically significant diarrhea of unexplained origin
- Intraoperative identification of a lesion not apparent at surgery (e. g., polypectomy site, location of a bleeding site)
- Treatment of bleeding from such lesions as vascular malformation, ulceration, neoplasia, and polypectomy site (e. g., electrocoagulation, heater probe, laser or injection therapy)
- Foreign-body removal
- Excision of colonic polyp
- Decompression of acute nontoxic megacolon or sigmoid volvulus
- Balloon dilation of stenotic lesions (e. g., anastomotic strictures)
- Palliative treatment of stenosing or bleeding neoplasms (e. g., laser, electrocoagulation, stenting)
- Marking a neoplasm for localization

Table 14.2 Colonoscopy is generally not indicated in the following circumstances

- Chronic, stable irritable bowel syndrome or chronic abdominal pain; there are unusual exceptions in which colonoscopy may be done once to rule out disease, especially if symptoms are unresponsive to therapy
- Acute diarrhea
- Metastatic adenocarcinoma of unknown primary site, in the absence of colonic signs or symptoms, when it will not influence management
- Routine follow-up of inflammatory bowel disease (except for cancer surveillance in chronic ulcerative colitis)
- Upper gastrointestinal bleeding or melena with a demonstrated upper gastrointestinal source

Table 14.3 Colonoscopy is generally contraindicated in the following circumstances

- Contraindications listed under general indications statements
- Fulminant colitis
- Documented acute diverticulitis

noscopic screening following curative resection for colorectal cancer has been shown to be ineffective. Anastomotic recurrence occurs in 2–3 % of cases, but is usually accompanied by incurable metastatic spread. A randomized trial of 325 patients after curative resection [9] compared routine follow-up (history, physical examination, fecal occult blood testing, and carcinoembryonic antigen) to routine follow-up plus annual computed tomography (CT) scanning and colonoscopy for 5 years. Annual colonoscopy failed to detect a single patient with a curable recurrence. Patients with colon cancer should have a clearing colonoscopy preoperatively or within 6 months of surgery, if obstructed. Thereafter, colonoscopic surveillance should be aimed at adenoma detection to prevent a second primary, with standard surveillance intervals at 3–6 years. A family history of CRC (in a first-degree relative) is a risk factor for developing cancer and warrants colonoscopic screening. Colonoscopic screening of those with known (from genetic testing) or suspected (strong family history) hereditary nonpolyposis colorectal cancer (HNPCC) has been shown to reduce both the incidence of and the mortality from CRC [10]. Surveillance in this group is usually offered at 1–3-yearly intervals, starting at age 25 or 5 years earlier than the index case. For individuals with one first-degree relative affected below the age of 60 years or with two first-degree relatives, screening at 5-yearly intervals starting 10 years before the index case is usually the preferred strategy. The large number of individuals with a single first-degree relative affected above the age of 60 should be encouraged to take part in population screening, the optimal strategy being 10-yearly colonoscopy from the age of 50. Patients with chronic inflammatory bowel disease are at increased risk of developing CRC, particularly if the colitis is extensive (beyond the splenic flexure), of long duration (> 8 years) or associated with sclerosing cholangitis or a family history of CRC [11]. Although there is no hard proof of the efficacy of colonoscopic surveillance, it is a reasonable strategy to offer 1–3-yearly examinations with multiple biopsies to look for dysplasia starting after 8 years of extensive colitis and after 15 years of left-sided colitis. An alternative and increasingly used strategy, which appears to be more effective at detecting dysplastic lesions, is to perform a pancolonic dye-spray examination. The dye helps highlight abnormal areas of mucosa that can be targeted, reducing the need for time-consuming multiple background random biopsies [12].

Contraindications

There are few absolute contraindications to colonoscopy, but it should be avoided when there is a severe inflammatory disease such as acute diverticulitis or severe inflammatory bowel disease, when the colonic wall may be thin and fragile with ulceration, making perforation more likely. Abdominal discomfort on manual palpation and the presence of deep ulceration in the rectum or distal sigmoid colon should warn endoscopists to abandon the procedure early. Flexible sigmoidoscopy with biopsy (to help differentiate from infectious colitis), accompanied by plain abdominal radiography, is often as informative and considerably safer than attempting total colonoscopy in the context of acute colitis. Colonoscopy appears to be safe and on the whole well-tolerated in pregnancy, although common sense suggests that it should be performed only if absolutely necessary. Within 3 weeks of a myocardial infarction, colono-

scopy is also best avoided, due to the risk of provoking cardiac arrhythmia.

Bowel Preparation

Before colonoscopy is started, patients must undergo full bowel preparation. This is often the most unpleasant part of the entire procedure and requires considerable patient compliance. Clear written instructions are essential, and a wise precaution is to ask patients who feel the preparation has not worked to attend the endoscopy unit 30 min before their scheduled appointment so that an enema can be administered. Persistent attempts to intubate a partially prepared colon are usually a mistake, as the procedure becomes technically difficult due to poor visibility and even if the cecum is reached, lesions may be missed during withdrawal. Diathermy in a partially prepared bowel is also potentially dangerous, due to the possible build-up of explosive gases such as hydrogen and methane. If air is used as the insufflating agent, it is a wise precaution to exchange the gas several times before using diathermy. Whatever the preparation regimen, it is optimal to stop iron tablets for 7 days and for the patient to adhere to a low-residue diet for 48 h before the examination. Constipating medications should be avoided. There is no evidence that low-dose aspirin significantly increases the risk of postpolypectomy bleeding, and this medication can therefore be continued. Guidelines for patients on long-term anticoagulation treatment are available [13,14]. Patients who are at low risk of thromboembolism (atrial fibrillation) can stop warfarin safely 3–4 days before colonoscopy, restarting immediately after the procedure, but patients who are at high risk (metal prosthetic valves, pulmonary emboli) will usually require conversion to heparin, which is then stopped 3 h before the procedure. Great care is needed when stopping antiplatelet therapy (clopidogrel and aspirin) soon after placement of a drug-eluting coronary stent, as there is a risk of in-stent thrombosis. In this context, close liaison with a cardiologist or deferment of the colonoscopy is advised.

There are many bowel preparation regimens, but no one preparation is ideal for all patients, as taste and colonic physiology vary widely. Most of the regimens involve the administration of strong oral laxatives as a purge on the day before colonoscopy. To avoid solid residue in the right colon, it is important that patients with an afternoon appointment should receive some of the preparation on the morning of the procedure. Clear fluids are encouraged at all times to avoid dehydration and to ensure a fluid return. The most widely used preparations currently are polyethylene glycol balanced electrolyte solution (PEG-ELS) and sodium phosphate (phosphosoda). PEG-ELS is a high-volume (3–4 L) oral lavage solution that provides a rapid bowel washout. Because it is osmotically balanced, it avoids dehydration and dramatic electrolyte shifts (although these can still occur), and it can therefore be used in patients with cardiac, hepatic, and renal disease. The main disadvantage of PEG-ELS is the volume of fluid that the patient has to drink and its inherently salty taste, which can induce vomiting in up to 10 % of cases. Problems with tolerability can be improved by chilling and flavoring the solution, reducing the sodium content [15], and by a split administration regimen [16]. A new 2-L PEG-based preparation containing ascorbic acid has also been introduced, with good initial results [17]. Phosphosoda is a highly osmotic cathartic that has the advantage of having a low volume, with two 45-mL doses. In several comparative trials, phosphosoda has been shown to be as effective at cleansing as PEG-ELS, but was better tolerated and preferred by patients [18–21]. However, there are concerns over the risk of dehydration and electrolyte disturbances. In healthy individuals, phosphosoda appears to cause clinically insignificant electrolyte changes [22], but it is absolutely contraindicated in patients with renal impairment, heart failure, or liver disease with ascites, where hyperphosphatemia and concomitant hypocalcemia/hypokalemia could induce life-threatening cardiac arrhythmia. Another effect of phosphosoda is the appearance of "aphthous ulcer-like" mucosal lesions, which may cause confusion in patients with suspected inflammatory bowel disease. These lesions are always normal on biopsy, but are present in up to 14% of patients who undergo preparation with phosphosoda [23]. Nephrocalcinosis is also a rare but severe side effect [24]. An alternative bowel preparation (tried and trusted at St. Mark's Hospital in London) is a combination containing magnesium citrate (osmotic laxative) and chocolate-flavored senna granules (13 g by weight).

▪ Instructions for Morning and Afternoon Appointments

- A sachet of senna granules and two sachets of magnesium citrate are enclosed. Please follow the instructions carefully to ensure a good result, which is essential for a proper examination.
- Seven days before colonoscopy:
  Stop taking iron tablets. If you are taking warfarin tablets or have diabetes, please ring the endoscopy unit.
- Four days before colonoscopy:
  Stop taking any constipating agents—e. g., Lomotil, codeine phosphate, etc., which you may be prescribed, but continue with all other medication and any laxatives until your appointment.
- Two days before your colonoscopy:
  Eat only food from the following list: boiled or steamed white fish, boiled chicken, egg, cheese, white bread, butter, margarine, rich tea biscuits, potato (no skin). Have plenty to drink.
- *Do not eat* high-fiber foods such as red meat, pink fish, fruit, vegetables, cereals, salad, mushrooms, nuts, sweet corn, wholemeal bread, etc.
- On the day before colonoscopy:
  - Have a good breakfast of foods taken from yesterday's permitted list.
  - After this, *do not eat any solid food until after your examination,* but drink plenty of clear fluids (tea, coffee, squash, alcoholic drinks, carbonated drinks, water, clear soups, Bovril, Oxo, etc). You may have small amounts of milk in tea and coffee. Clear jelly and ice cream are permitted.
- At 2 p.m.:
  Commence the bowel preparation as follows: Mix the sachet of senna granules with half a cup of warm water and drink. To help wash it down, drink more water.
- At 5 p.m.:
  Dissolve the contents of one sachet of magnesium citrate in 200 mL (8 fluid ounces) of hot water in a wide-mouthed measuring jug. Allow to cool for at least half an hour before pouring into a suitable glass, and drink. During the day, drink at least one and half liters of fluid.
- At 7 p.m.:
  Dissolve *half* the contents of the second sachet of magnesium citrate in 100 mL (4 fl. oz.) of water, and drink this solution. During the evening, drink at least one and a half liters of water.
- On the day of your examination:
  At 6–7 a. m. if you have a morning appointment, or at 9–10 a. m. if you have an afternoon appointment, dissolve the other *half* of the magnesium citrate as above and drink this solution as instructed above.
- You should expect frequent bowel actions and eventually diarrhea starting within 3 h of the first dose. Some intestinal cramping is normal. Please use a barrier cream such as zinc and caster oil on your bottom to prevent soreness. Stay within easy reach of a toilet after commencing the preparation.
- *Remember to drink plenty of clear fluids.* These can be continued until you arrive at the hospital.
- If at any stage you vomit the preparation mixtures, if you feel the preparation has not worked, or if you have any other concerns regarding this procedure, please telephone the endoscopy department. A member of the nursing team will be delighted to assist you.

Sedation (see also Chapter 6)

Patients attending for colonoscopy are understandably anxious about what might be found, may be embarrassed about the invasive nature of the examination, and often perceive that it will be painful. Every effort should be made to achieve a calm, relaxed atmosphere in the endoscopy unit. The benefits of talking to patients and reassuring them throughout the examination cannot be overemphasized and this contributes to greater patient satisfaction and willingness to repeat the examination if necessary in the future.

The endoscopist needs to develop a flexible approach to patient sedation, and patient expectations for sedation vary considerably. In France, for instance, most colonoscopies are performed under deep sedation with propofol or anesthesia, whilst in Germany many procedures are unsedated. Provided the technique is good and the "human" aspects of the examination are emphasized, most procedures can be performed successfully with little or no sedation. If patients choose to start the procedure without sedation, it is important to reassure them that if they feel they would like sedation at any time during the procedure, it is available. Factors associated with patients' willingness to undergo the procedure without sedation include male sex, increasing age, and absence of abdominal pain [25]. Small doses of midazolam (1–3 mg) and pethidine (25–75 mg) provide effective analgesia and mild sedation, with some retrograde amnesia. Pain during colonoscopy is almost always due to stretching of the colon mesenteries (occasionally due to overdistension with air), and good technique with frequent straightening of the instrument and minimal air insufflation is therefore the key to a well-tolerated procedure, rather than the use of "heavy" sedation. That said, some patients are so anxious that they will not consent to the procedure unless they are asleep. In this situation (perhaps 2–3 % of cases), intravenous propofol is used [26]. Propofol has a rapid onset of action and produces heavy sedation/anesthesia, necessitating the presence of an anesthetist or a clinician trained in airway management in case of respiratory depression and the need for assisted respiration. Propofol has a short duration of action and patients can therefore recover rapidly, so that list times are not unduly affected. Patient-controlled sedation/analgesia is an attractive concept, as this method does not rely on the endoscopist recognizing that the patient has discomfort. A nitrous oxide/oxygen mixture (50/50) inhaled on demand has an onset of action within 1 min and has been shown to produce analgesia equivalent to standard doses of intravenous sedation, with appreciably shorter recovery times [27]. In fit patients, this approach appears entirely safe, but it is contraindicated in patients with congestive heart disease, severe cardiopulmonary disease, and increased intracranial pressure. Nitrous oxide can be prebreathed before the examination starts and also on instruction from the endoscopist before pushing through a loop. Given the very short duration of action of nitrous oxide inhalation, it may be safe for patients to drive within a short time after the procedure. This requires definitive research, but if it is shown to be safe it would be a major advantage for patients and endoscopists alike.

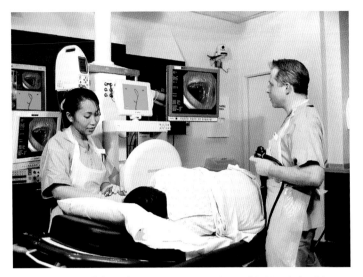

Fig. 14.1 One of the colonoscopy suites at St. Mark's Hospital, with pendant-mounted equipment, including high-definition flat-screen monitors for the endoscopist and patient.

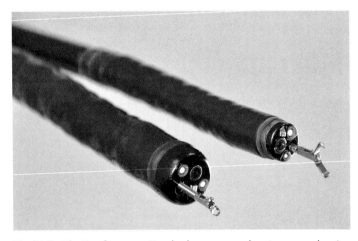

Fig. 14.2 The tip of a conventional colonoscope and gastroscope, showing the relative positions of the biopsy channel.

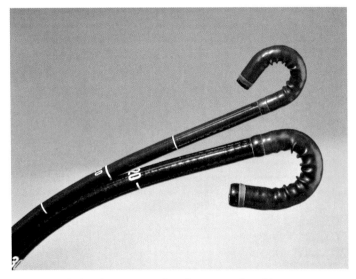

Fig. 14.3 The bending section of a colonoscope alongside a gastroscope.

Antispasmodics

Intravenous hyoscine (10–20 mg) or glucagon (1 mg) are both effective antispasmodics and can be used during colonoscopy to improve the endoscopic view and reduce the need for air insufflation, particularly in a hypercontractile colon. Routine use of antispasmodics at the beginning of the procedure is controversial, and some endoscopists believe they render the bowel atonic, leading to longer and more difficult examinations. However, the ability to see the lumen clearly without the need to overinsufflate, particularly in the 15–20% of Western patients with left-sided diverticular disease, is not to be underestimated, and in the author's experience this approach leads to a quicker insertion overall [28], with better views and possibly a higher pick-up rate for small polyps in the left colon. Studies assessing the ease of insertion with or without antispasmodics have, however, reported conflicting results [28–31].

Equipment for Colonoscopy

The equipment needed—in terms of video processor, light source, and connections for suction and water—is similar to that used in gastroscopy. It is helpful to have several monitors so that everyone in the endoscopy room can appreciate what is happening. Most patients are fascinated to watch the procedure and appreciate a running commentary, even if major pathology is detected. Flat-screen high-definition monitors (with over 1000 lines) are ideal for pendant mounting so that they can be accurately repositioned for the patient, endoscopist, or endoscopy assistants. Suspending the light source, processor, diathermy unit, and recording equipment on pendant mountings also has the advantage of removing electrical leads from the floor and makes the endoscopy suite easy to clean and an inherently safer operating environment (**Fig. 14.1**). Documentation, in terms of video print recording (usually video stills copied directly to the printed endoscopy report) and video recording are now mandatory, particularly for documenting complete colonoscopy and any significant pathology encountered. Modern endoscopy units have fully integrated electronic record systems that handle scheduling and generate printed or electronic reports sent directly to referring doctors via e-mail. The "electronic patient record" can be used for auditing, and this has become an invaluable tool for monitoring quality improvement in individual units.

Colonoscopes are basically similar in design to gastroscopes, but the instrument channel is at the 5–6-o'clock rather than the 7-o'clock position, a fact important for safe advancement of accessories out from the scope tip and when targeting lesions for therapy (**Fig. 14.2**). Colonoscopes have a longer bending section, which angulates equally in all directions, than gastroscopes, and this makes them more difficult to retroflex (**Fig. 14.3**). A long bending section facilitates passage around colonic bends, but it can lead to overangulation, the "walking-stick handle effect." If this occurs, inward force will simply push the whole colon upward rather than advance the tip. Particular care is required to avoid overangulation in the mid-sigmoid colon and at the splenic flexure. If it does occur, the colonoscope should be withdrawn and tension on the control wheels relaxed. Deflation of the distal colon often helps reduce an acute bend further up, as may a change in patient position or direct abdominal pressure. Further reinsertion applying torque to the shaft is then usually successful.

The shaft of a colonoscope is designed to be more flexible than that of a gastroscope, to allow for the looping that invariably occurs at some stage during a colonoscopy. A stiffer shaft results in more stretching of colonic loops and mesenteries and so more pain and greater danger of trauma. However, a degree of shaft "whip" or

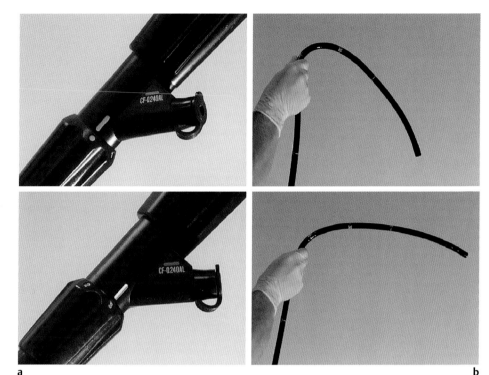

a

b

Fig. 14.4
a Dial of the variable-stiffness colonoscope, which is twisted anticlockwise to increase shaft stiffness and clockwise to decrease it.
b Benchtop demonstration of a variable-stiffness colonoscope in the stiff and floppy modes.

springiness is needed to transmit inward push pressure to the tip and complete torque stability is essential to allow twisting forces to be transmitted effectively down the length of the shaft to the tip. Standard colonoscopes are 1.3–1.5 cm in diameter, but thinner pediatric instruments (10 mm) are available. These have advantages in patients with fixed colons where the scope has to adapt to a fixed bend due to pericolic adhesions. Experienced colonoscopists learn to change instruments early during the procedure from an adult to pediatric instrument when a difficult sigmoid colon due to diverticulosis or previous pelvic surgery is encountered, to maintain patient comfort and reduce the risk of a traumatic complication. Most colonoscopists choose longer instruments, 160–170 cm in length, rather than intermediate, 130-cm colonoscopes. Although longer scopes are slightly more awkward to handle and take longer to pass accessories through, they make cecal intubation more likely even in the most redundant of colons. In a study of 100 consecutive colonoscopies, documented with magnetic imaging (see below), total colonoscopy was achieved in all patients, but in 6%, more than 140 cm of the colonoscope shaft was inserted at some point during intubation when pushing through a loop in a redundant colon [32].

Variable-stiffness instruments. A recent advance in colonoscope design is the variable-flexibility colonoscope (**Fig. 14.4**). This instrument has the same appearance as conventional instruments and has similar handling. The only difference is a control dial positioned just below the instrument head that differentially increases the shaft stiffness when it is twisted. The instrument can thus be used in floppy pediatric mode to negotiate tight or fixed bends and can then be stiffened to prevent recurrent looping. The variable-stiffness scope allows significantly quicker intubation times with less patient discomfort in comparison with conventional instruments, particularly if minimal or no sedation is used [33–36]. Manufacturers have been understandably cautious with the degree of maximum stiffness, recognizing that a "very stiff" mode in the scope could increase the risk of perforation if used inappropriately when the scope is looped. The ability to visualize the shaft configuration makes the use of the stiffening function safer and more intuitive. In a study assessing use of the variable-stiffness function under magnetic imaging

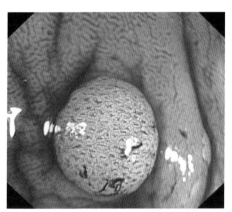

Fig. 14.5 A hyperplastic polyp with indigo carmine dye spray, showing a type 2 (non-neoplastic) pit pattern.

control (see below), the maximum stiffness function was found to be useful for passing around the splenic flexure by preventing recurrent sigmoid colon looping, and it speeded passage across the transverse colon [37].

High-resolution, magnification, and narrow-band imaging. In recent years, equipment manufacturers have achieved dramatic improvements in the quality of video images. Colonoscopes containing large video chips (> 800,000 pixels) produce a high-resolution image that can be digitally enhanced to improve definition further. High-definition flat-screen monitors allow the high-resolution image to be viewed in high definition and using magnifying colonoscopes. Endoscopists can now achieve in vivo images equivalent to those seen under low-powered (100 ×) light microscopy. Combined with dye spraying to define the mucosal pit pattern, magnification of the surface architecture of colonic polyps allows differentiation of neoplastic from nonneoplastic lesions (**Fig. 14.5**) [38,39]. Early prototype magnifying instruments were of intermediate length and proved difficult to maneuver around tight bends, as they had a long rigid section at the tip containing the lens array. Magnification was achieved by means of a dial mechanism on the instrument head, physically connected to the lens system in the scope tip. The latest magnifying instruments are almost as easy to use as conventional

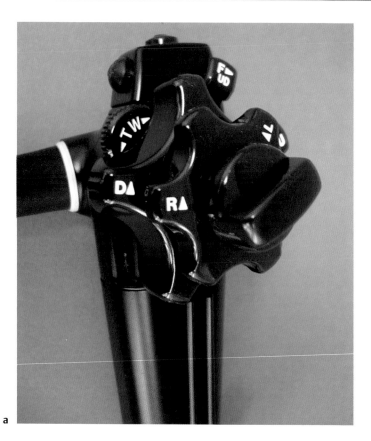

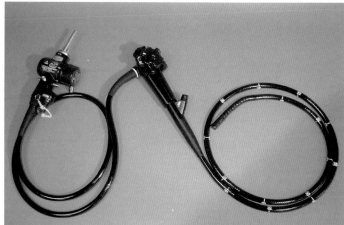

Figs. 14.6 a, b Olympus magnifying colonoscope. The dial attached between the head of the instrument and the control wheels is used for manual control of the degree of magnification.

colonoscopes and are 160 cm long, allowing total colonoscopy in nearly all patients, and have an electrically operated zoom-lens system controlled by a foot pedal or most conveniently a dial on the scope head, similar to the "bridge" on a side-viewing endoscope (**Figs. 14.6**).

Another innovation now reaching routine practice is narrow-band imaging (NBI). This is a push-button technology that allows visualization of the mucosal surface with narrowed bandwidth light from the blue and green parts of the light spectrum [40]. Although the image is significantly darker than with normal white light, the mucosal structures are enhanced, particularly superficial capillaries. When combined with magnification, extremely detailed views can be obtained and lesions can be classified according to the pit pattern and vascular pattern intensity (**Fig. 14.7**) [41]. Even in experienced hands, pit patterns can be difficult to interpret, but vascular intensity is easy (neoplastic lesions have a darker brown than the surrounding mucosa), and this technology will in the future offer the endoscopist the very real prospect of performing in-vivo histology (optical biopsy), avoiding the need for conventional histopathology in many cases [42].

Confocal endomicroscopy is another evolving imaging technology that provides real-time images similar in appearance to conventional histology [43]. Currently, a dedicated colonoscope containing the confocal endomicroscope is available and catheter probes that can be passed down the instrument channel of conventional instruments are under evaluation. Confocal endomicroscopy is the only current imaging technique that allows in-vivo cellular imaging below the mucosal surface. Although NBI, particularly with magnification, is probably sufficient for most routine optical diagnoses, confocal endomicroscopy may have particular advantages in diagnosing early submucosal invasion in early cancer.

Carbon Dioxide Versus Air Insufflation

During insertion and particularly during withdrawal, adequate distension of the colon is crucial to allow accurate steering and avoid missing abnormalities. This invariably means that at the end of the procedure, the colon and distal small bowel will contain residual gas even if the endoscopist has been careful to aspirate any excess during the procedure. Most colonoscopists use air as the insufflating agent, despite awareness of the potential advantages of CO_2. This is probably because of the misconception that CO_2 is expensive and troublesome to use. Cheap, low-pressure, metered-flow CO_2 delivery systems are now available, with easy-to-use scope connections. CO_2 has several potential advantages over air:
- When air is used, patients often experience abdominal bloating after the procedure. Abdominal radiographs taken several hours after colonoscopy with air have clearly demonstrated bowel distension [44]. By contrast, CO_2 is absorbed through the bowel wall into the circulation and is then excreted via the lungs in 15–20 min, so that postprocedural bloating is greatly reduced. Moreover, during examinations in patients with partial or complete stricture, CO_2 will minimize the risk of further distension. Although unproved, it is also likely to be a better-tolerated option when examining patients with irritable bowel syndrome and diverticulosis.
- CO_2, unlike air, does not support combustion and hence is safer to use during diathermy, particularly if bowel preparation is suboptimal. It is mandatory if mannitol bowel preparation has been used, because of the increased risk of hydrogen and methane build-up.
- If, for whatever reason, colonoscopy fails, a double-contrast enema can be performed soon after colonoscopy with CO_2, as the bowel is not excessively distended and is easier to coat with barium.

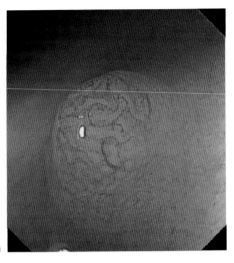

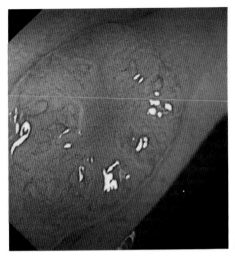

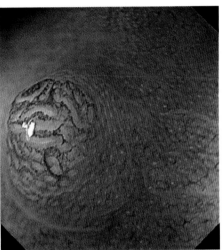

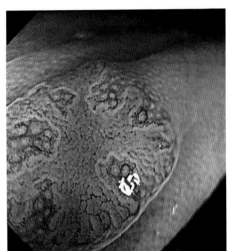

Fig. 14.7 a–d Examples of small tubular adenomas seen with white-light **(a, b)** and narrow-band **(c, d)** imaging. There is a type 3 pit pattern and an enhanced vascular pattern.

14

Accessories

It is important to check that all accessories are available before a colonoscopy is started. Biopsy forceps are mandatory for both cold and hot biopsy (very rarely used nowadays), as are snares for polypectomy (1 cm, 1.5 cm, and 2.5 cm) and a polyp trap for suction retrieval of small polyps. For defining subtle or flat lesions, topical indigo carmine (0.1 %) along with a dye-spray diffusion catheter is useful, and basic endoscopic mucosal resection (EMR) accessories include a long sclerotherapy needle (25 G) for submucosal injection and a supply of dilute epinephrine solution in 10-mL syringes (1 : 200 000). In addition, a 50-mL syringe for water-washing and for clearing the lens and a 30-mL syringe with dilute simethicone bubble breaker are essential. These are the basics, but it is also preferable to have readily at hand clipping and Endoloop devices in case of bleeding, as well as a range of balloons (5.5 cm in length and 8–20 mm in maximum diameter) for dilating strictures. Argon plasma coagulation is also invaluable for treating vascular abnormalities and stopping bleeding after therapy, for treating the telangiectasia of radiation colitis, and for completing polypectomy of sessile polyps after piecemeal resection.

Imaging during Colonoscopy

Fluoroscopy

The early pioneers of colonoscopy understood the advantages of being able to visualize the procedure (identification of the anatomical location of the colonoscope tip, correction of loops, and documentation of total colonoscopy) and routinely performed colonoscopy in the radiography suite with the benefit of fluoroscopy. With the expansion of endoscopy services during the 1970s and 1980s, dedicated endoscopy units were developed, often without access to fluoroscopy. By this time, colonoscopists had gained experience with the technique and some considered that imaging was only beneficial during the learning phase [45]. Today's generation of colonoscopists have developed skills without fluoroscopy and are therefore largely unaware of its potential advantages, particularly in the 10–20 % of patients in whom recurrent looping occurs and the endoscopist becomes effectively "lost." That said, fluoroscopy is fundamentally flawed as an imaging technique for colonoscopy.
- Fluoroscopy equipment is expensive, as is the initial financial outlay for lead-lining the room.
- The views are two-dimensional, fleeting, and localized, only showing a portion of the abdomen at any one time.
- There is a radiation risk, requiring staff to wear cumbersome protective clothing.

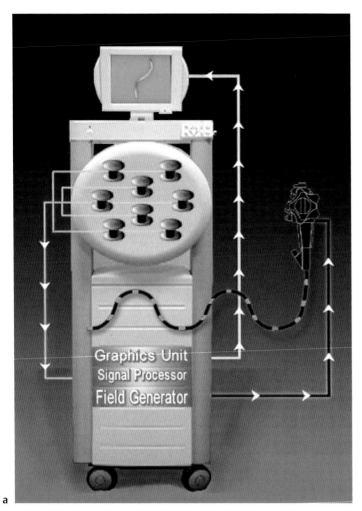

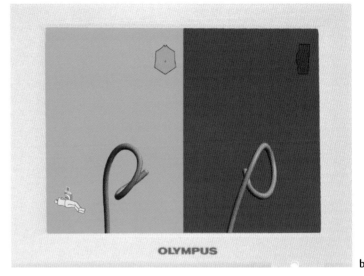

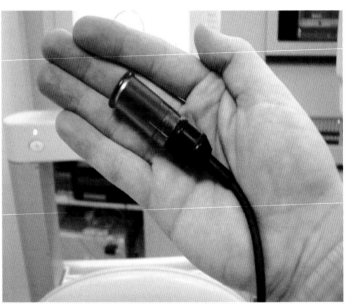

Fig. 14.8
a The ScopeGuide (Olympus) magnetic imaging system.
b A screen shot from the ScopeGuide, showing simultaneous lateral and anteroposterior views of an N spiral loop.
c The ScopeGuide hand pressure sensor.

Magnetic Endoscope Imaging

The clear advantage of being able to see what is happening and the inadequacies of fluoroscopy provided the impetus for the development of magnetic endoscope imaging (MEI) [46,47], which has been commercialized as ScopeGuide (Olympus Optical Company). MEI works by generating very low-strength magnetic fields (one-millionth that of a magnetic resonance scanner) by a series of tiny wire coils positioned at regular intervals along the length of the colonoscope (**Fig. 14.8 a**). Originally, these coils were fitted inside a plastic catheter that was introduced down the biopsy channel, but dedicated imager colonoscopes are now available with the coils and electronics in-built, underneath the metal casing of the shaft. Each coil along the colonoscope shaft sequentially generates a magnetic field, which induces a current in larger receiver coils contained within a box positioned alongside the patient. By calculating the strength of the current in each sensor coil, the exact distance from sensor coils to generator coils can be determined. The spatial position of each generator coil within the colonoscope is thus known. The generator coils are positioned only 10 cm apart, so that when a smooth line is drawn between each calculated point there is only one possible solution for the configuration of the colonoscope shaft. This is displayed on a separate computer monitor, or more conveniently can be placed adjacent to the endoscopic image on the video

monitor using a video card and mixer. The on-screen view is updated five times a second, so that the system is effectively real-time. Polygon rendering gives a cylindrical, colonoscope-like image, and differential shading (with light gray being nearest the viewer and dark gray furthest away) provides a three-dimensional effect. The system automatically produces an anteroposterior view of the scope within the abdomen, but can also provide a simultaneous lateral view (**Fig. 14.8 b**). An additional sensor coil is contained within a plastic button and can be attached to the endoscopy assistant's hand when applying abdominal compression, so that the hand can be seen in relation to the scope (**Fig. 14.8 c**).

Effect on performance and teaching of colonoscopy. The first results show that MEI has a considerable impact on performance of colonoscopy [48,49]. The real-time endoscope image on the screen gives the endoscopist exact feedback as to how far the endoscope tip has reached and what the shaft is doing. In some previously "difficult" examinations of patients with redundant colons, the confidence of seeing odd loops forming and the ability to apply appropriate shaft movements or targeted hand pressure makes the procedure substantially easier. Derotation and straightening of complex loops is made logical by using whichever of clockwise or anticlockwise twisting movements is relevant, as suggested by the three-dimensional display rather than simply by empirical trial and error. As a result, some previously exceedingly difficult cases have been made quick and easy using the imager, and in all cases, at all times, tip location and shaft configuration are obvious. For particular bends or loops, the manipulative dexterity and close-up visual judgement of the expert endoscopist are still fundamental, but the "extra dimension" provided by the imager information proves enormously helpful and reassuring.

As might be expected, the greatest impact of real-time imaging is on the learning process [50]. Inexperienced endoscopists see the folly of pushing in further when a loop is present and the patient has discomfort. The relevance of torque or twisting movements, and their maintenance during simultaneous insertion or withdrawal, becomes logical (rather than a mystical trick of the "experienced"). The endoscopist no longer needs to guess where the endoscope has reached, and this in some cases means that an examination can be terminated more quickly and in others that complete insertion can be assured, combining imager evidence with the endoscopic view in cases in which the anatomy is atypical. An initial randomized trial of imaging versus no imaging in trainees with intermediate experience (150–300 previous cases) demonstrated that insertion times, duration of endoscope looping, and number of straightening attempts once a loop had formed all improved with the benefit of imaging [49].

Formal evaluation of the imager is still in progress, but it is evident on using the system, or seeing others using it, that it represents a giant leap forward in the development of easier and more accurate colonoscopy.

Colonoscope Insertion: Technique

General Principles

In skilled hands, total colonoscopy and ileoscopy can be achieved safely and quickly in nearly all patients; however, the "art" of colonoscope insertion remains difficult to master. This is because essentially colonoscopy involves the passage of one flexible tube through another. The colon is of variable length, mobility, and fixation and moves around unpredictably under the influence of the colonoscope. Listening to the patient and responding appropriately to patient discomfort by straightening the instrument (not necessarily increasing the sedation) are fundamental to good technique and cannot be overemphasized. All too often, less experienced endoscopists, seeing a clear view on the monitor, simply push inward, making the loop bigger and the patient more uncomfortable.

Few areas in endoscopy provoke more debate than the technique of colonoscope insertion. Controversy exists because most examinations are performed "blindly," without the use of fluoroscopy or magnetic endoscope imaging. Thus, the endoscopist has to develop an instinctive feel for when the endoscope is looped and develop strategies for dealing with the many anatomical variations encountered. However, certain general principles are agreed by all:

- Use clockwise/anticlockwise torque on the instrument shaft to steer around bends and maximize inward force through the tip.
- Minimize air/CO_2 insufflation during insertion.
- Use frequent withdrawal movements to keep the shaft straight, keeping the length of scope inserted appropriate to the anatomical location of the tip (descending colon = 40 cm inserted; splenic flexure = 50 cm inserted; mid-transverse colon = 60 cm inserted; cecum = 70–80 cm inserted).
- Use light sedation wherever possible and maximize the view with changes in patient position.
- Respond to patient protests by pulling back and deflating.
- If the tip will not advance, try different combinations of position change, hand pressure, and shaft torque. Consider a change of endoscope—or even endoscopist!

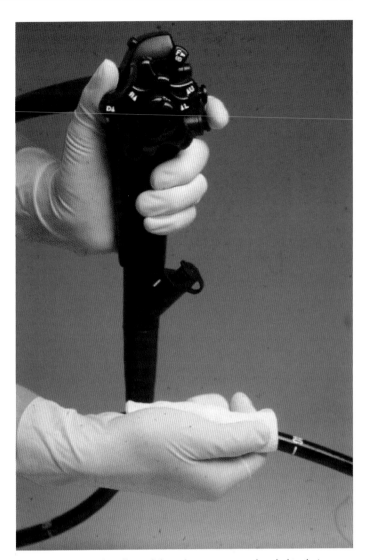

Fig. 14.9 Correct handling of the colonoscope: one-handed technique.

- Pushing through a loop should be a last resort. Warn the patient that there may be some discomfort for a few seconds and always push in slowly. Remember to straighten the shaft once the bend has been passed.

Instrument Handling

The heads of endoscopes were originally designed to be manipulated with two hands, with the left hand holding the instrument, the left thumb controlling the up/down control, and the right hand manipulating the lateral control. Whilst this is an acceptable arrangement for gastroscopy and endoscopic retrograde cholangiopancreatography (ERCP), where scope insertion is less problematic, colonoscopy requires simultaneous manipulation of the steering wheels and the instrument shaft. Most expert colonoscopists therefore use a "one-handed" in which the left hand controls both the up/down and lateral controls, leaving the right hand permanently on the colonoscope shaft. In the one-handed technique, the thumb stretches across to control both steering wheels, assisted by the left middle finger (**Fig. 14.9**). For many endoscopists, this one-handed grip seems impossible. With practice, however, even endoscopists with small hands can master the technique, much in the same way as "barring a chord" when playing the guitar.

If a two-handed technique is used, loss of control of the colonoscope shaft is inevitable when the right hand is removed to use the lateral control. This can be avoided by asking the endoscopy assistant to hold the shaft between maneuvers, or by allowing the colonoscope to trail alongside the endoscopy couch so that it can be trapped, and held in position, by pressure from the right thigh. A true two-person technique in which one operator inserts the shaft whilst another steers—although feasible if coordination is good— has largely been abandoned because of its impractical nature.

■ Ancillary Techniques for Colonoscope Insertion

Abdominal compression. The objective of abdominal compression is to help deflect inward force from a partially looped shaft toward the tip. When applied correctly (with firm continuous pressure from the palm of the hand over the apex of the loop), this technique may make insertion easier and less painful. Clearly, abdominal compression will only be effective if the part of the shaft that is starting to loop is anterior within the abdominal cavity and therefore accessible to the hand. Compression applied over the left lower abdomen, with pressure directed downward toward the pelvis, may help prevent looping in the sigmoid colon, whilst hand pressure in the mid- or lower abdomen directed upward may help reduce a deep transverse loop. Magnetic imaging has given a unique insight into the use of hand pressure. In a prospective audit of 100 consecutive colonoscopies in which the endoscopist and endoscopy assistant were blinded to the imager view, hand pressure was used on 239 separate occasions but was only effective in 100 (34%); loops were either deep within the abdomen, or the hand was misplaced and ineffective [32]. However, until MEI becomes widely available, the use of hand pressure, even performed blindly and on a trial-and-error basis, can be a very useful aid to intubation. Occasionally, it is beneficial in difficult cases for the endoscopist to palpate the abdomen whilst observing the video monitor for signs of forward progress. If the abdominal wall is lax, loops can be felt directly and a better idea of where to apply compression is achieved. If looping is a problem during insertion, it is generally advisable to try left lower quadrant pressure first, as sigmoid looping is common, followed by pressure at other locations, depending on the results of local palpation. Occasionally, when the colonoscope tip is at the hepatic flexure, asking the patient to hold the breath during deep inspiration can aid scope advancement; as the diaphragm contracts, it flattens and may push the scope tip downward into the ascending colon.

Changing the patient's position. Changing the patient's position is possibly of greater overall benefit than abdominal compression. Most examinations are commenced in the left lateral position, which is ideal for negotiating the rectum and distal sigmoid. However, the descending colon is usually fixed posteriorly on the left and therefore with the patient in the left lateral, both the sigmoid/ descending junction and the splenic flexure will tend to be acute, fluid-filled bends and hence difficult to pass under direct vision. Also, if a typical N-loop (see later) occurs during insertion through the sigmoid, an acute bend both in the mid-sigmoid and at the sigmoid/descending junction is created when the patient is in the left lateral position. The angles of these bends can be reduced, making insertion easier, by moving the patient to the supine position before the mid-sigmoid colon is reached. By moving the patient over even further to the right lateral position, the sigmoid/descending junction opens up as fluid runs away from it and air toward it under the influence of gravity. Laying the patient flat or even with the head slightly down on the endoscopy couch, rather than propped up, may also facilitate passage around an acute splenic flexure. As the colonoscope passes to the mid-transverse, there is an inevitable tendency for the transverse colon to bow downward and anteriorly toward the pelvis. Moving the patient into the supine position facilitates visualization, as fluid runs back toward the

splenic and hepatic flexures and air toward the mid-transverse. In the same way, movement back to the left lateral position when the tip is in the proximal transverse colon tends to open up the hepatic flexure, allowing easier steering into the ascending colon. It is important to remember that position changes are not only of value during insertion, but also crucial for maximizing views during withdrawal [51]. The right colon is examined optimally with the patient in the left lateral position, the transverse colon with the patient in the supine position, the splenic flexure and descending colon with the patient tipped slightly over to the right, and finally the sigmoid and rectum with the patient back in the left lateral position. Of course, these are general rules and because of the large variation in colonic anatomy and fixation, some degree of trial and error is often necessary to find the best patient position. Light sedation and close communication with the patient facilitate rapid changes in patient position and thus make the procedure easier and more tolerable for all concerned.

■ Anus and Rectum

Anatomy. The anal canal is 3 cm long and lined with pain-sensitive squamous epithelium as far as the dentate line. Continence is maintained by the internal and external anal sphincters, which are in tonic contraction. The endoscopist should be aware that the anal canal is liable to be deformed or scarred by any previous pathology, or after surgery. Fibroepithelial polyps, the remnants of shriveled hemorrhoids, should not be mistaken for adenomatous polyps. The rectum, although reaching only 15 cm proximal from the anal verge, may have a capacious "ampulla" in its mid-part, as well as prominent transverse folds (Houston folds), creating potential blind spots in which the endoscopist can miss significant pathology.

Insertion technique. Before inserting the colonoscope, most endoscopists still perform a digital rectal examination to detect pathology in the lower rectum. This also facilitates insertion of the "blunt" colonoscope tip through the lubricated anal canal as the examining finger is withdrawn. Having secured the scope tip inside the rectum, it is important to gently insufflate, pull back, and find the lumen. Often the lens view is partially obscured by adherent lubricant jelly or fecal matter, which should be washed off the scope tip before proceeding. The lens wash alone may be insufficient to clear the view. In this situation, high-pressure washing with water syringed down the biopsy channel whilst the colonoscope tip is held close to the rectal mucosa is usually successful. In the final analysis, it is better to withdraw the scope, manually clean the lens, and then start again than persist with a defective view. On finding the lumen, it is usual to encounter a sump of fluid in the rectum, which should be suctioned to avoid seepage during the procedure. The ability to rotate the scope to place fluid or polyps at the 5–6-o'clock position (opposite the biopsy/suction channel opening) is fundamental to good technique. Trainees should spend a few moments practicing coordination between the left and right hands to produce smooth tip rotation without losing the view in the rectum. When the fluid pool in the rectum is orientated correctly, all fluid can be suctioned without losing the view through air aspiration.

Because of its reservoir function, the rectum may contain semi-solid or particulate residue, which will tend to block the instrument suction channel. With many instruments, simply removing the suction button and occluding the hole with the gloved finger removes the source of blockage and results in audible passage of the blocked fecal residue. If suction is still not working, one can change the button on the instrument head and check for kinking in the suction tubing. If there is a perceptible decrease in background noise, the suction bottle may be full and need changing.

The rectum, because it can be so capacious, may be surprisingly difficult to examine properly. Retroversion may be needed to see the

IV

distal part adequately, and this is achieved by selecting the widest part of the ampulla, insufflating to distend the rectum, and then applying full upward angulation whilst gently pushing in. Once retroflexion has been achieved, application of the lateral wheel and scope torque allows 360° views of the distal rectum and dentate line (**Fig. 14.10**). Some rectums, especially if scarred because of previous inflammatory disease, deep radiotherapy, etc., are too narrow to allow the bending section to retroflex, but these are easy to examine anyway in the prograde view.

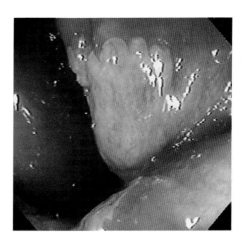

Fig. 14.10 Rectal retroflexion. The dentate line and hemorrhoidal cushions should be noted.

Sigmoid Colon

Anatomy. The sigmoid colon is 40–70 cm long when stretched during insertion, although contracted down to only 30–35 cm once the instrument is straightened fully—which is why careful inspection is important during insertion if lesions are not to be missed during the withdrawal phase. The distal sides of the sigmoid haustral folds, in particular, are best seen during insertion and all small polyps in this area should be removed whilst easily visible, as they can be frustratingly difficult to find during withdrawal. The sigmoid colon mesentery is inserted in a V-shape across the pelvic brim, but is variable in insertion and length and may also be modified by adhesions from previous inflammatory disease or surgery. In approximately 20% of Western patients, the sigmoid colon is narrowed and deformed internally by the thickened circular muscle rings of hypertrophic diverticular disease, and sometimes also rigidified and fixed externally by pericolic postinflammatory processes.

Insertion technique. Insertion through the sigmoid requires careful steering, ideally using single-handed "slalom" or "corkscrew" rotation to pass the sequential bends and haustral folds of the distal sigmoid. Use of clockwise or counterclockwise torque with the colonoscope tip slightly flexed allows passage around bends without excessive pushing or the need to use the lateral control. Careful steering is particularly important in the presence of diverticulosis, where the diverticular openings can look remarkably like the bowel lumen. A good general rule is that the correct direction of the lumen is always at 90° away from the diverticular openings (**Fig. 14.11**).

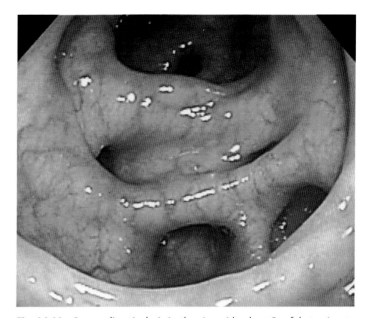

Fig. 14.11 Severe diverticulosis in the sigmoid colon. Careful steering to find the bowel lumen is essential.

When the colonoscope angles around the apex of the sigmoid, some pushing pressure and resultant upward looping is almost inevitable. The patient notices this stretching as an unpleasant sensation of "wind pain," similar to severe abdominal colic experienced during an episode of gastroenteritis. Pulling back the instrument, especially when it has just been angulated round a haustral fold or acute bend, will tend to reduce the loop, straighten the scope, and stop the discomfort. Often there is a mechanical advantage to moving the patient into the supine position when the mid-sigmoid is reached. This tends to flatten and reduce the often acute angle around the apex of the sigmoid. Occasionally, in a very long sigmoid or when the rectum is unusually capacious, bowing of the scope can be seen (using magnetic imaging) distal to the mid-sigmoid during application of inward pushing. In this situation, brief application of the stiffening device allows more inward force to be applied through the scope tip and subsequent easy passage to the proximal sigmoid colon. Great care should be taken when applying the stiffening device with the scope tip still in the sigmoid colon, and ideally with image guidance. By a combination of deft steering, minimal use of air, and short periods of inward push, each followed by withdrawal, the instrument can usually be coaxed up to the sigmoid/descending junction in at most 2–3 min (unless diverticular disease complicates things). With the patient in the left lateral position, the sigmoid/descending junction is heralded by the appearance of an acute, often fluid-filled, bend. To pass around this point, it is essential to try to straighten out the sigmoid as much as possible by pulling back, deflating, and reducing the degree of looping by the endoscopy assistant applying lower abdominal hand compression. That said, some degree of looping is inevitable and entirely understandable on anatomical grounds; the colonoscope has to pass from the back of the pelvis (rectum), then anteriorly into the abdominal cavity (sigmoid), and then posteriorly again into the fixed, retroperitoneal descending colon. This produces a spiral appearance, as seen using magnetic imaging, and is described as an "N" loop if the two-dimensional views of fluoroscopy are used. Forceful pushing through the sigmoid tends to produce a large spiral sigmoid loop and consequently an acute hairpin bend at the sigmoid/descending junction. Conversely, clockwise torque and withdrawal will tend to reduce the spiral loop. Thus, every attempt should be made using clockwise torque, withdrawal, deflation, and abdominal compression to produce a relatively shallow angle for easy passage around the sigmoid/descending junction.

Once at or near the sigmoid–descending colon junction, it is worth again deflating the colon and pulling back. Then, whilst maintaining assistant pressure from the outside, one can try clockwise rotation and slow insertion pressure to persuade the tip into the retroperitoneal part of the distal descending colon. It may be necessary to maneuver repeatedly to achieve this. Different combinations of angulation, rotation, and pushing/pulling are used, trying to slip into the distal descending colon without having to overangulate the tip. Ideally, this is achieved with the instrument straightened back to about 40–45 cm from the anus, and preferably

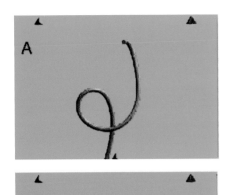
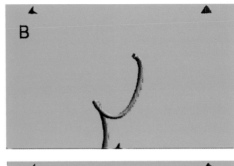
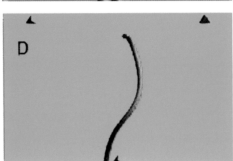

Fig. 14.12 Magnetic imager views showing straightening of an alpha loop.
a   The tip of colonoscope has passed just around the splenic flexure, but with an alpha loop.
b   Scope withdrawal with clockwise twisting reduces the alpha loop, converting it to an N sigmoid or spiral loop.
c   Continued clockwise torque straightens the remaining loop.
d   The colonoscope is now straight at the splenic flexure.

employing clockwise twisting to corkscrew in with minimum push pressure.

Once the tip is held retroperitoneally, clockwise shaft twisting tends to propel the instrument up the descending colon, without relooping and so without discomfort to the patient. This withdrawal and clockwise twist maneuver, described by Shinya as the "right turn shortening technique" [52], is the basic step in straight-scope insertion; when it succeeds, the rest of the insertion up the descending colon and on to the cecum can usually be completed very rapidly.

Alpha-loop formation (a relatively flat and large loop) should be presumed to have happened when the sigmoid loop is obviously long, as judged by the amount of instrument shaft inserted without particular discomfort, and because the alpha configuration allows the tip to run around the sigmoid loop smoothly up into the fluid-filled descending colon, without encountering any point of acute angulation. In the presence of an alpha loop, it is important not to pull back, but rather to push on to about 90 cm of insertion, which should represent the splenic flexure. At this point, straightening the sigmoid can be achieved by the application of clockwise torque and scope withdrawal. When reducing an alpha loop (**Fig. 14.12**), it is crucial to steer carefully in order always to maintain a luminal view, so that slippage of the scope tip can be recognized and corrected early. If the scope tip falls backward, it may be necessary to apply more clockwise torque during the withdrawal maneuver or to insert more scope and pass around the splenic flexure before pulling back. Occasionally, in patients with very long sigmoid mesenteries, the scope can be passed to the cecum rapidly and without discomfort whilst maintaining the alpha loop.

As the endoscopist is only guessing at the presence of the alpha loop and will be mistaken in some cases, the instrument tip may actually only be at the sigmoid–descending junction. If this happens, little has been lost except that passage of the supposed "splenic flexure" will prove harder than expected—requiring either aggressive straightening to pass around it directly (into the descending colon) or aggressive pressure to do so with a still-looped scope. Fortunately, as there is obviously a redundant colon and mesentery, the endoscopist may suffer more trauma in this than the patient.

The alpha loop is the longest form of spiral loop, the N-loop the intermediate variety, and the shortest is present when the direct "pull and twist" approach to the descending colon is easily successful. All of these loops are iatrogenic variations of each other, caused by the colonoscope stretching up the sigmoid loop from its normal, variably tortuous, configuration. The exact configuration adopted by the colonoscope depends on how it is pushed, pulled, and twisted, and so unless there are adhesions, the skilled endoscopist has the opportunity to manipulate the sigmoid into a shape conducive to passing the tip and bending section into the descending colon, preferably avoiding formation of an acute hairpin bend at the junction. Without external imaging, this process must be managed by empirical judgment, based on feel (of both shaft and controls) and results. Straightening a sigmoid colon loop simply involves pulling back on the shaft and simultaneously applying strong rotational twist—usually in a clockwise direction, for the reasons given above. Success in straightening a loop causes the responsive "feel" of the instrument to return, and in the process the tip may paradoxically run inward.

Assuming that there are no irreversible adhesions (a possibility to be treated with respect in anyone with a history of Crohn's disease, diverticulosis, or abdominal surgery), difficulty is usually due to lack of determination (not force) on the part of the endoscopist. The loop must first be considerably reduced in size before derotation, usually using clockwise twisting, and straightening suddenly starts to succeed. The splenic flexure is never more than 50 cm from the anus, but sometimes is so mobile that it will withdraw to 40 cm. Withdrawal to 60–70 cm is therefore always inadequate and indicative of a loop still being present. Larger or more complex loops may need several attempts before straightening is achieved. Typically, complex loops may need a combination of first anticlockwise and then clockwise twisting to resolve them, often finally straightening with a surprising jerk with only around 30–40 cm of shaft remaining inside the patient. Difficulty in passing the sigmoid–descending colon junction is normal, and may take some minutes and a number of attempts to resolve, but it can usually be overcome without resorting to force. Changing the patient's position to the supine or right lateral position is often helpful, probably because this aids visualization and also reduces the angle around this bend.

Approximately 10% of patients have the descending colon swinging free on a "descending mesocolon." In this situation, the colonoscope is enabled to push the sigmoid/descending colon (for they become one and the same) into a further variety of configurations. If the mesocolon is long and the sigmoid colon can be shortened, the colonoscope may progress straight up the midline. More often, an atypical loop will be formed, sometimes complex but usually in a

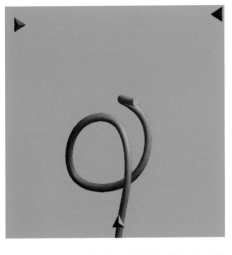

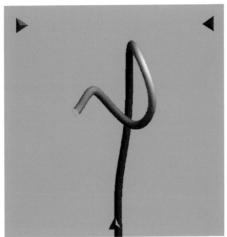

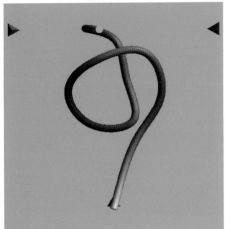

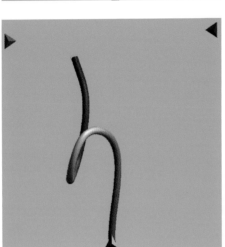

Fig. 14.13 Atypical loops with an anticlockwise spiral configuration.
a A reverse splenic flexure loop (3 % of all loops).
b A reverse alpha loop (5 % of all loops).
c A reverse sigmoid spiral (1 % of all loops).
d A transverse gamma loop (1 % of all loops).

14

"reversed alpha loop" or reversed splenic flexure in an *anti*clockwise spiral (**Fig. 14.13**). The endoscopist only recognizes this when attempting to straighten the loop and finding empirically that anticlockwise derotation works best. Unlike the more conventional colon with an alpha loop, straightening out the distal part of a mobile colon does not end the problems, for other atypical loops tend to form in the proximal colon also.

If the sigmoid feels fixed and angulated, then insertion may be impossible or unreasonable to persist with. Hysterectomy usually causes only a limited area of anterior adhesions low in the sigmoid, which although painful to pass, do not affect the examination thereafter. Diverticulitis typically causes fixation and angulation of the mid-sigmoid, which will sometimes not straighten, and then makes the rest of the insertion difficult. A pediatric instrument should be tried—preferably a floppy colonoscope if one is available—as this will adapt best to fixed bends without traumatization. A gastroscope will often pass too, but may not be long enough to reach the cecum thereafter. If in doubt, it is better to abandon in favor of referral to a more expert or better-equipped colonoscopist; even the most expert will abandon the attempt (perhaps in favor of CT colonography or barium enema) in the few percent of cases that prove too traumatic, rather than risk injury to the patient or damage to the instrument.

▓ Descending Colon and Splenic Flexure

Anatomy. The descending colon is a 20-cm long tubular structure running up the left paravertebral gutter. Usually it presents little difficulty to the endoscopist, other than being fluid-filled when viewed with the patient in the left lateral position. However, it may be considerably longer, with angulations and mobility resulting from the vagaries of retroperitoneal fixation or mesocolon mobility. The splenic flexure is situated—inconveniently from the endoscopist's point of view—behind the left costal margin, where it is inaccessible to palpation and not easily visible on transillumination. It is a relatively long flexure, made more acute in the left lateral position, probably due to dependency of the distal transverse colon; conversely, the splenic flexure is made less acute if the patient is supine and is almost erased in the right lateral position.

Insertion technique. Once the colonoscope has reached the descending colon, it will usually pass rapidly up to the splenic flexure. Then, either on reaching the flexure or passing just around it and emerging into the triangular, air-filled transverse colon, the instrument can be pulled back and straightened to between 40 and 50 cm according to its degree of fixation by the phrenicocolic ligament. Pulling the splenic flexure down maximally is the key to easy passage around into the transverse colon, but doing so and checking that the shortened shaft distance is appropriate (40–55 cm) is also an important guarantee that no sigmoid colon loop remains in place to complicate the rest of the insertion. Passing the splenic flexure requires a combination of small coordinated and additive actions. To avoid relooping of the sigmoid, clockwise twisting is applied, and then, since twisting loses the view of the transverse colon, the angulation controls are adjusted to obtain a partial view of the lumen ahead without overangling into the "walking-stick" configuration. In this scenario, inward push force is directed through the apex of the angulated bending section (the walking-stick handle) rather than toward the colonoscope tip, resulting in the splenic flexure being pushed up and down within the left upper quadrant.

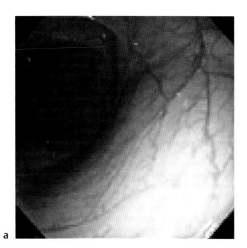
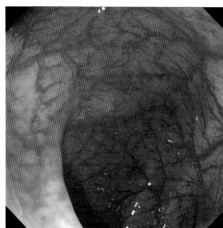

Fig. 14.14
a Endoscopic appearance of the hepatic flexure.
b Endoscopic appearance of the splenic flexure.

When the "handle" has been pushed up as far as it will go, there is a tendency for continued inward pressure to cause recurrent sigmoid looping, and paradoxically for the colonoscope tip to slip backward. Therefore, when passing the splenic flexure, one should push in slowly (too rapid pushing makes relooping of the sigmoid more likely), maintaining left iliac fossa pressure with clockwise twisting, and avoiding overangulation. If there is too much resistance at the flexure and the sigmoid reloops repeatedly, the patient should be moved to the supine or right lateral position and the rest of the formula should be repeated. If the splenic flexure is impassable in spite of all these maneuvers, then a change of instrument to the pediatric colonoscope or variable-stiffness instrument may prove successful. As a last resort, one can try pushing through any loop that may have formed, warning the patient that there may be a few seconds of discomfort. If all other measures have failed, a stiffening overtube, to splint the sigmoid colon, may very occasionally be invaluable, assuming that the tip really is at the splenic flexure and that the colon can be straightened. Even without full straightening of the sigmoid, a new shape-lock overtube can be applied to apparently good effect [53]. This device contains a flexible metal skeleton that can be rigidified once introduced over a looped colonoscope, thus directing subsequent inward pushing force away from the looped colon wall and toward the scope tip. It is important to remember that any overtube may cause trauma if passed through a narrowed or very acutely fixed sigmoid segment. If the instrument becomes "stuck" in the distal transverse colon, it is likely that the colon is mobile and a persistent descending mesocolon and long phrenicocolic ligament are combining to allow the scope to run up the midline and then pass around in a reversed splenic flexure loop. When this happens, and especially if external imaging is available, it is possible to twist *counter*clockwise when the scope tip is just around the splenic flexure; this swivels the tip around the axis of the phrenicocolic ligament to point back medially and simultaneously forces the descending colon back against the left abdominal wall, so that the scope configuration returns to normal and the rest of the insertion becomes easy. If the scope tip is already in the proximal transverse colon when this configuration is suspected, the reversed loop may be too large to derotate and it may be necessary to return to the splenic before derotating counterclockwise. Without imaging, these maneuvers are a matter of guesswork, but the message is to try withdrawal with counterclockwise twisting if things are going badly, before resorting to pushing alone.

Transverse Colon and Hepatic Flexure

Anatomy. The transverse colon, suspended on its transverse mesocolon and behind the greater omentum, is very variable in length and is longest in females. It runs across the anterior abdominal wall, so it can easily be indented with the finger and shows transillumination well. A triangular configuration is characteristic, and the longitudinal indentation of a tenia coli bundle is often visible, but the transverse colon may appear tubular, and occasionally the descending colon can be triangular. The blue-gray appearances of the left and/or right lobes of the liver adjacent to the transverse colon and hepatic flexure are suggestive, but not infallible, markers (**Fig. 14.14**). Aortic pulsation may be seen in the mid-transverse colon. The proximal transverse is often voluminous, so that deflation will make for easier passage, as the bowel collapses down with advancement of the colonoscope tip despite no scope insertion. The hepatic flexure is often acutely angled (less so with the patient in the left lateral position), and maximal application of both angling controls may be needed to steer around it. Because of its configuration, the hepatic flexure can be mistaken for the cecum, but apart from the absence of the ileocecal valve, the hepatic flexure is usually very clean (unlike the cecum, which is often fluid-filled). If there is any doubt, one can change the patient's position, insufflate, and give additional antispasmodic to confirm the presence of another bend.

Insertion technique. Provided that the splenic flexure and sigmoid colon have been passed with a "straight scope" configuration as described, passage of the instrument through the transverse colon should present little problem. It is almost inevitable that there will be some looping, but this is easily countered by withdrawal maneuvers, which need to be vigorously, and sometimes repeatedly, performed because of the length of instrument involved. The left lateral position is usually the most favorable for passing the proximal transverse colon, allowing deflation to collapse the hepatic flexure toward the instrument tip. However, other positions, including the supine, prone, and even right lateral (which causes the transverse colon to flop across to the right side) are all sometimes worth a try if looping seems uncontrollable and the hepatic flexure cannot be reached. In a proximal transverse colon of conventional length, counterclockwise twisting is a trick worth trying, which often helps somewhat in advancement, lifting and shortening the transverse colon by flattening out the counterclockwise spiral of the splenic flexure.

When the hepatic flexure is almost within reach, the endoscopist's best efforts (including deflation, shortening, and gentle pressure) may all tantalizingly fail to slide the endoscope up to the flexure. Trying additional "specific" abdominal pressure, empirically applied anywhere in the upper abdomen or in the low abdomen, pushing upward to lift the transverse colon as it loops around its apex, can be useful. Asking the patient to inspire will also depress the diaphragm, liver, and hepatic flexure in some patients and contribute to passage into the ascending colon.

If the scope feels looped and despite best efforts cannot be straightened to pass the hepatic flexure, there are three possibilities. Firstly, a reversed splenic flexure loop may have formed, as described earlier. In this scenario, the colonoscope has to be withdrawn to the distal transverse colon, followed by the application of counterclockwise torque to swing the descending colon back into its correct anatomical position. Secondly, a transverse gamma loop may have formed (Fig. 14.13 d). This can occur when the transverse is very long or when it is held by postsurgical adhesions. It is one of the most difficult loops to correct, even when imaging is available, but can be managed by withdrawal, suction to decompress the bowel, and reinsertion using torque (clockwise or counterclockwise twisting), with abdominal compression aimed at keeping the transverse high in the abdomen. Often it is not possible to completely derotate a gamma loop, and gentle inward pushing to go with the loop may therefore be the only option. Thirdly, there may be recurrent sigmoid looping, necessitating withdrawal to 50 cm and slow reinsertion with clockwise twisting and sigmoid abdominal compression.

Ascending Colon, Cecum, and Terminal Ileum

Anatomy. The ascending colon and cecum are always capacious, sometimes massively so. This can make endoscopic inspection of the interhaustral areas very demanding and uncertain. The variable positioning and mobility of this region is rarely apparent to the endoscopist relying on internal landmarks, but means that reliance on finger impression or transillumination alone is unreliable in comparison with positive identification of the ileocecal valve. The appendix orifice is usually a rather unimpressive curved slit at the pole of the cecum, where the three teniae coli fuse (although they are not always very visible). During colonoscopy, air refluxed into the ileum may cause a substantial, but soft, indenting deformity of the cecal pole.

The ileocecal valve almost invariably appears as a slight thickened bulge on the first large (ileocecal) fold distal to the pole (**Fig. 14.15**). Inconveniently for the endoscopist, the lips and slit-like orifice of the ileum most commonly appear on the proximal side of this fold, and so are rarely very obvious or easily entered straight on. The appearance of the valve varies substantially from individual to individual, and in some obese individuals it may appear enlarged or even frankly lipomatous. After long-standing inflammatory disease, the area can be considerably deformed, the valve opening being either stenosed or atrophic and widely patent, so that entry into the ileum may even happen with scarcely any obvious junction at all (**Fig. 14.16**). Using the light reflex to note the granular or lymphoid nodular appearance of the ileal surface in air, or the villi floating up under water, there is little difficulty in differentiating from colonic mucosa (**Fig. 14.17**). If, after disease or surgical anastomosis, the ileal villi are stunted and the difference is less obvious, it can be helpful to use dye spraying to enhance the surface detail and be certain which mucosal type is being examined.

The ascending colon appears as a dark void immediately after angling acutely around the hepatic flexure; immediate aspiration of some air is the best way of dropping the instrument down into it. Sometimes, with further deflation and gentle pushing, the instrument will easily slide down toward the cecum. In others, trying to push only loops the colon, but moving the patient to supine position and applying abdominal compression may help in coaxing it down. Occasionally, changing to a right lateral position facilitates pushing through a loop to reach the cecal pole before then straightening the

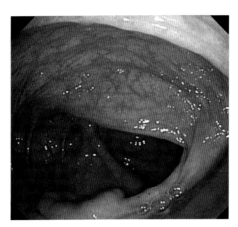

Fig. 14.15 Typical appearance of the cecum.

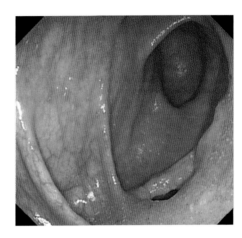

Fig. 14.16 A patent ileocecal valve in a patient with chronic ulcerative colitis.

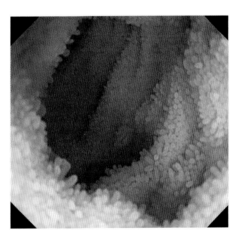

Fig. 14.17 Typical appearance of the terminal ileum.

14

colonoscope. In capacious colons, once the cecum is reached, retroversion is often possible and is helpful in examining behind haustra as far distally as the transverse colon when looking for small polyps, angiodysplasia, etc.

The ileocecal valve is often best seen from afar when the instrument is still in the ascending colon. If there is doubt about the site of the valve on the ileocecal fold, deflating will often cause it to bulge more obviously or to bubble. If it remains inapparent, it is sometimes possible to retrovert the scope tip in the cecal pole and locate the valve slit on the proximal side of the fold—although the long tip section of some video endoscopes may result in mechanical difficulty in retroversion and a poor view even when it is possible. Protruding the biopsy forceps to palpate for, and then lead into, the valve slit can be effective. The open forceps may also be used as a hook to pull open the valve; a "blind" biopsy of ileal mucosa can almost always be obtained through the valve even if the ileum cannot be intubated.

Entering the ileum with the instrument is reasonably easy and achievable in over 90% of cases. The key, as in all aspects of colonoscopy, is to have a straight scope (70–80 cm in the cecum) so that the valve fold can be positioned in the correct axis for scope insertion. After reaching the cecal pole, it is important to pull the scope tip back to the ascending colon so that the ileocecal valve fold can be clearly identified. Then the scope (or patient) should be rotated so that the ileocecal valve fold is at the 6-o'clock position. This is crucial, because entry into the valve then only necessitates use of the up–down control. Next, one should pass in over the valve fold, aspirate slightly to reduce the tension across the lips of the valve, and angle down whilst gently pulling back, to engage the distal lip of the valve. Often at this point the view is obscured, but as the ileum is entered, the endoscopist is rewarded with the typical close-up reflective pattern of the villi. To obtain a better view, the scope tip is then de-angled, with insufflation to find the lumen of the ileum. Anything up to 70 cm of ileum can then be examined, depending on the clinical indication and ease of access. Often, repeated attempts at ileal intubation are necessary and once the scope tip has slipped back, the entire procedure of lining up the valve has to be repeated. Occasionally, the valve is easier to enter with the scope retroflexed, when the scope tip is paradoxically pulled back into the valve.

Is Total Colonoscopy Achievable in All Patients?

With good bowel preparation and assuming that there is no obstruction, total colonoscopy is possible in approaching 100% of all patients. However, at least 20% of examinations are technically difficult even for experts, and it should always be remembered that for most patients virtual colonoscopy or barium enema are acceptable alternatives with very low complication rates (perforation in less than one in 25,000 examinations). Most difficulties at colonoscopy are related to recurrent looping of the colonoscope in a long and mobile colon or to a relatively fixed colon secondary to serosal adhesions, either from diverticular disease or previous surgery. Long and mobile colons can usually be intubated with any colonoscope, provided that good technique is applied with particular attention to straightening loops and appropriate use of position change and abdominal compression. Successful cecal intubation for particularly long and redundant colons has recently been described by using balloon-assisted intubation (double-balloon overtube for enteroscopy) [54]. Fixed colons, however, can make total colonoscopy impossible and even unsafe, particularly if the only instrument available is a standard adult colonoscope. When there is a fixed angulation that will not allow passage of a standard colonoscope, the thin (10-mm diameter), floppy (130 or 160 cm in length) pediatric instrument is ideal [55]. An alternative is a gastroscope, but as it is only 100 cm in length, total colonoscopy may not be possible. Occasionally, patients have the "dreaded" combination of a fixed, angulated sigmoid colon with a very long proximal colon. In this situation, the sigmoid can usually be negotiated using a pediatric instrument, but recurrent looping proximally can prevent total colonoscopy. The 160-cm pediatric variable-stiffness colonoscope is the ideal instrument here.

Examination Technique during Withdrawal

Although the major technical challenge of colonoscopy is to intubate as far as the cecum predictably, comfortably, and safely, the whole point of the procedure is to obtain an accurate diagnostic assessment. Many polyps and even some early cancers can be missed if a meticulous approach is not adhered to [56–58] (**Fig. 14.18**). A useful

proportion of visual assessment, and some biopsies and polypectomies, can best be achieved during the insertion phase when the colon is stretched out, but most diagnostic and therapeutic effort takes place during withdrawal. Rapid and scrupulous technique is required to scan the maximum area of the mucosa and to reduce the number of blind spots. Obsessiveness is needed to aspirate all fluid or irrigate any residue that may be obscuring the surface and to look behind prominent folds or rescan areas that have been poorly seen. Circular muscle spasticity can significantly reduce the view, so that use of antispasmodics may improve accuracy in the hunt for small polyps. It is also inevitable that some acute bends may require more than one pass for proper inspection, and that certain flexures may be best seen after a change of position. Turning the patient to the right oblique position to examine the splenic flexure and the descending colon, but then back to left lateral for examination of the sigmoid and rectum, improve visualization considerably. The process of accurate colorectal examination cannot be hurried. It is impossible to examine a colon adequately on withdrawal in less than 6 min; scanning carefully for small polyps should take nearer 10 min [59]. Adenoma detection rates (overall > 20%) have become established markers of quality performance [60,61] and techniques for enhancing adenoma detection, such as the use of dye spraying, narrow-band imaging, wide-angle colonoscopes, and an endoscope cap to hold down haustral folds, are all under evaluation. Too little emphasis in the past has been placed on quality withdrawal examination, although in the future it is likely that examination technique will be a standard and crucial part of colonoscopy accreditation and that all examinations will be recorded electronically for auditing and review purposes.

Complications

With the introduction of modern, flexible instruments, major complications at diagnostic colonoscopy have become infrequent [62]. Perforation may occur due to excessive force being applied during insertion, usually at the rectosigmoid junction, the apex of the sigmoid colon, or at the sigmoid/descending junction, particularly if the sigmoid colon is relatively fixed by adhesions. Abdominal pain after the procedure is usually due to excessive air insufflation, and all endoscopists using air should attempt to aspirate any excess during withdrawal. It should be remembered that pneumatic perforation is a possibility in the right colon if excessive air insufflation is used, particularly after EMR or any procedure has been performed that may weaken the bowel wall. Left upper quadrant pain, particularly if associated with a drop in hemoglobin, may indicate splenic trauma, easily diagnosed on abdominal scanning. Most serious complications are related to therapy, polypectomy, or dilation [62]. Hemorrhage occurs following 1–2% of polypectomies and may be delayed for up to 14 days. Perforation is less frequent (0.05–1.0% of polypectomies) and can also be delayed in presentation, and patients undergoing colonoscopy should therefore be warned to report immediately any significant bleeding, severe abdominal pain, or fever. Localized pain, fever, and leukocytosis are characteristic features of postpolypectomy syndrome, where there is localized peritonitis from a full-thickness burn but no frank perforation. With all significant complications, the immediate principle of management is to hospitalize the patient, with close observation of vital signs. Postpolypectomy syndrome and some small perforations can be managed conservatively with bed rest, fluids, and broad-spectrum antibiotics, whilst frank perforations require immediate repair with open or laparoscopic surgery.

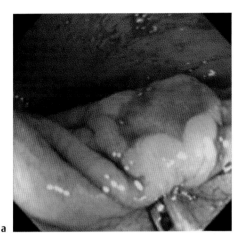
a

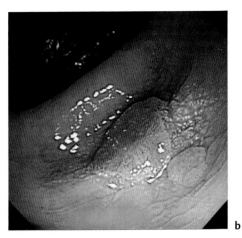
b

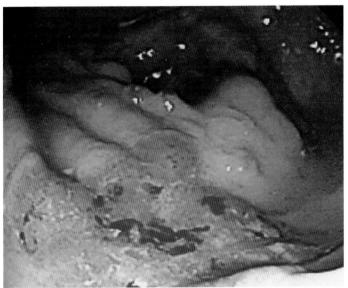
c

Fig. 14.18 a–c   Early flat cancers highlighted by indigo carmine dye spraying.

14

References

1. Wolff WI, Shinya H. Colonofiberoscopy. JAMA 1971;30:525–9.
2. Winawer SJ, Stewart ET, Zauber AG, Bond JH, Ansel H, Waye JD. A comparison of colonoscopy and double-contrast barium enema for surveillance after polypectomy. N Engl J Med 2000;342:1766–72.
3. U.S. Preventive Services Task Force. Screening for colorectal cancer: U.S. Preventive Services Task Force recommendation statement. Ann Intern Med 2008;149:627–37. [Summary for patients in Ann Intern Med 2008;149:I–44.]
4. Vader JP, Froehlich F, Dubois RW, Beglinger C, Wietlisbach V, Pittet V, et al. European Panel on the Appropriateness of Gastrointestinal Endoscopy (EPAGE): conclusion and WWW site. Endoscopy 1999;31:687–94.
5. Winawer SJ, Zauber AG, O'Brien MJ, Ho MN, Gottlieb L, Sternberg SS, et al. Randomized comparison of surveillance intervals after colonoscopic removal of newly diagnosed adenomatous polyps. The National Polyp Study Workgroup N Engl J Med 1993;328:901–6.
6. Winawer SJ, Zauber AG, Fletcher RH, Stillman JS, O'Brien MJ, Levin B, et al. Guidelines for colonoscopy surveillance after polypectomy: a consensus update by the US Multi-Society Task Force on Colorectal Cancer and the American Cancer Society. Gastroenterology 2006;130:1872–85.
7. Marbet UA, Bauerfeind P, Brunner J, Dorta G, Valloton JJ, Delcò F. Colonoscopy is the preferred colorectal cancer screening method in a population-based program. Endoscopy 2008;40:650–5.
8. Pox C, Schmiegel W, Classen M. Current status of screening colonoscopy in Europe and in the United States. Endoscopy 2007;39:168–73.
9. Schoemaker D, Black R, Gilles L, Toouli J. Yearly colonoscopy, liver CT, and chest radiography do not influence 5-year survival of colorectal cancer patients. Gastroenterology 1998;114:7–14.
10. Renkonen-Sinisalo L, Aarnio N, Mecklin JP, Jarvinen HJ. Surveillance improves survival of colorectal cancer in patients with hereditary nonpolyposis colorectal cancer. Gastroenterology 2000;24:137–42.
11. Rutter MD, Saunders BP, Wilkinson KH, Rumbles S, Schofield G, Kamm MA, et al. Thirty-year analysis of a colonoscopic surveillance program for neoplasia in ulcerative colitis. Gastroenterology 2006;130:1030–8.
12. Rutter MD, Saunders BP, Schofield G, Forbes A, Price AB, Talbot IC. Pancolonic indigo carmine dye spraying for the detection of dysplasia in ulcerative colitis. Gut 2004;53:256–60.
13. Veitch AM, Baglin TP, Gershlick AH, Harnden SM, Tighe R, Cairns S, et al. Guidelines for the management of anticoagulant and antiplatelet therapy in patients undergoing endoscopic procedures. Gut 2008;57:1322–9.
14. Guideline on the management of anticoagulation and antiplatelet therapy for endoscopic procedures. American Society for Gastrointestinal Endoscopy. Gastrointest Endosc 1998;48:672–5.
15. Froehlich F, Fried M, Schnegg JF, Gonvers JJ. Palatability of a new solution compared with standard polyethylene glycol solution for gastrointestinal lavage. Gastrintest Endosc 1991;37:325–8.
16. Rosch T, Classen M. Fractional cleansing of the large bowel with GoLytely for colonoscopic preparation: a controlled trial. Endoscopy 1987;19:198–200.
17. Worthington J, Thyssen M, Chapman G, Chapman R, Geraint M. A randomised controlled trial of a new 2 litre polyethylene glycol solution versus sodium picosulphate + magnesium citrate solution for bowel cleansing prior to colonoscopy. Curr Med Res Opin 2008;24:481–8.
18. Cohen SM, Wexner SD, Binderow SR, Nogueras JJ, Daniel N, Ehrenpreis ED, et al. Prospective, randomized, endoscopic-blinded trial comparing precolonoscopy cleansing methods. Dis Colon Rectum 1994;37:689–96.
19. Henderson JM, Barnett JL, Turgeon DK, Elta GH, Behler EM, Crause I, et al. Single-day, divided-dose oral sodium phosphate laxative versus intesti-

nal lavage as preparation for colonoscopy: efficacy and patient tolerance. Gastrointest Endosc 1995;42:238–43.

20. Kolts BE, Lyles WE, Achem SR, Burton L, Geller AJ, MacMath T. A comparison of the effectiveness and patient tolerance of oral sodium phosphate, castor oil, and standard electrolyte lavage for colonoscopy or sigmoidoscopy preparation. Am J Gastroenterol 1993;88:1218–23.

21. Vanner SJ, MacDonald PH, Paterson WG, Prentice RS, Da Costa LR, Beck IT. A randomized prospective trial comparing oral sodium phosphate with standard polyethylene glycol-based lavage solution (GoLytely) in the preparation of patients for colonoscopy. Am J Gastroenterol 1990;85: 422–7.

22. Huynh T, Vanner S, Paterson W. Safety profile of 5-h oral sodium phosphate regimen for colonoscopy cleansing: lack of clinically significant hypocalcemia or hypovolemia. Am J Gastroenterol 1995;90:104–7.

23. Zwas FR, Cirillo NW, El-Serag HB, Eisen N. Colonic mucosal abnormalities associated with oral sodium phosphate solution. Gastrointest Endosc 1996;43:463–6.

24. Ori Y, Herman M, Tobar A, Chernin G, Gafter U, Chagnac A, et al. Acute phosphate nephropathy—an emerging threat. Am J Med Sci 2008;336: 309–14.

25. Rex DK, Imperialo T, Portish VL. Patients willing to try colonoscopy without sedation: associated clinical factors and results of a randomized controlled trial. Gastrointest Endosc 1999;49:554–9.

26. Rex DK, Deenadayalu V, Eid E. Gastroenterologist-directed propofol: an update. Gastrointest Endosc Clin N Am 2008;18:717–25.

27. Saunders BP, Fukumoto M, Halligan S, Williams CB. Patient-administered nitrous oxide/oxygen inhalation provides effective sedation and analgesia for colonoscopy. Gastrointest Endosc 1994;40:418–21.

28. Saunders BP, Williams CB. Premedication with intravenous antispasmodic speeds colonoscope insertion. Gastrointest Endosc 1996;43: 209–11.

29. Froehlich F. Colonoscopy: antispasmodics not only for premedication, but also during endoscope withdrawal? Gastrointest Endosc 2000;51:379.

30. Cutler CS, Rex DK, Hawes RH, Lehman GA. Does routine intravenous glucagon administration facilitate colonoscopy? Gastrointest Endosc 1995;42:346–50.

31. Marshall JB, Patel M, Mahajan RJ, Early DS, King PD, Banerjee B. Benefit of intravenous antispasmodic (hyoscine sulfate) as premedication for colonoscopy. Gastrointest Endosc 1999;49:720–6.

32. Shah SG, Saunders BP, Brooker JC, Williams CB. Magnetic imaging of colonoscopy: an audit of looping, accuracy and ancillary maneuvers. Gastrointest Endosc 2000;52:1–8.

33. Brooker JC, Saunders BP, Shah SG, Williams CB. A new variable stiffness colonoscope makes colonoscopy easier: a randomised controlled trial. Gut 2000;46:801–5.

34. Othman MO, Bradley AG, Choudhary A, Hoffman RM, Roy PK. Variable stiffness colonoscope versus regular adult colonoscope: meta-analysis of randomized controlled trials. Endoscopy 2009;41:17–24.

35. Lee DW, Li AC, Ko CW, Chu DW, Chan KC, Poon CM, et al. Use of a variable-stiffness colonoscope decreases the dose of patient-controlled sedation during colonoscopy: a randomized comparison of 3 colonoscopes. Gastrointest Endosc 2007;65:424–9.

36. Shah SG, Saunders BP. Aids to insertion: magnetic imaging, variable stiffness, and overtubes. Gastrointest Endosc Clin N Am 2005;15:673–86.

37. Shah SG, Brooker JC, Williams CB, Thapar C, Suzuki N, Saunders BP. The variable stiffness colonoscope: assessment of efficacy by magnetic endoscope imaging. Gastrointest Endosc 2002;56:195–201.

38. Axelrad AM, Fleischer DE, Geller AJ, Nguyen CC, Lewis JH, Al-Kawas FH, et al. High-resolution chromoendoscopy for the diagnosis of diminutive colon polyps: implications for colon cancer screening. Gastroenterology 1996;110:1253–8.

39. Kim CY, Fleischer DE. Colonic chromoscopy: a new perspective on polyps and flat adenomas. Gastrointest Endosc Clin N Am 1997;7:423–7.

40. Gono K, Obi T, Yamaguchi M, Ohyama N, Machida H, Sano Y, et al. Appearance of enhanced tissue features in narrow-band endoscopic imaging. J Biomed Opt 2004;9:568–77.

41. East JE, Suzuki N, Bassett P, Stavrinidis M, Thomas HJ, Guenther T, et al. Narrow band imaging with magnification for the characterization of small and diminutive colonic polyps: pit pattern and vascular pattern intensity. Endoscopy 2008;40:811–7.

42. East JE, Saunders BP. Narrow band imaging at colonoscopy: seeing through a glass darkly or the light of a new dawn? Expert Rev Gastroenterol Hepatol 2008;2:1–4.

43. Goetz M, Kiesslich R. Confocal endomicroscopy: in vivo diagnosis of neoplastic lesions of the gastrointestinal tract. Anticancer Res 2008; 28(1B):353–60.

44. Hussein AM, Bartram CI, Williams CB. Carbon dioxide insufflation for more comfortable colonoscopy. Gastrointest Endosc 1984;30:68–70.

45. Waye JD. Colonoscopy without fluoroscopy. Gastrointest Endosc 1990; 36:72–3.

46. Williams CB, Guy C, Gilles D, Saunders B. Electronic three-dimensional imaging of intestinal endoscopy. Lancet 1993;341:724–5.

47. Bladen JS, Anderson AP, Bell GD, Rameh B, Evans B, Heatley DJ. Non-radiological technique for three-dimensional imaging of endoscopes. Lancet 1993;341:719–22.

48. Saunders BP, Bell GD, Williams CB, Anderson AP. First clinical results with a real-time, electronic imager as an aid to colonoscopy. Gut 1995;36: 913–7.

49. Shah SG, Brooker JC, Williams CB, Thapar C, Saunders BP. Effect of magnetic endoscope imaging on colonoscopy performance: a randomised controlled trial. Lancet 2000;356:1718–22.

50. Shah SG, Thomas-Gibson S, Lockett M, Brooker JC, Thapar CJ, Grace I, et al. Effect of real-time magnetic endoscope imaging on the teaching and acquisition of colonoscopy skills: results from a single trainee. Endoscopy 2003;35:421–5.

51. East JE, Suzuki N, Arebi N, Bassett P, Saunders BP. Position changes improve visibility during colonoscope withdrawal: a randomized, blinded, crossover trial. Gastrointest Endosc 2007;65:263–9.

52. Shinya H. Colonoscopy—diagnosis and treatment of colonic diseases. New York: Igaku-Shoin; 1982.

53. Hawari R, Pasricha PJ. Going for the loop: a unique overtube for the difficult colonoscopy. J Clin Gastroenterol 2007;41:138–40.

54. Gay G, Delvaux M. Double-balloon colonoscopy after failed conventional colonoscopy: a pilot series with a new instrument Endoscopy 2007;39: 788–92 e.

55. Bat L, Williams CB. Usefulness of pediatric colonoscopes in adult colonoscopy. Gastrointest Endosc, 1989;35:329–32.

56. van Rijn JC, Reitsma JB, Stoker J, Bossuyt PM, van Deventer SJ, Dekker E. Polyp miss rate determined by tandem colonoscopy: a systematic review. Am J Gastroenterol 2006;101:343–50.

57. Shehadeh I, Rebala S, Kumar R, Markert RJ, Barde C, Gopalswamy N. Retrospective analysis of missed advanced adenomas on surveillance colonoscopy. Am J Gastroenterol 2002;97:1143–7.

58. Bressler B, Paszat LF, Vinden C, Li C, He J, Rabeneck L. Colonoscopic miss rates for right-sided colon cancer: a population-based analysis. Gastroenterology 2004;127:452–6.

59. Barclay RL, Vicari JJ, Doughty AS, Johanson JF, Greenlaw RL. Colonoscopic withdrawal times and adenoma detection during screening colonoscopy. N Engl J Med 2006;355:2533–41.

60. Rex DK, Petrini JL, Baron TH, Chak A, Cohen J, Deal SE, et al. Quality indicators for colonoscopy. Am J Gastroenterol 2006;101:873–85.

61. Rex DK. Quality in colonoscopy: cecal intubation first, then what? Am J Gastroenterol 2006;101:732–4.

62. Waye JD, Kahn O, Auerbach ME. Complications of colonoscopy and flexible sigmoidoscopy. Gastrointest Endosc Clin N Am 1996;6:343–77.

IV

15 ERCP

Gregory B. Haber, Gurpal S. Sandha, and Meinhard Classen

Historical Background

Endoscopic retrograde cholangiopancreatography (ERCP) is a combined endoscopic and radiographic procedure that allows visualization of the biliary and pancreatic duct systems by direct cannulation of the papilla of Vater and retrograde contrast injection using a side-viewing duodenoscope. Endoscopic cannulation of the papilla was first described by McCune et al. in 1968 [1]. Since then, there have been numerous reports and accumulating experience in the technique of ERCP [2–13]. Extensive development of a variety of endoscopes and endoscopic accessories over the last four decades has established the applicability of ERCP for diagnostic and therapeutic indications in the pancreaticobiliary system. Specialized training is required to achieve competence and the necessary skills, with their increasing complexity [14,15].

With the increasing complexity of the techniques used, however, it soon became clear that ERCP and associated therapeutic techniques required dedicated and extensive facilities, properly trained physicians and gastroenterology assistants, and a multidisciplinary environment, all of which are available in referral centers. It was shown that outcomes after diagnostic and therapeutic endoscopy are influenced by the endoscopist's level of expertise (and the center's case volume), and this prompted the next generation to reconcentrate the most difficult cases in tertiary referral centers. The following description of ERCP therefore includes those techniques that should be available routinely (such as endoscopic sphincterotomy for acute cholangitis or acute gallstone pancreatitis) and those that should be performed in centers that have a sufficient volume for proper management. Diagnostic uses for ERCP are currently disappearing in the developed countries.

This chapter deals with the current standard of practice for ERCP, outlining the indications, technique, and complications of this widely available and clinically useful procedure.

Indications

The major indications for ERCP are listed in **Table 15.1**. The emergence of newer and less invasive modalities for visualizing the pancreatic and biliary ducts, such as magnetic resonance cholangiopancreatography (MRCP) and endoscopic ultrasonography (EUS), are replacing diagnostic ERCP in many clinical situations. However, because of its therapeutic capabilities, ERCP will remain the procedure of choice when intervention, tissue sampling, or more accurate anatomic detail is required. Details of the therapeutic techniques are discussed in other chapters of this book.

Facilities

An ERCP room should be dedicated for these procedures (and should also include standing equipment for therapeutic EUS). It should be large enough to accommodate all the necessary equipment to do ERCP, including a radiography table, storage space for ancillary devices, space for the endoscopist, two gastroenterology

Table 15.1 Indications for endoscopic retrograde cholangiopancreatography (ERCP)

Biliary tract disorders
Jaundice or cholestasis of suspected obstructive origin
Acute cholangitis
Biliary cholangitis
Biliary lesions seen on other imaging procedures
Biliary fistula or leak
Pancreatic disorders
Recurrent acute pancreatitis of uncertain etiology
Severe acute biliary pancreatitis
Pancreas cancer for tissue sampling and palliation
Pancreatic fistula or leak
Pancreatic insufficiency or malabsorption
Chronic pancreatitis with pain, jaundice, or leak for preoperative assessment or therapy
Pancreatic pseudocyst for preoperative assessment or therapy
Abdominal pain and laboratory tests or imaging studies suggesting pancreatic disease
Endoscopic therapy
Endoscopic papillotomy/sphincterotomy
Biliary/pancreatic duct drainage
Endoscopic tissue and fluid sampling
Biopsy, brush, fine-needle aspiration
Bile/pancreatic juice collection
Preoperative ductal mapping
Malignant tumors
Benign strictures
Chronic pancreatitis
Manometry
Sphincter of Oddi
Ductal stricture/stenosis

assistants, one radiography technician and anesthesia equipment and personnel [16].

Appropriate placement of fluoroscopic and endoscopic monitors is also important and may vary with the usual position preferred for the patients. Ideally, they should be mounted on movable booms so that the best positioning can be found for every case. When the patient is in the supine position, the best place for the monitors is on the same side as the endoscopist, while the opposite side may be more comfortable when working with the patient in prone position. A second fluoroscopic monitor that displays the most recently captured image is also useful in difficult procedures, to allow better appreciation of the anatomy.

In centers in which more advanced endoscopic procedures are performed, an EUS machine allowing the use of a linear therapeutic EUS scope should also be available when needed.

Equipment

Endoscopes

Side-viewing duodenoscopes, which should be regarded as standard and routine, are used as "therapeutic" scopes with a 4.2-mm channel. They make it possible to use the whole range of diagnostic and therapeutic accessories and have no disadvantages in comparison with the 2.8-mm "diagnostic" duodenoscopes. The therapeutic scopes can be used for almost all indications, including pediatric patients. Only neonates or infants under the age of 2 may require the use of pediatric scopes with a therapeutic channel of 2.2 mm. Forward-viewing scopes are preferred by some endoscopists for patients with Billroth II anatomy, although they do not facilitate access to the papilla [17] and make devices more difficult to manipulate, due to the lack of an elevator.

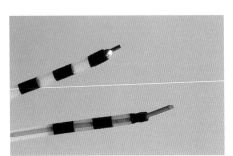

Fig. 15.1 *Top:* A small conical metal-tipped catheter with a 23-gauge needle for entry into the minor papilla. *Below:* A tapered catheter with guide wire.

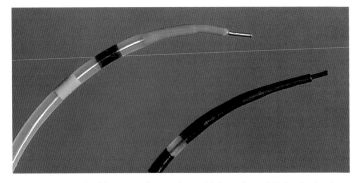

Fig. 15.2 Two highly tapered cannulas, which go from 5 Fr in the body to 3 Fr at the tip, with passage of a small-caliber 0.018-in Roadrunner metal-tipped wire or a 0.018-in hydrophilic Terumo wire.

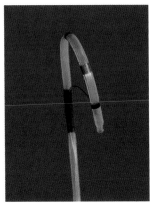
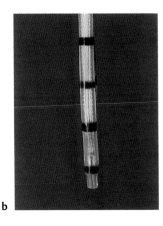

a   b

Fig. 15.3
a Close-up view of the KD-21Q Olympus non–wire-guided sphincterotome. The flat metal plate in the catheter should be noted.
b The flat metal plate has been preshaped to achieve an angled direction of the tip of the sphincterotome on bowing.

Cannulating Devices

Catheters. Cannulating catheters are usually made with Teflon tubing to provide adequate stiffness. The standard size is 5–7 Fr, with the tip tapered to 4 Fr and a lumen that accommodates a 0.035-inch wire. The tip has radiopaque material impregnated into it to allow fluoroscopic visualization, and colored surface markers to indicate the depth of insertion. Ultratapered catheters have 3-Fr tips and a lumen that allows a 0.021 or 0.018-inch wire. Dual-lumen tandem catheters allow wire insertion in one channel and contrast injection in the other. For wire-guided passage, a monorail-design system is used with specialized catheters, such as a perfused triple-lumen manometry catheter, in which the wire enters the tip of the catheter and exits from a side hole close to the tip. Some catheters are precurved by the manufacturer, although most are straight and require "grooming" to create a curve at the tip.

Catheter tips have been modified with the insertion of a metal ball or blunt needle tip. The ball tip is designed to prevent impaction of the catheter and to allow easy changes in direction between the biliary and pancreatic orifices. The conical needle tip provides a 22-gauge narrow tip to enter a tiny punctum, as with the minor papilla, or a stenotic pancreatic orifice in the major papilla (**Figs. 15.1, 15.2**).

Sphincterotomes. Sphincterotomes vary with regard to the length and type of the cutting wire, tip length, and caliber, as well as the presence of separate guide wire and injection channels.

Most manufacturers have phased out braided wires, which induce more coagulation than a comparable monofilament wire. The latter is also available in smaller diameters down to 0.010 in, minimizing the coagulative effect. Sphincterotome wire lengths vary from 15 to 35 mm, with the middle range being the more widely used lengths. The longer the cutting wire, the greater the radius of curvature, which increases the range of movement of the tip of the papillotome. The drawback of a longer wire is the need to back away from the papilla with the endoscope. Thus, a shorter wire is required when the endoscope tip enters a narrow duodenum, as with tumor infiltration. Our personal preference is for a 30–35-mm cutting wire, to maximize the maneuvers possibly needed with difficult cannulation (**Fig. 15.3**). The standard taper of the tip of a sphincterotome is 5 Fr, but diameters of 3.5 and 4.0 Fr are also available.

Sphincterotomes are now most often provided with a three-lumen design, allowing guide-wire manipulation and contrast injection. Various systems are now available to allow the endoscopist to manipulate the wire, the best known being the Rapid Exchange system) and the Fusion system (Cook Endoscopy, Winston-Salem, North Carolina, USA). The principle of the monorail system, which enables the endoscopist to control the guide wire and the exchange procedure, is similar in the two systems. They both have a dedicated locking device fixed on the endoscope, and they differ with regard to the distance of the side hole from the tip of the device, which is shorter in the Fusion system (6.0 or 2.5 cm), making it possible to carry out intraductal exchanges into the common bile duct (CBD) or main pancreatic duct—particularly useful when multiple stenting is indicated.

The V system (Olympus) also allows the guide wire to be manipulated by the endoscopist and is associated specifically with the V scope, which has an elevator design that makes it possible to fix the guide wire during exchanges.

Guide wires are the cornerstone of therapeutic ERCP. They are used to achieve and maintain access to the desired structure, and also to help advance the various accessories. The most frequently used can be divided into two categories :
- Those typically designed to obtain access to a specific structure. These consist of a coated wire covered with hydrophilic polymers. They may be angled or straight and are available in diam-

eters ranging from 0.020 to 0.035 inches. Typical examples are the Terumo (Terumo Corporation, Tokyo, Japan), the Jagwire or Hydrajag (Boston Scientific), the Tracer (Cook Endoscopy), and the X wire (ConMed, Utica, New York, USA). The Terumo, which is also available in smaller diameters, is often considered to be the most useful wire for difficult access, although it is slightly more difficult to manipulate during exchanges.

- The coiled and stiff standard wires (Teflon wires, Amplatz wires), which are used because of their rigidity to help advance devices through tight strictures or sharp angles.

A specialized sigmoid configuration for the papillotome, with the cutting wire on the convex curve, is designed to allow correct orientation of the wire in patients with Billroth II anatomy.

A needle tip rather than a bowed wire is used for precutting, cutting over a stent, and fistulotomy. The needle tip is a short, narrow, monofilament tip, and this device also has a separate wire-guide port.

Contrast Agents

Iodinated contrast agents are in standard use, with a maximum concentration of 60–65%. Full-strength contrast is used for maximum definition of ductal architecture—important for pancreatography or detection of subtle changes in the intrahepatic ducts in patients with early sclerosing cholangitis. Dense contrast can impair the detection of small stones, especially in a dilated duct with a thick column of contrast, and dilution to a 30% concentration or less is therefore helpful for cholangiography to detect stones.

Iodine allergy is not an absolute contraindication to the use of an iodinated agent for ERCP. The intraductal instillation of contrast and duodenal spill-over rarely cause a problem even when severe iodine allergies have been noted during previous intravenous use. We routinely administer intravenous antihistamine (Benadryl 50 mg) and steroid (Solu-Cortef 100 mg) before the procedure as prophylaxis. The alternative to this approach is simply to use a noniodinated contrast agent.

The hypertonicity of iodinated contrast has been implicated as a factor potentially associated with post-ERCP pancreatitis. However, its impact on the incidence of this complication appears to be marginal and of less importance than several other established risk factors. Since the alternative of a nonionic isoosmotic contrast agent is far more expensive, the increased cost does not appear to be justified.

Technique

Patient Preparation and Sedation

Preparation and consent. Informed consent is always important, but more so with ERCP, in view of the risks. In a tertiary care setting, many patients are seen for the first time just before their endoscopy. Consent is best obtained with a close relative or friend in attendance, to ensure that the patient understands the reasons for the test and the associated risks. A translator should be available or requested if needed. In an emergency situation, when a delay in obtaining informed consent may jeopardize the patient's health, we proceed with ERCP when the indication is clear. Patients or referring doctors are requested to provide pertinent records of prior investigations, and the onus is on the endoscopist to ascertain whether or not ERCP is appropriate for that patient. The history should include relevant comorbid problems, especially cardiorespiratory disease, prior surgery, medications, and allergies. The use of aspirin, anti-inflammatories, platelet inhibitors, or anti-coagulants

is noted. We do not defer ERCP when the patient has a history of recent ingestion of these drugs, with the exception of Coumadin or heparin. On the other hand, if the patient is seen in advance, we recommend stopping aspirin or antiplatelet drugs 7 days before the procedure. After sphincterotomy, we suggest re-starting these drugs 48–72 h later.

Outpatients are asked to bring someone to accompany them home. Patients change into a hospital gown, and venous access is obtained with a scalp needle or small intracatheter. Intravenous fluids are only given as needed for hydration or venous access in the unstable patient. Vital signs (heart rate, blood pressure, and oxygen saturation) are assessed before starting and throughout the entire procedure. After removing the patient's dentures, if present, we use lidocaine for topical anesthesia, either in the form of a spray or as a liquid for gargle. Local anesthesia is not common practice in every country, however.

Position. We prefer to have our patients in the semiprone position, with the left arm straight alongside the back and the right arm flexed in front. Other authors prefer the prone position, due to the improved image quality. In obese patients or those with respiratory compromise, care needs to be taken not to have the patient prone, since movement of the diaphragm may be impaired due to the abdominal compression. In those with hilar tumors, or occasionally when there is difficulty in passing the endoscope, the patient is placed supine.

Sedation. Sedation is generally deeper than for other endoscopic procedures. We do not routinely presedate. However, in the unduly anxious patient, or in those known to have sedation problems, an oral benzodiazepine or anxiolytic taken 2–4 h before the procedure with 100–150 mL of water often reduces the overall sedation requirements during the procedure. We use a combination of meperidine (or fentanyl when indicated due to meperidine allergy) and midazolam, both given intravenously. Usual starting doses are 50 mg of meperidine (Demerol) and 3 mg of midazolam (Versed), but the dose needs to be tailored to each individual patient. Due to a longer half-life, the full effect of the meperidine may not occur for several minutes. Incremental doses of meperidine should therefore be timed accordingly. In patients with a history of drug or alcohol abuse, regular use of narcotic analgesics, hypnotics, or sedatives, or with a prior history of difficult sedation, further measures are useful. These include the use of droperidol, propofol, or general anesthesia. The best agent in these situations is propofol, due to its rapid onset, deep sedation, and quick recovery. The principal side effect is respiratory depression, and the dose therefore needs careful adjustment and continuous monitoring. In most countries, an anesthetist has traditionally administered this drug. However, in western Europe and the United States, many endoscopists or trained nurses now give the propofol themselves, and this will undoubtedly become more the norm as understanding of the pharmacokinetics and complications becomes more widespread. For further details, see Chapter 6.

At our institutions, general anesthesia is rarely used in adults, other than those with severe respiratory compromise or prior failure of droperidol.

The narcotic antagonist naloxone (0.2–0.4 mg i.v.) and the benzodiazepine antagonist flumazenil (0.3–0.6 mg i.v.) must always be in the room and available for emergency use. Antimotility drugs are used to reduce duodenal peristaltic activity. Glucagon 0.25–1.0 mg i.v., or hyoscine butylbromide (Buscopan) 20–40 mg i.v. are the two drugs most commonly used to stop duodenal contractions. Some units administer atropine 0.6 mg subcutaneously or intravenously before the procedure to reduce the risk of aspiration in patients placed in the supine position.

15

Procedure

▦ Oropharyngeal Intubation

Intubation with a side-viewing duodenoscope is performed, observing the right side of the pharynx, the epiglottis, and the arytenoids. Difficulty may be encountered with fibrosis and narrowing after radiation, a Zenker's diverticulum, a cricopharyngeal bar, or a high esophageal web, stricture, or cancer. If resistance occurs, a small-caliber forward-viewing gastroscope should be used to inspect the pharynx and upper esophagus. Wire-guided dilation is performed as needed. With a spastic or thickened upper esophageal sphincter, empirical use of a 50–54-Fr Savary bougie often facilitates subsequent introduction of the duodenoscope. With Zenker's diverticulum, a 0.038-in stiff biliary wire can be placed in the stomach and then backloaded into the duodenoscope by advancing a 6-Fr catheter to the tip and inserting the stiff end of the wire up the catheter. The catheter is then advanced down the wire to stiffen the assembly. Even with the wire and catheter inserted, it may be difficult to maneuver the duodenoscope into the esophagus. A useful alternative is to insert a small 21-Fr Savary bougie, which holds the esophageal sphincter open, so that the duodenoscope can then be inserted alongside the bougie.

Positioning the endoscope in the second duodenum. The first landmark before gaining access to the duodenum is the upper part of the stomach, high on the lesser curvature, 2–5 cm distal to the cardia (**Fig. 15.4a**). At this time, the endoscopist has to insufflate slightly, making sure that the longitudinal folds are visualized and following them as the instrument is advanced. Between the cardia and the angle of the lesser curvature, the endoscopist and endoscope have to rotate clockwise to follow the gastric lumen against the greater curvature. To pass the pylorus, the tip is angled up, with the pylorus in a "setting-sun" fashion (**Fig. 15.4b**). This maneuver is easy if the instrument is in the central axis of the antrum. Lateral (right or left) deflection or twisting of the endoscope can be used to achieve the correct position facing the pyloric ring. After passing the pylorus, the endoscope is pushed into the distal bulb and subsequently slightly withdrawn (**Fig. 15.4c**). The tip is then angled right (with the brake in the right position) and upward while the instrument is rotated clockwise (for visualization of the second duodenal lumen) (**Fig. 15.4d**). The key point at this time is to pull back and straighten the endoscope, which "falls" into the second duodenum (**Fig. 15.4e**). This straightened "short route" position is the only one in which control of the distal tip is sufficient to achieve the maneuvers required for selective cannulation (**Fig. 15.4f**). The short route is usually achieved in adults when the tip is between 60 and 70 cm from the teeth. After straightening, the side-viewing scope is facing either the papilla or the third part of the duodenum. The papilla is then visualized by slowly pulling back the scope while rotating from left to right. The papilla is usually seen above a longitudinal fold or within several oblique folds. The orifice is sometimes covered by a transverse fold, which has to be lifted with a catheter to visualize the papilla.

Selective cannulation technique. The first step in cannulation is proper positioning of the scope, facing the papilla. It is much better to spend time ensuring a good position before any attempt at cannulation, as tangential access is doomed to failure and multiple manipulations make the procedure more difficult. The endoscope must face onto the papilla in the frontal axis, in the upper part of the image.

Either a guide-wire method or a contrast-injection technique can be used for selective cannulation. There is no definitive answer as to which is best, although recent studies have suggested that the cannulation success rate with the guide wire is superior, without altering the incidence of pancreatitis [18]. Debatable issues are the fact that the trials concerned were conducted by practitioners well versed in the guide-wire technique and that injection may be helpful for appreciating any difficult anatomy in the papilla.

Using a sphincterotome that can be bent in the biliary direction has also been shown to be superior to a standard catheter for selective biliary cannulation (**Fig. 15.1**) [19]. When the catheter is placed in the papillary orifice perpendicular to the duodenum, the pancreatic ducts are most often opacified. Biliary access requires more tangential access, between the 11-o'clock and 1-o'clock positions. Using a guide wire for initial cannulation may reduce physical pressure and distortion on the papilla, which might accentuate a tortuous distal duct. Whichever technique is used, however, it is important to bear in mind that the intrapapillary part of the bile duct (and the pancreatic duct) is not straight and that initial cannulation should follow the anatomy, which can only be appreciated using the injection technique. The roof of the orifice has to be approached from below and slightly from the right. Thereafter, the catheter has to go from the left to the right, by turning left the lateral wheel. The scope can also be pulled back for this second phase of cannulation. Finally, the catheter is introduced into the CBD by turning back the lateral wheel to the right and pushing back the scope (**Fig. 15.2**).

In difficult cases, combined injection of small volumes and careful manipulation of a hydrophilic guide wire are helpful, especially in cases of tortuous anatomy. Tapered-tip sphincterotomes (Minitome, Cook Endoscopy) manipulated with a 0.020-in Terumo guide wire are also useful for the small papilla, where it may be difficult to catch the orifice.

▦ Cannulating the Minor Papilla (Table 15.2)

The minor papilla is situated 2 cm proximal and 2 cm anterior or to the right of the major papilla. These distances are approximate, and the only certainty is that the minor papilla will be situated in the right upper quadrant of a circle with the major papilla at the center. In the absence of a pancreas divisum, the minor papilla is patent in only a small proportion of patients. An interesting facet of a patent minor papilla is that it protects against post-ERCP pancreatitis by allowing run-off of contrast injected through the major papilla. The hallmark of pancreas divisum is the filling of a small-caliber duct system limited to the head of the pancreas, with early acinarization on continued injection (**Figs. 15.6–15.8**). The ventral duct system may be difficult to fill, either due to the small orifice or a somewhat atretic ventral bud. Thus, failure to find the pancreatic duct at the major papilla is a further reason for identifying and attempting to cannulate the minor papilla. This can be quite challenging, considering the unstable position of the endoscope, in addition to the fact that the minor papilla may be difficult to find and cannulate. From its position at the major papilla, the endoscope should be withdrawn slowly, trying not to slide back into the duodenal cap. Just beyond the superior duodenal angle, slightly to the right of the major papilla, the minor papilla appears as a small nodule, barely recognizable at times (**Fig. 15.9**). If this is not apparent in a short

Table 15.2 A summary of tips for minor papilla cannulation

Inspection—inspection—inspection
Short scope position
Entry at the 9-o'clock position
Using a needle-tip catheter
3-Fr curved tip
? Secretin administration

IV

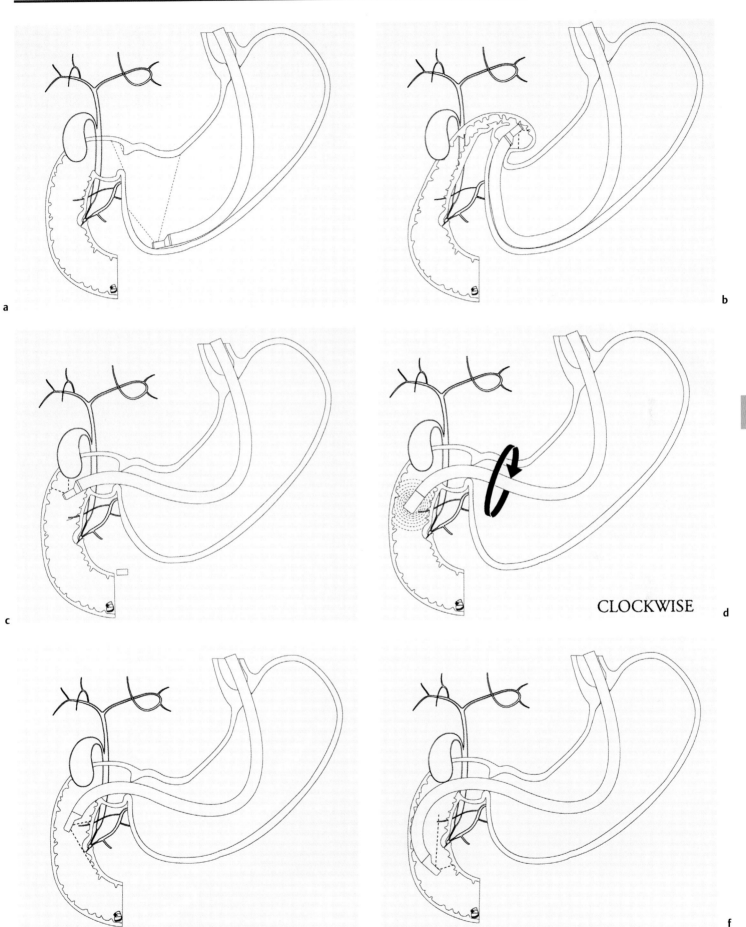

a

b

c

d

CLOCKWISE

e

f

Fig. 15.4 The landmarks in positioning the endoscope in the second duodenum. (Courtesy of J. Devière, Brussels)

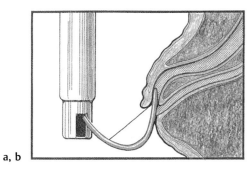
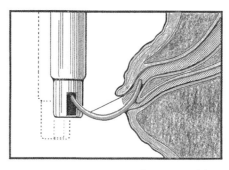
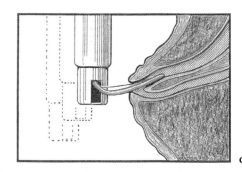

a, b   c

Fig. 15.5
a The sphincterotome tip is angled up to gain entry into the biliary orifice.
b Relaxation of the bowed sphincterotome wire allows the tip to advance across the intramural bile duct segment.

c Shortening of the endoscope position allows straightening of the sphincterotome tip for deep cannulation.

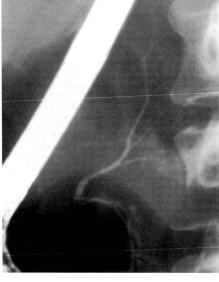

Fig. 15.6 Injection of an isolated ventral duct system in a patient with pancreas divisum. The fine, feathery, tapered termination of the branch ducts should be noted.

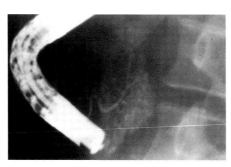

Fig. 15.7 Injection of an isolated ventral duct system from the major papilla in which early acinarization has occurred due to the small volume required to fill the entire duct system.

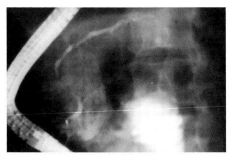

Fig. 15.8 Partial pancreas divisum. It should be noted that filling from the major papilla into the ventral duct shows acinarization, indicating a high filling pressure, followed by communication through a branch duct with the pancreatic duct in the body and tail.

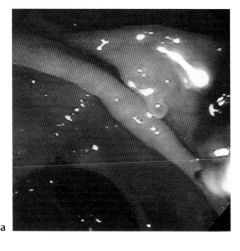

a

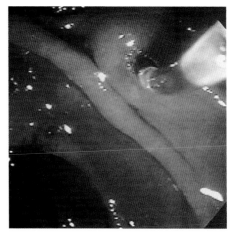

b

Fig. 15.9 a, b The approach to the minor papilla, seen from the short duodenoscope position, with a 9-o'clock direction of entry.

scope position, the duodenoscope should be withdrawn into the duodenal cap and pushed back into the descending duodenum for inspection prior to withdrawing into a short scope position.

The minor papilla is not distinctly visible on most occasions, unlike the papilla of Vater, and may have no sentinel folds to help localization. Once it is identified, some time should be taken simply to observe the papilla, with periodic suction to create negative pressure that may result in opening of a tiny punctum. This is important, as the orifice is more often eccentrically located. The small size of the aperture requires that small cannulating instruments be used. We begin attempts at cannulation with a needle-tipped catheter (Cremer catheter, Wilson-Cook) (**Fig. 15.1**). The other method is to use an ultratapered 3-Fr tip catheter with a wire of 0.018 or 0.021 inches (**Fig. 15.2**). Contrast is injected once the catheter has been advanced into the duct and the wire withdrawn. Minor duct cannulations should preferably be performed by an endoscopist who is experienced in this technically difficult maneuver (**Fig. 15.10**).

▥ Challenging Scenarios

Billroth II gastrojejunostomy. This surgery results in removal of the distal portion of the stomach and closure of the duodenal stump. A gastrojejunostomy is then created to form an afferent and an efferent loop. In order to reach the papillary orifice from the stomach, the endoscope has to be advanced in a retrograde fashion along the afferent loop. ERCP is challenging in this situation for two main reasons.

Firstly, the angle of the afferent loop with the stomach is generally acute, which makes it difficult to advance the side-viewing endoscope. It is usually the more difficult of the two loops to enter, with the opening often between the 2-o'clock and 5-o'clock positions on the gastrojejunostomy opening when viewed from within the stomach. The presence of bile aids in correctly identifying this loop. Fluoroscopy may also be helpful, especially if the endoscope is seen progressing toward the pelvis. This would suggest passage down the efferent loop. If this happens, taking a few biopsies from the efferent loop just inside the stoma will ensure prompt recognition of the wrong loop on subsequent attempts. Adhesions make the afferent loop less pliable and more prone to perforation, and adequate caution is therefore taken to avoid pushing when the endoscope is not seen to advance. There are usually no reliable landmarks in finding the papilla until it is finally reached. However, if the scope is passed to the closed end of the duodenal stump, the papilla will be found lying just proximal to it.

Secondly, cannulation may be difficult because everything is in the opposite of the normal ERCP position. The natural curve of cannulating devices is therefore not helpful, and instead a straight cannula is needed. The bile duct is found at the 5-o'clock position, rather than the normal 11-o'clock position (**Fig. 15.11**). To align the cannulating device in the correct axis, the tip of the endoscope may need to be kept at a little distance from the papilla, usually at the junction of the second and third parts of the duodenum. This makes the process of cannulating more challenging. Using a guide wire can facilitate cannulation in cases in which a straight cannula fails to achieve cholangiography.

If it is not possible to advance the side-viewer to the papilla, a small-caliber gastroscope is a feasible alternative to advance past a sharp angulation. In long afferent loops in which even a gastroscope does not reach the papilla, a pediatric colonoscope or enteroscope can be used, but the latter requires extra-long accessories that are custom-made for this scope.

As Billroth II gastrojejunostomies are technically challenging and not commonly seen in clinical practice, only endoscopists who have therapeutic experience in these difficult scenarios should attempt to perform ERCP [20–24].

Periampullary diverticula. The presence of the papilla of Vater within a diverticulum (periampullary) or adjacent to it (juxta-ampullary) is the commonest anomaly that presents difficulty in cannulating the common bile or pancreatic ducts. The ampulla can be situated anywhere along the inferior rim of the diverticulum, but in our experience it is seen most commonly at around the 3-o'clock position within the diverticular sac when seen *en face* from the duodenoscope. Proper alignment with the upstream duct may be

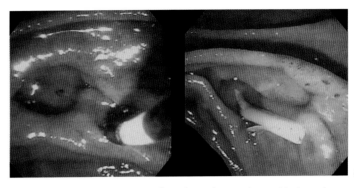

a, b

Fig. 15.10 a There is a tiny papilla within a diverticulum, with the red spot indicating the orifice after prior cannulation. **b** Note the placement of a pancreatic stent in the dorsal duct of the system and the angle of entry after stent placement.

difficult to achieve. Probing with a sphincterotome or cannula can usually accentuate the papilla by bringing it closer to the diverticular rim for better access. Cannulation with the tip of the duodenoscope within the sac is possible, but care needs to be taken to avoid perforation. A dual insertion of a wire used to evert and hold the papillary fold outside the diverticulum, along with a cannula, has been reported to facilitate access (**Fig. 15.11**).

Papillary distortion. A number of clinical entities can cause distortion or bulging of the papillary orifice. The most common of these are impacted common bile duct stones, ampullary tumors (adenoma or carcinoma), and choledochocele. A stone impacted in the ampulla is a potentially serious condition and requires early intervention to extract the stone. The papilla often looks slightly prominent and erythematous, and is usually dry, with no bile flow visible. Cannulation may be difficult, as the stone may prevent passage of the cannulating device into the bile duct. Ampullary tumors may be either benign or malignant. They appear as exophytic masses originating from the ampulla and may obscure the papillary orifice. Careful observation is necessary before probing, so as to avoid excessive bleeding from the friable surface of these lesions. The opening is usually situated around the center of the lesion, although it may prove impossible to find, especially if there is extensive necrosis and excoriation. A choledochocele is a congenital anomaly of the intrahepatic or extrahepatic bile ducts. Type III choledochocele is a sacculation of the intramural portion of the distal common bile duct and is seen endoscopically as a smooth bulge at the papillary orifice. The opening can occur anywhere on this bulge, but is most frequently seen at the lower part and may present technical difficulty in cannulation.

Advanced pancreatic tumors may infiltrate the duodenal wall and cause luminal narrowing, thereby limiting the passage of the duodenoscope. This also reduces compliance of the duodenal wall and prevents straightening of the endoscope, making it difficult to achieve an optimal position. In addition, the papilla itself may become infiltrated with the cancer and make ERCP improbable, if not impossible.

Complications

ERCP has a greater potential for procedure-related complications than other endoscopic procedures in the upper gastrointestinal tract [25]. The complications seen with diagnostic ERCP are discussed here; those relating to sphincterotomy are described in Chapter 34.

15

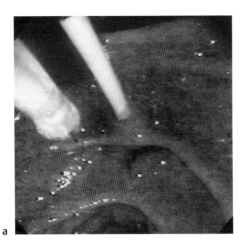

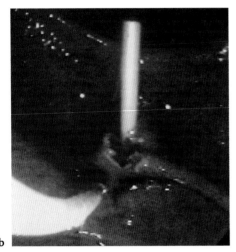

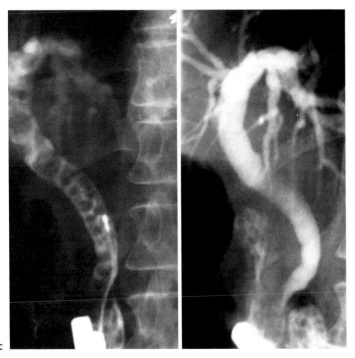

Fig. 15.11
a A view of the major papilla, with a biliary stent in place and a needle-knife catheter emerging from the tip of the duodenoscope.
b Use of the needle-knife to cut the sphincterotome over the tent in Billroth II anatomy.
c *Left:* Cholangiogram in a patient with Billroth II anatomy, showing a bile duct full of stones. *Right:* Clearance of the stones from the bile duct after sphincterotomy in Billroth II.

The complications of endoscopy include adverse effects of intravenous medications, oxygen desaturation, aspiration of gastroduodenal contents, and hemorrhage or perforation related to the traumatic passage of the endoscope.

Complications associated with manipulation of the ampulla and the pancreaticobiliary tree include pancreatitis and sepsis. A multicenter study by Loperfido et al. suggested significant differences in the morbidity and mortality rates between diagnostic and therapeutic ERCP (1.38% vs. 5.4% and 0.21% vs. 0.49%, respectively; $P < 0.0001$) [26,27]. Death is rare and is usually a result of multiple organ failure resulting from severe pancreatitis or sepsis, or from complications arising as a result of bowel perforation, as seen in Billroth II gastrojejunostomy.

▓ Pancreatitis

This is the most common complication of ERCP and is seen in 3–7% of procedures. Post-ERCP pancreatitis is defined as a clinical syndrome of abdominal pain occurring after ERCP, along with a rise in serum amylase (more than three times normal), leading to hospital admission for more than 24 h [28]. Based on the duration of the hospital stay, it is also classified into mild (<3 days), moderate (4–7 days), and severe (>7 days).

Various causative factors have been implicated in causing post-ERCP pancreatitis, including manipulative trauma to the ampulla leading to sphincter spasm and/or edema; multiple pancreatic duct injections; and high injection pressure, resulting in acinarization and hydrostatic injury [29]. The osmolality and ionic content of contrast agents has not been shown to be predictive in inducing pancreatitis [30]. Certain other factors have been predictive of increasing the risk of developing post-ERCP pancreatitis. The benefits of a large case load and extensive experience on the part of the endoscopist mean that tertiary referral centers that perform more than 200 ERCPs per endoscopist are the least likely to encounter significant problems [27]. Younger age, female sex, a previous history of pancreatitis, sphincter of Oddi dysfunction, and a normal-caliber bile duct devoid of stones are the most predictive risk factors [31–33].

A variety of agents have been investigated for their value in preventing post-ERCP pancreatitis. Trials of octreotide, somatostatin, corticosteroids, and interleukin-10 have shown conflicting results [34–40]. Other trials report that a protease inhibitor (gabexate mesylate) and an inhibitor of platelet-activating factor (lexipafant) are useful, but no definite conclusions can be drawn from these preliminary studies [41,42]. A meta-analysis included trials using octreotide, somatostatin, and gabexate and concluded that somatostatin and gabexate were significantly associated with improvements in various clinical parameters [43,44]. The clinical efficacy of these agents is still unclear. The incidence of pancreatitis tends to decrease with the introduction of protective pancreatic stents after manipulations or sphincterotomy of the pancreatic orifice. Regardless of this, we also recommend meticulous attention to careful selection of patients with the appropriate indications, and improving basic ERCP technique.

Future Directions

ERCP has evolved over the last 40 years to become the procedure of choice for the diagnosis and treatment of pancreaticobiliary disorders. Safety remains an issue of concern with this interventional procedure. Although many studies have shown that the risk of complications is significantly higher with therapeutic ERCP, the risk with a purely diagnostic procedure is not negligible and cannot be justified in the absence of appropriate indications. Recent research on newer diagnostic tools for biliary tract disease has led to challenges to the diagnostic role of ERCP. Magnetic resonance cholangiopancreatography has been shown to have efficacy comparable to that of ERCP in terms of sensitivity and specificity for choledocholithiasis, bile duct obstruction, and cystic lesions of the pancreaticobiliary tree [45–47]. In addition, MRCP is noninvasive and is safer for patients, especially when the indication for biliary tract imaging is less convincing. Endoscopic ultrasound has also been shown to have diagnostic and therapeutic capacities for biliary and pancreatic disorders. Patients requiring intervention for duct clearance, tissue sampling, and/or drainage have to be carefully selected for therapeutic ERCP or alternatives to it.

References

1. McCune WS, Shorb PE, Moscovitz H. Endoscopic cannulation of the ampulla of Vater: a preliminary report. Ann Surg 1968;167:752–6.
2. Oi I. Fiberduodenoscopy and endoscopic pancreatocholangiography. Gastrointest Endosc 1970;17:59–62.
3. Takagi K, Ikeda S, Nakagawa Y, Sakaguchi N, Takahashi T. Retrograde pancreatography and cholangiography by fiber duodenoscope. Gastroenterology 1970;59:445–52.
4. Kasugai T, Kuno N, Aoki I, Kizu M, Kobayashi S. Fiberduodenoscopy: analysis of 353 examinations. Gastrointest Endosc 1971;18:9–16.
5. Classen M. Fiberduodenoscopy of the intestines. Gut 1971;12:330–8.
6. Cotton PB, Blumgart LH, Davies GT, Pierce JW, Salmon PR, Burwood RJ, et al. Cannulation of papilla of Vater via fiber-duodenoscope: assessment of retrograde cholangiopancreatography in 60 patients. Lancet 1972;i:53–8.
7. Vennes JA, Silvis SE. Endoscopic visualization of the bile and pancreatic ducts. Gastrointest Endosc 1972;18:149–52.
8. Cotton PB. ERCP. Gut 1977;18:316–41.
9. Vennes JA. Technique of ERCP. In: Sivak MV, editor. Gastroenterologic endoscopy. Philadelphia: Saunders; 1987. p. 562–80.
10. Oi I. Technical guidance of endoscopic pancreatocholangiography. Int J Pancreatol 1991;9:1–6.
11. O'Mahony S, Lintott DJ, Axon A. Endoscopic retrograde cholangiopancreatography. Semin Laparosc Surg 1995;2:93–101.
12. Silvis SE, Meier PB. Technique for endoscopic retrograde cholangiopancreatography. In: Silvis SE, Rohrmann CA Jr, Ansel HJ, editors. Text and atlas of endoscopic retrograde cholangiopancreatography. New York: Igaku-Shoin, 1995; p. 22–50.
13. Waye JD. Basic techniques of ERCP. Gastrointest Endosc 2000;51:250–3.
14. American Society for Gastrointestinal Endoscopy. Principles of training in gastrointestinal endoscopy. Gastrointest Endosc 1992;38:743–6.
15. Jowell PS, Baillie J, Branch MS, Affronti J, Browning CL, Bute BP. Quantitative assessment of procedural competence: a prospective study of training in endoscopic retrograde cholangiopancreatography. Ann Intern Med 1996;125:983–9.
16. Kimmey MB. The ERCP room. In: Baron TH, Kozarek R, Carr-Locke DL, editors. ERCP. Philadelphia: Saunders/Elsevier; 2008. p. 13–8.
17. Kim MH, Lee SK, Lee MH, Myung SJ, Yoo BM, Seo DW, et al. Endoscopic retrograde cholangiopancreatography and needle-knife sphincterotomy in patients with Billroth II gastrectomy: a comparative study of the forward-viewing endoscope and the side-viewing duodenoscope. Endoscopy 1997;29:82–5.
18. Schwacha H, Allgaier HP, Deibert P, Olschewski M, Allgaier U, Blum HE. A sphincterotome-based technique for selective transpapillary common bile duct cannulation. Gastrointest Endosc 2000;52:387–91.
19. Schwacha H, Allgaier HP, Deibert P, Olschewski M, Allgaier U, Blum HE. A sphincterotome-based technique for selective transpapillary common bile duct cannulation. Gastrointest Endosc 2000;52:387–91.
20. Aabakken L, Holthe B, Sandstad O, Rosseland A, Osnes M. Endoscopic pancreaticobiliary procedures in patients with a Billroth II resection: a 10-year follow-up study. Ital J Gastroenterol Hepatol 1998;30:301–5.
21. Costamagna G. ERCP and endoscopic sphincterotomy in Billroth II patients: a demanding technique for experts only? Ital J Gastroenterol Hepatol 1998;30:306–9.
22. Faylona JMV, Qadir A, Chan ACW, Lau JYW, Chung SCS. Small-bowel perforations related to endoscopic retrograde cholangiopancreatography (ERCP) in patients with Billroth II gastrectomy. Endoscopy 1999;31:546–9.
23. Lin LF, Siauw CP, Ho KS, Tung JC. ERCP in post-Billroth II gastrectomy patients: emphasis on technique. Am J Gastroenterol 1999;94:144–8.
24. Siegal JH, Cohen SA, Kasmin FE. Experience and volume: the ingredients for successful therapeutic endoscopic outcomes, especially ERCP and postgastrectomy patients. Am J Gastroenterol 2000;95:133–4.
25. Aliperti G. Complications related to diagnostic and therapeutic endoscopic retrograde cholangiopancreatography. Gastrointest Endosc Clin N Am 1996;6:379–407.
26. Loperfido S, Angelini G, Benedetti G, Chilovi F, Costan F, De Berardinis F, et al. Major early complications from diagnostic and therapeutic ERCP: a prospective multicenter study. Gastrointest Endosc 1998;48:1–10.
27. Freeman ML. Toward improving outcomes of ERCP. Gastrointest Endosc 1998;48:96–102.
28. Cotton PB, Lehman G, Vennes J, Geenen JE, Russell RC, Meyers WC, et al. Endoscopic sphincterotomy complications and their management: an attempt at consensus. Gastrointest Endosc 1991;37:383–93.
29. Johnson GK, Geenen JE, Johanson JF, Sherman S, Hogan WJ, Cass O. Evaluation of post-ERCP pancreatitis: potential causes noted during controlled study of differing contrast media. Midwest Pancreaticobiliary Study Group. Gastrointest Endosc 1997;46:217–22.
30. Johnson GK, Geenen JE, Bedford RA, Johanson J, Cass O, Sherman S, et al. A comparison of nonionic versus ionic contrast media: results of a prospective, multicenter study. Midwest Pancreaticobiliary Study Group. Gastrointest Endosc 1995;42:312–6.
31. Chen YK, Abdulian JD, Escalante-Glorsky S, Youssef AI, Foliente RL, Collen MJ. Clinical outcome of post-ERCP pancreatitis: relationship to history of previous pancreatitis. Am J Gastroenterol 1995;95:2120–3.
32. Dickenson RJ, Davies S. Post-ERCP pancreatitis and hyperamylasaemia: the role of operative and patient factors. Eur J Gastroenterol Hepatol 1998;10:423–8.
33. Tarnasky P, Cunningham J, Cotton PB, Hoffman B, Palesch Y, Freeman J, et al. Pancreatic sphincter hypertension increases the risk of post-ERCP pancreatitis. Endoscopy 1997;29:252–7.
34. Sternlieb JM, Aronchick CA, Retig JN, Dabezies M, Saunders F, Goosenberg E, et al. A multicenter, randomized, controlled trial to evaluate the effect of prophylactic octreotide on ERCP-induced pancreatitis. Am J Gastroenterol 1992;87:1561–6.
35. Binmoeller KF, Harris AG, Dumas R, Grimaldi C, Delmont JP. Does the somatostatin analogue octreotide protect against ERCP induced pancreatitis? Gut 1992;33:1129–33.
36. Bordas JM, Toledo-Pimentel V, Llach J, Elena M, Mondelo F, Gines A, et al. Effects of bolus somatostatin in preventing pancreatitis after endoscopic pancreatography: results of a randomized study. Gastrointest Endosc 1998;47:230–4.
37. Poon RT, Yeung C, Lo CM, Yuen WK, Liu CL, Fan ST. Prophylactic effect of somatostatin on post-ERCP pancreatitis: a randomized controlled trial. Gastrointest Endosc 1999;49:593–8.
38. Devière J, LeMoine O, Van Laethem JL, Eisendrath P, Ghilain A, Severs N, et al. Interleukin 10 reduces the incidence of pancreatitis after therapeutic endoscopic retrograde cholangiopancreatography. Gastroenterology 2001;120:498–505.
39. De Palma GD, Catanzano C. Use of corticosteroids in the prevention of post-ERCP pancreatitis: results of a controlled prospective study. Am J Gastroenterol 1999;94:982–5.
40. Dumot JA, Conwell DL, O'Connor JB, Ferguson DR, Vargo JJ, Barnes DS, et al. Pretreatment with methylprednisolone to prevent ERCP-induced pancreatitis: a randomized, multicenter, placebo-controlled clinical trial. Am J Gastroenterol 1998;93:61–5.
41. Cavallini G, Tittobello A, Frulloni L, Masci E, Mariana A, Di Francesco V. Gabexate for the prevention of pancreatic damage related to ERCP. N Engl J Med 1996;335:919–23.
42. McKay CJ, Curran F, Sharples C, Baxter JN, Imrie CW. Prospective placebo-controlled randomized trial of lexipafant in predicted severe acute pancreatitis. Br J Surg 1997;84:1239–43.
43. Andriulli A, Leandro G, Niro G, Mangia A, Festa V, Gambassi G, et al. Pharmacological treatment can prevent pancreatic injury after ERCP: a meta-analysis. Gastrointest Endosc 2000;51:1–7.
44. Haber GB. Prevention of post-ERCP pancreatitis. Gastrointest Endosc 2000;51:100–3.
45. Varghese JC, Liddell RP, Farrell MA, Murray FE, Osborne H, Lee MJ. The diagnostic accuracy of magnetic resonance cholangiopancreatography and ultrasound compared with direct cholangiography in the detection of choledocholithiasis. Clin Radiol 1999;54:604–14.
46. Adamek HE, Albert J, Weitz M, Breer H, Schilling D, Riemann JF. A prospective evaluation of magnetic resonance cholangiopancreatography inpatients with suspected bile duct obstruction. Gut 1998;43:680–3.
47. Irie H, Honda H, Jimi M, Yokohata K, Chijiiwa K, Kuroiwa T, et al. Value of MR cholangiopancreatography in evaluating choledochal cysts. AJR Am J Roentgenol 1998;171:1381–5.

15

16 Peroral Cholangioscopy

Axel Eickhoff and Juergen F. Riemann

Introduction

Intraductal miniature endoscopes may have an increasingly important role in the diagnosis and nonsurgical treatment of biliary and pancreatic diseases. Early attempts to inspect the biliary and pancreatic ducts endoscopically were made in the mid-1970s, but were limited by technical problems with the instruments [1,2]. More recently, the development of fine-caliber flexible scopes (miniscopes), which also provide a biopsy channel, obviated many of these problems. These instruments have provided a valuable new tool for a growing number of indications.

Miniature endoscopes can be used intraoperatively during endoscopic retrograde cholangiopancreatography (ERCP) and percutaneous transhepatic cholangiography. This review focuses on peroral cholangioscopy performed during ERCP. Percutaneous transhepatic cholangioscopy and peroral pancreatoscopy are reviewed separately (see Chapter 17).

Procedure

Instruments and Technique

When performed during ERCP, intraductal endoscopy requires no additional preparation. We typically use a combination of midazolam hydrochloride plus propofol for intensive sedation, plus butylscopolamine to diminish intestinal motility (glucagon in the United States). Antibiotic prophylaxis is also recommended for patients undergoing intraductal endoscopy, to reduce the risk of bacterial cholangitis [3].

Peroral cholangioscopy is usually performed by two experienced endoscopists using a "mother–baby" scope system, in which a thin fiberscope is inserted into the channel of a large therapeutic duodenoscope [4]. Flexible miniscopes have significantly improved and are now smaller and more durable, featuring an accessory channel and providing better-quality images [5,6]. Traditionally, optical imaging in choledochoscopes was achieved using fiberglass technology (**Fig. 16.1**). Newer scopes combine fiberglass with charge-

coupled device (CCD) technology in a hybrid fashion, and recently purely CCD-based scopes have provided optical enhancement technologies such as narrow-band imaging (NBI) in the bile duct [7].

The current generation of miniscopes have an outer diameter of 2.0–3.5 mm and can be inserted through a normal therapeutic duodenoscope into the bile duct after endoscopic sphincterotomy. The biopsy channel of the miniscopes permits sampling for histological and cytological examination and the insertion of catheters for dye or probes for laser lithotripsy or electrohydraulic lithotripsy. Cholangioscopes can also be used for pancreatoscopy. New instruments that do not require a sphincterotomy are being evaluated and may be commercially available soon.

Choledochoscopy and pancreatoscopy are technically successful in the majority of patients. However, a number of anatomic features may restrict access to the biliary or pancreatic ducts, such as ductal or luminal strictures, previous gastric or bile duct surgery, high-grade stenosis due to proximal bile duct carcinoma (Klatskin tumor), and pancreas divisum. In one series, the procedure was not feasible for these technical reasons in 15 of 240 patients (6%) [5].

New Intraductal Endoscopy Techniques

The peroral cholangioscopic approach requires feeding a small-caliber (about 3 mm) scope (the "baby" scope) through the channel of a duodenoscope (the "mother" scope) and then advancing it into the common bile duct. Overall, this procedure continues to be expensive, time-consuming, cumbersome, and as mentioned above usually requires at least two experienced endoscopists, one to guide the duodenoscope and the other to guide the baby scope. The lack of separate water and air channels compromises visibility and requires the assembly of a cumbersome water irrigation system, adding time and effort to the procedure. Additional limitations include the extreme fragility of the baby scope (resulting in short durability and high repair costs) and the small caliber of the working channel (ranging from 0.5 mm to 1.2 mm), only allowing the use of small biopsy forceps capable of obtaining very small and often inadequate tissue samples. Because of these drawbacks and the small range of suitable indications, the popularity of peroral cholangioscopy has remained limited over the last decade. However, crucial technical improvements have been developed during the last few years.

These new devices are being developed and tested. In one report, it was possible to introduce a miniscope with an external diameter of 2.09 mm through a normal papilla of Vater in 97% of patients without the need for a sphincterotomy [8]. Another instrument (PolyDiagnost; **Fig. 16.2**) has an outer diameter of 2.3 mm, with a biopsy channel that is a little wider than the one previously mentioned [9]. In one report using this instrument, five of 11 patients did not require sphincterotomy and only one endoscopist was needed to perform the examination [9].

Ultrathin endoscopes for cholangioscopy and pancreatoscopy (external diameter 0.5–0.8 mm) can be inserted through a standard duodenoscope. However, they are not equipped with a biopsy channel and the tip cannot be angulated [5]. A peroral electronic pancreatoscope (with an external diameter of 2.1 mm), which can also be used as a choledochoscope, has been developed and provides an

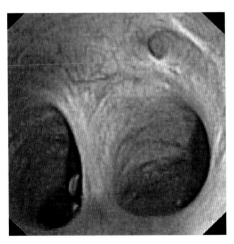

Fig. 16.1 A cholangioscopic view of normal intrahepatic bile ducts.

excellent optical resolution of 0.07 mm, compared with 0.2 mm with the standard fiberoptic pancreatoscope [10].

At present, optimal visualization of the bile duct lumen, allowing direct interventions through an adequate working channel, is still a dream. However, recent advances in endoscopic technology have expanded the horizons of both diagnostic and interventional biliary endoscopy. In individual cases, performing endoscopic direct cholangioscopy with an ultraslim upper endoscope originally designed for pediatric patients and transnasal applications appears to be feasible (**Fig. 16.3**). Larghi et al. performed ERCP and placed a 0.035-inch diameter super-stiff Jagwire in the common bile duct. The guide was left in place and the duodenoscope was replaced. They loaded an ultraslim endoscope (5.9 mm) onto the guide wire and pushed it under fluoroscopic and endoscopic control into the bile duct. This endoscopic "direct cholangioscopy" was successfully completed in three patients for diagnostic purposes [11]. Due to its larger size, the lack of stability, and the very long initial distance from the mouth to the papilla, this technique should be reserved for exceptional cases only [12].

Brand-new mini-endoscopes are now on the horizon and will probably become available in the near future. Prototypes of new "hybrid" ultrathin video choledochoscopes with integrated CCD chips can now provide accurate and brilliant images from the biliary system. This allows precise diagnosis and makes it possible to distinguish between benign and malignant lesions in the bile duct. The novel techniques of NBI and confocal laser microscopy for superficial tissue evaluation are now also available in mini-endoscopes. NBI is a new endoscopic system based on narrowing the bandwidth of the spectral transmittance of red, green, and blue optical filters. NBI makes it possible to enhance the imaging of certain features, such as mucosal structures and mucosal microvessels. Itoi and co-workers reported their initial experience with a standard peroral video choledochoscope with the newly available NBI system for the diagnosis of biliary tract diseases. Twelve patients with 21 benign and malignant lesions were evaluated. Identification of the surface structure and vessels in the lesions using NBI observation was significantly better than with conventional observation [7]. These initial results from a pilot study are promising, but larger studies are still required in order to clarify the benefit of these technologies in the biliary system (**Figs. 16.4, 16.5, 16.6, 16.7**).

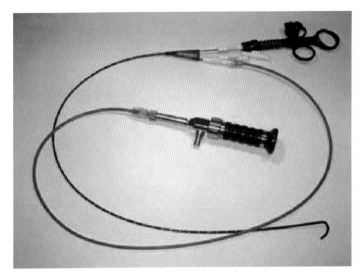

Fig. 16.2 The PolyDiagnost choledochoscope.

To overcome infectious problems, a new overtube-guided optical device has been developed. It features 6-megapixel fiberoptics with a diameter of 8 Fr and with four-way deflected steering and dedicated irrigation channels. This single-operator peroral cholangiopancreatoscopy system (SpyGlass; Boston Scientific, Natick, Massachusetts, USA) is now available and has been evaluated by Chen et al. in an initial clinical study including 35 patients (**Fig. 16.8**). The procedure was successfully performed in 91 % of the patients. For diagnosis of malignancy based on guided biopsies, the sensitivity and specificity of the system were 71 % and 100 % and thus within the range of previously published data [13]. Stone disintegration with electrohydraulic lithotripsy succeeded in five patients. The procedures were safe and well tolerated. In comparison with standard choledochoscopes and especially the new CCD and NBI scopes, optical images provided by the SpyGlass system appear to be less brilliant, as it only has 6000-pixel fiberoptics and inadequate illumination of dilated bile ducts.

16

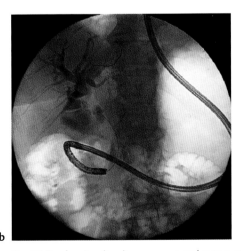

b

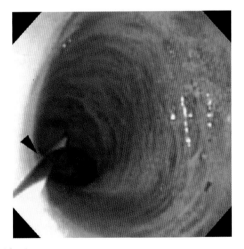

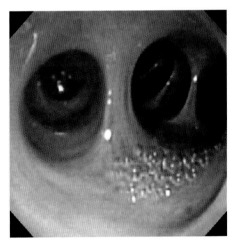

c

Fig. 16.3 a, b An ultraslim scope passed over a guidewire.
c The biliary bifurcation.

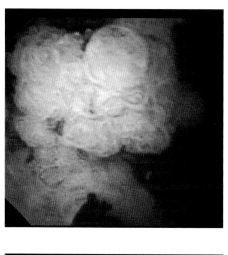

a

Fig. 16.4   Polypoid cholangiocarcinoma.
a   White-light mode.
b   Narrow-band imaging.

b

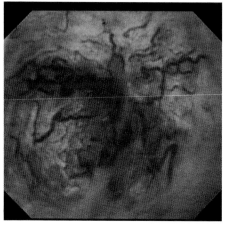

a

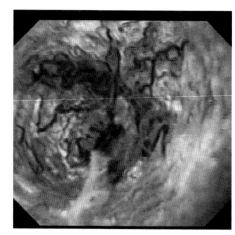

b

Fig. 16.5   Cholangiocarcinoma with a tumor vessel.
a   White-light mode.
b   Narrow-band imaging.

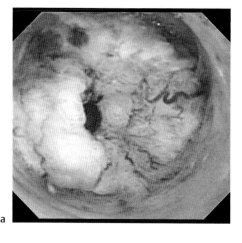

a

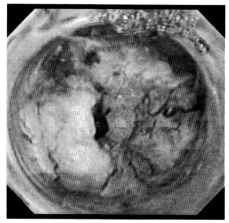

b

Fig. 16.6
a   Conventional cholangioscopy shows nodular polypoid lesion with tortuous tumor vessels.
b   NBI shows fine mucosal structure of the tumor. (Courtesy of Takao Itoi.)

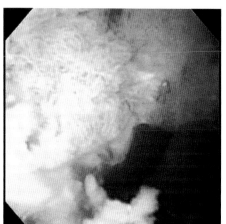

a

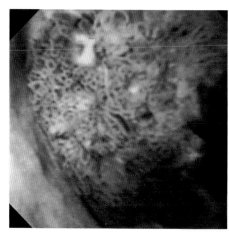

b

Fig. 16.7
a   Conventional cholangioscopy shows slightly redish tumor.
b   NBI shows fine grannular structure of surface of the tumor. (Courtesy of Takao Itoi.)

IV

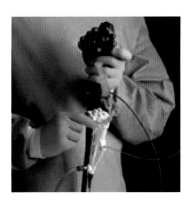

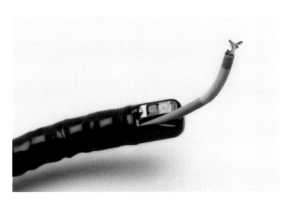

Fig. 16.8 The SpyGlass single-operator chole-dochoscope.

Complications

Risks in peroral cholangioscopy are mostly related to the ERCP procedure. In our experience with 255 patients, only three (1%) developed chills and short-term fever [3]. The rate of occult bacteremia may be higher, as illustrated in another report in which bacteremia was detected in 15 of 100 patients, six of whom developed cholangitis [14]. Endoscopic sphincterotomy of the pancreatic duct was associated with mild acute pancreatitis in two of 40 cases (5%). Two of 55 patients (4%) who underwent pancreatoscopy with the ultrathin miniscope developed mild to moderate pancreatitis. Small bile duct ulcers due to lithotripsy occurred rarely. Bile duct perforation may occur, particularly during lithotripsy, but is uncommon [15].

Clinical Applications

The role of peroral cholangioscopy is continuing to be clarified [16–18]. At present, it is only offered in a few centers worldwide, where it is most commonly used for tissue sampling of filling defects or strictures in the biliary system, and for extraction of intrahepatic stones or biliary parasites [19–21].

▦ Diagnostic Peroral Cholangioscopy

Confirmation of suspected malignant biliary lesions. Choledochoscopy can be used to obtain direct visualization and targeted tissue sampling in patients with filling defects suggestive of malignancy on standard cholangiography [3,22,23].Overall, cholangioscopy with and without biopsy yielded a sensitivity of up to 89%, a specificity of 96%, a positive predictive value of 89%, and a negative predictive value of > 95% [23]. Thus, cholangioscopy with and without biopsy appears to be highly accurate in diagnosing and excluding malignancy in patients with clinically and radiographically suspected biliary malignancy (**Table 16.1**) [13,22–25].

Despite this, however, a major limitation lies in the difficulty of confirming suspected malignant lesions. This is mainly due to the underlying biology of bile duct tumors (particularly hilar tumors), which expand in the subepithelial layers toward the intrahepatic bile ducts in such a way that malignant cells are often absent on superficial mucosal biopsies. Another problem is that the biopsy forceps cannot be opened within tight strictures. In this setting, combining brush cytology with biopsy improves the yield to approximately 50%. The benefit may be substantially greater with a transhepatic approach, which may be required in patients with hilar strictures and in whom the peroral approach produces negative results.

How can these problems be overcome? Chromoendoscopy using methylene blue is used to delineate neoplastic lesions in the gastrointestinal tract. After topical methylene blue application, characteristic surface staining patterns are seen in chronic inflammation, dysplasia, and ischemic-type biliary lesions. Nondysplastic mucosa appears homogeneously stained, whereas scarred strictures show weak uptake of methylene blue. These differences in the staining patterns can identify normal, dysplastic, and inflamed mucosa in the bile duct. Whereas homogeneous staining has been found to predict the presence of normal mucosa, absence of staining of circumscribed lesions or diffused staining of such lesions represents neoplastic changes or inflammation [24]. Chromocholedochoscopy may become very helpful in unmasking malignancy in patients with primary sclerosing cholangitis and ischemic lesions of the bile ducts (**Fig. 16.9**).

Primary sclerosing cholangitis (PSC). The role of peroral cholangioscopy in patients with PSC remains open and has yet to be clarified. Awadallah and co-workers assessed the benefit of cholangioscopy in terms of cholangioscopy-based biopsy, detection of stones not seen in cholangiography, and stone removal with cholangioscopy-directed lithotripsy. Sixty cholangioscopy procedures were performed in 41 patients. In 80% of the patients, cholangioscopy-directed biopsies were obtained. Extrahepatic cholangiocarcinoma was detected in one patient, 31 patients had negative/atypical findings, and one examination was inadequate. Stones were found in 23

16

Table 16.1 The accuracy of cholangioscopy in suspected bile duct stenosis

First author, ref.	Year	Patients (n)	Instruments	Sensitivity	Specificity
Wang [25]	2000	27	Pentax (3.1 mm)	70%	95%
Fukuda [22]	2005	97	Olympus (3.4 mm)	100%	86%
Shah [23]	2006	62		89%	96%
Authors' own data	2007	255	Olympus (3.1 mm)	68%	86%
Chen [13]	2007	35	SpyGlass (3.3 mm)	71%	100%
Hoffmann [24]	2008	24	Pentax (3.1 mm) + chromocholangioscopy	90%	

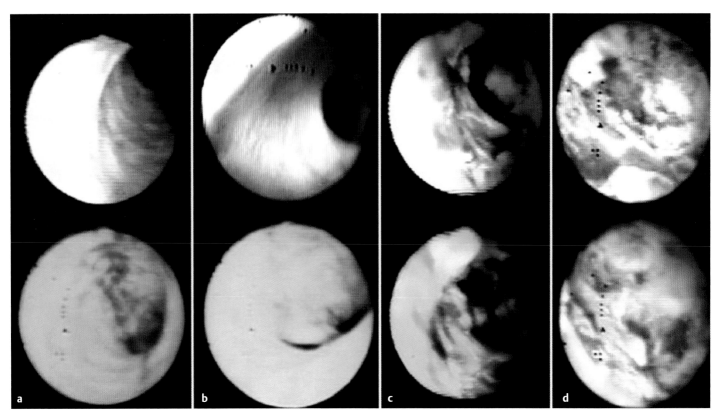

Fig. 16.9 Methylene blue chromocholedochoscopy, showing different staining patterns (courtesy of A. Hoffmann).
a Bile duct
b Scar tissue.
c Inflammation.
d Dysplastic tissue.

of the 41 (56%) patients, of which seven (30%) had been missed on cholangiography and were detected only by cholangioscopy. Nine of 23 patients (39%) underwent cholangioscopy-directed lithotripsy. Stone clearance was complete in 10 patients (seven underwent cholangioscopy-directed lithotripsy after failed conventional stone extraction), partial in seven, and was not attempted in six [26]. This study was the first series of patients with PSC who underwent cholangioscopy for evaluation of dominant strictures and cholangioscopy-directed stone therapy, showing demonstrable clinical benefits. In addition, stones detected on cholangioscopy were missed by cholangiography in nearly one in three patients. Cholangioscopy-directed lithotripsy was found to be superior to conventional ERCP for achieving complete stone clearance. Despite the use of cholangioscopy, however, the diagnosis of cholangiocarcinoma continues to be technically challenging, as cholangiocarcinoma was found to be present in the specimens from two of eight patients.

Recently, another study by a German group showed that cholangioscopy improves accuracy in differentiating indeterminate biliary strictures in PSC patients in comparison with cholangiography alone. Cholangioscopy was significantly superior to cholangiography in detecting malignancy in terms of its sensitivity (92% versus 51%), accuracy (93% versus 66%), positive predictive value (79% versus 29%), and negative predictive value (97% versus 84%) [27]. Peroral cholangioscopy thus increases the ability to distinguish between malignant and benign dominant biliary strictures in patients with PSC.

▪ Therapeutic Peroral Cholangioscopy

Bile duct stones. Peroral cholangioscopy (with intracorporeal lithotripsy) can also be used in patients with bile duct stones that are difficult to treat, including intrahepatic stones. Piraka et al. reported

their experience and the long-term follow-up with cholangioscopy-directed management of difficult bile duct stones. Peroral cholangioscopy-directed lithotripsy was performed in 32 patients with biliary stones, in whom conventional endoscopic extraction techniques had failed after a mean of 3.3 procedures. The stones were intrahepatic (n = 8), extrahepatic (n = 18), or both (n = 6). Biliary strictures were present in 20 patients. Cholangioscopy identified additional stones not seen at ERCP in nine patients (28%). A mean of 1.4 lithotripsy sessions achieved complete (81%) or partial (16%) stone clearance, or failed (3%). Follow-up was available in 88% of the patients for a mean of 29.2 months. Stones recurred in four of the 22 patients (18%) who had complete clearance and follow-up data. There were two minor periprocedural complications and one late complication [28]. Cholangioscopy-directed lithotripsy thus appears to be a safe and effective approach in patients in whom standard endoscopic stone extraction has failed. Stone recurrences in the study were found to be low in patients who had undergone complete stone clearance, except in those patients with PSC. Cholangioscopy can thus detect stones missed by cholangiography.

A number of reports have described the value of choledochoscopy with electrohydraulic and/or laser lithotripsy for removal of bile duct stones that cannot be extracted during ERCP (**Fig. 16.10**; **Table 16.2**) [15,28–34]. In one series including 65 patients, it was possible to clear the bile duct of stones after a mean of 1.2 sessions in all but one patient (in whom the cholangioscope could not be inserted into the bile duct) [15]. Bile duct perforation was observed in one patient and was managed conservatively.

Similar results were observed in another study including 125 patients, in whom combined treatment for intraductal stones was compared with surgical exploration of the common bile duct [29]. The combination of electrohydraulic lithotripsy, extracorporeal shock-wave lithotripsy, and laser lithotripsy was successful in 94% of the patients. Fragmentation rates appear to be increased using

IV

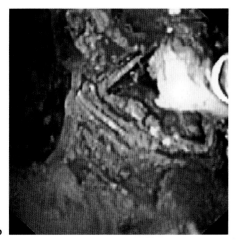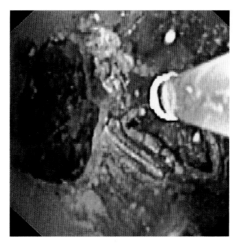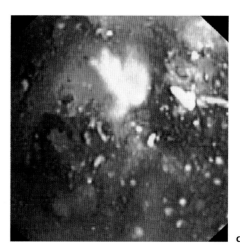

b c

Fig. 16.10 a–c Cholelithiasis: successful intraductal lithotripsy with electrohydraulic lithotripsy.

Table 16.2 Cholangioscopy-guided treatment of difficult bile duct stones using different techniques

First author, ref.	Year	Patients (n)	Technique	Success (%)	Complications (%)
Binmoeller [15]	1993	65	EHL	98%	1.5%
Adamek [29]	1996	125	EHL + laser + ESWL	94%	2%
Jakobs [30]	1997	17	Laser	91%	0%
Neuhaus [31]	1998	28	Laser	97%	0%
Farrell [32]	2005	52	EHL	100%	0%
Piraka [28]	2007	32	EHL	82%	6%
Jakobs [33]	2007	89	EHL + laser	98%	2%/

EHL, electrohydraulic lithotripsy; ESWL, extracorporeal shock-wave lithotripsy.

16

novel laser systems such as the holmium:yttrium–aluminum garnet (Ho:YAG) laser. Hazey et al. reported high rates for cracking complex and very large (> 2 cm) biliary calculi using the Ho:YAG laser system [35]. No severe complications occurred, and the 30-day mortality was zero. In one series, cholangioscopy allowed identification of stones that had not been visualized using conventional cholangioscopy in 30% of patients with primary sclerosing cholangitis [26]. Stone extraction has also been successful in patients with Mirizzi syndrome. Long-term success appears to be most likely in patients who do not have residual gallbladder stones [36]. Intrahepatic stones can be removed completely in up to 60% of patients [37]. Long-term follow-up of such patients suggests that stone clearance may be durable.

Conclusions

Peroral cholangioscopy with duodenoscopic assistance can allow direct visualization of the bile duct. Several large-scale clinical studies have suggested that peroral cholangioscopy is valuable in the management of various bile duct lesions. Direct visual observation is a useful adjunct to ERCP for distinguishing between malignant and benign bile duct lesions. The diagnostic accuracy of new optical imaging modalities such as NBI and chromocholedochoscopy needs to be further assessed in controlled clinical studies. Intracorporeal lithotripsy using a peroral cholangioscope appears to be a safe and effective method for bile duct stones that are difficult to treat, including intrahepatic stones. Preliminary data obtained with the new peroral video choledochoscopes, which provide excellent-quality images, are encouraging. This video scope is also expected to provide longer durability of the optical images and better manipulation than previous fiberscopes.

References

1. Roesch W, Koch H, Demling L. Peroral cholangioscopy. Endoscopy 1976;8:172–6.
2. Kawai K, Nakajima M, Akasaka Y, Shimamotu K, Murakami K. [A new endoscopic method: the peroral choledocho-pancreatoscopy (author's translation)]. Leber Magen Darm 1976;6:121–4. German.
3. Riemann JF. Transpapilläre Endoskopie (Cholangioskopie, Pankreatikoskopie). In: Fruehmorgen P, editor. Gastroenterologische Endoskopie. Berlin: Springer; 1999. p.151.
4. Bogardus ST, Hanan I, Ruchim M, Goldberg MJ. "Mother–baby" biliary endoscopy: the University of Chicago experience. Am J Gastroenterol 1996;91:105–10.
5. Riemann JF, Kohler B. Endoscopy of the pancreatic duct: value of different endoscope types. Gastrointest Endosc 1993;39:367–70.
6. Kodama T, Tatsumi Y, Sato H, Imamura Y, Koshitani T, Abe M, et al. Initial experience with a new peroral electronic pancreatoscope with an accessory channel. Gastrointest Endosc 2004;59:895–900.
7. Itoi T, Sofuni A, Itokawa F, Tsuchiya T, Kurihara T, Ishii K, et al. Peroral cholangioscopic diagnosis of biliary-tract diseases by using narrow-band imaging. Gastrointest Endosc 2007;66:730–6.
8. Soda K, Shitou K, Yoshida Y, Yamanaka T, Kashii A, Miyata M. Peroral cholangioscopy using new fine-caliber flexible scope for detailed examination without papillotomy. Gastrointest Endosc 1996;43:233–8.
9. Sander R, Poesl H. Initial experience with a new babyscope for endoscopic retrograde cholangiopancreaticoscopy. Gastrointest Endosc 1996;44:191–4.
10. Kodama T, Sato H, Horii Y, Tatsumi Y, Uehira H, Imamura Y, et al. Pancreatoscopy for the next generation: development of the peroral electronic pancreatoscope system. Gastrointest Endosc 1999;49:366–71.
11. Larghi A, Waxman I. Endoscopic direct cholangioscopy by using an ultraslim upper endoscope: a feasibility study. Gastrointest Endosc 2006;63:853–7.
12. Mori A, Sakai K, Ohashi N, Maruyama T, Tatebe H, Shibuya T, et al. Electrohydraulic lithotripsy of the common bile duct stone under transnasal direct cholangioscopy. Endoscopy 2008;40(Suppl 2):E63.

13. Chen YK, Pleskow DK. SpyGlass single-operator peroral cholangiopancreatoscopy system for the diagnosis and therapy of bile-duct disorders: a clinical feasibility study. Gastrointest Endosc 2007;65:832–41.

14. Chen MF, Jan YY. Bacteremia following postoperative choledochofiberoscopy—a prospective study. Hepatogastroenterology 1996;43:586–9.

15. Binmoeller KF, Brückner M, Thonke F, Soehendra N. Treatment of difficult bile duct stones using mechanical, electrohydraulic and extracorporeal shock wave lithotripsy. Endoscopy 1993;25:201–6.

16. Lew RJ, Kochman ML. Video cholangioscopy with a new choledochoscope: a case report. Gastrointest Endosc 2003;57:804–7.

17. Jung M, Zipf A, Schoonbroodt D, Herrmann G, Caspary WF. Is pancreatoscopy of any benefit in clarifying the diagnosis of pancreatic duct lesions? Endoscopy 1998;30:273–80.

18. Siddique I, Galati J, Ankoma-Sey V, Wood RP, Ozaki C, Monsour H, et al. The role of choledochoscopy in the diagnosis and management of biliary tract diseases. Gastrointest Endosc 1999;50:67–73.

19. Kohler B, Köhler G, Riemann JF. Pancreoscopic diagnosis of intraductal cystadenoma of the pancreas. Dig Dis Sci 1990;35:382–4.

20. Riemann JF, Kohler B, Weber J. [Differential indications for peroral pancreaticoscopy]. Z Gastroenterol 1991;29:134–6. German.

21. Leung JW, Yu AS. Hepatolithiasis and biliary parasites. Baillière's Clin Gastroenterol 1997;11:681–706.

22. Fukuda Y, Tsuyuguchi T, Sakai Y, Tsuchiya S, Saisyo H. Diagnostic utility of peroral cholangioscopy for various bile-duct lesions. Gastrointest Endosc 2005;62:374–82.

23. Shah RJ, Langer DA, Antillon MR, Chen YK. Cholangioscopy and cholangioscopic forceps biopsy in patients with indeterminate pancreaticobiliary pathology. Clin Gastroenterol Hepatol 2006;4:219–25.

24. Hoffman A, Kiesslich R, Bittinger F, Galle PR, Neurath MF. Methylene blue-aided cholangioscopy in patients with biliary strictures: feasibility and outcome analysis. Endoscopy 2008;40:563–71.

25. Wang HP, Chen JH, Wu MS, Wang HH, Chou AL. Application of peroral cholangioscopy in an endemic area with high prevalence of hepatocellular carcinoma and choledocholithiasis. Hepatogastroenterology 2000;47:1555–9.

26. Awadallah NS, Chen YK, Piraka C, Antillon MR, Shah RJ. Is there a role for cholangioscopy in patients with primary sclerosing cholangitis? Am J Gastroenterol 2006;101:284–91.

27. Tischendorf JJ, Krüger M, Trautwein C, Duckstein N, Schneider A, Manns MP, et al. Cholangioscopic characterization of dominant bile duct stenoses in patients with primary sclerosing cholangitis. Endoscopy 2006;38:665–9.

28. Piraka C, Shah RJ, Awadallah NS, Langer DA, Chen YK. Transpapillary cholangioscopy-directed lithotripsy in patients with difficult bile duct stones. Clin Gastroenterol Hepatol 2007;5:1333–8.

29. Adamek HE, Maier M, Jakobs R, Wessbecher FR, Neuhauser T, Riemann JF. Management of retained bile duct stones: a prospective open trial comparing extracorporeal and intracorporeal lithotripsy. Gastrointest Endosc 1996;44:40–7.

30. Jakobs R, Adamek HE, Maier M, Krömer M, Benz C, Martin WR, et al. Fluoroscopically guided laser lithotripsy versus extracorporeal shock wave lithotripsy for retained bile duct stones: a prospective randomised study. Gut 1997;40:678–82.

31. Neuhaus H, Zillinger C, Born P, Ott R, Allescher H, Rösch T, et al. Randomized study of intracorporeal laser lithotripsy versus extracorporeal shock-wave lithotripsy for difficult bile duct stones. Gastrointest Endosc 1998;47:327–34.

32. Farrell JJ, Bounds BC, Al-Shalabi S, Jacobson BC, Brugge WR, Schapiro RH, et al. Single-operator duodenoscope-assisted cholangioscopy is an effective alternative in the management of choledocholithiasis not removed by conventional methods, including mechanical lithotripsy. Endoscopy 2005;37:542–7.

33. Jakobs R, Pereira-Lima JC, Schuch AW, Pereira-Lima LF, Eickhoff A, Riemann JF. Endoscopic laser lithotripsy for complicated bile duct stones: is cholangioscopic guidance necessary? Arq Gastroenterol 2007;44:137–40.

34. Hixson LJ, Fennerty MB, Jaffee PE, Pulju JH, Palley SL. Peroral cholangioscopy with intracorporeal electrohydraulic lithotripsy for choledocholithiasis. Am J Gastroenterol 1992;87:296–9.

35. Hazey JW, McCreary M, Guy G, Melvin WS. Efficacy of percutaneous treatment of biliary tract calculi using the holmium:YAG laser. Surg Endosc 2007;21:1180–3.

36. Tsuyuguchi T, Saisho H, Ishihara T, Yamaguchi T, Onuma EK. Long-term follow-up after treatment of Mirizzi syndrome by peroral cholangioscopy. Gastrointest Endosc 2000;52:639–44.

37. Okugawa T, Tsuyuguchi T, Ando T, Ishihara T, Yamaguchi T, Yugi H, et al. Peroral cholangioscopic treatment of hepatolithiasis: long-term results. Gastrointest Endosc 2002;56:366–71.

IV

17 Percutaneous Transhepatic Cholangiography and Cholangioscopy

Jean-Pierre Charton, Chan-Sup Shim, and Horst Neuhaus

Introduction

Percutaneous transhepatic cholangiography (PTC) is indicated when noninvasive modalities or endoscopic retrograde cholangiography (ERC) are inconclusive. In patients with biliary obstruction, PTC is usually followed by percutaneous transhepatic cholangiographic drainage (PTCD) to achieve decompression of the biliary tree and to reduce the risk of cholangitis. The percutaneous approach is more invasive and time-consuming than ERC and should be restricted to patients in whom transpapillary procedures have failed—mainly due to difficult anatomy or large, impacted, or intrahepatic concrements. After establishment of PTCD, cholangioscopes can be inserted through the cutaneobiliary fistula to allow percutaneous transhepatic cholangioscopy (PTCS), particularly for target biopsies or intracorporeal lithotripsy of difficult bile duct stones. PTCD and PTCS can be combined with cholangioplasty, biliary stent placement, or photodynamic therapy (PDT).

Indications

Percutaneous procedures are considered when transpapillary procedures fail because of:
- Inaccessibility of the papilla of Vater due to previous surgery (Billroth II resection or Roux-en-Y anastomosis with a long afferent loop) or a difficult duodenal diverticulum
- Inaccessibility of a biliodigestive anastomosis—e.g., hepaticojejunostomy
- Bile duct strictures that cannot be passed or adequately dilated
- Unsuccessful lithotripsy of giant, impacted, or inaccessible stones

Detailed indications for various percutaneous transhepatic procedures are listed in **Table 17.1** [1].

Contraindications

Percutaneous procedures are contraindicated in patients with coagulopathy (prothrombin time < 50%, platelet count < 50×10^9/L). The risk of bleeding is high in patients with vascular tumors, arteriovenous malformations, and advanced liver cirrhosis. Ascites prevents establishment of a mature cutaneobiliary tract; in this case, the use of sheaths is required. Transhepatic interventions should not be performed in uncooperative or restless patients, as there is an increased risk of complications. A history of allergic reactions to iodinated contrast medium requires prophylactic treatment with corticosteroids and antihistamines.

Equipment

Accessories are listed in **Table 17.2** [2].

Table 17.1 Indications for percutaneous transhepatic procedures

Percutaneous transhepatic cholangiography (PTC)
- Differential diagnosis of ductal obstruction when less invasive methods are inconclusive
- Delineation of congenital abnormalities
- Detection of communication between a hepatic abscess and the biliary tract
- Visualization of ductal anatomy before PTCD

Percutaneous transhepatic cholangiographic drainage (PTCD)
- Palliation of malignant biliary obstruction
- Treatment of cholangitis
- Diversion of bile for treatment of biliary leakage
- Access for cholangioplasty, cholangioscopy, stent placement or photodynamic therapy

Cholangioplasty
- Dilation of benign and malignant biliary strictures with or without stent placement

Biliary stent placement
- Internal biliary drainage of malignant bile duct obstruction
- Temporary drainage after cholangioplasty of benign biliary strictures
- Permanent drainage of benign biliary strictures in selected cases—e.g., patients at high surgical risk

Diagnostic percutaneous transhepatic cholangioscopy (PTCS)
- Differentiation of undetermined bile duct lesions
- Biopsy under direct visual control
- Delineation of intraductal tumor spread

Therapeutic PTCS
- Treatment of extrahepatic or intrahepatic bile duct stones not amenable to endoscopic retrograde cholangiopancreatography (ERCP)
- Target cannulation of difficult bile duct strictures not amenable to radiographic techniques

Photodynamic therapy (PDT)
- Treatment of nonresectable cholangiocarcinoma

Table 17.2 Accessories for establishment of a transhepatic tract

Needles
- Chiba needle (diameter 0.6–0.7 mm, length 90–400 mm)
- Uni-Dwell needle with a Teflon sheath (outer diameter 1.0–1.3 mm; accepts 0.035-inch guide wire)

Guide wires
- Hydrophilic guide wires with straight or J-shaped tip
- Flexible and stiff kink-resistant torque guide wires with straight or J-shaped tip (outer diameter 0.035 inches, length 145–220 cm)

Catheters
- Vessel bougies (outer diameter 7, 8, 9, 10 or 12 Fr)
- Pigtail drainage catheters (diameter 7, 8.5, or 10 Fr; 16 or 32 side holes)
- Nimura-type bougies (outer diameter 10, 12, 14, 16 or 18 Fr)
- Yamakawa transhepatic tubes (diameter 10, 12, 14, 16 or 18 Fr) [2]

Stents
- Plastic endoprostheses (diameter 10–14 Fr)
- Self-expanding metal stents (outer diameter 8 or 10 mm), made of stainless steel (Gianturco–Rösch, Palmaz, Wallstent, Spiral-Z) or nitinol (ZA stent, Shim–Hanaro stent)

17

Table 17.3 Cholangioscopes for the percutaneous transhepatic approach

	Diameter of the distal end	Diameter of the channel	Tip bending up/ down	Field of view
Olympus				
CHF-160	5.2 mm	2.0 mm	180°/130°	120°
CHF-P160	4.9 mm	2.0 mm	180°/130°	120°
Pentax				
FCN-15X	4.8 mm	2.2 mm	180°/130°	125°
Polydiagnost				
PTC Scope	2.65 mm	1.2 mm	180° (one-sided)	70°

Cholangioscopes

Cholangioscopes of different companies are commercially available (**Table 17.3**). A cholangioscope with an outer diameter of 4.9 mm requires a transhepatic tract of at least 16 Fr. Ultraslim endoscopes can be inserted through smaller fistulas and are more flexible, making it easier to approach biliary side branches [3]. Most of the instruments have a two-way angulation system that allows easy maneuvering, particularly due to the short length of the insertion tube. The optical performance is excellent, with a clear image of the biliary tree that can be transmitted to a video display. The working channel of ultraslim instruments, of course, has a smaller diameter, and irrigation of the biliary tree is therefore less effective than with large-bore choledochofiberscopes, particularly after the insertion of lithotripsy probes.

Lithotriptors

Electrohydraulic lithotripsy. The electrohydraulic lithotripsy (EHL) system includes a shock-wave generator and probes with a minimum diameter of 0.8 mm for transmitting energy to the surface of the stone. A spark discharge from a bipolar coaxial electrode at the tip of the probe produces shock waves in a fluid medium. Absorption of the energy within the stone leads to a build-up of pressure gradients, subsequently causing stone fragmentation [4]. The frequency and intensity of shock-wave generation can be adjusted according to the size and composition of the stones. Although EHL probes with built-in balloon catheters are available, enabling the instrument to be positioned in the central axis of the bile duct, cholangioscopic control of shock-wave application is strongly recommended, since perforation or bleeding can occur when the ductal wall comes into direct contact with the probe [5–7].

Laser lithotripsy. Among laser systems in clinical application for biliary lithotripsy, a pulsed laser system is one of the most often used. The laser energy is transmitted via a flexible quartz fiber that is positioned directly on a biliary concrement. Pulses with a duration of approximately 1 μs can be applied at a repetition rate of 1–10 Hz, with an energy output of up to 150 mJ. A fluid medium is required to initiate a laser plasma leading to stone fragmentation. Although conventional laser lithotripsy is probably safer than EHL, direct visual control is recommended, since perforation of the bile duct can occur when the energy is applied to the ductal wall.

Intracorporeal cholangioscopic lithotripsy can alternatively be performed using a laser with an automatic stone-recognition system. This technique allows lithotripsy even when there is limited visual control or during fluoroscopy [8]. The system automatically cuts out in case of tissue contact, to exclude tissue damage. Unfortunately, this system is no longer manufactured.

Patient Preparation

Medical history, physical examination, and laboratory tests (particularly coagulation status) are required before initiation of transhepatic procedures. Abdominal ultrasound and/or magnetic resonance cholangiography (MRC) should be done to delineate the biliary tree and detect any anatomical variations, as well as intrahepatic masses. The patient must be informed of the planned interventions (standardized informed consent) at least 1 day before the procedure. In addition, the risks, duration of the procedures, and alternatives to the planned procedures must be explained. The patient should not ingest any solids or liquids for at least 6 h before PTC, to minimize the risk of aspiration. Sedatives and analgetics are administered intravenously, while general anesthesia is rarely required. Continuous monitoring of pulse oximetry, blood pressure, level of consciousness, and electrocardiographic monitoring are obligatory. Resuscitation equipment must be available. Sterilization of cholangioscopes by autoclaving is required in order to reduce the risk of cholangitis. Antibiotic prophylaxis (e.g., mezlocillin and metronidazole, or ciprofloxacin) should be given before and at least 48 hours after PTC.

Procedures

Percutaneous Transhepatic Cholangiography

Transabdominal ultrasound and/or MRC findings guide the site of the transhepatic approach. The right-lateral puncture site is selected in the midaxillary line, midway between the costophrenic angle and the lower margin of the liver—usually caudal to the tenth rib, to avoid the pleural space. After local anesthesia, a Chiba needle is inserted under fluoroscopic guidance toward the hilum of the liver, the position of which is estimated by observing the dome of the liver and the air in the duodenal bulb. The needle is directed in a plane parallel to the table top. Guidance with transabdominal ultrasound can be helpful in difficult cases, especially if the biliary tract is not dilated or when a left-sided/epigastric approach is required. After removal of the stylet, contrast medium is injected through the Chiba needle in small boluses to avoid paravascular effects. The needle is slowly withdrawn until contrast flow into the biliary system has been obtained. If puncture fails, the procedure has to be repeated by inserting the needle in a slightly different position. After successful puncture of the biliary tract, bile can be aspirated and examined for Gram staining, culture, and sensitivity tests. Further injection of contrast medium provides a complete cholangiogram (**Figs. 17.1, 17.2 a**). Distension of the biliary tree should be avoided, to reduce the risk of bacteremia. Tilting the table allows contrast to flow to distal parts of the common bile duct. Radiographs should be obtained at several oblique angles.

Percutaneous Transhepatic Cholangiographic Drainage

After PTC, the Chiba needle is left in place so that contrast medium can be reinjected if necessary. Next, a Uni-Dwell needle is inserted close to the puncture site of the Chiba needle into a selected biliary segment that allows easy transhepatic access and dilation procedures without sharp angulation. Puncture of the central part of the biliary tree should be avoided, due to the proximity of large vessels. After removal of the mandrel of the needle, a hydrophilic guide wire can be passed through the sheath into the biliary tree. These highly flexible guide wires usually can be manipulated even through angulated or tight strictures into the distal part of the common bile

IV

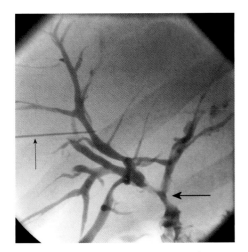
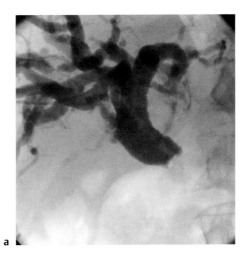
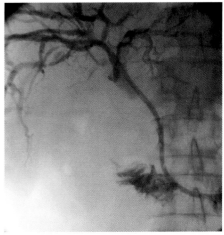

Fig. 17.1 A normal percutaneous transhepatic cholangiogram (right-sided puncture, small arrow) in a patient with a hepatobiliary anastomosis (large arrow).

Fig. 17.2
a Percutaneous transhepatic cholangiogram (right-sided puncture) in a 75-year-old patient with jaundice and stenosis of the common bile duct due to metastasis from a colorectal carcinoma.
b The same patient after transhepatic drainage and implantation of a Yamakawa-type prosthesis.

duct or through the papilla or a biliodigestive anastomosis. The hydrophilic wire is exchanged subsequently for a stiffer wire, and the transhepatic tract is sequentially widened with vessel bougies up to a diameter of 8–10 Fr. If a malignant stenosis is suspected during PTC, endobiliary brush cytology can be performed with high sensitivity [9].

The first session of percutaneous treatment is completed by placing a pigtail catheter for temporary extrahepatic drainage. On the following day, the catheter is capped to allow internal drainage only. If a guide wire cannot be passed through a biliary stenosis, a catheter is placed above the obstruction for external biliary drainage for 2–3 days. After decompression, the stenosis can usually be crossed, and an internal–external catheter is placed.

A mature large-bore cutaneobiliary fistula (sinus tract) is established for PTCS or placement of transhepatic tubes to provide long-term internal biliary drainage. For this purpose, the transhepatic tract is dilated every second day in one to three sessions by placing Nimura-type bougie catheters with inserted side holes or pigtail catheters with progressively increasing diameters [10]. This gradual sinus-tract technique is safer than performing dilation and cholangioscopy as a single-step procedure [5]. Yamakawa-type transhepatic tubes provide a flat stopcock at skin level and can be left in place for internal biliary drainage between treatment sessions (**Fig. 17.2 b**).

In some patients, peroral access can be achieved using a combined endoscopic and transhepatic procedure (rendezvous maneuver) [11,12]. A guide wire is inserted transhepatically and can be grasped endoscopically with a basket catheter or a snare. The endoscope is then advanced to the papilla or a biliodigestive anastomosis by applying traction to the percutaneous wire. Subsequently, an endoscopic approach to the biliary tract is achieved, and usually no further percutaneous interventions are required. Problems may arise when the endoscope slips back during further maneuvers and the combined procedure has to be repeated.

▥ Percutaneous Transhepatic Cholangioplasty, Biliary Stent Placement, and Photodynamic Therapy

A variety of balloon catheters are available for dilating benign and malignant biliary stenoses. The catheters are inserted over transhepatic guide wires and provide radiopaque markers for precise positioning. The balloon size should be approximately 30% larger

than the obstructed duct, and the balloon is gradually inflated (**Fig. 17.3**). After dilation, a temporary drainage catheter is placed to prevent early recurrent obstruction by edema or blood clots, if there is no indication for placement of a permanent biliary stent.

Stents provide biliary drainage without an external catheter and thus improve the patient's quality of life. The disadvantage of stents is the risk of obstruction, which may require difficult repeat interventions. Stents are most useful in patients with a limited life expectancy of less than a year. Various types of plastic and metal stent are in clinical use. Plastic endoprostheses require 12–14-Fr sheaths for placement, while metal stents can be introduced with 7–8-Fr delivery catheters. Some metal stents are released by a self-expansion mechanism and some are dilated with a delivery angioplasty balloon catheter. Plastic endoprostheses usually have to be replaced after 3 months due to blockage by sludge and debris. In contrast to plastic endoprostheses, there is no need to remove metal stents, so that the risk of additional transhepatic procedures is reduced.

If biliary obstruction extends into the hilum, isolating the right and left ducts, drainage of a single system usually provides adequate palliation in patients with symptomatic jaundice. Bilateral drainage is necessary when patients develop contralateral cholangitis, or if jaundice fails to resolve after unilateral decompression (**Fig. 17.4**). Bilateral drainage is most commonly accomplished by carrying out separate transhepatic punctures and inserting the stents in a parallel fashion. Decompression of isolated ducts through a single transhepatic access is technically demanding, but it is preferable to the dual-access approach, as it has a lower morbidity rate and is better tolerated by patients. Several techniques have been described for draining the contralateral biliary tree via an ipsilateral transhepatic access [13–16].

Recently, photodynamic therapy has been shown to be effective in nonresectable cholangiocarcinoma [17,18]. Intraluminal photoactivation can be carried out endoscopically or percutaneously after administration of a sensitizer such as porfimer sodium (Photofrin).

Percutaneous cholangioscopy–guided PDT can provide effective, homogeneous irradiation of the targeted lesion with the possibility of direct visual control. Nevertheless, the use of percutaneous PDT in treating bile duct cancer also poses some difficulties. The most important problem is that the percutaneous transhepatic biliary drainage (PTCD) tube is left permanently in place in order to maintain patency of the PTCD tract for repeated examination and retreatment; this can cause poor patient compliance due to bile drainage during the follow-up period (**Fig. 17.5**).

17

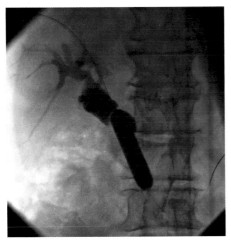

Fig. 17.3 Percutaneous balloon dilation of a benign stenosis of the common bile duct.

■ Percutaneous Transhepatic Cholangioscopy

PTCS is usually performed according to the techniques initially described by Nimura et al. [19]. Cholangioscopy can be carried out without using sheaths at the earliest 7–8 days after the initial PTCD through a 10–18-Fr sinus tract, depending on the outer diameter of the cholangioscope (**Table 17.3**). Contrast medium is injected directly through the cutaneous stoma to confirm that the fistula has matured without any leakage. A cholangioscope is inserted alongside a guide wire under visual control into the biliary system. Alternatively, a single-step approach can be used. For this technique, a thin endoscope is inserted through a sheath in a single session to minimize dilation and to avoid bile leakage.

Effective irrigation of the biliary tree is achieved by infusing saline through the instrumentation channel. Of course, large quantities of saline solution involve a risk for cardiovascular problems. Aspiration can be avoided by placing a nasogastric tube.

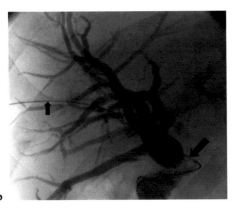
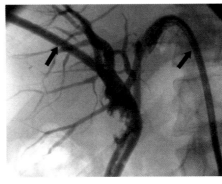

a, b

Fig. 17.4
a Percutaneous transhepatic cholangiogram (right-sided puncture, small arrow) of a 35-year-old patient with an R2-resected neuroendocrine carcinoma of the gallbladder (biliodigestive anastomosis). There is intrahepatic cholestasis due to a stenosis of the anastomosis, which has already been passed with a guide wire (large arrow). There is no communication between the two hepatic ducts (Bismuth type II stenosis), so that the left liver lobe has to be drained separately via an epigastric percutaneous approach.
b Internal biliary drainage by means of transhepatic Yamakawa-type prostheses from the left and from the right sides (arrows).

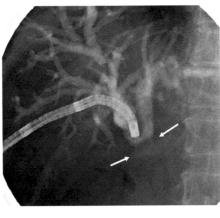
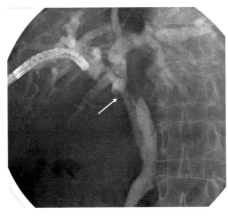

a

b

Fig. 17.5 Advanced bile duct adenocarcinoma.
a Percutaneous cholangioscopy, showing complete luminal obstruction of the common hepatic duct (arrow) before treatment.
b Four months after photodynamic therapy (PDT), complete recanalization of the common hepatic duct (arrow) is visible on percutaneous cholangioscopy.
c Cholangioscopy showed almost complete luminal obstruction of the bifurcation before PDT.
d At 4 months after PDT, cholangioscopy showed the recanalized bile duct.

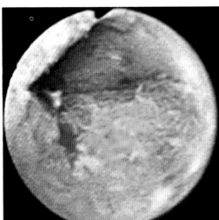
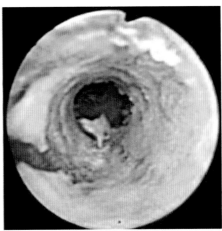

c

d

IV

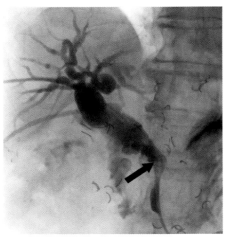
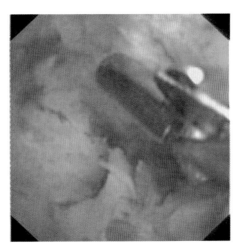
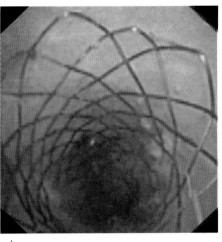

b

c

Fig. 17.6
a Percutaneous transhepatic cholangiogram of a 73-year-old patient with cholestasis and suspected benign stenosis of the common bile duct (arrow) after pancreatitis and with a history of gastrectomy due to gastric carcinoma (multiple intra-abdominal clips are visible).

b Percutaneous cholangioscopic image of the stenosis. Cholangioscopy-guided biopsies confirmed the benign origin of the stenosis.
c As the patient was at high surgical risk and refused placement of a percutaneous transhepatic tube, a metal stent was implanted. The figure shows the proximal end of the stent in the common bile duct.

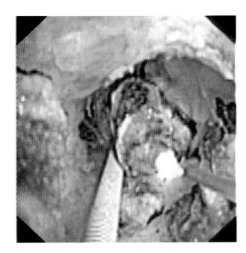

Fig. 17.7 Percutaneous cholangioscopic image of intrahepatic stones. Cholangioscopy-guided fragmentation of the stones is being carried out using laser lithotripsy. The wall of the bile duct shows chronic inflammatory changes.

PTCS miniscopes are suitable for brush cytology, biopsy (**Fig. 17.6**), laser (**Fig. 17.7**), electrocoagulation, and stone extraction with baskets. Difficult strictures not amenable to radiographic techniques can usually be cannulated under direct visual control with hydrophilic guide wires inserted through the instrumentation channel of the endoscope. Then the endoscope is removed, leaving the guide wire in place for subsequent dilation maneuvers and stent insertion (**Fig. 17.8**). Large-bore cholangioscopes are useful for biopsy studies, but they are less flexible than thinner devices. In addition, bougienage or dilation of the papilla can be performed, and in some cases transhepatic sphincterotomy is necessary (**Fig. 17.9**) [20–22]. The sinus tract can be preserved by leaving Yamakawa-type transhepatic tubes in place.

Percutaneous Stone Removal

Bile duct stones can be approached through a cutaneobiliary fistula using baskets or balloon catheters [21–24]. Unless the sinus tract was created at least 3 weeks before the procedure, percutaneous extraction of sharp stone fragments should be performed through

sheaths, as disruption of the fistula may otherwise occur. A safe, rapid, and effective alternative is prograde cholangioscopic removal of concrements through the papilla or a biliodigestive anastomosis, preferably after lithotripsy (**Fig. 17.9**) [5–7,25,26]. Intrahepatic stones in particular can often only be approached transhepatically. Forceful flushing through the instrumentation channel usually causes migration of the concrements into central parts of the biliary tree. Large and impacted stones can either be disintegrated using extracorporeal shock-wave lithotripsy (ESWL) before the endoscopic procedure, or with intracorporeal laser lithotripsy. The latter procedure is more promising and faster, due to the ease of the cholangioscopic approach and the option of complete bile duct clearance within a single session after the percutaneous tract has been established [26]. For this purpose, the tip of the EHL probe or the laser fiber is positioned on the surface of the stone (**Fig. 17.9**). Continuous intraductal irrigation is required to establish a fluid medium. Cholangioscopic vision may be limited due to stone fragments or biliary sludge. In contrast to ESWL, there is no upper limit on the number of pulses that can be applied during intracorporeal lithotripsy, provided that ductal lesions are avoided. However, the procedure should not last longer than approximately 2 h, as elderly patients do not tolerate longer treatment sessions well.

If complete bile duct clearance is not achieved within one treatment session, a transhepatic catheter must be inserted. Biliary sludge and small stone fragments usually pass spontaneously. After bile duct clearance, cholangioscopy may reveal further bile duct lesions or abnormalities.

Postprocedural Care of the Transhepatic Tract

After successful PTCS or stent placement, the transhepatic catheter is removed once adequate internal biliary drainage has been demonstrated. The cutaneobiliary fistula closes spontaneously within a few days. Continuous bile leakage indicates biliary obstruction and requires cholangiographic examination by injecting contrast medium through the unclosed fistula. In patients with benign bile duct strictures, transhepatic Yamakawa tubes are left in place for approximately 3 months to prevent early recurrent biliary stenosis after dilation [27–29]. Cholangiography is repeated after this period to decide whether further treatment is required due to a persistent stricture. Alternative methods—e.g., surgery or percutaneous implantation of metal stents—should be discussed in patients at high

17

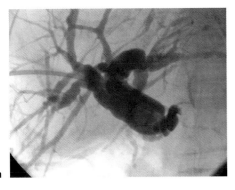

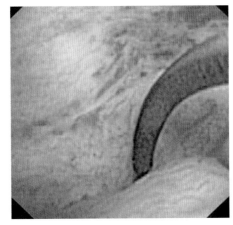

Fig. 17.8
a Percutaneous cholangiogram of a patient with centrally pronounced cholestasis and a history of Billroth II resection for gastric cancer. Internal biliary drainage failed due to complete obstruction of the common bile duct.
b Percutaneous cholangioscopy reveals an eccentric stenosis caused by recurrence of the gastric cancer. Cannulation of the difficult stenosis with a hydrophilic guide wire is being carried out under direct visual control.
c Percutaneous implantation of a metal stent.
d Balloon dilation of the metal stent is being carried out, due to a persistent stenosis and delayed drainage of contrast.

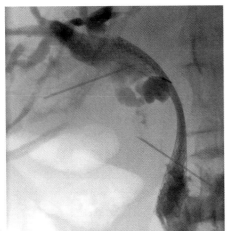

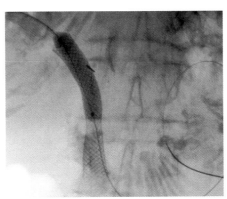

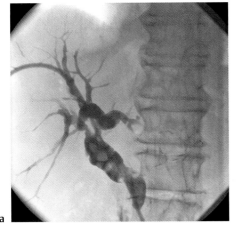

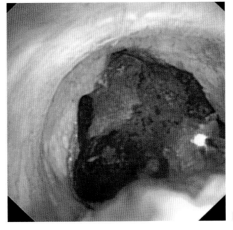

Fig. 17.9
a Percutaneous cholangiogram in a 77-year-old patient with a history of Billroth II surgery due to gastric cancer. The image shows multiple stones in the common bile duct (CBD).
b Percutaneous laser lithotripsy of stones in the CBD.
c The prograde view on the papilla of Vater, showing a benign stenosis. Radiography showed delayed contrast drainage.
d Prograde sphincterotomy.

Fig. 17.9e, f ▷

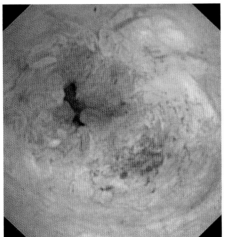

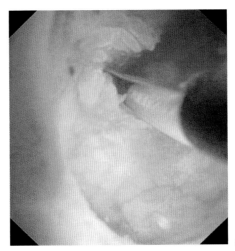

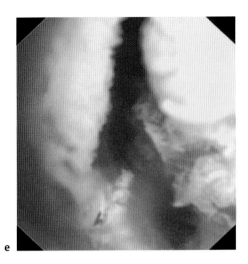
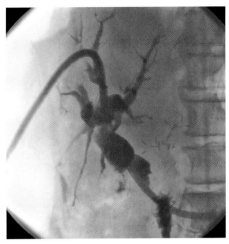

e

f

Fig. 17.9 (continued)
e The situation after the sphincterotomy.
f The final result, with passage of a percutaneous Yamakawa-type prosthesis (16 Fr) into the duodenum. The tube was left for 2 days to maintain access in case of delayed bleeding after sphincterotomy.

surgical risk, or in those with incurable malignant stenosis. Transhepatic tubes should be flushed once or twice a week with sterile saline solution to prevent blockage or the formation of stones.

Results

▦ PTC, PTCD, Cholangioplasty, and Stent Placement

Fine-needle PTC is successful in 91–98 % of patients with dilated bile ducts and in 70 % of patients with nondilated ducts [30–33]. The sensitivity (98–100 %) and specificity (89–100 %) rates for diagnosing biliary tract obstruction are comparable to those of endoscopic retrograde cholangiopancreatography (ERCP) [34]. PTC is technically demanding if there is no dilation of the intrahepatic bile ducts, and several passes with the needle are required. In these cases, ultrasound-guided puncture is helpful.

After successful cholangiography, PTCD is almost always feasible. In patients with malignant biliary obstruction, bilirubin levels fall quickly after decompression, and patients who receive drainage for sepsis show improvement within a few days. Failure can be caused by incomplete drainage, particularly in patients with multiple ductal stenoses. In these cases, further drains may be necessary to achieve complete biliary drainage.

Transhepatic balloon dilation is a safe procedure and achieves rapid reopening of obstructed bile ducts even when there are tight or rigid strictures. The long-term patency rates of cholangioplasty are 67–93 % for anastomotic strictures, 76–88 % for iatrogenic strictures, and 42–54 % after dilation of strictures due to primary sclerosing cholangitis [35–37]. Balloon dilation can also be successfully performed for biliary strictures in liver transplant recipients [38]. There is controversy regarding the value of stent placement after cholangioplasty for benign strictures. Removal of plastic prostheses can be technically difficult, but metal stents may obstruct later surgery.

The efficacy and safety of percutaneous transhepatic interventions have been examined in several studies. Our own data include 34 patients with anastomotic stenoses after hepaticojejunostomy. In 31 of these patients (91 %), PTCD was successfully performed. Transhepatic tubes were left in place until disappearance of the strictures or until surgery and could be removed in 23 of the 31 patients (74 %) after 212 ± 122 days, with no evidence of cholestasis during a follow-up period of 736 ± 479 days. Four patients received metal stents because of persistent strictures. Surgery had to be performed in five patients The 30-day morbidity and mortality rates were 23.5 % and 0 %, respectively [32]. In another study, PTCD was successful in 33 of 36 patients (92 %) with symptomatic benign bile duct stenoses [33]. Relief of the stricture was achieved in 72 % of the patients after a median stenting period of 14.5 months (6–34 months). This study documented a 27 % rate of long-term failures (10 of 36 patients) after a median follow-up of 48 months.

Permanent internal drainage is an effective method for palliative treatment of patients with malignant biliary obstruction [39]. Transhepatic tubes are inexpensive and effective for this purpose. Of course, stents are more convenient, because the patient is not disturbed by a foreign body at skin level, with the need for regular care to avoid infection. On the other hand, obstruction of plastic endoprostheses (by sludge or tumor) occurs within a mean of 5 months in common bile duct obstruction and 3 months in hilar stenoses after placement. In a series of 49 patients with hilar bile duct carcinoma, 45 % of the patients required repeat interventions due to blockage of percutaneously inserted endoprostheses [40]. Repeat interventions can be technically demanding and hazardous, because obstructed plastic stents have to be removed through the transhepatic tract.

The characteristics of metal stents are a small delivery catheter and large stent diameter, offering a longer period of patency, which may outweigh the high initial costs. Patients with malignant stenoses (e.g., cholangiocarcinoma) in particular benefit from the use of metal stents. In a study of 97 patients with obstructive jaundice (92 of malignant origin), 68 metallic stents were implanted in 66 patients [41]. Clinical improvement and a decrease in the serum bilirubin level were achieved in 61 patients (92.4 %). The metallic stents occluded in only nine patients (13.6 %), after a mean of 129 days. The survival time in patients with malignancy ranged from 6 to 485 days (mean 139 days), and no intervention-related deaths occurred.

The wire mesh of metallic endoprostheses allows stenting of multiple ducts; the stents can also be placed parallel to each other or in tandem fashion. One stent can even be placed through another by puncturing and dilating the mesh [15]. Percutaneous transhepatic insertion of metal stents may be associated with a lower complication rate in comparison with plastic endoprostheses (22 % versus 39 %) [42].

Burke et al. presented quality improvement guidelines for PTC and biliary drainage [43]. The guidelines suggest procedure-specific thresholds for success rates and complications. The authors recommend that internal processes should be reviewed if individual results differ significantly from the suggested thresholds.

17

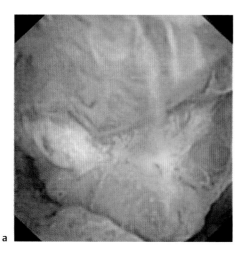
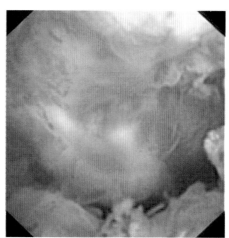

a

b

Fig. 17.10 a, b Percutaneous cholangioscopic images of the anastomosis in the patient with a history of neuroendocrine carcinoma of the gallbladder (compare **Fig. 17.4**). Histological evaluation of cholangioscopy-guided biopsies confirmed malignancy (neuroendocrine carcinoma).

Diagnostic Percutaneous Transhepatic Cholangioscopy

Percutaneous transhepatic cholangioscopy achieves excellent visualization of the biliary tree and of ductal lesions. Due to the short working length, easy access to the biliary tree, and the maneuverability of the instrument, target biopsies can be obtained precisely (**Figs. 17.6, 17.10**) [10,44–49]. The procedure is well tolerated and can be performed without general anesthesia [49]. PTCS allows early detection of small or multiple neoplastic foci; in particular, irregular dilated and tortuous vessels within the protruding or stenotic segment are characteristic of malignancy (**Fig. 17.8**) [45–47]. The accuracy for bile duct carcinoma is very high; positive results were obtained in 141 of 155 patients (sensitivity 96%) in a large series on PTCS [46]. PTCS is thus the most reliable nonsurgical diagnostic procedure for bile duct cancer. In addition, diagnostic PTCS together with selective cholangiography is used to evaluate the intrahepatic extent of biliary tumors. In particular, superficial spreading bile duct cancer with granular and papillary mucosa extending from a primary lesion can be differentiated from non-neoplastic bile duct mucosa [45,47,48]. Routine PTCS for preoperative staging of proximal bile duct carcinoma is therefore recommended in order to achieve high rates of curative resection and low surgical mortality rates [45,50]. A study by Seo et al. also underlined the impact of precise preoperative staging in 28 patients with hilar bile duct cancer [51]. Cholangioscopy revealed significantly more patients with advanced tumor stages than had been suspected using indirect imaging methods (14 vs. five patients with Bismuth type IV; $P < 0.05$). Sato et al. studied the sensitivity of PTCS for detecting intramural invasive carcinoma and showed that cholangioscopic diagnosis of the intramural extension of bile duct carcinoma limited to the adventitia is difficult [48]. Still, further prospective trials are needed to determine the impact of PTCS on the surgical treatment of bile duct cancer.

Biliary parasites are usually diagnosed using ERCP, and endoscopic papillotomy allows removal of echinococcal cysts obstructing the biliary tree. In selected cases, PTCS is indicated as a complementary procedure to detect minor lesions or intrahepatic findings not accessible with ERCP.

Therapeutic Percutaneous Transhepatic Cholangioscopy

PTCS is the nonsurgical method of choice for hepatolithiasis and extrahepatic stones that are not amenable to transpapillary procedures. The percutaneous approach is frequently combined with intracorporal lithotripsy. EHL and laser lithotripsy appear to be similarly effective, with success rates of 80–100% [5–7,25,26, 52,53]. The largest series have been reported in the Far East, owing to the high incidence of hepatolithiasis in this region.

Yeh et al. reported on 615 patients with hepatolithiasis, 450 of whom initially underwent surgery [28]. PTCS was the primary therapy in 165 patients because of the surgical risk, previous biliary surgery, or refusal of surgery. EHL was used for larger stones. A mean of 5.1 sessions of PTCS were needed for bile duct clearance, and complete clearance was achieved in 81% of the patients. One in five of the patients had at least one episode of cholangitis, and the mortality rate was 1.2%. In patients with difficult ductal strictures, transhepatic drainage catheters were left in place for several months to prevent recurrent stenosis. The stone recurrence rate was 33% after a mean of 58 months. All but one patient with recurrent stones were managed nonsurgically.

In another study, Huang achieved complete clearance of hepatolithiasis in 209 of 245 patients (85.3%) using a percutaneous transhepatic approach. This study group observed a higher rate of incomplete clearance in patients with intrahepatic duct stricture (24.6% vs. 5.5%; $P = 0.002$) [52]. The follow-up in this retrospective study was 1–22 years, and the overall recurrence rate of hepatolithiasis and/or cholangitis was 63.2%. The rate of major complications was 1.6% (four of 245) and included liver laceration (n = 2), intra-abdominal abscess (n = 1), and disruption of the percutaneous transhepatic biliary drainage fistula (n = 1). Other authors have reported comparable initial success rates of complete clearance of hepatolithiasis but observed recurrence rates of up to 100% in patients with severe intrahepatic strictures or advanced biliary cirrhosis [53].

The importance of the management of biliary strictures was also underlined by Jeng et al. [54]. This group performed 208 balloon dilations in 57 patients with ductal strictures and intrahepatic stones. The success rate for complete clearance increased from 0% before dilation to 95% after dilation. Temporary stenting was performed in only 14% of the patients. Recurrent strictures occurred in only 8% after 3 years.

Therapeutic PTCS can also be used to reopen difficult strictures that are not amenable to radiologic techniques. The tiny lumen of a

IV

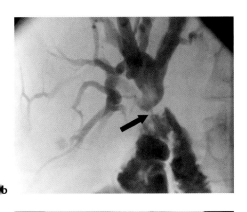

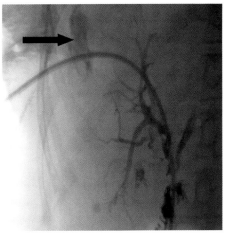

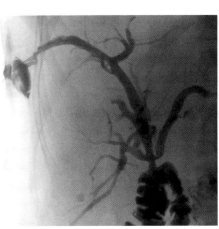

Fig. 17.11
a Cholangiogram in a 70-year-old patient with a history of Whipple's surgery due to pancreatic cancer (pT3 N1 M0 L 1 V1 G2) 5 years before. The patient presented with cholangitis, and a stenosis of the anastomosis (arrow) was diagnosed.
b After PTCD an unstable sinus tract with effusion of contrast media (arrow) was diagnosed, which resolved spontaneously. In addition, regression of the cholestasis is evident.
c Percutaneous cholangioscopy of the anastomosis revealed a stone that could be removed.
d After temporary placement of a percutaneous Yamakawa-type prosthesis, the stenosis resolved and the prosthesis was removed. There was no evidence of relapse of the pancreatic cancer (brush cytology and histology of percutaneous transhepatic cholangioscopy–guided biopsies were negative).

stenosis can often be visualized on PTCS even if cholangiography has suggested complete ductal obstruction. A guide wire is passed under visual control, and dilation or stent implantation is subsequently possible [55]. In addition, PTCS can be helpful for recovering migrated endoprostheses or for pulling guide wires to the contralateral liver lobe using biopsy forceps or snares.

PDT, which can be carried out percutaneously (under cholangioscopic control) or endoscopically, has been reported to be successful in patients with nonresectable cholangiocarcinoma [17,18]. Further studies are needed to establish this treatment option.

Complications and Management

PTC(D) is a relatively safe procedure for some biliary tract diseases in which transpapillary management is not possible. Complications of percutaneous interventions in particular occur in relation to the placement of transhepatic catheters and dilation of the sinus tract [10,56]. Cholangitis and hemobilia are the complications most often observed. The incidence of cholangitis is higher in patients with incomplete biliary drainage, particularly if multiple stones or bile duct strictures cause obstruction of several liver segments. Prophylactic antibiotic treatment is strongly recommended in these cases.

Hemobilia is mainly caused by biliovenous fistula and rarely by arterial hemorrhage into the biliary tract. Biliovenous fistulas usually close spontaneously after insertion of a transhepatic catheter that compresses the bleeding area. In cases of arterial bleeding, a transhepatic catheter can also be inserted for compression, but there is often recurrent hemorrhage after removal of the catheter. In these cases, selective angiographic embolization is the treatment of choice. To prevent hemorrhage or bile duct perforation, gradual dilation is preferable to the creation of a large-bore tract within a single session. A subcapsular liver hematoma usually disappears spontaneously within a few days; dilation procedures should be avoided during this time.

If a sinus tract has not been stabilized, migration of the catheter may cause bile leakage and biliary peritonitis. Immediate replacement of the drainage catheter or a repeated PTCD is required, which can be difficult, as the bile ducts usually narrow after decompression or as a result of continuous leakage. The risk of this serious complication appears to be lower when the tip of a transhepatic catheter is inserted through the papilla into the duodenum.

Another rare complication of PTCD/PTCS is the development of a biliopleural fistula (**Fig. 17.11**) [57]. In this case, effective biliary drainage must be guaranteed endoscopically or percutaneously. A significant pleural effusion has to be treated by insertion of a drainage tube. The overall mortality of PTCD is <2% in larger patient groups [31].

Cholangioscopic procedures rarely cause serious complications after a cutaneobiliary fistula has matured. Minor hemobilia was seen in up to 20% of patients treated with EHL, but conservative management is usually successful [5–7]. Laser lithotripsy is a safe procedure if the investigator concentrates on keeping the tip of the fiber on the stone and away from the biliary wall. The main complications of plastic and metal stents are bleeding, perforation, biliary fistula, cholangitis, and liver abscesses [42], as well as blockage and migration. Occlusion is usually caused by tumor growth or sludge. These long-term complications can usually be managed by implantation of additional stents. An analysis of PTCS-related complications was presented recently by Oh et al. [56].

17

Conclusions

PTC is a safe procedure and provides detailed information about the biliary tree, bile leakage, and intraductal lesions if this cannot be obtained by noninvasive diagnostic methods or ERC. PTCD achieves effective drainage in patients with malignant or benign biliary obstruction, but the morbidity is higher than with endoscopic procedures. Catheters can usually be advanced for internal biliary drainage. Cholangioplasty, with or without temporary placement of stents or transhepatic tubes, is an efficient technique for the treatment of postoperative or primary benign biliary strictures. Percutaneous implantation of internal stents is the method of choice for palliative treatment of malignant biliary obstruction not amenable endoscopically, while percutaneous (or transpapillary) PDT is a new treatment option for nonresectable cholangiocarcinoma. Metal stents are usually preferred to plastic endoprostheses, particularly due to their longer patency and greater comfort for the patient. PTCS provides important diagnostic information, allows visually guided biopsies to be taken, and promises to improve the preoperative staging of biliary tumors. Transhepatic treatment of bile duct stones offers an effective alternative to surgery when transpapillary procedures have failed or are not possible. Indications should always be discussed on an interdisciplinary basis. Extrahepatic stones are easy to approach, even with less flexible large-bore instruments. Intrahepatic stones are more difficult to access, but the approach is facilitated by cholangioscopes. Impacted or large stones can be fragmented by EHL or laser lithotripsy under direct visual control. In general, transhepatic lithotripsy is very effective; the short instruments have excellent optical resolution and are easy to maneuver toward the stones, and fragments are flushed in a prograde direction. Once a stable tract has been established, bile duct clearance can usually be achieved in a single session. Failures are mainly observed in difficult cases of oriental hepatolithiasis or excessively large stones. The long-term results of transhepatic treatment of biliary tract stone disease are promising. Recurrences are mainly caused by strictures of the bile duct or biliodigestive anastomoses. Temporary placement of large-bore transhepatic tubes may reduce the recurrence of strictures. Although transhepatic procedures appear to be technically easy, expertise is required in difficult cases and for the management of complications.

References

1. Pitt HA, Venbrux AC, Coleman J, Prescott CA, Johnson MS, Osterman FA Jr, et al. Intrahepatic stones. The transhepatic team approach. Ann Surg 1994;219:527–37.
2. Yamakawa T. Percutaneous cholangioscopy for management of retained biliary tract stones and intrahepatic stones. Endoscopy 1989;21(Suppl 1):333–7.
3. Neuhaus H, Hoffmann W, Classen M. Laser lithotripsy of pancreatic and biliary stones via 3.4 and 3.7 mm miniscopes: first clinical results. Endoscopy 1992;24:208–14.
4. Harrison J, Morris DL, Haynes J, Hitchcock A, Womack C, Wherry DC. Electrohydraulic lithotripsy of gall stones—in vitro and animal studies. Gut 1987;28:267–71.
5. Bonnel DH, Liguory CE, Cornud FE, Lefebvre JF. Common bile duct and intrahepatic stones: results of transhepatic electrohydraulic lithotripsy in 50 patients. Radiology 1991;180:345–8.
6. Chen MF, Jan YY. Percutaneous transhepatic cholangioscopic lithotripsy. Br J Surg 1990;77:530–2.
7. Jeng KS, Chiang HS, Shih SC. Limitations of percutaneous transhepatic cholangioscopy in the removal of complicated biliary calculi. World J Surg 1989;13:603–10.
8. Hochberger J, Tex S, Maiss J, Hahn EG. Management of difficult common bile duct stones. Gastrointest Endosc Clin N Am 2003;13:623–34.
9. Xing GS, Geng JC, Han XW, Dai JH, Wu CY. Endobiliary brush cytology during percutaneous transhepatic cholangiodrainage in patients with obstructive jaundice. Hepatobiliary Pancreat Dis Int 2005;4:98–103.
10. Neuhaus H, Hoffmann W, Classen M. [The benefits and risks of percutaneous transhepatic cholangioscopy]. Dtsch Med Wochenschr 1993;118:574–81. German.
11. Ponchon T, Valette PJ, Bory R, Bret PM, Bretagnolle M, Chavaillon A. Evaluation of a combined percutaneous–endoscopic procedure for the treatment of choledocholithiasis and benign papillary stenosis. Endoscopy 1987;19:164–6.
12. Fujita R, Yamamura M, Fujita Y. Combined endoscopic sphincterotomy and percutaneous transhepatic cholangioscopic lithotripsy. Gastrointest Endosc 1988;34:91–4.
13. Druy EM, Melville GE. Obstructed hepatic bifurcation: decompression via single percutaneous tract. AJR Am J Roentgenol 1984;143:73–6.
14. Becker CD, Fache JS, Gibney RG, Burhenne HJ. External–internal cross-connection for bilateral percutaneous biliary drainage. AJR Am J Roentgenol 1987;149:91–2.
15. Neuhaus H, Gottlieb K, Classen M. The stent through wire mesh technique for complicated biliary strictures. Gastrointest Endosc 1993;39:553–6.
16. Kubota Y, Seki T, Yamaguchi T, Tani K, Mizuno T, Inoue K. Bilateral internal drainage of biliary hilar malignancy via a single percutaneous track: role of percutaneous transhepatic cholangioscopy. Endoscopy 1992;24:194–8.
17. Ortner ME, Caca K, Berr F, Liebetruth J, Mansmann U, Huster D, et al. Successful photodynamic therapy for nonresectable cholangiocarcinoma: a randomized prospective study. Gastroenterology 2003;125:1355–63.
18. Shim CS, Cheon YK, Cha SW, Bhandari S, Moon JH, Cho YD, et al. Prospective study of the effectiveness of percutaneous transhepatic photodynamic therapy for advanced bile duct cancer and the role of intraductal ultrasonography in response assessment. Endoscopy 2005;37:425–33.
19. Nimura Y, Hayakawa N, Toyoda S. Percutaneous transhepatic cholangioscopy. Stomach Intestine 1981;16:681–9.
20. Itoi T, Shinohara Y, Takeda K, Nakamura K, Sofuni A, Itokawa F, et al. A novel technique for endoscopic sphincterotomy when using a percutaneous transhepatic cholangioscope in patients with an endoscopically inaccessible papilla. Gastrointest Endosc 2004;59:708–11.
21. Nagashima I, Takada T, Shiratori M, Inaba T, Okinaga K. Percutaneous transhepatic papillary balloon dilation as a therapeutic option for choledocholithiasis. J Hepatobiliary Pancreat Surg 2004;11:252–4.
22. Park YS, Kim JH, Choi YW, Lee TH, Hwang CM, Cho YJ, et al. Percutaneous treatment of extrahepatic bile duct stones assisted by balloon sphincteroplasty and occlusion balloon. Korean J Radiol 2005;6:235–40.
23. Mazzariello RM. A fourteen-year experience with nonoperative instrument extraction of retained bile duct stones. World J Surg 1978;2:447–55.
24. Han JK, Choi BI, Park JH, Han MC. Percutaneous removal of retained intrahepatic stones with a pre-shaped angulated catheter: review of 96 patients. Br J Radiol 1992;65:9–13.
25. Neuhaus H, Hoffmann W, Zillinger C, Classen M. Laser lithotripsy of difficult bile duct stones under direct visual control. Gut 1993;34:415–21.
26. Neuhaus H, Zillinger C, Born P, Ott R, Allescher H, Rösch T, et al. Randomized study of intracorporeal laser lithotripsy versus extracorporeal shockwave lithotripsy for difficult bile duct stones. Gastrointest Endosc 1998;47:327–44.
27. Neuhaus H, Zillinger C, Illek B, Hoffmann W, Classen M. Percutaneous transhepatic cholangioscopy (PTCS) for laser lithotripsy of bile duct stones: medium-term follow-up in 55 patients [abstract]. Gastroenterology 1994;106:A352.
28. Yeh YH, Huang MH, Yang JC, Mo LR, Lin J, Yueh SK. Percutaneous transhepatic cholangioscopy and lithotripsy in the treatment of intrahepatic stones: a study with 5-year follow-up. Gastrointest Endosc 1995;42:13–8.
29. Jan YY, Chen MF. Percutaneous transhepatic cholangioscopic lithotomy for hepatolithiasis: long-term results. Gastrointest Endosc 1995;42:19–24.
30. Harbin WP, Mueller PR, Ferrucci JT Jr. Transhepatic cholangiography: complications and use patterns of the fine needle technique. Radiology 1980;135:15–9.
31. Oberholzer K, Pitton MB, Mildenberger P, Lechner C, Düber C, Thelen M. [The current value of percutaneous transhepatic biliary drainage]. Rofo 2002;174:1081–8. German.
32. Schumacher B, Othman T, Jansen M, Preiss C, Neuhaus H. Long-term follow-up of percutaneous transhepatic therapy (PTT) in patients with definite benign anastomotic strictures after hepaticojejunostomy. Endoscopy 2001;33:409–15.

33. Eickhoff A, Schilling D, Jakobs R, Weickert U, Hartmann D, Eickhoff JC, et al. Long-term outcome of percutaneous transhepatic drainage for benign bile duct stenoses. Rocz Akad Med Bialymst 2005;50:155–60.

34. Teplick SK, Flick P, Brandon JC. Transhepatic cholangiography in patients with suspected biliary disease and nondilated intrahepatic bile ducts. Gastrointest Radiol 1991;16:193–7.

35. Mueller PR, van Sonnenberg E, Ferrucci JT Jr, Weyman PJ, Butch RJ, Malt RA, et al. Biliary stricture dilatation: multicenter review of clinical management in 73 patients. Radiology 1986;160:17–22.

36. Millis JM, Tompkins RK, Zinner MJ. Management of bile duct strictures: an evolving strategy. Arch Surg 1992;127:1077–81.

37. Williams HJ Jr, Bender CE, May GR. Benign postoperative biliary strictures: dilation with fluoroscopic guidance. Radiology 1987;163:629–34.

38. Sung RS, Campbell DA Jr, Rudich SM, Punch JD, Shieck VL, Armstrong JM, et al. Long-term follow-up of percutaneous transhepatic balloon cholangioplasty in the management of biliary strictures after liver transplantation. Transplantation 2004;77:110–5.

39. Radeleff BA, López-Benítez R, Hallscheidt P, Grenacher L, Libicher M, Richter GM, et al. [Treatment of malignant biliary obstructions via the percutaneous approach]. Radiologe 2005;45:1020–30. German.

40. Laméris JS, Hesselink EJ, Van Leeuwen PA, Nijs HG, Meerwaldt JH, Terpstra OT. Ultrasound-guided percutaneous transhepatic cholangiography and drainage in patients with hilar cholangiocarcinoma. Semin Liver Dis 1990;10:121–5.

41. Pappas P, Leonardou P, Kurkuni A, Alexopoulos T, Tzortzis G. Percutaneous insertion of metallic endoprostheses in the biliary tree in 66 patients: relief of the obstruction. Abdom Imaging 2003;28:678–83.

42. Beissert M, Wittenberg G, Sandstede J, Beer M, Tschammler A, Burghardt W, et al. Metallic stents and plastic endoprostheses in percutaneous treatment of biliary obstruction. Z Gastroenterol 2002;40:503–10.

43. Burke DR, Lewis CA, Cardella JF, Citron SJ, Drooz AT, Haskal ZJ, et al. Quality improvement guidelines for percutaneous transhepatic cholangiography and biliary drainage. J Vasc Interv Radiol 2003;14(9 Pt 2):S 243–6.

44. Maier M, Kohler B, Benz C, Körber H, Riemann JF. [Percutaneous transhepatic cholangioscopy (PTCS)—an important supplement in diagnosis and therapy of biliary tract diseases (indications, technique and results)]. Z Gastroenterol 1995;33:435–9. German.

45. Nimura Y. Staging of biliary carcinoma: cholangiography and cholangioscopy. Endoscopy 1993;25:76–80.

46. Nimura Y, Kamiya J. Cholangioscopy. Endoscopy 1998;30:182–8.

47. Nimura Y, Kamiya J, Hayakawa N, Shionoya S. Cholangioscopic differentiation of biliary strictures and polyps. Endoscopy 1989;21(Suppl 1):351–6.

48. Sato M, Inoue H, Ogawa S. Differences in fine mucosal structure between superficial spreading carcinoma and nonneoplastic bile duct mucosa detected by percutaneous transhepatic cholangioscopy. Dig Endosc 1997;9:43–7.

49. Van Steenbergen W, Van Aken L, Van Beckevoort D, Stockx L, Fevery J. Percutaneous transhepatic cholangioscopy for diagnosis and therapy of biliary diseases in older patients. J Am Geriatr Soc 1996;44:1384–7.

50. Nimura Y, Hayakawa N, Kamiya J, Kondo S, Shionoya S. Hepatic segmentectomy with caudate lobe resection for bile duct carcinoma of the hepatic hilus. World J Surg 1990;14:535–44.

51. Seo DW, Kim YS, Kim HJ. The usefulness of preoperative cholangioscopy in patients with Klatskin tumor [abstract]. Gastrointest Endosc 1998;47:AB 129.

52. Huang MH, Chen CH, Yang JC, Yang CC, Yeh YH, Chou DA, et al. Long-term outcome of percutaneous transhepatic cholangioscopic lithotomy for hepatolithiasis. Am J Gastroenterol 2003;98:2655–62.

53. Lee SK, Seo DW, Myung SJ, Park ET, Lim BC, Kim HJ, et al. Percutaneous transhepatic cholangioscopic treatment for hepatolithiasis: an evaluation of long-term results and risk factors for recurrence. Gastrointest Endosc 2001;53:318–23.

54. Jeng KS, Yang FS, Ohta I, Chiang HJ. Dilatation of intrahepatic biliary strictures in patients with hepatolithiasis. World J Surg 1990;14:587–93.

55. Neuhaus H, Hagenmüller F, Griebel M, Classen M. Percutaneous cholangioscopic or transpapillary insertion of self-expanding biliary metal stents. Gastrointest Endosc 1991;37:31–7.

56. Oh HC, Lee SK, Lee TY, Kwon S, Lee SS, Seo DW, et al. Analysis of percutaneous transhepatic cholangioscopy-related complications and the risk factors for those complications. Endoscopy 2007;39:731–6.

57. De Meester X, Vanbeckevoort D, Aerts R, Van Steenbergen W. Biliopleural fistula as a late complication of percutaneous transhepatic cholangioscopy. Endoscopy 2005;37:183.

17

18 Endoscopic Therapy in Obesity

Elisabeth M.H. Mathus-Vliegen

Introduction

(Morbid) obesity is a chronic, lifelong, multifactorial and genetically related life-threatening disease of excessive fat storage, which in addition to the way in which the fat is distributed places the individual at risk of premature death and obesity-associated comorbidities. Almost every organ system is affected by obesity, and the gastrointestinal tract is involved as well [1,2]. The world epidemic of overweight—body mass index (BMI) $\geq 25\,\mathrm{kg/m^2}$—is estimated to encompass about 1.7 billion individuals; more than 300 million people are obese [3,4]. In the United States, approximately 64% of individuals are overweight. The prevalence of obesity is approximately 30%. In 2002, 5.1% of U.S. adults had a BMI $\geq 40\,\mathrm{kg/m^2}$. In Europe, in most countries at least 40% of males and females are overweight and obese. The prevalence of morbid obesity (BMI $\geq 40\,\mathrm{kg/m^2}$) in the United Kingdom is 2.9% of women and 1.0% of men.

The National Heart, Lung, and Blood Institutes and the World Health Organization have documented that weight loss reduces many of the risk factors for increased death and obesity-related diseases [1,2]. The first approach should consist of a combination of energy-restricted diet, physical activity, and behavior modification. When motivated patients have seriously attempted but failed to achieve weight loss, pharmacotherapy is recommended. A surgical approach is restricted to very obese individuals (BMI $\geq 40\,\mathrm{kg/m^2}$ or BMI $\geq 35\,\mathrm{kg/m^2}$ with obesity-associated comorbidity), but there is an intermediate group of patients who do not respond to medical therapy but are not (yet) surgical candidates. For this group, endoscopic treatment might appear attractive. The disappointing results of current approaches to treat obesity and the lack of long-term effectiveness of nonsurgical treatments for clinically severe obesity has led to burgeoning interest in bariatric surgery ("bariatrics" is derived from the Greek *baros,* weight, and *iatreia,* medical treatment) [5]. Buchwald reported an increase in procedures from 40,000 in 1998 to 146,301 procedures in 2003 [6]. Yet only approximately 1% of eligible individuals with morbid obesity in the U.S. and around 1–3% of eligible patients in Britain receive bariatric surgery. In a meta-analysis, the operative mortality varied between 0.1% and 1.1% [3]. Significant risk reductions and resolution or improvement of obesity-associated diseases were noted [3,7]. When compared with age-matched and gender-matched severely obese patients who had not undergone weight-reduction surgery, digestive complaints and complications increased in the bariatric cohort—relative risk (RR) 1.48 (1.42/1.78) [8]. Endoscopic therapy thus has a role to play in the treatment of obesity, either as an alternative or as an adjunct to medical treatment or as a modality for treating complications after bariatric surgery.

Endoscopic Treatments for Obesity

▓ Intragastric Balloon Treatment

Intragastric balloon treatment had to be abandoned in the 1980s following a prohibitive number of complications and premature balloon deflations, mainly with the Food and Drug Administration (FDA)-approved Garren–Edwards Gastric Bubble (GEGB). In GEGB balloons, deflations occurred in 31% of cases, and surgical interventions were needed in 2.3%. Gastric ulcers were seen in 26% of cases, and the balloon was not tolerated in 7% [9]. In 1987, experts decided against recommending removal of existing intragastric balloons from the market, but urged that their use be discouraged outside of a controlled investigation [10]. However, this resulted in the withdrawal of balloons from the American market [11]. Notwithstanding this, research continued in Europe and Australia and resulted in a better understanding of balloon mechanics and a more straightforward definition of suitable patients [9,11–13]. It also became clear that the use of intragastric balloons had to be embedded in a weight-care program, which had to be continued after balloon removal in order to maintain the lost body weight. However, none of the existing balloons conformed to the fundamental requirements for optimal balloon design as formulated by the experts in 1987— i.e., being smooth, seamless, and constructed of long-lasting material with a low ulcerogenic and obstructive potential, with a radiopaque marker to allow appropriate follow-up in case of deflation and capable of being adjusted to a variety of sizes and filled with fluid rather than air (**Fig. 18.1 a**) [10]. Many years of research finally resulted in a balloon that met these requirements, the BioEnterics Intragastric Balloon (BIB™; Allergan, Irvine, California, USA) (**Fig. 18.1 b–d**).

Indications and Contraindications

Patients are eligible if they are 18 years or older, have failed to achieve weight loss within a supervised weight control program, and present with a BMI of at least $30\,\mathrm{kg/m^2}$ with comorbidities or $\geq 32\,\mathrm{kg/m^2}$ without comorbidities. Candidates are excluded if a hormonal or genetic cause for the obese state, malignancy within the last 5 years, (desire for) pregnancy, and alcohol or drug abuse is present. Contraindications more specifically related to the balloon consist of gastrointestinal lesions such as a large (> 3 cm) hiatal hernia, grade C–D esophagitis, peptic ulceration, varices, or angiodysplasias; or previous bariatric or abdominal surgery because of adhesions. Patients who are not cooperative at endoscopy or whose poor general health would preclude surgery if a complication should occur are also excluded. The use of anticoagulants or nonsteroidal anti-inflammatory drugs (NSAIDs) is prohibited. In severely obese patients, the intragastric balloon is used for the treatment of those with a BMI $\geq 40\,\mathrm{kg/m^2}$ who are poor surgical candidates and those with a BMI $\geq 50\,\mathrm{kg/m^2}$ who are surgical candidates, with the aim of achieving moderate weight loss before surgery to reduce anesthesia risks and surgical complications and to better visualize the operative field. Some surgeons use the balloon as a predictive instrument to single out patients who would not benefit

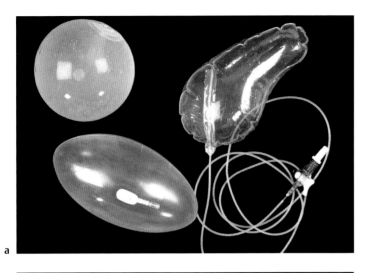
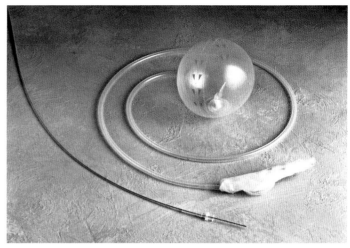
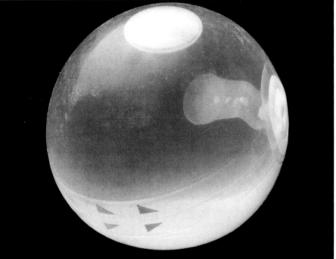
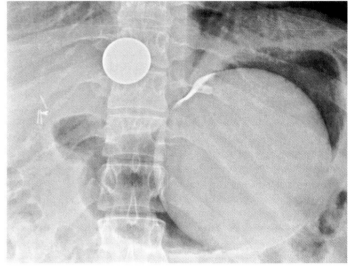

Fig. 18.1
a Three balloon designs have been used. *Top left:* the BioEnterics Intragastric Balloon (BIB™, Allergan, Irvine, California, USA). *Lower left:* the Danish Ballobes balloon. *Right:* the Wilson-Cook balloon, with an inflation catheter.
b The BIB inflated and the placement assembly, with the collapsed balloon and balloon fill tube.

c The smooth, spherical BIB with arrows at the middle that point toward the valve. The radiopaque self-sealing and repenetrable valve, with its Z-shaped configuration, is visible inside the balloon.
d A plain abdominal radiograph showing the balloon in the body of the stomach. A coin taped onto the lower sternum allows comparison of the balloon size during follow-up to detect premature deflation.

from gastric restrictive surgery (sweet eaters, snackers, grazers, compulsive eaters, and binge eaters), but in a prospective study no predictive value of balloon treatment prior to gastric banding was demonstrated [14].

Balloon Insertion and Removal

First, an endoscopy has to be performed to rule out abnormalities that preclude insertion. After removal of the endoscope, the placement assembly, which consists of a sheath with the collapsed balloon and a balloon fill tube, is inserted up to 10 cm beyond the distance from the incisors to the esophagogastric junction (**Fig. 18.1 b**). The endoscope is then reinserted into the stomach to observe the balloon-filling and releasing steps. With a syringe attached to the balloon fill tube and the balloon, the balloon is filled with the recommended initial volume of 500 mL saline. After the balloon has been filled, gentle suction applied by withdrawing the plunger of the syringe creates a vacuum that seals the valve. The balloon is released by a short pull at the fill tube, after which the fill tube and empty placement assembly are removed.

For balloon removal, a needle aspirator is available to puncture the balloon and remove as much fluid as possible by suction before the balloon is grasped with a snare or a two-pronged or three-pronged grasper. The endoscope and the grasped balloon are gently removed.

After insertion, nausea, vomiting, abdominal cramps, and acid reflux are to be expected for 72 h and require treatment with antiemetics, antispasmodics, analgesics as suppositories, or acid suppressants. Instructions for a 72-h liquid diet after insertion have to be provided. Thereafter, antacids or acid-suppressing drugs are given on request.

Results of Balloon Treatment

The greatest weight loss was observed in morbidly obese and preoperative patients (**Table 18.1**) [15–27]. In those studies that defined successful weight loss (7, 10, or 13 kg weight loss or 20 % excess weight loss), a failure rate of 15.3 % with no or insufficient weight loss was observed. Weight loss maintenance after balloon removal was reported in seven studies, with two studies having a balloon-

Table 18.1 Weight losses achieved by intragastric balloon treatment in different patient groups

	Age	Initial BMI	Change (kg)	Change (kg/m²)	Excess weight loss (%)
Nonmorbidly obese					
Five studies (n = 665) [15–19]	33.0–37.5	31.0–39.0	9.5–18.6	5.3–5.7	38.1–50.8
Morbidly obese					
Five studies (n = 573) [20–24]	31.0–43.0	41.0–46.6	13.0–15.0	4.8–5.3	18.7–35.0
Preoperative					
Two studies (n = 58) [25,26]	38.8–43.3	58.4–60.2	18.1–26.4	6.4–9.4	21.0–26.1
Three studies (n = 2573, including [27])	38.8–43.3	44.4–60.2		4.9–9.4	21.0–33.9

BMI, body mass index.

Table 18.2 Gastrointestinal symptoms and complications of intragastric balloon treatment

	16 studies, 1999–2006 [15–26,28,30–32] (n = 1402)		17 studies, 1999–2006, including Italian survey [27] (n = 3917)	
	n	%	n	%
Early vomiting	495	35.3	≈ 495	12.6
Late vomiting	139	9.9	158	4.0
Early reflux symptoms	52	3.7	≈ 52	1.3
Late reflux symptoms	62	4.4	≈ 62	1.6
Early abdominal discomfort	149	10.6	≈ 149	3.8
Late abdominal discomfort	82	5.8	101	2.6
Hypokalemia	22	1.6	≈ 22	0.6
Dehydration, (pre)renal insufficiency	39	2.8	≈ 39	1.0
Esophagitis	72	5.1	104	2.7
Peptic ulcer	12	0.86	17	0.40
Gastric erosions	7	0.50	≈ 7	0.18
Gastric perforation	3	0.20	8	0.20
Balloon intolerance	94	6.7	124	3.2
Weight loss failure	171/1115	15.3	?	?
Balloons (n)	1522		4037	
Balloon deflation	123	8.1	132	3.3
● In stomach	31	2.0	40	0.99
● Per rectum	87	5.7	≈ 87	2.2
● Removal by surgery	5	0.3	≈ 5	0.12
Problematic endoscopic removal	9	0.59	≈ 9	0.22
Overall major complication rate	77	5.5	121	3.1
Mortality	0	0	2	0.05

≈: Number approximately the same in the 17 studies in comparison with the 16 studies without the Italian survey, as these complications were not reported as such in the Italian survey.

free follow-up period of 12 months. The results showed that 28–40 % of the lost weight was regained. Two studies showed impressive beneficial changes in comorbidities, with resolution or improvement of hypertension, diabetes, respiratory disorders, and osteoarthritis in over 85 % of patients and resolution or improvement of dyslipidemia in 52 % [27,28]. All studies published between 1999 and 2006 were reviewed to extract data on balloon intolerance, balloon deflation, complaints and gastrointestinal complications [29]. Sixteen studies reported on 1402 patients, with early and late vomiting in 35.2 % and 9.9 % of cases, respectively; early and late gastroesophageal reflux in 3.7 % and 4.4 %; and early and late abdominal discomfort in 11.6 % and 5.8 %, respectively (**Table 18.2**) [15–28,30–32]. Hypokalemia and (prerenal) dehydration occurred in 1.6 % and 2.8 % of cases, respectively. Intolerance to such an extent that the balloon had to be removed occurred in 6.7 %.

Gastrointestinal complications consisted of esophagitis (5.0 %), peptic ulcer (0.86 %), gastric erosions (0.50 %), and gastric perfora-

tion (0.20 %). No deaths occurred. The overall complication rate was 5.5 %. All of these figures were halved when the Italian survey by Genco et al. was added to the 16 studies, including 3917 patients in total [27]. The Italian survey reported an additional five gastric perforations and mortality in two patients (0.05 %) [27]. The same 16 studies reported on 1522 balloons, combining with the Italian survey to provide data on 4037 balloons [27]. Deflation occurred in 8.1 %; balloons were retrieved in the stomach, were mainly evacuated per rectum, and needed emergency surgery in five patients (**Table 18.2**). Difficulties were encountered in the removal of nine balloons (0.59 %). The overall deflation rate was 8.1 %, with a need for surgical intervention in 0.3 %. The Italian survey added only nine deflated balloons [27]. Unfortunately, the Cochrane review, which was very negative in its conclusions, included many of older balloon studies [33].

18

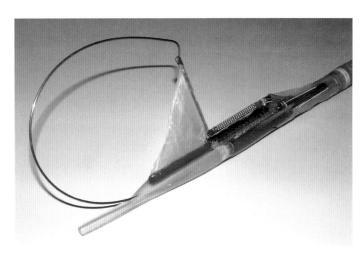

Fig. 18.2 The instrument for creating the gastroplasty, with the retraction wire, sail, and opened stapler device. (Reproduced courtesy of J. Devière, Erasmus Hospital, Brussels, Belgium.)

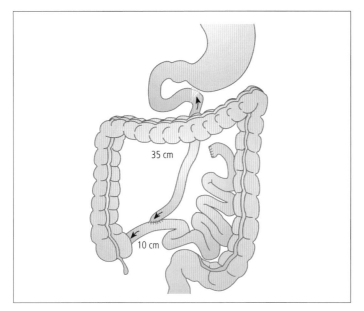

Fig. 18.3 Jejunoileal bypass: 35 cm of the jejunum is anastomosed to the terminal 10 cm of the ileum, with a blindly closed jejunal end. (Reproduced by permission from Int J Gastroenterol 2000;5:8–11.)

Other Endoscopic Modalities

Several new balloon designs are under development. A new endoscopically delivered device designed to produce weight loss is the Endobarrier (GI Dynamics, Watertown, Massachusetts, USA), a 60-cm long sleeve that is anchored in the duodenum, to create a duodenojejunal bypass [34].

Other developments are the creation of a vertical banded gastroplasty using an endoscopic suturing machine (EndoCinch; Bard, Inc., Murray Hill, New Jersey, USA) and endoluminal gastroplasty with an endoscopic suture device (Eagle Claw; Olympus, Tokyo, Japan [35]). Recently, Devière's group in Belgium have published their experience with the transoral gastroplasty (TOGA) system (Satiety Inc., Palo Alto, California, USA) (**Fig. 18.2**). After the creation of a gastric stapled restrictive pouch along the lesser curve of the stomach, patients lost an average of 13 kg (24 % of excess weight) in 6 months [36]. However, gaps in the staple lines were evident in 13 of 21 patients. Technical improvement of the device and refinement of

the method resulted in a more favorable outcome, with a 6-month weight loss of 24 kg (46 % excess weight loss) [37].

Endoscopic Treatment for Bariatric Surgery Complications

Surgical Procedures

There are several types of procedure: purely malabsorptive, such as the jejunoileal bypass (JIB); purely restrictive, such as horizontal gastroplasty; vertical banded gastroplasty (VBG); adjustable silicone gastric banding (ASGB) and laparoscopic adjustable silicone gastric banding (LASGB); and combined restrictive–malabsorptive procedures. The short-limb or proximal Roux-en-Y gastric bypass (RYGB) and the long-limb gastric bypass are the most restrictive operations in the latter group. Biliopancreatic diversion (BPD), biliopancreatic diversion with duodenal switch (BPD-DS), and the very long-limb or distal Roux-en-Y gastric bypass are the most malabsorptive procedures. Worldwide survey data from 2002 and 2003 show that gastric bypass is the most commonly performed weight loss procedure (65.1 %), and slightly more than half of gastric bypasses are done laparoscopically, followed by LASGB (24 %), VBG (5.4 %), and BPD (4.9 %) [6]. Apart from differences in obesity prevalence, the United States and Europe also differ in their choices of bariatric procedure. In the United States, gastric bypass is regarded as the first-line treatment for morbid obesity and represents more than 80–90 % of the surgical procedures [38]. In Europe, (L)ASGB is the preferred method. In France, for example, three types of surgical procedure cover 97 % of all procedures: VBG (7 %), RYGB (13.8 %), and (L)ASGB (76.9 %) [39].

Jejunoileal bypass (JIB). Bariatric surgery was first performed in 1954 with the introduction of the jejunoileal bypass by Kremen. Nearly a decade later, Payne and DeWind popularized the procedure, which became the mainstay for the surgical treatment of obesity for nearly two decades (**Fig. 18.3**). The jejunoileal bypass incorporates approximately 35 cm of jejunum anastomosed end-to-side to the terminal 10 cm of ileum. The remainder of the small intestine, with a blindly closed jejunal end, was separated from the food circuit. The jejunoileal bypass fell out of favor because of an unacceptable incidence of complications such as nephrolithiasis, renal insufficiency, cirrhosis, acute liver failure, and immune complex arthritis, mainly as a result of endotoxemia and bacterial overgrowth in the bypassed segment of intestine. The jejunoileal bypass has been largely abandoned since 1978.

Gastric bypass. The first gastric bypass was reported in 1967 by Mason and Ito. It combined the creation of a small gastric pouch with bypassing the remainder of the stomach, duodenum, and a portion of the upper small intestine using a side-to-side loop gastrojejunostomy. Additional modification due to severe alkaline reflux resulted in the Roux-en-Y gastric bypass (RYGB), an operation that is now common, which involves stapling the upper stomach into a small proximal 15–30-mL pouch along the lesser curvature, attached to the jejunum through a narrow (11-mm) anastomosis (stoma) (**Fig. 18.4**). The remainder of the stomach, duodenum, and a small part of the jejunum are anastomosed to the jejunum via a jejunojejunostomy. The Roux limb is the alimentary limb, which is attached to the stomach; the biliopancreatic limb is the tract through which the bile and pancreatic juices drain; and the common channel is the tract in which food is absorbed when mixed with the digestive juices—i.e., between the jejunojejunostomy and the ileocecal valve. To avoid gastrogastric fistula formation between the stapled portions of the stomach and to prevent gastric pouch dilation, the gastric bypass has been further modified to form a transected vertical banded gastric bypass with jejunal interposition, with a Silastic ring placed around the gastric pouch [40]. In most procedures, the biliopancreatic limb is 35–75 cm long; in the standard Roux-en-Y, the Roux limb is 75 cm long, and in the long-limb gastric bypass it is 150 cm. In a distal gastric bypass, the common channel is shortened, causing significantly greater weight loss but at the expense of nutritional deficiencies due to malabsorption. The RYGB procedure generates weight loss by limiting gastric capacity, causing mild malabsorption, causing dumping syndrome symptoms when high-calorie sweet foods are consumed, and inducing hormonal changes.

Gastroplasty. With the development of surgical staples came the introduction of gastroplasty procedures. In the early procedures, the upper portion of the stomach was stapled into a small gastric pouch with a narrow outlet (stoma) to the remaining distal stomach. The small pouch limited the size of the meal and induced early satiety; the narrow stoma delayed the emptying of the pouch into the distal stomach, thereby prolonging satiety after a small meal had been consumed. Early types of gastroplasty included the Pace–Carey gastroplasty, with the stoma in the middle of the horizontally applied staple line, and the horizontal greater-curvature Gomez gastroplasty, with a stoma at the greater curvature. These procedures were prone to staple-line breakdown or stoma enlargement and were modified by Mason in 1982 to form the vertical banded gastroplasty (VBG) (**Fig. 18.5**). A transgastric window is made 6–8 cm below the His angle using a circular stapler, and a linear stapler is placed to create a pouch of 30 mL. The narrow outlet of 10–11 mm is surrounded by a nondistensible collar of polypropylene mesh or polytetrafluoroethylene (PTFE), or a silicone ring (vertical ring gastroplasty), to avoid enlargement. The horizontal gastroplasty has been abandoned since the early 1980s.

Gastric banding was developed as an alternative to gastric stapling in the 1970s. Tight gastric bands around the upper stomach, creating small proximal pouches, functioned in a very similar fashion to the VBG. Significant complications related to the band included band migration, band erosion, and pouch dilation. In the late 1980s, gastric banding was rejuvenated with the introduction of the adjustable silicone gastric band (ASGB) by Kuzmak, implanted through laparotomy and followed in 1993 by a modified version of the gastric band that could be inserted laparoscopically (LASBG) (**Fig. 18.6**). The band is positioned on the upper stomach, just below the esophagogastric junction, where it acts to limit food intake by constricting the stomach. The upper chamber is a 15–20-mL gastric pouch. The band is connected to a reservoir by a thin tube. The reservoir is fixed below the skin on the abdominal wall. The band can be tightened by injecting saline into the reservoir, which fills the inner expandable band, and loosened by withdrawing saline. Further refinement of the method to avoid band slippage, pouch dilation, and band erosion, involves constructing a very small pouch (15 mL, or a "virtual" pouch) and the placement of the band in a suprabursal position (i.e., through the hepatogastric ligament; the "pars flaccida" technique) instead of through the lesser sac (the "perigastric" technique). Finally, seromuscular gastrogastric sutures on the anterior side of the stomach prevent slipping of the band [41]. The principles underlying the two bands that are available differ; the Swedish Adjustable Gastric Band (Obtech, Ethicon Endosurgery, Cincinnati, Ohio) is a low-pressure, high-volume band whereas the Lapband (Inamed, Allergan, Santa Barbara, California) is a high-pressure, low-volume band [42,43].

Biliopancreatic diversion (BPD), developed by Scopinaro in 1979, differs from the jejunoileal bypass in that it lacks the blind intestinal segment, thus avoiding the consequences of bacterial overgrowth. After an 80–90% partial gastrectomy has been carried out, the ileum is divided at 250 cm from the ileocecal valve and the end of this distal ileal segment (the alimentary limb) is anastomosed to the gastric remnant (**Fig. 18.7**). The duodenum, jejunum, and proximal ileum (the biliopancreatic limb) is anastomosed to the terminal

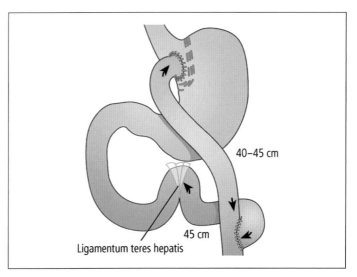

Fig. 18.4 Roux-en-Y gastric bypass: creation of a 15–30-mL gastric pouch, which is attached to the jejunum by a narrow 11-mm stoma while bypassing the remainder of the stomach, duodenum, and proximal jejunum. (Reproduced by permission from Int J Gastroenterol 2000;5:8–11.)

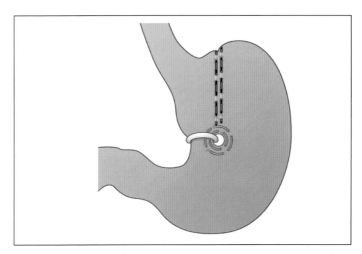

Fig. 18.5 Vertical banded gastroplasty. (Reproduced by permission from Int J Gastroenterol 2000;5.2:8–11.) A transgastric window is made 6–8 cm below the angle of His by a circular stapler, and a linear stapler is placed from the angle to His to the window to create a pouch of 30 mL, reinforced by a Silastic ring or a polypropylene mesh collar.

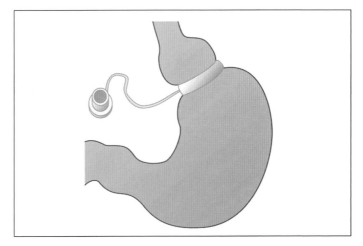

Fig. 18.6 Adjustable silicone gastric banding, with the inner inflatable silicone balloon connected by tubing to a reservoir. The band is positioned just below the esophagogastric junction to create a very small 15-mL or "virtual" pouch. (Reproduced by permission from Int J Gastroenterol 2000;5:8–11.)

18

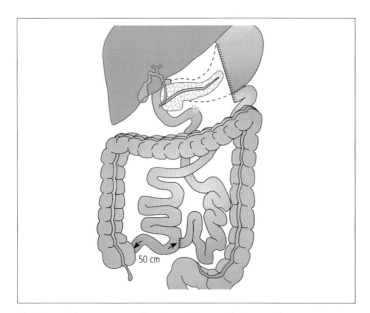

Fig. 18.7 Biliopancreatic diversion (Scopinaro). A partial gastrectomy is performed, and the ileum is divided at 250 cm from the ileocecal valve. The distal end of the transected ileum is anastomosed to the gastric remnant. The duodenum, jejunum, and remaining part of the ileum are anastomosed to the terminal ileum at a distance of 50–100 cm from the ileocecal valve. (Reproduced by permission from Int J Gastroenterol 2000;5:8–11.)

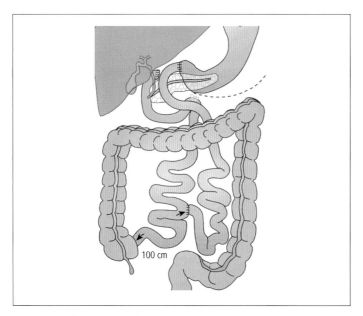

Fig. 18.8 Biliopancreatic diversion with duodenal switch. This operation involves a sleeve gastrectomy of the stomach, leaving the antrum and pylorus intact. The ileum is transected at 250 cm from the ileocecal valve. The distal end of the transected ileum is anastomosed to the duodenum, and the remainder of the duodenum, jejunum, and proximal part of the ileum are anastomosed to the terminal ileum at a distance of 100 cm from the ileocecal valve. (Reproduced by permission from Int J Gastroenterol 2000;5:8–11.)

ileum approximately 50–100 cm from the ileocecal valve, to create a common channel. The partial gastrectomy is thought to initiate weight loss as a result of nutrient restriction; the intestinal bypass is thought to maintain long-term weight loss. The most serious complications include protein-energy malnutrition, severe vitamin deficiency, and bone demineralization. Some of these complications have been reduced by extending the length of the common channel. The biliopancreatic diversion with duodenal switch (BPD-DS) involves a sleeve gastrectomy of the greater curvature of the stomach,

leaving the antrum pump and pyloric sleeve intact (**Fig. 18.8**). The ileum is anastomosed to the duodenum, and the remainder of the duodenum, jejunum, and ileum is anastomosed to the distal ileum. The antrum, pylorus, and bulb of the duodenum remain in continuity with the alimentary stream, thereby reducing the incidence of stomal ulceration and dumping.

Laparoscopy. Finally, the laparoscopic method is increasingly being used, with numerous advantages such as reduced postoperative pain, shorter hospitalization times, decreased impairment due to pulmonary complications, quicker recovery, reduced parameters of systemic injury, and a dramatic reduction in the frequency of wound infections and delayed ventral hernias [7,44].

Role of Endoscopy

The surgical options and the benefits of them are evident from six systemic reviews and meta-analyses [3,7,45–48] and two prospective longitudinal series [8,49]. Adverse effects on digestive symptoms are to be expected (RR 1.48; 95 % CI, 1.42 to 1.78) [8,50].

The common indications for endoscopy include the evaluation of symptoms, the management of a complication, and the evaluation of failure of weight loss [51,52]. The endoscopist should discuss the bariatric operation with the patient's surgeon, review the formal surgical report and perioperative records, review all available postoperative abdominal imaging studies, select the most appropriate type of endoscope and accessories needed, and recognize that specially designed accessories may be necessary [52,53].

Normal Endoscopic Findings

Laparoscopic adjustable silicone gastric banding. With a "virtual" pouch, no pouch at all can be visualized. The endoscopic appearance is that of an elongated cardia [54]. When the pouch volume is 15–60 mL, there is a visible separation between the impression made by the band and the cardia, and the distance between the cardia and the band is less than 3 cm. Sometimes some resistance can be met during introduction of the endoscope. In retroflexion, the band produces a bulging rosette encircling the endoscope (**Fig. 18.9**).

Horizontal gastroplasty and vertical banded gastroplasty. The endoscopist should read the surgical report to ascertain the location of the stoma in a horizontal gastroplasty. Because of the peculiar orientation of the greater curvature channel, it is sometimes difficult to negotiate the endoscope through the channel.

A normal appearance in vertical banded gastroplasty (VBG) consists of a clean gastric channel 6–8 cm long, with a rosette at 46.6 cm from the incisors and snug passage of an 11-mm scope without difficulty. The outlet of the VBG is formed by a calibrated channel (around a 32-Fr tube) and an externally restricted 5.0-cm outlet, 1.5 cm high. The internal diameter may vary due to the inherent thickness of the gastric wall and the amount of stomach wall puckered by the annular mesh band. Retroflexion of the tip of the endoscope in the distal stomach allows inspection of the caudal aspect of the staple-line partition and the remainder of the gastric fundus. As the endoscope passes the esophagogastric junction, the gastric channel should be clearly in view directly ahead of the end of the endoscope. It should not be necessary to angle the endoscope in any way to find the opening. If this is the case, the channel is angulated [55].

Roux-en-Y gastric bypass. The normal gastric pouch is small, so minimal air should be insufflated. Special attention should be paid to the gastrojejunostomy, which normally has a stoma measuring 10–12 mm in diameter. Being an end-to-side anastomosis, it gives the endoscopist a double-barrel view. There is typically a short

IV

(1–2 cm) blind limb of jejunum just distal to the gastrojejunostomy in addition to the Roux limb, which may be perforated easily by too much pressure by the endoscope or by wires and balloons [53,56]. The afferent biliopancreatic limb is outside the reach of a normal endoscope. For the construction of the gastrojejunostomy, a circular or linear stapler is used and staples can be recognized; hand-sewn anastomoses with absorbable sutures retain their tensile strength for about 4–6 weeks after surgery. Endoscopists should be aware of variation such as the loop gastrojejunostomy, which was part of the original gastric bypass procedure; here, the afferent limb can often be negotiated to search the proximal duodenum and distal stomach.

Biliopancreatic diversion and duodenal switch. In the biliopancreatic diversion, a larger (200 mL) gastric remnant is present, which is anastomosed end-to-side to the ileum, giving a double-barrel view when examined through the gastric lumen. In the BPD-DS, the stomach is a tube-like structure without the usual findings of a fundic pouch (**Fig. 18.10**). The pylorus is intact and the duodenum is stapled end-to-end to the ileum. After both operations, the biliopancreatic limb is beyond the reach of the endoscope.

Reported Complications

In general terms, the most common indications for endoscopy in bariatric surgical patients are for evaluation of symptoms, as many of the complications and side effects of weight-loss procedures are gastrointestinal and related to alterations in the gastrointestinal tract [8,57]. Monteforte and Turkelson reviewed 3568 restrictive procedures and 3626 gastric bypasses and reported vomiting after 8.5% of restrictive procedures and 2.6% of bypass procedures, whereas dumping was present after 0.28% and 14.6%, respectively [45]. In the restrictive procedures, the four most common major complications included gastric pouch/stoma dilation (2.4%), stoma stenosis/gastric outlet obstruction (2.2%), staple-line failure (1.5%), and stomach erosion/ulcer (1.2%; 0.56% of these were band erosions). The figures for gastric bypass were 0.47%, 2.7%, 5.9%, and 1.2% (with 0.06% band erosions), respectively. Chapman et al. studied in more detail the complications of LASGB in 64 studies and of RYGB and VBG in 57 studies [46]. They found that the reported rates were underestimates, as not every study that reported complications included all complications (**Table 18.3**) [46]. The most common complications related to LASGB were pouch dilation, displacement of the band, port rotation/movement, catheter/tube problems, band erosion, and infection of the band/reservoir. The most common complications of VBG were staple-line disruption, stomal stenosis, occluded/kinked stoma, failure to lose weight, gastrogastric fistula, enlarged stoma, band erosion, and anastomotic/gastric leak. The most common complications associated with RYGB were stenosis of the pouch outlet, marginal ulcer/ulcer disease, staple-line disruption, cholelithiasis, and small-bowel obstruction/necrosis. Vomiting and food intolerance showed a broad range of rates, with LASGB rates varying from 0% up to 60%, those for VBG ranging from 0.8% up to 76.5%, and those for RYGB from 4.7% up to 68.8%. In a meta-analysis of 128 studies reporting complications, Maggard et al. reported anastomotic leaks in 2.2% of RYGBs, 1.0% of VBGs, and 1.8% of BPDs [7]. Anastomotic/stomal stenosis was present in 4.6% of RYBGs and 6% of VBGs. Gastrointestinal symptoms were reported as adverse events in 16.9% of RYGB patients, 17.5% of VBG patients, 7.8% of LASGB pa-

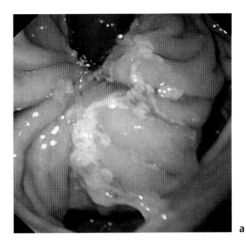

a

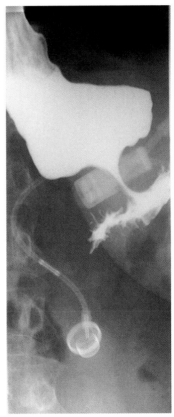
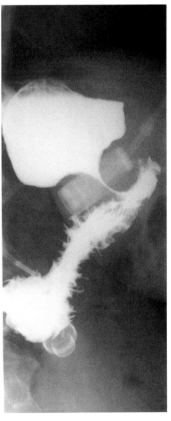

b

Fig. 18.9 Gastric banding.
a The normal appearance of a gastric band. In retroflexion, the band produces a bulging rosette encircling the endoscope.
b An excessively tight band, with gastric pouch dilation and esophageal dilation above the band. After 1 h, a small streak of contrast passing the band is seen. The tubing and the reservoir are also visible.

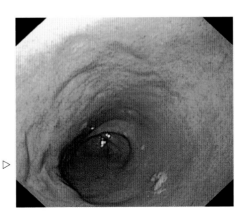

Fig. 18.10 The normal appearance of a gastric sleeve. The stomach is a ▷ tubular structure without the presence of a fundic pouch. (Reproduced courtesy of J.M. Jansen and M.L. van Ierland-van Leeuwen, Onze Lieve Vrouwe Gasthuis, Amsterdam, Netherlands.)

Table 18.3 Specific complications across 64 studies reporting complications for laparoscopic adjustable silicone gastric banding (LASGB) and 57 studies reporting complications for Roux-en-Y gastric bypass (RYGB) and vertical banded gastroplasty (VBG). Only the most prevalent gastrointestinal complications are mentioned in numbers and percentages [46].

Complications	LASGB (n = 8504)		VBG (n = 3849)		RYGB (n = 9413)	
	n	%	n	%	n	%
Total mortality	13	0.22	22	0.77	91	0.98
Morbidity (median %)		10.7		23.6		27.4
Stoma stenosis	10	0.12	76	1.97	448	4.76
Marginal ulcer/ulcer	1	0.01	5	0.13	386	4.10
Dilation	338	3.97	12	0.31	–	–
Staple-line disruption			113	2.94	229	2.43
Occluded/ kinked stoma	12	0.14	69	1.79	11	0.12
Cholelithiasis	16	0.19	6	0.16	164	1.74
Clinical failure	–	–	66	1.71	3	0.03
Displacement of band	138	1.62	–	–	–	–
Gastrogastric fistula			53	1.38	24	0.25
Esophagitis	12	0.14	43	1.12	9	0.10
Small bowel obstruction/ necrosis			1	0.03	99	1.05
Gastritis	1	0.01	8	0.21	89	0.95
Port rotation/ movement	74	0.87	–	–	–	–
Enlarged stoma			31	0.81	2	0.02
Tubing problems	68	0.80	–	–	–	–
Band erosion	50	0.59	10	0.26	6	0.06
Anastomotic/ gastric leak	–	–	12	0.31	36	0.38
Infection band/ reservoir Iatrogenic morbidity	31	0.36	2	0.05	–	–
Gastric perforation/ injury	68	0.80	6	0.16		
Splenic injury/ splenectomy			7	0.18	26	0.35

tients, and 37.7 % of BPD patients. Reflux was reported by 10.9 % of RYGB patients, 2.2 % of VBG patients, and 4.7 % of LASGB patients.

Endoscopic Findings and Therapy in the Early Postoperative Period

In the immediate postoperative period, it is unusual for patients to need endoscopy. A gastrointestinal leak or fistula, acute gastrointestinal hemorrhage, and early postoperative obstructive symptoms may be exceptions to the rule.

Gastrointestinal Leaks

Gastrointestinal leak is an early postoperative and often life-threatening complication [58]. Subtle signs such as unexplained tachycardia, tachypnea, dyspnea, increased fluid requirements, and the patient's feeling of impending doom are frequently the only warning of an intra-abdominal leak and may be confused with pulmonary embolism [58,59]. Emergency surgery is justified if the patient appears to be deteriorating, if the suspicion of a leak is high, and if a leak is detected [59,60].

If a leak is detected or large anastomotic leaks persist, an alternative treatment modality could be to bypass the leak endoscopically—a treatment that has been reported to be effective in Boerhaave's syndrome and in traumatic or anastomotic leaks in the esophagus [61–63]. Eisendrath et al. treated 21 patients endoscopically with partially covered nitinol self-expanding metal stents (SEMS), which are soft and most effective for closure of fistulas,

especially in the absence of associated strictures [64]. Development of tissue hyperplasia at both ends minimizes the risk of migration and should increase watertightness. On the other hand, hyperplasia makes removal difficult. Placement of self-expanding plastic stents (SEPS) inside SEMS can induce pressure necrosis in this hyperplasia, allowing subsequent removal of the stent. SEMS insertion led to primary closure in 62 % of cases (13 of 21). Complementary endoscopic treatment of sealant insertion (biological fibrin glue), surgical tissue adhesive injection (N-butyl-2-cyanonacrylate), or fistula bioprosthetic plug (Surgisis, an acellular matrix from porcine submucosa) and clip placement after stent removal led to four secondary closures, with a total success rate of 81 % (17 of 21). After stent insertion, 30 % of the patients reported transient thoracic pain, probably related to an inflammatory reaction due to expansion of the stent. Patients in whom the procedure was unsuccessful died. Endoscopic insertion of strips of Surgisis has been shown to be successful in the closure of 71 % (five of 7) and 92 % (12 of 13) of refractory esophagogastric fistulas that developed after bariatric surgery [65,66]. Successful closure of fistulas with fibrin sealant has also been reported [67].

Gastrointestinal Hemorrhage

Another emergency is an acute gastrointestinal hemorrhage [53]. Early gastrointestinal bleeding postoperatively usually arises from the staple lines of the gastrojejunostomy, gastric remnant, gastric pouch, or jejunojejunostomy, but peptic ulcer bleeding from the stomach or duodenum has to be considered as well. Some have advised against using therapeutic endoscopy in the acute setting,

IV

given the risk associated with early postoperative endoscopy, the risk of perforation at the surgical anastomosis, and the inaccessibility of the excluded stomach, duodenum, and jejunojejunostomy in case of RYGB.

Early Obstructive Symptoms

Signs of early postoperative obstruction may involve the jejunal Roux limb. At endoscopy, a normal-appearing gastrojejunostomy is recognized with a proximally dilated jejunum, which then leads to a stricture. Early dysphagia can also be caused by rotation of the limb inadvertently performed during surgery. The rotational stricture is visible. Both need surgical correction. Early obstruction of the gastroenterostomy is mainly caused by postoperative edema and should not be an indication for endoscopic dilation but should be managed by replacement of the nasogastric drain. If conservative treatment fails, early balloon dilation to a maximum of 12 mm may temporarily relieve the dysphagia.

▓ Endoscopic Findings and Therapy in the Late Postoperative Period and Follow-Up [51,53,57–59,68,69]

Nausea and vomiting are extremely common after bariatric surgery. A history should be taken regarding the types of food associated with vomiting, the amount of food eaten, the time over which the food is eaten, the consistency of the food and the extent to which it is chewed, and whether liquids were drunk immediately after eating solid food. Certain types of food such as red meat, sometimes poultry, and foods that tend to clump together after being chewed, such as fried or scrambled eggs and bread, are not tolerated by most patients. Another frequent cause of emesis is overfilling of the pouch with a large volume of food or drinking liquids immediately after eating certain solids. The addition of liquids results in acute overdistension of the pouch, which temporary blocks the outlet. Providing information and advice about eating behavior is of primary importance for prevention of vomiting [50].

Acute onset of vomiting is frequently due to ingestion of something that acts acutely to obstruct the outlet, such as uncooked beans, cherry stones, unpopped popcorn, or foreign material (bezoar). Endoscopy is expected to retrieve or push down the obstructing item, or to institute treatment to remove the bezoar. In the case of acute and repeated vomiting, as in viral gastroenteritis, the resulting edema and inability to tolerate solid foods may require a liquid diet for 4–7 days. Vomiting can also be associated with gallstones.

Vomiting after *gastric restrictive operations* can be related to gastric prolapse or pouch slippage superiorly through the band, producing obstruction at the band; a too tightly closed gastric band; a malpositioned gastric band; the erosion of the prosthetic material or the gastric band; a pouch dilation that "hangs over" and thereby obstructs the stoma; or angulation or kinking of the outlet. Chronic vomiting with stable weight or weight gain may suggest persistent pouch dilation. If there is an inflated gastric band, it should be deflated (**Fig. 18.9 b**).

Vomiting after Roux-en-Y *gastric bypass* (RYGB) and *BPD* can be due to anastomotic ulceration, stomal stenosis, erosion of the band in vertical banded gastric bypass, obstruction of the Roux limb, or partial or complete obstruction of the small bowel by adhesions or internal herniation. Patients with stomal stenosis will present with epigastric pain and vomiting of undigested food, followed by vomiting of liquids. Many of these patients will require dilation or surgery. Anastomotic ulceration may be treated with proton-pump inhibitors (PPIs), sucralfate, and *Helicobacter pylori* eradication. Nausea and vomiting can be symptoms of the dumping syndrome. Dumping is precipitated by ingestion of food and liquids with high sugar content, which enters immediately into the small bowel because of the reduced size of the stomach. Dumping syndrome can be seen in patients who are not compliant with their diet. It is common in the early postoperative period and subsides within 12–18 months after surgery. Prevention includes consumption of small, frequent meals, avoidance of foods with high sugar content, eating and drinking slowly, chewing food thoroughly, and drinking liquids between meals.

Delayed gastric emptying, inherently present or after surgical injury to the vagus nerves to the stomach, may become manifest as vomiting. Prokinetics may be tried.

Heartburn, reflux, epigastric or retrosternal pain, suggestive of gastroesophageal reflux, is often caused by an excessively tight band, gastric prolapse, pouch dilation, excessive eating with overfilling of the pouch, and gastric emptying disturbances in case of *gastric restrictive operations*, by stomal stenosis in *RYGB and BPD*, and by alkaline reflux in the presence of a *loop gastric bypass*.

Diarrhea can be multifactorial, due to the dumping syndrome, lactose intolerance, malabsorption, bacterial overgrowth and infection.

Constipation may be due to limited food, fiber, and fluid intake. Calcium and iron supplements can contribute.

Abdominal pain has many causes. In *gastric restrictive surgery*, the differential diagnosis includes gastric and duodenal ulcer, esophagitis, pouch outlet obstruction, gallstones, incisional hernia, abscess, or perforation at the site of the eroding band. A spontaneous disconnection between the tube and the port of the gastric band should be suspected in patients who report acute abdominal pain. After *gastric bypass surgery*, the afferent loop syndrome should be considered, sometimes with pancreatitis, efferent limb obstruction, anastomotic, stomal, or marginal ulcer (defined as an ulcer of the jejunal mucosa, near the gastrojejunostomy on the small-bowel side of the anastomosis), peptic ulcer in the bypassed stomach or duodenum, pouch outlet obstruction, incisional hernia, gallstones, and adhesions. Severe (crampy) abdominal pain and pain out of proportion to the physical examination suggest ischemia due to internal herniation or adhesions.

Hematemesis and melena suggest gastrointestinal bleeding, which may originate from the esophagus, gastric pouch, bypassed stomach and duodenum, gastrojejunostomy, or jejunojejunostomy [70]. Endoscopic accessibility will determine the therapeutic options for hemostasis, including epinephrine injection, cauterization with heater or gold probe, argon plasma coagulation, and hemoclipping.

Inadequate weight loss or weight gain may be the result of a large proximal pouch or erosion of the band with a loss of its restrictive function in LASGB; staple-line disruption with a gastrogastric fistula in VBG and RYGB; or an enlarged stoma in RYGB.

Endoscopic Therapeutic Interventions

Many of the above complications can either be diagnosed or therapeutically managed by endoscopy. Appropriate diagnosis and medical treatment is important in the case of marginal ulceration in RYGB and gastroesophageal reflux in VBG and LASGB. Whereas an increased gastric cancer risk in bariatric surgery has not been substantiated, the increased risk for reflux esophagitis (OR 1.94; 95 % CI, 1.47 to 2.57) and esophageal adenocarcinoma (OR 2.78; 95 % CI, 1.85 to 4.16) in the obese population per se is of concern [71]. So far, one adenocarcinoma in an area of Barrett's mucosa has been described in LASGB [72]. Näslund et al. found that Barrett's esophagus had developed in six of 140 patients (4.3 %), without clear symptoms and

18

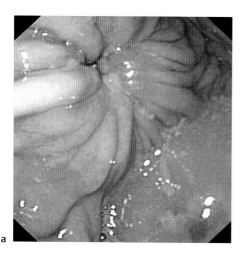

a

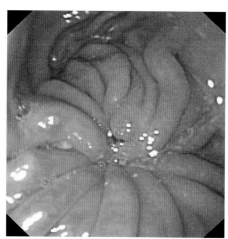

b

Fig. 18.11 a, b A clearly oversized, asymmetrical pouch due to the band slipping downward or slippage of the gastric wall upward.

despite the use of acid-reducing drugs, after 9 years' follow-up, with a slight difference in the risk of developing postoperative Barrett's esophagus (4 % in gastric banding, 0.5 % in VBG) [73]. Current series of LASGB are limited to 15 years of follow-up. Longer-term follow-up is needed to further define whether there will be an increased incidence of Barrett's mucosa or esophageal carcinoma in LASGB patients. Therapeutic interventions are discussed in more detail in this section.

Stomal Stenosis and Stoma/Outlet Obstruction

LASGB

Stoma obstruction is defined as an obstruction to the flow of food from the gastric pouch to the remainder of the stomach. Stoma obstruction in the *early* postoperative period has a number of causes. Stoma obstruction is usually caused by incorporation of too much tissue inside the band, or is associated with small bands applied over a thick gastrointestinal junction area [41]. In some cases, the band is positioned too distally, causing a large amount of fundus and stomach wall to be encompassed by the band. Early stoma obstruction also can be initiated by postoperative edema of the area incorporated by the band, or due to hematoma or postoperative reaction. The lumen can also be obstructed by insufficiently chewed food, pills, or stones; endoscopy can remove the items causing this.

Late stoma obstructions are usually related either to gastric pouch dilation, prolapse, or band erosion. Several terms (band slippage, slippage of the gastric wall, pouch slippage, gastric prolapse, pouch dilation) are used to describe what are ultimately similar findings, although with different etiologies—the postoperative development of an overly large upper gastric pouch that is characterized by food intolerance, epigastric pain, and reflux [41]. The size of the pouch can be estimated at endoscopy [54]. If the distance between the band and the cardia is 3–5 cm, the volume is approximately 60–100 mL; if the distance to the cardia is more than 5 cm and the pouch is large but symmetric, the volume is approximately 100–200 mL. A clearly oversized pouch is usually asymmetric (**Fig. 18.11**). Prolapse should be considered when patients who had a normal postoperative period begin to experience changes in their eating ability—e. g., an increase in the sense of restriction or obstruction. Gastric pouch dilation is due to overinflation of the band, combined with failure to comply with instructions regarding oral intake (**Fig. 18.9 b**) [74]. One cause of pouch dilation is excessive vomiting due to overeating and ingestion of sparkling drinks [75]. The first action should be to deflate the band, decompress the

stomach, give intravenous hydration as needed, and determine whether the patient can swallow liquids.

A matter of serious concern here is ischemia of the stomach or necrosis of the occluded tissue in case of an overtight band. True prolapse, as opposed to gastric pouch dilation, usually does not respond to conservative measures. The presence of a prolapse or gastric pouch dilation should be identified using an upper gastrointestinal barium study, which reveals the presence of a clearly dilated pouch with an "overhanging wall" relative to the band (**Fig. 18.12 a, b**) [76]. The endoscopist will find a relatively large pouch with no pouch outlet, and during air insufflation the pouch dilation will temporarily increase and occlude the outlet even more (**Fig. 18.12 c, d**). A word of caution is appropriate here: symptoms may be caused by an excessively tight band, and endoscopy in this setting may lead to perforation. Endoscopy should be performed if symptoms persist after band deflation.

VBG

In studies that have investigated the yield of endoscopy, 14 % of patients (28 of 199) were treated for food impaction or a bezoar [77–81]. Bezoars are a rare complication resulting from poor mastication, eating quickly, and stasis in the achlorhydric channel. They can be dissolved by sipping a half teaspoon of meat tenderizer (containing the proteolytic enzyme papain) in 250 mL of liquid, or can be extracted or fragmented during endoscopy [79].

Stenosis of the stoma has to be divided into the immediate postoperative, early postoperative (< 3 months), and late postoperative (> 3 months) periods, as edema or edema with early scar formation respond well to dilation and the outcome in late scarring is rather poor. Stomal obstruction in the initial postoperative period has been simply solved by waiting to see whether the stomal edema and swelling subside after replacement of a nasogastric tube [82]. Stenosis occurring later is believed to result from fibrosis or an inflammatory reaction occurring around the band (**Fig. 18.13**) [83]. If dilation becomes necessary, Eder–Puestow olive–tipped dilators and flexible polyvinyl tapered bougies (of the Savary–Gilliard type) have been used. Both are passed over a previously inserted guide wire; the plastic dilators allow longer, less traumatic stretching of the stoma. Fluoroscopy-guided balloons and endoscopic balloons have been used as well. Success rates vary from 85–88 % for the Eder–Puestow method and 46–68 % for the Savary–Gilliard bougie to 50–60 % for (fluoroscopy-guided) balloon dilation [55,79,80,84–86]. Dilators larger than 12 mm do not enhance the chances of response, but may increase the risk of rupturing the gastric band, thus eliminating the weight loss potential. Torsion of

IV

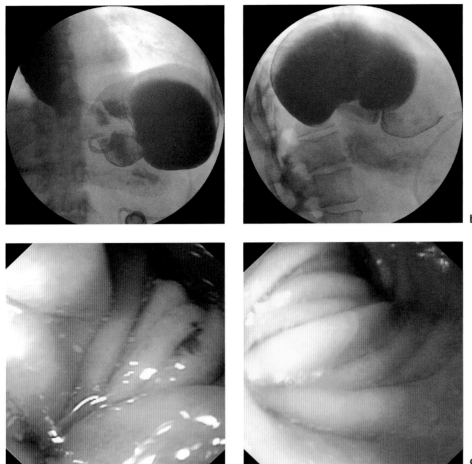

Fig. 18.12 Gastric prolapse or pouch dilation.
a, b Diagnosed by an upper gastrointestinal barium study. A clearly dilated pouch with an overhanging wall relative to the gastric band is seen.
c, d Diagnosed by upper gastrointestinal endoscopy. A relatively large pouch, with a barely visible pouch outlet that is impossible to pass.

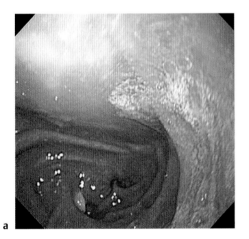
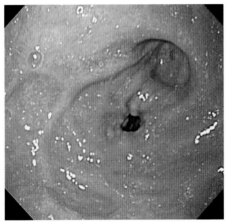

Fig. 18.13 a, b A vertical banded gastroplasty, with late stenosis of the stoma and pouch dilation and diverticular blow-out of the gastric wall.

the stoma or an angulated channel are predictive of failure. Outlet stenosis after VBG is evidently difficult to treat and often requires surgical intervention.

RYGB

In gastric bypass, the risk of stomal stenosis is highest in the first 2–3 months after surgery; thereafter, the risk declines dramatically to negligible levels by 8–10 months [87–90]. Dilation can be achieved by fluoroscopy-guided balloon dilation, with success rates of 50–60% [85,86]. Endoscopic dilation of stomal stenosis after bariatric surgery is safe, effective, and durable [53,57,91]. It can be performed successfully by several methods, including controlled radial expansion (CRE), through-the-scope (TTS) balloon dilation, and passage of dilators over a guide wire (Savary–Gilliard, Eder–Puestow). In gastric bypass surgery, mainly CRE balloons have been used (**Fig. 18.14**). Safe dilation was possible at the earliest 4 weeks after the operation [88,92]. In patients with stomal stenosis, endoscopic dilation can be attempted in the absence of ulceration at the stoma. If there is an ulcer, patients should be placed on an ulcer treatment regimen, as dilation of the stoma might cause a perforation [57,68].

The gastric pouch, which is small and extends just 5–7 cm from the Z-line, should be entered with the endoscope under continuous direct vision. If the stricture can be passed with a therapeutic endo-

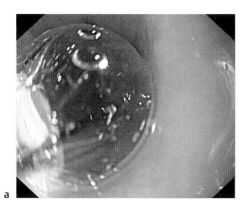

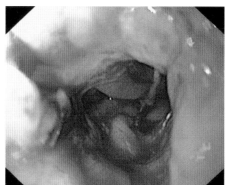

a

b

Fig. 18.14
a Through-the-scope controlled radial expansion (CRE) balloon dilation of a narrowed gastric bypass anastomosis. (Reproduced courtesy of J.M. Janssen and M.L. van Ierland-van Leeuwen, Onze Lieve Vrouwe Gasthuis, Amsterdam, Netherlands.)
b After balloon dilation, the endoscopist should evaluate the absence of ulceration distal to the stenosis. (Reproduced courtesy of J.M. Janssen and M.L. van Ierland-van Leeuwen, Onze Lieve Vrouwe Gasthuis, Amsterdam, Netherlands.)

scope (with a working channel of at least 2.8 mm), the balloon catheter is advanced via the working channel until the entire length of the balloon is in view. The endoscope and balloon are then withdrawn together until the balloon is in position for dilation. If the stricture cannot be passed with the endoscope, the endoscope is positioned above the stricture, and the balloon catheter is advanced until its tip freely cannulates the stricture. Next, it is slowly withdrawn into the stricture and inflated with water to its maximum pressure rating in three steps. Endoscopists should recognize that there is a short blind loop of jejunum beyond the gastrojejunostomy and should exercise caution when passing TTS balloon catheters through a tightly strictured stoma. In these conditions, some prefer cautious cannulation with the balloon guide wire first under fluoroscopy, followed by passing the balloon over the wire to prevent perforation.

The initial dilation should be only enough to accommodate an endoscope of 9–10 mm for evaluation, to ensure that there is no ulceration distal to the stenosis, which has to heal first before resuming the dilation [92]. The goal for the stomal diameter after dilation is 10–12 mm, up to a maximum of approximately 15 mm. Additional dilation should take account of the internal diameter of the encircling restrictive prosthetic band, with an additional margin for the thickness of the gastric wall, to prevent crushing the tissue within the band [57]. Dilation of a circular stapled anastomosis must be based on the internal diameter of the anastomosis, generally 7 mm smaller than the outside diameter of the circular stapler. In almost no case should dilation progress to dilators in excess of 15 mm diameter for fear of disrupting the anastomosis, resulting in leakage or progressive dilation and loss of restrictive function. Barba et al. recommended that all strictures should be dilated to at least 15 mm, as dilating to at least 15 mm decreased the chances of symptomatic recurrence [88]. If the scope was able to traverse the stricture, the latter was dilated to 18 mm. If a patient returned with recurrent symptoms and a stricture, dilation was always performed to 18 mm. This was confirmed by Ahmad et al., who mentioned that nearly 60% of patients had complete symptomatic resolution after a single balloon dilation session with a 15-mm balloon, suggesting that this size should be used initially; and by Peifer et al., who reported a significantly low rate of repeat endoscopic dilation of strictures dilated to at least 15 mm in comparison with those dilated to 12 mm or less [89,93]. Most patients require a single dilation; 5–10% of patients may require a second dilation, and a few may need three or more dilations.

Success rates have varied between 62.5% and 100% [87–90, 93–97]. The main concerns with dilation of the gastrojejunostomy are bleeding and perforation [92]. Perforation of the anastomosis is related to the size of the balloon and the amount of circular force exerted on the stricture, which is related to the initial narrowing and length of the stricture. Also, the tip of the balloon can perforate the jejunal Roux limb. Perforation can also be related to the timing of

the dilation after surgery. Schwartz et al. considered their outcomes unsatisfactory; they obtained a satisfactory result in only 62.5% (20 of 32); perforations occurred in four patients (12.5%), three of the four being at the first attempt, and eight patients (25%) required repeat surgery [96]. Perforations were reported infrequently by others groups, in 1.6–3.0% of cases [90,97,98]. Failure of dilation may be predicted in the presence of torsion or angulation of the stoma and marginal ulceration with edema [87,90,94].

Dilated Gastrojejunostomy after Gastric Bypass Surgery

Catalano et al. identified 28 patients with a dilated gastrojejunostomy during gastroscopy performed for symptoms of weight gain and increased volume tolerance [99]. Stimulated by the experience reported by Spaulding in eight patients, they performed sclerotherapy of the gastrojejunostomy with injections of sodium morrhuate, using a 25-gauge needle (1–2 mL per site) [100]. A total of one to three injection sessions were needed in an attempt to achieve a stoma diameter of 1.2 cm or smaller, which was obtained in 64.3% of cases. Twenty-one of the 28 patients (75%) had significant post-injection pain for the first 12–24 h. At the initial post-therapy endoscopy, 10 patients were noted to have shallow circumferential ulcers (36%). The presence of ulcer formation resulted in a higher rate of endotherapy success: the success rate was 80% (eight of 10) in comparison with 56% (10 of 18) in those without ulcers.

Staple-Line Dehiscence and Gastrogastric Fistula in VBG and RYGB

VBG

Weight gain and less restriction of food intake is the only symptom of staple-line disruption in VBG. The endoscopist will see two entrances to the stomach, but usually diagnosis is made by a barium swallow, which reveals the gastrogastric fistula.

RYGB

After staple-line failure, a leak develops with an abscess, which then drains into the distal stomach, forming the gastrogastric fistula—a communication between the proximal gastric pouch and the distal gastric remnant [101]. Early symptoms may mimic those of a perforation, including fever, tachycardia, abdominal pain, tachypnea, and shoulder pain. Failure to lose weight and a marginal ulcer are late clinical signs. At endoscopy, dehiscences are frequently small and easily overlooked and they may have an endoscopic appearance

IV

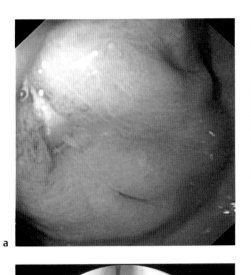

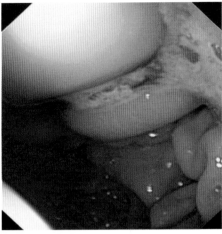

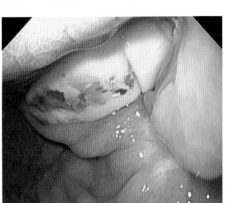

Fig. 18.15 Band erosion.
a At an early stage, with the whitish band merely visible.
b A large part of the band has eroded into the lumen and is discolored by bile. A pressure ulcer is visible underneath the band.
c The diagnosis of band erosion can sometimes be made on a plain abdominal radiograph, where the band and a thickened gastric fold are outside the normal gastric contours.
d The buckle of the gastric band is visible. If the band is to be removed endoscopically, cutting of the band should be done at the thinnest part of it, which is at the left of the buckle in this case.

18

similar to that of a diverticulum. Large dehiscences are identified easily and may allow passage of the endoscope into the bypassed stomach and duodenum. Barium contrast radiography is the preferred initial study for detecting staple-line dehiscence [53]. Patients with a gastrogastric fistula are usually treated with a 6–8-week course of PPIs and then undergo repeat endoscopy. Failure to document improvement in the gastrogastric fistula after 3 months is an indication for surgical therapy or endoscopic injection of fibrin glue [102]. Thompson et al. achieved complete closure of a gastrogastric communication in six of eight patients with a combination of endoscopic suturing, hemoclips, and argon plasma coagulation [103].

Band Erosion

Intraluminal migration or intrusion, usually known as band erosion, is a complication that may be caused by a too tightly placed band, resulting in necrosis and erosion, or ischemia from pressure of the gastric banding, especially when inflated too tightly; suturing the band to the stomach; infection; foreign-body reaction; exaggerated stress on the upper gastric pouch by forced endoscopy, excessively large food boluses, or excessive vomiting; or gastric lesions caused by aspirin, NSAIDs, alcohol, or smoking.

(L)ASGB

Acute erosion is characterized by free leakage of gastric contents into the peritoneum, similar to the clinical picture of gastric perforation with peritonitis [41]. In chronic band erosion, the migration process of the band is very slow. It induces significant perigastric localized inflammation and a cicatricial response, and the band is finally engulfed by the stomach, where it is exposed to the gastric contents. Many patients are asymptomatic and present only with a nonfunctioning band, with no restriction to the flow of food. They may gain weight, and band adjustment has no effect. In many cases, the first indication of possible erosion is infection at the access port by means of the connecting tube [104]. At endoscopy, the band is visible in the stomach, whitish when it has recently penetrated and black when discolored by the influence of bile (**Fig. 18.15**). Often, the band erosion is only detected in retroflexion. The band can be removed by endoscopy. To enhance the degree of migration and allow safer removal without the risk of perforation, some have advocated increasing the filling volume of the band and awaiting a more complete intragastric band migration before an attempt is made to remove the band. After extraction of the port and the maximum length of catheter tubing through a cutaneous exploration, the band can be removed by endoscopy by using scissors and diathermy, or a laser technique, or by cutting the small bridge of tissue holding the device to the gastric wall with a papillotome or argon plasma coagulation [105–109]. The band is extracted with the help of a polypectomy snare.

Regusci et al. and Sakai et al. used the tourniquet technique to cut the band [110,111]. A metallic thread is passed through the biopsy channel of the endoscope, introduced around the migrated band, and retracted back with a grip to the mouth. The two ends of the metallic thread are then introduced into an external narrow metal tube or sheath and passed into the tourniquet of the handle of the AMI gastric band cutter device (Agency for Medical Innovation, Feldkirch, Austria) (**Fig. 18.16**) or a Soehendra biliary mechanical lithotriptor. The metal tube or sheath containing the metallic threads looped around the intragastric band is passed through the esophagus to the stomach. By twisting the handle, the band is cut

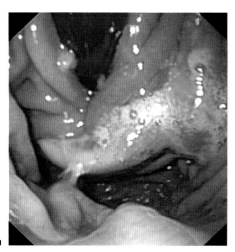
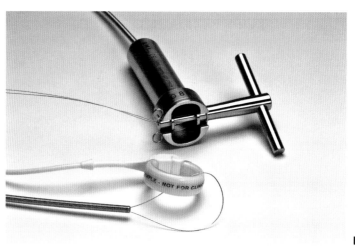

a
b

Fig. 18.16
a A gastric band that has eroded with its entire thickness through the gastric wall, which can be removed with the gastric band cutter.
b The gastric band cutter (AMI, Feldkirch, Austria). The soft flexible end of the cutting wire is introduced through the instrumentation channel of the endoscope, turned around the visible migrated gastric band, grasped, and pulled out together with the endoscope. The two external ends are inserted into the lumen of an external flexible metal sheath, and this is gently pushed down into the stomach until it comes to a stop on the migrated gastric band. Both external ends of the cutting wire are inserted into the distal opening of the handle and inserted into the opening of the lever. The lever is properly positioned in the bearing of the handle and turned, pulling in the cutting wire into the flexible metal sheath and thus cutting and dissecting through the migrated gastric band.

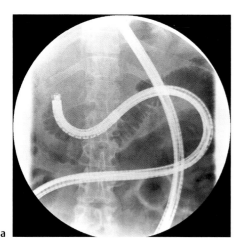
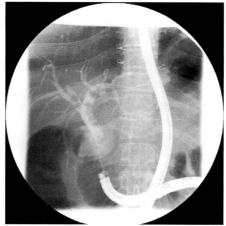

a
b

Fig. 18.17
a Successful retrograde endoscopy of bypassed segments with a pediatric colonoscope, in a patient with a Roux-en-Y gastric bypass. (Reproduced courtesy of B.L.A.M. Weusten, St. Antonius Ziekenhuis, Nieuwegein, Netherlands.)
b Successful bile duct cannulation and stone removal with a pediatric colonoscope, in a patient with a Roux-en-Y gastric bypass. (Reproduced courtesy of B.L.A.M. Weusten, St. Antonius Ziekenhuis, Nieuwegein, Netherlands.)

under direct vision by strangulation. A pneumoperitoneum, without evidence of esophageal or gastric perforation, complicated the procedure in only one of 14 patients (7.1%). Usually, the extensive tissue reaction prevents a gastric leak after removal of the band.

VBG

Generally, band erosions occur 1–3 years after surgery. An eroded Silastic ring can be removed by cutting the stay sutures that anchor it to the gastric wall. It is generally difficult to cut the ring itself. The Marlex mesh should be cut in two places as close to the gastric wall as possible. Endoscopic scissors are helpful for transecting and removing the Gortex band [112].

RYGB

Fobi et al. modified the gastric bypass to develop a transected vertical banded gastric bypass with jejunal interposition, with a Silastic ring band placed around the gastric pouch. Band erosion can be managed expectantly, by endoscopic band removal or open surgical intervention. Endoscopic band removal is the treatment of choice; 16 bands were removed without bleeding or leakage, eight patients had spontaneous extrusion of the band, and 26 required surgical revision [113].

▦ Endoscopic Access to the Bypassed Stomach and Duodenum and to the Papilla of Vater in RYGB

A need to examine the distal stomach arises when the patient reports epigastric or right upper quadrant pain, or when anemia with positive fecal guaiac occurs. The distal stomach and duodenum are not easily accessible for endoscopy because of the combined length of the esophagus (25 cm), proximal gastric pouch (5 cm), Roux limb (75–150 cm), biliopancreatic jejunal limb (35–70 cm), duodenum (20 cm), excluded stomach (10–15 cm)—with a total extent, therefore, in the range of 2–3 m. Retrograde endoscopy of the bypassed segments with a pediatric colonoscope was successful in 65% (33 of 51) [114] and 66% (45 of 68) of patients (**Fig. 18.17 a**) [115]. The most common reason for failure to enter the bypassed stomach was acute angulation at the jejunojejunostomy or ligament of Treitz and a gastroenterostomy that was too narrow for passage of the endoscope. It is occasionally difficult to determine at the jejunojejunostomy which of the two segments is the afferent limb.

When intubation fails, one may elect to construct a percutaneous gastrostomy and perform percutaneous endoscopy of the bypassed stomach after dilating the track [116]. Surgeons may tag the stomach to the anterior peritoneal wall and place radiopaque tubing during the Roux-en-Y procedure, to allow convenient radiologic localization for future percutaneous access [117]. A fairly new technology, the double-balloon endoscopy method—in which one balloon is attached to the tip of the endoscope and the other is at the distal end of the overtube, with repeated pushing and pulling maneuvers being used to straighten and shorten the bowel, allowing introduction well beyond the 2 m of the enteroscope—was carried out using the retrograde route, through the enteroenterostomy, via the duodenopancreatic limb up to the bypassed stomach. The excluded stomach was reached in a total of 40 of 46 cases (87%) [118,119].

Cholelithiasis occurs in 9–33% of patients after bariatric surgery, with symptomatic gallstones in approximately 10% of patients [57,58]. Endoscopic retrograde cholangiopancreatography (ERCP) in RYGB patients is an arduous task, but can be accomplished by several methods. Using an enteroscope or pediatric colonoscope, Elton et al. reported an 84% success rate in patients with a long-limb surgical bypass, including three RYGB patients (**Fig. 18.17 b**) [120]. Disadvantages of this technique were the lack of ERCP accessories of sufficient length compatible with the enteroscope, lack of an elevator, and the limitations of forward-viewing endoscopes in performing biliopancreatic therapy. Wright et al. described successful ERCP in six of 11 RYGB patients (55%) by advancing the duodenoscope under fluoroscopic evaluation over a stiff guide wire previously placed in the bypassed stomach with a forward-viewing endoscope, or pulling up the duodenoscope by means of a wire-guided biliary balloon anchored at the pylorus [121]. The main reason for failure was inability to advance the duodenoscope through the biliopancreatic limb to the region of the papilla. An alternative technique involves establishing percutaneous access to the bypassed stomach by means of a gastrostomy [122]. In BPD, the incidence of cholelithiasis is so high and the biliopancreatic limb is so far down the gastrointestinal tract that cholecystectomy forms part of the procedure.

Conclusions

The role of endoscopy in the treatment of obesity is rather limited. Today, only intragastric balloons are available, but surgical procedures via the endoscope are under development. More important roles for endoscopy lie in the evaluation of symptoms and failure to lose weight, as well as in managing complications after bariatric surgery. The endoscopist should discuss the operation with the bariatric surgeon and should be informed about the normal endoscopic appearance. In case of complications, he or she should consider the endoscopic treatment options and select the most appropriate type of endoscope and (specially designed) accessories.

References

1. World Health Organization. Obesity: preventing and managing the global epidemic. Report of a WHO Consultation on Obesity, Geneva, 3–5 June 1998. Geneva: World Health Organization, 1999 (Report no.: WHO/NUT/NCD/98.1, 1999).
2. National Institutes of Health, Heart, Lung and Blood Institutes. Clinical guidelines on the identification, evaluation, and treatment of overweight and obesity in adults—the evidence report. Obes Res 1998;6(Suppl 2):1–209 S.
3. Buchwald H, Avidor Y, Braunwald E, Jensen MD, Pories W, Fahrbach K, et al. Bariatric surgery: a systematic review and meta-analysis. JAMA 2004;292:1724–37.
4. Demaria EJ. Bariatric surgery for morbid obesity. N Engl J Med 2007;356:2176–83.
5. Deitel M, Melissas J. The origin of the word "bari." Obes Surg 2005;15:1005–8.
6. Buchwald H, Williams SE. Bariatric surgery worldwide 2003. Obes Surg 2004;14:1157–64.
7. Maggard MA, Shugarman LR, Suttorp M, Maglione M, Sugerman HJ, Livingston EH, et al. Meta-analysis: surgical treatment of obesity. Ann Intern Med 2005;142:547–59.
8. Christou NV, Sampalis JS, Liberman M, Look D, Auger S, McLean AP, et al. Surgery decreases long-term mortality, morbidity, and health care use in morbidly obese patients. Ann Surg 2004;240:416–23.
9. Mathus-Vliegen EMH. Gastric balloon revisited. Scientific Sessions Handouts, Digestive Disease Week, San Francisco, May 2002. p. 212–4.
10. Schapiro M, Benjamin S, Blackburn G, Frank B, Heber D, Kozarek R, et al. Obesity and the gastric balloon: a comprehensive workshop. Tarpon Springs, Florida, March 19–21, 1987. Gastrointest Endosc 1987;33:323–7.
11. [Editorial]. Who needs an intragastric balloon for weight reduction? Lancet 1988;ii:664.
12. Mathus-Vliegen EM, Tytgat GN. Intragastric balloons for morbid obesity: results, patient tolerance and balloon life span. Br J Surg 1990;77:76–9.
13. Mathus-Vliegen EM, Tytgat GN, Veldhuyzen-Offermans EA. Intragastric balloon in the treatment of super-morbid obesity. Double-blind, sham-controlled, crossover evaluation of 500-milliliter balloon. Gastroenterology 1990;99:362–9.
14. De Goederen-van der Meij S, Pierik RGJM, Oudkerk Pool M, Gouma DJ, Mathus-Vliegen LM. Six months of balloon treatment does not predict the success of gastric banding. Obes Surg 2007;17:88–94.
15. Hodson RM, Zacharoulis D, Goutzamani E, Slee P, Wood S, Wedgwood KR. Management of obesity with the new intragastric balloon. Obes Surg 2001;11:327–9.
16. Totté E, Hendrickx L, Pauwels M, Van Hee R. Weight reduction by means of intragastric device: experience with the BioEnterics intragastric balloon. Obes Surg 2001;11:519–23.
17. Sallet JA, Marchesini JB, Paiva DS, Komoto K, Pizani CE, Ribeiro ML, et al. Brazilian multicenter study of the intragastric balloon. Obes Surg 2004;14:991–8.
18. Roman S, Napoléon B, Mion F, Bory RM, Guyot P, D'Orazio H, et al. Intragastric balloon for "non-morbid" obesity: a retrospective evaluation of tolerance and efficacy. Obes Surg 2004;14:539–44.
19. Herve J, Wahlen CH, Schaeken A, Dallemagne B, Dewandre JM, Markiewicz S, et al. What becomes of patients one year after the intragastric balloon has been removed? Obes Surg 2005;15:864–70.
20. Doldi SB, Micheletto G, Di Prisco F, Zappa MA, Lattuada E, Reitano M. Intragastric balloon in obese patients. Obes Surg 2000;10:578–81.
21. Evans JD, Scott MH. Intragastric balloon in the treatment of patients with morbid obesity. Br J Surg 2001;88:1245–8.
22. Loffredo A, Cappuccio M, De Luca M, de Werra C, Galloro G, Naddeo M, et al. Three years experience with the new intragastric balloon, and a preoperative test for success with restrictive surgery. Obes Surg 2001;11:330–3.
23. Doldi SB, Micheletto G, Perrini MN, Librenti MC, Rella S. Treatment of morbid obesity with intragastric balloon in association with diet. Obes Surg 2002;12:583–7.
24. Al-Momen A, El-Mogy I. Intragastric balloon for obesity: a retrospective evaluation of tolerance and efficacy. Obes Surg 2005;15:101–5.
25. Weiner R, Gutberlet H, Bockhorn H. Preparation of extremely obese patients for laparoscopic gastric banding by gastric-balloon therapy. Obes Surg 1999;9:261–4.
26. Busetto L, Segato G, De Luca M, Bortolozzi E, MacCari T, Magon A, et al. Preoperative weight loss by intragastric balloon in super-obese patients treated with laparoscopic gastric banding: a case–control study. Obes Surg 2004;14:671–6.
27. Genco A, Bruni T, Doldi SB, Forestieri P, Marino M, Busetto L, et al. BioEnterics intragastric balloon: the Italian experience with 2,515 patients. Obes Surg 2005;15:1161–4.
28. Mathus-Vliegen EMH, Tytgat GNJ. Intragastric balloon for treatment-resistant obesity: safety, tolerance, and efficacy of 1-year balloon treatment followed by 1-year balloon-free follow-up. Gastrointest Endosc 2005;61:19–27.
29. Mathus-Vliegen EMH. Intragastric balloon treatment for obesity: what does it really offer? Dig Dis 2008;26:40–4.
30. Galloro G, De Palma GD, Catanzano C, De Luca M, de Werra C, Martinelli G, et al. Preliminary endoscopic technical report of a new silicone intragastric balloon in the treatment of morbid obesity. Obes Surg 1999;9:68–71.

18

31. Vandenplas Y, Bollen P, De Langhe K, Vandemaele K, De Schepper J. Intragastric balloons in adolescents with morbid obesity. Eur J Gastroenterol Hepatol 1999;11:243–5.

32. Genco A, Cipriano M, Bacci V, Cuzzolaro M, Materia A, Raparelli L, et al. BioEnterics Intragastric Balloon (BIB): a short-term, double-blind, randomised, controlled, crossover study on weight reduction in morbidly obese patients. Int J Obes (Lond) 2006;30:129–33.

33. Fernandes M, Atallah AN, Soares BG, Humberto S, Guimarães S, Matos D, et al. Intragastric balloon for obesity. Cochrane Database Syst Rev 2007;(1):CD004931.

34. Rodriguez-Grunert L, Neto MPG, Alamo M, Ramos AC, Baez PB, Tarnoff M. First human experience with endoscopically delivered and retrieved duodeno-jejunal bypass sleeve. Surg Obes Rel Dis 2008;4:55–59.

35. Hu B, Chung SCS, Sun LCL, Kawashima K, Yamamoto T, Cotton PB, et al. Transoral obesity surgery: endoluminal gastroplasty with an endoscopic suture device. Endoscopy 2005;37:411–414.

36. Devière J, Ojeda Valdes G, Cuevas Herrera L, Closset J, Le Moine O, Eisendrath P, et al. Safety, feasibility and weight loss after transoral gastroplasty: first human multicentre study. Surg Endosc 2008;22:589–98.

37. Moreno C, Closset J, Dugardeyn S, Baréa M, Mehdi A, Collignon L, et al. Transoral gastroplasty is safe, feasible, and induces significant weight loss in morbidly obese patients: results of the second human pilot study. Endoscopy 2008;40:406–13.

38. Demaria EJ, Jamal MK. Laparoscopic adjustable gastric banding: evolving clinical experience. Surg Clin North Am 2005;85:773–87.

39. Weber J, Azagra-Goergen M, Strock P, Azagra J. Endoscopy after bariatric surgery. Acta Endosc 2007;37:27–37.

40. Fobi MA, Lee H. The surgical technique of the Fobi-Pouch operation for obesity (the transected silastic vertical gastric bypass). Obes Surg 1998;8:283–8.

41. Spivak H, Favretti F. Avoiding postoperative complications with the LAP-BAND system. Am J Surg 2002;184(6B):31–7 S.

42. Fried M, Miller K, Kormanova K. Literature review of comparative studies of complications with Swedish band and Lap-Band. Obes Surg 2004;14:256–60.

43. Gravante G, Araco A, Araco F, Delogu D, De Lorenzo A, Cervelli V. Laparoscopic adjustable gastric bandings: a prospective randomized study of 400 operations performed with 2 different devices. Arch Surg 2007;142:958–61.

44. Podnos YD, Jimenez JC, Wilson SE, Stevens CM, Nguyen NT. Complications after laparoscopic gastric bypass: a review of 3464 cases. Arch Surg 2003;138:957–61.

45. Monteforte MJ, Turkelson CM. Bariatric surgery for morbid obesity. Obes Surg 2000;10:391–401.

46. Chapman AE, Kiroff G, Game P, Foster B, O'Brien P, Ham J, et al. Laparoscopic adjustable gastric banding in the treatment of obesity: a systematic literature review. Surgery 2004;135:326–51.

47. Colquitt J, Clegg A, Loveman E, Royle P, Sidhu MK. Surgery for morbid obesity. Cochrane Database Syst Rev 2005;(4):CD003641.

48. O'Brien PE, McPhail T, Chaston TB, Dixon JB. Systematic review of medium-term weight loss after bariatric operations. Obes Surg 2006;16:1032–40.

49. Sjöström L, Narbro K, Sjöström CD, Karason K, Larsson B, Wedel H, et al. Effects of bariatric surgery on mortality in Swedish obese subjects. N Engl J Med 2007;357:741–52.

50. Kalfarentzos F, Kechagias I, Soulikia K, Loukidi A, Mead N. Weight loss following vertical banded gastroplasty: intermediate results of a prospective study. Obes Surg 2001;11:265–70.

51. Greve JW. Surgical treatment of morbid obesity: role of the gastroenterologist. Scand J Gastroenterol Suppl 2000;(232):60–4.

52. Stellato TA, Crouse C, Hallowell PT. Bariatric surgery: creating new challenges for the endoscopist. Gastrointest Endosc 2003;57:86–94.

53. Huang CS, Farraye FA. Endoscopy in the bariatric surgical patient. Gastroenterol Clin North Am 2005;34:151–66.

54. Forsell P, Hellers G, Laveskog U, Westman L. Validation of pouch size measurement following the Swedish adjustable gastric banding using endoscopy, MRI and barium swallow. Obes Surg 1996;6:463–7.

55. Sataloff DM, Lieber CP, Seinige UL. Strictures following gastric stapling for morbid obesity. Results of endoscopic dilatation. Am Surg 1990;56:167–74.

56. Wetter A. Role of endoscopy after Roux-en-Y gastric bypass surgery. Gastrointest Endosc 2007;66:253–5.

57. Knol JA. Management of the problem patient after bariatric surgery. Gastroenterol Clin North Am 1994;23:345–69.

58. Byrne TK. Complications of surgery for obesity. Surg Clin North Am 2001;81:1181–8.

59. Livingston EH. Complications of bariatric surgery. Surg Clin North Am 2005;85:853–68.

60. Kim JJ, Tarnoff ME, Shikora SA. Surgical treatment for extreme obesity: evolution of a rapidly growing field. Nutr Clin Pract 2003;18:109–23.

61. Siersema PD, Homs MYV, Haringsma J, Tilanus HW, Kuipers EJ. Use of large-diameter metallic stents to seal traumatic nonmalignant perforations of the esophagus. Gastrointest Endosc 2003;58:356–61.

62. Gelbmann CM, Ratiu NL, Rath HC, Rogler G, Lock G, Schölmerich J, et al. Use of self-expandable plastic stents for the treatment of esophageal perforations and symptomatic anastomotic leaks. Endoscopy 2004;36:695–9.

63. Radecke K, Gerken G, Treichel U. Impact of a self-expanding, plastic esophageal stent on various esophageal stenoses, fistulas, and leakages: a single-center experience in 39 patients. Gastrointest Endosc 2005;61:812–8.

64. Eisendrath P, Cremer M, Himpens J, Cadiere GB, Le Moine O, Devière J. Endotherapy including temporary stenting of fistulas of the upper gastrointestinal tract after laparoscopic bariatric surgery. Endoscopy 2007;39:625–30.

65. Maluf-Filho F, Moura E, Sakai P. Endoscopic treatment of esophagogastric fistulae with an acellular matrix. Gastrointest Endosc 2004;59:P151.

66. Raju GS, Thompson C, Zwischenberger JB. Emerging endoscopic options in the management of esophageal leaks (videos). Gastrointest Endosc 2005;62:278–86.

67. Papavramidis ST, Eleftheriadis EE, Apostolidis DN, Kotzampassi KE. Endoscopic fibrin sealing of high-output non-healing gastrocutaneous fistulas after vertical gastroplasty in morbidly obese patients. Obes Surg 2001;11:766–9.

68. Ukleja A, Stone RL. Medical and gastroenterologic management of the post-bariatric surgery patient. J Clin Gastroenterol 2004;38:312–21.

69. Eisenberg D, Duffy AJ, Bell RL. Update on obesity surgery. World J Gastroenterol 2006;12:3196–203.

70. Nguyen NT, Longoria M, Chalifoux S, Wilson SE. Gastrointestinal hemorrhage after laparoscopic gastric bypass. Obes Surg 2004;14:1308–12.

71. Hampel H, Abraham NS, El Serag HB. Meta-analysis: obesity and the risk for gastroesophageal reflux disease and its complications. Ann Intern Med 2005;143:199–211.

72. Snook KL, Ritchie JD. Carcinoma of esophagus after adjustable gastric banding. Obes Surg 2003;13:800–2.

73. Näslund E, Stockeld D, Granström L, Backman L. Six cases of Barrett's esophagus after gastric restrictive surgery for massive obesity: an extended case report. Obes Surg 1996;6:155–8.

74. Busetto L, Segato G, De Marchi F, Foletto M, De Luca M, Caniato D, et al. Outcome predictors in morbidly obese recipients of an adjustable gastric band. Obes Surg 2002;12:83–92.

75. Busetto L, Valente P, Pisent C, Segato G, de Marchi F, Favretti F, et al. Eating pattern in the first year following adjustable silicone gastric banding (ASGB) for morbid obesity. Int J Obes Relat Metab Disord 1996;20:539–46.

76. Niville E, Dams A. Late pouch dilation after laparoscopic adjustable gastric and esophagogastric banding: incidence, treatment, and outcome. Obes Surg 1999;9:381–4.

77. Strodel WE, Knol JA, Eckhauser FE. Endoscopy of the partitioned stomach. Ann Surg 1984;200:582–6.

78. Scapa E, Negri M, Halpern Z, Bogokowsky H, Eshchar J. Endoscopic diagnosis and management of complications after vertical banded gastroplasty. Endoscopy 1988;20:11–2.

79. Deitel M, Bendago M. Endoscopy of vertical banded gastroplasty. Am Surg 1989;55:287–90.

80. Wayman CS, Nord JH, Combs WM, Rosemurgy AS. The role of endoscopy after vertical banded gastroplasty. Gastrointest Endosc 1992;38:44–6.

81. Verset D, Houben JJ, Gay F, Elcheroth J, Bourgeois V, Van Gossum A. The place of upper gastrointestinal tract endoscopy before and after vertical banded gastroplasty for morbid obesity. Dig Dis Sci 1997;42:2333–7.

82. Paulk SC. Formal dilation after gastric partitioning. Surg Gynecol Obstet 1983;156:502–4.

83. Bowersox JC, Pearce WA, Carter PL. Acute pouch obstruction after vertical banded gastroplasty. Gastrointest Endosc 1990;36:146–7.

84. Al Halees ZY, Freeman JB, Burchett H, Brazeau-Gravelle P. Nonoperative management of stomal stenosis after gastroplasty for morbid obesity. Surg Gynecol Obstet 1986;162:349–54.

85. Holt PD, de Lange EE, Shaffer HA Jr. Strictures after gastric surgery: treatment with fluoroscopically guided balloon dilatation. AJR Am J Roentgenol 1995;164:895–9.

IV

86. Vance PL, de Lange EE, Shaffer HA Jr, Schirmer B. Gastric outlet obstruction following surgery for morbid obesity: efficacy of fluoroscopically guided balloon dilation. Radiology 2002;222:70–2.

87. Sanyal AJ, Sugerman HJ, Kellum JM, Engle KM, Wolfe L. Stomal complications of gastric bypass: incidence and outcome of therapy. Am J Gastroenterol 1992;87:1165–9.

88. Barba CA, Butensky MS, Lorenzo M, Newman R. Endoscopic dilation of gastroesophageal anastomosis stricture after gastric bypass. Surg Endosc 2003;17:416–20.

89. Ahmad J, Martin J, Ikramuddin S, Schauer P, Slivka A. Endoscopic balloon dilation of gastroenteric anastomotic stricture after laparoscopic gastric bypass. Endoscopy 2003;35:725–8.

90. Go MR, Muscarella P, Needleman BJ, Cook CH, Melvin WS. Endoscopic management of stomal stenosis after Roux-en-Y gastric bypass. Surg Endosc 2004 18:56–9.

91. Saeed ZA, Winchester CB, Ferro PS, Michaletz PA, Schwartz JT, Graham DY. Prospective randomized comparison of polyvinyl bougies and through-the-scope balloons for dilation of peptic strictures of the esophagus. Gastrointest Endosc 1995;41:189–95.

92. Nguyen NT, Stevens CM, Wolfe BM. Incidence and outcome of anastomotic stricture after laparoscopic gastric bypass. J Gastrointest Surg 2003;7:997–1003.

93. Peifer KJ, Shiels AJ, Azar R, Rivera RE, Eagon JC, Jonnalagadda S. Successful endoscopic management of gastrojejunal anastomotic strictures after Roux-en-Y gastric bypass. Gastrointest Endosc 2007;66:248–52.

94. Wolper JC, Messmer JM, Turner MA, Sugerman HJ. Endoscopic dilation of late stomal stenosis. Its use following gastric surgery for morbid obesity. Arch Surg 1984;119:836–7.

95. Kretzschmar CS, Hamilton JW, Wissler DW, Yale CE, Morrissey JF. Balloon dilation for the treatment of stomal stenosis complicating gastric surgery for morbid obesity. Surgery 1987;102:443–6.

96. Schwartz ML, Drew RL, Roiger RW, Ketover SR, Chazin-Caldie M. Stenosis of the gastroenterostomy after laparoscopic gastric bypass. Obes Surg 2004;14:484–91.

97. Carrodeguas L, Szomstein S, Zundel N, Lo ME, Rosenthal R. Gastrojejunal anastomotic strictures following laparoscopic Roux-en-Y gastric bypass surgery: analysis of 1291 patients. Surg Obes Relat Dis 2006;2:92–7.

98. Goitein D, Papasavas PK, Gagne D, Ahmad S, Caushaj PF. Gastrojejunal strictures following laparoscopic Roux-en-Y gastric bypass for morbid obesity. Surg Endosc 2005;19:628–32.

99. Catalano MF, Rudic G, Anderson AJ, Chua TY. Weight gain after bariatric surgery as a result of a large gastric stoma: endotherapy with sodium morrhuate may prevent the need for surgical revision. Gastrointest Endosc 2007;66:240–5.

100. Spaulding L. Treatment of dilated gastrojejunostomy with sclerotherapy. Obes Surg 2003;13:254–7.

101. Filho AJ, Kondo W, Nassif LS, Garcia MJ, Tirapelle RA, Dotti CM. Gastrogastric fistula: a possible complication of Roux-en-Y gastric bypass. JSLS 2006;10:326–31.

102. Gumbs AA, Duffy AJ, Bell RL. Management of gastrogastric fistula after laparoscopic Roux-en-Y gastric bypass. Surg Obes Relat Dis 2006;2:117–21.

103. Thompson CC, Carr-Locke DL, Saltzman J. Peroral endoscopic repair of staple-line dehiscence in Roux-en-Y bypass: a less invasive approach [abstract]. Gastroenterology 2004;126(Suppl 2):A810.

104. Carbajo Caballero MA, Martin del Olmo JC, Blanco Alvarez JI, de la CC, Guerro Polo JA, Sanchez RA. Intragastric migration of laparoscopic adjustable gastric band (Lap-Band) for morbid obesity. J Laparoendosc Adv Surg Tech A 1998;8:241–4.

105. Jess P, Fonnest G. Gastroscopic treatment of gastric band penetrating the gastric wall. Dan Med Bull 1999;46:428.

106. Weiss H, Nehoda H, Labeck B, Peer-Kuhberger R, Lanthaler M, Aigner F. Deflated adjustable gastric band: migration through anterior gastric wall. Endoscopy 2000;32:S 35.

107. Weiss H, Nehoda H, Labeck B, Peer R, Aigner F. Gastroscopic band removal after intragastric migration of adjustable gastric band: a new minimal invasive technique. Obes Surg 2000;10:167–70.

108. Baldinger R, Mluench R, Steffen R, Ricklin TP, Riedtmann HJ, Horber FF. Conservative management of intragastric migration of Swedish adjustable gastric band by endoscopic retrieval. Gastrointest Endosc 2001;53:98–101.

109. Meyenberger C, Gubler C, Hengstler PM. Endoscopic management of a penetrated gastric band. Gastrointest Endosc 2004;60:480–1.

110. Regusci L, Groebli Y, Meyer JL, Walder J, Margalith D, Schneider R. Gastroscopic removal of an adjustable gastric band after partial intragastric migration. Obes Surg 2003;13:281–4.

111. Sakai P, Hondo FY, Almeida Artifon EL, Kuga R, Ishioka S. Symptomatic pneumoperitoneum after endoscopic removal of adjustable gastric band. Obes Surg 2005;15:893–6.

112. Evans JA, Williams NN, Chan EP, Kochman ML. Endoscopic removal of eroded bands in vertical banded gastroplasty: a novel use of endoscopic scissors (with video). Gastrointest Endosc 2006;64:801–4.

113. Fobi M, Lee H, Igwe D, Felahy B, James E, Stanczyk M, et al. Band erosion: incidence, etiology, management and outcome after banded vertical gastric bypass. Obes Surg 2001;11:699–707.

114. Sinar DR, Flickinger EG, Park HK, Sloss RR. Retrograde endoscopy of the bypassed stomach segment after gastric bypass surgery: unexpected lesions. South Med J 1985;78:255–8.

115. Flickinger EG, Sinar DR, Pories WJ, Sloss RR, Park HK, Gibson JH. The bypassed stomach. Am J Surg 1985;149:151–6.

116. Sundbom M, Nyman R, Hedenstrom H, Gustavsson S. Investigation of the excluded stomach after Roux-en-Y gastric bypass. Obes Surg 2001;11:25–7.

117. Fobi MA, Chicola K, Lee H. Access to the bypassed stomach after gastric bypass. Obes Surg 1998;8:289–95.

118. Sakai P, Kuga R, Safatle-Ribeiro AV, Faintuch J, Gama-Rodrigues JJ, Ishida RK, et al. Is it feasible to reach the bypassed stomach after Roux-en-Y gastric bypass for morbid obesity? The use of the double-balloon enteroscope. Endoscopy 2005;37:566–9.

119. Kuga R, Safatle-Ribeiro AV, Faintuch J, Ishida RK, Furuya CK Jr, Garrido AB Jr, et al. Endoscopic findings in the excluded stomach after Roux-en-Y gastric bypass surgery. Arch Surg 2007;142:942–6.

120. Elton E, Hanson BL, Qaseem T, Howell DA. Diagnostic and therapeutic ERCP using an enteroscope and a pediatric colonoscope in long-limb surgical bypass patients. Gastrointest Endosc 1998;47:62–7.

121. Wright BE, Cass OW, Freeman ML. ERCP in patients with long-limb Roux-en-Y gastrojejunostomy and intact papilla. Gastrointest Endosc 2002;56:225–32.

122. Pimentel RR, Mehran A, Szomstein S, Rosenthal R. Laparoscopy-assisted transgastrostomy ERCP after bariatric surgery: case report of a novel approach. Gastrointest Endosc 2004;59:325–8.

18

19 Magnifying Chromocolonoscopy and Tattooing

Shin-ei Kudo, Hideyuki Miyachi and Shungo Endo

Introduction

Observation of the pit structure of colorectal lesions using magnifying endoscopy is a useful method for diagnosing the quality of the lesions and depth of invasion. Since the release of the Olympus CF-200Z electronic magnifying scope (Olympus Medical Systems Corporation, Tokyo) in 1993, magnifying scopes have been steadily improving. Recent models have operating characteristics and an image quality far superior to those of earlier products, providing a significant advance in the quality of diagnosis possible in clinical applications.

Over the years, detailed clinicopathological studies including large numbers of patients have provided accumulating data, to a point at which consensus has been reached on the indications for the treatment of submucosal colorectal carcinoma [1,2]. The degree of submucosal invasion (**Fig. 19.1**) is classified into three stages, based on the depth of invasion—sm1, sm2, and sm3. The sm1 stage is subclassified into 1 a, 1 b, and 1 c, according to the horizontal extension of the invaded area. Cancers with a grade of sm1 a or 1 b (slightly invasive submucosal cancers) without vessel involvement never metastasize to the lymph nodes, liver, or other organs. In contrast, sm1 c and sm2 or sm3 lesions (massively invasive submucosal cancers) are associated with nodal metastasis in a substantial proportion of cases (approximately 10 %) [3,4]. Slightly invasive submucosal cancers are not considered to have a potential for metastasis, and endoscopic resection is therefore indicated for these lesions. With massively invasive submucosal cancers, however, surgical resection accompanied by lymph-node dissection is indicated, as they do have a potential for lymph-node metastasis. Adequate preoperative diagnosis is therefore mandatory in order to determine the optimal treatment policy. To obtain an accurate diagnosis, the present authors carry out magnifying endoscopic examinations of colorectal lesions and decide on the treatment policy on the basis of a qualitative diagnosis that is largely based on the pit pattern [3,5].

The orifices of the crypts in the colonic mucosa are called "pits," and the form and arrangement of the pits is referred to as the "pit pattern" (**Fig. 19.2**) [6]. The introduction of the CF-200Z instrument made it possible to obtain images of colorectal tissue with 100× magnification instantly. In-vivo observation of the fine surface pattern of tumorous lesions and one-to-one comparison of the magnified scope image with the stereomicroscopic image or pathological tissue from an excised sample allow much more precise endoscopic diagnosis than was previously possible [7,8]. Improved understanding of the morphological development of colorectal cancers, and establishing treatment indications according to the precise diagnosis of the invasion depth, have also made it possible to avoid unnecessary biopsies and polypectomies [9]. There has been remarkable recent progress in endoscopic treatment and in minimally invasive surgical methods such as laparoscopy-assisted procedures. Choosing the appropriate treatment method is very important both in terms of the patient's quality of life and cost–benefit considerations.

This chapter describes how to diagnose colorectal neoplastic lesions using pit pattern diagnosis, as well as the vascular pattern classification that can be obtained using magnification with narrow-

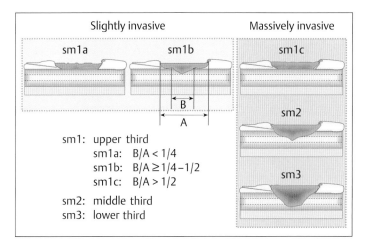

Fig. 19.1 Classification of the degree of submucosal invasion. The submucosa is divided into three equal layers. In sm1 a lesions, cancer invasion limited to the upper third of the submucosal layer and the ratio of the diameters B:A is less than 1:4. In sm1 b, the B:A ratio is 1:4 to 1:2. In sm1 c, the B:A ratio is more than 1:2. In sm2 lesions, cancer invasion is limited to the middle third of the submucosal layer. In sm3, cancer invasion is limited to the lower third of the submucosal layer.

band imaging (NBI) or similar methods—Fujinon intelligent chromoendoscopy (FICE) or iScan (Pentax) [10,11].

Practical Aspects of Diagnosis Based on Magnifying Endoscopy

We carry out colonoscopies using a magnifying scope in all cases. When a lesion is discovered with conventional imaging, we perform NBI observation to distinguish between neoplasms and nonneoplastic lesions, and then carry out a magnifying dye-spray examination to determine the treatment plan. During the initial careful observation procedure using standard white-light imaging, the aim is to localize the lesion and assess its size and visible shape as well as its color tone, surface properties, firmness, the fold concentration and the presence of white spots [12,13]. If the lesion is diagnosed as an epithelial neoplasm, we then switch the imaging method to NBI and use magnifying observation to differentiate between neoplasms and non-neoplasms. NBI highlights the capillaries near the mucosal surface in a brownish tone. NBI examination of lesions abundant in blood vessels makes it possible to assign the lesions to the following categories (**Fig. 19.3**) [14] referring to the Sano et al. classification [15,16]:

- *Normal pattern:* in the normal colorectal mucosa, vessels appear as a regularly arranged web around the gland duct.
- *Faint pattern:* in a hyperplastic polyp, the vessels are not clearly imaged and have a faint color tone.
- *Network pattern:* in a tubular adenoma, vessels with a regular thickness appear in a network pattern located around oval pits.
- *Dense pattern:* in a villous or tubulovillous adenoma, densely concentrated vessels produce an appearance resembling severe hyperemia in the superficial epithelium of the adenoma.

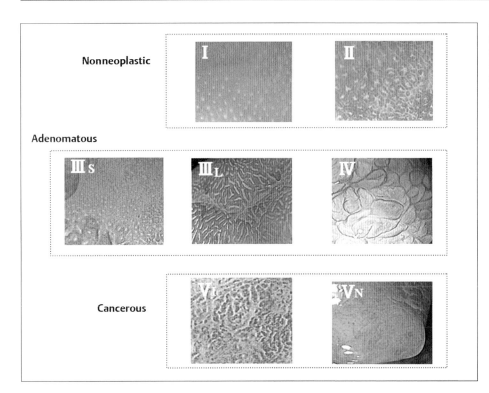

Fig. 19.2 Pit pattern classification. Pit patterns are classified into seven types. Type I and II pit patterns are characteristic of nonneoplastic lesions. Type III$_L$, III$_S$, and IV represent dysplasia (adenomas). Types V$_I$ and V$_N$ are cancerous. Type V$_N$ pit patterns show a desmoplastic reaction associated with deeply invasive submucosal cancer.

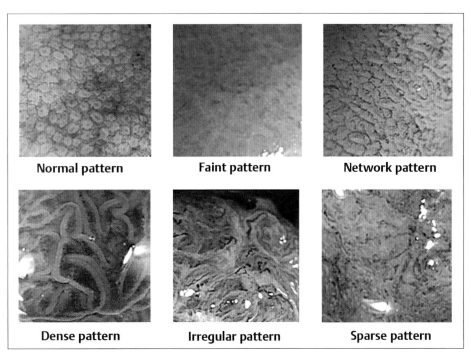

Fig. 19.3 Classification of the vascular pattern. These six patterns are used as the basis for diagnoses. Lesions with normal or faint patterns are judged to be nonneoplastic. Those with the network, dense, irregular, or sparse patterns are considered to be neoplastic and undergo magnifying dye-spraying examination for detailed qualitative diagnosis.

- *Irregular pattern:* in a flat and protruding submucosal carcinoma, thick and very serpentine vessels are observed.
- *Sparse pattern:* in a depressed-type submucosal carcinoma, the vessels in the depressed region tend to be sparse.

These six pattern categories are used as the basis for diagnosis. Lesions with normal or faint patterns are classified as nonneoplastic, and the patients are scheduled for follow-up monitoring. Lesions with the network, dense, irregular, or sparse patterns are judged to be neoplastic. Particularly when the irregular or sparse patterns are observed, it is necessary to keep the possibility of submucosal invasion in mind and carry out a magnifying dye-spraying examination for detailed qualitative diagnosis.

There are two ways of performing magnifying dye-spraying endoscopy: the contrast method, in which the dye forms pools in the depressed surface or crypt orifices, to enhance the contrast; and the dyeing method, in which the surface of the lesion is stained. The contrast method is suitable for assessing the shape and depression of lesions. It uses 0.2 % indigo carmine and often allows pit pattern diagnosis. In the dyeing method, 0.05 % crystal violet is usually used, and this method is suitable for detailed examination of the pit pattern [13,17]. The pit pattern is usually classified into six types: I, II, IIIS, IIIL, IV, and V. **Figure 19.2** shows the pit pattern classification that we use [18]. Pit pattern diagnosis is based on magnified examination of the structural arrangement of the gland ducts, and we regard it as useful because it corresponds well with the pathological diagnoses (**Table 19.1**) [19,20].

- *Type I:* this presents the pit pattern of normal mucosa, with round pits. It is also seen on the surface of inflammatory polyps.

Table 19.1 Pit patterns and histology of the lesions (April 2001–June 2008)

Pit pattern	Dysplasia (adenoma)		Submucosal cancer	Total
	Low-grade	High-grade		
III$_L$	5562 (84.6%)	1015 (15.4%)	0	6577
IV	947 (50.4%)	879 (46.8%)	53 (2.8%)	1879
III$_S$	50 (58.8%)	33 (38.8%)	2 (2.4%)	85
V$_I$	57 (9.8%)	322 (55.7%)	200 (34.5%)	579
V$_N$	0	12 (8.9%)	123 (91.1%)	135

- *Type II:* the pits have star-shaped or open circular patterns. This pit pattern is observed with most hyperplastic polyps.
- *Type III$_L$* ("L" stands for "large" or "long"): The pits are linear and thin. This pit pattern is usually seen in polyp-shaped tubular adenomas with a relatively small diameter.
- *Type III$_S$* ("S" stands for "small" or "short"): The pits are compactly arranged and are smaller than the normal ones. The small pits reflect the straight and compactly arranged glands of the lesion [8,21]. This is the pattern seen in depressed-type lesions, which tend to be early cancers.
- *Type IV:* The pits are linear, as in type IIIL, but are gyrated and accompanied by branches. This pit pattern is observed mostly with tubular adenomas, but a coralloid pattern with a shaggy appearance is characteristic of villous adenomas. This pattern is often observed in protruding polyps with relatively large diameters and sometimes accompanied by submucosal carcinoma.
- *Type V:* This pit pattern reflects the structural atypia of the superficial gland duct and is usually associated with carcinomas.

Although the actual treatment policy is also determined by taking into account the results of conventional observations such as the localization, size and visual shape of a lesion, the pit pattern classification described above generally leads to the following treatment policies. When a hyperplastic polyp has a type II pit pattern, it can also be diagnosed using the vascular pattern diagnosis possible with magnifying NBI observation [16]; this type of polyp does not receive treatment. The type III–V pit patterns indicate neoplastic lesions, which should be treated. However, the type III$_L$ pit pattern is the basic pattern for tubular adenomas. Some authors consider that small-diameter tubular adenomas can receive follow-up only, as their growth is very slow, but this view is controversial. The type III$_S$ pit pattern is typical of depressed neoplasms. Lesions of type III$_S$ are not often detected, but they are candidates for precursor lesions of "de novo" cancers. Depressed-type lesions have a marked tendency to invade the submucosa. As depressed-type lesions may be accompanied with massively invasive submucosal cancers even when less than 5 mm in diameter, surgical treatment may be indicated even for small ones. Early detection and timely treatment of these lesions are critical for improving the morbidity and mortality rates associated with colorectal cancer [22,23]. Lesions with the type IV pit pattern undergo endoscopic resection, but caution is required here, as these lesions are often submucosal carcinomas accompanied by the type V pit pattern. A lesion that has the type V pit pattern is subjected to endoscopic resection when it is diagnosed as high-grade dysplasia or slightly invasive submucosal carcinoma, or to surgical resection when it is diagnosed as a massively invasive submucosal carcinoma. The following section describes in detail the subclassification of the type V pit pattern, providing an index for depth diagnosis.

Recent Trends in Endoscopic Diagnosis of the Type V Pit Pattern

In general, the type V pit pattern signifies carcinoma, as it reflects structural atypia in the superficial gland ducts. It is subclassified into type V$_I$, indicating high-grade dysplasia or slightly invasive submucosal carcinoma; and type V$_N$, indicating deeply invasive submucosal carcinoma or advanced carcinoma. When the cancerous tissue is infiltrating into the deep submucosal layer, the desmoplastic reaction on the superficial layer of the lesion causes a decrease in the density of the gland ducts [13,22]. The magnifying dye-spraying examination of this type of lesion shows a surface that has no structure, or almost none. The type V$_N$ pit pattern (N stands for "nonstructure") indicates massively invasive submucosal carcinoma or advanced carcinoma. When a pit pattern shows atypical features such as irregular size, asymmetry, abnormal branching or derangement, but does not present a clear type V$_N$ pattern, it is classified as having a type V$_I$ pit pattern (I stands for "irregular"), indicating high-grade dysplasia or slightly invasive submucosal carcinoma [3,24].

However, imprecision in these diagnostic criteria led to assessment variations between different institutes, and the criteria also proved difficult for beginners to grasp. To deal with these problems, a research project on the significance and clinical application of pit pattern analysis in diagnosing colorectal neoplastic lesions was started in 2002, with funding from the Japanese Ministry of Health, Labor and Welfare (MHLW). Consensus meetings were held to resolve the differences between institutions in diagnosing type V pit patterns.

At the Hakone Pit Pattern Symposium held in April 2004, the participants attempted to formulate a unified definition of the type V pit pattern, the main objectives being to achieve simplicity, comprehensibility, a meaningful classification (with guidelines for depth diagnoses and treatment policies), and to reflect the information and experience gathered in many years of research. The symposium eventually reached the following consensus:
- Pit patterns that clearly have nonstructure surfaces should be classified as type V$_N$.
- Irregular duct structures should be classified as type V$_I$.
- In addition, the presence of an invasive pattern, scratch sign, and gland duct groups with a high degree of irregularity can also be noted as indicating deep submucosal invasion.

This consensus, known the Hakone Consensus, clarified the boundary between types V$_I$ and V$_N$ with a classification method that is easier to understand even for beginners than the previous classification one.

In fact, all of the lesions that were diagnosed as type V$_N$ in accordance with the Hakone Consensus classification were found to be deeply invasive submucosal cancers or advanced cancers, so that identifying a type V$_N$ lesion was a clear sign of deep invasion [22,25]. However, this meant that the invasion depths included in the type V$_I$ pit pattern covered a wider range than before, including lesions from high-grade dysplasia to deeply invasive submucosal carcinoma. This made it necessary to gather more data about the type V$_I$ pit pattern findings to serve as evidence of deeply invasive submucosal carcinoma. At a meeting held at the Japanese MHLW in December 2005 to discuss the subclassification of the type V$_I$ pit pattern, a new definition of "type V$_I$ high-grade" was established on the basis of studies of a large number of cases [9,25–28].

Type V$_I$ high-grade is defined as a condition in which the existing pits have been destroyed or damaged (**Fig. 19.4**). It is specifically accompanied by:
- A narrowed lumen
- Rough margins
- Unclear boundaries

19

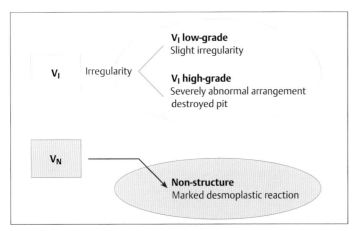

Fig. 19.4 Subclassification of the type V pit pattern. All lesions diagnosed as type V_N in accordance with the Hakone Consensus criteria were found to be massively invasive submucosal cancers, so that a finding of type V_N is a clear sign of deep invasion. A variety of tumor types ranging from dysplasia to invasive cancer may show type V_I. In depressed lesions, surgery is indicated when type V_I high-grade is observed. In flat or protruding lesions, those with type V_I high-grade sometimes represent slightly invasive submucosal carcinoma, for which endoscopic resection is initially indicated.

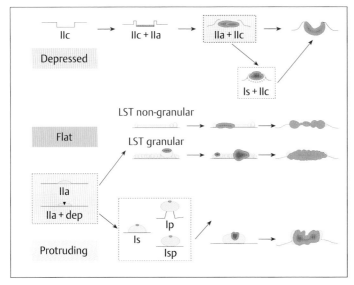

Fig. 19.6 The gross appearance of the development and progression of colorectal neoplasms. This classification is a slight modification of the Paris endoscopic classification and the Japanese system. The diagnostic characteristics of deep submucosal invasion vary depending on the morphological development of colorectal cancers. The red area indicates the cancerous portion.

- Reduced or absent staining of the stromal area between pits
- Scratch sign

This definition means that type V_I high-grade is a sign of deeply invasive submucosal carcinoma, allowing clearer, more objective depth diagnosis.

The basic treatment policy resulting from the above classifications is that surgical resection is carried out when a type V_N pit pattern is observed; treatment with surgical resection is considered when a type V_I high-grade pattern is observed; and endoscopic resection is considered when a type V_I low-grade pattern is observed [26,29].

Treatment Policies Based on Morphological Development and Pit Patterns

Almost all lesions with a type V_N pit pattern are deeply invasive submucosal carcinomas or advanced carcinomas. However, surgical resection is not absolutely indicated for type V_I high-grade lesions. The diagnostic characteristics of deep submucosal invasion vary depending on the gross appearance (**Figs. 19.5, 19.6**) [4,13,30], which is assessed using the Paris endoscopic classification [31] and Japanese rule [32]. According to our study, the specificity of type V_I high-grade cases for deep submucosal invasion was 73.3% overall. It was 100% with depressed lesions (IIc, IIa + IIc, Is + IIc), 68.4% with flat lesions and 71.4% with protruding lesions. The positive predictive value (PPV) was 82.8% overall, 100% for depressed lesions, 68.4% for flat lesions, and 86.4% for protruding lesions. It is therefore important to reach a well-balanced judgment that takes into account both the morphological (Paris) classification of colorectal cancers and the pit pattern diagnosis [5,23,29].

To avoid unnecessary surgery, we use the following treatment policies. In de novo depressed lesions with rapid growth and a high degree of malignancy, the pit pattern on the depressed surface typically progresses from type III_S to V_I to V_N, and surgery is indicated if type V_I high-grade is observed. In flat or protruding lesions, growth in the adenoma–carcinoma sequence is slow and the pit pattern progresses from type III_L to IV to V_I to V_N. Even when this type of lesion shows type V_I high-grade findings and has a large diameter, it is sometimes a slightly invasive submucosal carcinoma, for which endoscopic resection is initially indicated; surgical colectomy and lymph-node dissection can be considered in addition after histological analysis of the excised specimen. In noninvasive or slightly invasive lesions (sm1 a or 1 b) without vessel infiltration, observation and monitoring is sufficient (**Fig. 19.7**) [3,22].

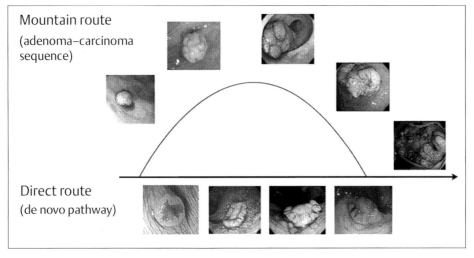

Fig. 19.5 The adenoma–carcinoma sequence and de novo theory. There are two routes for the development of colorectal neoplasms—the adenoma–carcinoma sequence and the de novo pathway. In the adenoma–carcinoma sequence, lesions grow with a protruding shape and finally develop into ulcerative forms. This is called the "mountain route." Depressed lesions develop on the de novo pathway, which is called the "direct route."

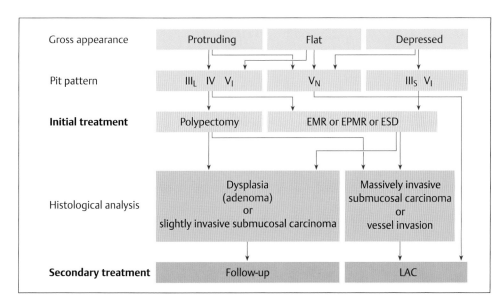

Fig. 19.7 The strategy for the treatment of colorectal neoplasms, showing the pit pattern diagnosis and gross appearance. Pit pattern diagnosis together with consideration of the development and progression of the lesion is useful for decision-making regarding the treatment of colorectal neoplasms. Type V_N lesions should receive surgical treatment. EMR, endoscopic mucosal resection; EPMR, endoscopic piecemeal resection; ESD, endoscopic submucosal dissection; LAC, laparoscopy-assisted or standard colectomy.

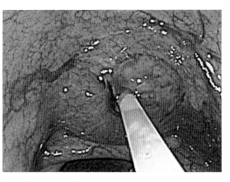
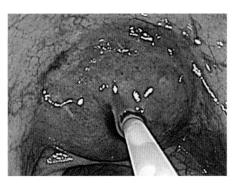
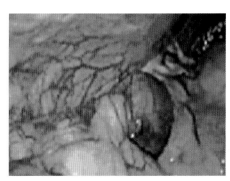

a   b   c

Fig. 19.8 a–c The prior saline injection tattooing technique.
a To begin with, 3 mL of saline is injected into the submucosal layer to ensure adequate elevation of the submucosa.
b The saline syringe is then replaced with another syringe containing India ink, and 0.2 mL India ink is injected. The India ink syringe is then replaced with

the initial saline syringe again, and approximately 2 mL of saline is added to flush out any India ink left in the needle device.
c The resulting tattoos are easily detected during laparoscopic surgery.

The path to a standardized subclassification of type V pit patterns has not been straight, but the current system has certainly made endoscopic diagnosis of colorectal lesions easier and has succeeded in linking examination findings directly to treatments. The history of endoscopy involves not just ever-advancing technology, but also constantly developing diagnostic procedures. In the future, further progress in the diagnosis of colorectal neoplasia can be expected as a result of regular scientific discussions about diagnosis using optical filtering methods such as NBI, FICE, or iScan and endomicroscopic methods such as confocal laser endomicroscopy and endocytoscopy. The diagnosis of lesions due to inflammatory bowel diseases and diagnosis based on the pit pattern classification [33] will also continue to become more sophisticated and precise. The most important aspect is to provide patients with the optimal treatment based on accurate diagnosis. The choice between endoscopic resection and surgical treatment depends entirely on the diagnosis.

Endoscopic Tattooing Technique

Accurate identification of the location of colorectal lesions is necessary to ensure adequate margins for resection and lymphadenectomy. During laparoscopic surgery, small submucosal cancers or postpolypectomy sites are difficult to identify using palpation [34]. In these cases, other methods of location such as intraoperative colonoscopy or preoperative marking are necessary. Options for preoperative marking include fluoroscopic localization, application

of metal clips, and preoperative colonic tattooing using India ink or another dye solution. Intraoperative colonoscopy is time-consuming, expensive and troublesome to carry out, and it may distend the bowel, increasing the risk of contamination [35]. Measurements of the distance of lesions from the anal verge during colonoscopy and localization of them using barium enemas or fluoroscopy may be unreliable. Metal clips may become dislodged and are expensive; in addition, special equipment is needed to identify them during laparoscopic surgery [36].

Colorectal tattooing with India ink is considered to be effective for preoperative marking or follow-up studies of colonic polyps [37,38]. We favor the use of India ink for preoperative tattooing, as it is a simple, safe, inexpensive and long-lasting technique, and because localization during surgery is prompt and accurate [37]. Initially, we injected the India ink directly into the colonic wall. However, complications such as silent local peritonitis and reactive lymph-node swelling may occur [39]. To achieve adequate submucosal injection and avoid spillage of the ink into the peritoneal cavity, we now use a technique with previous saline injection tattooing [36,40,41]. Firstly, 3 mL of saline is injected into the submucosal layer to ensure elevation of the submucosa. The saline syringe is then replaced with another syringe containing India ink, and 0.2 mL India ink is injected. The India ink syringe is then replaced again with the first saline syringe, and approximately 2 mL of saline is added to flush out any India ink remaining in the needle. The tattoos are easier to detect during laparoscopic surgery and ensure adequate resection margins (**Fig. 19.8**).

19

This endoscopic tattooing technique using India ink, with saline injections into the submucosa before and after, is more effective and safer than the direct injection technique both for identifying the lesion and in relation to complications, and it is less expensive and easier than other preoperative marking options.

References

1. Kudo S, Lambert R, Allen JI, Fujii H, Fujii T, Kashida H, et al. Nonpolypoid neoplastic lesions of the colorectal mucosa. Gastrointest Endosc 2008; 68 (4 Suppl): S 3–47.
2. Bianco MA, Rotondano G, Marmo R, Garofano ML, Piscopo R, de Gregorio A, et al. Predictive value of magnification chromoendoscopy for diagnosing invasive neoplasia in nonpolypoid colorectal lesions and stratifying patients for endoscopic resection or surgery. Endoscopy 2006; 38: 470–6.
3. Kashida H, Kudo SE. Early colorectal cancer: concept, diagnosis, and management. Int J Clin Oncol 2006; 11: 1–8.
4. Kudo S, Kashida H, Tamura T, Kogure E, Imai Y, Yamano H, et al. Colonoscopic diagnosis and management of nonpolypoid early colorectal cancer. World J Surg 2000; 24: 1081–90.
5. Kudo SE, Kashida H. Flat and depressed lesions of the colorectum. Clin Gastroenterol Hepatol 2005; 3 (7 Suppl 1): S 33–6.
6. Kudo S, Hirota S, Nakajima T, Hosobe S, Kusaka H, Kobayashi T, et al. Colorectal tumours and pit pattern. J Clin Pathol 1994; 47: 880–5.
7. Ajioka Y, Watanabe H, Kazama S, Hashidate H, Yokoyama J, Yamada S, et al. Early colorectal cancer with special reference to the superficial nonpolypoid type from a histopathologic point of view. World J Surg 2000; 24: 1075–80.
8. Tamura S, Furuya Y, Tadokoro T, Higashidani Y, Yokoyama Y, Araki K, et al. Pit pattern and three-dimensional configuration of isolated crypts from the patients with colorectal neoplasm. J Gastroenterol 2002; 37: 798–806.
9. Kato S, Fu KI, Sano Y, Fujii T, Saito Y, Matsuda T, et al. Magnifying colonoscopy as a non-biopsy technique for differential diagnosis of non-neoplastic and neoplastic lesions. World J Gastroenterol 2006; 12: 1416–20.
10. Gono K, Obi T, Yamaguchi M, Ohyama N, Machida H, Sano Y, et al. Appearance of enhanced tissue features in narrow-band endoscopic imaging. J Biomed Opt 2004; 9: 568–77.
11. Sano Y, Muto M, Tajiri H, Ohtsu A, Yoshida S. Optical/digital chromoendoscopy during colonoscopy using narrow-band imaging system. Dig Endosc 2005; 17: 43–8.
12. Nakahara T, Aoyama N, Maekawa S, Tamura T, Shirasaka D, Kuroda K, et al. Diagnostic significance of gently sloping depression and irregular margin in superficial elevated colorectal tumors. Int J Colorectal Dis 2007; 22: 25–31.
13. Kudo S. Early colorectal cancer: detection of depressed types colorectal carcinomas. Tokyo/New York: Igaku-Shoin; 1996
14. Wada Y, Kashida H, Ikehara N, et al. The diagnosis of colorectal lesions with magnifying narrow band imaging system [abstract]. Gastrointest Endosc 2008; 67: AB311–AB312.
15. Katagiri A, Fu KI, Sano Y, Ikematsu H, Horimatsu T, Kaneko K, et al. Narrow band imaging with magnifying colonoscopy as diagnostic tool for predicting histology of early colorectal neoplasia. Aliment Pharmacol Ther 2008; 27: 1269–74.
16. Machida H, Sano Y, Hamamoto Y, Muto M, Kozu T, Tajiri H, et al. Narrow-band imaging in the diagnosis of colorectal mucosal lesions: a pilot study. Endoscopy 2004; 36: 1094–8.
17. Fujii T, Hasegawa RT, Saitoh Y, Fleischer D, Saito Y, Sano Y, et al. Chromoscopy during colonoscopy. Endoscopy 2001; 33: 1036–41.
18. Kudo S, Rubio CA, Teixeira CR, Kashida H, Kogure E. Pit pattern in colorectal neoplasia: endoscopic magnifying view. Endoscopy 2001;73.
19. Kudo S, Tamura S, Nakajima T, Yamano H, Kusaka H, Watanabe H. Diagnosis of colorectal tumorous lesions by magnifying endoscopy. Gastrointest Endosc 1996; 44: 8–14.
20. Hurlstone DP, Cross SS, Adam I, Shorthouse AJ, Brown S, Sanders DS, et al. Efficacy of high magnification chromoscopic colonoscopy for the diagnosis of neoplasia in flat and depressed lesions of the colorectum: a prospective analysis. Gut 2004; 53: 284–90.
21. Kudo S, Tamure S, Nakajima T, Hirota S, Asano M, Ito O, et al. Depressed type of colorectal cancer. Endoscopy 1995; 27: 54–7.
22. Kudo SE, Takemura O, Ohtsuka K. Flat and depressed types of early colorectal cancers: from East to West. Gastrointest Endosc Clin N Am 2008; 18: 581–93.
23. Kudo S, Kashida H, Tamura T. Early colorectal cancer: flat or depressed type. J Gastroenterol Hepatol 2000; 15: D 66–70.
24. Togashi K, Konishi F. Magnification chromo-colonoscopy. ANZ J Surg 2006; 76: 1101–5.
25. Onishi T, Tamura S, Kuratani Y, Onishi S, Yasuda N. Evaluation of the depth score of type V pit patterns in crypt orifices of colorectal neoplastic lesions. J Gastroenterol 2008; 43: 291–7.
26. Kanao H, Tanaka S, Oka S, Kaneko I, Yoshida S, Arihiro K, et al. Clinical significance of type V_I pit pattern subclassification in determining the depth of invasion of colorectal neoplasms. World J Gastroenterol 2008; 14: 211–7.
27. Tobaru T, Mitsuyama K, Tsuruta O, Kawano H, Sata M. Sub-classification of type V_I pit patterns in colorectal tumors: relation to the depth of tumor invasion. Int J Oncol 2008; 33: 503–8.
28. Matsuda T, Fujii T, Saito Y, Nakajima T, Uraoka T, Kobayashi N, et al. Efficacy of the invasive/non-invasive pattern by magnifying chromoendoscopy to estimate the depth of invasion of early colorectal neoplasms. Am J Gastroenterol. 2008; 103: 2700–6.
29. Hurlstone DP, Cross SS, Adam I, Shorthouse AJ, Brown S, Sanders DS, et al. Endoscopic morphological anticipation of submucosal invasion in flat and depressed colorectal lesions: clinical implications and subtype analysis of the Kudo type V pit pattern using high-magnification-chromoscopic colonoscopy. Colorectal Dis 2004; 6: 369–75.
30. Kudo S, Tamura S, Hirota S, Sano Y, Yamano H, Serizawa M, et al. The problem of de novo colorectal carcinoma. Eur J Cancer 1995; 31A: 1118–20.
31. [No authors listed.] The Paris endoscopic classification of superficial neoplastic lesions: esophagus, stomach, and colon: November 30 to December 1, 2002. Gastrointest Endosc 2003; 58 (6 Suppl): S 3–43.
32. Japanese Society for Cancer of the Colon and Rectum. [General rules for clinical and pathological studies on cancer of the colon, rectum and anus]. 7th ed. Tokyo: Kanehara; 2006. p. 40. Japanese.
33. Kudo SE. New frontiers of endoscopy from the large intestine to the small intestine. Gastrointest Endosc 2007; 66 (3 Suppl): S 3–S 6.
34. Togashi K, Shimura K, Konishi F, Miyakura Y, Koinuma K, Horie H, et al. Prospective observation of small adenomas in patients after colorectal cancer surgery through magnification chromocolonoscopy. Dis Colon Rectum 2008; 51: 196–201.
35. Coman E, Brandt LJ, Brenner S, Frank M, Sablay B, Bennett B. Fat necrosis and inflammatory pseudotumor due to endoscopic tattooing of the colon with india ink. Gastrointest Endosc 1991; 37: 65–8.
36. Endo S, Kato S, Yoshimatsu H, et al. [A new technique of endoscopic tattooing for localization of the lesions during laparoscopic-assisted colectomy]. J Jpn Soc Coloproctol 1999; 52: 372–3. Japanese.
37. Arteaga-González I, Martín-Malagón A, Fernández EM, Arranz-Durán J, Parra-Blanco A, Nicolas-Perez D, et al. The use of preoperative endoscopic tattooing in laparoscopic colorectal cancer surgery for endoscopically advanced tumors: a prospective comparative clinical study. World J Surg 2006; 30: 605–11.
38. Aboosy N, Mulder CJ, Berends FJ, Meijer JW, Sorge AA. Endoscopic tattoo of the colon might be standardized to locate tumors intraoperatively. Rom J Gastroenterol 2005; 14: 245–8.
39. Yano H, Okada K, Monden T. Adhesion ileus caused by tattoo-marking: unusual complication after laparoscopic surgery for early colorectal cancer. Dis Colon Rectum 2003; 46: 987.
40. Park JW, Sohn DK, Hong CW, Han KS, Choi DH, Chang HJ, et al. The usefulness of preoperative colonoscopic tattooing using a saline test injection method with prepackaged sterile India ink for localization in laparoscopic colorectal surgery. Surg Endosc 2008; 22: 501–5.
41. Fu KI, Fujii T, Kato S, Sano Y, Koba I, Mera K, et al. A new endoscopic tattooing technique for identifying the location of colonic lesions during laparoscopic surgery: a comparison with the conventional technique. Endoscopy 2001; 33: 687–91.

IV

20 Tissue and Fluid Sampling

Koji Matsuda and Hisao Tajiri

Introduction

Tissue sampling is very important in endoscopy, as the pathological findings in the specimen obtained can have a direct influence on the management of the patient. This chapter describes tissue and fluid sampling devices and the sampling techniques and analysis methods used in esophagogastroduodenoscopy (EGD), enteroscopy, colonoscopy, endoscopic retrograde cholangiopancreatography (ERCP), and endoscopic ultrasonography (EUS).

Devices

▦ Biopsy Forceps

Biopsy forceps basically consist of a pair of sharpened cups, a spiral metal cable, and a control handle. The maximum diameter is limited by the size of the working channel, and the length of the cups is limited by the radius of curvature through which they have to pass in the instrument tip. The jaws of the biopsy cups may be round, oval, or elongated, fenestrated or nonfenestrated, and smooth or serrated. Other variations include swing-jaw, rotatable, and angled forceps (**Fig. 20.1**).

Biopsy forceps that have a needle spike at the center of the two biopsy cups are commonly used. Spikes improve directed lesion sampling by impaling the tissue and stabilizing the forceps cups. They also provide deeper biopsies than nonneedle designs [1]. Forceps designed to allow multiple-bite sampling during a single pass have been developed, but a practicable solution for multiple-bite sampling is still a technological challenge.

At ERCP, small-caliber or normal-sized forceps are used to carry out intraductal biopsies in the pancreatic and biliary ducts. An alternative wire-guided intraductal biopsy device has a conical-tipped circumferential cutting rim that deposits the sampled tissue into a cylindrical retrieval chamber [2,3].

Some manufacturers supply disposable single-use forceps in sterile packages. The advantages of these devices include convenience, variety, lower cost per unit, the potential for customized design, consistent performance, and a low risk of infection during the procedure. Their disadvantages include potentially higher costs per procedure and higher cumulative costs, the need for disposal after use, and the impact of the disposal on the environment [4]. Their cost-effectiveness depends on the current cost of the devices in comparison with the reprocessing costs and durability of reusable ones.

Biopsy forceps can be used for polypectomy in the form of what is known as a "hot biopsy" with electrodes, which provide simultaneous tissue biopsy and electrocautery. These devices theoretically provide improved hemostasis and more effective ablation of neoplastic tissue. Monopolar forceps, which are the ones most commonly used, involve the application of electrocautery between the two cups in contact with the polyp, with the return current passing through the patient's body to a distant return electrode or grounding pad. The most effective technique is to grasp the polyp superficially in the forceps, tent the mucosa, and apply energy to achieve a white coagulated area adjacent to the forceps. With the bipolar forceps, the two opposing cups serve as opposite electrodes, so that electrocautery is primarily applied to the tissue captured within the bite of the device and its penetration into neighboring tissue is extremely shallow. Bipolar forceps are preferably used in patients who have cardiac pacemakers.

▦ Polypectomy Snare

Polypectomy snares usually consist of a monopolar wire loop electrode that is advanced beyond a plastic insulating catheter to encircle the target lesion, which is then transected using mechanical and electrosurgical cutting as the loop is pulled back into the catheter. The snares are usually made of monofilament or braided wires of various gauges. The catheters vary in caliber and length to accommodate the working channel. All snares are designed for use with electrocautery, but either hot or cold snare techniques can be used with any device. Small or mini-monofilament snares are commonly used in the cold snare technique. Both single-use and reusable snares are available. Snares are made in a wide variety of sizes and shapes, designed to fit the anatomic requirements for ensnaring a given lesion. Endoscopic bipolar snares have been designed and studied, but they are not so widely available [5]. Bipolar snares are for use in patients who have cardiac pacemakers. Rotatable snares are useful for changing the orientation of the wire loop relative to the lesion [6]. Barbed and needle-tipped snares facilitate positioning and grasping of tissue without slipping away from the target lesion. Combination devices incorporating snares with injection needles are now available, and these are useful for saline injection-assisted polypectomy or endoscopic mucosal resection.

▦ Brush Cytology

A cytology brush basically consists of a covering plastic sleeve to protect the specimen during withdrawal, with or without a guidewire port. Cytology specimens are taken under direct vision with a sleeved brush, which is passed through the endoscope's working channel. The head of the brush is advanced out of its sleeve and rubbed and rolled repeatedly across the surface of the lesion. The brush is pulled back into the sleeve, and the brush and sleeve are then withdrawn together. After this, the brush is removed and wiped over two or three glass slides, which are then rapidly fixed before drying damages the cell walls.

▦ Fine-Needle Aspiration Cytology

The fine-needle aspiration (FNA) technique is used during ERCP and EUS. At ERCP, a small-caliber needle with a guidewire port is used to obtain tissue from the pancreaticobiliary tract. At EUS, single-use or partially reusable EUS-FNA needles with different sizes (19, 22, 25 G) and different tip shapes (needle, Tru-Cut, brush, and spray type) are available (**Fig. 20.2**). Most needle devices consist of a hollow needle with a solid removable stylet, a protective sheath, and a handle with a port for stylet insertion or withdrawal, as well as

IV

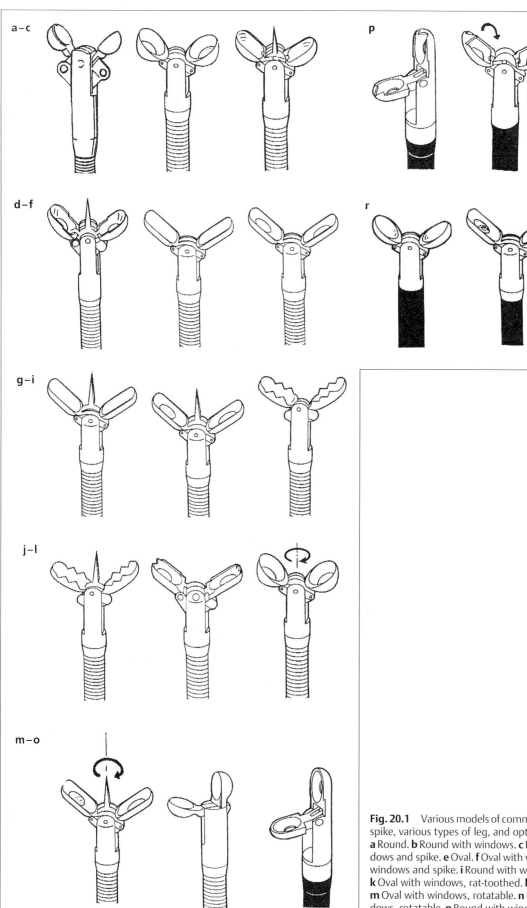

Fig. 20.1   Various models of commercially available forceps with a central spike, various types of leg, and optional "hot biopsy."
a Round. **b** Round with windows. **c** Round with spike. **d** Round with windows and spike. **e** Oval. **f** Oval with windows. **g** Oval with spike. **h** Oval with windows and spike. **i** Round with windows, rotatable. **j** Oval, toothed. **k** Oval with windows, rat-toothed. **l** Round with windows, rotatable. **m** Oval with windows, rotatable. **n** Round, alligator. **o** Round with windows, rotatable. **p** Round with windows, rat-toothed. **q** Round with windows, swiveling. **r** Round, hot biopsy. **s** Oval with windows, hot biopsy.

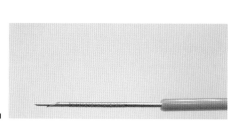

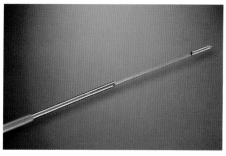

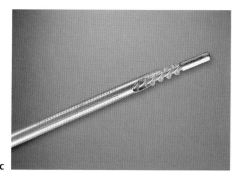

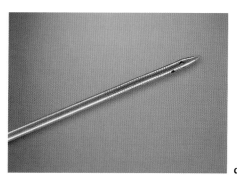

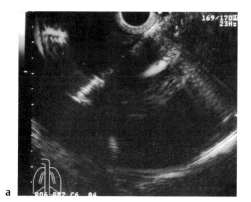

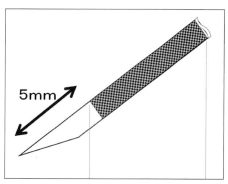

5mm

Fig. 20.3 Comparison between the endosonographic image and the "real" image of the needle.
a Endoscopic image.
b Scheme.

20

an attachment for a vacuum syringe to provide negative pressure inside the needle. The tip of the needle usually has dimpling, laser etching, or a sandblasted area to enhance its echogenicity for clear visualization on ultrasound. It is important to remember, especially with very small lymph nodes, that the real tip of the needle is typically 5 mm ahead of the hyperechoic bar of the needle tip on the EUS image (**Fig. 20.3**).

It is generally accepted that vacuum syringes should be used to provide negative pressure inside the needle. One study reported that vacuum syringes may increase the red blood cell content of the sample, especially in "juicy" tissue such as lymph nodes, although this does not alter the diagnostic yield [7].

A spring-loaded FNA needle is also available, which may be appropriate for relatively hard masses in the pancreas or mobile submucosal tumors in the gastrointestinal tract [8].

A core biopsy needle consists of a hollow, 19-gauge, metal cutting sheath enclosing a needle that has a tissue specimen tray which is 18 mm long. The spring-loaded mechanism cuts the specimen inside the lesion like a guillotine. The specimen obtained can usually serve for both cytological evaluation and histopathological evaluation. This device is suitable for pancreatic lesions, lymph nodes, hepatic lesions, submucosal lesions, mediastinal lesions, celiac ganglia, pancreatic parenchyma, and autoimmune pancreatitis [9–13]. A unique needle device for cytology consists of a 19-gauge needle and a stylet with a 5-mm brush at its leading end. This device may be useful for evaluation in patients with pancreatic cystic lesions [14]. A spray-type needle especially designed for EUS-guided celiac plexus block and neurolysis is also available. The tip of this needle has side holes for radial delivery of the desired agent into the celiac plexus and/or perineural space.

To allow more accurate diagnosis with EUS-FNA, it is very important for a cytopathologist to be present, as this can minimize the number of passes required and can ensure that at the completion of the procedure, adequate specimens have been obtained [15]. The sample obtained is squirted onto a slide and prepared with Diff-Quik staining [16], or modified Papanicolaou staining. Each specimen is checked by an experienced cytopathologist carefully at the time it is obtained, and further scrutiny of the samples is also carried out later in the pathology laboratory. One retrospective study showed that the discrepancy between rapid onsite evaluation and final cytology interpretation was very low of 2% (6 out of 300 suspicious malignant lesions) [17].

EGD

Esophagus

Malignant tumors of the esophagus can be diagnosed by biopsy alone in most cases. Additional brush cytology may enhance the accuracy of the diagnosis [18].

Barrett's esophagus is a condition in which the normal squamous mucosa is replaced by metaplastic specialized intestinal epithelium. Endoscopic biopsy is essential to detect the presence of intestinal metaplasia, confirming Barrett's esophagus, and is also helpful for ruling out infectious or inflammatory lesions that may mimic gastroesophageal reflux disease [19]. The critical role for biopsy in Barrett's esophagus is in detecting dysplasia and early carcinoma. In patients with Barrett's esophagus who have no evidence of dysplasia at the initial endoscopy, a repeat endoscopy should be performed with biopsy within 1 year. If dysplasia is not then confirmed, the patients are considered to be at low risk for progression of the condition and/or development of cancer. The recommended interval for further surveillance examinations used to be every 3 years [20], but recently the period has been extended up to 5 years [21].

Patients with high-grade dysplasia (HGD) are at significant risk for adenocarcinoma [22]. Surveillance endoscopy may be acceptable for patients with HGD without carcinoma, particularly in patients with contraindications to surgery and those who decline surgery. In these cases, frequent surveillance examinations should be carried out (e. g., every 3 months) with an extensive biopsy protocol (e. g., four-quadrant jumbo biopsies every 1 cm, with additional biopsies of macroscopic abnormalities) [23,24]. One study of patients with high-grade dysplasia reported that a 2-cm biopsy protocol missed 50 % of cancers that were detected with a 1-cm protocol [25]. If no dysplasia is found at two consecutive examinations, the interval can be lengthened to every 6 months, for example, for 1–2 years and then yearly unless dysplasia recurs [23]. Surveillance (e. g., every 1 year) has also been recommended in patients with Barrett's esophagus and low-grade dysplasia [19].

The usefulness of chromoendoscopy and magnifying endoscopy in detecting dysplasia still appears to be a matter of controversy, due to the poor reproducibility of the findings [26–29]. Flow cytometry and molecular markers may be promising methods for distinguishing patients with a low cancer risk from those with a high cancer risk for further follow-up [30]. One recent study suggested that narrow-band imaging detected significantly more patients with dysplasia and higher grades of dysplasia with fewer biopsy samples in comparison with white-light endoscopy at the standard resolution [31]. This method may provide a high dysplasia detection rate with fewer biopsies.

Endoscopic submucosal dissection (ESD), cap-assisted endoscopic mucosal resection (EMR-C), and ligation-assisted EMR (EMR-L) are often used for superficial esophageal squamous cell carcinoma, high-grade dysplasia in Barrett's esophagus, and superficial adenocarcinoma [32–34].

Brush cytology is of limited value, but may be useful as an adjunct to punch biopsy, particularly in patients with esophageal squamous cell carcinoma and esophageal candidiasis.

Stomach

Gastric neoplasia may be ulcerated, polypoid, flat, submucosal, or involve thickening of the gastric folds. Adequate tissue sampling is necessary to diagnose the lesion type [35]. If the suspicious lesion is ulcerated, multiple biopsy specimens should be obtained from the edge of each quadrant and from the base [36]. Polypoid lesions should be biopsied, and polyps larger than 2 cm in diameter should be removed if technically feasible [37].

The EMR technique is applied not only as a method of tissue sampling, but also as a curative treatment for early gastric cancer if the lesion is confined to the mucosa. ESD allows more accurate en bloc resection for larger superficial gastric cancers [38].

Duodenum

Benign periampullary lesions are usually removed with a standard polypectomy snare, without the submucosal injection. The technical success rates for endoscopic papillectomy of adenomas vary from 50 % to 100 % [39]. Endoscopic removal of malignant ampullary tumors is sometimes inadequate, and careful follow-up with endoscopy and/or additional surgical resection is therefore required.

Enteroscopy

It used to be difficult to obtain direct access to the small intestine in order to obtain tissue samples. Double-balloon endoscopy has now made it possible to access the entire small intestine via either the oral or anal routes and to obtain tissue specimens with direct endoscopic visualization [40]. Although this method requires fluoroscopic guidance and is relatively time-consuming (the procedure may take more than 1 h), it is useful for tissue acquisition as well as for assessing mid-gastrointestinal bleeding, diagnosing and treating stenoses, and removing foreign bodies [41].

Colonoscopy

Endoscopic biopsy at colonoscopy is also very important for distinguishing between different causes of colitis (infectious, ischemic, Crohn's disease, ulcerative colitis, etc.), assisting in the management of inflammatory bowel disease, and establishing the extent of lesions. Surveillance colonoscopy for dysplasia in patients with ulcerative colitis is recommended 8 years after the onset of the disease, when the cancer risk starts to increase [42]. In patients with the total type of ulcerative colitis, four-quadrant biopsy specimens are taken every 10 cm. In those with the left-sided type, specimens should also be taken in the right colon to reevaluate the extent of disease involvement [43].

For routine colon polyps, the cold snare technique is useful for removing polyps up to 10 mm in size, with few complications [44,45]. For larger, pedunculated polyps, cauterized snare techniques are typically used to reduce the risk of bleeding and ablate any neoplastic tissue not trapped within the snare. In comparison with standard polypectomy snares, rotatable snares appear to make it easier to snare polyps, reducing the total procedure time. Saline-assisted polypectomy was first reported by Deyhle et al. [46]. This technique is often used for relatively large, sessile polyps and laterally spreading tumors [47]. Details of endoscopic mucosal resection and endoscopic submucosal dissection will be precisely described in Chapter 30.

ERCP

During ERCP procedures, biopsy forceps, fine-needle aspiration, cytology of the bile and pancreatic juice, and brush cytology are commonly used for tissue sampling. From the technical point of view, bile and pancreatic juice cytology and brush cytology are the easiest sampling methods [48,49]. The pancreatic duct can be biopsied using small forceps through a catheter, if it is possible to

IV

advance a guide wire up to the level of the suspicious lesion. Biliary lesions located as far as the hilum of the liver can be biopsied with normal forceps, usually after sphincterotomy. The procedure is performed with real-time fluoroscopic or direct endoscopic guidance using the mother–baby scope system, which can be advanced through the working channel of a larger-channel duodenoscope. With forceps biopsy or FNA, most endoscopists first place a guide wire across the stricture to maintain access and to assist positioning of the forceps or needle catheter. These maneuvers can be technically challenging, and this is one reason why most practitioners prefer to perform brush cytology alone, as the device can be easily passed over a guidewire [48]. Forceps biopsy has the highest diagnostic yield, along with needle aspiration, and fluid cytology has the lowest sensitivity [50,51]. A combination of different methods of tissue sampling can enhance the diagnostic sensitivity [52]. However, dilating strictures before brush cytology does not improve the diagnostic yield [3]. Repeated brushing with consecutive brushes may enhance cancer detection. Brush cytology and forceps biopsy have a higher sensitivity for cholangiocarcinoma (44–100%) than for pancreatic cancer (30–65%) [2].

In spite of combination sampling with brush cytology, FNA, and biopsy, the sensitivity for all three methods combined is as low as 62%, with a negative predictive value of 39% [51]. In addition, multiple sampling is difficult and time-consuming unless the endoscopist is very familiar with the techniques. Moreover, maintaining guide-wire access through the stricture is quite challenging, especially when the devices are being changed. Forceps biopsy also generally requires sphincterotomy, which theoretically increases the risk of bleeding and perforation. For reasons of time and technical considerations, most practitioners only perform brush cytology, although this has a sensitivity as low as 30% [51].

Tissue sampling techniques during ERCP are gradually being replaced with EUS-FNA, except when the tumor is in a location that is not easily visualized using echoendoscope (e. g., in the upper part of the common bile duct and the hilum of the liver).

EUS-FNA

EUS makes it possible to obtain tissue from suspicious lesions with real-time ultrasound guidance, and EUS-FNA is now playing an important role in the diagnosis of mediastinal masses and lymph nodes [53], lymph-node metastases from esophageal tumors [54], and pancreaticobiliary tumors. The technique has a sensitivity of 88% and a specificity of 100% for detecting malignancies [55].

To allow both cytological diagnosis and histopathological diagnosis, larger needles of up to 19 gauge and Tru-Cut biopsy needles are used. The advantage of these devices is that immunological staining is possible with the specimens obtained, and they are particularly useful for the diagnosis of malignant lymphomas and gastrointestinal stromal tumors (GISTs). The cytomorphologic and immunohistochemical staining features of GISTs can be reliably diagnosed using cytological material (cell blocks) and core tissue specimens from EUS-FNA or core biopsy (e. g., Tru-Cut biopsy), respectively [56–58]. The typical immunohistochemical stains used to diagnose GISTs are c-*kit* (CD 117), CD 34, and smooth muscle actin. Positive staining for c-*kit* is considered diagnostic of GIST. Other markers, such as desmin and S-100 protein, can differentiate GIST from smooth-muscle tumors (leiomyoma, leiomyosarcoma, leiomyoblastoma) and schwannoma [59]. Although GISTs can be diagnosed on FNA, assessment of their malignant potential based on the mitotic count requires histology and is not possible from cytologic specimens alone. It is also important to recognize that not all GISTs are c-*kit*-positive [57]. In one recent study, a total of 62 patients with solid pancreatic masses (51 pancreatic cancers and 11 chronic pancreatitis) underwent EUS-FNA; p53 protein overexpres-

sion was observed in 67% of patients with pancreatic cancer, but not in patients with chronic pancreatitis [60].

Sampling of Body Fluids

The value of fluid sampling during EGD and colonoscopy is lower than that of tissue biopsy. The main role of this method is to assist the diagnosis of infectious diseases such as bacterial overgrowth in the small bowel or gastric juice aspiration when pulmonary tuberculosis is suspected.

At ERCP, it is usually possible to aspirate bile or pancreatic juices selectively without any major difficulties. In one study, investigators reported the presence of *TP53* gene mutations in pancreatic juice samples and in brush cytology specimens from 40–50% of patients with pancreatic cancer [61]. The detection and quantification of aberrantly methylated DNA in pancreatic fluid can also be a promising approach to the diagnosis of pancreatic cancer. The prevalence of pancreatic juice methylation in patients with chronic pancreatitis was lower than in patients with pancreatic cancer but higher than in control individuals [62].

Tumor markers in the fluid may be helpful for diagnosing pancreatic cystic lesions. A prospective multicenter study including 112 cysts diagnosed after surgical resection or biopsy found an optimal carcinoembryonic antigen (CEA) cutoff value of 192 ng/mL for differentiating mucinous tumors from other cystic lesions, with a sensitivity of 75% and a specificity of 84% [63]. Malignant tumors tend to have the highest CEA levels, but there are no obvious cutoff values that provide sufficient accuracy for clinical use [63–65]. When morphologic criteria (associated hypoechoic mass and/or macrocystic septations), cytology, and CEA levels (cutoff value 192 ng/mL) were taken together, EUS was able to differentiate mucinous from non-mucinous lesions with a sensitivity of 91% and a specificity of 31%. Cytology and CEA assessment without morphologic criteria had a better specificity value (71%), but the sensitivity fell to 82% [63].

EUS-guided paracentesis in patients with ascites identified malignancies missed using other imaging modalities, although negative ascitic fluid cytology from EUS-FNA did not exclude possible peritoneal carcinomatosis [66].

Summary

The various techniques for obtaining tissue and fluid samples in endoscopy are listed in **Table 20.1**. Tissue and fluid sampling is useful for differentiating between malignant and benign lesions and infectious disease, and various endoscopic devices and techniques are available for the purpose. Tissue and fluid sampling should be carried out whenever the results from the specimens obtained have the potential to influence the management of the patients. Even in the era of virtual endoscopy, tissue acquisition using endoscopy is still a safer and more accurate procedure than using other modalities. Close communication between gastroenterologists and pathologists is essential for more accurate diagnosis, as histology and cytology, as well as bacteriology and cytology of aspiration biopsies, are fundamental components of oncological diagnosis that provide the basis for later therapeutic decisions.

Table 20.1 Various techniques for obtaining tissue and fluid samples in endoscopy

	Biopsy	Cytology	Fluid analysis
EGD and colonoscopy	Yes	Seldom	Seldom
Enteroscopy	Yes	Seldom	Seldom
ERCP	Yes	Yes	Yes
EUS	Yes	Yes	Yes

References

1. Bernstein DE, Barkin JS, Reiner DK, Lubin J, Phillips RS, Grauer L. Standard biopsy forceps versus large-capacity forceps with and without needle. Gastrointest Endosc 1995; 41: 573–6.
2. De Bellis M, Sherman S, Fogel EL, Cramer H, Chappo J, McHenry L Jr, et al. Tissue sampling at ERCP in suspected malignant biliary strictures (part 1). Gastrointest Endosc 2002; 56: 552–61.
3. De Bellis M, Sherman S, Fogel EL, Cramer H, Chappo J, McHenry L Jr, et al. Tissue sampling at ERCP in suspected malignant biliary strictures (part 2). Gastrointest Endosc 2002; 56: 720–30.
4. Raltz SL, Kozarek RA. Overview of the problem: reprocessing versus disposal of endoscopic accessories. Gastrointest Endosc Clin N Am 2000; 10: 329–39.
5. Tucker RD, Platz CE, Sievert CE, Vennes JA, Silvis SE. In vivo evaluation of monopolar versus bipolar electrosurgical polypectomy snares. Am J Gastroenterol 1990; 85: 1386–90.
6. Yang R, Mabansag R, Laine L. Rotatable polypectomy snares: a randomized, prospective comparison with standard snares [abstract]. Gastrointest Endosc 2003; 57: T1480.
7. Wallace MB, Kennedy T, Durkalski V, Eloubeidi MA, Etamad R, Matsuda K, et al. Randomized controlled trial of EUS-guided fine needle aspiration techniques for the detection of malignant lymphadenopathy. Gastrointest Endosc 2001; 54: 441–7.
8. Binmoeller KF, Jabusch HC, Seifert H, Soehendra N. Endosonography-guided fine-needle biopsy of indurated pancreatic lesions using an automated biopsy device. Endoscopy 1997; 29: 384–8.
9. Levy MJ, Jondal ML, Clain J, Wiersema MJ. Preliminary experience with an EUS-guided trucut biopsy needle compared with EUS-guided FNA. Gastrointest Endosc 2003; 57: 101–6.
10. Varadarajulu S, Fraig M, Schmulewitz N, Roberts S, Wildi S, Hawes RH, et al. Comparison of EUS guided 19-gauge Trucut needle biopsy with EUS-guided fine-needle aspiration. Endoscopy 2004; 36: 397–401.
11. Larghi A, Verna EC, Stavropoulos SN, Rotterdam H, Lightdale CJ, Stevens PD. EUS-guided trucut needle biopsies in patients with solid pancreatic masses: a prospective study. Gastrointest Endosc 2004; 59: 185–90.
12. Levy MJ, Smyrk TC, Reddy RP, Clain JE, Harewood GC, Kendrick ML, et al. Endoscopic ultrasound-guided trucut biopsy of the cyst wall for diagnosing cystic pancreatic tumors. Clin Gastroenterol Hepatol 2005; 3: 974–9.
13. Levy MJ, Reddy RP, Wiersema MJ, Smyrk TC, Clain JE, Harewood GC, et al. EUS-guided trucut biopsy in establishing autoimmune pancreatitis as the cause of obstructive jaundice. Gastrointest Endosc 2005; 61: 467–72.
14. Al-Haddad M, Raimondo M, Woodward T, Krishna M, Pungpapong S, Noh K, et al. Safety and efficacy of cytology brushings versus standard FNA in evaluating cystic lesions of the pancreas: a pilot study. Gastrointest Endosc 2007; 65: 894–8.
15. Klapman JB, Logrono R, Dye CE, Waxman I. Clinical impact of on-site cytopathology interpretation on endoscopic ultrasound-guided fine needle aspiration. Am J Gastroenterol 2003; 98: 1289–94.
16. Hirschowitz SL, Mandell D, Nieberg RK, Carson K. The alcohol-fixed Diff-Quik stain. A novel rapid stain for the immediate interpretation of fine needle aspiration specimens. Acta Cytol 1994; 38: 499–501.
17. Eloubeidi MA, Tamhane A, Jhala N, Chhieng D, Jhala D, Crowe DR, et al. Agreement between rapid onsite and final cytologic interpretations of EUS-guided FNA specimens: implications for the endosonographer and patient management. Am J Gastroenterol. 2006; 101:2841–7.
18. Winawer SJ, Sherlock P, Belladonna JA, Melamed M, Beattie EJ Jr. Endoscopic brush cytology in esophageal cancer. JAMA 1975; 232: 1358.
19. Ippoliti AF. Esophageal biopsy. Gastrointest Endosc Clin N Am 2000; 10: 713–22.
20. Sampliner RE; Practice Parameters Committee of the American College of Gastroenterology. Updated guidelines for the diagnosis, surveillance, and therapy of Barrett's esophagus. Am J Gastroenterol 2002; 97: 1888–95.
21. Wang KK, Wongkeesong M, Buttar NS; American Gastroenterological Association. American Gastroenterological Association medical position statement: role of the gastroenterologist in the management of esophageal carcinoma. Gastroenterology 2005; 128: 1468–70.
22. Headrick JR, Nichols FC 3 rd, Miller DL, Allen MS, Trastek VF, Deschamps C, et al. High-grade esophageal dysplasia: long-term survival and quality of life after esophagectomy. Ann Thorac Surg 2002; 73: 1697–702.
23. Reid BJ, Weinstein WM, Lewin KJ, Haggitt RC, VanDeventer G, DenBesten L, et al. Endoscopic biopsy can detect high-grade dysplasia or early adenocarcinoma in Barrett's esophagus without grossly recognizable neoplastic lesions. Gastroenterology 1988; 94: 81–90.
24. Schnell TG, Sontag SJ, Chejfec G, Aranha G, Metz A, O'Connell S, et al. Long-term nonsurgical management of Barrett's esophagus with high-grade dysplasia. Gastroenterology 2001; 120: 1607–19.
25. Reid BJ, Blount PL, Feng Z, Levine DS. Optimizing endoscopic biopsy detection of early cancers in Barrett's high-grade dysplasia. Am J Gastroenterol 2000; 95: 3089–96.
26. Canto MI, Setrakian S, Willis J, Chak A, Petras R, Powe NR, et al. Methylene-blue directed biopsies improve detection of intestinal metaplasia and dysplasia in Barrett's esophagus. Gastrointest Endosc 2000; 51: 560–8.
27. Sharma P, Weston AP, Topalovski M, Cherian R, Bhattacharyya A, Sampliner RE. Magnification chromoendoscopy for the detection of intestinal metaplasia and dysplasia in Barrett's oesophagus. Gut 2003; 52: 24–7.
28. Dave U, Shousha S, Westaby D. Methylene blue staining: is it really useful in Barrett's esophagus? Gastrointest Endosc 2001; 53: 333–5.
29. Egger K, Werner M, Meining A, Ott R, Allescher HD, Höfler H, et al. Biopsy surveillance is still necessary in patients with Barrett's oesophagus despite new endoscopic imaging techniques. Gut 2003; 52: 18–23.
30. Reid BJ, Levine DS, Longton G, Blount PL, Rabinovitch PS. Predictors of progression to cancer in Barrett's esophagus: baseline histology and flow cytometry identify low- and high-risk patient subsets. Am J Gastroenterol 2000; 95: 1669–76.
31. Wolfsen HC, Crook JE, Krishna M, Achem SR, Devault KR, Bouras EP, et al. Prospective, controlled tandem endoscopy study of narrow band imaging for dysplasia detection in Barrett's esophagus. Gastroenterology 2008; 135: 24–31.
32. Fujishiro M, Yahagi N, Kakushima N, Kodashima S, Muraki Y, Ono S, et al. Endoscopic submucosal dissection of esophageal squamous cell neoplasms. Clin Gastroenterol Hepatol 2006; 4: 688–94.
33. Inoue H, Endo M, Takeshita K, Yoshino K, Muraoka Y, Yoneshima H. A new simplified technique of endoscopic esophageal mucosal resection using a cap-fitted panendoscope (EMRC). Surg Endosc 1992; 6: 264–5.
34. Fleischer DE, Wang GQ, Dawsey S, Tio TL, Newsome J, Kidwell J, et al. Tissue band ligation followed by snare resection (band and snare): a new technique for tissue acquisition in the esophagus. Gastrointest Endosc 1996; 44: 68–72.
35. Graham DY, Schwartz JT, Gain GD, Gyorkey F. Prospective evaluation of biopsy number in the diagnosis of esophageal and gastric carcinoma. Gastroenterology 1982; 82: 228–31.
36. Hatfield ARW, Slavin G, Segal AW, Levi AJ. Importance of the site of endoscopic gastric biopsy in ulcerating lesions of the stomach. Gut 1975; 16: 884–6.
37. Ginsberg GG, Al-Kawas FH, Fleischer DE, Reilly HF, Benjamin SB. Gastric polyp: relationship of size and histology to cancer risk. Am J Gastroenterol 1996; 91: 714–7.
38. Ono H, Kondo H, Gotoda T, Shirao K, Yamaguchi H, Saito D, et al. Endoscopic mucosal resection for treatment of early gastric cancer. Gut 2001; 48: 225–9.
39. Standards of Practice Committee, Adler DG, Qureshi W, Davila R, Gan SI, Lichtenstein D, et al. The role of endoscopy in ampullary and duodenal adenomas. Gastrointest Endosc 2006; 64: 849–54.
40. Yamamoto H, Sekine Y, Sato Y, Higashizawa T, Miyata T, Iino S, et al. Total enteroscopy with a nonsurgical steerable double-balloon method. Gastrointest Endosc 2001; 53: 216–20.
41. Yamamoto H, Ell C, Binmoeller KF. Double-balloon endoscopy. Endoscopy 2008; 40: 779–83.
42. Kornbluth A, Sachar DB. Ulcerative colitis practice guidelines in adults. American College of Gastroenterology, Practice Parameters Committee. Am J Gastroenterol 1997; 92: 204–11.
43. Bernstein CN, Riddell RH. Colonoscopy plus biopsy in the inflammatory bowel diseases. Gastrointest Endosc Clin N Am 2000; 10: 755–74.
44. Tappero G, Gaia E, De Giuli P, Martini S, Gubetta L, Emanuelli G. Cold snare excision of small colorectal polyps. Gastrointest Endosc 1992; 38: 310–3.
45. McAfee JH, Katon RM. Tiny snares prove safe and effective for removal of diminutive colorectal polyps. Gastrointest Endosc 1994; 40: 301–3.
46. Deyhle P, Largiader F, Jenny S, Fumagalli I. A method for endoscopic electroresection of sessile colonic polyps. Endoscopy 1973; 5: 38–40.
47. Kudo S, Tamegai Y, Yamano H, Imai Y, Kogure E, Kashida H. Endoscopic mucosal resection of the colon: the Japanese technique. Gastrointest Endosc Clin N Am 2001; 11: 519–35.
48. Foutch PG, Kerr DM, Harlan JR, Manne RK, Kummet TD, Sanowski RA. Endoscopic retrograde wire-guided brush cytology for diagnosis of patients with malignant obstruction of the bile duct. Am J Gastroenterol 1990; 85: 791–5.
49. Iituska Y, Hiraoka H, Kimura A, Kodoh H, Koga S. Diagnostic significance of bile cytology in obstructive jaundice. Jpn J Surg 1984; 14: 207–11.

IV

50. Howell DA, Beveridge RP, Bosco J, Jones M. Endoscopic needle aspiration biopsy at ERCP in the diagnosis of biliary strictures. Gastrointest Endosc 1992; 38: 531–5.

51. Kubota V, Takaoka M, Tani K, Ogura M, Kin H, Fujimura K, et al. Endoscopic transpapillary biopsy for the diagnosis of patients with pancreaticobiliary ductal strictures. Am J Gastroenterol 1993; 88: 1700–4.

52. Jailwala J, Fogel EL, Sherman S, Gottlieb K, Flueckiger J, Bucksot LG, et al. Triple-tissue sampling at ERCP in malignant biliary obstruction. Gastrointest Endosc 2000; 51: 383–90.

53. Vilmann P, Hancke S, Henriksen FW, Jacobsen GK. Endosonographically-guided fine needle aspiration biopsy of malignant lesions in the upper gastrointestinal tract. Endoscopy 1993; 25: 523–7.

54. Eloubeidi M, Wallace M, Reed C, Hadzijahic N, Lewin DN, Van Velse A, et al. The utility of EUS and EUS-guided fine-needle aspiration in detecting celiac lymph node metastasis in patients with esophageal cancer: a single-center experience. Gastrointest Endosc 2001; 54: 714–9.

55. Hünerbein M, Dohmoto M, Haensch W, Schlag PM. Endosonography-guided biopsy of mediastinal and pancreatic tumors. Endoscopy 1998; 30: 32–6.

56. Rader AE, Avery A, Wait CL, McGreevey LS, Faigel D, Heinrich MC. Fine-needle aspiration biopsy diagnosis of gastrointestinal stromal tumors using morphology, immunocytochemistry, and mutational analysis of c-*kit*. Cancer 2001; 93: 269–75.

57. Gu M, Ghafari S, Nguyen PT, Lin F. Cytologic diagnosis of gastrointestinal stromal tumors of the stomach by endoscopic ultrasound-guided fine-needle aspiration biopsy: cytomorphologic and immunohistochemical study of 12 cases. Diagn Cytopathol 2001; 25: 343–50.

58. Levy MJ, Wiersema MJ. EUS-guided Trucut biopsy. Gastrointest Endosc 2005; 62: 417–26.

59. Davila RE, Faigel DO. GI stromal tumors. Gastrointest Endosc 2003; 58: 80–8.

60. Itoi T, Takei K, Sofuni A, Itokawa F, Tsuchiya T, Kurihara T, et al. Immuno-histochemical analysis of p53 and MIB-1 in tissue specimens obtained from endoscopic ultrasonography-guided fine needle aspiration biopsy for the diagnosis of solid pancreatic masses. Oncol Rep 2005; 13: 229–34.

61. Sturm PD, Hruban RH, Ramsoekh TB, Noorduyn LA, Tytgat GN, Gouma DJ, et al. The potential diagnostic use of K-ras codon 12 and p53 alterations in brush cytology from the pancreatic head region. J Pathol 1998; 186: 247–53.

62. Matsubayashi H, Canto M, Sato N, Klein A, Abe T, Yamashita K, et al. DNA methylation alterations in the pancreatic juice of patients with suspected pancreatic disease. Cancer Res 2006; 66: 1208–17.

63. Brugge WR, Lewandrowski K, Lee-Lewandrowski E, Centeno BA, Szydlo T, Regan S, et al. Diagnosis of pancreatic cystic neoplasms: a report of the cooperative pancreatic cyst study. Gastroenterology 2004; 126: 1330–6.

64. Le Borgne J, de Calan L, Partensky C. Cystadenomas and cystadenocarcinomas of the pancreas: a multi-institutional retrospective study of 398 cases. Ann Surg 1999; 230: 152–61.

65. Frossard JL, Amouyal P, Amouyal G, Palazzo L, Amaris J, Soldan M, et al. Performance of endosonography-guided fine needle aspiration and biopsy in the diagnosis of pancreatic cystic lesions. Am J Gastroenterol 2003; 98: 1516–24.

66. DeWitt J, LeBlanc J, McHenry L, McGreevy K, Sherman S. Endoscopic ultrasound-guided fine-needle aspiration of ascites. Clin Gastroenterol Hepatol 2007; 5: 609–15.

20

21 The Contribution of Histopathology to Endoscopy

Karel Geboes

Introduction

Endoscopy and histology are diagnostic techniques that evaluate biological structures using optical methods. They rely on basic knowledge of the normal anatomy and histology, and through objective description of the morphology of an organ or tissue they can detect abnormalities and reach a definite diagnosis. The optical resolution provided by the two methods is different. Classical endoscopy uses essentially naked-eye observation of the tissue, which allows diagnosis of a polyp, for instance, while histopathology uses larger magnification that reaches the cellular and subcellular level and makes it possible to identify a polyp as an adenoma. Histopathology is thus an extension of endoscopy. The major contributions of histopathology to endoscopy are in connection with the diagnosis and treatment of inflammatory and neoplastic diseases. Histopathology can be an essential element in the diagnosis, as illustrated by Barrett's esophagus and gluten-sensitive enteropathy. Histopathology can also be important for confirming a diagnosis, and very often it can also provide a more precise diagnosis by determining the etiology of inflammation, as illustrated by *Helicobacter pylori*–positive and autoimmune gastritis, or by identifying the type of a tumor (adenocarcinoma or lymphoma). While a precise diagnosis is already essential for adequate treatment, the contribution made by histopathology goes further. Histopathology can provide essential elements for establishing the further treatment strategy by demonstrating the presence or absence of risk factors for residual tumor in polypectomy or endoscopic mucosal resection. Indirectly, it offers the possibility of using additional techniques such as biomarkers for dysplasia and cancer, or the demonstration of mutations such as K-*ras* in colorectal cancer [1]. These applications can have important therapeutic consequences. It has been shown, for instance, that activating mutations of the *KRAS* gene are associated with poor response to anti-epidermal growth factor receptor (EGFR) therapies.

Endoscopy and the Diagnostic Yield of Histopathology

The diagnostic yield of histopathology depends on several factors, including the pathologist's level of experience and also the quality of the biopsy samples and sampling error. The quality of the samples is influenced by a variety of elements, such as the size and shape of the biopsy forceps, the nature and location of the disease, the endoscopist's level of experience, and the number of samples. During endoscopy, samples can be obtained by way of different techniques. These include punch biopsy, suction biopsy with a multipurpose tube (which provides larger samples), brush cytology, endoscopic fine-needle aspiration (offering material from deep areas in the lesion) and snare excision or strip biopsy.

Punch biopsy is the most common technique. Several types of biopsy forceps are available. A distinction can be made between those with elliptical cups and those with round cups. Generally, the samples obtained with elliptical cups are larger. Round cups may thus be more appropriate in children, in order to avoid complications. The size of the biopsy forceps determines partly the size (surface and depth) of the samples. The small forceps has a width of 1.8 mm when opened. The average forceps has a diameter of 2.4 mm and makes it possible to obtain samples containing the muscularis mucosae (and upper submucosa) in 60% of the cases. The larger jumbo forceps has a diameter of 3.4 mm. Samples obtained with this forceps are larger, but they do not necessarily contain more submucosa and the risk of complications (perforation and bleeding) may be greater, whereas it is minimal with the smaller forceps (if the patient has normal coagulation). A forceps can have a central spike so that it stays in position in the mucosa during the procedure. The spike can induce artefacts, which should not be confused with erosions.

The anatomic location of certain types of lesion may be the reason why samples are of poorer quality or superficial in nature. This is often so in areas immediately distal to a stricture, and at the papilla of Vater in the duodenum. The extrahepatic bile ducts and the pancreatic duct are other areas in which biopsies are more difficult to obtain and they are therefore usually smaller. If biopsies from the papilla are taken after sphincterotomy, coagulation artefacts are likely to be present. This is also true with the hot biopsy forceps used for small polypoid lesions, although the quality of the biopsies obtained with a hot forceps is usually no poorer than in those obtained with the classical method. However, the hot forceps procedure is no longer widely used or recommended.

In order to obtain samples of appropriate depth, air insufflation during the endoscopic examination should be limited. When over-insufflation occurs, the mucosa is stretched and pushed toward the underlying submucosa and the samples are likely to be superficial.

The samples obtained with a forceps are usually small and limited to the mucosa. Normally they are not suitable for assessing submucosal or deeper lesions. This means that they are not good, for instance, for a diagnosis of "vasculitis," except for small vessel disease. By using a "burrowing technique," in which several biopsies are taken in the same area, information about deeply situated lesions can eventually be obtained. An alternative is provided by samples obtained with endoscopic ultrasound–guided fine-needle aspiration. These are usually smaller, but they allow both morphologic and cytologic analysis of lesions within or adjacent to the gastrointestinal tract. They can be used to assess neoplastic lesions, but because of their small size they are not good for conditions such as vasculitis [2].

Larger samples are obtained with endoscopic mucosal resection (EMR) and polypectomy. These samples have to be handled appropriately by the endoscopist and in the pathology laboratory. The histopathological interpretation of these samples is the most important consideration for subsequent management. Various microscopic features can help predict the risk for residual cancer and the need for further treatment. A correct diagnostic process involves adequate determination of the area of transection. Identification of this area is easy if the lesion is adequately oriented. The endoscopist can identify the point of transection with India ink or with a pin if the lesion is removed in one piece. If the resection has been performed in piecemeal fashion and the specimen is received in two or more fragments, it may be impossible to determine the true margin of resection if the endoscopist has not attempted to identify the true margin or has not placed a fragment with the true margin in a separate container [3].

Table 21.1 Recommendations for biopsy strategies in inflammatory conditions of the gastrointestinal tract

Organ	Disease	Location	Area for biopsies	Evidence
Esophagus	GERD/NERD	Distal esophagus	Z-line 2 cm above Z-line Cardia Stomach (antrum), *H. pylori*	?
	Eosinophilic esophagitis	Entire esophagus	Proximal, mid Distal esophagus	+
	Barrett's esophagus	Distal esophagus	Four-quadrant biopsy Every 1 cm (short) Every 2 cm (long) (Seattle protocol)	++
Stomach	Gastritis	Entire stomach	Corpus: 2 Antrum 2 Angular incisure 1 (Sydney protocol) + Duodenum	++
Small intestine	Celiac disease	Descending Duodenum	Multiple (4)	++
Colon	Colitis Crohn's disease Ulcerative colitis Microscopic colitis	Ileum Entire colon	Multiple	+

GERD, gastroesophageal reflux disease; NERD, nonerosive reflux disease.

Several studies have shown that the diagnostic yield of histopathology is increased and sampling error is decreased by increasing the number of biopsies. This has been demonstrated for inflammatory diseases such as chronic idiopathic inflammatory bowel disease (IBD) and for neoplastic diseases [4]. Different guidelines for endoscopic sampling in various diseases have therefore been developed (**Table 21.1**) [5–7]. These guidelines remain very important in clinical practice. However, the introduction of new technologies and modern endoscopes in recent years, including zoom endoscopy, high-magnification endoscopy, and more sophisticated techniques such as laser scanning confocal endoscopy and endocytoscopy (in which the microscope is incorporated into the endoscope) may change practices in the future by offering the possibility of targeted biopsies. These techniques are narrowing the gap between endoscopy and pathology. Laser scanning endoscopy provides a microscopy-level image without the need to take a biopsy specimen. Endocytoscopy is based on the technology of light contact microscopy. The tip of an endoscope is placed in direct contact with a dye-stained surface, and the surface is then scanned with condensed normal white light, producing cellular-level imaging. Laser endoscopy increases the real-time diagnostic yield and can be used to confirm intraepithelial neoplasia with a high degree of accuracy. Bioendoscopy is another technique under consideration. It involves the use of monoclonal antibodies labeled with a fluorescent tag or reporter probes (molecules that enter cells) or fluorescent DNA probes for fluorescence in situ hybridization (FISH) in order to detect in situ molecular changes or chromosomal instability [8–11].

While these new techniques can offer real-time imaging and diagnosis, the interpretation of the images is generally still dependent on the morphological features of the lesions as observed with microscopy. The endoscopist therefore has to have a thorough knowledge of pathology. Histopathology remains important for the study of the basic lesions, and there is a continuing need for collaboration between the pathologist and the endoscopist. The two

techniques are indeed complementary if used properly. Endoscopy can provide a real-time diagnosis in some cases, but it mainly makes it possible to obtain targeted biopsies rather than random samples, or biopsies according to well-established guidelines. Targeted biopsies can increase the diagnostic yield and decrease the workload of pathology laboratories. In addition, microscopy can explain the images observed during endoscopy and can clarify the nature of the images and confirm the endoscopic diagnosis or elaborate the diagnosis. It can also still provide a diagnosis when endoscopy remains negative, and it makes it possible to test a variety of markers on tissue samples.

Specimen handling should be done carefully in order to allow optimal diagnostic work-up. It includes proper identification of the patient, including age, specification of the site of origin, fixation, and in some instances orientation. Adequate fixation with an appropriate fixative is central to any histologic preparation. Tissue that is inadequately fixed will lead to difficulties in microtomy, staining, and performing ancillary tests. These problems are not correctable in a later stage. Unfortunately, there is no "all-purpose" fixative. The choice of the appropriate fixative is based on the type of tissue being fixed and on the expected need for ancillary tests such as special stains, immunohistochemistry, in situ hybridization, and electron microscopy. Routine hematoxylin–eosin staining is adequate in most cases but insufficient in particular situations such as a diagnosis of Hirschsprung's disease or metabolic storage disorders. For such indications, freshly frozen tissue for enzyme histochemistry for the demonstration of acetylcholinesterase activity in nerves or the identification of fat is needed, or tissue has to be fixed in glutaraldehyde for transmission electron microscopy. If possible, the endoscopist should be aware of the clinical indication for the biopsy and if necessary should contact the pathology laboratory in order to know whether a special fixation is needed. In general, formalin (10% neutral buffered formalin—i.e., a 10% v/v solution of 40% formaldehyde gas in water) allows good fixation and application of immunohistochemistry as well as molecular analyses. Formaldehyde fixes by cross-linking protein molecules, a relatively slow process. However, prolonged storage of the tissue in formaldehyde solutions can lead to excessive hardening and loss of routine and immune staining potential. The effectiveness of immunohistochemistry depends on the integrity, stability, and availability of the target antigen. Antigenicity may be affected by fixation. Frozen sections will allow application of most ancillary techniques. Freezing must be done properly (by immersion in liquid nitrogen, for instance) and quickly in order to avoid the formation of ice crystals. Rapid adequate freezing and prevention of tissue degeneration are equally essential when molecular techniques based on DNA analysis are considered.

Proper orientation of the tissue samples is important for a diagnosis of malabsorptive states such as celiac disease, where the ratio of villous height to crypt depth has to be assessed, and for specimens from endoscopic resections of polyps or early neoplastic lesions.

Immunohistochemistry and Other Ancillary Techniques

In most instances, histopathology identifies the nature of the lesion or tumor. Neoplastic (malignant) tumors are most frequently epithelial. A smaller number of lesions are neoplastic but nonepithelial, including lymphoproliferative disorders and soft-tissue tumors. Histopathology is an adequate tool for resolving differential diagnostic problems and for classifying tumor types. The differential diagnosis between anaplastic carcinomas, large-cell lymphomas, epithelioid stromal tumors, and neuroendocrine tumors can be difficult, but immunohistochemical staining with antibodies against cytokeratins (a marker for epithelial cells), CD 117 (a marker for

IV

gastrointestinal stromal tumors), chromogranin (a marker for endocrine cells) and a common leukocyte marker can solve the problem. Antibodies to intermediate filaments such as the cytokeratins (CKs) can be potentially useful in other situations. CKs comprise a subfamily of more than 20 members. The relatively limited distribution of some CKs such as CK7 and CK20 and examination of coordinate expression of these two CKs can help in the differential diagnosis of carcinomas of unknown primary site (**Table 21.2**).

Immunohistochemistry and cytogenetic analysis are essential for the management of lymphomas. Primary intestinal lymphomas should be subtyped into B cell and T cell malignancies and classified according to internationally validated classifications such as the one recently published by the World Health Organization. Most B cell lymphomas correspond to diffuse large B cell lymphoma. More rarely, an intestinal B cell lymphoma is composed of small B cells. In this case, differential diagnosis between mucosa-associated lymphoid tissue (MALT)-type lymphoma, mantle cell lymphoma, and follicular lymphoma is mandatory. The latter is recognized by its nodular growth, mimicking the B follicle, and its cellular composition. Most follicular lymphomas are associated with t(14;18) translocations resulting in *BCL2* gene rearrangement. The resulting gene overexpression and aberrant Bcl2 protein production can be identified by immunohistochemistry or by molecular techniques. As a primary gastrointestinal lymphoma, mantle cell lymphoma is the principal lesion presenting as lymphomatous polyposis (**Fig. 21.1**).

Evaluating the proliferation fraction of the tumor cells using a marker such as Ki67 or MIB1 may provide some additional information on the biological behavior of lymphomas. This is also true for endocrine tumors and gastrointestinal stromal tumors.

Histochemistry (using special histological stains) to search for mucins or other substances, and occasionally electron microscopy and genetic markers, can also be applied to biopsy samples. Many types of staining can be performed on routinely formalin-fixed material. However, there is no universal fixative that is ideal for all applications. In special situations such as abetalipoproteinemia, a fat malabsorption disorder, freshly snap-frozen samples will be needed. Electron microscopy also requires an appropriate fixative. Increasingly, there is some overlap between immunohistochemistry and molecular techniques, as genetic markers can also be demonstrated using immunohistochemistry. This is true, for instance, for large-bowel cancers with microsatellite instability (MS), in which the products of the DNA repair genes *hMLH1, hMSH2* and *MSH6,* or the lack of them, can be demonstrated immunohistochemically. However, these products do not cover the whole range of MS. DNA or RNA extraction and genetic analysis continue to be important and there may even be a growing need for them.

Role of Pathology in the Esophagus

Inflammatory Conditions

The role of biopsies in the diagnosis of esophagitis continues to be a problem, due to the relative lack of a gold standard for the diagnosis of gastroesophageal reflux disease (GERD), and there is sometimes a lack of correlation between symptoms, endoscopic appearance, and histology. At present, there is no ideal scenario for a biopsy series for the detection of GERD. In general, it is accepted that changes in the squamous mucosa are usually found close to the squamocolumnar junction (the Z-line). Biopsies from the squamous mucosa should be supplemented with biopsies from the cardia. Histologic changes indicative of gastroesophageal reflux are in fact found on both sides of the squamocolumnar junction (Z-line) [12–15]. The diagnosis of this condition, known as carditis, which occurs in the absence of signs of gastritis in the antrum and gastric body due to *H. pylori* or other causes of gastritis, also means that biopsies from the antrum

Table 21.2 Cytokeratin CK7 / CK20 immunophenotypes in carcinomas; the immunophenotypes are not absolute, but give an indication. Percentages of positive cases are included as examples

CK7 +/CK20 +
Transitional cell carcinoma Pancreatic carcinoma (64%) Ovarian mucinous carcinoma Liver, cholangiocarcinoma (65%)
CK7–/CK20 +
Colorectal adenocarcinoma (90%)
CK7 +/CK20–
Breast carcinoma Lung (non–small cell) Mesothelioma (epithelial) Thymoma Endometrial adenocarcinoma Ovarian serous carcinoma
CK7–/CK20–
Hepatocellular carcinoma Renal cell carcinoma Prostate carcinoma Squamous cell carcinoma Small cell carcinoma

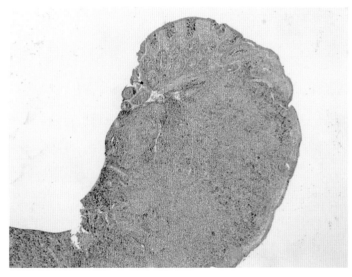

Fig. 21.1 Colon biopsy showing a massive, diffuse and monotonous infiltrate of lymphocytes, suggestive of lymphomatous polyposis.

and gastric body are required in order to exclude the presence of these causes. A biopsy run for GERD should therefore probably include samples from the distal esophagus, particularly from the Z-line and at 2 cm above (probably preferable from the right esophageal wall), from the cardia distal to the Z-line, and from the stomach [16,17]. However, in most cases, peptic esophagitis due to GERD—the most common inflammatory condition in the esophagus—does not require biopsy diagnosis in patients who present with typical symptoms and changes that are macroscopically visible on endoscopy [18].

Biopsies are mainly useful in patients presenting with normal endoscopy and abnormal acid exposure (nonerosive reflux disease, NERD), in patients with typical symptoms and normal endoscopy and pH-metry, and in patients with atypical symptoms. The presence of dilated intercellular spaces (DIS) or of a combination of DIS with other microscopic features such as basal zone hyperplasia observed in GERD may confirm the suspected diagnosis of reflux

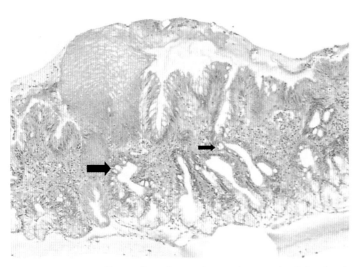

Fig. 21.2 A mucosal biopsy from the esophagus, showing glands lined with goblet cells (arrow) and squamous epithelium. The distal esophagus is lined with columnar epithelium with intestinal metaplasia—Barrett's esophagus.

[16]. However, there are also several other types of esophagitis. The presence of an intense eosinophil infiltration must suggest a diagnosis of eosinophilic esophagitis. Eosinophilic esophagitis can present a typical endoscopic pattern, known as ringed esophagus, but the esophagus can appear normal in up to 20 % of the patients. It is important to recognize that the eosinophilic infiltration may have a heterogeneous distribution within the esophagus. Therefore, when considering eosinophilic esophagitis, it is critical to have biopsies from multiple areas, including the distal, middle, and proximal esophagus [19]. Other possible conditions that can be refractory to the usual therapy for GERD and should be considered are skin disorders such as lichen planus and pemphigoid, which can affect the esophagus. Biopsies of the esophagus are also indicated in the presence of esophageal ulcers, erosions, or an atypical appearance or topography, and whenever an infectious etiology is suspected.

Barrett's esophagus poses a special problem. As indicated above, it is a classic example of a disorder in which the diagnosis depends on cooperation between the pathologist and the endoscopist. The current definition involves endoscopic abnormalities suggestive of Barrett's esophagus (endoscopically suspected esophageal metaplasia) and the presence of columnar epithelium in biopsies. Barrett's esophagus is a preneoplastic condition [20]. Effective management of the risk for esophageal adenocarcinoma in Barrett's esophagus requires sensitive detection of intestinal-type metaplasia and dysplasia (**Fig. 21.2**). The detection of intestinal metaplasia is subject to significant sampling error. Intestinal (specialized) columnar epithelium is the most abundant epithelium found in Barrett's esophagus, but nonintestinal tongues of columnar epithelium extending more

than 2 cm into the lower esophagus are found in approximately 1 % of cases studied [21]. Intestinal metaplasia increases with the length of the Barrett's mucosa segment, and detection improves with number of biopsies taken [22]. When only one or two biopsies are obtained, intestinal metaplasia can easily be missed. It has therefore been proposed that multiple, closely spaced biopsies should be taken. The best-researched biopsy protocol is four-quadrant biopsies every 1 cm for circumferential metaplastic segments (in short-segment Barrett's esophagus) or 2 cm (in long-segment Barrett's esophagus)—known as the Seattle protocol. In another study, it was proposed that eight random biopsies should be obtained to diagnose intestinal metaplasia. With one to four biopsies, the yield was 35 % [22,23]. The detection of intestinal metaplasia in biopsies could be increased by using mucin histochemistry or immunohistochemistry. It has been suggested that the presence of acidic mucins (which appear blue on Alcian blue staining) is a characteristic feature even in the absence of goblet cells. However, this theory has not been confirmed. Comparable disputed results have been obtained with immunohistochemical stains for CKs and MUC antigens (**Fig. 21.3**).

Neoplastic Conditions

As the major risk in patients with Barrett's esophagus is the development of adenocarcinoma, there has been considerable interest in ways of identifying a subgroup of patients who are at risk. At present, the identification of dysplasia in endoscopic mucosal biopsies is the standard method of detecting these patients. Systematic four-quadrant biopsy is also considerably more effective for the detection of dysplasia in Barrett's than nonsystematic biopsy sampling [24]. Nonadherence to a protocol during surveillance leads to underdiagnosis or missed diagnoses, due to sampling error [25]. Histopathological evaluation of mucosal biopsy specimens remains the foundation of clinical decision-making in patients with Barrett's esophagus and dysplasia (**Fig. 21.4**). However, problems with reproducibility of diagnoses of Barrett's esophagus–related neoplasms and with interobserver agreement regarding biopsy specimens, particularly in relation to low-grade dysplasia, have raised concerns in clinical circles about the ability of pathologists to provide a consistent and accurate diagnosis on which management decisions can be based [26,27]. Guidelines for surveillance have been established by national and international societies in order to reduce sampling errors. However, the diagnostic yield for dysplasia can be fundamentally improved and sampling errors reduced using targeted biopsies. These can be obtained with the help of endoscopic procedures such as chromoendoscopy and light-induced or laser-induced fluoroscopy [28,29].

High-grade intraepithelial neoplasia and early cancer can be treated by techniques that destroy or ablate the mucosa. Some techniques, such as photodynamic therapy and laser therapy, do

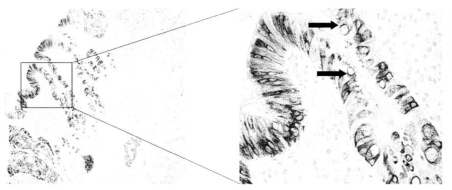

Fig. 21.3 Distal esophagus. Immunohistochemistry with antibodies directed against MUC 2, showing positive staining in foveolar epithelial cells, which are goblet cells (as confirmed on high magnification).

not allow any histological study, as the goal is complete destruction of the neoplastic tissue. However, follow-up biopsies can show remnants of metaplastic and even neoplastic tissue buried underneath squamous epithelium. The frequency of buried metaplastic glands may be as high as 51 % of cases. These glands may be difficult to identify on small endoscopic biopsies.

Endoscopic mucosal resection (EMR) is an ablative technique that was originally developed as a diagnostic procedure (strip-off biopsy) in the early 1980s, but has now gained considerable attention as a potentially curative form of therapy for patients with high-grade dysplasia and superficial cancers. It is also a good tool for histological staging, as the procedure makes it possible to remove intact mucosa and submucosa, allowing complete evaluation of mucosal and submucosal invasion. EMR has been shown to be superior to mucosal biopsy as a diagnostic tool, and interobserver agreement on Barrett's esophagus–related neoplasia is significantly higher in comparison with biopsy specimens [30]. Ideally, the specimen should be oriented, pinned, and stretched on cardboard in the endoscopy unit. If the specimen is not removed in one piece, reconstruction of the specimens should be attempted. Painting of the base and margins is useful, as tumor extension to the deep margin is an indication for surgery and remnants of the neoplastic epithelium at the lateral margins are indications for reexcision or postoperative destruction. It has been shown that there is a high rate of incomplete endoscopic resection in some series [23]. Good communication between the pathologist and the clinicians is important for assessing the efficacy of the treatment and for designing the strategy for additional treatment, which is based on the depth of invasion of the lesion. It has been shown that the presence of a double layer of muscularis mucosae, which is a hallmark of Barrett's esophagus, is an important landmark. It is only when invasion extends beyond the deeper layer (the genuine muscularis mucosae) that a diagnosis of submucosal invasion is justified [31]. Endoscopic biopsies are also commonly used for diagnosing cancer of the esophagus and distinguishing between squamous cell carcinoma and adenocarcinoma. It has been shown that two biopsies can provide a positive diagnosis in 95.8 % of cases. The addition of four samples increases the positive yield to 100 %. There is no statistically significant difference in the yield depending on the site and type of growth [32]. However, diagnosis can be difficult in strictures. In this situation, the additional use of brush cytology may increase the diagnostic yield. Soft-tissue tumors and lymphomas are less common in the esophagus. Fine-needle aspiration biopsy could be used for the tumors, although most soft-tissue tumors in the esophagus are not malignant.

Role of Pathology in the Stomach

▪ Inflammatory Conditions

Features such as redness, edema, swelling, erosions, and ulcers may be present throughout the gastrointestinal tract. They reflect inflammation and tissue damage, as well as mucosal atrophy and metaplasia. Metaplasia is most readily detected endoscopically in the distal esophagus, but it is also common in the stomach. In the latter, it may appear as small red depressions simulating erosions or aphthoid ulcers, as an irregular nodular area, or as larger geographic red areas. The red color and a depressed or nodular appearance can be explained by thinning of the mucosa due to atrophy and metaplasia and increased visibility of the vessels. Pathology is useful to confirm an endoscopic abnormality or exclude such abnormalities, or to provide another explanation. A depressed red spot may indeed be a genuine erosion, but it may also represent a vascular ectasia or a small area of mucosal atrophy. Mucosal atrophy is usually the result of gastritis. Inflammatory conditions in the stomach include gastritis

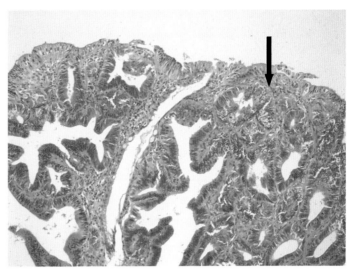

Fig. 21.4 The distal esophagus is lined with columnar epithelium showing features of high-grade dysplasia (arrow).

Table 21.3 Classification of chronic gastritis

Autoimmune gastritis
Infectious ● Bacterial: *Helicobacter pylori*–related gastritis ● Other infections: *H. heilmannii* ● Viral: cytomegalovirus ● Parasitic: *Strongyloides* ● Fungal: *Candida*
Chemical or reactive gastropathy (gastritis) ● Drug: bile reflux, other ● Postgastrectomy
Lymphocytic gastritis
Granulomatous gastritis
Eosinophilic gastritis
Collagenous gastritis
Focal active (enhanced) gastritis
Hypertrophic gastritis: large folds

21

and gastropathy. The latter is characterized by epithelial damage and a minimal inflammatory cell reaction. Several types of gastritis can be distinguished, and histopathology plays a major role in differentiating them (**Table 21.3**). An etiology-based classification was proposed in the Sydney system at the World Congress of Gastroenterology in 1990 and was updated in 1994 [33,34]. The Sydney system also established the need to take different biopsies of the gastric mucosa [33]. The guidelines require:

● Two biopsies from the gastric body and two from the antrum, for an overall assessment of the distribution of the gastritis and the distinction between antral gastritis, gastric body gastritis, and pangastritis.
● One biopsy from the angular incisure, as atrophic gastritis and intestinal metaplasia are related to the development of gastric cancer and occur most commonly at the incisure.
● The same area is also the most appropriate area to look for intraepithelial neoplasia if a macroscopically visible lesion is not present.

In small children, this approach may not be appropriate, however. Two samples from the stomach may be sufficient. Biopsy diagnosis should include the morphological site or sites, the morphological lesions present, and any potential cause. The sensitivity and specif-

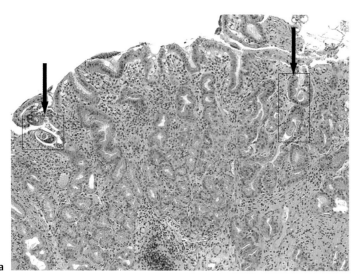

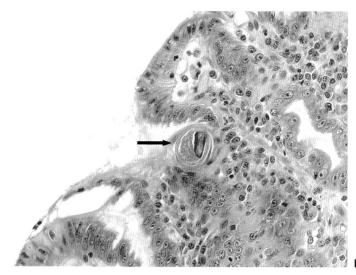

Fig. 21.5
a Gastric biopsy showing infection with Strongyloides stercoralis, also known as the threadworm, a nematode that can affect humans, especially those living in or traveling to endemic areas (Africa, Central America).

b A high-magnification image of a transverse section of the parasite.

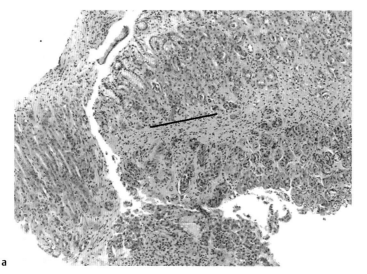

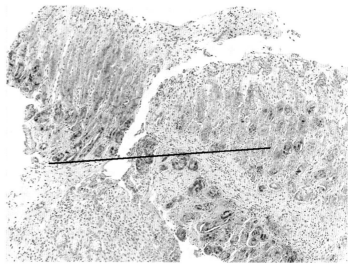

Fig. 21.6 Gastric glandular siderosis (**a**, hematoxylin–eosin, **b**, Perls stain). There is diffuse pigmentation of gastric gland cells, which occurs in systemic iron overload and portal hypertension. In iron pill–induced gastritis, the iron pigment (blue on the Perls stain) is in the lamina propria.

icity for the diagnosis of *H. pylori* gastritis are high (sensitivity 88–99%, specificity 90–100%). The negative predictive value is near 100% for antral biopsies. The necessity for the grading of severity is a matter of controversy. In general, reproducibility in grading the inflammation is good, but it is not very relevant clinically. Active gastritis, or gastritis with neutrophils, is often *H. pylori*–positive and will imply treatment whether activity is mild, moderate, or severe. Grading of atrophy and intestinal metaplasia is less reproducible [35]. Staging of gastritis has been proposed, but this may be difficult to apply in routine practice [36]. Grading and staging could be useful for identifying patients who are at risk for cancer, but evidence-based guidelines need to be developed. In addition to gastric biopsies, it seems reasonable during the first diagnostic examination also to obtain duodenal biopsies to look for the presence of mucous surface (gastric) metaplasia, a requirement for *H. pylori* colonization of the duodenum, which can induce duodenal ulcers, or for epithelial lymphocytosis. If the gastric biopsies are normal and duodenitis is found on histopathology, *H. pylori*-induced duodenitis is highly unlikely. If the patient has lymphocytic gastritis of the antrum and epithelial lymphocytosis in the duodenum, a diagnosis of celiac disease should be suspected. Follow-up biopsies for gastritis can be considered after treatment for *H. pylori* has been given in order to assess eradication, or when intestinal metaplasia and atrophy are very extensive.

Whenever special forms of gastritis are suspected, multiple biopsies are useful. Histopathology can identify the presence of pigments in iron (pill)–induced gastritis and gastric siderosis and a variety of pathogens in infectious gastritis (**Figs. 21.5, 21.6**). Many of the special types lack endoscopic abnormalities or present with different patterns. Lymphocytic gastritis can present as a hypertrophic variant with erosions and thickening of the mucosa, suggestive of Ménétrier's disease, but it can also be limited to the antrum. There are indeed variants of lymphocytic gastritis, including those associated with celiac disease, *H. pylori,* and Crohn's disease. The histopathology of gastroduodenal Crohn's disease includes a wide spectrum of changes, including the presence of granulomas as well as focally enhanced (active) gastritis [37]. A correct diagnosis of Crohn's disease of the stomach can be reached more accurately when multiple samples from the suspected sites (n = 5) and from normal sites are available. Granulomas can be detected in biopsies from macroscopically abnormal mucosa, as well as in biopsies from normal mucosa. The frequency of detecting granulomas varies from 4.6 % to 26 %, depending on the presence of endoscopic lesions, the number of biopsies, and the number of sections examined. Multiple biopsies will increase the diagnostic yield. Focally enhanced or focally active gastritis is typified by small collections of lymphocytes and histiocytes surrounding a small group of foveolae or gastric glands, often with infiltrates of neutrophils. Several studies have found that focally enhanced gastritis is common in adult patients with Crohn's disease. However, studies that used control groups have reported a prevalence of focally enhanced gastritis of up to 19.4 % in non-IBD patients. This type of gastritis may therefore not be a good marker for the diagnosis of IBD or IBD-related gastritis in adults [38,39]. It may still be a good marker in children, although it may not reliably distinguish between Crohn's disease and ulcerative colitis. Some studies have found that focally enhanced gastritis is present in up to 20 % of pediatric ulcerative colitis patients, suggesting that this type of gastritis is a marker of IBD in general in children.

Biopsies are less indicated for the diagnosis of vascular abnormalities. However, they may be useful for the diagnosis of gastric antral vascular ectasia (GAVE). GAVE is a rare condition (with a prevalence of approximately three in 10,000 upper endoscopies), characterized by red spots in linear array in the antrum of the stomach. On the basis of the striped features from the antrum at endoscopy, the disorder has also been called "watermelon stomach." The histological lesion consists of numerous dilated vessels in the mucosa, often with microthrombi, with fibromuscular hyperplasia and fibrohyalinosis of the perivascular lamina propria. The mucosa shows no or mild chronic inflammation or atrophy with intestinal metaplasia [40]. GAVE has to be distinguished from portal hypertensive gastropathy and from gastric vascular ectasia [41].

Neoplastic Conditions

In patients with marked atrophic gastritis or pernicious anemia, the possibility of endocrine cell hyperplasia and dysplasia needs to be considered, and immunostains can readily answer this question. In patients with endocrine tumors (carcinoids), the issue is whether the lesions are sporadic, associated with atrophic gastritis, or may represent multiple endocrine neoplasia (MEN) and Zollinger–Ellison syndrome. Biopsies of adjacent gastric body mucosa will show whether there is hyperplasia of parietal cells without atrophy as seen in Zollinger–Ellison and MEN, atrophy as seen in pernicious anemia, or normal mucosa as seen in sporadic endocrine tumors.

A macroscopic differential diagnosis between benign and malignant ulcers of the stomach can be made on average in 75 % of cases (52–94 % of cases, depending on the series reported in the literature). Consequently, the differential diagnosis often depends on the biopsies. Chromoendoscopy with targeted biopsies will change the guidelines in the future.

In the series reported in the literature, the proportion of cancer-positive biopsies is in the range of 49–56 %, and about 25 % of the biopsies are considered inadequate. A method of biopsy by quadrants with a technique that prevents the lesion from being covered by bleeding from earlier biopsies reduces the number of unusable biopsies to 5.7 % and increases the proportion of cancer-positive biopsies to 67 %. An average of seven to 10 biopsies is required in order to provide sufficient sensitivity and avoid false-negative results [42,43]. When gastric lymphoma is suspected, multiple biopsies are also required. If the lesion presents as an ulcer, biopsies from the edge (as for carcinoma) and from the ulcer base should be obtained. Proper fixation (in order to allow additional tests such

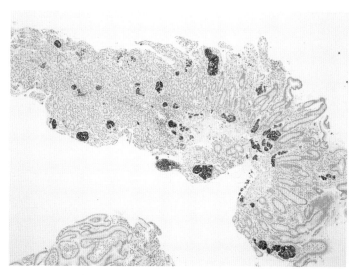

Fig. 21.7 Duodenal biopsy showing a CK7-positive metastasis from a breast carcinoma.

as immunohistochemistry and polymerase chain reaction) is an absolute requirement.

Histopathology is also very useful for identifying metastases or secondary malignant involvement in the gastrointestinal tract—a problem that is becoming more common. Approximately one metastasis is observed per 3847 upper gastrointestinal endoscopies and one metastasis per 1871 colonoscopies. The stomach and duodenum are the most common locations. Immunohistochemistry for cytokeratin patterns and other markers can help identify the origin of the primary lesion, if needed (**Fig. 21.7**).

Overall, a microscopic diagnosis of polyps (elevated lesions) depends on the type of lesion and on the size and number of biopsies. Polyps of epithelial origin can be diagnosed using classical punch biopsies. They include benign lesions such as fundic gland polyps and neoplastic lesions such as adenomas. A complete evaluation may require larger snare biopsies and implies orientation. This is also needed for EMR specimens from early superficial gastric cancer and adenomas. As in Barrett's esophagus, good orientation is needed for assessment of the risk factors for residual tumor and the need for additional surgery. In the stomach, there may also be soft-tissue tumors, especially gastrointestinal stromal tumors (GISTs). These tumors show positive staining with antibodies directed against CD 117 and often also for CD 34 (87 % positive cases in the stomach). They produce polypoid lesions with a smooth or ulcerated surface as a result of a submucosal process. This type of process can be inflammatory or tumoral and will often not be diagnosed adequately when the surface is intact and only mucosal biopsies are available (due to the superficial nature of these biopsies).

Role of Pathology in the Duodenum

Inflammatory Conditions

In the duodenum, inflammatory lesions include *Helicobacter*-associated disease, malabsorptive states, atrophic states, drug-associated disease, and the pathology of the papilla of Vater. Many gastrointestinal diseases and systemic diseases (*H. pylori*, Crohn's disease, vasculitis, eosinophilic infiltrates) affect both the stomach and duodenum. If duodenal biopsies are taken for any reason, it is therefore good to include biopsies of the antrum as well. Any duodenitis inevitably raises the question of whether the condition may be associated with *H. pylori* or drugs, and biopsies of the antrum can

21

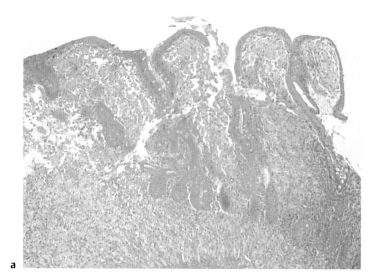

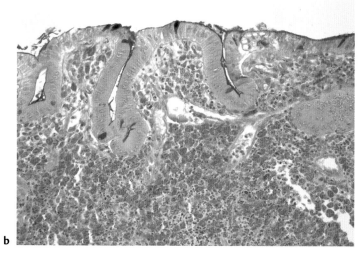

Fig. 21.8 Mycobacterium avium–intracellulare infection. The duodenal biopsy shows pale histiocytes in the lamina propria (**a**), which stain intensely positive on periodic acid–Schiff (PAS) staining (**b**).

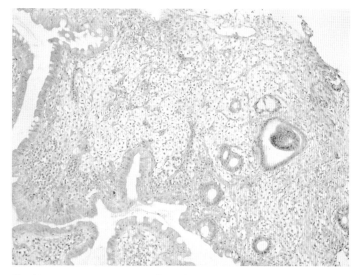

Fig. 21.9 Mastocytosis. Biopsy from the terminal ileum, showing large pale cells in the lamina propria. These cells were positive for CD 117 and tryptase.

Table 21.4 Differential diagnosis of small-bowel villous flattening or crypt hyperplasia

- Allergies to proteins other than gluten (e. g., chicken, cow's milk, eggs, fish and soy also cause epithelial lymphocytosis
- Celiac disease
- Autoimmune enteropathy
- Collagenous celiac disease
- Common variable immunodeficiency
- Drug-induced
- Ischemia
- Hypogammaglobulinemic sprue
- Radiation therapy
- T cell lymphoma–associated enteropathy
- Zollinger–Ellison syndrome

solve this issue readily. Histopathology of the duodenum alone is less useful for the diagnosis of *H. pylori.* Cytology is superior, with a sensitivity in the range of 56–100% and a specificity of 58–93%, depending on the coloring (modified Giemsa staining appears to be superior). Cytology can be performed in the endoscopy room [44].

Biopsy of the small intestine is still the gold standard for celiac disease and is superior for the diagnosis of Whipple's disease. However, whenever pale histiocytes are discovered, a differential diagnosis must be considered. This includes Whipple's disease, infections with Mycobacterium avium–intracellulare in patients with acquired immunodeficiency syndrome (AIDS) and also mastocytosis (**Figs. 21.8, 21.9**). Special stains and immunohistochemistry can solve the diagnosis. Biopsies from the descending duodenum rather than the more distal intestine appear to be sufficient for the diagnosis of celiac disease. Jumbo forceps do not have any marked advantages over standard-sized biopsies [45]. Due to the patchy nature of villous changes, multiple biopsies are necessary. It has been suggested that at least four endoscopic biopsies must be taken [46,47]. Ideally, the specimens are oriented properly in order to allow adequate assessment of villous height and crypt depth. The specimens can therefore be immersed in the fixative after being placed on a Millipore filter paper, with the luminal side upward. A major pitfall in the diagnosis is overinterpretation of villous morphology due to tangential sectioning. However, it is unclear whether orientation before fixation is capable of alleviating this problem.

The Marsh classification and modifications of it for recognizing the spectrum of histological changes seen in celiac disease have provided a major diagnostic advantage. The earliest lesions have still a normal villous architecture but show intraepithelial lymphocytosis. Intraepithelial lymphocytosis is not, however, specific for celiac disease and may be seen in infective enteropathies, Crohn's disease, nonsteroidal anti-inflammatory drug usage, giardiasis, and other conditions. In addition, celiac disease is not the only possible cause of subtotal or total villous atrophy (**Table 21.4**). Other possibilities such as autoimmune enteropathy and food intolerance need to be considered—especially in neonates, but also in adults. Serology is therefore still an important diagnostic tool. Histopathology is also essential for the diagnosis of rare congenital disorders such as microvillous inclusion disease and "tufting enteropathy" (also known as "intestinal epithelial dysplasia," with the term dysplasia being used in its etymological sense of malformation; the condition is due to defects in cell adhesion resulting from defects in the *EPCAM* gene).

Neoplastic Conditions

Refractory celiac disease is a condition that appears to consist of several diseases, including collagenous sprue and enteropathy-type T-cell lymphoma (ETL). Histology can help identify these [48].

Duodenal biopsies are also indicated in patients presenting with duodenal polyps. Many of these, especially in the first part of the duodenum, are benign lesions and represent inflammatory polyps or ectopic gastric tissue.

The small intestine constitutes 75% of the total length of the gastrointestinal tract and over 90% of its mucosal surface. Small-bowel tumors are rare, but approximately two-thirds of them are malignant. Malignant small-bowel tumors represent less than 5% of gastrointestinal malignancies. Four major different histological types of malignant small-bowel tumor can be distinguished: adenocarcinomas, endocrine tumors, lymphomas, and soft-tissue tumors. Adenocarcinoma is the most common type. As in the large bowel, most adenocarcinomas arise from preexisting adenomas that occur sporadically or in the context of familial adenomatous polyposis (FAP), hereditary nonpolyposis colorectal cancer (HNPCC), or variant syndromes. In patients with FAP, hyperplastic polyps and adenomas are most commonly found in the duodenum. In a prospective study of 100 patients, upper gastrointestinal endoscopy revealed adenomatous polyps in the duodenum in 33 cases. The lesions occur mainly in the second part of the duodenum, but may also involve the first and third parts. The severity of the duodenal lesions can be assessed using different methods, including video analysis and histology. A special staging system for duodenal polyposis has been designed in which the lesions are subdivided into different stages according to the number, size, and histological type of polyp. The histological part of this system distinguishes the various types of polyp and grades of dysplasia. The types are: tubular/ hyperplastic/inflammatory polyp, 1 point; tubulovillous, 2 points; and villous, 3 points. Dysplasia is graded into mild, 1 point; moderate, 2; and severe, 3 [49]. Other polyps that may occur in the duodenum include sporadic hamartomas or Peutz–Jeghers polyps, and polyps observed in other nonadenomatous polyposis syndromes.

Endocrine tumors of the small intestine include well-differentiated and malignant large-cell neuroendocrine carcinomas. In the gastrointestinal tract, most endocrine tumors occur in the small bowel (29% of the total) with the highest frequency in the ileum. Endoscopic biopsies are often negative, because of the superficial nature of the samples.

Lymphomatous infiltrates in the gastrointestinal tract are frequently found as part of a disseminated disease. Primary gastrointestinal lymphoma, defined as an extranodal lymphoma arising in the gastrointestinal tract with the bulk of the lesion in this site, is a rare disorder. These lymphomas represent 5–10% of all non-Hodgkin's lymphomas. Despite the fact that the small intestine is the preferential part of the gut in which mucosa-associated lymphoid tissue (MALT) is localized, less than 25% of gastrointestinal lymphomas affect the small intestine.

The duodenum is also the site of the papilla of Vater, where the extrahepatic bile and pancreatic ducts end. Tissue histopathology can be obtained during endoscopic retrograde cholangiopancreatography (ERCP) by brushing, biopsy, bile aspiration, or a combination of these. Biopsies of the bile ducts have a specificity of between 90% and 100%, with a sensitivity between 43% and 81% for the diagnosis of cholangiocarcinoma. Brush cytology has a similarly high specificity of nearly 100%, but the sensitivity is lower, ranging from 18% to 60%. The low sensitivity is linked to the low cellularity of many of these tumors. Repeated brushing may increase the yield. During ERCP, miniature cholangioscopes can be used, with which directed tissue biopsies can be obtained. The biopsies are usually

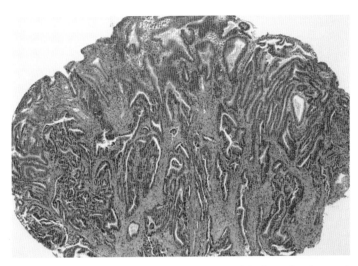

Fig. 21.10 A biopsy obtained from the common bile duct, showing carcinoma.

smaller than standard forceps biopsies of the gastrointestinal tract and may be inadequate in up to 28% of the samples [50]. However, adequate tissue for examination can be obtained with more modern equipment (**Fig. 21.10**) [51].

Role of Pathology in the Terminal Ileum and Colon

Inflammatory Conditions

Ileocolonoscopy with biopsies is an important tool for the diagnosis of colitis. Patients with chronic diarrhea, with or without the passage of blood, are likely to be fully investigated, including one or other form of endoscopy with biopsy. Several studies have shown that colonoscopy and biopsy are useful in the investigation of patients with chronic diarrhea, yielding a histological diagnosis in 22–31% of patients who had a macroscopically normal colon at colonoscopy [52–55]. Histological diagnosis includes a variety of conditions such as spirochetosis, pseudomelanosis coli, collagenous colitis, and lymphocytic colitis and variant forms (**Figs. 21.11, 21.12**). The correct diagnosis of collagenous colitis implies multiple biopsies from different segments, as thickening of the collagen layer

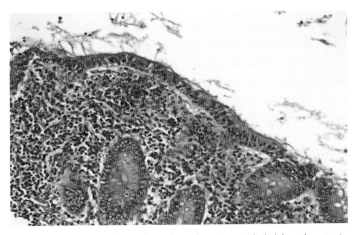

Fig. 21.11 A biopsy from the colon, showing epithelial lymphocytosis, cuboidal surface epithelial cells, and an increase in lamina propria cellularity suggestive of lymphocytic colitis.

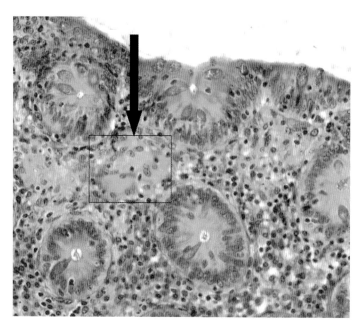

Fig. 21.12 A biopsy from the colon, showing the presence of several giant cells underneath the surface epithelium (arrow) and increased subepithelial collagen deposition: giant cell colitis.

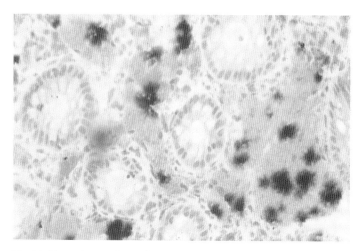

Fig. 21.13 A biopsy from the colon, showing lipid-laden macrophages staining bright red with Oil Red O stain, performed on freshly frozen samples. The patient was subsequently found to have Tangier disease (analphalipoproteinemia).

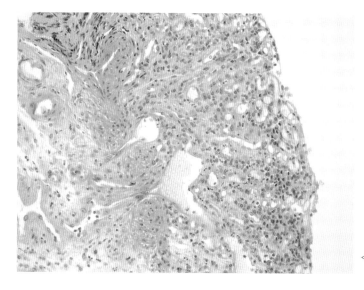

can be discontinuous [56]. Histopathology can also help identify amyloidosis and rare metabolic lysosomal or storage disorders such as Tangier disease (analphalipoproteinemia) and systemic diseases such as mastocytosis (**Fig. 21.13**) [4].

In inflammatory diarrhea, a precise diagnosis and differential diagnosis between infections and IBD and between ulcerative colitis and Crohn's disease is important for therapy and follow-up. Histopathology can identify a variety of pathogens such as amebas, schistosomes, and cytomegalovirus. In immune-depressed patients, a diagnosis of graft-versus-host disease can be confirmed and graded (**Fig. 21.14**). A correct diagnosis of ulcerative colitis can be made by the pathologist without clinical information in 64% of cases with rectal biopsies alone, and in 74% of the cases when multiple biopsies from different segments of the colon, including the ileum, are available [5,57]. With clinical information, a correct diagnosis is reached in more than 90% of cases. A diagnosis of Crohn's disease based on endoscopic samples from the colon relies particularly on the analysis of multiple biopsies from different segments of the colon, including the ileum [58]. For reliable diagnosis, biopsies from five sites in the colon (including the rectum) and ileum should be obtained. Biopsies should be obtained in diseased and uninvolved areas. Analysis of multiple biopsies yields a positive diagnosis of Crohn's disease in 64% of cases, in comparison with 24% for a single rectal biopsy [56,59]. Biopsies from the terminal ileum can be particularly useful, but this does not mean that such biopsies should be obtained systematically during each endoscopy. They are mainly useful in patients with inflammatory diarrhea [60,61]. The differential diagnosis between infections and IBD relies on the distribution of the inflammatory infiltrate in the lamina propria and the presence of architectural changes. Focal or diffuse basal plasmacytosis is a strong predictor for the diagnosis of IBD, especially ulcerative colitis (occurring in over 70% of the patients). It is only rarely observed in infectious colitis (approximately 3% of the patients). Structural epithelial changes include the presence of an irregular surface, sometimes called a pseudovillous or villiform surface, and a disturbed crypt architecture. Overall, an irregular surface is present in approximately 60% of cases of ulcerative colitis. Crypt alterations are more common and more widespread. They are observed in 57–100% of cases. Their widespread appearance enables the pathologist to differentiate ulcerative colitis from Crohn's disease, in which similar alterations are less common (27–71%) and less diffuse [62–64].

Atypical presentations such as ulcerative colitis with left-sided colitis and periappendicular inflammation or cecal patch are occasionally observed. However, the major clinical conditions in which endoscopic and histological lesions may not be characteristic include initial onset of the disease, inflammatory diarrhea in children, patients with liver disease and IBD, patients receiving treatment, and patients presenting with severe, fulminant disease. Colonic biopsies from children between 1 and 10 years of age presenting with new-onset ulcerative colitis show significantly less crypt branching, plasma cells in the lamina propria, cryptitis, crypt abscesses, and epithelial injury in comparison with samples from adults. In 4–8% of cases, the initial biopsy samples are completely normal. Rectal sparing has been well documented [65,66]. Rectal sparing and patchy and focal inflammation are also more common in patients with primary sclerosing cholangitis (PSC) without clinically overt colitis, in comparison with patients with ulcerative colitis without PSC [67,68].

◁ **Fig. 21.14** A small intestinal biopsy, showing severe loss of surface and crypt epithelial cells in graft-versus-host disease.

When the differential diagnosis between ulcerative colitis and Crohn's disease cannot be resolved with endoscopic biopsies, the patient should be categorized as "IBD unclassified" [69]. Clinical and histopathological follow up will eventually lead to a diagnosis in most cases.

During follow-up of IBD, histopathology can identify persistent active inflammation in ulcerative colitis more reliably than endoscopy [70]. Persistent microscopic inflammation may be important in the pathogenesis of dysplasia in IBD.

Neoplastic Conditions

An increased cancer risk has been established for Crohn's disease and ulcerative colitis. A sequence of colitis–dysplasia–cancer has been identified, and this allows surveillance of patients who are at increased risk (e.g., those with long-standing disease, extensive colitis, ulcerative colitis with primary sclerosing cholangitis). It has been estimated that 33 to 64 biopsies are required to detect dysplasia with probabilities of 90% and 95%, respectively. However, with 20–40 biopsies, less than 0.1% of the colorectal mucosa is covered [71,72]. Current practice guidelines recommend that four biopsy specimens be taken from every 10 cm (0.05% of the entire area of the colon) of diseased bowel, in addition to macroscopically atypical lesions [73]. However, the detection rate of IBD-related intraepithelial neoplasia or dysplasia can be substantially improved with targeted biopsies obtained with the newly developed endoscopic techniques, and this procedure will most probably replace the random biopsy approach in the future [8]. Dysplasia in IBD can appear as polypoid lesions or as flat lesions. Polypoid lesions can occur in mucosa with signs of colitis, or in mucosa with flat dysplasia. Biopsies should therefore be obtained from the elevated lesion and from the surrounding tissue. The microscopic diagnosis of dysplasia is based on the presence of "cytological and architectural abnormalities showing unequivocal, noninvasive (confined within the basement membrane), neoplastic transformation of the epithelium, excluding all reactive changes" [74]. Biopsies positive for dysplasia can be subdivided into low-grade and high-grade. The grade of dysplasia is determined by the features of the most dysplastic portion. The two-grade classification appears to be reproducible, although agreement is generally better for high-grade dysplasia. Because of the diagnostic problems related to dysplasia, ancillary techniques can be applied to the tissue samples in order to improve the diagnosis.

Sporadic adenomas and polypoid "dysplasia" in IBD can be managed with endoscopic techniques, and complete local excision appears to be adequate.

Endoscopic resection specimens of IBD-related neoplasia should be handled properly, like all polypectomy specimens. They should be removed entirely if possible. Sporadic small polyps can be handled with a cold or hot biopsy forceps. While the latter can induce coagulation artefacts, the damage does not usually prevent adequate histological interpretation. Larger polyps should be oriented (**Fig. 21.15**). The pathologist identifies the origin of the lesion (whether or not it is epithelial), and its type (whether or not it is neoplastic).

In recent years, it has become clear that hyperplastic polyps are a heterogeneous group of lesions, now reported as "serrated lesions." They include benign polyps, so-called (traditional) hyperplastic polyps, which can be subdivided into several types and lesions with neoplastic potential. Among the latter, traditional serrated adenomas with cytological dysplasia and sessile serrated adenomas or polyps have been identified. Both of these lesions have neoplastic potential, through the serrated neoplastic pathway. In sessile serrated polyps, the epithelial cells show some atypia, but not the classical features of dysplasia (**Fig. 21.16**) [75].

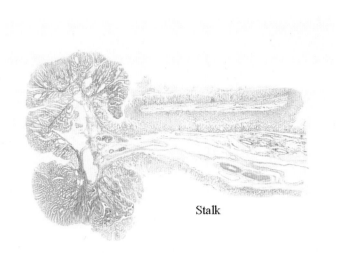

Fig. 21.15 A stalked tubular adenoma resected in the colon. Staining with antibodies against smooth muscle actin. The specimen is well-oriented, showing the stalk covered by normal mucosa and the thickened mucosa of the polyp.

Stalk

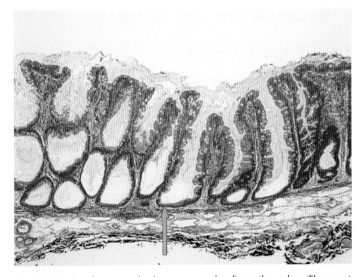

Fig. 21.16 Sessile serrated adenoma or polyp from the colon. The crypt lumen has a serrated aspect over the entire length of the crypt, with basal dilation. Epithelial cells are well-differentiated. The section margin is marked with India ink.

Histopathology allows grading of the dysplasia that is present in polyps and determination of the tubular or villous nature of the lesion. Tubular adenomas are by definition dysplastic and hence at least low-grade dysplastic lesions. Identification of high-grade dysplasia and intramucosal carcinoma is important. Endoscopic surveillance of patients with so-called "advanced adenoma" may need to be different from that provided in patients without advanced adenomas. In polyps, the presence of invasive cancer needs to be differentiated from high-grade dysplasia, intramucosal cancer, and entrapped (pseudoinvasive) mucosa. It is only when cancer invades the submucosa that it is considered to have the potential to metastasize, although lymphangiogenesis can occur in the mucosa, as shown in ulcerative colitis [76]. The established histopathological criteria that determine the choice of treatment between polypectomy or subsequent surgical resection, because of the risk of residual tumor, are the status of the resection margin, the histological grade, lymphovascular invasion, budding of cells, and invasion into the submucosa below the stalk of the polyps but above the muscularis propria (Haggitt level 4) [3,77].

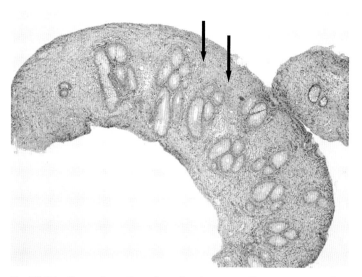

Fig. 21.17 Biopsy from the colon, showing a ganglioneuroma. Ganglion cells are indicated with arrows.

As in the stomach and small intestine, lymphomas and mesenchymal tumors can also occur in the colon, and it is appropriate to take biopsies to allow accurate diagnosis (**Fig. 21.17**).

Conclusions

Histopathology plays a critical role in gastrointestinal practice. Endoscopic biopsies are used to establish, confirm, or exclude a diagnosis that is suspected clinically or endoscopically, with or without the presence of endoscopic abnormalities. Biopsy diagnosis is greatly facilitated when the endoscopist provides adequate samples and understands the criteria used for histological diagnosis.

References

1. Amado RG, Wolf M, Peeters M, Van Cutsem E, Siena S, Freeman DJ, et al. Wild-type *KRAS* is required for panitumumab efficacy in patients with metastatic colorectal cancer. J Clin Oncol 2008;26:1626–34.
2. Geboes K. La collaboration entre l'endoscopiste et le pathologiste. Acta Endosc 2005;36:245–56.
3. Cooper HS. Pathology of the endoscopically removed malignant colorectal polyp. Curr Diagn Pathol 2007;13:423–7.
4. Dejaco C, Oesterreicher C, Angelberger S, Püspök A, Birner P, Poetzi R, et al. Diagnosing colitis: a prospective study on essential parameters for reaching a diagnosis. Endoscopy 2003;35:1004–8.
5. Stange EF, Travis SP, Vermeire S, Beglinger C, Kupcinkas L, Geboes K, et al. European evidence-based consensus on the diagnosis and management of Crohn's disease: definitions and diagnosis. Gut 2006;55(Suppl 1):i1–15.
6. Faller G, Berndt R, Borchard F, Ell C, Fuchs KH, Geddert H, et al. Histopathological diagnosis of Barrett's mucosa and associated neoplasias. Results of a consensus conference of the Working Group for "Gastroenterological Pathology of the German Society for Pathology" on 22 September 2001. Pathology 2003;24:9–14.
7. Stein HJ. Esophageal cancer: screening and surveillance. Results of a consensus conference held at the VIth World Congress of the International Society for Diseases of the Esophagus. Dis Esophagus 1996;9:S 3–19.
8. Kiesslich R, Fritsch J, Holtmann M, Koehler HH, Stolte M, Kanzler S, et al. Methylene blue-aided chromoendoscopy for the detection of intraepithelial neoplasia and colon cancer in ulcerative colitis. Gastroenterology 2003;124:880–8.
9. Kiesslich R, Neurath MF. Potential of new endoscopic techniques: intravital staining and in vivo confocal endomicroscopy for the detection of premalignant lesions and early cancer in patients with ulcerative colitis. Acta Endosc 2004;34:189–97.
10. Kiesslich R, Burg J, Vieth M, Gnaendiger J, Enders M, Delaney P, et al. Confocal laser endoscopy for diagnosing intraepithelial neoplasias and colorectal cancer in vivo. Gastroenterology 2004;127:706–13.
11. Inoue H, Kudo S, Shiokawa A. Technology Insight: laser-scanning confocal microscopy and endocytoscopy for cellular observation of the gastrointestinal tract. Nat Clin Pract Gastroenterol Hepatol 2005;2:31–7.
12. Riddell RH. The biopsy diagnosis of gastroesophageal reflux disease, "carditis," and Barrett's esophagus, and sequelae of therapy. Am J Surg Pathol 1996;20(Suppl 1):S 31–50.
13. Glickman JN, Fox V, Antonioli DA, Wang HH, Odze RD. Morphology of the cardia and significance of carditis in pediatric patients. Am J Surg Pathol 2002;26:1032–9.
14. Dent J. Microscopic esophageal mucosal injury in nonerosive reflux disease. Clin Gastroenterol Hepatol 2007;5:4–16.
15. Tytgat G. The value of esophageal histology in the diagnosis of gastroesophageal reflux disease in patients with heartburn and normal endoscopy. Curr Gastroenterol Rep 2008;10:231–4.
16. Vieth M. Contribution of histology to the diagnosis of reflux disease. Best Pract Res Clin Gastroenterol 2008;22:625–38.
17. Takubo K, Honma N, Aryal G, Sawabe M, Arai T, Tanaka Y, et al. Is there a set of histologic changes that are invariably reflux associated? Arch Pathol Lab Med 2005;129:159–63.
18. [No authors listed.] An evidence-based appraisal of reflux disease management—the Genval Workshop Report. Gut 1999;44(Suppl 2):S 1–16.
19. Chang F, Anderson S. Clinical and pathological features of eosinophilic oesophagitis: a review. Pathology 2008;40:3–8.
20. Vakil N, Van Zanten SV, Kahrilas P, Dent J, Jones R. The Montreal definition and classification of gastroesophageal reflux disease: a global evidence-based consensus. Am J Gastroenterol 2006;101:1900–20.
21. Weinstein WM, Ippoliti AF. The diagnosis of Barrett's esophagus: goblets, goblets, goblets. Gastrointest Endosc 1996;44:91–5.
22. Gatenby PA, Ramus JR, Caygill CP, Shepherd NA, Watson A. Relevance of the detection of intestinal metaplasia in non-dysplastic columnar-lined esophagus. Scand J Gastroenterol 2008;43:524–30.
23. Flejou JF. Histological assessment of oesophageal columnar mucosa. Best Pract Res Clin Gastroenterol 2008;22:671–86.
24. Abela J, Going JJ, Mackenzie JF, Mckernan M, O'Mahoney S, Stuart RC. Systematic four-quadrant biopsy detects Barrett's dysplasia in more patients than non-systematic biopsy. Am J Gastroenterol 2008;103:850–5.
25. Peters FP, Curvers WL, Rosmolen WD, de Vries CE, Ten Kate FJ, Krishnadath KK, et al. Surveillance history of endoscopically treated patients with early Barrett's neoplasia: nonadherence to the Seattle biopsy protocol leads to sampling error. Dis Esophagus 2008;21:475–9.
26. Reid BJ, Haggitt RC, Rubin CE. Criteria for dysplasia in Barrett's esophagus: a cooperative consensus study [abstract]. Gastroenterology 1985;88:AB1552.
27. Sagan C, Fléjou JF, Diebold MD, Potet F, Le Bodic MF. Reproductibilité des critères histologiques de dysplasie sur muqueuse de Barrett. Gastroenterol Clin Biol 1994;18:31–4.
28. Gossner L, Pech O, May A, Vieth M, Stolte M, Ell C. Comparison of methylene blue–directed biopsies and four-quadrant biopsies in the detection of high-grade intraepithelial neoplasia and early cancer in Barrett's esophagus. Dig Liver Dis 2006;38:724–9.
29. Curvers WL, Kiesslich R, Bergman JJGHM. Novel imaging techniques in the detection of oesophageal neoplasia. Best Pract Res Clin Gastroenterol 2008;22:687–720.
30. Mino-Kenudson M, Hull MJ, Brown I, Muzikansky A, Srivastava A, Glickman J, et al. EMR for Barrett's esophagus-related superficial neoplasms offers better diagnostic reproducibility than mucosal biopsy. Gastrointest Endosc 2007;66:660–6.
31. Geboes K, Ectors N, Geboes KP, Lambert R. Intraepithelial neoplasia, dysplasia and early cancer of the digestive tract: Modifications in terminology. Curr Cancer Ther Rev 2005;1:145–55.
32. Lal N, Bhasin DK, Malik AK, Gupta NM, Singh K, Mehta SK. Optimal number of biopsy specimens in the diagnosis of carcinoma of the oesophagus. Gut 1992;33:724–6.
33. Price AB. The Sydney System: histological division. J Gastroenterol Hepatol 1991;6:209–22.
34. Dixon MF, Genta RM, Yardley JH, Correa P. Classification and grading of gastritis: the updated Sydney System. Am J Surg Pathol 1996;20:1161–81.
35. Nichols L, Sughayer M, DeGirolami PC, Balogh K, Pleskow D, Eichelberger K, et al. Evaluation of diagnostic methods for *Helicobacter pylori* gastritis. Am J Clin Pathol 1991;95:769–73.
36. Rugge M, Correa P, Di Mario F, El-Omar E, Fiocca R, Geboes K, et al. OLGA staging of gastritis: a tutorial. Dig Liver Dis 2008;40:650–8.

IV

37. Oberhuber G, Püspök A, Oesterreicher C, Novacek G, Zauner C, Burghuber M, et al. Focally enhanced gastritis: a frequent type of gastritis in patients with Crohn's disease. Gastroenterology, 1997;112:698–706.

38. Xin W, Greenson JK. The clinical significance of focally enhanced gastritis. Am J Surg Pathol, 2004;28:1347–51.

39. Yao K, Yao T, Iwashita A, Matsui T, Kamachi S. Microaggregate of immunostained macrophages in noninflamed gastroduodenal mucosa: a new useful histological marker for differentiating Crohn's colitis from ulcerative colitis. Am J Gastroenterol 2000;95:1967–73.

40. Gilliam JH 3 rd, Geisinger KR, Wu WC, Weidner N, Richter JE. Endoscopic biopsy is diagnostic in gastric antral vascular ectasia. The "watermelon stomach." Dig Dis Sci 1989;34:885–8.

41. Misra V, Misra SP, Dwivedi M, Gupta SC. Histomorphometric study of portal hypertensive enteropathy. Am J Clin Pathol 1997;108:652–7.

42. Vyberg M, Hougen HP, Tonnesen K. Diagnostic accuracy of endoscopic gastrobiopsy in carcinoma of the stomach. Acta Path Microbiol Immunol Scand (A), 1983;91:483–7.

43. Misiewicz JJ, Tytgat GNJ, Goodwin CS, Price AB, Sipponen P, Strickland RG. The Sydney system: a new classification of gastritis. Proceedings of the 9th World Congress of Gastroenterology. Sydney, Australia, 1990, 1–10.

44. Debongnie JC, Delmee M, Mainguet P, Beyaert C, Haot J, Legros G. Cytology: a simple, rapid, sensitive method in the diagnosis of *Helicobacter pylori*. Am J Gastroenterol 1992;87:20–3.

45. Mee AS, Burke M, Vallon AG, Newman J, Cotton PB. Small bowel biopsy for malabsorption: comparison of diagnostic adequacy of endoscopic forceps and capsule biopsy specimens. Br Med J 1985;291:769–72.

46. Green PHR, Rostami K, Marsh MN. Diagnosis of coeliac disease. Best Pract Res Clin Gastroenterol 2005;19:389–400.

47. Dickson BC, Streutker CJ, Chetty R. Coeliac disease: an update for pathologists. J Clin Pathol 2006;59:1008–16.

48. Brousse N, Meijer JWR. Malignant complications of coeliac disease. Best Pract Res Clin Gastroenterol 2005;19:401–12.

49. Spigelman AD, Williams CB, Talbot IC, Domizio P, Phillips RKS. Upper gastrointestinal cancer in patients with familial adenomatous polyposis. Lancet 1989;ii:783–5.

50. Van Caillie MA, Geboes K, Van Eyken P, Van Steenbergen W. The diagnostic value of intraductal biopsy of the extrahepatic bile ducts. Tijdschr Geneeskd 2006;62:1035–43.

51. Nguyen K, Sing JT Jr. Review of endoscopic techniques in the diagnosis and management of cholangiocarcinoma. World J Gastroenterol 2008;14:2995–9.

52. Prior A, Lessels AM, Whorwell PJ. Is biopsy necessary if colonoscopy is normal? Dig Dis Sci 1987;32:673–6.

53. Whithead R. Colitis: problems in definition and diagnosis. Virchows Archiv Pathol Anat 1990;417:187–90.

54. Marshall JB, Singh R, Diaz-Arias AA. Chronic, unexplained diarrhea: are biopsies necessary if colonoscopy is normal? Am J Gastroenterol 1995;90:372–6.

55. Shah RJ, Fenoglio-Preiser C, Bleau BL, Giannella RA. Usefulness of colonoscopy with biopsy in the evaluation of patients with chronic diarrhea. Am J Gastroenterol 2001;96:1091–5.

56. Geboes K. Lymphocytic, collagenous and other microscopic colitides: pathology and the relationship with idiopathic inflammatory bowel diseases. Gastroenterol Clin Biol 2008;32:689–94.

57. Bentley E, Jenkins D, Campbell F, Warren BF. How could pathologists improve the initial diagnosis of colitis? Evidence from an international workshop. J Clin Pathol 2002;55:955–60.

58. Dejaco C, Oesterreicher C, Angelberger S, Püspök A, Birner P, Poetzi R, et al. Diagnosing colitis: a prospective study on essential parameters for reaching a diagnosis. Endoscopy 2003;35:1004–8.

59. Stange EF, Travis SPL, Vermeire S, Beglinger C, Kupcinkas L, Geboes K, et al. European evidence based consensus on the diagnosis and management of Crohn's disease: definitions and diagnosis. Gut 2006;55:1–15.

60. McHugh JB, Appelman HD, McKenna BJ. The diagnostic value of endoscopic terminal ileum biopsies. Am J Gastroenterol 2007;102:1084–9.

61. Geboes K. The strategy for biopsies of the terminal ileum should be evidence based. Am J Gastroenterol 2007;102:1090–2.

62. Schumacher G, Kollberg B, Sandstedt B. A prospective study of first attacks of inflammatory bowel disease and infectious colitis. Histologic course during the 1st year after presentation. Scand J Gastroenterol 1994;29:318–32.

63. Jenkins D, Balsitis M, Gallivan S, Dixon MF, Gilmour HM, Shepherd NA, et al. Guidelines for the initial biopsy diagnosis of suspected chronic idiopathic inflammatory bowel disease. The British Society of Gastroenterology Initiative. J Clin Pathol 1997;50:93–105.

64. Seldenrijk CA, Morson BC, Meuwissen SG, Schipper NW, Lindeman J, Meijer CJ. Histopathological evaluation of colonic mucosal biopsy specimens in chronic inflammatory bowel disease: diagnostic implications. Gut 1991;32:1514–20.

65. Markowitz J, Kahn E, Grancher K, Hyams J, Treem W, Daum F. Atypical rectosigmoid histology in children with newly diagnosed ulcerative colitis. Am J Gastroenterol 1993;88:2034–7.

66. Robert ME, Tang L, Hao LM, Reyes-Mugica M. Patterns of inflammation in mucosal biopsies of ulcerative colitis: perceived differences in pediatric populations are limited to children younger than 10 years. Am J Surg Pathol 2004;28:183–9.

67. Loftus EV Jr, Harewood GC, Loftus CG, Tremaine WJ, Harmsen WS, Zinsmeister AR, et al. PSC-IBD: a unique form of inflammatory bowel disease associated with primary sclerosing cholangitis. Gut 2005;54:91–6.

68. Perdigoto R, Wiesner RH, LaRusso NF. Inflammatory bowel disease associated with primary sclerosing cholangitis: incidence, severity and relationship to liver disease [abstract]. Gastroenterology 1991;100:A238.

69. Geboes K, Colombel JF, Greenstein A, Jewell DP, Sandborn WJ, Vatn MH, et al. Indeterminate colitis: a review of the concept—what's in a name? Inflamm Bowel Dis 2008;14:850–7.

70. Geboes K, Riddell R, Öst Ä, Jensfelt B, Persson T, Löfberg R. A reproducible grading scale for histological assessment of inflammation in ulcerative colitis. Gut 2000;47:404–9.

71. Rosenstock E, Farmer RG, Petras R, Sivak MV Jr, Rankin GB, Sullivan BH. Surveillance for colonic carcinoma in ulcerative colitis. Gastroenterology 1985;89:1342–6.

72. Rubin CE, Haggitt RC, Burmer GC, Brentnall TA, Stevens AC, Levine DS, et al. DNA aneuploidy in colonic biopsies predicts future development of dysplasia in ulcerative colitis. Gastroenterology 1992;103:1611–20.

73. Kornbluth A, Sachar DB. Ulcerative colitis practice guidelines in adults. American College of Gastroenterology, Practice Parameters Committee. Am J Gastroenterol 1997;92:204–11.

74. Riddell RH, Goldman H, Ransohoff DF, Appelman HD, Fenoglio CM, Haggitt RC, et al. Dysplasia in inflammatory bowel disease: standardized classification with provisional clinical applications. Hum Pathol 1983;14:931–68.

75. Yantiss RK. Serrated colorectal polyps and the serrated neoplastic pathway: emerging concepts in colorectal carcinogenesis. Curr Diagn Pathol 2007;13:456–66.

76. Kaiserling E, Kröber S, Geleff S. Lymphatic vessels in the colonic mucosa in ulcerative colitis. Lymphology 2003;36:52–61.

77. Ueno H, Mochizuki H, Hashiguchi Y, Shimazaki H, Aida S, Hase K, et al. Risk factors for an adverse outcome in early invasive colorectal carcinoma. Gastroenterology 2004;127:385–94.

21

22 Diagnostic Endoscopic Ultrasonography

Abdel M. Kassem, Thomas Rösch

Introduction

The rationale of combining ultrasonography with endoscopy is to allow more detailed imaging of the pancreas and gut wall. With the transducer positioned within the bowel lumen, mounted on the tip of the endoscope, high ultrasound frequencies can be used that allow higher-resolution images of the layers of the bowel wall in comparison with conventional abdominal ultrasound. This technique of intraluminal ultrasonography was initially used in the rectum, where blind and rigid ultrasound probes were applied, before the method was adapted for use in combination with flexible endoscopes. In the instruments currently available, a small ultrasound transducer is mounted at the tip of either side-viewing endoscopes (for the upper gastrointestinal tract) or forward-viewing instruments. Even higher frequencies and hence higher resolution, although with limited penetration, can be obtained with miniature ultrasound probes, which can be passed through the working channel of endoscopes.

The introduction of endoscopic ultrasonography (EUS) into gastroenterologic endoscopic practice opened up new avenues in the field of diagnosis as well as therapeutic interventions in gastroenterology. Organs such as the pancreas have become more accessible, and structural changes in the wall of the gastrointestinal tract can be more accurately delineated and interpreted. With technological advances in competing imaging tools such as computed tomography (CT), magnetic resonance imaging (MRI), and positron-emission tomography (PET), it might have been thought that EUS was a method doomed to extinction. However, the widespread use of EUS in many countries and endoscopy centers argues the contrary. An important reason for this apparent contradiction is that there have also been technical improvements and developments in EUS equipment, leading to a wider range of uses for EUS, including therapeutic interventions.

Available Instruments and Scanning Principles

Endoscopic ultrasonography (EUS) is a combination of endoscopy and high-frequency ultrasound. A small ultrasound transducer (diameter 11–13 mm) is mounted onto the tip of either side-viewing endoscopes (for the upper gastrointestinal tract) or forward-viewing instruments (such as the echo colonoscope). The technique of intraluminal ultrasonography was initially used in the rectum, where blind and rigid ultrasound probes were applied, before the method was adapted for use in combination with flexible endoscopes. Ultrasound generation with EUS is either mechanical or electronic, depending on the type of instrument used. The shift toward using electronic transducers for EUS is considered a milestone in its development. Electronic transducers allow applications such as harmonic imaging, Doppler and power Doppler imaging, three-dimensional imaging, and real-time tissue elastography. In addition, curvilinear electronic transducers are used for interventional diagnostic and therapeutic procedures. Miniaturization of the ultrasound components resulted in the development of miniprobes, which can be introduced through the working channel of conventional upper and lower gastrointestinal endoscopes. These can operate at high frequencies, resulting in higher-resolution images of the wall layers. However, due to their limited penetration depth (owing to the small diameter and higher ultrasound frequencies), miniprobes have not yet universally replaced conventional echo endoscopes. An overview of the instrument types currently in use for upper gastrointestinal tract EUS is given in **Table 22.1**; examples of instruments and probes are shown in **Figs. 22.1–22.11**.

The ultrasound transducer in echo endoscopes and blind probes either generates a radial image of 360°, oriented perpendicular to the shaft axis of the instrument, or a linear-type image directed

Table 22.1 Overview of instrument types in use for upper gastrointestinal endoscopic ultrasonography

Radially scanning echo endoscopes	
Mechanically rotating transducer, 360° ultrasonic plane perpendicular to the shaft axis, frequencies between 5 and 20 MHz	Olympus GF-UM20, JF-UM20, GF-UM2000, GF-UM160, GF-UM240, GF-UM130, GF-UMQ240, GF-UMQ130
Electronic transducer, 360° ultrasonic plane perpendicular to the shaft axis, frequencies between 5 and 10 MHz	Pentax: EG-3670URK
Electronic transducer, 360° ultrasonic plane perpendicular to the shaft axis, frequencies between 5 and 12 MHz	Fujinon: EG-530UR
Slim nonoptical probe (7 mm in diameter), introduced over a guide wire for use in esophageal stenoses (frequency 7.5 MHz)	Olympus: MH-908
Rigid rectal probes (frequency 7.5 MHz)	Olympus RU-75M-R1, RU-12M-R1
Linear-scanning echo endoscopes	
Frequencies between 5 and 10 MHz	Olympus: GF-UC240P-AL5, GF-UC140P-AL5, GF-UCT240P-AL5, GF-UCT140P-AL5, Pentax/Hitachi:EG-3870UTK
Frequencies between 5 and 12 MHz	Fujinon: EG-530UT
Frequencies between 5 and 7.5 MHz	Pentax/Hitachi FG-32UA, FG-34UX, FG-36UX and FG-38UX
Frequency 7.5 MHz	Olympus: GF-UC2000P-OL5, GF-UC160P-OL5, GF-UCT2000-OL5, GF-UCT160-OL5

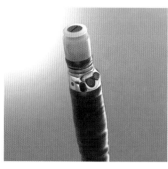

Fig. 22.1 The Olympus GF-UM160 upper gastrointestinal endoscope, with broadband frequencies ranging from 5 to 20 MHz. Four frequencies can be selected.

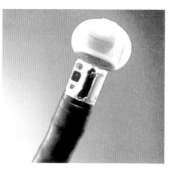

Fig. 22.2 A water-filled balloon around the tip of the Olympus JF-UM20 echo endoscope.

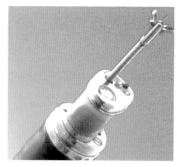

Fig. 22.3 The tip of the Olympus CF-UM20 echo colonoscope, with a forward-viewing lens and biopsy forceps introduced through the instrumentation channel.

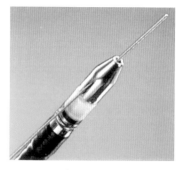

Fig. 22.4 The tip of the Olympus MH-908 blind probe, with an 8-mm distal tip, to be introduced over a guide wire for use in stenotic esophageal lesions.

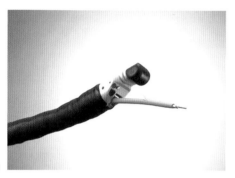

a

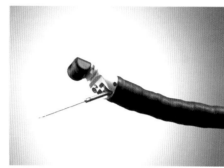

Fig. 22.5 Olympus longitudinal echo endoscopes.
a The Olympus GF-UCT160-AL5 (with a 3.7-mm channel) for endoscopic ultrasound–guided cyst drainage.
b The Olympus GF-UC160P-AL5 (with a 2.8-mm channel) for endoscopic ultrasound–guided puncture. Compatible with the Olympus EU-C60 processor. (Also available are the GF-UCT140-AL5 and GF-UC140P-AL5, compatible with the Aloka SSD5500 and SSD5000 ultrasound scanners).

b

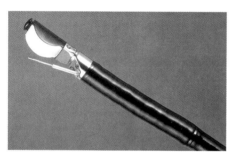

Fig. 22.6 The Pentax/ Hitachi longitudinal FG-32UA echo endoscope, with a distal needle tip for endoscopic ultrasound–guided puncture.

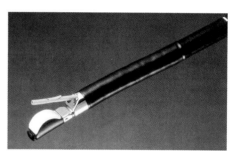

Fig. 22.7 The Pentax/ Hitachi FG-38UX therapeutic echo endoscope, with a stent introduced through the instrument channel (e.g., for endoscopic ultrasound–guided puncture and drainage of pancreatic pseudocysts; see text).

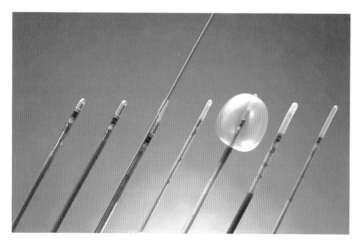

Fig. 22.8 The Olympus miniprobe range: radial-scanning probes with various frequencies from 12 to 30 MHz, a special guide wire, and balloon probes and dual-plane probes (radial and linear) with frequencies of 12 MHz and 20 MHz.

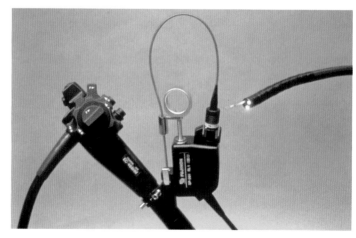

Fig. 22.9 The Fujinon SP-701 miniprobe, available with various ultrasound frequencies (12–20 MHz), with radial and longitudinal scanning capabilities.

IV

parallel to the shaft axis of the endoscope or probe. As mentioned above, curvilinear echo endoscopes are increasingly being used, particularly for diagnostic procedures (e.g., fine-needle aspiration) and therapeutic interventions. In contrast to radial instruments, in which a 360° view is generated (sometimes less with electronic radial transducers), which allows better orientation and provides a better overview of the gastrointestinal wall and surrounding structures, orientation with linear instruments is more difficult, as only a narrower segment can be visualized at one time. A systematic approach should therefore be sought during examination, with orientation toward key landmarks. During imaging of a target lesion, clockwise and anticlockwise rotation of the instrument can ensure complete assessment of the lesion and its surrounding structures. The accuracy with the two types of scanning appears to be equivalent [1,2].

As the gastrointestinal hollow organs contain air, acoustic coupling of the ultrasound transducer to the gastrointestinal wall requires either the use of a water-filled balloon around the instrument tip (for narrower organs such as the esophagus and bowel) or additional water instillation, especially into the stomach and occasionally into the colon. Perpendicular scanning should be attempted for target lesions, since oblique scanning may lead to broadening and blurring of normal and pathological structures and can give rise to erroneous diagnoses. An adequate focal distance is also essential (for practical reasons usually 0.5–1.0 cm, depending on the ultrasound frequencies used) in order to visualize small and discrete intramural lesions appropriately. It may be necessary to use higher frequencies for structures and lesions close to the transducer. Once a lesion has been identified and located by endoscopy, or by positioning the echo endoscope at a point from which the structure is usually visible (especially for extraluminal pathology—e.g., in the pancreas), the instrument should only be moved slightly and slowly backward and forward, with even, fine movements of the instrument tip, in order to depict the full extent of the lesion and its relation to neighboring organs and structures.

Basics of EUS-Guided Puncture Techniques

The introduction of thin steel needles through the working channel of echo endoscopes allows for puncture of intramural or paramural lesions. This is much more safely done with linear-type instruments, since these allow the entire course of the needle to be visualized on the ultrasound image. The needles used are guided through a plastic and metal-reinforced sheath in order to protect the instrumentation channel of the puncture echo endoscopes. The sheath extends out of the channel by approximately 1 cm with the same needle, whereas this distance can be modified with other needle types. Thereafter, the lesion to be punctured is brought into the focus of the needle passageway, which may be modifiable with the help of an elevator built into some types of instrument (**Fig. 22.12**). The shorter the distance between the tip of the echo endoscope and the target lesion, the more effective the procedure will be. Color Doppler imaging can be used to avoid puncturing intervening vascular structures that may lie in the path of the needle. Once the target lesion is in focus, the needle is pushed into and/or through the gastrointestinal wall to reach the lesion. A stopper is available with the same needle, to avoid unforeseen deep penetration into underlying vessels or other structures. The stylet in the needle is pulled back a little before the puncture is initiated, and it is then fully removed when

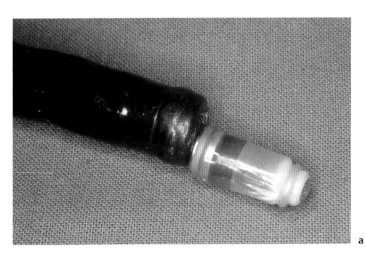

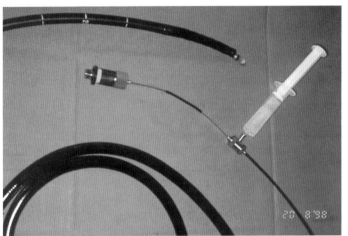

Fig. 22.10a, b The Fujinon probe (diameter 7.3 mm) to be attached to the tip of a conventional endoscope coupled to a 2.6-mm probe, which is introduced through the working channel. A water-filled balloon around the 7 mm transducer provides acoustic coupling.
a The tip of the instrument.
b The whole assembly.

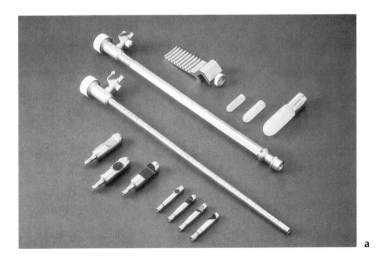

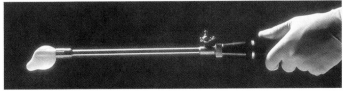

Fig. 22.11 The Bruel & Kjaer medical rigid rectal ultrasound probe, with a ▷ diameter of 13 mm.
a The whole set needed for endorectal scanning.
b The instrument with a balloon around the tip.

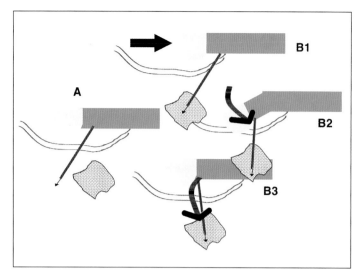

Fig. 22.12 Schematic drawing of endoscopic ultrasound–guided puncture. Since the lesion (L) does not lie ideally in the focus of the needle tract (A), the position of either the instrument (withdrawal, B1; tip modification, B2) or the needle (with the help of an elevator, B3) has to be modified so that the lesion can be reached with the needle.

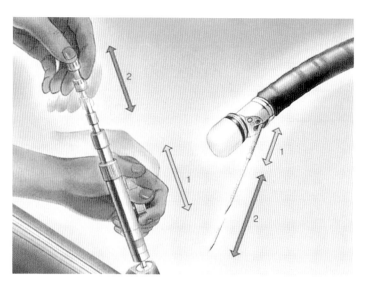

Fig. 22.13 The Olympus NA-10J-1 needle (22 gauge), which has a facility for gradually advancing the spiral sheath out of the instrumentation channel before the needle is extended to puncture a lesion.

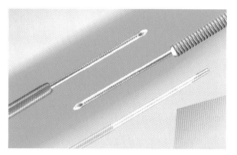

Fig. 22.14 The Vilmann-type needle (Sonotip; GIP).

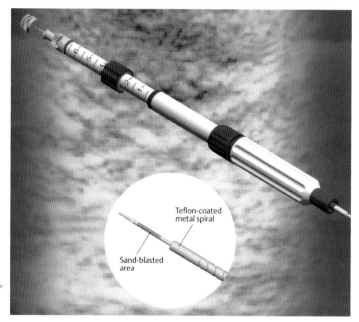

Fig. 22.15 The tip of the Wilson-Cook puncture needle. This single-use ▷ needle has a stop mechanism (not shown here), allowing the needle length exiting through the sheath to be exactly determined before puncture.

the needle tip has reached the lesion. Under continuous suction, the needle is moved forward and backward inside the lesion in order to obtain representative material. Care should be taken to avoid suction of blood or blood-tinged fluid into the needle, as this may substantially compromise cytopathological assessment. Some cytopathologists recommend flushing the needle with heparin before the procedure in order to prevent it from becoming clogged with blood clots [3]. Ten or more back-and-forth movements are required to obtain adequate samples. The number of punctures varies depending on the target lesion. In mediastinal lymph nodes, two or three punctures may be sufficient; five punctures are needed for abdominal lymph nodes and seven punctures for pancreatic masses. The path of each stroke within the target lesion should be changed as much as possible to obtain representative samples, and it should be borne in mind that the periphery of the lesion usually provides a

better cytological yield [4]. Examples of commercially available needles are shown in **Figs. 22.13–22.15**.

After each puncture, the material is smeared onto glass slides for cytological analysis. The use of slides with frosted margins is recommended. The slide should be labeled with a pencil on the frosted margin before the aspiration biopsy, to prevent incorrect assignment. It is important to deposit the aspirate as a single drop at one end of the slide; this is best achieved by bringing the tip of the needle into contact with the slide. Otherwise the aspirate will be diffusely distributed over the slide in the form of tiny droplets, which dry very rapidly. The drop is then spread along the slide in a single stroke using a glass cover-slip. Larger tissue particles are subsequently dispersed by applying slight pressure with a flatly applied slide or cover-slip.

Depending on the staining technique, the aspirate smears are either air-dried or fixed in alcohol. May–Grünwald staining is preferred by many cytologists, due to its better contrast; for this type of staining, the slides should be delivered air-dried. Smears to be stained using the Papanicolaou method must be fixed immediately in 95% ethanol or with a spray fixative before they dry. Small samples for histopathology can be also obtained, particularly with a 19-gauge Tru-Cut needle biopsy device with a spring-loaded handle [5]. Two to three needle passes usually need to be carried out. Rapid on-site evaluation of specimens by an in-room cytopathologist has been shown to increase the accuracy of this procedure. Rapid on-site evaluation may enhance the yield of fine-needle puncture (FNP) and may reduce unnecessary sampling [6,7].

Clinical Background and Prerequisites of EUS and EUS-Guided Fine-Needle Puncture

EUS is almost never a primary examination for gastrointestinal and pancreaticobiliary disorders, nor is it a screening test. In the gastrointestinal tract, there is usually a diagnosis or at least a strong suspicion of a lesion at endoscopy, often confirmed by bioptic histopathology. EUS then provides more detailed information about the lesion's extent and depth of penetration. In gastrointestinal cancers, EUS provides information about the locoregional tumor stage. In submucosal lesions, EUS examination should be carried out directly after the endoscopic (or occasionally radiological) diagnosis, in order to differentiate between intramural tumors and extramural compressions, and it can be used for follow-up of submucosal tumors. In the pancreas, EUS is used to search for endocrine tumors in patients in whom this diagnosis has been established previously by specific clinical signs and symptoms, as well as laboratory tests. In pancreatic cancer, some suspicion has almost always been raised by other imaging tests before EUS is used to visualize and stage the tumor. The indications for EUS agreed in consensus statements and publications of gastrointestinal endoscopy societies are shown in **Table 22.2**.

The following prerequisites should be fulfilled before the use of EUS is considered:

- The clinical consequences of the EUS diagnosis should be clear (e.g., decision between surgery and palliation, or between a diagnosis that needs no further diagnostic and therapeutic steps and a diagnosis that requires further tests).
- Other imaging tests should have established at least a tentative diagnosis that can be better characterized using EUS.
- The lesion should be reachable by endoscopy; i.e., one should make sure that it is within the reach of the echo endoscope—which is not the case in nontraversable strictures or in postoperative anatomic conditions (e.g., pancreatic head in patients with Billroth II operations). It is still a matter of debate whether dilation of malignant esophageal strictures to allow full evaluation of the entire tumor length is mandatory, or whether this is too risky.

The same applies to EUS-guided FNP. It is obvious that, as with other puncture techniques, EUS-guided FNP is mainly used to differentiate between benign and malignant conditions, or to allow cytological/histological characterization of a lesion that is strongly suspected to be malignant on imaging tests including EUS, but in which different tissue diagnoses (e.g., carcinoma versus lymphoma) result in different treatment approaches. It is also evident that in most cases, only a positive diagnosis of malignancy counts, whereas there is a 15–20% chance that a negative one is a false-negative. The clinical consequences must therefore be clear before EUS-guided FNP is performed. If a pancreatic mass is resectable and will also be operated on even if EUS-guided FNP is negative, it might be argued

Table 22.2 Indications for endoscopic ultrasonography [11]

	Expected benefit of EUS
Gastrointestinal tract	
Locoregional cancer staging	
• Esophagus	+++
• Stomach	++
• Rectum	+
• Colon	?
Follow-up of cancer after chemoradiotherapy	?
Detection of anastomotic recurrence	+(+)
Gastric lymphoma	
• Differential diagnosis of large folds	++
• Staging of gastric lymphoma	++
• Re-staging after chemoradiotherapy	++
Diagnosis of submucosal tumors	
• Differentiation from extraluminal compressions	+++
• Characterization of submucosal tumors	++
Varices and portal hypertension	?
Benign esophageal strictures	?
Achalasia	?
Differential diagnosis of gastric ulcers	–
Differential diagnosis of large gastric folds	+++
Pancreaticobiliary tract	
Diagnosis of small pancreatic cancer	++
Staging of ampullopancreatic and distal biliary cancer	++
Staging of proximal biliary cancer (miniprobes?)	?
Differential diagnosis of pancreatic masses	–
Differential diagnosis of indeterminate biliary strictures	?
Differential diagnosis of pancreatic cysts	?
Localization of pancreatic endocrine tumors	+++
Diagnosis of chronic pancreatitis	+
Diagnosis of common bile duct stones	++(+)
Colorectum	
Staging of rectal cancer	+++
Staging of colonic cancer	+
Differential diagnosis of large adenomas	+
Diagnosis and differentiation of inflammatory bowel disease	?
Detection of abscesses (and fistulas) in IBD**	++
Detection of anal sphincter defects	++(+)
EUS-guided fine-needle puncture	
Mediastinal tumors	+++
Mediastinal lymph nodes of bronchial cancer	++(+)
Distant mediastinal and paragastric lymph nodes due to gastrointestinal cancer (M1)	++
Indeterminate pancreatic masses	?
Unresectable pancreatic tumors before chemotherapy	++
Submucosal tumors	+
Large gastric folds	?

EUS, endoscopic ultrasonography; IBD, inflammatory bowel disease.
+++, strong benefit; ++, moderate benefit; +, benefit; –, no benefit; ?, questionable benefit.

22

that the procedure will be irrelevant unless another type of malignancy is discovered on tissue acquisition or the patient insists on histopathological confirmation before accepting the risks of a major surgical intervention. EUS-guided FNP is, however, also beneficial when other puncture methods have failed (e.g., because the lesion is too small or is in a difficult location) or when they are more invasive or risky. This is the case in mediastinal masses, where EUS-guided FNP competes with mediastinoscopy.

Examination Technique and Normal Findings

■ Preparation, Sedation, and Complications

The preparation for upper and lower (rectal and colonic) EUS is the same as for upper and lower gastrointestinal endoscopy. After an overnight fast, complemented by a rectal enema for rectal EUS or bowel cleansing as preparation for colonic EUS, upper and lower EUS are performed in most centers with the patient under conscious sedation [8,9], or with heavier sedation with propofol, or a combination of the two.

Complications are very rare in EUS. Those related to sedation include oxygen desaturation, which is usually clinically insignificant [8]. In an Italian multicenter study including 11,539 patients undergoing EUS, 808 of whom had interventional EUS, complications occurred in only 14 patients. The complications were related to bleeding, perforation, and infection, and there were no mortalities [10].

The positioning of the patient is the same in colorectal EUS as in colorectal endoscopy. In upper gastrointestinal EUS, the left lateral position is usually preferred, and occasionally the patient has to be turned into the supine position for better visualization of some gastric lesions at the angular fold or lesser curvature. However, this should be done with caution, since gastric fluid instillation is associated with a risk of aspiration. The same is true with water filling of the esophagus, which may be necessary for scanning flat and small lesions, especially with high-frequency ultrasound miniprobes.

■ Upper Gastrointestinal Tract

In the esophagus, balloon filling is usually sufficient to achieve proper ultrasound contact with the wall. Small and flat intramural lesions may require the use of higher frequencies and/or water

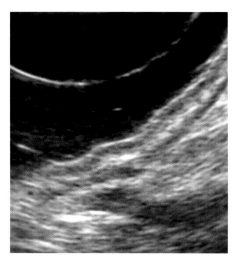

Fig. 22.16 Ultrasound image of the gastrointestinal wall (see text).

filling of the lumen, as balloon compression can lead to impaired visualization, with lesions potentially being either missed or overstaged. The problem of missing small lesions may be greater with linear scanning instruments unless clockwise and anticlockwise rotation of the scope is done in each segment being examined. Esophageal peristalsis can cause misinterpretation of wall thickening.

The instrument is introduced into the upper esophagus and then into the stomach, and EUS scanning is carried out as the scope is withdrawn. The perigastric area needs to be scanned, especially in cases of esophageal tumor, to search for distant lymph-node metastases—e.g., around the celiac axis. When the endoscope with a water-filled balloon is being withdrawn through the lower esophageal sphincter, the sphincter may resist easy passage of the instrument and sphincter spasm may even occur. Again, this can result in pseudothickening and blurring of the layers in this area. This region is therefore best scanned as the instrument is reintroduced slowly and carefully, and some views of the gastrointestinal junction may be better obtained using linear-type instruments; however, there are no precise data on this.

The gastrointestinal wall consists of five distinct layers (**Fig. 22.16**); the two inner layers (hyperechoic and hypoechoic) represent the interface/superficial mucosa and deep mucosa/muscularis mucosa. The third, hyperechoic, layer corresponds to the submucosa, the fourth (hypoechoic) to the muscularis propria, and the fifth (hyperechoic) to the adventitia or serosa, which is usually not easily distinguishable from the surrounding hyperechoic tissue. The diameter of the ultrasound layers does not exactly match the histological layers, but for practical purposes, the distinctions described work well for assessing the depth of tumor invasion in cancer staging. Needless to say, perpendicular scanning is required for proper diagnosis, avoiding the artifacts mentioned above. Perpendicular scanning is not always possible over 100% of the circumference with radial scanners, so different parts of the gastrointestinal lumen, especially in the stomach (lesser curvature with angular fold and subcardiac region), may require different tip positions for adequate visualization. There are no established values for the normal gastrointestinal wall, but a figure of 2–3 mm is usually considered to be the normal range, as well as a 1 : 1 : 1 relationship between the mucosa, submucosa, and muscularis propria.

The wall pattern described is easily seen in the stomach and colon with water filling. The esophageal and duodenal wall may be slightly compressed by the balloon, so that the balloon echo fuses with the inner three layers, giving a three-layered image (balloon–mucosa, submucosa, and muscularis). Additional layers appear to be visible with higher ultrasound frequencies; for example, the two layers of the muscularis propria may be seen, with a hyperechoic septum in between them.

The surrounding organs, vessels, and other structures are important for orientation and for diagnosing the depth of tumor invasion. Around the esophagus, the left atrium, spine, the aorta up to the aortic arch, the azygos vein, and the neck vessels can be seen (**Fig. 22.17**). Around the stomach, the pancreatic body and tail, parts of the liver (particularly the left lobe), and parts of the left kidney and spleen are seen, together with vessels such as the aorta, vena cava (proximal stomach), celiac trunk, and the splenic and left renal veins (**Figs. 22.18–22.22**). From the duodenum, the pancreatic head with the distal bile duct and gallbladder is seen, together with parts of the liver and right kidney and large vessels such as the aorta and vena cava, the portal vein with the confluence to the splenic and superior mesenteric veins, as well as the hepatic artery (**Figs. 22.23–22.25**). Details of the EUS examination technique are described elsewhere [11].

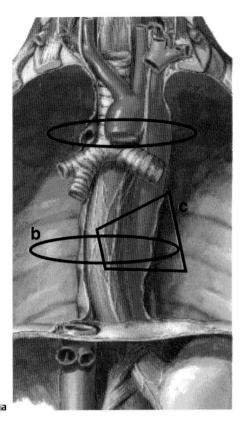

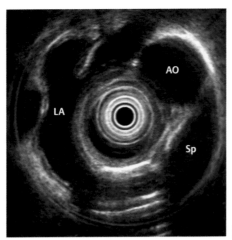

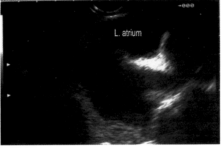

Fig. 22.17
a Esophageal and periesophageal anatomy, showing the levels of several ultrasound cross-sections; "b" denotes the instrument position of the radial and linear scanners shown in **b** and **c**.
b This section shows a distal cross-section with the aorta (AO), the left atrium (LA), and the spine (Sp) around the esophageal wall.
c This cross-section shows the same area scanned with a linear echo endoscope.

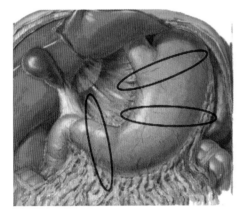

Fig. 22.18 Gastric and perigastric anatomy, showing three different endoscopic ultrasound sections through the distal (cf. **Fig. 22.19**), middle (cf. **Fig. 22.20**), and proximal stomach.

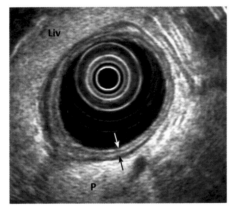

Fig. 22.19 An endoscopic ultrasound section through the gastric antrum (the wall lies between the arrows), with surrounding organs such as the liver (Liv) and pancreas (P).

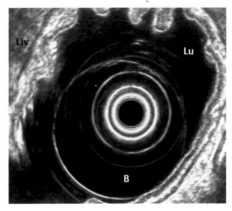

Fig. 22.20 An endoscopic ultrasound section through the gastric body, with close-up views of the gastric wall (for the layer structure, see **Fig. 22.17**). Both the water-filled balloon (B) and water filling of the gastric lumen (Lu) are used to provide acoustic coupling. A small section of the left liver lobe (Liv) is also seen.

■ Mediastinum

EUS plays an important role in the assessment of mediastinal lesions, particularly the posterior mediastinum. Mediastinal tumors and enlarged lymph nodes can be visualized and readily accessed for fine-needle puncture, as the echo endoscope in the esophagus is in a straight position. Benign lymph nodes are triangular or oval structures that are commonly encountered at the subcarina (20–25 cm from incisors), with a sonographically hyperechoic hilum commonly visible. These should be differentiated from malignant lymph nodes, which are rounded, well-demarcated, and hypoechoic, with no sonographic evidence of a hilum. As not all lymph nodes can be accessed with EUS, endobronchial ultrasound is an important adjunct in this respect.

■ Pancreas and Biliary Tract

The pancreas is scanned while the instrument is gradually being withdrawn from the starting position in the descending duodenum, at or below the papilla (uncinate process, periampullary area) to the upper duodenal curve and duodenal bulb (pancreatic head, pancreatic genu), and finally to the gastric body (pancreatic body) and fundus (pancreatic tail between the left kidney and spleen) (**Figs. 22.22–22.25**). The landmark vessels for defining the different parts of the organ are mainly the components of the portal venous system. The echo pattern of the pancreas is usually homogeneous. It is more hyperechoic than the liver and shows more or less well-defined margins relative to the surrounding tissue. Particularly in obese and older patients, however, the borders of the pancreas are

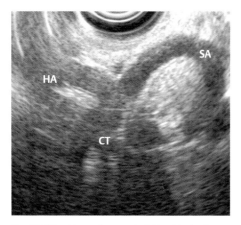

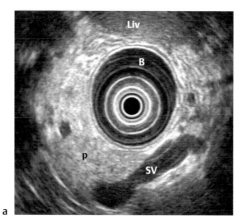

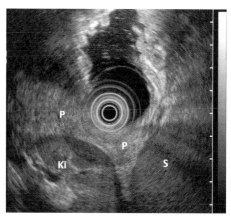

Fig. 22.21 The celiac trunk (CT) with the hepatic artery (HA) and splenic artery (SA), visualized close to the gastric body area.

Fig. 22.22 Perigastric anatomy from the gastric body, with the gastric wall close to the water-filled balloon (B).
a Parts of the pancreatic body (P) with the splenic vein (SV) and a small part of the liver (Liv) are seen.
b Higher up the gastric body, the pancreatic tail (P) is visualized, with the upper pole of the left kidney (Ki) and the spleen (S).

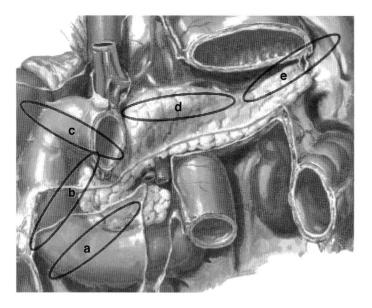

Fig. 22.23 The pancreas as visualized from different echo endoscope positions. Positions and regions of interest: a, the uncinate process, aorta, vena cava, and superior mesenteric vein; b, the papilla, distal common bile duct and pancreatic duct, pancreatic head, and portal vein; c, the pancreatic head, portal vein, and confluence; d, the pancreatic body, splenic vein, and celiac trunk; e, the pancreatic tail, splenic vein, left kidney, and spleen.

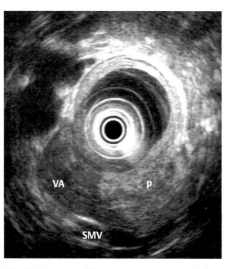

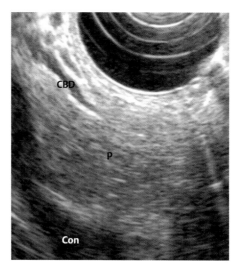

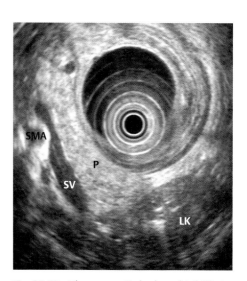

Fig. 22.24 Two different sections through the pancreatic head.
a A section with the echo endoscope positioned below the papilla. The pancreatic head with the ventral anlage (VA), more hypoechoic than the rest of the parenchyma (P), is demonstrated with the superior mesenteric vein (SMV).
b Here, the echo endoscope is in the so-called "long scope position" in the descending duodenum, above or at the papilla. The distal common bile duct (CBD) is seen running through the pancreatic head (P), with the confluence (Con).

Fig. 22.25 The pancreatic body and tail (P) visualized from the upper gastric body. Landmarks include the splenic vein (SV), superior mesenteric artery (SMA) in cross-section, and the upper pole of the left kidney (LK).

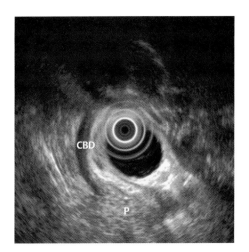

Fig. 22.26 A normal common bile duct (CBD) surrounded by pancreatic parenchyma (P).

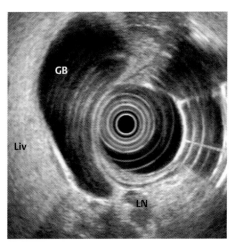

Fig. 22.27 A normal gallbladder (GB) with neighboring liver (Liv), seen from the duodenal bulb. A subhepatic inflammatory lymph node (LN) is also visible.

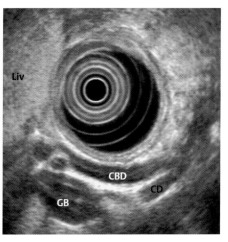

Fig. 22.28 Another view at the upper duodenal curve shows a small part of the gallbladder (GB) with the common bile duct (CBD) and the cystic duct (CD). Liv, liver.

less well seen, and here the landmark vessels are of the utmost importance in locating the organ correctly. Paragastric loops of small bowel can sometimes imitate the pancreas and should not be confused with it, and the caudate lobe of the liver can be confused with pancreatic tumor when scanned from the gastric fundus. The ventral part of the pancreas is seen in most, if not almost all, patients with a normal pancreas as a triangle-like part of the head, which is more hypoechoic than the rest of the organ. This can also be misinterpreted as a pathological lesion. The pancreatic duct is seen in parts as a tubular, anechoic structure lined by a thin, hyperechoic wall; nondilated side branches are usually not seen.

The bile duct (**Figs. 22.24b, 22.26**) is seen from its entrance to the papilla (endoscope position at the papilla), along its course through the pancreatic head (descending duodenum to upper duodenal curve), and up to the hilum (duodenal bulb). The proximal bile duct system, including the hilum and intrahepatic ducts, is visualized less regularly and less well on EUS (**Figs. 22.26–22.28**). Gallbladder visualization is from either the descending duodenum, the duodenal bulb, or the antrum, depending on its position [11,12] (**Fig. 22.22**).

With curvilinear instruments, complete scanning of the pancreaticobiliary system also requires scanning from the second part of the duodenum, where the aorta and inferior vena cava are landmarks for orientation; the duodenal bulb, from which the portal vein confluence, pancreatic head, and gallbladder can be visualized and taken as landmark structures; and finally from the stomach, where the abdominal aorta, celiac trunk, and splenic vessels, as well as the liver and left kidney, can be used as landmarks for orientation.

▦ Colorectum

Scanning is carried out using a water-filled balloon or with additional water filling of the rectum during withdrawal from the most proximal point of introduction. The echo colonoscope, with its forward-viewing lens, is handled like a normal colonoscope after adequate bowel preparation. Passing angulated or narrow parts of the colon may be more difficult due to the rigid tip of the instrument. Neighboring organs to be visualized on colorectal EUS are parts of the liver, kidneys, pancreas, and large vessels (depending on the relative position of the colon), and the bladder and prostate/seminal vesicles or vagina for rectal EUS. The same scanning principles apply,

and the same wall structure can be seen in the colorectum, as described above for the upper gastrointestinal tract.

Pathological Findings: General Principles

▦ Tumor Staging in the Gastrointestinal Tract

Gastrointestinal malignancies appear as hypoechoic, inhomogeneous wall thickening, localized or diffuse, involving deeper layers, growing outside of the wall, and eventually invading other structures, depending on the tumor stage (**Figs. 22.29–22.34**). Stage T1 is characterized by involvement of the inner two layers (T1 mucosa) or inner three layers (T1 submucosa), whereas flat lesions may not be visible. The balloon may compress discrete ulcers or elevations, and water filling and the use of higher frequencies is therefore recommended in this type of situation. Microscopic invasion can be missed (understaging), and peritumoral inflammation can lead to overstaging, especially with ulcerated cancers [13,14].

Differentiation between T1 tumors confined to the mucosa and those invading the submucosa is very important, particularly with the use of endoscopic mucosal resection as a therapeutic option in early malignancies [15–19]. There have been contradictory reports on the accuracy of EUS here—for example, in the accuracy of staging for early adenocarcinoma of the esophagus—with figures as low as 61% and as high as 95% being reported in Barrett's esophagus and early adenocarcinoma, irrespective of the use of conventional echo endoscopes or high-frequency miniprobes. Generally speaking, high-frequency miniprobes (12–30 MHz) can provide high-resolution images even of superficial lesions, with visualization of a seven-layered or even nine-layered structure in the esophagus.

More advanced cancer stages involve all of the wall layers, with a layer structure not being visible; smooth outer margins are seen in stage T2, whereas stage T3 is characterized by irregular outer margins. In stage T4, the boundary between the tumor and other organs (e.g., the tracheobronchial system, liver, or pancreas) or large vessels (e.g., the aorta) cannot be recognized. The absence of relative movements between organs and the tumor (e.g., between the liver and a gastric cancer) on respiration can be used as an indirect sign of tumor invasion. Lymph-node metastases are seen on EUS as roundish, hypoechoic lesions, either close to the tumor (stage N1) or at distant sites, and in some tumors these are regarded as distant

22

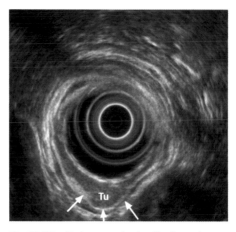

Fig. 22.29 Early cancer in the distal esophagus, in a patient with Barrett's esophagus. The superficial lesion (Tu) is somewhat compressed by the balloon, as is the underlying submucosal layer, which is well preserved (arrows).

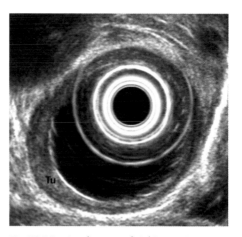

Fig. 22.30 Another superficial Barrett's cancer, which was flat and not visible on conventional endoscopic ultrasonography (EUS), due to balloon compression. Only the area of the tumor (Tu) was known, by placing the balloon precisely on the flat lesion. The absence of a visible abnormality on EUS is taken as sign of superficial cancer (T1m).

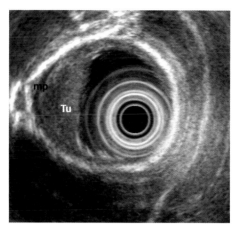

Fig. 22.31 Esophageal cancer in stage T2, with tumorous thickening (Tu), but no invasion through the muscularis propria (mp).

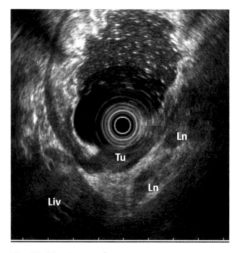

Fig. 22.32 Proximal gastric cancer in stage T3 (Tu), infiltrating through the wall and metastasizing into adjacent lymph nodes (Ln). Liv, part of the left liver.

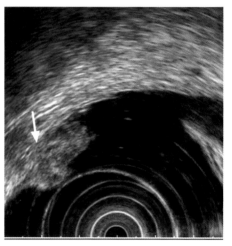

Fig. 22.33 A small polypoid rectal cancer infiltrating through the wall (arrow), thus corresponding to stage T3.

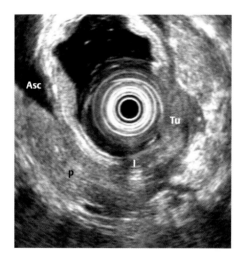

Fig. 22.34 Advanced gastric cancer (Tu) with peritoneal carcinomatosis and ascites (Asc), and with invasion (I) into the pancreas (P).

Table 22.3 Results of endoscopic ultrasonography in the locoregional staging of esophageal, gastric, pancreatic, and rectal cancer

Tumor site	Stage	Accuracy	References[*]
Esophagus	T	81%	[20]
	N	77%	
Stomach	T	77%	[33]
	N	71%	
Pancreas[†]	T	81%	[42]
	N	70%	
Rectum	T	84%	[11]
	N	74%	

* See text for further updates.
† See text for further details on accuracy in vascular invasion.

metastases (e.g., stage M1a in esophageal cancer). Although EUS is not reliable in differentiating between benign and malignant lesions in individual nodes, the likelihood of lymph-node metastases increases with their size and the concomitant T stage (with an 80% likelihood in stage T3 lesions versus 5% in stage T1m tumors). **Table 22.3** provides an overview of the literature results [11,14,20–74]. The results for the accuracy of EUS in staging gastroesophageal malignancies have been confirmed in systematic reviews [75,76].

The high level of accuracy of EUS in locoregional staging of esophageal tumors means that the technique is suitable for use in the diagnostic work-up, to avoid unnecessary surgical intervention in patients with advanced carcinoma, to depict early cases suitable for endoscopic mucosal resection, and to decide on preoperative therapy in patients with nodal involvement.

In the esophagus, nontraversable tumor stenoses may limit the assessment, but almost all squamous-cell cancers and most adenocarcinomas are in stages T3 or T4 if they are not traversable [77]. Endoscopic dilation should be carried out in order to pass the stricture with an endoscope and assess its length and any stomach

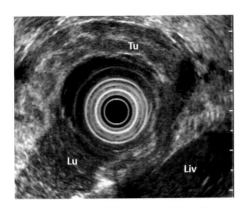

Fig. 22.35 Gastric linitis plastica (Tu), with massive wall thickening involving all layers; the layer structure is barely recognizable. Lu, gastric lumen; Liv, liver. This type of finding could also be due to advanced lymphoma, but it should always prompt further attempts at tissue diagnosis if initial biopsies are negative (see text).

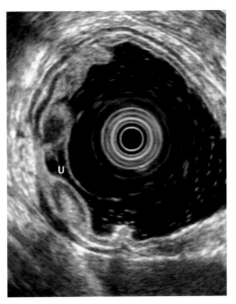

Fig. 22.36 Gastric lymphoma, seen as an ulcer (U) with massive thickening of the inner wall layers around it.

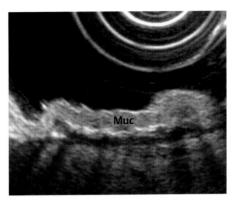

Fig. 22.37 Early gastric lymphoma (MALT lymphoma), evident only as a thickening of the mucosa (Muc), whereas the underlying submucosa and muscularis propria are intact.

22

pathology, as mentioned above. It is a matter of debate whether dilation should be carried out to a diameter sufficient to allow passage of the echo endoscope. The perforation risk appears to be increased, especially if forceful dilation and endosonography are performed in one session [78,79]—although this has been doubted by other authors [80]. Slimmer instruments, such as the blind probe introduced over a guide wire, or miniprobes (these have a limited penetration depth, however), are also available for this purpose, and are likely to carry a lower perforation risk [21,31,32]. Endobronchial echo endoscopes, which are slimmer than gastrointestinal echo endoscopes, can also be used in nontraversable strictures [81] Another limitation of EUS in esophageal tumor staging is re-staging following neoadjuvant therapy, due the to inability to distinguish between inflammatory or necrotic tissues and tumor tissue [82].

In the stomach, some locations (the lesser curvature, especially at the angular fold, and the subcardial region) are more difficult to cover with EUS, and lesions in these areas may be more difficult to visualize and stage. The TNM system differentiates between subserosal (T2) and serosal (T3) gastric cancer invasion, and this differentiation cannot reliably be made by EUS. In addition, not all of the gastric surface is covered by serosa. Despite this, the same staging criteria as for other tumor locations are used in the stomach, although the staging results are substantially poorer for stage T2 [33].

Diffuse gastric cancers (linitis plastica, scirrhous carcinoma) are seen as diffuse wall thickening. Some of the layered structure (with thickened and distorted layers) can often still be recognized here, and the outer margin is irregular, but relatively well preserved (Fig. 22.35). A similar picture can be seen with advanced gastric lymphoma, the early forms of which are either invisible—as in mucosa-associated lymphoid tissue (MALT) lymphoma diagnosed by subtle endoscopic abnormalities, or only on routine gastric biopsy—or manifest as thickening of the inner two or three layers [83] (Figs. 22.36, 22.37). However, the interobserver agreement in staging gastric MALT lymphoma has been questioned by some authors [84]. The differential diagnosis of enlarged gastric folds also includes benign conditions, which are discussed below.

EUS may be reliable for predicting and assessing the response to chemotherapy (and Helicobacter pylori eradication) for gastric lymphoma [85–87], but its value is controversial, both for re-staging after chemoradiotherapy of esophagogastric cancer [88–90] and rectal cancer [91] and for detecting recurrences after curative surgery in patients with esophageal cancer [92] and rectal carcinoma [93–95].

Submucosal Lesions

EUS plays a substantial role in the diagnosis of submucosal lesions, primarily to differentiate between true submucosal tumors (i.e., intramural tumors) and extraluminal compressions caused by either normal or pathological structures (Figs. 22.38, 22.39). If EUS shows that a suspected submucosal bulge is an impression caused by a normal organ (e.g., the spleen or gallbladder), further diagnostic steps are superfluous. If the lesion is intramural, tumors can be differentiated from cysts or vessels. Tumors can be further characterized by their layer of origin, echo pattern, and margin (Figs. 22.40–22.43).

The most frequent myogenic tumors are characteristically located in the second or fourth hypoechoic layer; they have a hypoechoic pattern and are more or less homogeneous and more or less well demarcated. Other lesions (granular cell tumors, aberrant pancreas, fibroma, lipoma) have different echo patterns and originate in the submucosa [96–100]. Several endosonographic criteria have been suggested in the effort to identify submucosal tumors with malignant potential (size > 3 cm, inhomogeneous echo pattern, irregular margins, presence of lymph nodes) [101,102]. Improved understanding of the origin and biological behavior of gastrointestinal stromal cell tumors (GISTs) is changing the scope of EUS in the management of submucosal tumors. GISTs appear endosonographically as hypoechoic masses in continuity with the muscle layer of the gut, and are thus endosonographically indistinguishable from true leiomyomas or leiomyosarcomas. Every GIST should be considered to be potentially malignant, even if small. The diagnosis is now

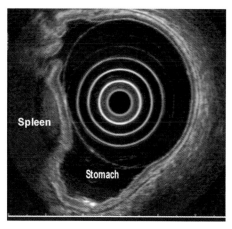

Fig. 22.38 An impression made on the stomach by the spleen, mimicking a submucosal tumor.

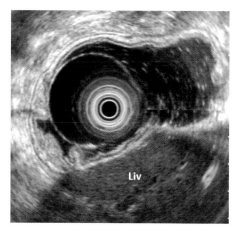

Fig. 22.39 A flat impression on the gastric wall made by the left liver lobe (Liv). No submucosal or extraluminal tumor was identified on endoscopic ultrasonography.

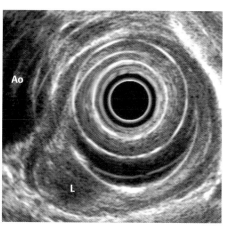

Fig. 22.40 A small (1-cm) leiomyoma in the distal esophagus. It originates in the muscularis mucosa, since the underlying submucosa and muscularis propria are intact. Ao, aorta.

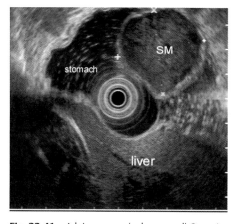

Fig. 22.41 A leiomyoma (submucosal) 3 cm in diameter, originating in the muscularis propria. This type of tumor could also be malignant, and this cannot be determined from the endoscopic ultrasound appearance alone.

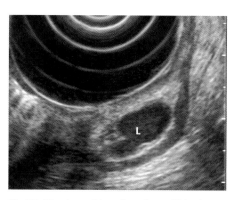

Fig. 22.42 A small lymphangioma (L) in the gastric wall. This tumor is almost anechoic and originates in the submucosal layer.

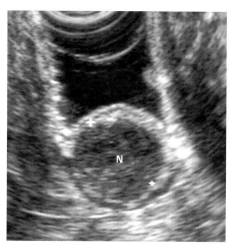

Fig. 22.43 A 2-cm neurinoma in the gastric wall. This type of lesion could be misinterpreted as a leiomyoma, but it is clearly seen to originate in the submucosa, as it is covered by a thin hyperechoic layer on all sides. Other tissue diagnoses (fibroma, aberrant pancreas, etc.) might also be possible.

based on immunohistochemical examination of specimens for c-*kit* (CD117), CD34, smooth muscle actin, and S100 protein [103–106].

Tumor Diagnosis and Staging in the Pancreaticobiliary Tract

Pancreatic tumors are visualized on EUS as more or less well-demarcated hypoechoic lesions, which—depending on their histological nature and size—are homogeneous or inhomogeneous, with hyperechoic spots or cystic spaces. EUS can suggest a cystic tumor with these features, but obviously does not allow reliable differentiation between the different forms of cystic tumor (**Fig. 22.44**). Small tumors, especially of the endocrine type, are hypoechoic and well-demarcated (**Fig. 22.45**), whereas small pancreatic cancers may either look like the endocrine lesions or display a pattern of focal inhomogeneity, which is much more difficult to diagnose on EUS (**Fig. 22.46**). With more advanced tumor stages, pancreatic cancers become more inhomogeneous and start to invade into neighboring organs, especially into large parapancreatic vessels

(**Figs. 22.47–22.48**). This latter issue is becoming increasingly important with advances in the treatment of pancreatic cancer with neoadjuvant chemotherapy. The endosonographic criteria for vascular invasion are:

- Venous collaterals in an area of a mass that obliterates the normal anatomic location of a major portal confluence vessel
- Tumor within the vessel lumen
- Abnormal vessel contour, with loss of the vessel–parenchymal sonographic interface [107].

These criteria have been extensively studied [108–111], and the value of EUS has been documented in a systematic review in which the pooled results showed an overall sensitivity of 73% and a specificity of 93% [112]. Basically, the accuracy of EUS in detecting splenic and portal venous involvement is greater than its accuracy in detecting arterial and superior mesenteric venous invasion. A recent study confirmed the superiority of EUS over abdominal ultrasound, angiography, and single-slice CT. It still remains to be investigated whether multislice CT can yield results comparable to those of EUS [113]. On the basis of the current state of knowledge, CT and

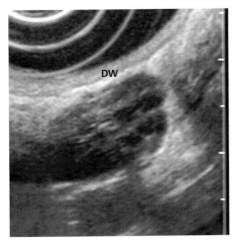

Fig. 22.44 A 2-cm pancreatic cystic tumor (cystadenoma) in the pancreatic head, close to the duodenal wall (DW). Endoscopic ultrasonography cannot differentiate reliably between the different forms of cystic pancreatic tumor, particularly between benign and malignant ones.

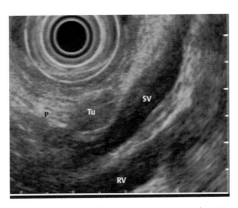

Fig. 22.45 A small (1 cm) pancreatic endocrine tumor (Tu) in the pancreatic body/tail area, surrounded by pancreatic tissue (P). SV, splenic vein; RV, left renal vein.

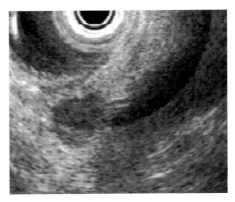

Fig. 22.46 A small (1.5 cm) pancreatic cancer in the area of the pancreatic head.

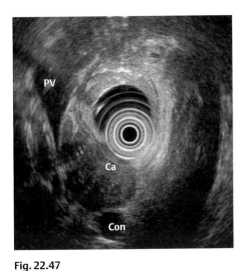

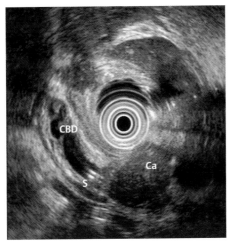

Fig. 22.47
a A large pancreatic head cancer, with compression of the portal vein (PV) in the confluence area (Con) by the tumor.
b In another section, occlusion of the common bile duct (CBD) with a stent (S) in situ can be seen.

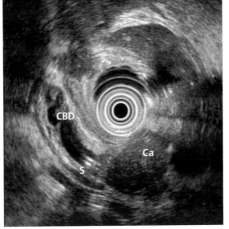

Fig. 22.48 A large pancreatic head cancer (Tu), more hyperechoic and inhomogeneous than the tumor in **Fig. 22.47**. Vascular invasion into the portal vein at the confluence level (Con) is clearly seen here.

EUS should be regarded as complementary in the assessment of pancreatic tumors.

EUS has a role in suggesting the nature of pancreatic cystic lesions. These are increasingly being diagnosed as imaging modalities improve. Serous cystadenoma, mucinous cystadenoma/cystadenocarcinoma, and intraductal papillary mucinous neoplasia can be differentiated from each other on the basis of endosonographic criteria, as well as chemical and cytological analysis of aspirates. Serous cystadenomas appear as microcystic lesions with little fluid; mucinous cystadenomas are more often unilocular and filled with viscous material; intraductal papillary mucinous neoplasia varies sonographically, with either a uniloculate or multiloculate cyst and pseudocysts with a rather thick, well-circumscribed wall. Aspirates from intraductal papillary neoplasia and mucinous cystadenoma show mucinous viscous material, with elevated carcinoembryonic antigen (CEA) concentrations in both types of lesion and an elevated amylase level in intraductal papillary neoplasia. Serous cystadenomas are characterized by an aspirate that has low amylase and CEA

levels. Aspirates from pseudocysts show an increased amylase level and relatively lower CEA [114].

Like other imaging tests, EUS is not able to differentiate between focal inflammatory masses and pancreatic cancer [115] (**Fig. 22.49**), although it has been suggested that contrast-enhanced EUS with power Doppler may be valuable here [116]. The results of [18]fluorodeoxyglucose PET-CT were found not to be superior to those of EUS in evaluating small pancreatic masses [117]. Different EUS imaging methods are being investigated (see "Further Developments," below) that may allow more accurate characterization of pancreatic lesions. This may help in depicting early carcinoma, particularly in patients with chronic pancreatitis. Although these are still investigational and not yet in routine clinical use, they may be available at least to guide tissue sampling in the near future.

EUS is of particular importance for preoperative localization of neuroendocrine pancreatic tumors. These tumors are often clinically evident and exact localization of the site of the tumor is mandatory before surgical removal. Other imaging modalities that

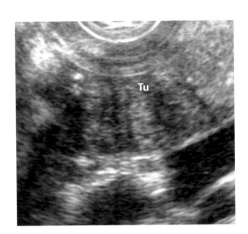

Fig. 22.49 A large pancreatic head mass (TU), found to be focal chronic pancreatitis at surgery. Endoscopic ultrasonography cannot distinguish this type of tumor from a malignant mass as in **Fig. 22.48**.

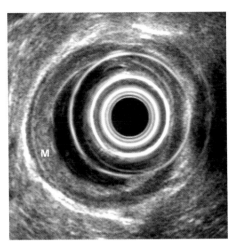

Fig. 22.50 Reflux stricture, seen on endoscopic ultrasound as mucosal thickening (M), with the underlying submucosa and muscularis propria remaining intact. In more advanced cases of inflammation and scarring, a concentric diffuse wall thickening with a loss of the layer structure can be seen, which is more difficult to distinguish from intramural malignancies.

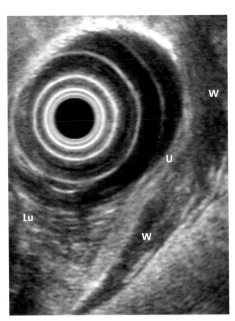

Fig. 22.51 A chronic benign and flat gastric ulcer (U) with massive wall thickening (w), especially involving the deeper layers of the gastric wall. Endoscopic ultrasonography is not capable of providing a reliable differential diagnosis between benign and malignant gastric ulcers. Lu, the gastric lumen, filled with food residues.

can be used here include transabdominal ultrasound, CT, MRI, PET, and somatostatin-receptor scintigraphy. Relatively high detection rates have been achieved with EUS (up to 93%) in patients with insulinomas [118,119], particularly in comparison with somatostatin-receptor scintigraphy, as the tumors have no somatostatin-2 or somatostatin-5 receptors, or a much lower density of these receptors [120], making them scintigraphically undetectable, and also due to the presence of the tumor within the pancreas in most cases. In patients with gastrinomas, the EUS localization rates are lower, particularly when the lesions are extrapancreatic.

Intraductal ultrasound using miniprobes that can be inserted over a guide wire into the common bile duct at endoscopic retrograde cholangiopancreatography (ERCP) have been used to assess biliary strictures. Although sonographic criteria for diagnosing malignancy have been proposed, such as hypoechoic nature, disruption of the duct wall, irregularity of the outer border, and a heterogenous internal echo pattern, these criteria are not reliable. The technique can be used only to improve the results of tumor staging in comparison with conventional EUS, particularly for hilar and mid-common bile duct strictures [121,122].

Benign Lesions and Differential Diagnosis

The place of EUS in the diagnosis of nonneoplastic conditions is much less well established. As a general rule, EUS has not been very successful in the differential diagnosis between benign and malignant conditions, such as indeterminate esophageal strictures and gastric ulcers (**Figs. 22.50, 22.51**), in indeterminate pancreatic masses (see above), or in common bile duct (CBD) strictures.

In patients with achalasia, EUS has also been used to depict muscular thickening in achalasia and to direct therapy if necessary, as with EUS-guided injection of botulinum toxin [123]. In portal hypertension, EUS can delineate intramural vessels and their feeding veins, as well as collateral vessels surrounding the gut wall

(**Fig. 22.52**) [124,125]. The azygos vein and periazygos collaterals can be visualized, and hemodynamic studies can be performed on azygos blood flow using Doppler. This tempted researchers to use EUS in studies on optimizing the management of varices and predicting bleeding and recurrence [126–129]. EUS-guided injection of varices, particularly gastric varices, has also been attempted [130,131]. Although the research data are interesting, EUS is still far from being a routine clinical utilization in patients with portal hypertension [132].

In the differential diagnosis of enlarged gastric folds, EUS is useful for ruling out intramural vessels as one of the differential diagnoses, and especially before large-particle biopsy is considered. Benign conditions such as hyperplastic gastritis or Ménétrier's disease (**Fig. 22.53**) show exclusive thickening of the inner two (mucosal) layers, but this feature can also be observed in early lymphoma [83]. However, it has been argued that if EUS shows only mucosal abnormalities, the diagnosis should be established by mucosal (or large-particle) biopsy. If deeper layers or all layers are involved, or if the layer structure becomes distorted or destroyed, the diagnosis of malignancy (lymphoma or linitis plastica) becomes very likely, and this may prompt the endoscopist to make further aggressive attempts at tissue diagnosis.

In patients with inflammatory bowel disease, EUS is of limited value in differentiating between Crohn's disease and ulcerative colitis [133]. Other areas in which EUS is still being investigated are the prediction of response to medical therapy in patients with ulcerative colitis and in the diagnosis of rectal fistulas [134,135]. In anal disorders, EUS is valuable in diagnosing internal and external anal sphincter defects and is as accurate as electromyography [136].

The diagnosis of CBD stones appears to be one of the domains of EUS (**Fig. 22.54**); both in retrospective and in prospective series, EUS has been shown to have a sensitivity and specificity of more than 90%. This is better than the accuracy of abdominal ultrasound, CT, and even ERCP or magnetic resonance cholangiopancreatography (MRCP). A negative EUS for CBD stones appears to be very reliable,

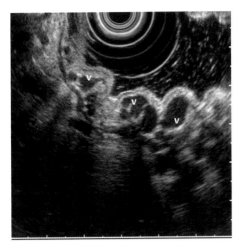

Fig. 22.52 Portal hypertension, with multiple vascular structures (v) in the gastric wall.

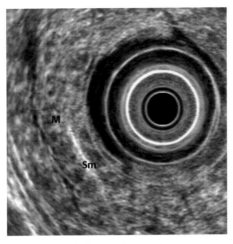

Fig. 22.53 Ménétrier's disease of the stomach. Massive thickening of the mucosa (M) with tiny hypoechoic spots can be seen, whereas the underlying submucosa and muscularis propria are intact. The enlarged fold is compressed by the balloon, with only a small luminal space between them. A thin submucosal layer (Sm) is also seen on the fold close to the transducer.

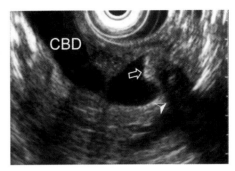

Fig. 22.54 Stone (open arrow) in the dilated distal common bile duct (CBD), with acoustic shadowing (arrowhead).

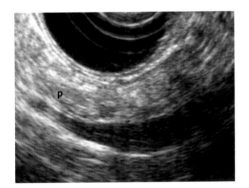

Fig. 22.55 Early chronic pancreatitis, with a slightly inhomogeneous echo pattern in the pancreatic parenchyma (P). The duct is not seen on this section, but was not dilated.

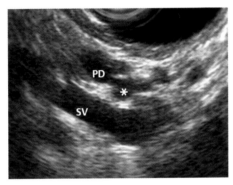

Fig. 22.56 Chronic pancreatitis with atrophic parenchyma, showing an inhomogeneous echo pattern and a dilated main pancreatic duct (PD), with grossly dilated side branches (*). SV, splenic vein.

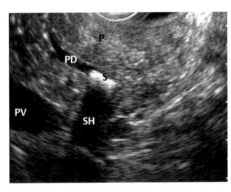

Fig. 22.57 Chronic pancreatitis with intraductal stone (S), showing acoustic shadowing (SH), leading to total ductal obstruction in the pancreatic head. The duct (PD) proximal to the stone is not dilated. The pancreatic parenchyma (P) is only slightly inhomogeneous. PV, portal vein.

with an almost negligible rate of false-negative results. This fact, together with the relatively low invasiveness of EUS, with no need for radiation exposure or contrast administration, makes the procedure very attractive. Only MRCP can be regarded as a competitive method here [137].

EUS is very sensitive and specific for detecting moderate to advanced disease in the diagnosis of chronic pancreatitis (**Figs. 22.55–22.57**). There have been several reports on the EUS features of early chronic pancreatitis [12]. However, there are no standardized criteria for an EUS diagnosis of pancreatitis. A panel of experts therefore agreed on the "Rosemont criteria" as a basis for EUS diagnosis of chronic pancreatitis. The EUS features are categorized into major and minor criteria. Major criteria for chronic pancreatitis are: A, hyperechoic foci with shadowing and main pancreatic duct calculi; and B, lobularity with honeycombing. Minor criteria consist of cysts, dilated ducts > 3.5 mm, irregular pancreatic duct contour, dilated side branches > 1 mm, hyperechoic duct wall, strands, nonshadowing hyperechoic foci, and lobularity with noncontiguous lobules. **Table 22.4** summarizes the suggested diagnosis based on the weighted diagnostic criteria. The Rosemont criteria

Table 22.4 The Rosemont criteria for endoscopic ultrasound diagnosis of pancreatitis

Most consistent with chronic pancreatitis	Suggestive of chronic pancreatitis	Indeterminate for chronic pancreatitis	Normal
A			
1 major A feature (+) > 3 minor features	1 major A feature (+) > 3 minor features	> 2 minor features, < 5 minor features	≤ 2 minor features
B			
1 major A feature (+) 1 major B feature	1 major B feature (+) 3 minor features	1 major B feature alone	
C			
2 major A features	≥ 5 minor features (any)		

Major features: A, hyperechoic foci with shadowing and main pancreatic duct calculi; B, lobularity with honeycombing.
Minor features: cysts, dilated ducts > 3.5 mm, irregular pancreatic duct contour, dilated side branches > 1 mm, hyperechoic duct wall, strands, nonshadowing hyperechoic foci, and lobularity with noncontiguous lobules.

still have to be evaluated in prospective studies [138]. In patients with pancreatitis, EUS is of course not only of diagnostic value, but can also be used for therapeutic interventions such as pseudocyst drainage. A recently published randomized clinical trial confirmed the importance of drainage and stenting with endosonographic guidance [139]. The development of echo endoscopes with wide working channels allows direct stenting under endosonographic and radiographic control.

Fine-Needle Puncture: Accuracy, Pitfalls, and Limitations

EUS-guided FNP has established itself as an important adjunct to diagnostic EUS. It is now part of the management algorithms in various types of mediastinal and gastrointestinal neoplasia. In addition, developments in EUS-FNP have opened up new horizons for therapeutic EUS. Developments in echo endoscopes, needles, and growing experience with the technique, as well as advances in the management protocols for various tumors, have contributed to this progress. Clear indications for EUS-FNP include pancreatic mass lesions, particularly when other methods of tissue sampling have failed, mediastinal masses, celiac lymphadenopathy, and submucosal masses. In these lesions, EUS-FNP has a specificity of almost 100%, with extremely few false-positive results. The reported sensitivity ranges from 60% to 95% in most studies [140,141].

As mentioned earlier, the clinical consequences and the impact on decision-making have to be clearly defined before one embarks on such a procedure. This may be expected to change, depending on developments in treatment protocols for various lesions, and it should be always a subject of discussion at a multidisciplinary level (e.g., among gastroenterologists, oncologists, and surgeons, etc.). For example, a still-controversial issue is whether or not to carry out puncture in patients with suspected pancreatic masses that are judged to be resectable. Negative FNP would not exclude malignancy, but exposes the patient to the risk of tumor seeding. The procedure will therefore add no clear benefit, as the patient will undergo surgery in any case, unless the patient insists on a histological diagnosis before undergoing a major surgical intervention.

Molecular markers have added a new dimension to the interpretation of EUS fine-needle aspirates. The higher level of CEA in aspirates from pancreatic cysts suggest a mucinous cystadenoma/cystadenocarcinoma. The detection of K-*ras* and p53 mutations in

aspirates from pancreatic masses has been investigated [142]. Fluorescent in-situ hybridization (FISH) to quantify nuclear DNA content has been used in the diagnosis of cholangiocarcinoma. Epidermal growth factor receptor is investigated in patients with non–small cell lung cancer in order to predict the response to kinase inhibitors [143].

An issue of concern is the limitation of the technique in patients with chronic pancreatitis. Although the accuracy of EUS-FNP in the diagnosis of pancreatic neoplasia can be up to 95%, the sensitivity and specificity of the method decline in the presence of underlying chronic pancreatitis. It has yet to be determined whether techniques such as detecting K-*ras* mutation in tissues can be of further value in these cases [144–147].

Further Developments

The field of endoscopic ultrasonography has seen many developments in recent years and is expected to develop further. Some of these developments have not yet found their way into routine clinical practice. Laparoscopic ultrasonography is one of the various combinations of endoscopy and ultrasound, and increasing numbers of reports have demonstrated the potential value of this method in defining the anatomy during minimally invasive surgery, as well as for staging gastroenterological malignancies [148,149].

Three-dimensional EUS, with volume data reconstruction, has been investigated in several studies, and new applications are expected [150,151]. Three-dimensional intraductal ultrasonography has been used in the diagnostic work-up of biliary diseases. It has been reported that this method allows more accurate assessment of the depth of tumor invasion and of portal vein and pancreatic invasion [152]. Doppler and power Doppler ultrasonography have been investigated in attempts to differentiate between benign and malignant lesions [116,153].

Contrast agents are continuing to be developed to improve the diagnostic accuracy of EUS. Levovist and sonicated serum albumin have been used to enhance EUS imaging, including color and power Doppler imaging, and Sonazoid is a recently introduced ultrasound contrast agent that enhances B-mode imaging. It consists of perflubutane microbubbles with a median diameter of 2–3 μm [154]. An echo endoscope was recently developed to allow contrast-enhanced harmonic EUS. It features a broadband transducer and has been used in pancreatic lesions to visualize parenchymal perfusion [155].

Tissue characterization using EUS spectral analysis has been investigated for differentiating between pancreatic adenocarcinoma and the normal pancreas. This would be an interesting technique if it can help differentiate between tumorous tissue and chronic pancreatitis [156].

Elastography is an advanced technique that has been recently introduced into ultrasonography (**Fig. 22.58**). With developments in ultrasound technology, it is possible to produce images showing the elasticity of tissues. The elasticity coefficient (Young's modulus, Y) is calculated from two variables—stress (defined as force per unit area) and strain (defined as change in length per unit length). To measure the strain, the reflected ultrasound frequencies before and after exertion of pressure by the transducer are compared. Identical frequency peaks denote no displacement (hardness), whereas an increased distance between peaks indicates soft tissue. Malignant tumors tend to be harder than benign lesions or normal tissues. Hypothetically, elastography could provide an important adjunct to imaging, as it allows virtual palpation of inaccessible organs and can even provide quantitative information about the degree of hardness. EUS elastography is a development in the field of tissue characterization that depends on the ultrasound consistency of tissues.

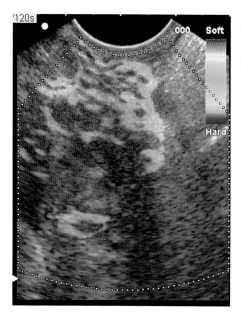

Fig. 22.58 Tissue elasticity can be mapped using EUS elastography, which may prove useful in guiding tissue sampling.

The technique will not replace histopathology, but may be useful for guiding tissue sampling [157–159].

With developments in small-intestinal endoscopy and the introduction of double-balloon and single-balloon enteroscopes, it became clear that ultrasound devices for examining the small bowel are also needed. A prototype miniprobe operating at 20 MHz has been developed and tested in a small series [160].

Training in EUS

EUS is a relatively difficult technique that requires extended and dedicated training and involves a difficult learning curve. The interpretation of EUS images is strongly dependent on the operator's level of experience. Models have therefore been developed to facilitate EUS training. One of these consists of porcine viscera in placed in a phantom model, with ultrasound gel. This showed encouraging results when tested on a small group of participants [161]. Live animal models (pigs) are also used for training, as well as computer-based endoscopy simulators that have an EUS module [162]. Nevertheless, difficulties in providing adequate training in EUS were still evident in a recent study in the United States, in which most gastroenterology fellows received less training than the minimum number of EUS examinations required by the American Society of Gastrointestinal Endoscopy (190 total supervised procedures, including 75 pancreaticobiliary cases, 75 mucosal tumors, and 40 submucosal abnormalities) [163].

References

1. Catalano MF, Kaul V, Hernandez LV, Pezanoski JP, Nalini M, Guda NM, et al. Diagnosis of chronic pancreatitis (CP) by endoscopic ultrasound (EUS)—radial vs. linear endosonography (EUS) [abstract]. Gastrointest Endosc 2008;67:AB204.
2. Stevens T, Vargo JJ, Zuccaro G, Dumot JA, Parsi MA, Lashner B, et al. Prospective comparison of radial and linear endoscopic ultrasound (EUS) for the diagnosis of chronic pancreatitis (CP) using secretin pancreatic function test (PFT) as reference standard [abstract]. Gastrointest Endosc 2008;67:AB210.
3. Savides TJ. Tricks for improving EUS-FNA accuracy and maximizing cellular yield. Gastrointest Endosc 2009;69(Suppl 1):S130–3.
4. Irisawa A, Hikichi T, Bhutani MS, Ohira H. Basic technique of FNA. Gastrointest Endosc 2009;2:S125–9.
5. Larghi A, Verna EC, Stavropoulos SN, Rotterdam H, Lightdale CJ, Stevens PD. EUS-guided Tru-Cut needle biopsies in patients with solid pancreatic masses: a prospective study. Gastrointest Endosc 2004;59:185–90.
6. Wiersema MJ, Vilmann P, Giovannini M, Chang KJ, Wiersema LM. Endosonography-guided fine-needle aspiration biopsy: diagnostic accuracy and complication assessment. Gastroenterology 1997;112:1087–95.
7. Eloubeidi MA, Tamhane A, Jhala N, Chhieng D, Jhala D, Crowe DR, et al. Agreement between rapid onsite and final cytologic interpretations of EUS-guided FNA specimens: implications for the endosonographer and patient management. Am J Gastroenterol 2006;101:2841–7.
8. Rösch T, Dennig V. A prospective assessment of complications and patient acceptance of upper gastrointestinal endoscopic ultrasonography: a multicenter study in 2500 patients [abstract]. Gastrointest Endosc 2000;51:AB177.
9. Ono Y, Shimizu Y, Kato M, Yoshida T, Hata T, Hirota J et al. Sedation for endoscopic ultrasonography: propofol with low-dose midazolam versus midazolam [abstract]. Gastrointest Endosc 2006;63:AB271.
10. Buscarini E, De Angelis C, Arcidiacono PG, Rocca R, Lupinacci G, Manta R, et al. Multicentre retrospective study on endoscopic ultrasound complications. Dig Liver Dis 2006;38:762–7.
11. Rösch T, Classen M. Gastroenterologic endosonography. New York: Thieme; 1992.
12. Kassem AM, Rösch T. Endosonographic imaging in pancreatic disease. Tech Gastrointest Endosc 2000;2:94–100.
13. Fein J, Gerdes H, Karpeh M. Overstaging of ulcerated gastric cancer by endoscopic ultrasonography [abstract]. Gastrointest Endosc 1993;39:A274.
14. Massari M, Cioffi U, De Simone M, Bonavina L, D'Elia A, Rosso L, et al. Endoscopic ultrasonography for preoperative staging of gastric carcinoma. Hepatogastroenterology 1996;43:542–6.
15. Akahoshi K, Chijiiwa Y, Hamada S, Sasaki I, Maruoka A, Kabemura T, et al. Endoscopic ultrasonography: a promising method for assessing the prospects of endoscopic mucosal resection in early gastric cancer. Endoscopy 1997;29:614–9.
16. Ohashi S, Segawa K, Okamura S, Mitake M, Urano H, Shimodaira M, et al. The utility of endoscopic ultrasonography and endoscopy in the endoscopic mucosal resection of early gastric cancer. Gut 1999;45:599–604.
17. Nakamura K, Morisaki T, Sugitani A, Ogawa T, Uchiyama A, Kinukawa N, et al. An early gastric carcinoma treatment strategy based on analysis of lymph node metastasis. Cancer 1999;85:1500–5.
18. Waxman I, Saitoh Y. Clinical outcome of endoscopic mucosal resection for superficial GI lesions and the role of high-frequency US probe sonography in an American population. Gastrointest Endosc 2000;52:322–7.
19. Canto MI. Barrett's esophagus. Gastrointest Endosc Clin N Am 2005;15:83–92.
20. Rösch T. Endosonographic staging of esophageal cancer: a review of literature results. Gastrointest Endosc Clin North Am 1995;5:537–47.
21. Binmoeller KF, Seifert H, Seitz U, Izbicki JR, Kida M, Soehendra N. Ultrasonic esophagoprobe for TNM staging of highly stenosing esophageal carcinoma. Gastrointest Endosc 1995;41:547–52.
22. Fekete F, Sauvanet A, Zins M, Berthoux L, Amouyal G. Imaging of cancer of the esophagus: ultrasound-endoscopy or computed tomography? Ann Chir 1995;49:573–8.
23. Chandawarkar RY, Kakegawa T, Fujita H, Yamana H, Toh Y, Fujitoh H. Endosonography for preoperative staging of specific nodal groups associated with esophageal cancer. World J Surg 1996;20:700–2.
24. Fockens P, Van den Brande JH, van Dullemen HM, van Lanschot JJ, Tytgat GN. Endosonographic T-staging of esophageal carcinoma: a learning curve. Gastrointest Endosc 1996;44:58–62.
25. Hasegawa N, Niwa Y, Arisawa T, Hase S, Goto H, Hayakawa T. Preoperative staging of superficial esophageal carcinoma: comparison of an ultrasound probe and standard endoscopic ultrasonography. Gastrointest Endosc 1996;44:388–93.
26. Natsugoe S, Yoshinaka H, Morinaga T, Shimada M, Baba M, Fukumoto T, et al. Ultrasonographic detection of lymph-node metastases in superficial carcinoma of the esophagus. Endoscopy 1996;28:674–9.
27. Yanai H, Yoshida T, Harada T, Matsumoto Y, Nishiaki M, Shigemitsu T, et al. Endoscopic ultrasonography of superficial esophageal cancers using a thin ultrasound probe system equipped with switchable radial and linear scanning modes. Gastrointest Endosc 1996;44:578–82.
28. Luketich JD, Schauer P, Landreneau R, Nguyen N, Urso K, Ferson P, et al. Minimally invasive surgical staging is superior to endoscopic ultrasound in detecting lymph node metastases in esophageal cancer. J Thorac Cardiovasc Surg 1997;114:817–21.
29. Hiele M, De Leyn P, Schurmans P, Lerut A, Huys S, Geboes K, et al. Relation between endoscopic ultrasound findings and outcome of patients with tumors of the esophagus or esophagogastric junction. Gastrointest Endosc 1997;45:381–6.
30. Hunerbein M, Ghadimi BM, Haensch W, Schlag PM. Transendoscopic ultrasound of esophageal and gastric cancer using miniaturized ultrasound catheter probes. Gastrointest Endosc 1998;48:371–5.
31. Bowrey DJ, Clark GW, Roberts SA, Maughan TS, Hawthorne AB, Williams GT, et al. Endosonographic staging of 100 consecutive patients with esophageal carcinoma: introduction of the 8-mm esophagoprobe. Dis Esophagus 1999;12:258–63.
32. Menzel J, Hoepffner N, Nottberg H, Schulz C, Senninger N, Domschke W. Preoperative staging of esophageal carcinoma: miniprobe sonography versus conventional endoscopic ultrasound in a prospective histopathologically verified study. Endoscopy 1999;31:291–7.
33. Rösch T. Endosonographic staging of gastric cancer: a review of literature results. Gastrointest Endosc Clin North Am 1995;5:549–57.
34. Grimm H, Hamper K, Henne-Bruns D, Kremer B. Preoperative locoregional staging of stomach carcinoma with endosonography. Zentralbl Chir 1995;120:123–7.
35. Motoo Y, Okai T, Songur Y, Watanabe H, Yamaguchi Y, Mouri I, et al. Endoscopic therapy for early gastric cancer: utility of endosonography and evaluation of prognosis. J Clin Gastroenterol 1995;21:17–23.
36. Hunerbein M, Dohmoto M, Rau B, Schlag PM. Endosonography and endosonography-guided biopsy of upper-GI-tract tumors using a curved array echoendoscope. Surg Endosc 1996;10:1205–9.
37. Yanai H, Tada M, Karita M, Okita K. Diagnostic utility of 20-megahertz linear endoscopic ultrasonography in early gastric cancer. Gastrointest Endosc 1996;44:29–33.

22

38. Yanai H, Matsumoto Y, Harada T, Nishiaki M, Tokiyama H, Shigemitsu T, et al. Endoscopic ultrasonography and endoscopy for staging depth of invasion in early gastric cancer: a pilot study. Gastrointest Endosc 1997;46:212–6.
39. Akahoshi K, Chijiiwa Y, Sasaki I. Pre-operative TN staging of gastric cancer using a 15 MHz ultrasound miniprobe. Br J Radiol 1997;70:703–7.
40. Wang JY, Hsieh JS, Huang YS, Huang CJ, Hou MF, Huang TJ. Endoscopic ultrasonography for preoperative locoregional staging and assessment of resectability in gastric cancer. Clin Imaging 1998;22:355–9.
41. Willis S, Truong S, Gribnitz S, Fass J, Schumpelick V. Endoscopic ultrasonography in the preoperative staging of gastric cancer: accuracy and impact on surgical therapy. Surg Endosc 2000;14:951–4.
42. Rösch T. Staging of pancreatic cancer: analysis of literature results. Gastrointest Endosc Clin North Am 1995;5:735–9.
43. Nattermann C, Dancygier H. Endoscopic ultrasound in detection of locoregional lymph node metastases of gastrointestinal tumors. Ultraschall Med 1994;15:202–6.
44. Tio TL, Sie LH, Kallimanis G, Luiken GJ, Kimmings AN, Huibregtse K, et al. Staging of ampullary and pancreatic carcinoma: comparison between endosonography and surgery. Gastrointest Endosc 1996;44:706–13.
45. Howard TJ, Chin AC, Streib EW, Kopecky KK, Wiebke EA. Value of helical computed tomography, angiography, and endoscopic ultrasound in determining resectability of periampullary carcinoma. Am J Surg 1997;174:237–41.
46. Cellier C, Cuillerier E, Palazzo L, Rickaert F, Flejou JF, Napoleon B, et al. Intraductal papillary and mucinous tumors of the pancreas: accuracy of preoperative computed tomography, endoscopic retrograde pancreatography and endoscopic ultrasonography, and long-term outcome in a large surgical series. Gastrointest Endosc 1998;47:42–9.
47. Legmann P, Vignaux O, Dousset B, Baraza AJ, Palazzo L, Dumontier I, et al. Pancreatic tumors: comparison of dual-phase helical CT and endoscopic sonography. AJR Am J Roentgenol 1998;170:1315–22.
48. Akahoshi K, Chijiiwa Y, Nakano I, Nawata H, Ogawa Y, Tanaka M, et al. Diagnosis and staging of pancreatic cancer by endoscopic ultrasound. Br J Radiol 1998;71:492–6.
49. Milsom JW, Lavery IC, Stolfi VM, Czyrko C, Church JM, Oakley JR, et al. The expanding utility of endoluminal ultrasonography in the management of rectal cancer. Surgery 1992;112:832–40.
50. Derksen EJ, Cuesta MA, Meijer S. Intraluminal ultrasound of rectal tumours: a prerequisite in decision making. Surg Oncol 1992;1:193–8.
51. Goldman S, Arvidsson H, Norming U, Lagerstedt U, Magnusson I, Frisell J. Transrectal ultrasound and computed tomography in preoperative staging of lower rectal adenocarcinoma. Gastrointest Radiol 1991;16:259–63.
52. Waizer A, Powsner E, Russo I, Hadar S, Cytron S, Lombrozo R, et al. Prospective comparative study of magnetic resonance imaging versus transrectal ultrasound for preoperative staging and follow-up of rectal cancer: preliminary report. Dis Colon Rectum 1991;34:1068–72.
53. Lindmark G, Elvin A, Pahlman L, Glimelius B. The value of endosonography in preoperative staging of rectal cancer. Int J Colorectal Dis 1992;7:162–6.
54. Houvenaeghel G, Delpero JR, Giovannini M, Orsoni P, Seitz JF, Rosello R, et al. Staging of rectal cancer: a prospective study of digital examination and endosonography before and after preoperative radiotherapy. Acta Chir Belg 1993;93:164–8.
55. Scialpi M, Andreatta R, Agugiaro S, Zottele F, Niccolini M, Dalla Palma F. Rectal carcinoma: preoperative staging and detection of postoperative local recurrence with transrectal and transvaginal ultrasound. Abdom Imaging 1993;18:381–9.
56. Nielsen MB, Qvitzau S, Pedersen JF. Detection of pericolonic lymph nodes in patients with colorectal cancer: an in vitro and in vivo study of the efficacy of endosonography. AJR Am J Roentgenol 1993;161:57–60.
57. Thaler W, Watzka S, Martin F, La Guardia G, Psenner K, Bonatti G, et al. Preoperative staging of rectal cancer by endoluminal ultrasound vs. magnetic resonance imaging: preliminary results of a prospective, comparative study. Dis Colon Rectum 1994;37:1189–93.
58. Harnsberger JR, Charvat P, Longo WE, Vernava AM III, Salimi Z, Arends T, et al. The role of intrarectal ultrasound (IRUS) in staging of rectal cancer and detection of extrarectal pathology. Am Surg 1994;60:571–6.
59. Rafaelsen SR, Kronborg O, Fenger C. Digital rectal examination and transrectal ultrasonography in staging of rectal cancer: a prospective, blind study. Acta Radiol 1994;35:300–4.
60. Fleshman JW, Myerson RJ, Fry RD, Kodner IJ. Accuracy of transrectal ultrasound in predicting pathologic stage of rectal cancer before and after preoperative radiation therapy. Dis Colon Rectum 1992;35:823–9.
61. Starck M, Bohe M, Fork FT, Lindstrom C, Sjöberg S. Endoluminal ultrasound and low-field magnetic resonance imaging are superior to clinical examination in the preoperative staging of rectal cancer. Eur J Surg 1995;161:841–5.
62. Joosten FB, Jansen JB, Joosten HJ, Rosenbusch G. Staging of rectal carcinoma using MR double surface coil, MR endorectal coil, and intrarectal ultrasound: correlation with histopathologic findings. J Comput Assist Tomogr 1995;19:752–8.
63. Yoshida M, Tsukamoto Y, Niwa Y, Goto H, Hase S, Hayakawa T, et al. Endoscopic assessment of invasion of colorectal tumors with a new high-frequency ultrasound probe. Gastrointest Endosc 1995;41:587–92.
64. Fedyaev EB, Volkova EA, Kuznetsova EE. Transrectal and transvaginal ultrasonography in the preoperative staging of rectal carcinoma. Eur J Radiol 1995;20:35–8.
65. Meyenberger C, Huch Boni RA, Bertschinger P, Zala GF, Klotz HP, Krestin GP. Endoscopic ultrasound and endorectal magnetic resonance imaging: a prospective, comparative study for preoperative staging and follow-up of rectal cancer. Endoscopy 1995;27:469–79.
66. Nielsen MB, Qvitzau S, Pedersen JF, Christiansen J. Endosonography for preoperative staging of rectal tumours. Acta Radiol 1996;37:799–803.
67. Detry RJ, Kartheuser AH, Lagneaux G, Rahier J. Preoperative lymph node staging in rectal cancer: a difficult challenge. Int J Colorectal Dis 1996;11:217–21.
68. Zagoria RJ, Schlarb CA, Ott DJ, Bechtold RI, Wolfman NT, Scharling ES, et al. Assessment of rectal tumor infiltration utilizing endorectal MR imaging and comparison with endoscopic rectal sonography. J Surg Oncol 1997;64:312–7.
69. Maier AG, Barton PP, Neuhold NR, Herbst F, Teleky BK, Lechner GL. Peritumoral tissue reaction at transrectal US as a possible cause of overstaging in rectal cancer: histopathologic correlation. Radiology 1997;203:785–9.
70. Lindmark GE, Kraaz WG, Elvin PA, Glimelius BL. Rectal cancer: evaluation of staging with endosonography. Radiology 1997;204:533–8.
71. Osti MF, Padovan FS, Pirolli C, Sbarbati S, Tombolini V, Meli C, et al. Comparison between transrectal ultrasonography and computed tomography with rectal inflation of gas in preoperative staging of lower rectal cancer. Eur Radiol 1997;7:26–30.
72. Kulling D, Feldman DR, Kay CL, Bohning DE, Hoffman BJ, Van Velse AK, et al. Local staging of anal and distal colorectal tumors with the magnetic resonance endoscope. Gastrointest Endosc 1998;47:172–8.
73. Massari M, De Simone M, Cioffi U, Rosso L, Chiarelli M, Gabrielli F. Value and limits of endorectal ultrasonography for preoperative staging of rectal carcinoma. Surg Laparosc Endosc 1998;8:438–44.
74. Blomqvist L, Machado M, Rubio C, Gabrielsson N, Granqvist S, Goldman S, et al. Rectal tumour staging: MR imaging using pelvic phased-array and endorectal coils vs. endoscopic ultrasonography. Eur Radiol 2000;10:653–60.
75. Kelly S, Harris KM, Berry E, Hutton J, Roderick P, Cullingworth J, et al. A systematic review of the staging performance of endoscopic ultrasound in gastroesophageal carcinoma. Gut 2001;49:534–9.
76. Puli SR, Reddy JB, Bechtold ML, Antillon D, Ibdah JA, Antillon MR. Staging accuracy of esophageal cancer by endoscopic ultrasound: a meta-analysis and systematic review. World J Gastroenterol 2008;14:1479–90.
77. Hordijk ML, Zander H, van Blankenstein M, Tilanus HW. Influence of tumor stenosis on the accuracy of endosonography in preoperative T staging of esophageal cancer. Endoscopy 1993;25:171–5.
78. Van Dam J, Rice TW, Catalano MF, Kirby T, Sivak MV Jr. High-grade malignant stricture is predictive of esophageal tumor stage: risks of endosonographic evaluation. Cancer 1993;71:2910–7.
79. Catalano MF, Van Dam J, Sivak MJ. Malignant esophageal strictures: staging accuracy of endoscopic ultrasonography. Gastrointest Endosc 1995;41:535–9.
80. Pfau PR, Ginsberg GG, Lew RJ, Faigel DO, Smith DB, Kochman ML. Esophageal dilation for endosonographic evaluation of malignant esophageal strictures is safe and effective. Am J Gastroenterol 2000;95:2813–5.
81. Murad FM, Gupta K, Li R Mallery S. GI applications of the endobronchial ultrasound device: a report of 12 patient cases. Gastrointest Endosc 2009;69(Suppl):S252.
82. Kalha I, Kaw M, Fukami N, Patel M, Singh S, Gagneja H, et al. The accuracy of endoscopic ultrasound for restaging esophageal carcinoma after chemoradiation therapy. Cancer 2004;101:940–7.
83. Songur Y, Okai T, Watanabe H, Motoo Y, Sawabu N. Endosonographic evaluation of giant gastric folds. Gastrointest Endosc 1995;41:468–74.
84. Fusaroli P, Buscarini E, Peyre S, Federici T, Parente F, De Angelis C, et al. Interobserver agreement in staging gastric malt lymphoma by EUS. Gastrointest Endosc 2002;55:662–8.
85. Levy M, Hammel P, Lamarque D, Marty O, Chaumette MT, Haioun C, et al. Endoscopic ultrasonography for the initial staging and follow-up in pa-

tients with low-grade gastric lymphoma of mucosa-associated lymphoid tissue treated medically. Gastrointest Endosc 1997;46:328–33.

86. Nakamura S, Matsumoto T, Suekane H, Takeshita M, Hizawa K, Kawasaki M, et al. Predictive value of endoscopic ultrasonography for regression of gastric low grade and high grade MALT lymphomas after eradication of *Helicobacter pylori*. Gut 2001;48:454–60.

87. El-Zahabi LM, Jamali FR, El-Hajj II, Naja M, Salem Z, Shamseddine A, et al. The value of EUS in predicting the response of gastric mucosa-associated lymphoid tissue lymphoma to *Helicobacter pylori* eradication. Gastrointest Endosc 2007;65:89–96.

88. Laterza E, de Manzoni G, Guglielmi A, Rodella L, Tedesco P, Cordiano C. Endoscopic ultrasonography in the staging of esophageal carcinoma after preoperative radiotherapy and chemotherapy. Ann Thorac Surg 1999;67:1466–9.

89. Zuccaro G Jr, Rice TW, Goldblum J, Medendorp SV, Becker M, Pimentel R, et al. Endoscopic ultrasound cannot determine suitability for esophagectomy after aggressive chemoradiotherapy for esophageal cancer. Am J Gastroenterol 1999;94:906–12.

90. Beseth BD, Bedford R, Isacoff WH, Holmes EC, Cameron RB. Endoscopic ultrasound does not accurately assess pathologic stage of esophageal cancer after neoadjuvant chemoradiotherapy. Am Surg 2000;66:827–31.

91. Rau B, Hunerbein M, Barth C, Wust P, Haensch W, Riess H, et al. Accuracy of endorectal ultrasound after preoperative radiochemotherapy in locally advanced rectal cancer. Surg Endosc 1999;13:980–4.

92. Catalano MF, Sivak MV, Rice TW, Van Dam J. Postoperative screening for anastomotic recurrence of esophageal carcinoma by endoscopic ultrasonography. Gastrointest Endosc 1995;42:540–4.

93. Hunerbein M, Dohmoto M, Haensch W, Schlag PM. Evaluation and biopsy of recurrent rectal cancer using three-dimensional endosonography. Dis Colon Rectum 1996;39:1373–8.

94. Rotondano G, Esposito P, Pellecchia L, Novi A, Romano G. Early detection of locally recurrent rectal cancer by endosonography. Br J Radiol 1997;70:567–71.

95. Lohnert MS, Doniec JM, Henne-Bruns D. Effectiveness of endoluminal sonography in the identification of occult local rectal cancer recurrences. Dis Colon Rectum 2000;43:483–91.

96. Yasuda K, Nakajima M, Kawai K. Endoscopic ultrasonography in the diagnosis of submucosal tumor of the upper digestive tract. Scand J Gastroenterol Suppl 1986;123:59–67.

97. Rösch T, Lorenz R, Dancygier H, von Wickert A, Classen M. Endosonographic diagnosis of submucosal upper gastrointestinal tract tumors. Scand J Gastroenterol 1992;27:1–8.

98. Rösch T. Endoscopic ultrasonography in upper gastrointestinal submucosal tumors: a literature review. Gastrointest Endosc Clin North Am 1995;5:609–14.

99. Chak A, Canto MI, Rösch T, Dittler HJ, Hawes RH, Tio TL, et al. Endosonographic differentiation of benign and malignant stromal cell tumors. Gastrointest Endosc 1997;45:468–73.

100. Kawamoto K, Yamada Y, Utsunomiya T, Okamura H, Mizuguchi M, Motooka M, et al. Gastrointestinal submucosal tumors: evaluation with endoscopic US. Radiology 1997;205:733–40.

101. Nickl N, Gress F, McClave S, Fockens P, Chak A, Savides T, et al. Hypoechoic intramural tumor study: final report [abstract]. Gastrointest Endosc 2002;55:AB98.

102. Rösch T, Kapfer B, Will U, Baronius W, Strobel M, Lorenz R, et al. Accuracy of endoscopic ultrasonography in upper gastrointestinal submucosal lesions: a prospective multicenter study. Scand J Gastroenterol 2002; 37:856–62.

103. Fletcher CD, Berman JJ, Corless C, Gorstein F, Lasota J, Longley BJ, et al. Diagnosis of gastrointestinal stromal tumors: a consensus approach. Hum Pathol 2002;33:459–65.

104. Miettinen M, Sobin LH, Lasota J. Gastrointestinal stromal tumors of the stomach: a clinicopathologic, immunohistochemical, and molecular genetic study of 1765 cases with long term follow-up. Am J Surg Pathol 2005;29:52–68.

105. Ando N, Goto H, Niwa Y, Hirooka Y, Ohmiya N, Nagasaka T, et al. The diagnosis of GI stromal tumors with EUS-guided fine needle aspiration with immunohistochemical analysis. Gastrointest Endosc 2002;55: 37–43.

106. Akahoshi K, Sumida Y, Matsui N, Oya M, Akinaga R, Kubokawa M, et al. Preoperative diagnosis of gastrointestinal stromal tumor by endoscopic ultrasound-guided fine needle aspiration. World J Gastroenterol 2007;13:2077–82.

107. Kochman ML. EUS in pancreatic cancer. Gastrointest Endosc 2002;56(4 Suppl):S6–12.

108. Rösch T, Braig C, Gain T, Feuerbach S, Siewert JR, Schusdziarra V, et al. Staging of pancreatic and ampullary carcinoma by endoscopic ultrasonography: comparison with conventional sonography, computed tomography, and angiography. Gastroenterology 1992;102:188–99.

109. Snady H, Bruckner H, Siegel J, Cooperman A, Neff R, Kiefer L. Endoscopic ultrasonographic criteria of vascular invasion by potentially resectable pancreatic tumors. Gastrointest Endosc 1994;40:326–33.

110. Brugge WR, Lee MJ, Kelsey PB, Schapiro RH, Warshaw AL. The use of EUS to diagnose malignant portal venous system invasion by pancreatic cancer. Gastrointest Endosc 1996;43:561–7.

111. Rösch T, Dittler HJ, Strobel K, Meining A, Schusdziarra V, Lorenz R, et al. Endoscopic ultrasound criteria for vascular invasion in the staging of cancer of the head of the pancreas: a blind reevaluation of videotapes. Gastrointest Endosc 2000;52:469–77.

112. Puli SR, Singh S, Hagedorn CH, Reddy J, Olyaee M. Diagnostic accuracy of EUS for vascular invasion in pancreatic and periampullary cancers: a meta-analysis and systematic review. Gastrointest Endosc 2007;65: 788–97.

113. Buchs NC, Frossard JL, Rosset A, Chilcott M, Koutny-Fong P, Chassot G, et al. Vascular invasion in pancreatic cancer: evaluation of endoscopic ultrasonography, computed tomography, ultrasonography, and angiography. Swiss Med Wkly 2007;137:286–91.

114. Levy MJ. Pancreatic cysts. Gastrointest Endosc 2009;69(2 Suppl):S110–6.

115. Rösch T, Lorenz R, Braig C, Feuerbach S, Siewert JR, Schusdziarra V, et al. Endoscopic ultrasound in pancreatic tumor diagnosis. Gastrointest Endosc 1991;37:347–52.

116. Becker D, Strobel D, Bernatik T, Hahn EG. Echo-enhanced color and power-Doppler EUS for the discrimination between focal pancreatitis and pancreatic carcinoma. Gastrointest Endosc 2001;53:784–9.

117. Schick V, Franzius C, Beyna T, Oei ML, Schnekenburger J, Weckesser M, et al. Diagnostic impact of ^{18}F-FDG PET-CT evaluating solid pancreatic lesions versus endosonography, endoscopic retrograde cholangiopancreatography with intraductal ultrasonography and abdominal ultrasound. Eur J Nucl Med Mol Imaging 2008;35:1775–85.

118. Zimmer T, Scherübl H, Faiss S, Stölzel U, Riecken EO, Wiedenmann B. Endoscopic ultrasonography of neuroendocrine tumours. Digestion 2000;62(Suppl 1):45–50.

119. Rösch T, Lightdale CJ, Botet JF, Boyce GA, Sivak MV Jr, Yasuda K, et al. Localization of pancreatic endocrine tumors by endoscopic ultrasonography. N Engl J Med 1992;326:1721–6.

120. Gibril F, Jensen RT. Diagnostic uses of radiolabelled somatostatin-receptor analogues in gastroenteropancreatic endocrine tumors. Dig Liver Dis 2004;36(Suppl 1):S106–20.

121. Tamada K, Ueno N, Tomiyama T, Oohashi A, Wada S, Nishizono T, et al. Characterization of biliary strictures using intraductal ultrasonography: comparison with percutaneous cholangioscopic biopsy. Gastrointest Endosc 1998;47:341–9.

122. Menzel J, Poremba C, Dietl KH, Domschke W. Preoperative diagnosis of bile duct strictures—comparison of intraductal ultrasonography with conventional endosonography. Scand J Gastroenterol 2000;35:77–82.

123. Hoffman BJ, Knapple WL, Bhutani MS, Verne GN, Hawes RH. Treatment of achalasia by injection of botulinum toxin under endoscopic ultrasound guidance. Gastrointest Endosc 1997;45:77–9.

124. Miller LS, Schiano TD, Adrain A, Cassidy M, Liu JB, Ter H, et al. Comparison of high-resolution endoluminal sonography to video endoscopy in the detection and evaluation of esophageal varices. Hepatology 1996;24: 552–5.

125. Leung VK, Sung JJ, Ahuja AT, Tumala IE, Lee YT, Lau JY, et al. Large paraesophageal varices on endosonography predict recurrence of esophageal varices and rebleeding. Gastroenterology 1997;112:1811–6.

126. Salama ZA, Kassem AM, Giovannini M, Hunter MS. Endoscopic ultrasonographic study of the azygos vein in patients with varices. Endoscopy 1997;29:748–50.

127. Kassem AM, Salama ZA, Rösch T. Endoscopic ultrasonography in portal hypertension. Endoscopy 1997;29:399–406.

128. Kassem AM, Salama ZA, Zakaria MS, Hassaballah M, Hunter MS. Endoscopic ultrasonographic study of the azygos vein before and after endoscopic obliteration of esophagogastric varices by injection sclerotherapy. Endoscopy 2000;32:630–4.

129. Nishida H, Giostra E, Spahr L, Mentha G, Mitamura K, Hadengue A. Validation of color Doppler EUS for azygos blood flow measurement in patients with cirrhosis: application to the acute hemodynamic effects of somatostatin, octreotide, or placebo. Gastrointest Endosc 2001;54:24–30.

130. Lee YT, Chan FK, Ng EK, Leung VK, Law KB, Yung MY, et al. EUS-guided injection of cyanoacrylate for bleeding gastric varices. Gastrointest Endosc 2000;52:168–74.

22

131. Romero-Castro R, Pellicer-Bautista FJ, Jimenez-Saenz M, Marcos-Sanchez F, Caunedo-Alvarez A, Ortiz-Moyano C, et al. EUS-guided injection of cyanoacrylate in perforating feeding veins in gastric varices: results in 5 cases. Gastrointest Endosc. 2007;66:402–7.

132. El-Saadany M, Jalil S, Irisawa A, Shibukawa G, Ohira H, Bhutani MS. EUS for portal hypertension: a comprehensive and critical appraisal of clinical and experimental indications. Endoscopy 2008;40:690–6.

133. Lew RJ, Ginsberg GG. The role of endoscopic ultrasound in inflammatory bowel disease. Gastrointest Endosc Clin N Am 2002;12:561–71.

134. Yoshizawa S, Kobayashi K, Katsumata T, Saigenji K, Okayasu I. Clinical usefulness of EUS for active ulcerative colitis. Gastrointest Endosc 2007;65:253–60.

135. Spradlin NM, Wise PE, Herline AJ, Muldoon RL, Rosen M, Schwartz DA. A randomized prospective trial of endoscopic ultrasound to guide combination medical and surgical treatment for Crohn's perianal fistulas. Am J Gastroenterol 2008;103:2527–35.

136. Schwartz DA, Harewood GC, Wiersema MJ. EUS for rectal disease. Gastrointest Endosc 2002;56:100–9.

137. Tse F, Barkun JS, Romagnuolo J, Friedman G, Bornstein JD, Barkun AN. Nonoperative imaging techniques in suspected biliary tract obstruction. HPB (Oxford) 2006;8:409–25.

138. Hernandez LV, Sahai A, Brugge WR, Wiersema MJ, Catalano MF. Standardized weighted criteria for EUS features of chronic pancreatitis: the Rosemont classification [abstract]. Gastrointest Endosc 2008;67: AB96–AB97.

139. Varadarajulu S, Christein JD, Tamhane A, Drelichman ER, Wilcox CM. Prospective randomized trial comparing EUS and EGD for transmural drainage of pancreatic pseudocysts. Gastrointest Endosc 2008;68: 1102–11.

140. Brugge WR. Endoscopic ultrasound-guided pancreatic fine-needle aspiration: a review. Tech Gastrointest Endosc 2000;2:149–54.

141. Erickson RA. EUS-guided FNA. Gastrointest Endosc 2004;60:267–79.

142. Pellisé M, Castells A, Ginès A, Solé M, Mora J, Castellví-Bel S, et al. Clinical usefulness of KRAS mutational analysis in the diagnosis of pancreatic adenocarcinoma by means of endosonography-guided fine-needle aspiration biopsy. Aliment Pharmacol Ther 2003;17:1299–307.

143. Levy MJ, Baron TH, Clayton AC, Enders FB, Gostout CJ, Halling KC, et al. Prospective evaluation of advanced molecular markers and imaging techniques in patients with indeterminate bile duct strictures. Am J Gastroenterol 2008;103:1263–73.

144. Buchler P, Conejo-Garcia JR, Lehmann G, Muller M, Emrich T, Reber HA, et al. Real-time quantitative PCR of telomerase mRNA is useful for the differentiation of benign and malignant pancreatic disorders. Pancreas 2001;22:331–40.

145. Tada M, Komatsu Y, Kawabe T, Sasahira N, Isayama H, Toda N, et al. Quantitative analysis of K-ras gene mutation in pancreatic tissue obtained by endoscopic ultrasonography guided fine needle aspiration: clinical utility for diagnosis of pancreatic tumor. Am J Gastroenterol 2002;97: 2263–70.

146. Wallace MB, Block M, Hoffman BJ, Hawes RH, Silvestri G, Reed CE, et al. Detection of telomerase expression in mediastinal lymph nodes of patients with lung cancer. Am J Respir Crit Care Med 2003;167:1670–5.

147. Chhieng DC, Benson E, Eltoum I, Eloubeidi MA, Jhala N, Jhala D, et al. MUC1 and MUC2 expression in pancreatic ductal carcinoma obtained by fine-needle aspiration. Cancer 2003;99:365–71.

148. Siperstein A, Pearl J, Macho J, Hansen P, Gitomirsky A, Rogers S. Comparison of laparoscopic ultrasonography and fluorocholangiography in 300 patients undergoing laparoscopic cholecystectomy. Surg Endosc 1999;13:113–7.

149. Long EE, Van Dam J, Weinstein S, Jeffrey B, Desser T, Norton JA. Computed tomography, endoscopic, laparoscopic, and intra-operative sonography for assessing resectability of pancreatic cancer. Surg Oncol 2005;14: 105–13.

150. Yoshino J, Nakazawa S, Inui K, Katoh Y, Wakabayashi T, Okushima T, et al. Surface-rendering imaging of gastrointestinal lesions by three-dimensional endoscopic ultrasonography. Endoscopy 1999;31:541–5.

151. Sumiyama K, Suzuki N, Kakutani H, Hino S, Tajiri H, Suzuki H, et al. A novel 3-dimensional EUS technique for real-time visualization of the volume data reconstruction process. Gastrointest Endosc 2002;55:723–8.

152. Inui K, Miyoshi H. Cholangiocarcinoma and intraductal sonography. Gastrointest Endosc Clin N Am 2005;15:143–55.

153. Săftoiu A, Popescu C, Cazacu S, Dumitrescu D, Georgescu CV, Popescu M, et al. Power Doppler endoscopic ultrasonography for the differential diagnosis between pancreatic cancer and pseudotumoral chronic pancreatitis. J Ultrasound Med 2006;25:363–72.

154. Hirooka Y, Itoh A, Goto H. New diagnostic technique of EUS using contrast-enhanced agents. In: Niwa H, Tajiri H, Nakajima M, Yasuda K, editors. New challenges in gastrointestinal endoscopy. Tokyo: Springer; 2008. p. 489–498.

155. Kitano M, Sakamoto H, Matsui U, Ito Y, Maekawa K, von Schrenck T, et al. A novel perfusion imaging technique of the pancreas: contrast-enhanced harmonic EUS. Gastrointest Endosc 2008;67:141–50.

156. Faulx AL, Kumon RE, Pollack MJ, Wong RCK, Isenberg GB, Wolf B, et al. Validation of tissue characterization by endoscopic ultrasound spectrum analysis in differentiating pancreatic adenocarcinoma from normal pancreas. Gastrointest Endosc 2009;69(Suppl 1):S241.

157. Kassem AM, Prinz C, Schmid R, Meining A. Endoscopic ultrasonographic elastography: a novel endoscopic application. Arab J Gastroenterol 2005;6:113–8.

158. Giovannini M, Hookey LC, Bories E, Pesenti C, Monges G, Delpero JR. Endoscopic ultrasound elastography: the first step towards virtual biopsy? Preliminary results in 49 patients. Endoscopy 2006;38:344–8.

159. Hirche TO, Ignee A, Barreiros AP, Schreiber-Dietrich D, Jungblut S, Ott M. Indications and limitations of endoscopic ultrasound elastography for evaluation of focal pancreatic lesions. Endoscopy 2008;40:910–7.

160. Kobayashi K, Haruki S, Yokoyama K, Sada M, Kida M, Saigenji K. Clinical usefulness of a prototype ultrasound probe for single-balloon enteroscopy. Gastrointest Endosc 2009;69(Suppl 1):S248.

161. Yusuf TE, Matthes K, Lee Y, Goodman AJ, Robbins DH, Stavropoulos S, et al. Evaluation of the EASIE-R simulator for the training of basic and advanced EUS. Gastrointest Endosc 2009;6969(Suppl 1):S264.

162. Bar-Meir S. Simbionix simulator. Gastrointest Endosc Clin N Am 2006;16:471–8.

163. Azad JS, Verma D. Can U.S. GI fellowship programs meet American Society for Gastrointestinal Endoscopy recommendations for training in EUS? A survey of U.S. GI fellowship program directors. Gastrointest Endosc 2006;64:235–41.

IV

23 Laparoscopic, Natural Orifice, and Laparoscopy-Assisted Surgery: New Paradigms in Minimally Invasive Therapy

Robert H. Hawes, Stefan von Delius, D. Nageshwar Reddy, and Hubertus Feußner

Introduction

Robert H. Hawes

The development of laparoscopic cholecystectomy has had a significant influence on the practice of surgery, as well as on surgeons' mindset, making them more aware of new ways of operating less invasively. Endoscopists—both physicians and surgeons—have always taken a less invasive approach, as therapeutic endoscopy primarily developed as an alternative to more invasive surgical procedures. As a result, the introduction of natural orifice surgery by Kalloo et al. in 2000 [1,2] created excitement in both disciplines. For surgeons, natural orifice transluminal endoscopic surgery (NOTES) offers new opportunities for less invasive procedures, while for endoscopists it has the potential to allow transluminal therapy and also promises to accelerate the development of devices facilitating a whole range of new endoluminal procedures.

Since the first description of NOTES, there has been considerable speculation—and indeed concern—about how it will develop. The chaos in the early days of laparoscopic cholecystectomy is still vivid in our memories. Although natural orifice surgery is considered to have great potential, guidance and direction in its implementation is needed in order to ensure that patients are protected and that it develops in a responsible way. Toward this end, the Society of American Gastrointestinal Endoscopic Surgeons (SAGES) and the American Society for Gastrointestinal Endoscopy (ASGE) established a joint committee to support basic research, promote education, and create a registry for human NOTES procedures. In addition, an organization called the Natural Orifice Surgery Consortium for Assessment and Research (NOSCAR) was formed, with its membership drawn from teams of laparoscopy and flexible-endoscopy experts from around the world. The joint ASGE/SAGES committee, in cooperation with the NOSCAR group, was charged with setting standards for conduct in the field of NOTES—such as insisting that all human NOTES procedures be conducted under the guidance and oversight of institutional review boards—and establishing guidelines for practice when appropriate. Groups with organizational structures and goals similar to those of NOSCAR have also emerged in Europe, Asia, and South America. This paradigm of cooperation between societies to provide leadership in the development of new techniques will surely be one of the most powerful legacies of natural orifice surgery.

It is very important to view natural orifice surgery as a movement toward less invasive therapies, rather than as a series of new surgical procedures. It has already had a significant influence and will undoubtedly continue to have an impact on therapeutic endoscopy for many years to come:

- It has brought endoscopists and laparoscopic surgeons together—each with their own unique perspectives. Together, they will accelerate innovation in endoscopy.
- It has brought representatives of medical-device manufacturers together—including companies that had previously concentrated on innovative devices only in their own markets. Now, companies specializing in laparoscopic devices, flexible endoscopes, and accessories for flexible endoscopes are exploring opportunities outside their own markets and are leveraging their knowledge and experience in order to solve the unique problems faced in natural orifice surgery.
- The improved relationship between surgeons and endoscopists, combined with innovative technologies from industry, will greatly accelerate the development of intraluminal therapies for obesity management, reflux disease, full-thickness resection of intramural tumors, and endoscopic submucosal dissection.

These direct effects of the NOTES movement will create a legacy that goes well beyond the new generation of minimally invasive surgical procedures. To appreciate the real impact of NOTES, these developments should be seen as a whole, without focusing exclusively on an announcement of the NOTES equivalent of laparoscopic cholecystectomy, for example. There is no question that procedures will eventually be performed using natural orifices as access points. Medical historians will look back and document the broad influence that the introduction of natural orifice surgery had on therapeutic endoscopy.

This trend toward procedures with access via natural orifices has tremendous implications for future practice and may well stimulate the development of a "comprehensive digestivist"—an individual trained in minimally invasive gastrointestinal therapy, regardless of whether it involves a laparoscope or a flexible endoscope, and one who is equally comfortable with intraluminal, transluminal, and transabdominal access. While the future may see the development of combined medical/surgical specialists in gastrointestinal therapy, this will take time. At present, speculation is continuing on whether it will be surgeons or gastroenterologists who will take the lead with NOTES. Initially, teams combining endoscopists and surgeons were the driving force in basic NOTES research. Even now, most research is being conducted with close cooperation between gastroenterology and surgery. However, the first NOTES procedures in humans have been carried out with laparoscopic assistance. Access has been primarily transvaginal, with dissection and organ removal via a natural orifice but with traction, insufflation, clipping (of the cystic duct and artery)—and in the case of transgastric access, closure—accomplished with laparoscopic access. Surgeons have clearly taken the lead in these developments and in the end it is likely that natural orifice surgery will be performed, with few exceptions, by surgeons who either already possess or have acquired skills in flexible endoscopy. This development has several important implications for the practice of natural orifice surgery.

Firstly, surgeons are developing a greater appreciation of therapeutic endoscopy. As they acquire the skills in flexible endoscopy needed to perform natural orifice surgery, they will probably also take advantage of the opportunities developing for intraluminal therapies such as antireflux procedures, obesity therapies, full-thickness resection, and mucosal resection.

Secondly, gastroenterologists must not be discouraged if they are excluded from performing NOTES, but instead should seize the remarkable opportunity to leverage their endoscopic skills and take advantage of the new devices and techniques that are developing as part of the NOTES movement. There will be abundant opportunities for intraluminal therapies such as those mentioned above.

Thirdly, these opportunities in intraluminal treatment need to be recognized in training programs. Over the last decade, there has been an explosion in knowledge and available treatments in the fields of hepatology, inflammatory bowel disease, and gastrointestinal motility. As a result, these topics are now taking up more training time during the 3 years of gastroenterology fellowship. The direct consequence of this is that techniques in "advanced endoscopy"—mainly endoscopic retrograde cholangiopancreatography (ERCP) and endoscopic ultrasonography (EUS)—have been displaced from standard fellowships, and in most programs it is considered that they should be part of a fourth "advanced" endoscopy year. However, only a limited number of fourth-year advanced endoscopy positions are available, and they fall outside the normal funding systems. As a result, the future generation of gastroenterologists will not be trained in the advanced techniques that will serve as a springboard for learning the new intraluminal techniques developing in the NOTES movement. It is time to follow the lead of cardiology and create different tracks within gastroenterology training. Some trainees will concentrate on diagnosis, while others will sacrifice training in areas such as hepatology in favor of therapeutic endoscopy training. If this does not occur, then the future of gastroenterology will lie exclusively in the field of diagnosis, and physicians with surgical training will become the therapeutic endoscopists of the future.

Laparoscopic Cholecystotomy

Stefan von Delius

Laparoscopic cholecystectomy is considered the treatment of choice for patients with symptomatic gallbladder stones [3]. Since its first description by the German surgeon Mühe in 1985 and the French gynecologist Mouret, the technique of laparoscopic cholecystectomy has been rapidly accepted by the general population and is one of the most frequent abdominal operations performed today [4]. Although laparoscopic cholecystectomy can be regarded as a remarkably safe surgical procedure, it does carry a certain risk. Complications include hematoma in the gallbladder bed, infection (usually of the hematoma), bile leak, inadvertent injury to the bowel, and retained stones in the bile duct. The most serious complication is injury of the bile duct, occurring at a rate of 0.2% in both laparoscopic and open surgery [5]. This may necessitate endoscopic stent therapy or further surgery to repair the bile duct, or to join the bile duct to the bowel by anastomosis. Laparoscopic cholecystectomy includes resection of the gallbladder. However, some patients decline loss of the organ when it is still functioning well.

A multitude of conservative treatment modalities for cholecystolithiasis have been developed in recent decades, but none has proved to be successful over the longer term [6]. Oral bile acid dissolution therapy, with or without prior extracorporeal shockwave treatment, is effective only in highly selected patients who represent only approximately 10% of all patients with symptomatic gallstone disease. Laparoscopic cholecystotomy (LCT) with primary closure of the organ was first described by Frimberger in 1989, as an alternative gallbladder-preserving treatment for cholecystolithiasis [7].

Patient Selection

LCT may be offered to selected patients with symptomatic cholecystolithiasis who want to preserve the gallbladder and decline cholecystectomy. The procedure is restricted to patients with a functioning gallbladder and an ability to tolerate general anesthesia. Previous upper abdominal surgery may prevent access to the gallbladder. Thickening of the gallbladder wall or obstruction of the cystic duct should be excluded before the procedure. Preoperative abdominal ultrasonography should also confirm gallbladder function, which is demonstrated by an emptying volume of at least 30% of the fasting volume after consumption of a test meal.

Technique

LCT is carried out with the patient under general anesthesia. Patients are placed in the supine position and receive antibiotics for single-shot prophylaxis. LCT starts with establishing a pneumoperitoneum and placement of three trocars. Cannula 1 is introduced through the umbilicus; cannula 2 in the right paramedian position; and cannula 3 is lateral to cannula 1 (**Fig. 23.1 a**). For exposure of the gallbladder, a pivot-arm laparoscope (**Fig. 23.1 b**) with the arm retracted is introduced through the umbilical cannula [8]. The gallbladder is exposed by elevation of the right hepatic lobe, with the extended arm of the laparoscope placed medially to the gallbladder (**Fig. 23.1 a**). The angle of the extended arm can be adjusted according to the individual anatomy. The gallbladder can be seen in the optical field of the 30° viewing angle of the instrument, which is connected to a monitor. The fundus of the gallbladder is grasped with an atraumatic forceps (via cannula 3) and then punctured with a 2.2-mm trocar (via cannula 2). Following removal of the mandrin of that trocar, a tube with lateral holes is introduced. Bile is aspirated. After this, the gallbladder is rinsed several times with saline solution. A longitudinal incision into the gallbladder is carried out with a needle-knife inserted through cannula 2 (**Fig. 23.2 a**). The length of the incision is based on the objective of the laparoscopic cholecystotomy—i. e., in most cases, the size of the stones to be extracted.

A flexible cholecystoscope fixed in a rigid shaft, sparing the bending section of the instrument, is inserted into the gallbladder through cannula 2. During cholecystoscopy, saline is instilled through the endoscope channel for distension of the gallbladder (**Fig. 23.2 b**). Stones are extracted with a basket or a grasper through cannula 2 (**Fig. 23.2 c**). If the stones are too large to pass through cannula 2, a plastic bag is introduced into the abdominal cavity and placed on the liver surface. The stone is extracted with the bag at the end of the procedure.

Polypectomy of gallbladder polyps can also be carried out with a diathermy snare.

After extraction of the stone or stones, the interior of the gallbladder is thoroughly inspected with the flexible cholecystoscope, up to the opening of the cystic duct, to ensure complete removal of all stones. Finally, the incision is closed with titanium clips (**Fig. 23.2 d**). The margins can be adapted as needed by pulling the incision caudally with a small hook (cannula 3) or a grasping forceps. Starting from the cranial part of the incision, clips are set separately every 4 mm using an applicator introduced through the laparoscope. In addition, the incision is sealed with fibrin glue.

If a large stone was deposited in the bag, the open end of the bag is pulled into cannula 2 with a forceps. The cannula is extracted, and the opening of the bag is pulled to the exterior, leaving the bottom of the bag with the stone inside the abdominal cavity. The stone is grasped using a basket introduced into the bag. Medium-sized stones can be retrieved with a bag directly through the opening

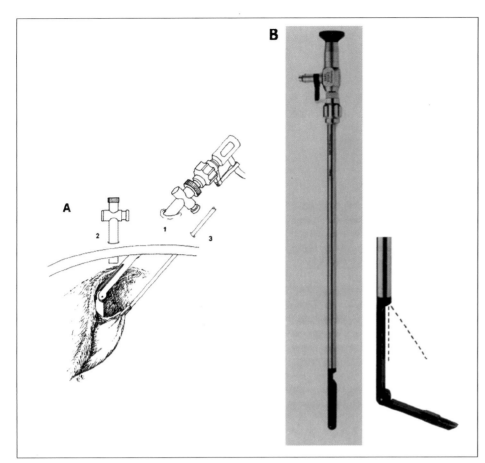

Fig. 23.1
a Position of the three cannulae and diagram of laparoscopic cholecystotomy. The gallbladder is exposed by elevating the right liver lobe with the pivot-arm laparoscope.
b The pivot-arm laparoscope. The arm of the laparoscope can be elevated to any angle required for elevation of the liver.

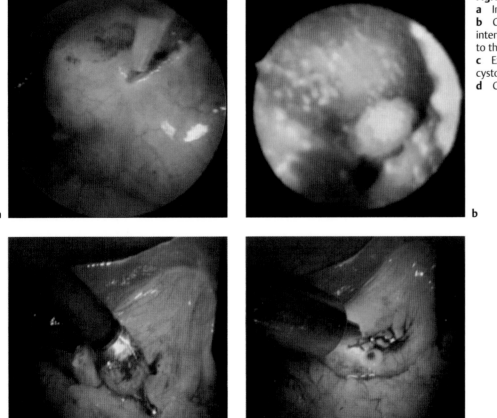

Fig. 23.2 Laparoscopic cholecystotomy.
a Incision of the gallbladder with a needle-knife.
b Cholecystoscopy with a flexible endoscope. The interior of the gallbladder is thoroughly inspected up to the cystic duct opening, to check for stones.
c Extraction of a gallbladder stone with the cholecystoscope.
d Closure of the incision with titanium clips.

23

left behind by the extracted trocar. The elasticity of the abdominal wall allows extraction of stones that are too large to pass through the rigid cannula. Very large stones are fragmented before extraction, using a lithotripsy basket or other lithotriptic devices.

The operative field is thoroughly rinsed with saline and the fluid is aspirated. A 12-Fr drain is placed close to the gallbladder through cannula 3. The drain is extracted on the first or second postoperative day. Beginning on the second postoperative day, the patients are given ursodeoxycholic acid (UDCA; 10 mg/kg body weight p. o.) for 4 weeks.

Effectiveness of LCT

LCT with primary closure of the gallbladder by clips was successfully applied in a series of 64 patients. One bile leak from the gallbladder requiring cholecystectomy was observed in these 64 procedures. No other relevant complications were encountered [9]. In particular, injury to the common bile duct cannot occur in LCT. In contrast, laparoscopic cholecystectomy–related bile duct injuries are severe and potentially life-threatening complications [10,11].

However, the long-term effectiveness of LCT has not yet been demonstrated. A significant drawback of LCT is the possibility of gallstone recurrence, as the gallbladder is left in place and the underlying cause of gallstone formation is not corrected. Stone recurrence has been studied in a series of 50 patients undergoing LCT with a follow-up period of 1–5 years (median 3.6 years). Stones recurred in 10 patients. No recurrent stones were observed in patients either with pigment stones or with a crystal formation time of more than 2 days [12]. However, the clinical importance of the latter observation is limited, as preoperative analysis of patients' bile would require aspiration of bile by puncture of the gallbladder. The stone recurrence rate is even higher with other gallbladder-preserving treatment modalities. It is about 10 % annually for up to 5 years after medical therapy for gallstones [13] and up to 69 % after more than 5 years of follow-up after extracorporeal shock-wave lithotripsy [14]. Maintenance therapy with low-dose UDCA has been reported to decrease the recurrence rate, but it is costly [15]. Patients with multiple primary stones have an increased recurrence rate. Additional factors that have been reported to predict recurrence after successful lithotripsy are obesity [16], poor gallbladder emptying [17], an increased deoxycholic acid pool [18], and an apolipoprotein E4 genotype [19].

However, gallstone recurrence may be absent in a group of patients in whom the initial lithogenic process is transient. Pregnancy, rapid weight loss, and convalescence from abdominal surgery are recognized transient risk factors [20,21]. Trying to identify and characterize patients with transient lithogenicity is an important challenge for future studies.

Percutaneous Cholecystostomy

Percutaneous cholecystostomy can be used when the patient presents with severe acute cholecystitis and in cases in which conservative treatment alone has failed, especially in patients who are poor candidates for surgery. With this technique, the gallbladder is not closed primarily but is drained for several days with a balloon catheter. Percutaneous cholecystostomy is performed with the patient under local anesthesia, with radiologic or ultrasound guidance, and the procedure has a high technical success rate and low complication rate [22–24]. It usually leads to resolution of acute cholecystitis [25]. However, in a randomized trial in high-risk patients, routine percutaneous cholecystostomy was not found to be superior to conservative measures followed by percutaneous cholecystostomy when needed [26]. Drainage may be followed by delayed cholecystectomy or percutaneous stone extraction in patients who are poor candidates for surgery.

Endoscopic Gallbladder Drainage

In patients with acute cholecystitis in whom a percutaneous transhepatic approach is contraindicated or anatomically impossible, endoscopic transpapillary gallbladder drainage by means of ERCP is safe and effective as an alternative method of gallbladder drainage for acute cholecystitis [27–33]. After successful selective deep cannulation of the common bile duct and treatment of stones or obstructions in the common bile duct, a guide wire is inserted via the cystic duct into the gallbladder. Following successful gallbladder cannulation, either an internal plastic stent (from the gallbladder to the duodenum) or a nasocholecystic drainage catheter is negotiated into position under fluoroscopic guidance.

Recently, it has been suggested that endosonography-guided transmural cholecystostomy may provide initial, interim, or even definitive treatment of severe acute cholecystitis in patients who are at high surgical risk. The puncture site is located in the prepyloric antrum or the superior duodenal angle and is chosen in such a way as to access the gallbladder body or neck and avoid visible vessels. The gallbladder is then punctured under combined EUS and fluoroscopic guidance, with a 19-gauge needle. Fluid is aspirated for microbacterial culture, and contrast is injected to confirm the position. The EUS needle is exchanged over the wire for a cystoenterostome or cystotome, and a tract is created by passage of the cystoenterostome into the gallbladder using cutting current. Alternatively, the transmural tract can be dilated with a 6-Fr or 7-Fr bougie. A single pigtail nasocholecystic drain is then placed over the guide wire [34,35]. The technique appears to be safe and effective. However, only a few patients have been treated using EUS-guided drainage so far.

Natural Orifice Transluminal Endoscopic Surgery

D. Nageshwar Reddy

Introduction

Natural orifice transluminal endoscopic surgery (NOTES) is a novel technique that combines flexible endoscopic instruments and surgical techniques to accomplish therapeutic interventions without an incision on the anterior abdominal wall. It essentially involves the insertion of a flexible endoscopic device through a natural orifice (the mouth, anus, vagina, urethra), followed by a transvisceral incision to gain access to the peritoneal cavity, where surgery is performed. The first successful attempt in a porcine model was reported by Kalloo et al. in 2000; they explored the peritoneal cavity transgastrically and performed a liver biopsy [1,2]. The first experience in humans was in a procedure conducted by Rao et al., who reported on transgastric appendectomy [36]. The publication in 2005 of a white paper by the Natural Orifice Surgery Consortium for Assessment and Research (NOSCAR) highlighted the challenges and limitations in implementing NOTES and set guidelines for future development and progress [37]. Since then, many experimental porcine procedures have been described and more recently some very encouraging highly selective procedures in humans have been successfully completed, with no reported morbidity [38,39]. We describe here the techniques used to obtain access through different natural orifices, highlighting their advantages and disadvantages.

Transgastric Appendectomy

The peroral transgastric route was chosen in the initial trials because of the experience that endoscopists have in performing safe gastrotomy during percutaneous endoscopic gastrotomy procedures [36]. The potential risk of injury to adjacent organs remains minimal when the gastrotomy is sited by observing the indentation on the gastric wall produced by palpation of the anterior abdominal wall [40]. Also, the risk of peritoneal contamination remains negligible, given the relative sterility of the stomach in comparison with other access routes. A recent study has shown that although transgastric access does contaminate the peritoneal cavity, the pathogenic load is too small to cause any clinically significant infection [41].

The procedure is carried out with the patient under general anesthesia, with nasotracheal intubation. Antibiotics are administered preoperatively and continued for 48 h postoperatively. The stomach is also lavaged with antibiotic solution preoperatively. An overtube is used to facilitate repeated passages of the endoscope. The use of double overtubes has been reported to further reduce the chances of contamination being carried in from the oral flora [42]. The relatively avascular area midway between the two gastric curvatures on the anterior wall of the body of the stomach is chosen for the gastrotomy [43]. Stretching of the vessels in the gastrohepatic ligament and the short gastric vessels while the endoscope is continuously passing forward and backward is avoided. A double-channel endoscope passed through an overtube is used to suck out the gastric contents. A stab gastrotomy is created using a needle-knife with blended current. The CO_2 insufflator is then connected to the sheath after withdrawal of the knife, to create the pneumoperitoneum. The pneumoperitoneum can be monitored via a separate Veress needle passed transabdominally [44]. Alternatively, introduction of a pressure monitor via the accessory channel of the scope has been described [45]. Once an adequate pneumoperitoneum has been created, a CRE balloon dilator is passed through the stab, using the railroading technique—withdrawing the needle-knife and using a guide wire. The gastrostoma is widened by inflating the balloon (**Fig. 23.3**). The endoscope balloon assembly is passed into the peritoneal cavity, and the balloon is withdrawn after deflation (**Fig. 23.4**). Alternatively, a sphincterotome has been used to widen the stab, which is reported to be quicker than balloon dilation; in addition, as there is no tendency for the hole to spontaneously close because muscle is cut, this is advantageous if speed and repeated gastric crossing are required [40]. In two animal studies, a submucosal endoscopy with mucosal flap (SEMF) safety valve technique was used in a bid to control peritoneal contamination [46,47]. This involved creating a submucosal working space using high-pressure CO_2 injection and balloon dissection to allow resection of the muscle layer, while allowing the overlying gastric mucosa to control contamination from a perforating muscle layer resection.

An abdominal exploration is first performed to rule out any damage that may have occurred during performance of the gastrotomy. The table is tilted to a head-down, left lateral position. The small-bowel loops fall away from the right iliac fossa, allowing easier access to the appendix. A rat-toothed forceps is used to lift the appendix, and a hot biopsy forceps is used to dissect the mesoappendix (**Fig. 23.5**). After the base of the appendix has been exposed, it is secured with an Endoloop. The appendix is then transected using a polypectomy snare. The right iliac fossa is irrigated with povidone–iodine solution and fluid-suctioned with the endoscope. The appendix is held with a grasping forceps, withdrawn through the gastrotomy into the stomach, and retrieved transorally.

Since peritonitis is not acceptable even in a minor percentage of cases, given its rarity in conventional surgery, perfect closure of the gastrotomy has become a sine qua non for a successful NOTES

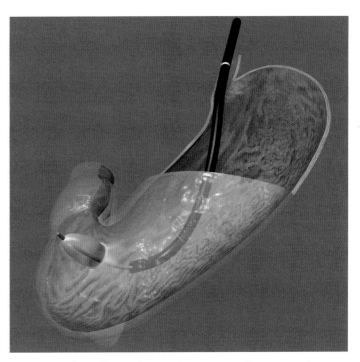

Fig. 23.3 Balloon dilation of an anterior gastrotomy for transgastric access.

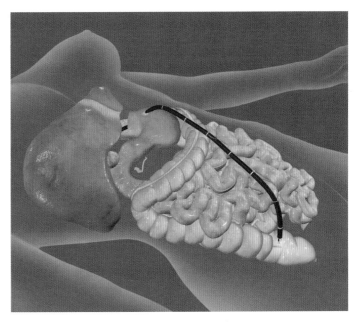

Fig. 23.4 The transgastric approach for appendectomy.

procedure [37]. However, gastric injuries heal quickly due to the good vascularization of the stomach and its thick organ wall [48,49]. Endoscopic sutures and clips were used in the earlier reports [50,51]. Now, various stapling devices, including the NDO Plicator [52] originally designed for endoscopic plication for gastroesophageal reflux disease, endoscopic tissue plicating devices [53], and automated flexible stapling devices (SurgASSIST) [54], among many others, have been evaluated and their safety has been confirmed in various studies. Fluid and air leak tests are simple techniques that can be used to evaluate the adequacy of transluminal access site closure in vivo after NOTES procedures [55].

23

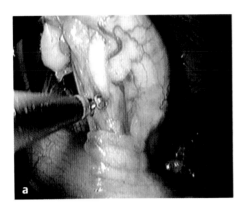

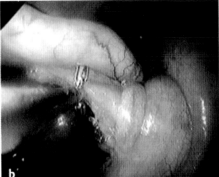

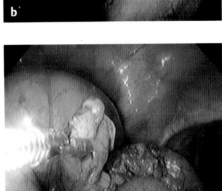

Fig. 23.5 Transgastric appendectomy.
a, b Division of the mesoappendix with electro-cautery.
c Division of the appendix with loop cautery after ligation of the base with an Endoloop.
d Extraction of the divided appendix.

IV

Transgastric Tubal Occlusion

A similar transgastric approach can be used for tubal occlusion (**Fig. 23.6**). A transvaginal uterine elevator is used to assist the procedure [38]. The procedure is done using a single-channel 9-mm gastroscope. Resolution clips are doubly applied over the fallopian tubes, which are divided in between using a needle-knife. Alternatively, an Endoloop can be used to occlude the tubes. Methylene blue is injected at the end of the procedure to confirm tubal occlusion on the table.

The hybrid technique. Hybrid procedures involve performing NOTES with laparoscopic assistance [56]. While some groups have limited the assisting laparoscopic port to an independent visualization port [57] in the form of a needlescope to monitor the pneumoperitoneum, others have used it as a retraction port [58] or even as a working port [59]. The hybrid technique provides better visual information independently of the endoscope that is being used to carry out the procedure. During dissection with the working instruments, the endoscopic image is constantly in motion and even shifts away from the operative field. The laparoscopic image, however, is stable and the operated field can always be kept at the center of it. In particular, this ensures the safety of the initial puncture and incision and greatly facilitates advanced NOTES procedures, as it provides a wide field of vision and sufficient illumination. The hybrid technique is also a useful bridge to performing "pure" NOTES procedures.

Natural orifice (transvaginal or transanal) extraction of a laparoscopically dissected specimen has also been described as a modification of hybrid NOTES [60]. The dual-lumen or rendezvous technique [61,62] is another variant of hybrid NOTES. The transgastric and transvaginal routes are used simultaneously here to provide the same advantages of the hybrid technique while avoiding an external scar.

Transvaginal Cholecystectomy

The transgastric route for cholecystectomy requires the scope to be positioned in a retroflexed position. The resulting difficulties in working with a retroflexed scope can be avoided by using a more direct transvaginal route. The other advantage of this route is that it is easy to close the colpotomy using manual suturing under vision [63]. The richness of the vaginal flora in comparison with the gastric flora is a cause for concern. From the gynecological point of view, other potential disadvantages of this route include the formation of adhesions, spread of preexisting endometriosis, infertility, and dyspareunia [64].

The patient receives preoperative antibiotics, which are continued for 48 h postoperatively. The vagina is disinfected with povidone–iodine. The patient is placed in a lithotomy position, with the surgeon positioned between her legs. The cholecystectomy is usually assisted with a needlescope placed transabdominally to guide the initial puncture and to monitor the pneumoperitoneum. Some surgeons have also used the laparoscopic port for organ retraction and clip placement [65]. A triangular area between the uterosacral ligaments, which is avascular and without innervation, is chosen for port placement [38] (**Fig. 23.7**). An incision is sited on the posterior vaginal cul-de-sac [66]. A double-channel endoscope is introduced into the peritoneum after adequate pneumoperitoneum has been achieved (**Fig. 23.8**). The dissection is commenced in the Calot triangle, separating the peritoneum off the cystic duct. The combination of grasping and cutting with the endoscopic instruments and the deflection movements of the tip of the endoscope are used to accomplish the dissection (**Fig. 23.9**). Once sufficiently skeletonized, the cystic duct and artery are clipped and divided with endoscopic scissors. The gallbladder is then dissected from the liver and placed in a retrieval bag. The gallbladder bed is checked for hemostasis. The specimen is then removed transvaginally. The colpotomy is closed with absorbable sutures transvaginally.

A recent systematic review shows that the NOTES operation performed most often to date in humans is transvaginal cholecys-

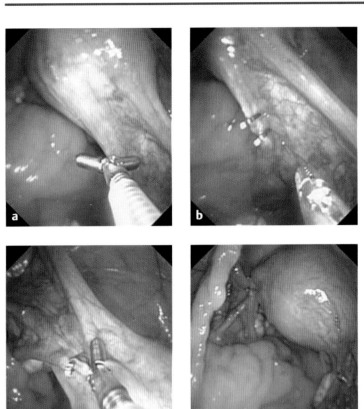

Fig. 23.6 Transgastric tubectomy.
a Clip application on the right fallopian tube.
b Two clips have been applied to the right fallopian tube.
c Clip application on the left fallopian tube.
d Completed tubectomy of both the tubes.

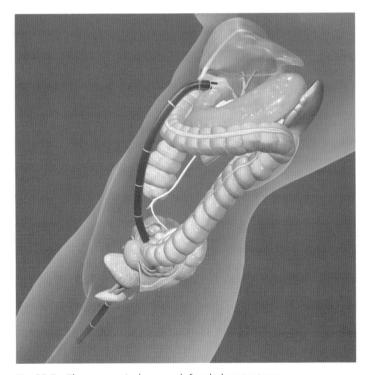

Fig. 23.7 The transvaginal approach for cholecystectomy.

tectomy [67]. Previous experience and the proven relative safety of transvaginal access by gynecologists have made this a natural first operation to perform. The experience gained with this convenient route has also allowed more complex procedures to be carried out.

Recently, Lacy et al. reported the first transvaginal minilaparoscopy-assisted natural orifice radical sigmoidectomy [68].

▦ Other Access Routes

Gettman et al. described a case of transvesical peritoneoscopy before robotic prostatectomy using a flexible ureteroscope [69]. They reported good visualization of all intraperitoneal structures and maintenance of pneumoperitoneum using the ureteroscope alone.

With the exception of a single instance of pelvic abscess drainage, the transcolonic/rectal/anal route has not yet been implemented in humans [70]. This approach requires preoperative bowel cleansing. The incision is sited 50 cm from the anal verge [71] (**Fig. 23.10**). The experience gained with transanal endoscopic microsurgery instrumentation has been transferred to transanal NOTES procedures. As the anorectum is more compliant and capacious than the pharynx or esophagus, it may allow passage of larger-diameter instruments and retrieval of larger specimens. The potential disadvantages of the transanal route are also significant and include issues of sterility, the risk of inadvertent trauma to adjacent organs during transmural puncture, and the risk of colonic wall shearing [72].

Procedures performed through a single port placed transumbilically, with the umbilicus serving an embryonic natural orifice, have also been described in NOTES [73]. As the scar is buried within the umbilicus, scarless status is achieved.

Transesophageal NOTES in animal models has provided excellent visualization of structures that are difficult to visualize via traditional cervical mediastinoscopy and thoracoscopy [74]. A complete Heller myotomy of the gastroesophageal junction has also been performed with this approach, without complications [75].

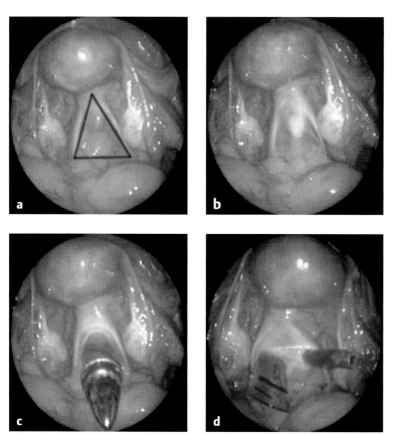

Fig. 23.8   Needlescope images of transvaginal access.
a   The "safe triangle" (marked with a black outline), with boundaries formed by the two uterosacral ligaments.
b   Puncture of the triangle with a trocar.
c   Single-trocar transvaginal access.
d   Two-trocar transvaginal access.

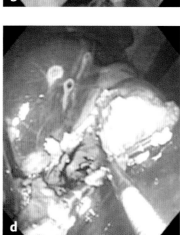

Fig. 23.9   Transvaginal cholecystectomy.
a   Dissection of the Calot triangle.
b   Division of the cystic artery after clipping.
c   Dissection of the cystic duct.
d   Division of the cystic duct.

Benefits and Pitfalls

The lack of a surface incision means that NOTES has a number of potential benefits in comparison with traditional surgical techniques. Apart from the obvious cosmetic advantage of the absence of a visible scar [76], the chance of surgical-site infections and incisional hernias is eliminated. Other advantages of minimally invasive surgery over laparotomy can be extrapolated to NOTES, such as a reduced insult to the immune system and less adhesion formation. Although well-controlled clinical trials are still needed in order to demonstrate these benefits, the data from studies on animals are encouraging [77,78]. By avoiding subcutaneous fatty tissue, NOTES procedures may have an advantage in patients with morbid obesity [79,80]. As the procedure can potentially be performed with minimal anesthesia or with the patient under conscious sedation, the advantages multiply. This may also allow NOTES to be carried out as a bedside procedure, especially in very sick patients for whom transport from the intensive-care unit to the operating room may be detrimental [81]. The transvisceral approach might also allow better access to retroperitoneal structures, sparing the deep dissection required for an open procedure.

As it is a new concept, with techniques and instruments borrowed from other fields, NOTES still has a number of challenges to overcome, foremost among which is the risk of organisms being transferred from the natural orifices into the peritoneal cavity [82]. Periprocedural antibiotics, lavage and disinfection of the site of entry, and the use of sterile overtubes have so far prevented any serious infectious complications in the human procedures that have been carried out [67]. As NOTES involves the use of a flexible scope in a large abdominal cavity, with operating instruments in line with the light source, difficulties associated with poor visibility, maintenance of spatial orientation, maneuverability, and grasping are evident. Effective and safe closure of the viscerotomy is another obstacle to the implementation of NOTES in everyday clinical practice. However, it is expected that technological advances in laparoscopic and endoscopic devices, including user-friendly platforms, safe pneumoperitoneum insufflator devices, and endoscope-friendly anastomotic devices, will lead to further advances in NOTES.

Conclusion

NOTES has attracted increasing interest among surgeons and endoscopists all over the world. The outcomes obtained in the human studies conducted so far indicate that NOTES can in fact be used to perform some intra-abdominal procedures. However, the enthusiasm needs to be tempered by an appreciation that there is still a great deal to do and many hurdles to be overcome before the new technology can enter mainstream practice. Further detailed studies comparing NOTES procedures with existing surgical interventions are required in order to assess the safety and efficacy of this novel approach.

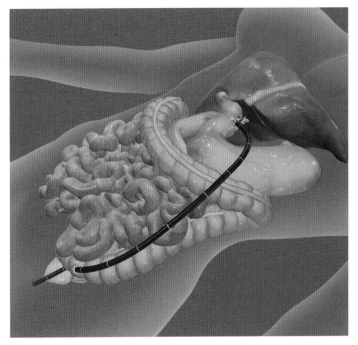

Fig. 23.10 The transcolonic approach for cholecystectomy.

23

Combined Laparoscopic and Endoscopic Interventions and Transcolonic/Transgastric NOTES Procedures

Hubertus Feußner

Introduction

Both flexible therapeutic endoscopy and laparoscopic surgery have specific limitations. Large, broad-based lesions and lesions located behind folds or sharp bends may be associated with increased risk if they are removed using flexible endoscopy, and complete removal of such lesions may be impossible. The limitations of flexible endoscopy are difficult to define, of course, as they partly depend on the endoscopist's level of experience and the aggressiveness of the treatment, but it can be assumed that some 5 % of gastric and colonic lesions are not suitable for endoscopic resection.

On the other hand, it may be difficult for a surgeon maneuvering within the peritoneal cavity to assess the precise location of small lesions and to verify the completeness with which the lesion has been excised. In recent years, a combination of intracavitary (laparoscopic) and endoluminal (endoscopic) techniques during the same procedure has therefore become increasingly important as a way of compensating for the shortcomings of each separate technique. This type of combined laparoscopic–endoscopic procedure (LEP) or hybrid (rendezvous) procedure was first introduced in the early 1990s [83,84]. More recently, a combination of flexible endoscopy with laparoscopic support has been further encouraged by efforts to develop what is known as "scarless surgery" in clinical practice.

Originally, natural orifice transluminal endoscopic surgery (NOTES) was conceived as an intervention performed with flexible endoscopes alone. However, it soon became evident that this type of "pure NOTES" is not yet ready for clinical application. Hybrid procedures have therefore been advocated, in which the endoscopist

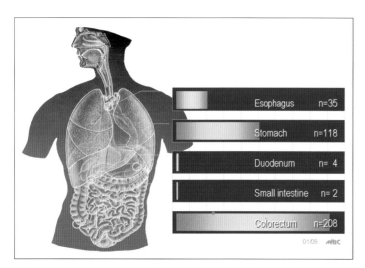

Fig. 23.11   The distribution of 367 combined laparoscopic–endoscopic procedures.

Table 23.1   Indications for combined laparoscopic–endoscopic procedures in early gastric cancer

T1 tumor (mucosal), well differentiated, with no vascular or lymphatic invasion [86]

Parts of stomach inaccessible to endoscopic mucosal resection (e. g., fundus, posterior body, cardia)
   Elevated less than 2.5 cm
   Depressed less than 1.5 cm (not ulcerated)

Any part of the stomach
   Elevated 2.5–4.5 cm
   Depressed 1.5–2.5 cm (not ulcerated)

performing the NOTES procedure is assisted by a (small-bore) laparoscope and transabdominal instruments.

Indications

LEP can be used for lesions in which local excision is adequate but cannot be achieved using peroral or transanal flexible endoscopy, due to the lesion's size and location. Another indication for LEP is lesions requiring local full-thickness resection of the gastrointestinal wall (**Fig. 23.11**).

Esophagus. LEP mainly focuses on intramural lesions such as benign leiomyomas, lipomas, and neurinomas. In contrast to other parts of the gastrointestinal tract, LEP is very rarely suitable for endoluminal lesions.

Stomach. In the stomach, lesions that are suitable for LEP are gastric wall tumors such as benign gastric stromal tumors (leiomyomas) [85] and carcinoids, epithelial growths such as adenomas, and early gastric cancer (**Table 23.1**) [86]. Bleeding gastric lesions such as ulcers, Mallory–Weiss tears, and Dieulafoy lesions can be treated by intragastric laparoscopy if peroral endoscopy does not achieve control of bleeding [87,88].

Duodenum. Symptomatic duodenal diverticula, duodenal carcinoid tumors, and adenomas may be indications for LEP.

Colon. Indications for LEP in the colon are similar to those in the stomach—in particular, adenomas, early cancers with invasion no

deeper than the mucosa and superficial layer of the submucosa (sm1), and benign submucosal lesions [89].

Contraindications

Lesions with a malignant appearance and a high probability of advanced disease should not be considered for local excision using LEP. Conventional or laparoscopic surgical resection should be performed in these cases.

LEP is contraindicated in patients who are unfit to undergo anesthesia and in those with clotting disorders.

General Principles

The respective contributions of the endoscopist and laparoscopist to LEP depend on the lesion being treated. Either the endoscopist or the laparoscopist may take the leading role.

In laparoscopy-assisted endoscopy, the endoscopist resecting the lesion is assisted by the laparoscopist, who helps expose the site and is easily able to close a transmural defect inadvertently caused by the endoscopist's intervention. Vice versa, in endoscopy-assisted laparoscopy, the laparoscopist resecting the lesion is supported by the intraluminal endoscopist.

Positioning, anesthesia, and equipment. Simultaneous performance of laparoscopy and endoscopy is more demanding than doing either of these procedures alone. When LEP is carried out in an operating room, the endoscopist will not be working in familiar conditions. The patient may be placed in a different position, and access to the patient may be impaired by drapes and the intubation tube. The endoscopist may not be assisted by an experienced endoscopic assistant, but instead by surgical personnel. Conversely, the surgical team have to accept more limited access to the patient. Fortunately, what are known as "integrated operating room systems" are available today which alleviate the technical restrictions of LEP.

LEPs are carried out with the patient under general anesthesia. The patient is placed in a supine position. For colonoscopy, the endoscopist sits between the patient's abducted legs (lithotomy position). The monitor for the video colonoscope is placed on the patient's right side (**Fig. 23.12**). The positions of the laparoscopist, endoscopist, assistants, and equipment depend on the site of the lesion to be treated. For treatment of lesions in the right colon, the laparoscopist's position is on the patient's left side, and the monitor is placed on the right side. For left-sided lesions, the position is vice versa. For LEP in the upper abdomen (stomach, duodenum), the endoscopist is positioned at the patient's head. The surgeon stands on the right side of the table (**Fig. 23.13**).

General Technical Aspects

Establishing the pneumoperitoneum and placing the trocars should be carried out before the flexible endoscope is inserted; distension of the hollow visceral organs caused by the insufflation necessary for flexible endoscopy enhances the risks related to the placement of the Veress needle and trocars.

Colonoscopy in patients who have been prepared for surgery is more difficult than conventional colonoscopy. Maneuvers such as external fixation and changing the patient's position are not feasible. As a substitute for external compression, the surgeon can carry out adequate intracavitary maneuvers using blunt instruments. When the colonoscopist has reached a proximally located lesion, the endoscope should be straightened to eliminate loops impairing

IV

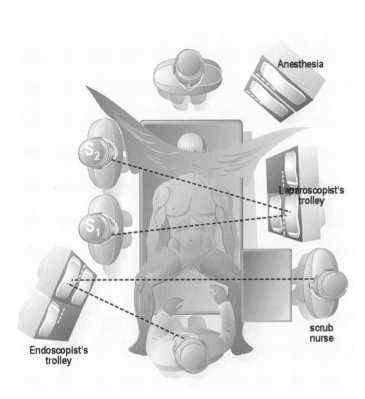

Fig. 23.12 Positioning of the equipment and of the operating-room team for colonic interventions.

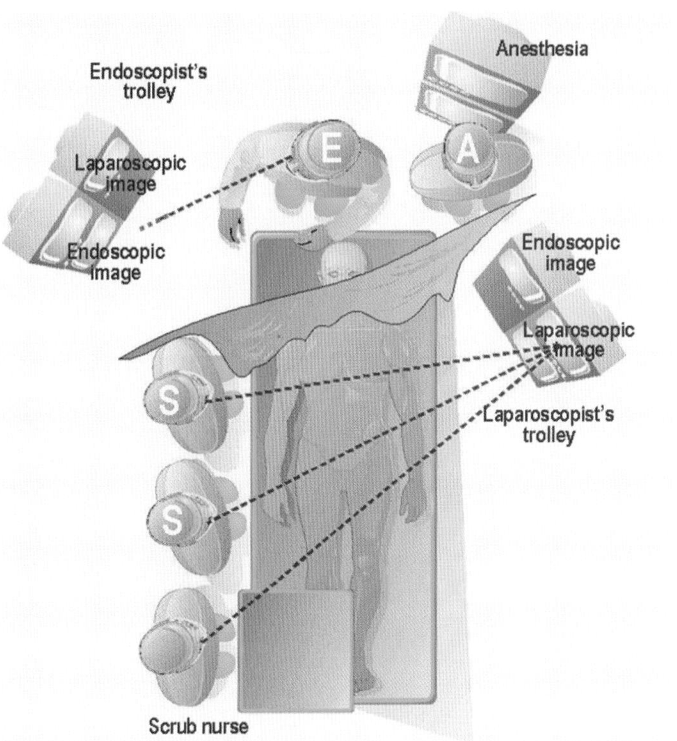

Fig. 23.13 Positioning of the equipment and of the operating-room team for upper abdominal surgery.

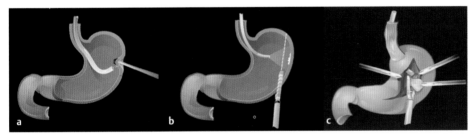

Fig. 23.14 Three different variants of laparoscopic–endoscopic procedures.
a Laparoscopy-assisted endoscopic resection.
b Endoscopy-assisted laparoscopic wedge resection.
c Endoscopy-assisted laparoscopic transluminal (transgastric/transcolonic) resection.

the laparoscopist's vision. After a lesion has been removed and the resulting defect has been closed, the site is checked for leakage by instilling methylene blue.

LEP Variants

Different forms of LEP can be used, depending on the type and location of the lesion to be treated. The principles of the various LEP modalities are similar, independently of whether they are used for lesions in the upper or lower gastrointestinal tract (**Fig. 23.14**).

Laparoscopy-assisted endoscopic resection. This technique is the least invasive variant of LEP. It is used if a lesion is in principle accessible to intraluminal (flexible) endoscopy, but cannot be completely visualized or would involve a substantial risk of perforation if removed endoscopically.

Under endoscopic intraluminal vision, the gastrointestinal segment in which the lesion is located is manipulated laparoscopically from outside in order to achieve better exposure of the lesion and its surroundings, facilitating complete endoscopic removal. In case of perforation or imminent perforation, the gastrointestinal wall can easily be reinforced by means of laparoscopic sutures, or by applying a linear stapler.

Endoscopy-assisted laparoscopic wedge resection. Laparoscopic wedge resection can be used for lesions that are accessible to the linear stapling device. An essential prerequisite for adequate resection is precise localization of the lesion, which is achieved by intraluminal flexible endoscopy. In segments in which stenoses may result after partial removal of the wall, the endoscope protects the lumen during wedge resection. For this purpose, the endoscope is advanced beyond the resection area. In resections in the cecal region, the endoscope has to be passed into the terminal ileum.

Endoscopy-assisted transluminal (transgastric/transcolonic) resection. Lesions located on the posterior wall of the stomach can be removed via a gastrotomy in the anterior wall. The gastroscope is inserted perorally, and the lesion is visualized. The anterior gastric wall is lifted up by means of two stay sutures passed through the seromuscular layer. A gastrotomy is made using cutting diathermy, providing direct access to the lesion. The lesion is grasped with grasping forceps and pulled through the gastrotomy. Delivery of the tumor everts the posterior gastric wall, forming a pedicle of normal gastric tissue. Sequential application of the laparoscopic linear stapler at the pedicle of the lesion transects and staples the posterior gastric wall [85]. After removal of the specimen, the gastrotomy is closed with single stitches or with the linear stapler.

When colonic lesions are not accessible to wedge resection because they are located near the mesenteric side of the colon, a small colostomy to reach the lesion is made laparoscopically. For this purpose, the exact position of the lesion has to be indicated by the operator of the flexible endoscope. The lesion is removed as described above for lesions in the posterior gastric wall.

▦ Results of Laparoscopic–Endoscopic Procedures

Esophagus. Submucosal tumors in the esophagus (gastrointestinal stromal tumors) are not rare. Usu ally, these tumors are resected using an open transthoracic approach. Several reports, as well as our own experience [89–91], have clearly demonstrated that thoracoscopic removal is feasible in most cases. Postoperative pain and morbidity and the overall hospitalization period can be markedly reduced.

However, precise intraoperative localization of the tumor site may be difficult due to the extraesophageal position of the thoracoscope. Simultaneous endoscopy is able to unequivocally demonstrate the position of the lesion with endoscopic diaphanoscopy. Endoscopy also helps avoid mucosal damage through careful intraluminal inspection.

The operation is usually performed through the right thoracic cavity. One-lung ventilation is helpful to create the appropriate space. Three to four trocars are required. The position of the tumor is precisely demonstrated endoscopically, facilitating mobilization of the appropriate segment by transillumination.

The muscular layer is split, and the submucosal tumor is gradually developed by blunt and sharp dissection while the endoscopist monitors the integrity of the mucosa. After removal of the tumor lesion, the muscular layer is closed with single stitches. The intraluminal endoscopist may instill methylene blue to confirm that no leakage is present. A chest tube is inserted for 2–3 days. Oral nutrition can be started after 2–3 days.

The difference in the postoperative recovery is striking, as in this type of operation, postoperative complaints and morbidity are mainly caused by the thoracic incision [92]. In our own series, the hospital stay was reduced from 11 to 7 days [90].

Stomach. Combined laparoscopic–endoscopic procedures may have a place here in between purely endoscopic (e. g., endoscopic mucosal resection) and genuinely open surgical approaches (partial, subtotal, or total gastric resection). In the case of benign lesions, invasiveness should be minimal. Accordingly, endoscopic procedures are always preferable. In malignant cases, a compromise between invasiveness and the required radicality has to be found. Again, three different approaches are conceivable.

Laparoscopy-assisted endoscopic resection. Lesions on the borderline between a need for endoscopic resection and more aggressive full-thickness resection can be treated by means of laparoscopy-assisted endoscopic resection. Under endoscopic guidance, the tumor site is protruded into the gastric lumen by means of a pushing rod under laparoscopic vision. This provides very good exposure of the lesion and its surroundings, making it easier to apply the snare and excise the lesion in total, including safe margins. If there is perforation or imminent perforation at the site, the gastric wall can easily be reinforced by means of laparoscopic sutures or by applying a linear stapler.

Endoscopy-assisted laparoscopic wedge resection. Laparoscopic wedge resection is easy and safe provided that the tumor is located in an area suitable for tangential resection. Lesions in the anterior gastric wall and on the greater curvature are ideally suited for wedge resection. An essential precondition for this, however, is very precise localization of the tumor, which can only be achieved by means of intraoperative endoscopy. The center of the lesion is elevated by the endoscopist using grasping forceps. The laparoscopist applies oral and caudal stay sutures. The relevant area of the gastric wall is now elevated and the linear stapler is applied. Finally, the endoscopist is able to check the closure of the gastric wall by insufflating air or instilling methylene blue.

Laparoscopic transgastric resection. If the lesion is located on the posterior wall of the stomach, wedge resection may be technically difficult. In these cases, it is easier to perform a gastrotomy on the anterior wall (between stay sutures and to remove the tumor transgastrically). In these cases, too, it is extremely helpful to use the endoscope to locate the lesion. This makes it easier to carry out the gastrotomy at an appropriate site. After removal of the specimen, the gastrotomy is closed again by means of single stitches or with the linear stapler.

It has been demonstrated that these three different procedures allow minimally invasive treatment for almost all submucosal gastric lesions [93], and this has been confirmed in several similar studies (**Table 23.2**) [94–101].

Duodenum. Minimally invasive treatment of duodenal lesions is a particular challenge. Infrequently, they are not accessible for the endoscopist. On the other hand, the laparoscopic approach is sometimes difficult because of the partial retroperitoneal position of the duodenum. However, by combining the endoscopic approach with a laparoscopic operation, a considerable number of lesions may be treatable without the need for laparotomy.

A prerequisite for this is that the duodenum, including the pancreatic head, is first mobilized with a laparoscope (Kocher maneuver). The lesion should then be localized precisely using the endoscope, and the distance to the papilla has to be defined exactly. The resection can now be performed in the same way as described above

Table 23.2 Recent studies on combined laparoscopic–endoscopic resection of submucosal lesions in the stomach

First author [ref.]	Year	Patients (n)	Mean age (y)	Operating time (min)	Hospitalization (days)	Conversion (%)	Complications (%)
Choi [94]	2000	32	51.4	80–180	6	3.1	6.2
Shimizu [95]	2002	11	64.2	145	13.2	0	0
Ludwig [96]	2003	44	65.3	58.4	6.6Z	4.5	13.6
Bouillot [97]	2003	65	56.7	104	6.5	16.9	3.7
Hindmarsh [98]	2005	30	64.2	73.8	5	23.3	3.3
Schubert [99]	2005	26	67.2	53–83	5.6	11.5	7.7
Mochizuki [100]	2006	12	60	100	7	0	16.7
Novitsky [101]	2006	50	60	135	3.8	0	(8)
Present series	2007	93	58	90	7.4	6.5	7.5

IV

in the stomach. After successful removal of the lesion, the endoscopist finally has to check the width of the lumen (ensuring there is no stenosis) and should confirm that there is no alteration in the papilla.

However, locally resectable lesions are rare and the majority of them are removed using flexible endoscopy. Practical experience with LEP in the duodenum is therefore limited, although a number of case reports and our own experience confirm that LEP is feasible and safe.

Colorectum. The majority of LEP series are performed in the colorectum. Colonic lesions, again, can be removed endoscopically with laparoscopic support, or using laparoscopic wedge or transluminal resection with endoluminal endoscopic assistance. Precise localization of the lesion is a major issue. Attempts have been made to mark lesions by applying metal clips or by injecting dye solutions [102–105]. Problems reported with these methods include inaccurate localization, dislodgment of clips, and serious complications including peritonitis and phlegmonous gastritis [106–108]. Combined procedures are therefore coming into increasingly widespread use throughout the world [109]. In our own experience [110], combined laparoscopic–endoscopic resection is an efficient, safe and minimally invasive alternative to open or laparoscopic resection for selected patients with difficult polyps, but it should be restricted to benign disease.

Laparoscopic–Endoscopic Procedures as "Pseudo-NOTES"

Most "scarless" procedures have so far involved transvaginal cholecystectomy. Rigid instruments are used, and the procedure is facilitated by combination with a transumbilical approach [65]. However, transgastric and transrectal approaches using flexible endoscopes have also been attempted. With laparoscopic visualization, the abdomen can be entered safely with the endoscope. Manipulations carried out by the endoscopist can be monitored by the laparoscopist, who can also check the closure of the gastrointestinal incision as soon as the operation is finished. This does not yet represent a "pure" NOTES procedure, but it is a safe and feasible intermediate step until NOTES advances sufficiently for it to enter the clinical routine.

References

1. Kalloo AN, Kantsevoy SV, Singh VK, et al. Flexible transgastric peritoneoscopy: a novel approach to diagnostic and therapeutic interventions in the peritoneal cavity [abstract]. Gastroenterology 2000;118:A1039.
2. Kalloo AN, Singh VK, Jagannath SB, Niiyama H, Hill SL, Vaughn CA, et al. Flexible transgastric peritoneoscopy: a novel approach to diagnostic and therapeutic interventions in the peritoneal cavity. Gastrointest Endosc 2004;60:114–7.
3. Strasberg SM. Clinical practice. Acute calculous cholecystitis. N Engl J Med 2008;358:2804–11.
4. Reynolds W Jr. The first laparoscopic cholecystectomy. JSLS 2001;5: 89–94.
5. Keus F, de Jong JA, Gooszen HG, van Laarhoven CJ. Laparoscopic versus open cholecystectomy for patients with symptomatic cholecystolithiasis. Cochrane Database Syst Rev 2006;(4):CD006231.
6. Konikoff FM. Gallstones—approach to medical management. MedGenMed 2003;5:8.
7. Frimberger E. Operative laparoscopy: cholecystotomy. Endoscopy 1989;21(Suppl 1):367–72.
8. Frimberger E, Kühner W, Klann H. Schwenkarm-Laparoskop: ein neues Instrument zur Inspektion von Organunterflächen und zur Kompression von Punktionsstellen bei der Laparoskopie. In: Henning H, editor. Fortschritte der gastroenterologischen Endoskopie, vol. 13. Gräfelfing [Germany]: Demeter; 1983. p.26–8.
9. Frimberger E. Laparoscopic cholecystotomy. Baillière's Best Pract Res Clin Gastroenterol 1999;13:199–205.
10. Strasberg SM, Hertl M, Soper NJ. An analysis of the problem of biliary injury during laparoscopic cholecystectomy. J Am Coll Surg 1995;180: 101–25.
11. Clavien PA, Sanabria JR, Strasberg SM. Proposed classification of complications of surgery with examples of utility in cholecystectomy. Surgery 1992;111:518–26.
12. Jüngst D, del Pozo R, Dolu MH, Schneeweiss SG, Frimberger E. Rapid formation of cholesterol crystals in gallbladder bile is associated with stone recurrence after laparoscopic cholecystotomy. Hepatology 1997; 25:509–13.
13. Lanzini A, Jazrawi RP, Kupfer RM, Maudgal DP, Joseph AE, Northfield TC. Gallstone recurrence after medical dissolution. An overestimated threat? J Hepatol 1986;3:241–6.
14. Cesmeli E, Elewaut AE, Kerre T, De Buyzere M, Afschrift M, Elewaut A. Gallstone recurrence after successful shock wave therapy: the magnitude of the problem and the predictive factors. Am J Gastroenterol 1999;94: 474–9.
15. Villanova N, Bazzoli F, Taroni F, Frabboni R, Mazzella G, Festi D, et al. Gallstone recurrence after successful oral bile acid treatment. A 12-year follow-up study and evaluation of long-term postdissolution treatment. Gastroenterology 1989;97:726–31.
16. Sackmann M, Niller H, Klueppelberg U, von Ritter C, Pauletzki J, Holl J, et al. Gallstone recurrence after shock-wave therapy. Gastroenterology 1994;106:225–30.
17. Pauletzki J, Althaus R, Holl J, Sackmann M, Paumgartner G. Gallbladder emptying and gallstone formation: a prospective study on gallstone recurrence. Gastroenterology 1996;111:765–71.
18. Berr F, Mayer M, Sackmann MF, Sauerbruch T, Holl J, Paumgartner G. Pathogenic factors in early recurrence of cholesterol gallstones. Gastroenterology 1994;106:215–24.
19. Portincasa P, van Erpecum KJ, van De Meeberg PC, Dallinga-Thie GM, de Bruin TW, van Berge-Henegouwen GP. Apolipoprotein E4 genotype and gallbladder motility influence speed of gallstone clearance and risk of recurrence after extracorporeal shock-wave lithotripsy. Hepatology 1996;24:580–7.
20. O'Leary DP, Johnson AG. Future directions for conservative treatment of gallbladder calculi. Br J Surg 1993;80:143–7.
21. Gilat T, Konikoff FM. Pregnancy and the biliary tract. Can J Gastroenterol 2000;14:55–9.
22. Verbanck JJ, Demol JW, Ghillebert GL, Rutgeerts LJ, Surmont IP. Ultrasound-guided puncture of the gallbladder for acute cholecystitis. Lancet 1993;341:1132–3.
23. Leveau P, Andersson E, Carlgren I, Willner J, Andersson R. Percutaneous cholecystostomy: a bridge to surgery or definite management of acute cholecystitis in high-risk patients? Scand J Gastroenterol 2008;43:593–6.
24. Silberfein EJ, Zhou W, Kougias P, El Sayed HF, Huynh TT, Albo D, et al. Percutaneous cholecystostomy for acute cholecystitis in high-risk patients: experience of a surgeon-initiated interventional program. Am J Surg 2007;194:672–7.
25. McGahan JP, Lindfors KK. Percutaneous cholecystostomy: an alternative to surgical cholecystostomy for acute cholecystitis? Radiology 1989;173: 481–5.
26. Hatzidakis AA, Prassopoulos P, Petinarakis I, Sanidas E, Chrysos E, Chalkiadakis G, et al. Acute cholecystitis in high-risk patients: percutaneous cholecystostomy vs conservative treatment. Eur Radiol 2002;12: 1778–84.
27. Tamada K, Seki H, Sato K, Kano T, Sugiyama S, Ichiyama M, et al. Efficacy of endoscopic retrograde cholecystoendoprosthesis (ERCCE) for cholecystitis. Endoscopy 1991;23:2–3.
28. Johlin FC Jr, Neil GA. Drainage of the gallbladder in patients with acute acalculous cholecystitis by transpapillary endoscopic cholecystostomy. Gastrointest Endosc 1993;39:645–51.
29. Feretis C, Apostolidis N, Mallas E, Manouras A, Papadimitriou J. Endoscopic drainage of acute obstructive cholecystitis in patients with increased operative risk. Endoscopy 1993;25:392–5.
30. Baron TH, Farnell MB, LeRoy J. Endoscopic transpapillary gallbladder drainage for closure of calculous gallbladder perforation and cholecystoduodenal fistula. Gastrointest Endosc 2002;56:753–5.
31. Nakatsu T, Okada H, Saito O. Endoscopic transpapillary gallbladder drainage (ETGBD) for the treatment of acute cholecystitis. J Hepatobiliary Pancreat Surg 1997;4:31–5.
32. Kjaer DW, Kruse A, Funch-Jensen P. Endoscopic gallbladder drainage of patients with acute cholecystitis. Endoscopy 2007;39:304–8.

23

33. Itoi T, Sofuni A, Itokawa F, Tsuchiya T, Kurihara T, Ishii K, et al. Endoscopic transpapillary gallbladder drainage in patients with acute cholecystitis in whom percutaneous transhepatic approach is contraindicated or anatomically impossible (with video). Gastrointest Endosc 2008;68:455–60.

34. Kwan V, Eisendrath P, Antaki F, Le Moine O, Devière J. EUS-guided cholecystenterostomy: a new technique (with videos). Gastrointest Endosc 2007;66:582–6.

35. Lee SS, Park do H, Hwang CY, Ahn CS, Lee TY, Seo DW, et al. EUS-guided transmural cholecystostomy as rescue management for acute cholecystitis in elderly or high-risk patients: a prospective feasibility study. Gastrointest Endosc 2007;66:1008–12.

36. Rao GV, Reddy DN, Banerjee R. NOTES: human experience. Gastrointest Endosc Clin N Am 2008;18:361–70; x.

37. ASGE; SAGES. ASGE/SAGES Working Group on Natural Orifice Transluminal Endoscopic Surgery white paper, October 2005. Gastrointest Endosc 2006;63:199–203.

38. Giday SA, Kantsevoy SV, Kalloo AN. Principle and history of natural orifice transluminal endoscopic surgery (NOTES). Minim Invasive Ther Allied Technol 2006;15:373–7.

39. Al-Akash M, Boyle E, Tanner WA. N.O.T.E.S.: The progression of a novel and emerging technique. Surg Oncol 2009;18:95–103.

40. Sumiyama K, Gostout C. Techniques for transgastric access to the peritoneal cavity. Gastrointest Endosc Clin N Am 2008;18:235–44; vii.

41. Narula VK, Happel LC, Volt K, Bergman S, Roland JC, Dettorre R, et al. Transgastric endoscopic peritoneoscopy does not require decontamination of the stomach in humans. Surg Endosc 2009;23:1331–6.

42. Hondo FY, Giordano-Nappi JH, Maluf-Filho F, Matuguma SE, Sakai P, Poggetti R, et al. Transgastric access by balloon overtube for intraperitoneal surgery. Surg Endosc 2007;21:1867–9.

43. Rao GV, Sriram PV, Santosh D. Endoscopic transgastric peritoneoscopy as a potential alternative to laparoscopy [abstract]. Gastrointest Endosc 2003;57:AB396.

44. Ko CW, Shin EJ, Buscaglia JM, Clarke JO, Magno P, Giday SA, et al. Preliminary pneumoperitoneum facilitates transgastric access into the peritoneal cavity for natural orifice transluminal endoscopic surgery: a pilot study in a live porcine model. Endoscopy 2007;39:849–53.

45. McGee MF, Rosen MJ, Marks J, Chak A, Onders R, Faulx A, et al. A reliable method for monitoring intraabdominal pressure during natural orifice transluminal endoscopic surgery. Surg Endosc 2007;21:672–6.

46. Sumiyama K, Gostout CJ, Rajan E, Bakken TA, Knipschield MA, Chung S, et al. Transgastric cholecystectomy: transgastric accessibility to the gallbladder improved with the SEMF method and a novel multibending therapeutic endoscope. Gastrointest Endosc 2007;65:1028–34.

47. Sumiyama K, Gostout CJ, Rajan E, Bakken TA, Knipschield MA, Marler RJ. Submucosal endoscopy with mucosal flap safety valve. Gastrointest Endosc 2007;65:688–94.

48. Reddy DN, Rao GV. Transgastric approach to the peritoneal cavity: are we on the right tract? Gastrointest Endosc 2007;65:501–2.

49. Stadlhuber RJ, Yano F, Mittal SK, Hunt B, Filipi CJ. Anatomy of NOTES gastrotomy in human tissue. Surg Innov 2008;15:253–9.

50. Merrifield B, Wagh M, Thompson C. Peroral transgastric organ resection in the abdomen: a feasibility study in pigs. Gastrointest Endosc 2006;63:693–7.

51. Jagannath SB, Kantsevoy SV, Vaughn CA, Chung SS, Cotton PB, Gostout CJ, et al. Peroral transgastric endoscopic ligation of fallopian tubes with long-term survival in a porcine model. Gastrointest Endosc 2005;61:449–53.

52. McGee MF, Marks JM, Onders RP, Chak A, Jin J, Williams CP, et al. Complete endoscopic closure of gastrotomy after natural orifice transluminal endoscopic surgery using the NDO Plicator. Surg Endosc 2008;22:214–20.

53. McGee MF, Marks JM, Jin J, Williams C, Chak A, Schomisch SJ, et al. Complete endoscopic closure of gastric defects using a full-thickness tissue plicating device. J Gastrointest Surg 2008;12:38–45.

54. Meireles OR, Kantsevoy SV, Assumpcao LR, Magno P, Dray X, Giday SA, et al. Reliable gastric closure after natural orifice transluminal endoscopic surgery (NOTES) using a novel automated flexible stapling device. Surg Endosc 2008;22:1609–13.

55. Dray X, Gabrielson KL, Buscaglia JM, Shin EJ, Giday SA, Surti VC, et al. Air and fluid leak tests after NOTES procedures: a pilot study in a live porcine model. Gastrointest Endosc 2008;68:513–9.

56. Mintz Y, Horgan S, Cullen J, Ramamoorthy S, Chock A, Savu MK, et al. NOTES: the hybrid technique. J Laparoendosc Adv Surg Tech A 2007;17:402–6.

57. Pearl JP, Marks JM, Ponsky JL. Hybrid surgery: combined laparoscopy and natural orifice surgery. Gastrointest Endosc Clin N Am 2008;18:325–32; ix.

58. Palanivelu C, Rajan PS, Rangarajan M, Parthasarathi R, Senthilnathan P, Praveenraj P. Transumbilical flexible endoscopic cholecystectomy in humans: first feasibility study using a hybrid technique. Endoscopy 2008;40:428–31.

59. Branco AW, Branco Filho AJ, Kondo W, Noda RW, Kawahara N, Camargo AA, et al. Hybrid transvaginal nephrectomy. Eur Urol 2008;53:1290–4.

60. Franklin ME Jr, Kelley H, Kelley M, Brestan L, Portillo G, Torres J. Transvaginal extraction of the specimen after total laparoscopic right hemicolectomy with intracorporeal anastomosis. Surg Laparosc Endosc Percutan Tech 2008;18:294–8.

61. Mintz Y, Horgan S, Cullen J, Falor E, Talamini MA. Dual-lumen natural orifice transluminal endoscopic surgery (NOTES): a new method for performing a safe anastomosis. Surg Endosc 2008;22:348–51.

62. Auyang ED, Vaziri K, Volckmann E, Martin JA, Soper NJ, Hungness ES. NOTES: cadaveric rendezvous hybrid small bowel resection. Surg Endosc 2008;22:2277–8.

63. Branco Filho AJ, Noda RW, Kondo W, Kawahara N, Rangel M, Branco AW. Initial experience with hybrid transvaginal cholecystectomy. Gastrointest Endosc 2007;66:1245–8.

64. Thele F, Zygmunt M, Glitsch A, Heidecke CD, Schreiber A. How do gynecologists feel about transvaginal NOTES surgery? Endoscopy 2008;40:576–80.

65. Zornig C, Mofid H, Emmermann A, Alm M, von Waldenfels HA, Felixmüller C. Scarless cholecystectomy with combined transvaginal and transumbilical approach in a series of 20 patients. Surg Endosc 2008;22:1427–9.

66. Harlaar JJ, Kleinrensink GJ, Hop WC, Stark M, Schneider AJ. The anatomical limits of the posterior vaginal vault toward its use as route for intra-abdominal procedures. Surg Endosc 2008;22:1910–2.

67. Sodergren MH, Clark J, Athanasiou T, Teare J, Yang GZ, Darzi A. Natural orifice transluminal endoscopic surgery: critical appraisal of applications in clinical practice. Surg Endosc 2009;23:680–7.

68. Lacy AM, Delgado S, Rojas OA, Almenara R, Blasi A, Llach J. MA-NOS radical sigmoidectomy: report of a transvaginal resection in the human. Surg Endosc 2008;22:1717–23.

69. Gettman MT, Blute ML. Transvesical peritoneoscopy: initial clinical evaluation of the bladder as a portal for natural orifice transluminal endoscopic surgery. Mayo Clin Proc 2007;82:843–5.

70. Abbas MA, Falls G. Transanal endoscopic drainage of abdominopelvic sepsis. JSLS 2008;12:347–50.

71. Ryou M, Thompson C. Techniques for transanal access to the peritoneal cavity. Gastrointest Endosc Clin N Am 2008;18:245–60.

72. Whiteford MH, Spaun GO. A colorectal surgeon's viewpoint on natural orifice transluminal endoscopic surgery. Minerva Chir 2008;63:385–8.

73. Zhu JF, Hu H, Ma YZ, Xu MZ, Li F. Transumbilical endoscopic surgery: a preliminary clinical report. Surg Endosc 2009;23:813–7.

74. Gee DW, Willingham FF, Lauwers GY, Brugge WR, Rattner DW. Natural orifice transesophageal mediastinoscopy and thoracoscopy: a survival series in swine. Surg Endosc 2008;22:2117–22.

75. Pauli EM, Mathew A, Haluck RS, Ionescu AM, Moyer MT, Shope TR, et al. Technique for transesophageal endoscopic cardiomyotomy (Heller myotomy): video presentation at the Society of American Gastrointestinal and Endoscopic Surgeons (SAGES) 2008, Philadelphia, PA. Surg Endosc 2008;22:2279–80.

76. Hagen ME, Wagner OJ, Christen D, Morel P. Cosmetic issues of abdominal surgery: results of an enquiry into possible grounds for a natural orifice transluminal endoscopic surgery (NOTES) approach. Endoscopy 2008;40:581–3.

77. Pham BV, Morgan K, Romagnuolo J, Glenn J, Bazaz S, Lawrence C, et al. Pilot comparison of adhesion formation following colonic perforation and repair in a pig model using a transgastric, laparoscopic, or open surgical technique. Endoscopy 2008;40:664–9.

78. Fong D, Pai R, Thompson C. Transcolonic endoscopic abdominal exploration: a NOTES survival study in a porcine model. Gastrointest Endosc 2007;65:312–8.

79. Fuchs KH, Breithaupt W. [Natural orifice transluminal endoscopic surgery in future obesity treatment]. Chirurg 2008;79:837–42. German.

80. Ramos AC, Zundel N, Neto MG, Maalouf M. Human hybrid NOTES transvaginal sleeve gastrectomy: initial experience. Surg Obes Relat Dis 2008;4:660–3.

81. Onders RP, McGee MF, Marks J, Chak A, Rosen MJ, Ignagni A, et al. Natural orifice transluminal endoscopic surgery (NOTES) as a diagnostic tool in the intensive care unit. Surg Endosc 2007;21:681–3.

82. Kantsevoy S. Infection prevention in NOTES. Gastrointest Endosc Clin N Am 2008;18:291–6.

IV

83. Ohgami M, Otani Y, Kubota T, Kumai K, Kitajima M. [Laparoscopic curative surgery for early gastric cancer]. Nippon Rinsho 1996;54:1307–11. Japanese.

84. Ohashi S. Laparoscopic intraluminal (intragastric) surgery for early gastric cancer: a new concept in laparoscopic surgery. Surg Endosc 1995;9:169–71.

85. Hepworth CC, Menzies D, Motson RW. Minimally invasive surgery for posterior gastric stromal tumors. Surg Endosc 2000;14:349–53.

86. Mittal SK, Filipi CJ. Indications for endo-organ gastric excision. Surg Endosc 2000;14:318–25.

87. Hannon JK, Snow LL, Weinstein LS, Lane DR. Balloon-tipped cannulas for use in laparoscopic diagnosis and treatment of acute upper GI bleeding. Surg Endosc 2000;14:123–6.

88. Lee LS, Singhal S, Brinster CJ, Marshall B, Kochman ML, Kaiser LR, et al. Current management of esophageal leiomyoma. J Am Coll Surg 2004;198:136–46.

89. von Rahden BHA, Stein HJ, Feussner H, Siewert JR. Enucleation of submucosal tumors of the esophagus. Surg Endosc 2004;18:924–30.

90. Vallböhmer D, Hölscher AH, Brabender J, Bollschweiler E, Gutschow C. Thoracoscopic enucleation of esophageal leiomyomas: a feasible and safe procedure. Endoscopy 2007;39:1097–9.

91. Palanivelu C, Rangarajan M, Madankumar MV, John SJ, Senthilkumar R. Minimally invasive therapy for benign tumors of the distal third of the esophagus—a single institute's experience. J Laparoendosc Adv Surg Tech A 2008;18:20–6.

92. Wilhelm D, von Delius S, Burian M, Schneider A, Frimberger E, Meining A, et al. Simultaneous use of laparoscopy and endoscopy for minimally invasive resection of gastric subepithelial masses—analysis of 93 interventions. World J Surg 2008;32:1021–8.

93. Botoman VA, Pietro M, Thirlby RC. Localization of colonic lesions with endoscopic tattoo. Dis Colon Rectum 1994;37:775–6.

94. Choi YB, Oh ST. Laparoscopy in the management of gastric submucosal tumors. Surg Endosc 2000;14:741–5.

95. Shimizu S, Noshiro H, Nagai E. Laparoscopic wedge resection of gastric submucosal tumors. Dig Surg 2002;19:169–73.

96. Ludwig K, Weiner R, Bernhardt J. [Minimally invasive resections of gastric tumors]. Chirurg 2003;74:632–7. German.

97. Bouillot JL, Bresler L, Fagniez PL, Samama G, Champault G, Parent Y, et al. [Laparoscopic resection of benign submucosal stomach tumors. A report of 65 cases]. Gastroenterol Clin Biol 2003;27(3 Pt 1):272–6. French.

98. Hindmarsh A, Koo B, Lewis MP, Rhodes M. Laparoscopic resection of gastric gastrointestinal stromal tumors. Surg Endosc 2005;19:1109–12.

99. Schubert D, Kuhn R, Nestler G, Kahl S, Ebert MP, Malfertheiner P, et al. Laparoscopic–endoscopic rendezvous resection of upper gastrointestinal tumors. Dig Dis 2005;23:106–12.

100. Mochizuki Y, Kodera Y, Fujiwara M, Ito S, Yamamura Y, Sawaki A, et al. Laparoscopic wedge resection for gastrointestinal stromal tumors of the stomach: initial experience. Surg Today 2006;36:341–7.

101. Novitsky YW, Kercher KW, Sing RF, Heniford BT. Long-term outcomes of laparoscopic resection of gastric gastrointestinal stromal tumors. Ann Surg 2006;243:738–47.

102. Hammond DC, Lane FR, Welk RA. Endoscopic tattooing of the colon: an experimental study. Am Surg 1989;55:457–61.

103. Salamon P, Berner JS, Waye JD. Endoscopic India ink injection: a method for preparation, sterilization, and administration. Gastrointest Endosc 1993;39:803–5.

104. Tabibian N, Michaletz PA, Schwartz JT, Heiser MC, Dixon WB, Smith JL, et al. Use of an endoscopically placed clip can avoid diagnostic errors in colonoscopy. Gastrointest Endosc 1988;34:262–4.

105. Coman E, Brandt LJ, Brenner S, Frank M, Sablay B, Bennett B. Fat necrosis and inflammatory pseudotumor due to endoscopic tattooing of the colon with india ink. Gastrointest Endosc 1991;37:65–8.

106. Hornig D, Kuhn H, Stadelmann O, Botticher R. Phlegmonous gastritis after India ink marking. Endoscopy 1983;15:266–9.

107. Park SI, Genta RS, Romeo DP, Weesner RE. Colonic abscess and focal peritonitis secondary to India ink tattooing of the colon. Gastrointest Endosc 1991;37:68–71.

108. Franklin MR Jr, Leyva-Alvizo A, Abrego-Medina D, Glass JL, Treviño J, Arellano PP, et al. Laparoscopically monitored colonoscopic polypectomy: an established form of endoluminal therapy for colorectal polyps. Surg Endosc 2007;21:1650–3.

109. Wilhelm D, von Delius S, Weber L, Meining A, Schneider A, Friess H, et al. Combined laparoscopic–endoscopic resections of colorectal polyps: 10-year experience and follow-up. Surg Endosc 2009;23:688–93.

110. Saitoh Y, Obara T, Watari J, Nomura M, Taruishi M, Orii Y. Invasion depth diagnosis of depressed type early colorectal cancers by combined use of videoendoscopy and chromoendoscopy. Gastrointest Endosc 1998;48:362–70.

23

24 Liver Biopsy

Andrew K. Burroughs, Marco Senzolo, and Evangelos Cholongitas

Introduction

Modern diagnosis and management of liver diseases began with the widespread application of needle biopsy of the liver, and today still largely depends on the results of liver biopsies. Wider use of liver biopsy did not occur until Menghini reported a quick "one-second" method of taking a needle biopsy of the liver in the late 1950s [1,2]. The low mortality rate (0.01–0.17%) and the relatively low morbidity associated with this procedure have meant that liver biopsy has become widely used [3]. Advances in medical technology, particularly in imaging, together with advances in drug therapy and recently the use of noninvasive tests for fibrosis—both serum tests and transient elastography—have changed diagnostic algorithms and as a consequence have altered the indications for liver biopsy.

Indications

The principal indications for liver biopsy are listed in **Table 24.1**. Prominent among these is the evaluation of otherwise unexplained abnormalities in liver function tests, with or without associated hepatomegaly [3–7]. In chronic viral hepatitis, liver biopsy is useful for assessing those patients who will benefit from treatment, as well as assessing the response to treatment.

The use of percutaneous liver biopsy in the diagnosis of focal liver lesions depends on the clinical picture. In most patients with hepatocellular carcinoma (HCC), ultrasound scanning, spiral computed tomography (CT), and α-fetoprotein concentration allow the diagnosis to be made. Liver biopsy has a documented risk of seeding tumors down the biopsy track [8–10]. Modern imaging techniques can also help define other types of focal hepatic lesion, such as hemangioma and focal nodular hyperplasia. Fine-needle aspiration biopsy may be a safer option if material for histological examination is required in cases of suspected angioma [5].
Other indications for liver biopsy include:

- Evaluation of unexplained fever [7]. For example, in patients with acquired immunodeficiency syndrome (AIDS), liver biopsy is the fastest method of diagnosing viral and mycobacterial liver involvement.
- Diagnosis of drug-induced liver injury.
- Granulomatous liver disease.
- Infiltrative processes such amyloidosis.
- Quantitation of the level of iron in a patient with suspected genetic hemochromatosis, or copper in a patient with Wilson disease, which remain important diagnostic tests in these diseases.

In liver transplantation, liver biopsy is essential for diagnosing acute rejection and assessing disease recurrence. There is a dispute as to whether prophylactic antibiotics are required in liver transplant recipients who have a biliary–enteric anastomosis [11–13], with several centers showing that prophylactic antibiotics are not needed if there is no biliary obstruction [13–15].

The routine use of liver biopsy is being questioned as a result of the use of noninvasive markers for the evaluation of fibrosis. In addition, recent studies have tried to determine optimal standards

24.1 Indications for liver biopsy

- Evaluation of abnormal liver function tests
- Grading and staging of chronic hepatitis
- Identification and staging of alcoholic liver disease
- Recognition of systemic inflammatory or granulomatous disorders
- Evaluation of fever of unknown origin
- Evaluation of the extent and type of drug-induced liver injury
- Identification and diagnosis of space-occupying lesions
- Diagnosis of multisystem infiltrative disorders
- Evaluation of cholestatic liver disease (primary biliary cirrhosis, primary sclerosing cholangitis)
- Diagnosis and follow-up of treatment of heritable disorders (hemochromatosis, Wilson disease)
- After liver transplantation

for the length and number of complete portal tracts (CPTs) for accurate evaluation of grading and staging in patients with chronic viral hepatitis [14,15].

The coagulation profile, presence of ascites, and results of previous imaging techniques dictate the choice of liver biopsy approach—percutaneous, transvenous, or laparoscopic. The needles used can be classified as large—i.e., with an external diameter ≥ 1.0 mm (14–19 G); or thin, with an external diameter of < 1.0 mm (≥ 20 G) [16]. Depending on the technique being used in the procedure, they may be suction needles (Menghini) or cutting needles (Tru-Cut).

Percutaneous Liver Biopsy

Procedure. Percutaneous liver biopsy (PLB) should be performed in a hospital setting by physicians experienced in the technique. According to data obtained from the 1991 British Society of Gastroenterology audit, the frequency of complications was slightly higher if the operator had performed fewer than 20 PLBs, at 3.2%, in comparison with 1.1% if the operator had performed more than 100 biopsies [6]. The experience of operators is also an important factor for the length of liver specimens obtained with PLB. In our own systematic review of reported PLB series [17], the mean length of liver samples in studies with ≥ 100 PLBs was 20.4 mm, compared with 16 mm in those with < 100 PLBs (P = 0.026) Experience was an important factor, particularly with Menghini PLB, since the samples were significantly longer in studies with ≥ 100 PLBs in comparison with those with < 100 PLBs (24 mm vs. 16.1 mm; P = 0.005). Interestingly, ultrasound guidance was also not helpful in enabling less experienced operators to obtain longer specimens [17].

Outpatient biopsies should only be carried out in centers where they are performed routinely and when patients can be observed for at least 6 h, as most of the complications occur during the first few hours after the procedure [18,19]. Before a biopsy is carried out, it is necessary to ensure that there are clearly defined indications for the biopsy, with the risk to the patient not outweighing the potential benefit; and that the risks of the procedure have been explained to the patient.

Ultrasound examination of the liver should have been performed in every patient before liver biopsy and is part of the diagnostic

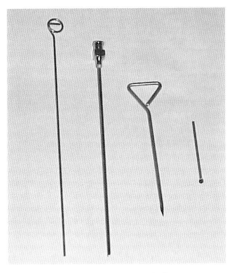

Fig. 24.1 A Menghini disposable biopsy set (1.9 × 110 mm).

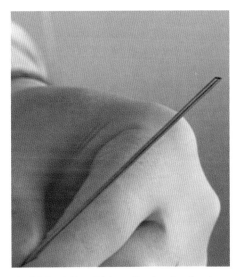

Fig. 24.2 A Menghini needle, showing the sharp bevel tip.

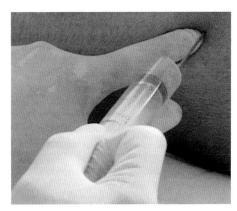

Fig. 24.3 The intercostal space is verified and the instrument is pushed through the skin at the previously chosen site into the subcutaneous tissue to a depth of 4–5 mm. The needle is pushed inward roughly at right angles to the skin surface.

work-up for a patient with liver disease. Information provided by ultrasound helps in selecting the procedure for liver biopsy, and it is essential for recognizing two contraindications to blind liver biopsy—namely, dilation of the intrahepatic bile ducts and the presence of hydatid cysts. The size of the right lobe of the liver, an absence of vascular tumors (hemangiomas), and the position of the gallbladder can also be assessed using ultrasonography. Postbiopsy ultrasound is not necessary and is usually only indicated if complications are suspected [20].

Other requirements are:
- The patient's platelet count and prothrombin time should be checked in the week before the percutaneous liver biopsy, provided the patient's liver disease is stable.
- The patient's blood group should be known.
- Transfusion facilities should be available.
- Hemoglobin should be over 10 g/dL.
- The platelet count should be at least 60 000/mm³.
- Prothrombin time should be prolonged no more than 3 s. The bleeding time should be checked if drugs affecting platelet function have been taken. If vitamin K, 10 mg i. m./day for 2 days, does not improve the prothrombin time sufficiently, fresh frozen plasma may be tried prior to biopsy. If this is successful, it can be used to cover the procedure, but there is no evidence that it reduces the risk of bleeding.

Contraindications to liver biopsy include [21]:
- An uncooperative patient
- Extrahepatic biliary obstruction
- Bacterial cholangitis
- Abnormal coagulation indices
- Tense ascites
- Cystic lesions
- Hypervascular tumors
- Amyloidosis
- Congestive liver

Technique. The patient is placed supine, with the right side close to the edge of the bed and the right hand behind the head. Intravenous midazolam is useful in anxious patients. Careful explanation and instructions should be given, particularly on holding the breath at full expiration; the patient must be able to carry this out satisfactorily.

The point of maximum dullness to percussion at full expiration in the right midaxillary line in the eighth to tenth intercostals space is marked. After skin antisepsis, 1 % lignocaine (without epinephrine) is infiltrated, firstly subcutaneously, then into the intercostal area, and finally down the diaphragm and capsule of the liver, with care being taken to infiltrate each layer adequately. Some centers advocate an ultrasound immediately before the biopsy, but the benefit of this is still debated.

Menghini Technique

The Menghini technique is the easiest to teach and perform. A skin incision facilitates penetration with a standard 1.9-mm diameter Menghini needle; the disposable type is preferred, as the bevel is consistently sharp (**Figs. 24.1, 24.2**). A 20-mL syringe containing 10 mL of isotonic sterile saline is attached to the proximal end of the needle after the 3-cm nail has been inserted, to prevent aspiration of the specimen into the syringe; 1 mL of saline is injected to clear any tissue after insertion down to the parietal pleura. Aspiration is started and maintained with the right thumb, while the left thumb is placed on the proximal end of the needle as a guard (**Fig. 24.3**). The needle is rapidly introduced perpendicular to the skin, and immediately removed with a single smooth motion while the patient holds his or her breath at full expiration. It remains in the liver for little more than 1 s. Occasionally, small fragmented specimens are obtained from cirrhotic livers; a second pass usually yields sufficient tissue, although this is associated with higher complication rate [21–26]. No further passes should be attempted [1,2].

Tru-Cut Needle Biopsy

The Tru-Cut needle consists of an inner solid needle and an outer hollow needle (**Fig. 24.4**), the cannula. The obturator has a pointed end for tissue penetration, and immediately behind this there is a notch for the biopsy specimen (**Fig. 24.5**). The needle is inserted perpendicular to the skin. When it reaches the intercostal space, the patient holds his or her breath in expiration. The needle in the closed position is advanced 4–5 cm into the right lobe. The obturator, with its biopsy slot, is thus advanced further into the liver parenchyma to its full extent (2 cm). Liver tissue prolapses into the biopsy slot (**Fig. 24.6**). With the obturator being kept firmly in position, the cannula, with its cutting surface, is advanced over the obturator, separating a core of the liver in the slot (**Fig. 24.7**). The needle is now in the fully closed position, and is withdrawn. The total time in the liver is 2–8 s. If no specimen is obtained at the first pass, a second attempt can be made after a careful reappraisal of the point of entry and depth of penetration [27,28]. The likelihood of complications increases with the number of punctures made.

It is considered that the Tru-Cut needle produces larger and less fragmented samples in comparison with the Menghini needle [6,26,29,30], particularly in patients with advanced fibrosis or cirrhosis [31]. However, in our review on the quality of PLB, we found that the Menghini technique yielded significantly longer samples (19.9±6.6 mm) in comparison with Tru-Cut (14.3±3.2 mm; P = 0.016), which may be related to the fact that the maximum length of sample provided by the Tru-Cut needle is determined by the notch in the needle shaft (usually 20–25 mm). Theoretically, a new Tru-Cut needle with a larger notch (more than 30 mm) might overcome this, but it could result in more complications. Finally, there are conflicting results regarding the safety of these two techniques [30,32]: a retrospective study [11] reported a higher rate of major complications with the Tru-Cut needle as a consequence of its longer intrahepatic phase, but a prospective study [33] found no significant differences in complication rates in relation to the type of needle used [34].

Aftercare. The patient should be kept in hospital for at least 6 h after the procedure. Vital signs should be monitored every 15 min for the first 2 h, and then every 30 min for 2 h, and then hourly for the rest of the remaining period. Mild oral analgesics, and occasionally parenteral analgesia, are required for pain at the puncture site or referred to the shoulder. If discharged within 24 h, the patient should be advised to remain within easy reach of the hospital overnight, and should be provided with the hospital's telephone number and the name of the member of staff to contact should severe pain, syncope, or other symptoms develop.

Complications. Other factors related to the complication rate in PLB are:
- Technical factors, including larger size needles [6,16], more than one pass [21–26], and the use of ultrasonography either before or at the time of the liver biopsy [29,35,36]
- Impaired coagulation beyond current safe limits [19]

However, the reduction in the complication rate when ultrasound is used has not been shown consistently [21,23,37–40]. The most important complication is bleeding. Major and minor complications occur in up to 6% of patients undergoing PLB, and in 0.04–0.11% of cases these can be life-threatening [19,41,42]—including puncture of the gallbladder or major bile ducts, and hemorrhage [11,23,26,43]. The mortality rate is approximately 0.017%. Bile leakage causes immediate severe abdominal pain, which rapidly progresses to biliary peritonitis unless the leak seals itself.

Hemorrhage from capsular tears usually takes a few hours to become apparent. Hemobilia causes biliary colic, with melena and bilirubinuria a few days later. Cholangitis may occur, particularly in bile duct obstruction. Puncture of the kidney or colon usually has no sequelae, but pancreatic puncture may be serious. Intrahepatic hematomas and arteriovenous fistulas are seldom clinically significant and resolve spontaneously [3,6,23,43].

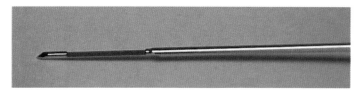

Fig. 24.4 A Tru-Cut needle, showing the obturator with the specimen notch advanced.

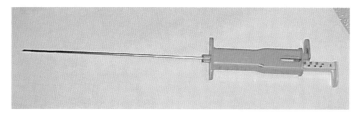

Fig. 24.5 A 14-gauge Tru-Cut cutting needle, 11.4 cm (4.5 in) long (Sherwood Medical).

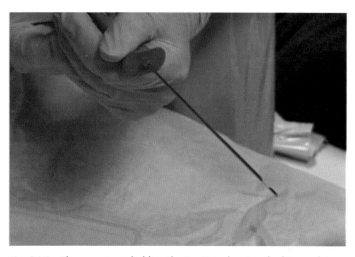

Fig. 24.6 The operator is holding the Tru-Cut, showing the biopsy slot.

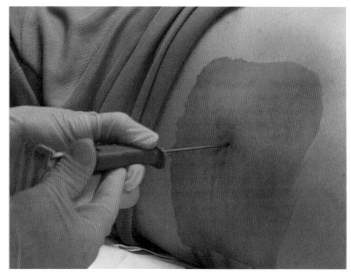

Fig. 24.7 In closed position, the needle is advanced 4–5 cm into the right lobe.

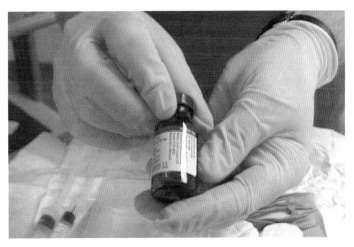

Fig. 24.8 Embolization particles (polyvinyl formaldehyde foam) (Ultra Ivalon-Nycomed, Amersham, England).

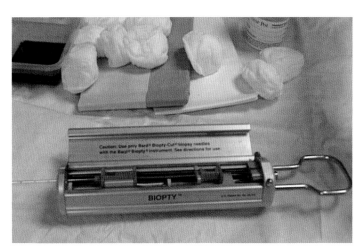

Fig. 24.9 A Biopty gun (Bard) assembled with the Tru-Cut needle.

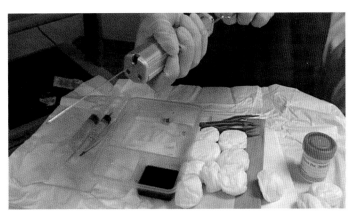

Fig. 24.10 The Biopty gun firing system with an 18-gauge Tru-Cut needle.

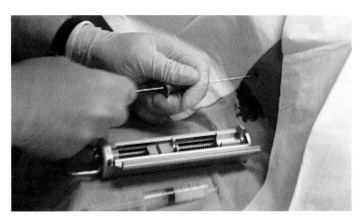

Fig. 24.11 The Tru-Cut needle is removed, leaving the needle track ready for injection of the embolization particles.

Plugged Percutaneous Liver Biopsy

There are various versions of this technique, but the basic principle underlying it is performing the biopsy through a sheath, followed by embolization of the biopsy track (Fig. 24.8). The needle used is usually of the Tru-Cut type. The most extensive published experience with this technique is that of Tobin and Gilmore [44], who successfully performed plugged liver biopsies in 100 patients with impaired blood coagulation. Our own center has reported a randomized controlled trial comparing the safety and efficacy of transjugular and plugged percutaneous liver biopsy techniques in patients with impaired blood coagulation [45]. Both methods of liver biopsy were associated with a high success rate and a low incidence of complications. Plugged percutaneous liver biopsy provides larger biopsies, but may be associated with an increased risk of bleeding (3.5%) [45].

Plugged percutaneous liver biopsy is easier and quicker than transjugular liver biopsy and can be readily applied to the biopsy of focal lesions in patients with impaired coagulation if ultrasound or CT imaging is available. The average time required for a plugged liver biopsy, including scanning, is 15 min. The average time required for a transjugular liver biopsy is 45 min. When coagulation disorders do not allow conventional percutaneous biopsy, and when the transvenous approach is not available or has been unsuccessful, the plugged liver biopsy is recommended [46].

Technique. An 18-gauge Biopty-Cut needle mounted in a firing system (Radiplast, Inc., Uppsala, Sweden) is introduced through a 16-gauge plastic sheath (Figs. 24.9, 24.10).The assembly is passed into the liver during held expiration (Fig. 24.11). This technique allows the biopsy apparatus to be positioned, fired, and withdrawn with one hand. The needle track, occupied by a flexible plastic sheath, is held with the other hand and injected with gelatin sponge from a prefilled syringe as the sheath is withdrawn (Fig. 24.12). A maximum of two biopsy passes is recommended.

Fine-Needle Aspiration Biopsy of the Liver

Fine-needle aspiration biopsy (FNAB) (with a needle caliber of < 1 mm) can be used to evaluate liver lesions. Although primarily applied to malignant disease, it is also used to evaluate benign conditions. Liver biopsy is an important tool in the diagnostic work-up, especially for nodules between 1 and 2 cm in size in which hepatocellular carcinoma is suspected [47,48]. Fine-needle PLB should be avoided for grading and staging in patients with chronic viral hepatitis, due to the inadequacy of the liver sample specimens [17]. Biopsy complications, although rare, are possible. They are limited largely to hemorrhage, which may be due to the vascularity of the lesion, the location of the lesion, or the needle size. Follow-up studies have indicated a very low rate of serious complications and a 0.006–0.1% mortality rate [49]. The estimated rate of needle-track seeding following FNAB of all abdominal organs ranges from 0.003%

to 0.009% [50]. Louha et al. [51], using molecular techniques with reverse transcriptase polymerase chain reaction for α-fetoprotein messenger RNA, showed that needle biopsies of hepatocellular carcinoma are associated with evidence of tumor dissemination into the circulation. A recent review [10] showed that the median seeding rate was 2.29% for biopsy alone and 0.95% when associated with ablation techniques. This was confirmed by another review, in which the risk of malignant seeding was estimated as up to 2.7% [52], Using current guidelines for the diagnosis of HCC [53], biopsy is limited to tumors between 1 and 2 cm diameter that do not have both arterial hypervascularity and portal venous wash-out. Similar imaging diagnosis can be achieved for metastases [52,54], but tissue diagnosis is still important for planning optimal chemotherapy. Torzilli et al. [54] have recently shown that evaluating the findings of standard imaging techniques without using FNAB can achieve an overall accuracy of 98.2% for preoperative diagnosis of each single nodule identified—a rate comparable with the best results reported with FNAB. With this approach, the diagnostic accuracy for HCC nodules was 99.6%, with a sensitivity of 100% and a specificity of 98.9%, with similar results for liver metastases [52,54].

Technique. Fine-needle biopsy can be performed by aspiration followed by cytological examination. This can be achieved using a needle with a long bevel, such as a spinal needle. Modifying the needle tip to give it a short bevel instead of a long one allows larger specimens to be aspirated, so that histological examination is possible. This technique is known as "fine-needle cutting liver biopsy." Fine-needle Tru-Cut biopsy is also available, which combines the safety of the fine needle with the better sample quality of a large-bore needle biopsy technique. Almost all liver FNAB procedures use an imaging method to guide biopsy—primarily ultrasonography and computed tomography.

Three basic biopsy techniques are frequently used. An individual puncture requires experience and skill and can only be carried out with real-time ultrasound guidance. It uses freehand motion, with a biopsy guide attached to the transducer. The coaxial biopsy technique can be used with either CT or ultrasonography, and a 17-gauge or 20-gauge cannula is generally used, through which the smaller aspiration and core biopsy needles are passed. This technique is best for small lesions in difficult locations in which there is very little margin of error for placing the needle tip. The tandem needle biopsy technique can also be used with either CT or ultrasonography. This method uses a reference needle that serves as a guide for the biopsy needle. After the reference needle has been placed in the lesion, its parameters are marked on the biopsy needle, allowing multiple aspirations without repeat imaging [44,49].

Ultrasound-Guided Liver Biopsy

Ultrasound-guided percutaneous liver biopsy is used extensively for investigating focal liver lesions; however, its use in diffuse liver disease is more controversial. Although ultrasound has not been rigorously tested, it is reasonable to use it to try to prevent complications in those patients in whom the landmarks of the liver are difficult to ascertain by physical examination—e.g., in obesity. In patients with suspected tumor, the use of ultrasound-guided or CT-guided biopsy is the safest and has the highest diagnostic yield. Prebiopsy ultrasonography, if easily available, can rule out any anatomical abnormalities. Recently, Riley [55] reported that ultrasound altered the positioning of the biopsy in 15% of cases by demonstrating intervening structures. Most commonly, the gallbladder and lung were the reasons for altering a position chosen on the basis of percussion. In this study of 165 patients, there were no complications and a 100% first-pass success rate. However, using the criteria of difficult percussion, obesity, and unusual chest shape,

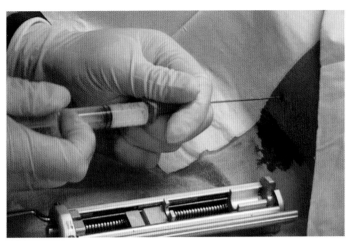

Fig. 24.12 The needle track, occupied by a flexible plastic sheath, is injected with the embolization particles (Ivalon, 3–5 mL) as the sheath is withdrawn.

it was not possible to predict when ultrasound would be useful. The lower complication rate with ultrasound guidance [29,35,36] can also be explained by the lower number of passes needed to obtain an adequate sample [21,23]. A recent study failed to show that real-time ultrasound guidance had an advantage in terms of safety in comparison with ultrasound performed within the previous 24 h to mark an optimal puncture site [20]. Although in some studies ultrasound guidance has been reported to decrease minor and major complications [29,35,36,56], other studies comparing it with blind PLB have suggested that it is still debatable whether ultrasound guidance is cost-effective [29,35,38,39,56–60]. PLB is more often performed with ultrasound guidance, although in France ultrasound guidance is used by 56% of gastroenterologists and hepatologists [25].

Transvenous (Jugular) Approach

The transjugular route is used for liver biopsy if there is impaired hemostasis, if gross ascites is present, or if measurement of hepatic venous pressures is needed. Liver transplantation has increased the demand for transjugular liver biopsies, as histology is frequently required in these patients, who initially have coagulation disorders. Liver biopsy may also have a role in assessing the prognosis in patients with fulminant hepatic failure, and the transjugular route may be the safest approach [61]. The main advantage of transjugular liver biopsy (TJLB) is that there is no penetration of the Glisson capsule unless there is a technical error, and bleeding is therefore extremely rare [34,37,42,62].

The transjugular biopsy can be part of a combined procedure. In our center, a day-case procedure can be performed as a "one-stop liver shop," during which hepatic venography, wedge hepatic venous pressure measurements, caval pressure measurements, and carbon dioxide portography are performed using the same minimal access (**Figs. 24.13, 24.14**) [63,64]. The hepatic venous pressure gradient might be a better end point than histology for assessing the therapeutic benefit of antiviral therapy [65]. The transjugular approach has also facilitated antegrade embolization of gastro-esophageal varices via the portal vein, and the creation of transjugular intrahepatic portosystemic shunts [65]. In some cases in which the jugular veins are not available because the patient has indwelling lines or thrombosed jugular veins, the transfemoral route can be used.

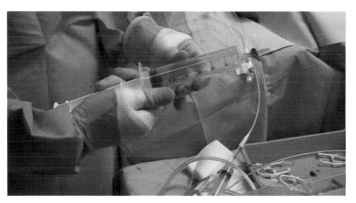

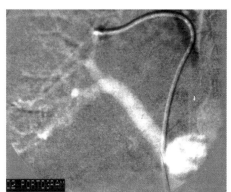

Fig. 24.14 CO_2 portography (subtraction film), showing the hepatic vein approach from the femoral route. Note the occluded balloon, behind which carbon dioxide is being injected to give a clear outline of the portal vein.

Fig. 24.13 A syringe filled with 100 mL of CO_2, which is to be injected via the transjugular route to evaluate the patency of the portal vein.

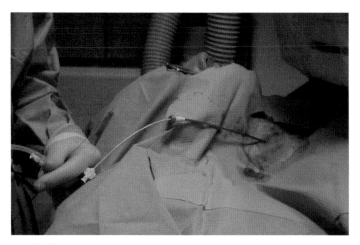

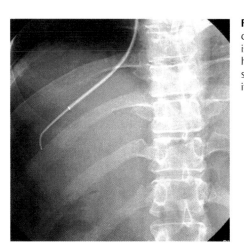

Fig. 24.16 A 7-Fr cobra catheter (Cordis Europa) is introduced into the hepatic vein, and a sheath is advanced over it.

Fig. 24.15 A 7-Fr sheath introducer (Arrow International, Inc.) is introduced into the right internal jugular vein using the Seldinger technique with the patient under local anesthesia.

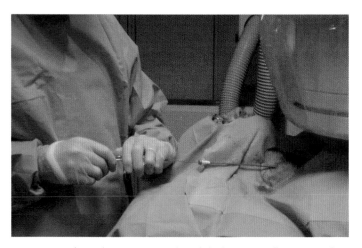

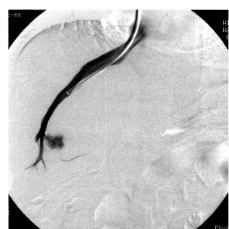

Fig. 24.18 The hepatic vein is outlined for positioning of the transjugular liver biopsy needle.

Fig. 24.17 The catheter is removed, and the biopsy needle is inserted via the sheath into the hepatic vein.

Technique. Transvenous liver biopsy must be performed in a vascular catheterization laboratory equipped with fluoroscopy. During the biopsy procedure, vital signs must be closely monitored. The patient is placed in the supine position, with the head rotated to the side opposite that of the internal jugular vein to be punctured. Intravenous sedation with a benzodiazepine is often useful. The right internal jugular vein is punctured under local anesthesia. When venous blood is aspirated, a 7-Fr or 10-Fr sheath is introduced (Arrow International, Inc.) using a Seldinger technique (**Fig. 24.15**).

A 7-Fr cobra catheter is introduced into the sheath and guided into the superior vena cava, the right atrium, the inferior vena cava, and the right hepatic vein, and the sheath is advanced over it (**Fig. 24.16**). The catheter is removed, and the biopsy needle is inserted via the sheath into the hepatic vein (**Fig. 24.17**). The correct position has to be confirmed by injecting contrast medium into the needle, visualizing either a junction of two small veins or liver parenchyma (**Fig. 24.18**). The latter position must be centrally placed, and not too close to the liver capsule [62]. At our center,

IV

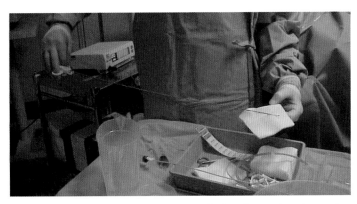

Fig. 24.19 The full length of the transjugular liver biopsy (Quick-Core Tru-Cut type).

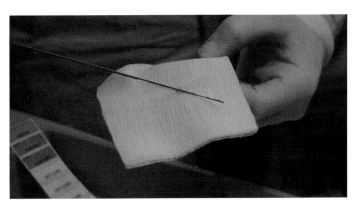

Fig. 24.20 The tip of the transjugular needle.

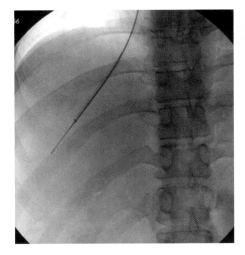

Fig. 24.21 The biopsy needle (Tru-Cut type) in the hepatic vein.

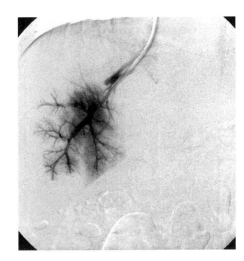

Fig. 24.22 Contrast medium has been injected into the hepatic vein in order to detect possible capsular perforation and leaking blood vessels. In such cases, embolization coils (Wilson-Cook Europe) are injected via the transjugular catheter.

24

we use a Quick-Core Tru-Cut type biopsy needle (**Figs. 24.19, 24.20**). When the correct position of the tip of the needle is confirmed, the patient is asked to hold his or her breath, and the needle is rapidly advanced 1–2 cm beyond the tip of the catheter and withdrawn (**Fig. 24.21**). After each pass, contrast medium is injected (**Fig. 24.22**). If the hepatic tissue specimen is absent or inadequate, other attempts can be made in the same manner or at another site until success is achieved, without any increase in the complication rate. The total complication rate is 7.1 % [66]. Minor complications are reported in 6.6 % of cases and include abdominal pain, supraventricular arrhythmias, and complications from the neck. The latter are significantly fewer with ultrasound guidance [66]. Major complications have occurred in 0.6 % of cases and include hepatic hematoma and intraperitoneal hemorrhage. The latter is the most common major complication (0.2 %), as a result of capsular perforation. This occurs particularly in patients with small livers, but it can be detected and treated during the procedure by injecting gelatin material or coils at the site of leakage [63]. Deaths have occurred in 0.09 % of TJLBs due to intraperitoneal hemorrhage (0.06 %) or ventricular arrhythmia (0.03 %). In comparison with adult series, pediatric series have shown significantly higher total complication rates [66]. Although uncommon, unsuccessful transjugular liver biopsy may occur for a number of reasons. These failures are generally related to anatomical problems preventing the puncture of the internal jugular vein, catheterization of the hepatic vein, or retrieval of liver tissue [67].

The use of TJLB has expanded with the development of an automated Tru-Cut needle, which has improved the effectiveness of the procedure (with reduced fragmentation and larger specimens) [68,69]. At our center, we use a Quick-Core 19-G Tru-Cut needle.

In our review of TJLB [66], it was found that Tru-Cut needles provide better samples (longer and more adequate for histological diagnosis) than Menghini needles. In addition, Tru-Cut may result in a lower complication rate in comparison with the aspiration (Menghini) technique, as it is easier to control the depth of puncture [66].

Quality of Liver Biopsies for Accurate Histological Interpretation

Adequate biopsy specimens are crucial for accurate histological interpretation [14,15]. However, liver biopsy tissue represents approximately 1/50,000 of the total liver mass [42]. According to recent studies, a liver specimen should be at least 20–25 mm long and/or contain ≥ 11 CPTs for reliable assessment of grading and staging in chronic viral hepatitis. The CPT number is the most suitable parameter for comparing different kinds of liver biopsy specimen (e. g., percutaneous versus transjugular, or Menghini versus Tru-Cut, or using different needle sizes) [17]. Similarly, adequate liver sample size is important for elimination of heterogeneity and intraobserver and interobserver variation in liver biopsy interpretation. A recent study has shown that that sample variability could be eliminated using liver specimens longer than 20 mm. In addition, Rousselet et al. [70] confirmed that longer specimens with more portal tracts can improve interobserver agreement, which is also confirmed in the literature [17].

However, often it is not feasible to obtain optimal PLBs routinely and safely [17]. In our review of PLB series [17], the mean length and number of CPTs were lower than the optimal standard (17.7 ± 5.8 mm and 7.5 ± 3.4, respectively) for accurate histological interpretation [14,15]. This means that using a standard percutaneous approach, more than one pass is often needed to obtain sufficient tissue, but this is known to increase complications [21–23,25].

On the other hand, although TJLB has been considered to be a second-line procedure in comparison with PLB [30,42], the quality of biopsies documented in our review[66] showed that the mean length and number of CPTs obtained with TJLB after an average of 2.5 passes were 12.8 ± 4.5 mm and 6.8 ± 2.3, respectively. In our center, using TJLB with Tru-Cut needles and three passes as a standard, we obtained a mean length and number of CPTs of 22 ± 7 mm and 8.7 ± 5, respectively—comparable with PLB specimens and without any serious complications [71]. In addition, three-core TJLB provides lower sample variability in comparison with one or two cores with TJLB [72]. Thus, in contrast to the risks of PLB with multiple passes, TJLB allows multiple passes [21–23,73] with a far lower likelihood of increasing the complication rates [63,74] and with reduced sample variability. Moreover, we have shown that four-pass TJLB provides liver specimens with a significantly larger number of CPTs in comparison with three passes (median CPTs: nine versus eight, respectively; $P = 0.04$) [75] and without an increase in complications in comparison with a previous series [63]. TJLB with sufficient passes is therefore an alternative and safe approach for obtaining an optimal liver biopsy, particularly in clinical trials. Operators should be aware that the optimal standard of liver biopsy has been estimated on formalin-fixed liver specimens. However, the size of liver samples is reduced by 7 % during the fixation process [76]. The degree of fragmentation affects the number of CPTs, thus affecting the quality of the biopsy and makes interpretation more difficult. Liver specimens become more fragmented at the time of handling just after they have been obtained, and in a randomized study fragmentation was not found to improve when the liver biopsy cores were placed in a cassette for transport [75].

Laparoscopic Biopsy of the Liver

Diagnostic laparoscopy with liver biopsy is as safe as blind percutaneous liver biopsy [77,78], but is more specific for staging chronic liver diseases [79,80]. Several studies have suggested that laparoscopic liver biopsy can serve as the gold standard for diagnosing cirrhosis [32]. Laparoscopic biopsy can be directed at focal disease, whilst inspection of the liver surface provides additional information. It allows application of direct pressure or the heater probe to obtain hemostasis in the event of bleeding from a biopsy site, and can also be carried out safely despite hematological abnormalities (international normalized ratio > 1.5, platelets < 60) that are routinely contraindications for a percutaneous liver biopsy [81]. The recent introduction of minilaparoscopy with miniature instruments has reduced the invasive nature of these procedures to a minimum [82], and it is therefore feasible in patients with significantly impaired coagulopathy. It could be particularly helpful in cholestatic liver disease, in which the sampling variability of biopsies is increased [32].

Indications. The indications for laparoscopic liver biopsy are:
- Patients in whom the laboratory examination or imaging procedures do not allow a definitive diagnosis to be made.
- Evaluation of chronic liver diseases [79,83].
- Staging of malignancies [84–86].
- Diagnosis of peritoneal disease [87,88].

Laparoscopy allows a highly guided liver biopsy to be performed with little risk [89]. Adequate biopsies are usually obtainable, and multiple specimens can easily be taken. However, wedge biopsy in patients with diffuse liver disease may overestimate the extent of fibrosis (for staging), due to fibrous septa that spread from the Glisson capsule, as well as the degree of necroinflammation [90]. Needle biopsies should thus be used when laparoscopic liver biopsy is performed to assess grading and staging. Further discussion of laparoscopy is given in Chapter 23.

References

1. Menghini R. One-second needle biopsy of the liver. Gastroenterology 1958;35:190–9.
2. Menghini G. One-second biopsy of the liver–problems of its clinical application. N Engl J Med 1970;283:582–5.
3. Sherlock S, Dick R, Van Leeuwen D. Liver biopsy: the Royal Free experience. J Hepatol 1984;1:75–85.
4. Alberti A, Morsica G, Chemello L, Cavalletto D, Noventa F, Pontisso P, Ruol A. Hepatitis C viraemia and liver disease in symptom-free individuals with anti-HCV. Lancet 1992;340:697–8.
5. Caldironi MW, Mazzucco M, Aldinio MT, Paccagnella D, Zani S, Pontini F, et al. [Echo-guided fine-needle biopsy for the diagnosis of hepatic angioma. A report on 114 cases]. Minerva Chir 1998;53:505–9.
6. Gilmore IT, Burroughs A, Murray-Lyon IM, Williams R, Jenkins D, Hopkins A. Indications, methods, and outcomes of percutaneous liver biopsy in England and Wales: an audit by the British Society of Gastroenterology and the Royal College of Physicians of London. Gut 1995;36:437–41.
7. Holtz T, Moseley RH, Scheiman JM. Liver biopsy in fever of unknown origin. A reappraisal. J Clin Gastroenterol 1993;17:29–32.
8. Vergara V, Garripoli A, Marucci MM, Bonino F, Capussotti L. Colon cancer seeding after percutaneous fine needle aspiration of liver metastasis. J Hepatol 1993;18:276–8.
9. Schotman SN, de Man RA, Stoker J, Zondervan PE, Ijzermans JN. Subcutaneous seeding of hepatocellular carcinoma after percutaneous needle biopsy. Gut 1999;45:626–7.
10. Stigliano R, Marelli L, Yu D, Davies N, Patch D, Burroughs AK. Seeding following percutaneous diagnostic and therapeutic approaches for hepatocellular carcinoma. What is the risk and the outcome? Seeding risk for percutaneous approach of HCC. Cancer Treat Rev 2007;33:437–47.
11. Dillon JF, Simpson KJ, Hayes PC. Liver biopsy bleeding time: an unpredictable event. J Gastroenterol Hepatol 1994;9:269–71.
12. Larson AM, Chan GC, Wartelle CF, McVicar JP, Carithers RL Jr, Hamill GM, et al. Infection complicating percutaneous liver biopsy in liver transplant recipients. Hepatology 1997;26:1406–9.
13. Ben-Ari Z, Neville L, Rolles K, Davidson B, Burroughs AK. Liver biopsy in liver transplantation: no additional risk of infections in patients with choledochojejunostomy. J Hepatol 1996;24:324–7.
14. Colloredo G, Guido M, Sonzogni A, Leandro G. Impact of liver biopsy size on histological evaluation of chronic viral hepatitis: the smaller the sample, the milder the disease. J Hepatol 2003;39:239–44.
15. Bedossa P, Dargere D, Paradis V. Sampling variability of liver fibrosis in chronic hepatitis C. Hepatology 2003;38:1449–57.
16. Sherlock S, Dooley J. Diseases of the liver and biliary system. 10th ed. London: Blackwell Science; 1997.
17. Cholongitas E, Senzolo M, Standish R, Marelli L, Quaglia A, Patch D, et al. A systematic review of the quality of liver biopsy specimens. Am J Clin Pathol 2006;125:710–22.
18. Montalto G, Soresi M, Carroccio A, Bascone F, Tripi S, Aragona F, et al. Percutaneous liver biopsy: a safe outpatient procedure? Digestion 2001;63:55–60.
19. Gunneson TJ, Menon KV, Wiesner RH, Daniels JA, Hay JE, Charlton MR, et al. Ultrasound-assisted percutaneous liver biopsy performed by a physician assistant. Am J Gastroenterol 2002;97:1472–5.
20. Manolakopoulos S, Triantos C, Bethanis S, Theodoropoulos J, Vlachogiannakos J, Cholongitas E, et al. Ultrasound-guided liver biopsy in real life: comparison of same-day prebiopsy versus real-time ultrasound approach. J Gastroenterol Hepatol 2007;22:1490–3.
21. Grant A, Neuberger J. Guidelines on the use of liver biopsy in clinical practice. British Society of Gastroenterology. Gut 1999;45(Suppl 4): IV1–IV11.
22. Robles-Diaz G, Chavez M, Lopez M, Dehesa M, Centeno F, Wolpert E. [Critical analysis of 1263 percutaneous hepatic biopsies carried out over a 12-year period (1970–1981) in the Salvador Zubiran National Institute of Nutrition]. Rev Gastroenterol Mex 1985;50:13–7.
23. McGill DB, Rakela J, Zinsmeister AR, Ott BJ. A 21-year experience with major hemorrhage after percutaneous liver biopsy. Gastroenterology 1990;99:1396–1400.

IV

24. Maharaj B, Bhoora IG. Complications associated with percutaneous needle biopsy of the liver when one, two or three specimens are taken. Postgrad Med J 1992;68:964–7.

25. Cadranel JF, Rufat P, Degos F. Practices of liver biopsy in France: results of a prospective nationwide survey. For the Group of Epidemiology of the French Association for the Study of the Liver (AFEF). Hepatology 2000;32:477–81.

26. Piccinino F, Sagnelli E, Pasquale G, Giusti G. Complications following percutaneous liver biopsy. A multicentre retrospective study on 68,276 biopsies. J Hepatol 1986;2:165–73.

27. Westaby D, Williams R. How to biopsy the liver. Br J Hosp Med 1980;23:527–9.

28. Maharaj B, Pillay S. "Tru-Cut" needle biopsy of the liver: importance of the correct technique. Postgrad Med J 1991;67:170–3.

29. Lindor KD, Bru C, Jorgensen RA, Rakela J, Bordas JM, Gross JB, et al. The role of ultrasonography and automatic-needle biopsy in outpatient percutaneous liver biopsy. Hepatology 1996;23:1079–83.

30. Guido M, Rugge M. Liver biopsy sampling in chronic viral hepatitis. Semin Liver Dis 2004;24:89–97.

31. Sherman M, Goodman ZD, Sullivan S, Faris-Young S, Gilf Study Group. Liver biopsy in cirrhotic patients. Am J Gastroenterol 2007;102:789–93.

32. Strassburg P, Manns M. Approaches to liver biopsy techniques—revisited. Semin Liver Dis 2006;26:318–27.

33. Forssell P, Bonkowsky H, Anderson P, Howell D. Intrahepatic hematoma after aspiration liver biopsy. A prospective randomized trial using two different needles. Dig Dis Sci 1981;26:631–5.

34. Tobkes AI, Nord HJ. Liver biopsy: review of methodology and complications. Dig Dis 1995;13:267–74.

35. Younossi ZM, Teran JC, Ganiats TG, Carey WD. Ultrasound-guided liver biopsy for parenchymal liver disease: an economic analysis. Dig Dis Sci 1998;43:46–50.

36. Farrell RJ, Smiddy PF, Pilkington RM, Tobin AA, Mooney EE, Temperley IJ, et al. Guided versus blind liver biopsy for chronic hepatitis C: clinical benefits and costs. J Hepatol 1999;30:580–7.

37. Burroughs AK, Dagher L. Liver biopsy. In: Classen M, Tytgat G, Lightdale C, editors. Gastrointestinal endoscopy. New York: Thieme Medical, 2002:252–9.

38. Papini E, Pacella CM, Rossi Z, Bizzarri G, Fabbrini R, Nardi F, Picardi R. A randomized trial of ultrasound-guided anterior subcostal liver biopsy versus the conventional Menghini technique. J Hepatol 1991;13:291–7.

39. Muir AJ, Trotter JF. A survey of current liver biopsy practice patterns. J Clin Gastroenterol 2002;35:86–8.

40. Stotland BR, Lichtenstein GR. Liver biopsy complications and routine ultrasound. Am J Gastroenterol 1996;91:1295–6.

41. Mayoral W, Lewis JH. Percutaneous liver biopsy: what is the current approach? Results of a questionnaire survey. Dig Dis Sci 2001;46:118–27.

42. Bravo AA, Sheth SG, Chopra S. Liver biopsy. N Engl J Med 2001;344:495–500.

43. Froehlich F, Lamy O, Fried M, Gonvers JJ. Practice and complications of liver biopsy. Results of a nationwide survey in Switzerland. Dig Dis Sci 1993;38:1480–4.

44. Tobin MV, Gilmore IT. Plugged liver biopsy in patients with impaired coagulation. Dig Dis Sci 1989;34:13–5.

45. Sawyer AM, McCormick PA, Tennyson GS, Chin J, Dick R, Scheuer PJ, et al. A comparison of transjugular and plugged-percutaneous liver biopsy in patients with impaired coagulation. J Hepatol 1993;17:81–5.

46. Riley SA, Ellis WR, Irving HC, Lintott DJ, Axon AT, Losowsky MS. Percutaneous liver biopsy with plugging of needle track: a safe method for use in patients with impaired coagulation. Lancet 1984;2:436.

47. Bruix J, Sherman M, Llovet JM, Beaugrand M, Lencioni R, Burroughs AK, et al. Clinical management of hepatocellular carcinoma. Conclusions of the Barcelona-2000 EASL conference. European Association for the Study of the Liver. J Hepatol 2001;35:421–30.

48. Llovet JM, Fuster J, Bruix J. The Barcelona approach: diagnosis, staging, and treatment of hepatocellular carcinoma. Liver Transpl 2004;10:S115–20.

49. Pitman MB. Fine needle aspiration biopsy of the liver. Principal diagnostic challenges. Clin Lab Med 1998;18:483–506, vi.

50. Smith EH. Complications of percutaneous abdominal fine-needle biopsy. Review. Radiology 1991;178:253–8.

51. Louha M, Nicolet J, Zylberberg H, Sabile A, Vons C, Vona G, et al. Liver resection and needle liver biopsy cause hematogenous dissemination of liver cells. Hepatology 1999;29:879–82.

52. Silva MA, Hegab B, Hyde CJ, Guo B, Buckels JA, Mirza DF. Needle track seeding following biopsy of liver lesions in the diagnosis of hepatocellular cancer: a systematic review and meta-analysis. Gut 2008;7:1592–6.

53. Bruix J, Sherman D. Management of hepatocellular carcinoma. Hepatology 2005;42:1208–36.

54. Torzilli G, Minagawa M, Takayama T, Inoue K, Hui AM, Kubota K, et al. Accurate preoperative evaluation of liver mass lesions without fine-needle biopsy. Hepatology 1999;30:889–93.

55. Riley TR III. How often does ultrasound marking change the liver biopsy site? Am J Gastroenterol 1999;94:3320–2.

56. Al Knawy B, Shiffman M. Percutaneous liver biopsy in clinical practice. Liver Int 2007;27:1166–73.

57. Pasha T, Gabriel S, Therneau T, Dickson ER, Lindor KD. Cost-effectiveness of ultrasound-guided liver biopsy. Hepatology 1998;27:1220–6.

58. Celle G, Savarino V, Picciotto A, Magnolia MR, Scalabrini P, Dodero M. Is hepatic ultrasonography a valid alternative tool to liver biopsy? Report on 507 cases studied with both techniques. Dig Dis Sci 1988;33:467–71.

59. Caturelli E, Giacobbe A, Facciorusso D, Bisceglia M, Villani MR, Siena DA, et al. Percutaneous biopsy in diffuse liver disease: increasing diagnostic yield and decreasing complication rate by routine ultrasound assessment of puncture site. Am J Gastroenterol 1996;91:1318–22.

60. Shah S, Mayberry JF, Wicks AC, Rees Y, Playford RJ. Liver biopsy under ultrasound control: implications for training in the Calman era. Gut 1999;45:628–9.

61. Donaldson BW, Gopinath R, Wanless IR, Phillips MJ, Cameron R, Roberts EA, et al. The role of transjugular liver biopsy in fulminant liver failure: relation to other prognostic indicators. Hepatology 1993;18:1370–6.

62. Lebrec D. Various approaches to obtaining liver tissue–choosing the biopsy technique. J Hepatol 1996;25(Suppl 1):20–4.

63. Papatheodoridis GV, Patch D, Watkinson A, Tibballs J, Burroughs AK. Transjugular liver biopsy in the 1990s: a 2-year audit. Aliment Pharmacol Ther 1999;13:603–8.

64. Senzolo M, Burra P, Cholongitas E, Lodato F, Marelli L, Manousou P, et al. The transjugular route: the key hole to the liver world. Dig Liver Dis 2007;39:105–16.

65. Burroughs AK, Groszmann R, Bosch J, Grace N, Garcia-Tsao G, Patch D, et al. Assessment of therapeutic benefit of antiviral therapy in chronic hepatitis C: is hepatic venous pressure gradient a better end point? Gut 2002;50:425–7.

66. Kalambokis G, Manousou P, Vibhakorn S, Marelli L, Cholongitas E, Senzolo M, et al. Transjugular liver biopsy—indications, adequacy, quality of specimens, and complications—a systematic review. J Hepatol 2007;47:284–94.

67. McAfee JH, Keeffe EB, Lee RG, Rosch J. Transjugular liver biopsy. Hepatology 1992;15:726–32.

68. Gamble P, Colapinto RF, Stronell RD, Colman JC, Blendis L. Transjugular liver biopsy: a review of 461 biopsies. Radiology 1985;157:589–93.

69. Lebrec D, Goldfarb G, Degott C, Rueff B, Benhamou JP. Transvenous liver biopsy: an experience based on 1000 hepatic tissue samplings with this procedure. Gastroenterology 1982;83:338–40.

70. Rousselet MC, Michalak S, Dupre F, Croue A, Bedossa P, Saint-Andre JP, et al. Sources of variability in histological scoring of chronic viral hepatitis. Hepatology 2005;41:257–64.

71. Cholongitas E, Quaglia A, Samonakis D, Senzolo M, Triantos C, Patch D, et al. Transjugular liver biopsy: how good it is for accurate histological interpretation? Gut 2006;55:1789–94.

72. Cholongitas E, Quaglia A, Samonakis D, Mela M, Patch D, Dhillon AP, et al. Transjugular liver biopsy in patients with diffuse liver disease: comparison of three cores with one or two cores for accurate histological interpretation. Liver Int 2007;27:646–53.

73. Demetris AJ, Ruppert K. Pathologist's perspective on liver needle biopsy size? J Hepatol 2003;39:275–7.

74. Smith TP, Presson TL, Heneghan MA, Ryan JM. Transjugular biopsy of the liver in pediatric and adult patients using an 18-gauge automated core biopsy needle: a retrospective review of 410 consecutive procedures. AJR Am J Roentgenol 2003;180:167–72.

75. Vibhakorn S, Cholongitas E, Kalambokis G, Manousou P, Quaglia A, Marelli L, et al. A comparison of four- versus three-pass transjugular biopsy using a 19-G Tru-Cut needle and a randomized study using a cassette to prevent biopsy fragmentation. Cardiovasc Intervent Radiol 2008 Aug 13. [Epub ahead of print].

76. Riley TR, III, Ruggiero F. The effect of processing on liver biopsy core size. Dig Dis Sci 2008;53:2775–7.

77. Haydon GH, Hayes PC. Diagnostic laparoscopy by physicians: we should do it. QJM 1997;90:297–304.

78. Knauer CM. Percutaneous biopsy of the liver as a procedure for outpatients. Gastroenterology 1978;74:101–2.

24

79. Jalan R, Harrison DJ, Dillon JF, Elton RA, Finlayson ND, Hayes PC. Laparoscopy and histology in the diagnosis of chronic liver disease. QJM 1995;88:559–64.

80. Poniachik J, Bernstein DE, Reddy KR, Jeffers LJ, Coelho-Little ME, Civantos F, et al. The role of laparoscopy in the diagnosis of cirrhosis. Gastrointest Endosc 1996;43:568–71.

81. Sharma P, McDonald GB, Banaji M. The risk of bleeding after percutaneous liver biopsy: relation to platelet count. J Clin Gastroenterol 1982;4:451–3.

82. Nader AK, Jeffers LJ, Reddy RK, Molina E, Leon R, Lavergne J, et al. Small-diameter (2 mm) laparoscopy in the evaluation of liver disease. Gastrointest Endosc 1998;48:620–3.

83. Orlando R, Lirussi F, Okolicsanyi L. Laparoscopy and liver biopsy: further evidence that the two procedures improve the diagnosis of liver cirrhosis. A retrospective study of 1,003 consecutive examinations. J Clin Gastroenterol 1990;12:47–52.

84. Lightdale CJ. Laparoscopy for cancer staging. Endoscopy 1992;24:682–6.

85. Brady PG, Peebles M, Goldschmid S. Role of laparoscopy in the evaluation of patients with suspected hepatic or peritoneal malignancy. Gastrointest Endosc 1991;37:27–30.

86. Sans M, Andreu V, Bordas JM, Llach J, Lopez-Guillermo A, Cervantes F, et al. Usefulness of laparoscopy with liver biopsy in the assessment of liver involvement at diagnosis of Hodgkin's and non-Hodgkin's lymphomas. Gastrointest Endosc 1998;47:391–5.

87. Mimica M. Usefulness and limitations of laparoscopy in the diagnosis of tuberculous peritonitis. Endoscopy 1992;24:588–91.

88. Shakil AO, Korula J, Kanel GC, Murray NG, Reynolds TB. Diagnostic features of tuberculous peritonitis in the absence and presence of chronic liver disease: a case control study. Am J Med 1996;100:179–85.

89. Friedman IH, Wolff WI. Laparoscopy: a safer method for liver biopsy in the high risk patient. Am J Gastroenterol 1977;67:319–23.

90. Imamura H, Kawasaki S, Bandai Y, Sanjo K, Idezuki Y. Comparison between wedge and needle biopsies for evaluating the degree of cirrhosis. J Hepatol 1993;17:215–9.

IV

V Therapeutic Procedures

Section editors:
Guido N.J. Tytgat, Meinhard Classen, and Charles J. Lightdale

25 Hemostasis

Sandy H.Y. Pang and James Y.W. Lau

Overview

Endoscopic therapy now has a central role in the management of upper gastrointestinal hemorrhage. After initial volume resuscitation, the management algorithm has evolved from medical management alone to providing prompt endoscopic intervention. Adjunctive use of pharmacotherapy further improves outcomes. Endoscopic therapy can be broadly categorized into injection, thermal, and mechanical methods. For practical purposes, the causes of upper gastrointestinal bleeding are classified into variceal and nonvariceal in origin. Both of these carry varying prognoses and require different modes of endoscopic intervention. This chapter discusses the use of endoscopic therapy in the two clinical entities separately.

Nonvariceal Hemorrhage

Injection Therapy

Injection therapy is still the most widely practiced method of endoscopic hemostasis. A wide range of agents are used, including diluted epinephrine, sclerosants, absolute alcohol, thrombin, and fibrin sealant.

Diluted epinephrine. Diluted epinephrine (1 : 10 000–1 : 100 000) is the most commonly used agent in injection therapy. Submucosal injection of diluted epinephrine works principally by volume tamponade of the artery. Epinephrine appears to have a local vasoconstrictive effect as well. Lai et al. found that endoscopic injections of water or diluted epinephrine were similarly effective in treating bleeding ulcers [1]. It has been reported that larger volumes of 13–20 mL resulted in less recurrent bleeding in high-risk ulcers in comparison with smaller volumes of 5–10 mL [2]. As epinephrine does not damage tissue, a larger volume of 10–20 mL can be injected submucosally. A transient rise in plasma catecholamines is seen following submucosal injection of diluted epinephrine (1 : 10 000) [3]. Absorbed epinephrine is then rapidly metabolized by the liver. Submucosal injection of epinephrine is generally safe, except for transient tachycardia following injection of a large volume, but should probably be used with caution in patients with marginal hepatic reserve and those with severe ischemic heart disease.

A disposable 23-gauge or 25-gauge sclerotherapy needle with a short bevel is used. The needle protrudes about 5 mm beyond the sheath. In chronic ulcers with a fibrotic base, a metallic needle is used for better tissue penetration. A metallic needle is also recommended if a side-viewing duodenoscope is used, as the elevator in a duodenoscope may compress on the plastic sheath and prevent the needle from protruding. A dual-channel therapeutic endoscope is preferred, as it allows simultaneous delivery of therapy and suctioning (**Fig. 25.1 a**). The additional channel also provides an alternate angle of access. Aliquots of 0.5–1 mL are injected around the bleeding vessel. In actively bleeding ulcers, cessation of bleeding represents a treatment end point (**Fig. 25.1 b**). Mucosal edema and blanching should be seen following epinephrine injection. If this is not immediately evident, it could be due to the presence of a heavily fibrotic ulcer base, or the needle being pushed too far into the

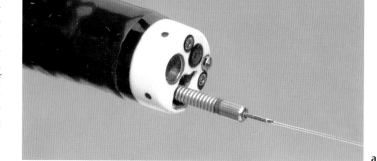

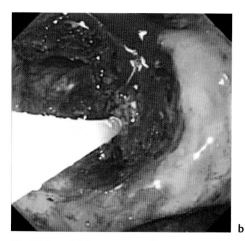

Fig. 25.1 a A 21-gauge metallic injection sclerotherapy needle in a dual-channel therapeutic scope (Olympus 2 T-240) with 3.7-mm and 2.8-mm channels. The additional channel allows simultaneous suctioning and an alternate angle of access.
b Injection treatment of an actively bleeding gastric ulcer at the angular incisure.

visceral wall. In the latter case, one should withdraw the needle slightly until the needle lies within the submucosa, and tissue edema should ensue. In nonbleeding visible vessels (defined as a protuberant discoloration), the treatment end point is less distinct. Often a volume of up to 10 mL is injected around the vessel.

Sclerosants. Sclerosants such as polidocanol, ethanolamine, sodium tetradecyl sulfate (STD), and absolute ethanol have fallen out of favor during the last 10 years. Absolute ethanol and sclerosants cause tissue necrosis and ulceration—the former by tissue dehydration and fixation, and the latter by acute inflammation and sclerosis. These agents cause tissue damage in a dose-dependent manner. Only a small volume can therefore be injected. They are used as an adjunct to injection with diluted epinephrine. Several trials compared the addition of a sclerosant after epinephrine injection to epinephrine injection alone. The pooled risk difference in recurrent bleeding was small [4–7]. There have also been rare

V

reports of gastric necrosis in the literature [8,9]. For this reason, and in view of the marginal benefit of adding a sclerosant to epinephrine injection, injection sclerosis is not now commonly practiced.

Thrombin and fibrin sealant. Thrombin is a component of the clotting cascade and represents the most physiologic agent for injection therapy. When reconstituted, thrombin is watery and can be injected with a standard injection catheter. In a randomized controlled trial of 140 patients with high-risk ulcers, Kubba et al. showed that the added injection of high-dose human thrombin (600–1000 IU) to epinephrine was superior to the injection of epinephrine alone with regard to the rebleeding rate, transfusion requirements, and mortality rate [10]. Fibrin sealant consists of two components: fibrinogen and thrombin (reconstituted with calcium chloride solution and aprotinin, respectively). A dual-channel injection catheter is required for the injection. Because of the higher viscosity of fibrinogen, one of the channels is wider for the injection. Mixing of the two components occurs at the tip of the injection catheter, deep in the submucosal tissue. Clogging of the needle is a frequent problem.

The technique of fibrin sealant injection is referred to as the "plug technique." In ulcers with active bleeding, preinjection with epinephrine is required. Considerable abutment of the dual-channel injector is required to advance the needle sufficiently deep into the submucosa. Four quadrants around the bleeding point are injected, each with 0.5 mL of fibrinogen and thrombin (a total of 1 mL fibrin sealant). After each injection, with the needle remaining in tissue, the reconstituted sealant is immediately followed by 1.0–1.5 mL of normal saline in order to drive the sealant submucosally. Following four-quadrant injection, the bleeding point is then injected. As the glue is being injected, the needle is slowly withdrawn, leaving a central fibrin plug. Both thrombin and fibrin sealant are derived from pooled human plasma. There is a theoretical concern regarding the transmission of viral agents, anaphylaxis (especially with the use of bovine thrombin), and intra-arterial injection causing systemic thrombosis. However, none of these complications has been reported in the literature. In a European multicenter trial, patients with actively bleeding ulcers and ulcers with nonbleeding visible vessels were randomly assigned to receive endoscopic injection of polidocanol alone, a single epinephrine and fibrin sealant treatment, and daily epinephrine and fibrin sealant treatment until complete fading of bleeding stigmata from the ulcer floors. Less recurrent bleeding was seen in the group receiving a single fibrin treatment (51 of 266, 19.2%) and in the group with repeated fibrin treatments (41 of 270, 15.2%) in comparison with the group receiving a polidocanol injection alone (58 of 254, 22.8%) [11]. The difference reached statistical difference only between polidocanol and repeated fibrin sealant treatment. The cost of fibrin sealant is substantial, especially after repeated injections.

Thermal Methods

Thermal devices can be divided into contact methods such as the heater probe and the multipolar probe, and noncontact methods such as neodymium:yttrium-aluminum-garnet (Nd:YAG) laser and argon plasma coagulation. In canine mesenteric arteries, Johnston and co-workers studied the effects of different thermal devices on arterial coagulation [12]. Laser results in the heating of tissue protein, contraction of the arterial wall, and vessel shrinkage. However, there is a "heat-sink" effect from flowing arterial blood, leading to the dissipation of thermal energy. In an experimental setting, laser was effective only for the direct coagulation of 0.25 mm exposed arteries. Contact thermal devices such as the heater probe and bipolar probe are more effective than laser electrocoagulation in coagulating medium-sized arteries, and can consistently seal ar-

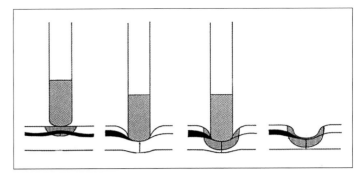

Fig. 25.2 The principle of coaptive thermocoagulation. The artery is compressed firmly, reducing the "heat-sink" effect. The two walls of the artery are then sealed using thermal energy.

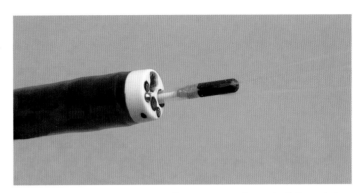

Fig. 25.3 A 3.2-mm heat probe (Olympus CD-10Z) in a dual-channel therapeutic endoscope (Olympus GIF-2T240). Three irrigation ports are located 1 cm proximal to the Teflon-coated tip, allowing targeted irrigation of an ulcer bed.

teries of up to 2 mm in diameter. Johnston et al. emphasized the importance of vascular compression and tamponade. The group introduced the term "coaptive coagulation" (the use of a hemostat to tamponade blood flow and coapt the vessel walls, followed by the application of cautery to thermally seal the vessel) (**Fig. 25.2**). Coagulation of arteries is ineffective if only a light touch is applied.

Contact method. Either the heat probe or the bipolar probe is used. The heater probe (Heat Probe Unit HPU-20; Olympus America, Inc., Central Valley, Pennsylvania, USA) consists of a heat coil inside a Teflon-coated copper tip. The probe is heated to 250 °C and can be programmed to deliver a fixed amount of energy directly onto tissue in contact with the probe. There are three irrigation ports to the side 1 cm from the probe tip. This allows simultaneous irrigation with the probe tip whilst it is in contact with the tissue (**Fig. 25.3**). Irrigation of the ulcer bed washes off clots and debris, allowing accurate positioning of the probe. The Teflon tip prevents coagulum from sticking to the tip after vessel coagulation, but it wears thin with repeated use, so that bleeding may be provoked if the coagulum is lifted off as the probe is withdrawn. Activation of the irrigation ports and "floating" of the probe off the tissue bed after vessel coagulation may reduce this risk. Jensen recommended the following settings for the treatment of a bleeding peptic ulcer: 1, firm tamponade; 2, four 30-J pulses given per tamponade station before repositioning [13] (**Fig. 25.4**). The mean bond strengths in canine mesenteric arteries sealed by heater probe coagulation were similar for 120 and 240 J. The depth of coagulation associated with 14 s of 30-J pulses was found to be 2.1 mm, increasing to 3.7 mm with doubling of the contact time. The heater probe can be applied tangentially and is available in two sizes (2.4 mm and 3.2 mm). Morris et al. compared the use of two probes in animal experiments

25

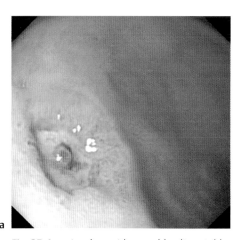
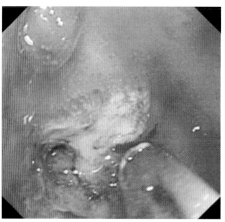

Fig. 25.4 a An ulcer with a nonbleeding visible vessel (protuberant discoloration).
b Coaptive coagulation is applied with a heat probe, leaving a "footprint" or cavitation in the ulcer bed. Irrigation is activated, and the tip of the heat probe is "floated off" the ulcer bed to prevent provocation of bleeding.

Fig. 25.5 An angiodysplasia in the small bowel, with typical "spider-like" vascular projections.

Fig. 25.6 a, b Antral vascular ectasia, before and after argon plasma coagulation treatment.

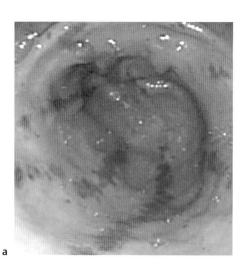
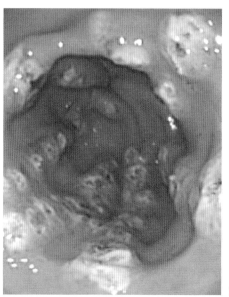

and found that the larger probe was better in securing hemostasis, without increasing the depth of coagulation [14]. In clinical situations, the 3.2-mm heater probe is generally preferred in a twin-channeled endoscope.

The bipolar probe (e. g., Injection Gold Probe, Boston Scientific, Natick, Massachusetts, USA) has positive and negative electrodes located at the tip of the probe, and it heats contacted tissue as an electrical current passes between the electrodes. Coagulum is formed at the tip of the probe when the temperature exceeds 60 °C. Once the superficial tissue has been desiccated, there is increasing resistance to coagulation in the deeper tissue, and the procedure is thus associated with a reduced risk of thermal injury and tissue perforation. A 3.2-mm probe is again preferred. Some probes also have built-in irrigation ports, as well as an injection needle. For securing hemostasis, the recommendations are: 1, firm tamponade over the bleeding point; 2, a low power setting of 12–16 W; and 3, continuous coagulation for 7–10 s per tamponade station before repositioning the probe.

Noncontact thermal method. Argon plasma coagulation (APC) and laser deliver thermal energy without contacting the tissue. Laser is no longer commonly used, as laser units are expensive and cum-

bersome to transport. Argon plasma coagulation works by using ionized argon gas to deliver a plasma of evenly distributed thermal energy to a field of tissue adjacent to the probe. It coagulates tissue to a depth of 2–3 mm and can be used to treat mucosal lesions. It is particularly useful in the treatment of vascular malformations such as angiodysplasia (**Fig. 25.5**). and gastric antral vascular ectasia (GAVE) (**Fig. 25.6**). It can also be used to obliterate residual post-polypectomy tissue, and in selected cases for limited palliative resection of tumors. There is a small risk of tissue perforation and submucosal emphysema if the catheter is in contact with the tissue for prolonged periods. There have been two randomized trials comparing APC with heater probe treatment and injection sclerotherapy, respectively, in patients with bleeding ulcers. The two trials did not demonstrate any difference in treatment outcomes [15].

Hemoclips

Three single-use clipping devices are currently available: 1, Quick-Clip2, with standard sizes of 9 mm or 11 mm open (Olympus America Inc., Central Valley, Pennsylvania, USA); 2, TriClip, which is three-pronged, with 12 mm open between the prongs (Cook Endoscopy,

Winston-Salem, North Carolina, USA); and 3, Resolution Clip, which is 11 mm open (Microvasive, Boston Scientific, Natick, Massachusetts, USA). E2 Clip (Olympus America, Inc., Central VAlley, Pennsylvania, USA) is a reusable system, utilizing cartridge-housed clips (**Fig. 25.7**). Clips can now be rotated or torqued into the desired axis. The Resolution Clip has a grasping and releasing mechanism that allows repositioning of the clip before final deployment. Clipping is conceptually closest to a surgical method of hemostasis. It does not damage tissue. In practice, deploying a clip tangentially through a duodenoscope or in a retroflexed endoscope can be difficult. High-risk ulcers such as those located at the posterior bulb and on the lesser curvature of the stomach are therefore difficult to treat using hemoclipping. In the treatment of ulcers, clips are applied to the two ends of a "sentinel clot"—a term synonymous with "nonbleeding visible vessel." In an ulcer with a fibrotic ulcer base, considerable abutment is required to ensure that the jaws of a clip grasp onto the ulcer base (**Fig. 25.8**). Jensen compared the above three clipping devices in a randomized controlled canine study, and reported similar learning curves, initial hemostasis rates, and safety profiles, although the Resolution Clip appeared to have the longest retention rates [16]. The use of smaller clips may be an advantage when they are deployed within a limited space such as the bulbar duodenum. In the authors' experience, the prongs of the TriClip are soft; deploying a TriClip onto an ulcer with a fibrotic base can be difficult.

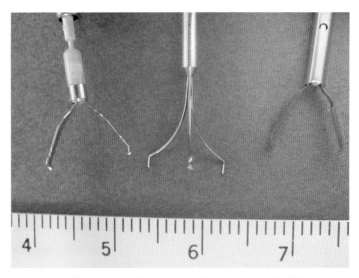

Fig. 25.7 Different types of hemoclip. *Left to right:* EZ Clip (Olympus HX-610–135), TriClip (Cook Endoscopy TC-7–12-S), Resolution Clip (Boston Scientific).

▤ Heater Probe vs. Hemoclips

A meta-analysis of 15 randomized trials that compared hemoclips to thermocoagulation, with or without injection, found no significant differences between the two modalities in terms of initial and definitive hemostasis, rebleeding rate, and mortality rate [17]. In one trial, the initial hemostasis rate was lower with the use of hemoclips in comparison with thermocoagulation. This was thought to be partially due to "difficult-to-approach" lesions [18]. The two modalities should not be used exclusively of each other.

▤ Monotherapy versus Combination Treatment

From pooled analyses, it is now clear that endoscopic injection of diluted epinephrine alone is an inferior treatment. A second treatment modality should be added to the vessel. The combination approach was shown to significantly reduce the rates of recurrent bleeding, surgery, and death in comparison with epinephrine injection alone [19]. In actively bleeding ulcers, prior injection of diluted epinephrine slows down bleeding and allows precise localization of the bleeding vessel. A second modality can then be targeted to the vessel to induce thrombosis. Preinjection with diluted epinephrine also has the theoretical benefit of reducing the heat-sink effect if a thermal device is to follow. In ulcers with a non-bleeding visible vessel and an adherent clot, preinjection may reduce the risk of provoking bleeding. We would recommend the use of hemoclips and/or thermocoagulation as a second modality.

▤ Endoscopic Signs of Bleeding

Forrest and Finlayson divided the endoscopic appearances of bleeding ulcers into those with active bleeding; those with stigmata of recent bleeding; and those with a clean base [20]. A modified version of the Forrest classification has since been in widespread use in the endoscopy literature for the description of endoscopic signs in bleeding peptic ulcers (**Table 25.1**). These signs represent stages of the development of a bleeding artery into an ulcer. Ulcer

25

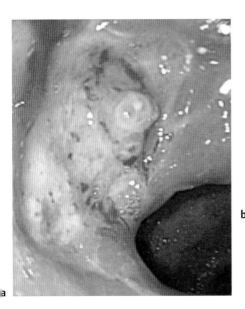
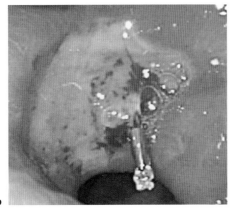
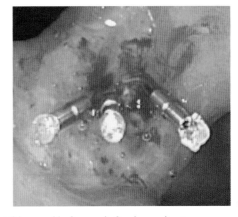

Fig. 25.8 a–c A gastric ulcer with a nonbleeding visible vessel before and after hemoclipping.

Table 25.1 Prevalence of characteristic peptic ulcer stigmata, corresponding to the Forrest criteria and spontaneous rebleeding rates [25,35]

Endoscopic characteristics	Forrest class	Prevalence % (range)	Rebleeding % (range)
Active bleeding	I	18 (4–26)	55 (17–100)
Nonbleeding visible vessel	IIa	17 (4–35)	43 (0–81)
Adherent clot	IIb	17 (0–49)	22 (12–36)
Flat spot	IIc	20 (0–42)	10 (0–13)
Clean base	III	42 (19–52)	5 (0–10)

bleeding starts with an eroded artery. A fibrin clot or a larger clot may plug the artery, giving rise to a nonbleeding visible vessel or a clot. Johnston et al. used the term "sentinel clot" synonymously with "nonbleeding visible vessel" [12]. As the ulcer heals, a flat pigment and then a clean base are seen. The natural evolution takes less than 72 h in the majority of ulcers. These endoscopic signs can predict the risk of continued or recurrent bleeding (**Fig. 25.1**). Active bleeding ulcers seen at endoscopy clearly mandate endoscopic treatment. Ulcers with a nonbleeding visible vessel also warrant therapy. The correct approach to a clot is a matter of controversy. Most would attempt to wash off the clot in order to examine the ulcer base. Reports varied in descriptions of the vigor used for clot irrigation before clots were declared to be adherent. Some use focal irrigation of a large thermal probe for up to 5 min. Some use mechanical devices such as snares to "cheese-wire" the clot. A meta-analysis of six studies including 240 patients favored clot removal by focal irrigation or using the "guillotine-snare" technique, and treating the underlying lesion endoscopically [21]. Whether or not a clot should be removed remains controversial, especially when powerful proton-pump inhibitors are available.

Limitations of Endoscopic Therapy

Swain et al. studied bleeding arteries in gastrectomy specimens of recurrent bleeding gastric ulcers and in postmortem examinations of patients who had succumbed to bleeding peptic ulcers [22]. In the surgical specimens, the mean external diameter of the bleeding artery was 0.7 mm (range 0.1–1.8 mm). Serosal arteries were significantly larger than submucosal arteries (mean 0.88 mm vs. 0.50 mm). In patients who died of exsanguination from bleeding ulcers, the artery was as large as 3.85 mm in external diameter [23]. In vitro experiments suggested that arteries larger than 2 mm in size could not be controlled using contact thermal probes. In the clinical setting, conditions are less ideal, and it has been suggested that bleeding from arteries over 1 mm in size is difficult to control endoscopically. The main trunk of the gastroduodenal artery, for instance, is estimated to be 3–6 mm in size. Large deep ulcers in the posterior wall of the duodenal bulb or the lesser curvature may erode into the gastroduodenal artery complex or the left gastric artery, respectively. Erosions into major arteries are not amenable to endoscopic therapy. Immediate surgery or angiographic embolization should be considered in such cases. A pooled analysis of studies examining factors predictive of endoscopic treatment failures consistently identified large ulcers (> 2 cm in size) located at the above sites as sources of recurrent bleeding [24].

Other Nonvariceal Bleeding Sources

Mallory–Weiss tears frequently occur after excessive vomiting and retching, and account for 3–15 % of nonvariceal upper gastrointestinal bleeds. These often run a benign course and generally do not require any endoscopic treatment. Bleeding from Mallory–Weiss tears can occasionally be severe. Injection with diluted epinephrine, hemoclipping, band ligation, and the use of thermal devices have been described in the treatment of actively bleeding Mallory–Weiss tears in anecdotal reports.

A Dieulafoy's lesion is a caliber-persistent submucosal artery associated with a minute mucosal defect [25]. It is still a rare but important cause of upper gastrointestinal hemorrhage. The lesions can be difficult to detect in massive bleeding episodes, which may be life-threatening. Most of them are found in the fundus, usually within 6 cm of the esophagogastric junction, although they can occur in any part of the gastrointestinal tract. The treatment of a bleeding Dieulafoy's lesion is similar to that of a bleeding peptic ulcer. Banding ligation as a treatment modality has also been reported.

Variceal Hemorrhage

Endoscopic Variceal Ligation

Endoscopic variceal ligation (EVL) is now the standard treatment in patients with acute esophageal variceal bleeding. It is also used in secondary prophylaxis against recurrent bleeding. There is now evidence to support its use in primary prophylaxis against a first bleed in patients with large esophageal varices who are intolerant to selective beta-blocker and/or nitrate treatment. Stiegmann et al. first introduced a rubber band ligation device in 1986 [26] (**Fig. 25.9**). The concept was derived from the banding of hemorrhoids. Multiple-firing devices have replaced single-shot ligators. Before the ligation device is loaded, a careful examination of the esophagus and stomach should be carried out to identify the site, location, and appearance of the varices. During endoscopy, varices are aspirated by suction into a cap until a complete red-out is seen. Rubber bands are then released over the varices (**Fig. 25.10**). The strangulated varices then undergo thrombosis, inflammation, and necrosis, and then slough off within a week, leaving shallow ulcerations. These heal during the following weeks, resulting in fibrosis and scarring in the mucosa and submucosa.

The use of multiple-firing devices avoids the need for an esophageal overtube, which is necessary for multiple scope passage with single-shot devices. Overtubes were associated with several complications, including esophageal perforation, laceration, and pinch injury of the esophageal wall in the gap between the overtube and the endoscope.

Treatment begins with ligation of the most distal variceal columns in the esophagus, just above the esophagogastric junction, and continues in a helical fashion for 5–8 cm proximally. The bleeding point or a fibrin clot can be aspirated directly into the cap and a band can then be applied. In situations in which the exact bleeding point cannot be seen, we recommend that the scope be passed first into the stomach and then slowly withdrawn. Variceal columns are then banded at their most distal portions, usually just caudal to or at the esophagogastric junction. As patients with an initial variceal bleed are at high risk for rebleeding, a second banding session should be scheduled 3–7 days after the initial bleeding episode. Repeated sessions are needed weekly until obliteration of the varices is achieved.

Complications associated with EVL include transient dysphagia and chest discomfort. Bleeding from postbanding ulcerations can occur in a small proportion of patients. Administration of proton-pump inhibitor therapy for 10 days after EVL can reduce ulcer-related bleeding.

V

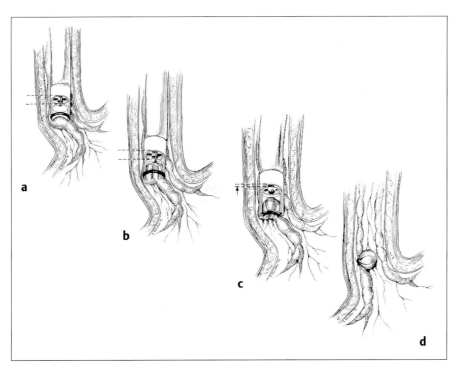

Fig. 25.9 Esophageal variceal ligation using a single ligator, as originally described by Stiegmann and Goff. (Reproduced with permission from Stiegmann GV. Endoscopic management of esophageal varices. In: Cameron JL, editor. *Advances in Surgery.* Chicago: Mosby Year Book, 1993.)
a Full contact between the suction cylinder and the varix to be ligated.
b Aspiration of the varix into suction cylinder. This produces a total "red-out" in the endoscopic view.
c Pulling the tripwire withdraws the inner cylinder, releasing the rubber band around the varix.
d The ligated varix.

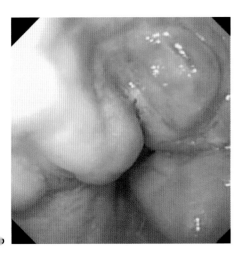 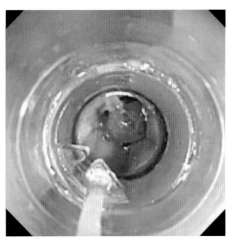 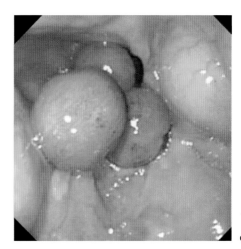

Fig. 25.10 a–c Esophageal varices before, during, and after band ligation.

Endoscopic Injection Sclerotherapy

Endoscopic injection sclerotherapy (EIS) is used both in the control of acute bleeding and in the elective obliteration of varices and is effective in stopping 80–90 % of variceal bleeds. It works by inducing variceal thrombosis and scarring through the injection of a variety of sclerosing agents (e. g., polidocanol, absolute alcohol, sodium tetradecyl sulfate, 5 % ethanolamine oleate).

The technique of EIS can be variable. It can be divided into paravariceal and intravariceal injection. We use a freehand method, injecting sclerosant intravariceally. Aliquots of 2 mL are injected into each varix at esophagogastric junction, then 2.5 and 5 cm cephalad. A total of less than 50 mL is injected at each session. Weekly injection is then continued until eradication. EIS is associated with a complication rate as high as 20 %. Local complications include stricture formation, ulceration, bleeding, and rarely perforation. Bacteremia, sepsis, and pleural effusion are some of the systemic complications. Because of its risk of local complications, injection sclerotherapy should not be used as a means of primary prophylaxis, especially with the advent of endoscopic band ligation therapy, which has proved to be safer and more effective in the management of esophageal varices.

Band Ligation versus Endoscopic Injection Sclerotherapy

There have been many trials comparing band ligation to injection sclerotherapy in the treatment of esophageal varices. In the original Denver trial studying 129 patients, band ligation was associated with fewer complications—principally esophageal strictures, pneumonia, and other infections (2 % vs. 22 %) [27]. Fewer treatment sessions were required with band ligation to eradicate varices, and less recurrent bleeding was observed. A survival benefit was seen in patients with Child–Pugh A and B cirrhosis who were treated with band ligation. In a subsequent meta-analysis of seven randomized controlled trials comparing sclerotherapy with banding, an absolute difference of 13 % (95 % CI, –18 % to –6 %) in the risk of bleeding was shown for banding [28]. Band ligation was also associated with less frequent and less severe complications. Fewer sessions are needed with EVL to achieve eradication of varices. Although EVL is preferred over sclerotherapy, repeated banding causes fibrosis and scarring, which may make further banding difficult. Sclerotherapy may have a role in treating residual varices in these situations.

Combining Banding Ligation and Sclerotherapy

In an effort to hasten variceal eradication, many groups have administered small-volume sclerotherapy proximal to bands. This synchronous approach theoretically reduces the volume of sclerosants used and the associated local side effects. Venous stasis induced by band ligation enhances the effect of a sclerosant. There is also a theoretical advantage of obliterating perforating channels between submucosal varices and larger paraesophageal varices. Combination treatment is performed by injecting a sclerosant immediately after elastic band ligation. Ligation of individual esophageal varices is first done near the gastroesophageal junction. Intravariceal injection is then performed using 1 mL of sclerosant per varix at sites 1–3 cm cephalad to the site of ligation. Alternately, some endoscopists apply two bands above and below a varix and inject sclerosant intravariceally between the two bands. Two meta-analyses that evaluated trials studying the benefit of adding sclerotherapy to EVL found no differences in mortality rates, risk of rebleeding, or number of endoscopic sessions required to achieve complete variceal eradication [29,30]. Patients who received combination therapy also had a significantly higher incidence of esophageal stricture.

EVL is less effective in smaller varices and in situations in which fibrosis induced by previous band ligation makes suction of residual varices difficult. A randomized study suggested that a sequential approach may be worthwhile. Following a course of weekly EVL, small residual varices were then treated with injection sclerotherapy. This approach reduced the rates of recurrence of varices and rebleeding during a median follow-up period of 2 years [31].

Tissue Adhesives

N-butyl-2-cyanoacrylate (Histoacryl) is a watery substance that polymerizes and hardens instantaneously when it comes into contact with blood. This unique property makes it attractive for use in obliterating varices. It is particularly useful in the treatment of fundic varices. Histoacryl is reconstituted with Lipiodol (0.7 mL in 0.5 mL), an oil-based radiopaque contrast agent. The therapeutic channel of the endoscope is first flushed with 2 mL of Lipiodol. The injection needle is then filled with 2 mL of the Lipiodol/Histoacryl mixture. The varix is punctured, and the Lipiodol/Histoacryl mixture is injected. Before retraction of the needle, the residual glue is pushed into the varix with a further 2 mL of Lipiodol. The needle is then retracted, and the catheter is rinsed with water. It is important at this juncture not to activate suction in the endoscope, and to continue irrigation to avoid contact between the glue and the lens.

There have been few randomized studies comparing Histoacryl to sclerotherapy or banding in the treatment of esophagogastric varices. In esophageal varices, we reserve Histoacryl glue for rescue treatment when band ligation fails to control bleeding. Histoacryl glue should not be used for elective obliteration of esophageal varices, as significant complications such as strictures and ulcerations can occur. In the literature, there have been reports of distal embolization into the pulmonary and cerebral vasculature.

Histoacryl glue is particularly useful in the endoscopic treatment of gastric varices. EVL is not effective in this situation, as gastric

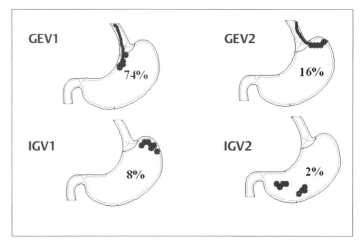

Fig. 25.11 Classification of gastric varices and their relative frequency, adapted from Sarin et al. [32]. GEV, gastroesophageal varix; IGV, isolated gastric varix.

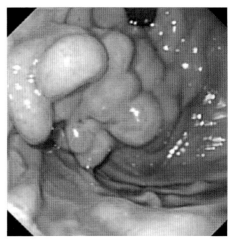

Fig. 25.12 An example of a conglomerate of fundic varices.

varices tend to be large. Application of rubber bands with the endoscope in a retroflexed position is difficult, and the bands often come off, leading to recurrent bleeding. Sarin et al. classified gastric varices into four types on the basis of their anatomic location: gastroesophageal varices types 1 and 2, and isolated gastric varices types 1 and 2 [32]. Type 1 gastroesophageal varices extend along the lesser curvature into the stomach, whereas type 2 gastroesophageal varices extend into the gastric fundus (**Fig. 25.11**). Gastroesophageal varices should probably be treated as esophageal varices, with band ligation close to the esophagogastric junction. Isolated gastric varices (type 1) are located in the gastric fundus and carry a high risk of bleeding and death (**Fig. 25.12**). Histoacryl glue is probably the only effective endoscopic treatment for controlling acute bleeding. Ectopic gastric varices (type 2) are uncommon and can occur in any part of the stomach.

Endoloops and Detachable Mini-Snares

Mini-Endoloops and detachable snares are useful alternatives to rubber bands for variceal ligation. Using the same principle as suction band ligation, the varix is sucked into a transparent cap mounted on the tip of the endoscope and is ligated with the loop. The cap contains an inner ridge that captures the opened loop. To ensure optimal orientation of the Endoloop within the ridge of the cap, it is positioned at right angles to the shaft so that it can ensnare

V

tissue. Mini-Endoloops appear to be able to grasp larger amounts of tissue, and in theory may remain in place longer after they have been applied. Like Endoloops, detachable snares can also grasp a large amount of tissue. Yoshida et al. and Cipolleta et al. used detachable snares in the treatment of large fundic gastric varices [33,34]. Varices up to 5 cm in size are said to be suitable for snaring. It can be difficult to use Endoloops in ulcer bleeding, as the ulcer bases are often fibrotic, and aspiration of the tissue into the suction chamber is difficult if not impossible. However, Endoloops may be suitable for other lesions, such as Dieulafoy's lesions.

References

1. Lai KH, Peng SN, Guo WS, Lee FY, Chang FY, Malik U, et al. Endoscopic injection for the treatment of bleeding ulcers: local tamponade or drug effect? Endoscopy 1994;26:338–41.
2. Lin HJ, Hsieh YH, Tseng GY, Perng CL, Chang FY, Lee SD. A prospective, randomized trial of large- versus small-volume endoscopic injection of epinephrine for peptic ulcer bleeding. Gastrointest Endosc 2002;55: 615–9.
3. Sung JY, Chung SC, Low JM, Cocks R, Ip SM, Tan P, et al. Systemic absorption of epinephrine after endoscopic submucosal injection in patients with bleeding peptic ulcers. Gastrointest Endosc 1993;39:20–2.
4. Chung SC, Leong HT, Chan AC, Lau JY, Yung MY, Leung JW, et al. Epinephrine or epinephrine plus alcohol for injection of bleeding ulcers: a prospective randomized trial. Gastrointest Endosc 1996;43:591–5.
5. Villanueva C, Balanzó J, Espinós JC, Fábrega E, Sáinz S, González D, et al. Endoscopic injection therapy of bleeding ulcer: a prospective and randomized comparison of adrenaline alone or with polidocanol. J Clin Gastroenterol 1993;17:195–200.
6. Choudari CP, Palmer KR. Endoscopic injection therapy for bleeding peptic ulcer: a comparison of adrenaline alone with adrenaline plus ethanolamine oleate. Gut 1994; 35: 608–10.
7. Lin HJ, Perng CI, Lee SD. Is sclerosant injection mandatory after an epinephrine injection for arrest of peptic ulcer haemorrhage? A prospective, randomised, comparative study. Gut 1993;34:1182–5.
8. Loperfido S, Patelli G, La Torre L. Extensive necrosis of gastric mucosa following injection therapy of bleeding peptic ulcer [letter]. Endoscopy 1990;22:285–6.
9. Chester JF, Hurley PR. Gastric necrosis: a complication of endoscopic sclerosis for bleeding peptic ulcer [letter]. Endoscopy 1990;22:287.
10. Kubba KA, Murphy W, Palmer KR. Endoscopic injection for bleeding peptic ulcer: a comparison of adrenaline alone with adrenaline plus human thrombin. Gastroenterology 1996;111:623–8.
11. Rutgeerts P, Rauws E, Wara P, Swain P, Hoos A, Solleder E, et al. Randomised trial of single and repeated fibrin glue compared with injection of polidocanol in treatment of bleeding peptic ulcer. Lancet 1997;350: 692–6.
12. Johnston JH, Jensen DM, Auth D. Experimental comparison of endoscopic yttrium-aluminum-garnet laser, electrosurgery, and heater probe for canine gut arterial coagulation: importance of compression and avoidance of erosion. Gastroenterology 1987;92:1101–8.
13. Jensen DM. Heat probe for hemostasis of bleeding peptic ulcers: techniques and results of randomized controlled trials. Proceedings of the Consensus Conference on Therapeutic Endoscopy in Bleeding Peptic Ulcers. Gastrointest Endosc 1990;30:42–9.
14. Morris DL, Brearley S, Thompson H, Keighley MR. A comparison of the efficacy and depth of gastric wall injury with 3.2- and 2.3-mm bipolar probes in canine arterial hemorrhage. Gastrointest Endosc 1985;31: 361–3.
15. Havanond C, Havanond P. Argon plasma coagulation therapy for acute non-variceal upper gastrointestinal bleeding. Cochrane Database Syst Rev 2005;(2):CD 003 791.
16. Jensen DM, Machicado GA, Hirabayashi K. Randomized controlled study of 3 different types of hemoclips for hemostasis of bleeding canine acute gastric ulcers. Gastrointest Endosc 2006;64:768–73.
17. Sung JJ, Tsoi KK, Lai LH, Wu JC, Lau JY. Endoscopic clipping versus injection and thermo-coagulation in the treatment of non-variceal upper gastrointestinal bleeding: a meta-analysis. Gut 2007;56:1364–73.
18. Lin HJ, Hsieh YH, Tseng GY, Perng CL, Chang FY, Lee SD. A prospective, randomized trial of endoscopic hemoclip versus heater probe thermocoagulation for peptic ulcer bleeding. Am J Gastroenterol 2002;97: 2250–4.
19. Vergara M, Calvet X, Gisbert JP. Epinephrine injection versus epinephrine injection and a second endoscopic method in high risk bleeding ulcers. Cochrane Database Syst Rev 2007;(2):CD 005 584.
20. Forrest JA, Finlayson ND, Shearman DJ. Endoscopy in gastrointestinal bleeding. Lancet 1974;2:394–7.
21. Kahi CJ, Jensen DM, Sung JJ, Bleau BL, Jung HK, Eckert G, et al. Endoscopic therapy versus medical therapy for bleeding peptic ulcer with adherent clot: a meta-analysis. Gastroenterology 2005;129:855–62.
22. Swain CP, Storey DW, Bown SG, Heath J, Mills TN, Salmon PR, et al. Nature of the bleeding vessel in recurrently bleeding gastric ulcers. Gastroenterology 1986;90:595–608.
23. Lai KC, Swain CP. The size of vessel in patients dying from bleeding gastric ulcer [abstract]. Gastroenterology 1993;104:A202.
24. Barkun A, Bardou M, Marshall JK; Nonvariceal Upper GI Bleeding Consensus Conference Group. Consensus recommendations for managing patients with nonvariceal upper gastrointestinal bleeding. Ann Intern Med 2003;139:843–57.
25. Juler GL, Labitzke HG, Lamb R, Allen R. The pathogenesis of Dieulafoy's gastric erosion. Am J Gastroenterol 1984;79:195–200.
26. Stiegmann GV, Cambre T, Sun JH. A new endoscopic elastic band ligating device. Gastrointest Endosc 1986;32:230–3.
27. Stiegmann GV, Goff JS, Michaletz-Onody PA, Korula J, Lieberman D, Saeed ZA, et al. Endoscopic sclerotherapy as compared with endoscopic ligation for bleeding esophageal varices. N Engl J Med 1992; 326: 1527–32.
28. Laine L, Cook D. Endoscopic ligation compared with sclerotherapy for treatment of esophageal variceal bleeding: a meta-analysis. Ann Intern Med 1995;123:280–7.
29. Karsan HA, Morton SC, Shekelle PG, Spiegel BM, Suttorp MJ, Edelstein MA, et al. Combination endoscopic band ligation and sclerotherapy compared with endoscopic band ligation alone for the secondary prophylaxis of esophageal variceal hemorrhage: a meta-analysis. Dig Dis Sci 2005;50: 399–406.
30. Singh P, Pooran N, Indaram A, Bank S. Combined ligation and sclerotherapy versus ligation alone for secondary prophylaxis of esophageal variceal bleeding: a meta-analysis. Am J Gastroenterol 2002;97:623–9.
31. Lo GH, Lai KH, Cheng JS, Lin CK, Huang JS, Hsu PI, et al. The additive effect of sclerotherapy to patients receiving repeated endoscopic variceal ligation: a prospective, randomized trial. Hepatology 1998;28:391–5.
32. Sarin SK, Lahoti D, Saxena SP, Murthy NS, Makwana UK. Prevalence, classification and natural history of gastric varices: a long-term follow-up study in 568 portal hypertension patients. Hepatology 1992;16: 1343–9.
33. Yoshida T, Hayashi N, Suzumi N, Miyazaki S, Terai S, Itoh T, et al. Endoscopic ligation of gastric varices using a detachable snare. Endoscopy 1994;26:502–5.
34. Cipolletta L, Bianco MA, Rotondano G, Piscopo R, Prisco A, Garofano ML. Emergency endoscopic ligation of actively bleeding gastric varices with a detachable snare. Gastrointest Endosc 1998;47:400–3.
35. Laine L, Petersen WL. Bleeding peptic ulcer. N Engl J Med 1994;331: 717–27.
36. Stiegmann GV. Endoscopic management of esophageal varices. Adv Surg 1994;3:209–31.

25

26 Laser Application

Hugh Barr

Physics and Principles of Laser Therapy

The word "laser" is an acronym for *l*ight *a*mplification by the *s*timulated *e*mission of *r*adiation. Light has a dual nature, behaving both as a wave and as a quantum-mechanical particle (photon). Its wave nature gives light a wavelength and an oscillation frequency. Its particle aspect allows it to carry a discrete amount of energy. Both wave and particle viewpoints are helpful in understanding the principles involved in lasers, although the concept of a particle is more important.

Quantum mechanics limits atoms and molecules to discrete states of energy, with instantaneous transitions between energy levels occurring when energy is absorbed or released. This transition energy is often manifest as a photon. The electrons orbiting the nucleus of an atom have specific energy levels, with electrons further away from the nucleus having a higher energy state and lower-orbiting electrons remaining in the ground state. Consider an incoming photon with a specific quantum of energy that matches the difference between the two energy levels of the atom. This photon can be absorbed to produce an excited atom, with an electron moving to a higher energy (orbital) level. Spontaneous emission occurs if the electron spontaneously returns to a lower orbital, releasing a photon. Stimulated emission occurs if an atom is already in an excited state when struck by another photon. Absorption cannot occur, and instead a second photon of equal frequency, energy, and direction as the stimulating photon is released.

Atoms will always tend to arrange themselves in such a way that there are more in lower than in higher energy states. Thus, in ordinary circumstances, absorption always occurs. Stimulated emission can occur if more atoms are in the higher energy state—a condition known as a population inversion. This excited state is necessary for laser action, and it can be achieved by "pumping" the laser medium with light, heat, or chemical reactions. Stimulated emission produces light that travels in the same direction, but it is a weak effect that can only build to high powers after the light has traveled long distances in an optical resonator.

Light from a laser has several very special properties. It is coherent, with photons traveling in the same direction and being in step with each other in both time (temporal coherence) and space (spatial coherence). The high spatial coherence means that the divergence of the laser beam is very small (the output is collimated). The light is monochromatic, polarized, and the irradiance of the beam is very high. Most notably for the endoscopist, it can be focused down optical fibers with very high powers.

Interaction of Laser Light with Tissue

On striking an air–tissue interface, some photons are reflected from the surface (specular reflection). On penetrating the tissue, some photons are "back-scattered" and escape the tissue (diffuse reflection). In order for a biological reaction to occur, light must be absorbed by components of tissue. Nonspecific absorption results in heating of the tissue. The temperature reached is dependent on the thermal conduction, diffusion, and storage properties of the tissue, and the vascular supply. Local heating of malignant tissue up to 45 °C may produce selective hyperthermic destruction of more heat-sensitive neoplastic cells. At greater temperatures, all cells are rapidly killed, and as the temperature rises above 60 °C, thermal contraction and coagulation of tissue occur, with small vessels being sealed. Thrombosis of the occluded vessel is a secondary event. This hemostatic effect of laser light is best when the volume of tissue heated is relatively large (5 mm). The neodymium:yttrium–aluminum garnet (Nd:YAG) laser is able to seal vessels up to 1 mm in diameter. If more energy is used, tissue necrosis occurs, with vaporization at water's boiling temperature of 100 °C.

In certain circumstances, thermal effects of the laser beam are not required, but photons are required to generate a photochemical reaction, similar in many ways to photosynthetic and photodestructive reactions in plants. Photodynamic therapy involves the activation of administered or generated photosensitizers in tissue by light to produce tumor and tissue destruction.

"Nonlinear" laser–tissue interactions occur when tissue is exposed to pulsed laser light. The Excimer (ultraviolet light) laser produces a beam in which the individual photon energy is very high and highly absorbed. Thus, the laser beam is capable of breaking interatomic bonds, and photoablation occurs. The important biological feature is the very sharp cut between normal and ablated tissue, with no charred zone as occurs with photothermal ablation.

A further nonlinear effect is exploited for laser lithotripsy. When directed at a hard stone, a pulsed laser beam can shatter it. Most biliary and pancreatic calculi can be removed at endoscopic sphincterotomy. However, mechanical lithotripsy may fail if the baskets fail to capture large stones in collapsed ducts. A flashlamp-pumped dye laser with a repetition rate of 1–10 Hz delivering 60–150 mJ energy in pulses of 2.5 ms can disintegrate most biliary stones. It is possible to incorporate an optical detection system based on the back-scattered light to ensure that the laser fiber is in contact with the stone [1]. The holmium:yttrium–aluminium garnet (Ho:YAG) laser is also a promising laser for lithotripsy. It has a repetition frequency of 5 Hz and a pulse energy of 114–159 mJ/pulse. Five pulses with this laser will perforate biliary epithelium, making the need for a stone recognition system an important safety feature.

Types of Lasers

Several lasers are used for the thermal effects that they produce. The commonly used lasers for endoscopic photothermal applications are Nd:YAG (1064 nm), frequency-doubled Nd:YAG or potassium titanyl phosphate (KTP, 532 nm), argon ion laser (514.5 nm), and the diode laser (805 nm). The carbon dioxide (CO_2, wavelength 10 600 nm) laser is not used with flexible endoscopy because of the difficulty in transmitting the beam through fiberoptics. The beam from the CO_2 laser produces a very localized effect being rapidly absorbed by water, causing vaporization with very small areas of coagulation (0.1 mm). In contrast, the Nd:YAG beam produces coagulation up to 6 mm into tissue, with only superficial vaporization. The reason is that the photon from the Nd:YAG laser is ten times more likely to be scattered than absorbed, so that it will travel further into tissue before absorption occurs. The KTP and argon ion lasers have a penetration depth of 0.3 mm in stomach tissue and will produce 1 mm of histological damage lateral to and below the incident beam. Their wavelength of light is well absorbed by vascular tissue and is very effective for the treatment of angiodysplasia. The diode laser will penetrate to a greater depth, but less than that of the Nd:YAG laser.

Endoscopic photodynamic therapy usually uses a dye laser or a diode laser (630 nm, 654 nm). The most important feature in this form of treatment is matching the wavelength of light to the action spectrum of the absorbing photosensitizer. In order to penetrate deeply into tissue, photosensitizers activated in the red end of the spectrum are usually chosen. Lithotripsy requires a pulsed Nd:YAG or dye laser.

Endoscopic Laser Therapy

■ Hemostasis

The use of lasers is now being overtaken by the widespread application of lower-cost thermal devices for controlling acute hemorrhage. The Nd:YAG laser has been predominantly used for the management of acute peptic ulcer hemorrhage. It is highly effective, with a significantly lower rebleeding rate and mortality in comparison with control patients and those treated with the heater probe only. However, local injection therapy with epinephrine has been shown to be equally effective and has superseded laser therapy. There is now no rationale for laser treatment for variceal hemorrhage.

Argon ion, KTP, diode, and Nd:YAG lasers have been used to coagulate gastrointestinal angiodysplasias. Initial data from the treatment with the argon ion laser for vascular abnormalities in the stomach indicated that often the bulk of the abnormality was not destroyed and was preserved in the submucosa. The Nd:YAG laser coagulates vessels at a greater depth (1.75 mm in the stomach wall) and will control hemorrhage in over 80% of patients. There is recurrent bleeding in approximately 10% of patients with isolated vascular lesions, but in over 60% of patients with multiple abnormalities (e. g., Osler–Weber-Rendu disease). The Nd:YAG laser is set to deliver 60–80 W in pulses of 0.5–1.0 s. The fiber is usually used in noncontact mode, with the fiber tip being placed 1–2 cm away from the tissue. Visible whitening of the tissue indicates coagulation, with destruction of the lesion. Complications of laser photocoagulation include perforation in 3–4% of patients. There is also a risk of delayed hemorrhage. Argon plasma coagulation is now more widely used for thermal control of hemorrhagic lesions.

Palliative treatment for advanced bleeding gastric cancer is much more difficult. Palliative radiotherapy to the stomach is proving to be highly effective. Most tumors do not bleed from a specific site, but ooze diffusely from the exposed surface. It is necessary to completely coagulate the entire surface of the tumor in order to achieve hemostasis. Often, in these large tumors, the entire surface is not accessible and is covered with blood, preventing direct coagulation of the surface. Tumors greater than 8–10 cm in diameter may be impossible to treat endoscopically. However, low-powered interstitial laser hyperthermia has proved to be useful. The Nd:YAG laser is set to deliver 1–5 W of power for 200–1000 s (100 J). The laser fiber is then inserted into the center of the tumor. The core of the lesion is photocoagulated. Several areas can be treated, controlling the bleeding and reducing transfusion requirements for the remainder of the patient's life [2].

■ Palliation of Malignant Dysphagia

Obstructing esophageal cancer usually presents with malignant dysphagia. Many patients are unsuitable for radical curative therapy, and the main effort is directed at relieving dysphagia and prolonging symptom-free life. Laser therapy is highly effective in recanalizing the esophageal lumen (**Figs. 26.1–26.3**). The endoscopic results are often very satisfactory, and most patients can be restored to swallowing a near-normal diet. The effect is often short-lived, and repeated treatments need to be performed at intervals of 4–6 weeks to prevent recurrent dysphagia. The mortality is approximately 2%, with the major complication being perforation. This is usually best managed with immediate intubation with a covered self-expanding stent, and aggressive conservative therapy with antibiotics and intravenous feeding. Attempting radical surgical resection is highly dangerous in this group of patients and is associated with increased mortality.

The laser is a method of applying heat, and there are several other thermal methods of tumor destruction. The overall effect is similar whether a laser or a lower-cost device such as an argon plasma coagulator (APC) is used. Tissue is vaporized and coagulated, either to remove obstruction or arrest bleeding. The APC is generally considered to be less efficient than laser coagulation, and more treatments may be required to produce the same effect [3].

An important large randomized comparison (including 236 patients) of thermal Nd:YAG laser with photodynamic therapy (PDT) showed that the two methods were equally effective. PDT was associated with temporary photosensitivity, but was easier to per-

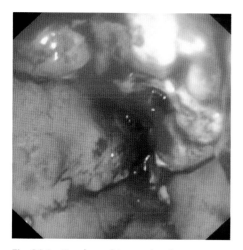

Fig. 26.1 Esophageal tumor. An obstructing esophageal cancer arising in Barrett's esophagus.

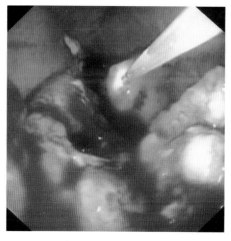

Fig. 26.2 Nd:YAG laser therapy, starting distally and working more proximally.

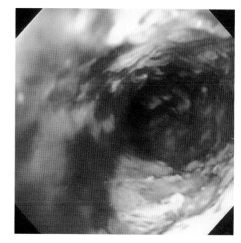

Fig. 26.3 The esophageal lumen is widely open.

form and associated with less perforations (PDT 1 %, thermal laser 7 %) [4]. Injection of alcohol and intratumoral chemotherapy can also be very useful. As with PDT and thermal therapy treatment, it has to be repeated.

A combination of endoscopic laser therapy with intraluminal radiotherapy has been used in an attempt to prolong the dysphagia-free interval. There are undoubtedly some beneficial effects, with the time to repeat treatment being between 9 and 11 weeks [5]. There is a worrying incidence of recurrent dysphagia, due to radiotherapy-induced fibrous stricture (34 %) and a combination of intraluminal tumor with fibrous stricture (37 %), with only 29 % of patients requiring no further intervention [6].

The development of self-expanding metal prostheses has allowed intubation of esophageal carcinoma with a low risk of perforation and other complications, similar to the risks associated with laser therapy. The advantage is that this is regarded as a definitive single procedure that may not need to be repeated, although repeat intervention is unfortunately often necessary. The use of covered prostheses is vital for the treatment of tracheo-esophageal fistula. A randomized comparison of endoscopic laser therapy and self-expanding metal prosthesis insertion showed very similar overall results, although the laser therapy was repeated at monthly intervals until death to maintain esophageal patency (**Table 26.1**).

Ampullary and Duodenal Neoplasia

Although ampullary and duodenal carcinoma are unusual tumors, they continue to be a challenging clinical problem. In addition, there is the increasing problem of adenomatous polyp and carcinoma development in patients with familial adenomatous polyposis. Nd:YAG laser photocoagulation of the tumor may aid local control, preventing bleeding and duodenal obstruction (**Figs. 26.4, 26.5**). The median survival period in these patients, who are unsuitable for surgery or decline surgical resection, was 20 months. This compares with a median survival of 12 months in historical series of patients treated with sphincterotomy or stent insertion alone [7].

Colorectal Cancer

Nd:YAG laser therapy still has a role in the treatment of colorectal cancers and large adenomas (up to 12 cm) that may be unsuitable for snare resection [8]. A large multicenter review demonstrated that the symptoms of obstruction, bleeding, and abnormal discharge could be effectively controlled in 80–100 % of patients, mostly those with rectal cancer. Comparison of endoscopic transanal resection with endoscopic laser therapy, specifically for rectal cancer, has demonstrated that endoscopic laser therapy is safer and that symptom control is similar (**Table 26.2**) [9,10]. Usually, transanal resection is performed with the patient under general or regional anesthesia and is limited to the lower rectum.

Early Gastrointestinal Cancer and Precancer

Radical surgical excision of upper gastrointestinal cancers is a procedure with high rates of morbidity and mortality. Surveillance of patients with columnar-lined (Barrett's) esophagus and previous squamous cell carcinomas of the upper aerodigestive tract is now becoming accepted. This results in the early detection of very small neoplastic changes in asymptomatic patients. The detection of these lesions in the lining of the gastrointestinal tract must be matched with methods of endoscopic therapy to destroy the lesion and cure the patient. Endoscopic laser therapy is clearly an option.

Table 26.1 Randomized comparison of endoscopic laser therapy and self-expanding metal prosthesis insertion. The stricture size was measured at radiological screening by the ability of barium-dissolving wax spheres (2–18 mm) to pass through the stricture. Dysphagia grades: 0, saliva; 1, water; 2, milk; 3, custard; 4, jelly; 5, scrambled egg; 6, baked fish; 7, bread/cake; 8, apple/fruit; 9, meat

	Laser (n = 10)	Self-expanding metal prosthesis (n = 10)
Mean stricture size		
• Pretreatment (mm)	4.9	5.3
• Post-treatment (mm)	9.8	9.7
Mean dysphagia grade		
• Pretreatment	2.7	2.9
• Post-treatment	5.9	5.7
Mean survival (weeks)	17 (4–36)	15 (2–28)
Complications	2 *	2 †

* Fistula, resistant stricture.
† Food bolus obstruction and tumor overgrowth.

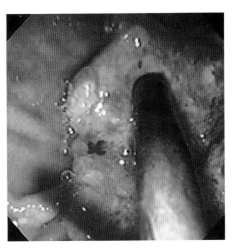

Fig. 26.4 View of a periampullary tumor.

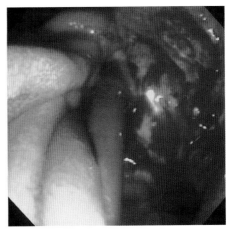

Fig. 26.5 The area has been completely destroyed with the laser.

On theoretical grounds, the potassium titanyl phosphate (KTP) laser has tissue penetration characteristics that should allow safe thermal treatment of mucosal disease. Photothermal laser ablation is nonspecific, targeting dysplastic, metaplastic, and normal tissue equally. This may be of little consequence provided that the depth of damage does not risk perforation and that healing occurs without fibrosis and a risk of stricture formation.

26

Table 26.2 Comparative studies of endoscopic laser therapy performed under sedation, and endoscopic transanal resection, usually performed under general anesthetic, in palliative treatment for rectal cancer

	Barr 1995 [9]		Tacke et al. 1993 [10]	
	Endoscopic laser therapy	Endoscopic transanal resection	Endoscopic laser therapy	Endoscopic transanal resection
Patients	65	41	37	26
Symptom control (%) *	94	88	95	100
Median survival (months)	8	11	8	14
Mortality (%)	3	10	0	4
Morbidity (%)	4.5	12	0	4

Mainly bleeding and obstruction.

Three types of laser have been compared for the thermal destruction of superficial areas of nondysplastic mucosa in the esophagus: Nd:YAG (1064 nm), KTP (532 nm), and diode (805 nm). Irradiation with the KTP laser (power 15–20 W for a pulse of 1 s) produced mucosal temperatures of more than 65 °C, with a temperature of 21 °C on the outer surface of the esophagus. It was extremely difficult to generate high temperatures on the external surface of the esophagus using the KTP laser. The diode laser (25 W for 5 s) was able to produce surface temperatures of 90 °C, but with an external temperature of 38 °C. The Nd:YAG laser tended to produce worrying temperatures through to the external surface at energy levels that were sufficient to produce thermal destruction on the mucosa. For the clinical application of laser photodestruction for the eradication of dysplastic and nondysplastic Barrett's esophagus, the KTP laser is often chosen as the safest method and as the one most likely to produce intense superficial destruction only. It has proved to be highly effective for the treatment of dysplasia and early cancer [11]. The Nd:YAG laser has been used very effectively, but the risk of perforation and full-thickness damage is greater. Using the KTP laser, mucosal ablation of metaplastic Barrett's accompanied by profound acid suppression with proton-pump inhibitor therapy often results in satisfactory endoscopic results (**Figs. 26.6, 26.7**). However, the histological appearance of the esophagus reveals residual glands in many patients.

Attempts to target the dysplastic and metaplastic mucosa are possible using photodynamic therapy after endogenous photosensitization with aminolevulinic acid (5-ALA). There are extensive data on the uptake and distribution of photosensitizers in the gastrointestinal mucosa. In the esophageal mucosa, protoporphyrin IX (PpIX) is generated in the epithelial cells, whether squamous or columnar, with maximum levels occurring 3 h after oral administration of 5-ALA. The uptake in the mucosa was 3.5 times greater than in the muscularis propria. There was little difference between oral or parental administration of the 5-ALA. Following the accumulation of PpIX, a photodynamic action will only occur after light irradiation, usually from a dye laser.

There have been two major clinical studies of 5-ALA photodynamic therapy for the ablation of high-grade dysplasia. Both have

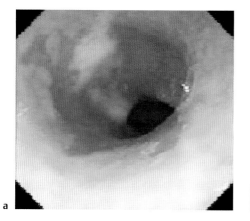
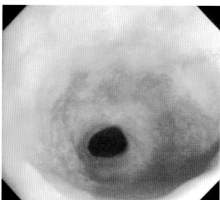

Fig. 26.6 Thermal ablation using the Nd:YAG laser to eradicate Barrett's esophagus.
a There is clear reflux injury.
b The endoscopic examination 12 weeks later shows some residual areas of Barrett's, which were ablated at the next endoscopic examination.

a, b

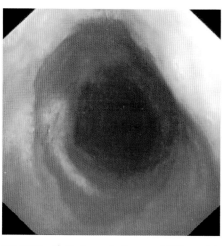
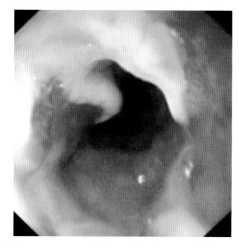
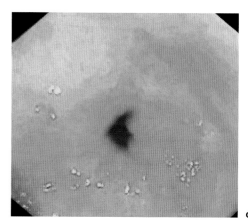

Fig. 26.7 Photodynamic therapy (PDT) used to ablate a segment of Barrett's esophagus with intramucosal carcinoma.
a The initial appearance.
b Forty-eight hours after PDT, with extensive necrosis of the lining of the esophagus.
c The result after 6 weeks, showing extensive squamous reepithelialization, with some residual areas of Barrett's that require ablation with the KTP laser.

V

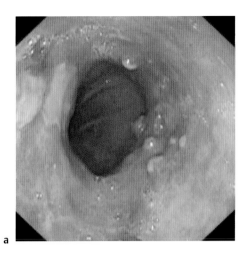
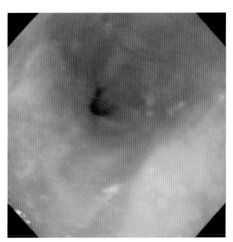

a b

Fig. 26.8 An area of multifocal dysplasia in the esophagus before (**a**) and after (**b**) treatment over an extensive area using thermal laser therapy with the Nd:YAG and KTP laser.

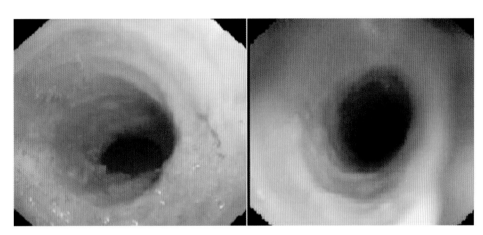

Fig. 26.9 An area of elevated and nodular squamous dysplasia that has been destroyed using the KTP laser. The image shows the endoscopic appearance 6 weeks later.

26

demonstrated eradication of the dysplasia, and one series demonstrated successful eradication of T1 tumors that were less than 2 mm in depth. A prospective randomized trial of treatment for low-grade dysplasia using ALA and irradiation with green light, rather than the usual 630 nm red light, has again confirmed how effective this treatment is in reversing both dysplasia and metaplasia. Healing proceeded with the regeneration of neosquamous epithelium. A variation of 5-ALA photodynamic therapy involves direct endoscopic spraying of the agent, combined with sodium bicarbonate as a mucolytic, onto dysplastic Barrett's esophagus. A period of time is allowed for local absorption, and then the area is irradiated with light. The response following this technique was variable, with two of nine patients failing to show any response [12].

Photodynamic therapy for early cancer and high-grade dysplasia can also be carried out using intravenously administered photosensitizers. Great encouragement for this technique was received when Sibille et al. published a large series of patients with early squamous cell carcinoma and adenocarcinoma treated with photodynamic therapy using a hematoporphyrin derivative [13]. These patients had comorbid disease and were considered unsuitable for surgery. Sixty-one patients were staged using endosonography as uT1, and 27 patients had uT2 tumors. The 5-year disease-specific survival was 74%. The complete response rate did not differ between patients treated with photodynamic therapy alone or with a combination of chemotherapy, radiotherapy, and photodynamic therapy. This gave a clear indication that if the cancer was local to the esophagus, then local therapy could eradicate the disease and lead to prolonged survival. At present, photodynamic therapy and photothermal therapy are equally effective in eradicating dysplastic lesions and early cancer (**Fig. 26.8**).

The most important randomized and controlled trial in this area has been a partially blinded study of the prevention of cancer in Barrett's esophagus, in which 208 patients with confirmed high-grade dysplasia were examined. It is very instructive to note that over 485 patients (with a diagnosis of high-grade dysplasia) had to be screened for 208 patients with confirmed high-grade dysplasia to be included. The patients were randomly assigned (2 : 1) in such a way that 138 received PDT and omeprazole and 70 received omeprazole alone. At the end of the minimum 24-month follow-up period, ablation of all areas of high-grade dysplasia was noted in 76.8% of patients in the PDT plus omeprazole group, versus 38.6% in the omeprazole group ($P < 0.0001$). After a mean follow-up period of 24.2 months, 13.0% of patients in the PDT plus omeprazole group had disease progression to cancer, in comparison with 28% in the omeprazole group after a mean follow-up of 18.6 months. Strictures occurred in 37.1% of patients following PDT [14]. These data establish that photodynamic therapy is now a highly effective treatment for the eradication of high-grade dysplasia in Barrett's esophagus (**Fig. 26.9**). The data have been used to show that photodynamic therapy is the most cost-effective solution for treatment of photodynamic therapy [15], and a report on the long-term efficacy of the method has shown that these excellent results are maintained after 5 years of follow-up [16]. Radiofrequency ablation has also recently come into widespread use for the ablation of Barrett's esophagus. A recent comparative study demonstrated that 83% of patients had endoscopic resolution following PDT, in comparison with 63% in the radiofrequency group [17]. Strictures occurred in both groups.

A randomized trial compared ALA photodynamic therapy following continuous light and fractionated irradiation and APC thermal coagulation for ablation in patients with low-grade dysplasia and no dysplasia in Barrett's esophagus [18]. The results showed that the mean endoscopic reduction of Barrett's esophagus at 6 weeks was 51 % for ALA with continuous irradiation, 86 % following fractionated irradiation, and 93 % following APC treatment. A comparison of endoscopic devices, argon plasma coagulation, and multipolar thermocoagulation has shown that the latter resulted in fewer treatment sessions, with significantly more patients achieving histological ablation. The study included 52 patients with Barrett's esophagus segments 2–7 cm in length, without cancer or high-grade dysplasia, who were followed up with 6-monthly endoscopies for up to 4 years [19].

Biliary Tract

The most important application for laser is the treatment of cholangiocarcinoma using endoscopic photodynamic therapy. A very important randomized multicenter study compared stent insertion with stent insertion plus photodynamic therapy for the treatment of unresectable cholangiocarcinoma. A standard dose of porfimer sodium (2 mg/kg) was given by intravenous injection 2 days before intraluminal irradiation with 630-nm laser light at 180 J/cm^2. There was a striking statistically significant survival advantage for those treated with photodynamic therapy (493 days) in comparison with those who received stenting alone (98 days) [20]. These findings have been confirmed, with the PDT/stent group surviving 16 months in comparison with 7.4 months for those with stenting alone, with very minimal side effects of skin phototoxicity [21].

Extrahepatic and intrahepatic common bile duct and pancreatic ductal stones can be shattered using a high-power density focused Ho:YAG laser beam, a frequency-doubled YAG laser, or a pulsed dye laser. The stone can be accessed using endoscopic retrograde cholangiopancreatography (ERCP), choledochoscopy, pancreatoscopy, or a combination of methods, and the laser energy can be directed via a long optical fiber. There is minimal risk of damage to surrounding ductal tissue, and the lithotripsy is targeted very accurately to the stone. Complications are unusual, with few occurring in comparison with mechanical lithotripsy. Overall, there is a 7–9 % complete procedural complication rate, often associated with the ERCP; the most common complications are hemobilia, cholangitis, and very rarely ductal perforation. There are randomized trial data showing that laser lithotripsy can achieve complete bile duct clearance in 92 % of patients, in comparison with only 66 % of those treated with extracorporeal shock-wave lithotripsy (EWSL). Patients treated using the latter technique have a 30–40 % complication rate, most commonly with biliary colic [22].

Conclusions

Endoscopic laser therapy with thermal ablation and photodynamic therapy has an established role in the treatment of both advanced and early neoplastic lesions of the gastrointestinal tract. It is clear that the use of lasers is being overtaken by endoscopic mucosal resection [23,24] and argon beam coagulation [25] for the management of early disease. The use of lasers to control hemorrhage from angiodysplasia is also highly successful. It is rarely necessary to use the laser to treat peptic ulcers or variceal bleeding. Photodynamic therapy for cholangiocarcinoma is proving to be highly effective, with prolonged survival. Currently, laser therapy is most widely used in the treatment of cancer, either with photodynamic therapy or thermal ablation.

References

1. Neuhaus H, Hoffman W, Gottlieb K, Classen M. Endoscopic lithotripsy of bile duct stones using a new laser with automatic stone recognition. Gastrointest Endosc 1995;40:708–15.
2. Barr H, Krasner N. Interstitial laser photocoagulation for treating bleeding gastric cancer. BMJ 1989;299:659–60.
3. Gossner L, Ell C. Malignant stricture thermal treatment. Gastrointest Endosc Clin North Am 1998;8:493–501.
4. Lightdale CJ, Heier SK, Marcon NE, McCaughan JS Jr, Gerdes H, Overholt BF, et al. Photodynamic therapy with porfimer sodium versus thermal ablation therapy with Nd:YAG laser for palliation of esophageal cancer: a multicenter randomized trial. Gastrointest Endosc 1995;42:507–12.
5. Spencer GM, Thorpe SM, Sergeant IR, Blackman GM, Solanao J, Tobias JS, et al. Laser and brachytherapy in the palliation of adenocarcinoma of the oesophagus and cardia. Gut 1996;39:726–31.
6. Shumeli E, Srivastava, Dawes PJ, Claque M, Matthewson K, Record CO. Combination of laser treatment and intraluminal radiotherapy for malignant dysphagia. Gut 1996;38:803–5.
7. Fowler A, Barham PB, Britton BJ, Barr H. Laser ablation of ampullary cancer Endoscopy 1999;31:745–7.
8. Hyser MJ, Gau FC. Endoscopic Nd:YAG laser therapy for villous adenomas of the colon and rectum. Am Surg 1996;62:577–81.
9. Barr H. Laser phototherapy for gastrointestinal cancer [master of surgery thesis]. Liverpool, United Kingdom: University of Liverpool, 1995; 160–9.
10. Tacke W, Peach S, Kruis W, Stuetzer H, Mueller JM, Ziegenhagen DJ, et al. Comparison between endoscopic laser and different surgical treatments for palliation of advanced rectal cancer. Dis Colon Rectum 1993;36:377–82.
11. Gossner L, May A, Stolte M, Seitz G, Hahn EG, Ell C. KTP laser destruction of dysplasia and early cancer in columnar-lined Barrett's esophagus. Gastrointest Endosc 1999;49:8–12.
12. Ortner M, Zumbusch K, Liebetruth J. Photodynamic therapy in Barrett's esophagus after local administration of 5-aminolevulinic acid [abstract]. Gastroenterology 1997;112:A633.
13. Sibille A, Lambert R, Souquet JP, Sabben G, Descos F. Long-term survival after photodynamic therapy for esophageal cancer. Gastroenterology 1995;108:337–44.
14. Overholt BF, Lightdale CJ, Wang KK, Canto MI, Burdick S, Haggitt RC, et al. Photodynamic therapy with porfimer sodium for ablation of high-grade dysplasia in Barrett's esophagus: international, partially blinded, randomized phase III trial. Gastrointest Endosc 2005;62:488–98.
15. Vij R, Triadafilopoulos G, Owens DK, Kunz P, Sanders GD. Cost-effectiveness of photodynamic therapy for high-grade dysplasia in Barrett's esophagus. Gastrointest Endosc 2004;60:739–56.
16. Overholt BF, Wang KK, Burdick JS, Lightdale CJ, Kimmey M, Nava HR, et al. Five-year efficacy and safety of photodynamic therapy with Photofrin in Barrett's high-grade dysplasia. Gastrointest Endosc 2007;66:460–8.
17. Seth A, Gross SA, Gill KR, Wolfsen HC. Comparative outcomes of photodynamic therapy and radiofrequency ablation for treatment of Barrett's esophagus with high-grade dysplasia [abstract]. Gastrointest Endosc 2008;67:AB179.
18. Hage M, Sieresma PD, van Dekken H, Steyerberg EW, Haringsma J, van de Vrie W, et al. 5-Aminolevulinic acid photodynamic therapy versus argon plasma coagulation for ablation of Barrett's oesophagus: a randomised trial. Gut 2004;53:785–90.
19. Kelty CJ, Ackroyd R, Brown NJ, Stephenson TJ, Stoddard CJ, Reed MW. Endoscopic ablation of Barrett's oesophagus: a randomized-controlled trial of photodynamic therapy vs. argon plasma coagulation. Aliment Pharmacol Ther 2004;20:1289–96.
20. Ortner ME, Caca K, Berr F, Liebetruth J, Mansmann U, Huster D, et al. Successful photodynamic therapy for nonresectable cholangiocarcinoma: a randomized prospective study. Gastroenterology 2003;125: 1355–63.
21. Kahaleh M, Mishra R, Shami VM, Northup PG, Berg CL, Bashlor P, et al. Unresectable cholangiocarcinoma: comparison of survival in biliary stenting alone versus stenting with photodynamic therapy. Clin Gastroenterol Hepatol 2008;6:290–7.
22. DiSario J, Chuttani R, Croffie J, Liu J, Mishkin D, Shah R, et al. Biliary and pancreatic lithotripsy devices. Gastrointest Endosc 2007;65:750–6.
23. Barr H, Stone N, Rembacken B. Endoscopic therapy for Barrett's oesophagus. Gut 2005;54:875–84.
24. American Society for Gastrointestinal Endoscopy Technology Committee. Mucosal ablation devices. Gastrointest Endosc 2008;68:1031–42.
25. Basu KK, Pick B, Bale R, West KP, de Caestecker JS. Efficacy and one year follow-up of argon plasma coagulation therapy for ablation of Barrett's oesophagus: factors determining persistence and recurrence of Barrett's epithelium. Gut 2002;51:776–80.

V

27 Argon Plasma Coagulation

James A. DiSario

Technology

Argon plasma coagulation (APC) is a noncontact monopolar technology that allows electrical energy to be delivered to the target tissue as ionized argon gas (argon plasma). Argon plasma that transfers energy to tissue occurs in an electrical field that completes the monopolar circuit via the path of least resistance. The beam can travel at any angle to the target tissue, be it en face or lateral to the electrode. Electrical resistance in tissue increases with coagulation, and the beam moves to adjacent tissue with lower electrical resistance. This helps maintain a relatively constant coagulation depth and confluent tissue destruction [1–5].

The unit consists of an argon source, an electrical generator, a probe that connects to the generator and passes through the endoscope, a grounding pad to complete the monopolar circuit, and an activation pedal. The probe is a flexible Teflon tube that allows argon flow and contains an electrode recessed in the distal tip that ionizes the argon when activated.

The basic generator has wattage controls and induces proportional changes in high-frequency voltage and applies continuous energy over time. Second-generation electrical generators are available that have unique APC modes based on electrical waveforms. The "forced" mode (**Fig. 27.1**) is similar to the first-generation system, but with increased efficiency. Pulsed effects 1 and 2 have discontinuous energy delivery using two frequencies (**Fig. 27.2**). In contrast to forced mode, the pulsed effects have constant high-frequency voltage over the entire setting range. The "precise" mode provides continuous application of energy with an automatic adjustment control that modifies the argon plasma regardless of the impedance of the overall system (**Fig. 27.3**) [6].

APC probes are available in various lengths and diameters and can fire straight, sideways, or circumferentially (**Fig. 27.4**). There may be a mark 10 mm from the tip of the probe, and manufacturers recommend that the probe be extended at least 10 mm outside the endoscope to prevent thermal damage to the instrument. However, this is unlikely, as the endoscope will not transmit the electrical current to complete the monopolar circuit. However, some probes have ceramic tips that may become very hot and could cause direct thermal damage when in contact with the endoscope.

Tissue Effects

The tissue effects of APC are shown in **Fig. 27.5**. Carbonization (charring) is due to combustion in the presence of oxygen and is not clinically beneficial. It may be minimized by suctioning out the oxygen and instilling the inert argon. Factors influencing coagulation depth, in order of decreasing importance, are: 1, duration of application—a longer duration causes deeper burns; 2, power setting in watts or effect in precise mode—higher wattage causes deeper burns; 3, distance from the probe to target tissue—closer positioning causes deeper burns. In vivo porcine studies show that burns often occur through to the muscular propria at standard generator settings [2–4,7].

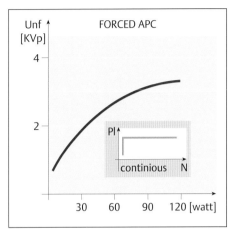

Fig. 27.1 Argon plasma coagulation (APC) in forced mode. The high-frequency voltage (red line) increases as the output setting (W) increases. There is continuous energy output over time (insert). (Reproduced with permission from Erbe Elektromedizin Ltd.)

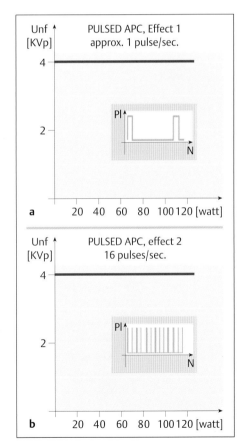

Fig. 27.2 APC in pulsed mode. The voltage for the pulsed APC effect 1 (**a**) and pulsed APC effect 2 (**b**) modes remains constant (red line). Effect 1 produces a higher energy output per pulse, with a longer interval, and effect 2 produces a greater number of pulses with lower energy output per pulse. There is consistent firing from 10 W, with application distances of up to 7 mm from the probe tip to the tissue. High-frequency energy output can be adjusted between 1 and 20 W. (Reproduced with permission from Erbe Elektromedizin Ltd.)

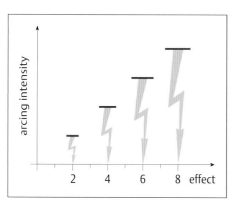

Fig. 27.3 APC in precise mode. There is continuous energy application. The intensity of the ionized plasma increases with effect settings 1–8. The tissue effect is relatively independent of the distance between the probe and tissue up to 5 mm. (Reproduced with permission from Erbe Elektromedizin Ltd.)

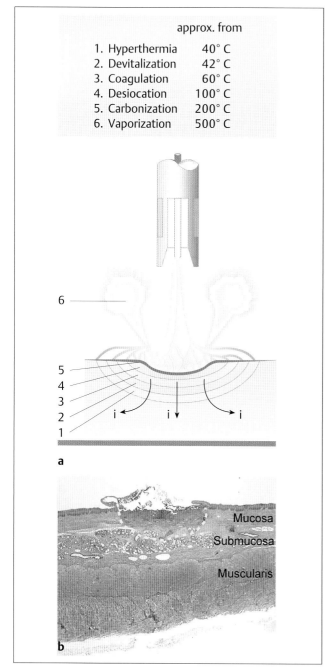

	approx. from
1. Hyperthermia	40° C
2. Devitalization	42° C
3. Coagulation	60° C
4. Desiocation	100° C
5. Carbonization	200° C
6. Vaporization	500° C

Fig. 27.5 Tissue effects of APC. (Reproduced with permission from Erbe Elektromedizin Ltd.)

a Temperature-dependent tissue effects; "i" indicates the direction of argon plasma flow.

b In this porcine histological specimen, the dashed yellow line shows the radial spread of coagulation after application of precise APC effect 1 for 1 s. (Reproduced with permission from Erbe Elektromedizin Ltd.)

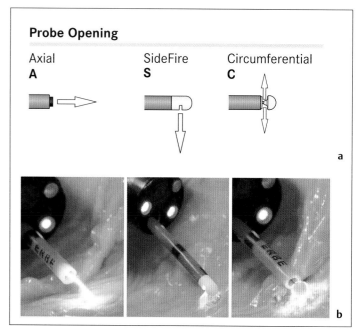

Probe Opening

| Axial | SideFire | Circumferential |
| A | S | C |

Fig. 27.4 a, b Argon plasma coagulation probes. The direction of the argon gas flow depends on the probe tip design and on the position in the lumen. (Reproduced with permission from Erbe Elektromedizin Ltd.)

Clinical Techniques

It is best to begin with the shortest activation time for the desired effect, particularly in thin-walled organs. The optimal power setting or precise effect depends on the location and size of the lesion, and one should follow the manufacturer's recommendations. Typically, lower settings are suitable for very superficial small lesions and in thin-walled organs. Mid-range settings are used for many lesions in which hemostasis, devitalization, and/or tissue reduction are desired. Very high settings are for tissue destruction—for example, debulking tissue and restoring lumen patency. Generally, the penetration depth decreases as the distance from the probe to the tissue increases. However, in Precise mode, the tissue effect remains fairly constant up to a probe distance of 5 mm, and deeper burns may occur at more than 5 mm from the target tissue (**Fig. 27.3**) [6–11]. **Table 27.1** outlines the characteristics, applications, and appropriate organs for each of the modes.

One should insert the probe to protrude about 10 mm from the endoscope, position the tip at the greatest effective distance from the target, keep the endoscope and probe tip in motion when activated to achieve a spray-paint–like effect, and continually suction to minimize distension and to clear fluid and smoke from the field. An effort should be made to avoid touching the mucosa with the probe, to prevent pneumatosis and perforation (**Fig. 27.6**). Blood should be irrigated and suctioned from the field, as the surface blood can be coagulated without stopping the underlying bleeding. The coagulum may be seen to bulge and crack, and blood may ooze from below (**Fig. 27.7**). To minimize electrical interference with video equipment, the grounding pad should be placed as close to the working area as possible and the distance from the probe to the target should be reduced. Thin-walled structures may be thickened by injecting saline to minimize the risk of perforation due to transmural coagulation [3,12].

Table 27.1 Characteristics, applications, and appropriate organs for each of the modes of argon plasma coagulation

Mode	Characteristics	Applications	Organs
Forced	Highest energy output	Hemostasis of small, diffuse areas	Stomach
	Continuous ionized plasma	Debulking	Rectum
	Burns deep and wide	Lumen restoration	Esophagus
	Rapid tissue destruction	Cutting metal stents	Left colon
Pulsed	Less energy output than forced	Hemostasis of diffuse areas	Any
	Not continuous ionized plasma	Devitalization for thinner lesions	Preferable for: right colon, small bowel
	More controlled and superficial effects		
	Long activations—more tissue injury		
• Effect 1	Higher, more focused energy delivery	Static delivery for *small*, superficial lesions	Thin-walled organs
• Effect 2	Lower, more frequent energy delivery	Static delivery for *diffuse*, superficial lesions	Thin-walled organs
Precise	Low energy output	Hemostasis for superficial lesions	Right colon
	Superficial effects	When it is difficult to keep the probe off the lumen (e.g., in enteroscopy)	Small bowel
	Effect independent of distance to tissue		Thin walls

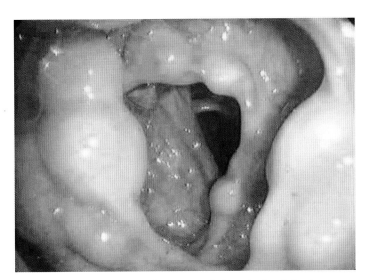

Fig. 27.6 Endoscopic view of pneumatosis intestinalis of the transverse colon, 3 months after argon plasma coagulation treatment for polyps. Argon gas is inert and is not absorbed, and it may persist in the body for long periods of time.

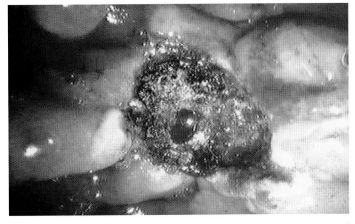

Fig. 27.7 Endoscopic image of a bleeding polypectomy site after an initial argon plasma coagulation treatment that only coagulated the surface blood, but not the underlying bleeding source. The dark coagulated crust is cracking under pressure from the uncoagulated blood oozing from below.

Clinical Applications and Outcomes

Tissue Ablation

Barrett's Esophagus

Barrett's esophagus is a premalignant metaplastic change in the esophageal mucosa caused by chronic reflux of gastric acid and duodenal secretions. Progression to high-grade dysplasia is associated with a significant cancer risk, and esophagectomy has historically been the treatment of choice. However, the associated morbidity, mortality, and impaired quality of life are significant detractors. Newer therapies that destroy or remove the metaplastic epithelium, in conjunction with potent acid reduction using proton-pump inhibitors or fundoplication, may lead to the restoration of a seemingly normal neosquamous epithelium. Such technologies include thermal, photochemical, and/or cryotherapy ablation, and/or endoscopic mucosal resection of the Barrett's epithelium. However, the value of this approach is limited by incomplete ablation and serious morbidity. There are no randomized studies comparing ablation with surgery, and the long-term data are limited [5].

Photodynamic therapy reduces the risk of cancer following the ablation of Barrett's epithelium with high-grade dysplasia [13]. The American College of Gastroenterology recommends endoscopic therapy only with mucosal resection and only for high-grade dysplasia, with no firm position on ablation therapies [14].

APC has been used for ablation of Barrett's epithelium and is best suited to short, flat, easily accessible lesions. Longer segments require multiple procedures and are associated with greater post-treatment discomfort, complications, and increased recurrence rates. Multifocal high-grade dysplasia imparts an increased cancer risk and is more difficult to ablate [15]. Nodular disease is likely to require mucosal resection, with or without adjuvant ablation. Other technologies, especially radiofrequency ablation, may have better outcomes and should be considered in these circumstances [16].

Anticoagulants and antiplatelet drugs should be discontinued in accordance with the unit's protocol. Most authorities recommend high-dose (double-dose) proton-pump inhibitors or fundoplication. Endoscopy can usually be done with standard sedation on an outpatient basis and usually requires 5–20 min. The technique involves identification of the columnar epithelium, which can be facilitated by chromoendoscopy with Lugol solution, narrow-band imaging, or electronic adjustment of the optical wavelengths, with high-resolution or magnification endoscopy. The 7-Fr or 10-Fr straight or side-

27

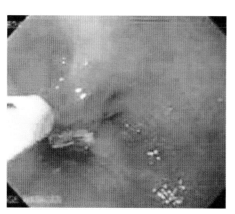

Fig. 27.8 Argon plasma coagulation of short-segment Barrett's esophagus with high-grade dysplasia. White coagulum is seen following treatment.

firing APC probe is inserted through the endoscope and positioned tangentially 5–10 mm from the selected Barrett's segment. Using power settings of 15–90 W and argon flow of about 1.5–2.0 L/min in the forced mode, the device is energized. Coagulation is generally done from distal to proximal in overlapping longitudinal stripes that give a white coagulum with moderate depth. It is important to keep the endoscope and probe in constant motion, overlapping the margins to achieve confluent ablation. Frequent suctioning to minimize abdominal distension should be done to remove smoke, keeping the visual field clear. Short segments and small areas can be treated in a single session (**Fig. 27.8**). More extensive disease requires repeated sessions. No more than 50 % of the circumference of the esophagus should be coagulated in a single session, to minimize potential dysphagia, chest pain, and stricture formation. Endoscopy should be repeated every 4–8 weeks until ablation is complete. Topical or systemic analgesics may be provided for large treatments. The patient will require continued endoscopic surveillance, with biopsies of visualized Barrett's and neosquamous epithelium to look for buried columnar epithelium.

From a total of 22 series including 781 patients with mostly nondysplastic Barrett's esophagus who were followed for a mean of 28 months (range 2–78 months), it appears that a mean of 3.7 (range 1–10) endoscopies with APC using a mean of 63 W (range 30–90 W) resulted in complete eradication (visual or histological) of Barrett's epithelium in a mean of 72 patients (range 62–100 patients; 10.8 %). Recurrences, including buried glands, advanced dysplasia, and cancer were found in a mean of 20 patients (range 0–68 patients; 39 %), a rate of about 3–6 % per year. Circumferential disease and longer segments are associated with incomplete ablation and recurrence. Morbidity occurred in a mean of eight patients (range 0–43 patients; 97.6 %) and included pain, fever, pleural effusions, pneumomediastinum, dysphagia, bleeding, perforation, stenoses requiring dilation, and death [17–38]. A recent meta-analysis shows that APC is more effective than photodynamic therapy in the treatment of endoscopic and histological regression of Barrett's esophagus (OR 3.46; 95 % CI, 1.67 to 7.81; $P = 0.008$), but there was no statistically significant difference between APC and multipolar electrocautery (OR 2.01; 95 % CI, 0.77 to 5.23; $P = 0.15$) [39].

Esophageal Cancer

Early esophageal cancers are less than 2 cm in diameter, moderately differentiated or well differentiated, and show no lymph-node involvement on endoscopic ultrasound. The lesions have a minimal risk of lymphovascular involvement and may be amenable to endoscopic therapy. There are limited data on APC ablation, and its role as a sole therapy is uncertain. Endoscopic mucosal resection can be carried out to remove the lesion and associated Barrett's epithelium, providing tissue for staging. Complete remission of neoplastic tissue

is reported in more than 90 % of patients, with relapse in 11–28 %, which is usually endoscopically treated. Morbidity is usually mild and occurs in 6–13 % of cases, with bleeding, stenosis, and perforation. There is rare mortality [40–42]. Adjunct ablation therapy with photodynamic therapy or APC is effective in treating residual dysplastic tissue, eradicating Barrett's epithelium and minimizing relapses [9,15,41–44]. APC ablative therapy alone for early cancer has been reported in six patients, with initial complete remission and a recurrence in one patient, who received successful repeat treatment [34,45].

APC is useful for palliative debulking and recanalizing luminal obstruction due to unresectable cancer. The technique is to use high power settings (60–90 W) and flow rates (1.6–2.0 L/min). The endoscope is passed into the stomach, which may require esophageal dilation. It is best to use a large-channel or dual-channel endoscope for continual fluid and smoke suctioning. The cardia can be coagulated in a retroflexed fashion with little if any potential for the argon beam to damage the endoscope, as it will not transmit electricity to complete the monopolar circuit. However, contact between the heated probe tip and the endoscope could cause thermal damage. Esophageal lesions are treated from distal to proximal by slowly retracting the endoscope with the protruding probe, using continued coagulation in overlapping longitudinal stripes, and/or by coagulating particular targets in a static position for several seconds before moving. Coagulated tissue can be pushed into the stomach with the endoscope, and more tissue will slough within 48 h. Results from three series including 123 patients who were treated with approximately two procedures each (range 1–18 procedures) show that luminal patency in dysphagic patients was achieved in a mean of 87 procedures (range 71–100; 70 %), while 10 perforations occurred (8 %), leading to one death. The overall survival was a mean of 98–190 days (range 5–612 days) [46–48]. APC has also been used to ablate tumor ingrowth or overgrowth causing stent obstruction [49–51].

Gastric Cancer

Early gastric cancers are confined to the mucosa or submucosa, with no lymph-node metastases. Factors associated with lymphovascular involvement include a diameter larger than 3 cm and histopathological ulceration [52]. The standard endoscopic approach is mucosal resection, but APC can be used in patients who are unfit for mucosal resection. Results from four series including 87 patients who were treated with one to three sessions of APC at about 60 W and 2 L/min, and who were followed for up to means of 21–30 months, show initial ablation in 99 % of cases. Relapse occurs in 27 % of cases, depending on the size and morphology of the lesion and the depth of invasion [53–55]. APC has also been applied as adjuvant therapy after mucosal resection, and to debulk large gastric tumors and restore luminal patency after malignant gastric outlet obstruction [49].

Small-Bowel and Ampullary Adenomas

APC therapy applied to the resection margins of large colorectal adenomas after snare resection reduces recurrence rates [56]. It can also be used for primary therapy and as an adjuvant to endoscopic resection of small-bowel and ampullary adenomas that occur sporadically or in familial adenomatous polyposis (FAP). APC can be applied in the duodenum, jejunum, ileum, and ileal pouches using gastroscopes, duodenoscopes, and push and balloon enteroscopes. APC is also useful for ablating the numerous small to medium-sized polyps found in FAP patients (**Fig. 27.9**). APC was used as the sole therapy in 15 patients with sporadic duodenal polyps. With a me-

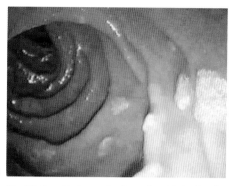
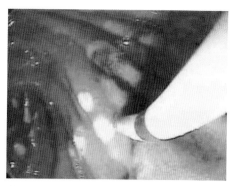
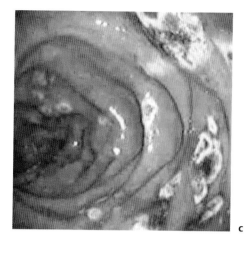

Fig. 27.9 a Endoscopic view of multiple duodenal polyps in a patient with familial adenomatous polyposis.
b A 7-Fr APC probe, extending from a duodenoscope, is applying pulsed mode with effect 1.
c Ablated polyps after APC.

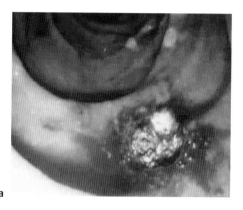
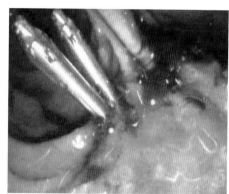

Fig. 27.10 a Duodenal perforation after argon plasma coagulation
b Successful closure of the perforation with endoscopic clips.

27

dian of 1.8 procedures, ablation was achieved in 61% after a single session and in 92% after a second procedure over a mean of 40 months (range 26–68 months). There was no progression to cancer and only one episode of bleeding (3%) [57]. There are four series including 126 patients with sporadic duodenal and periampullary polyps with mean diameters of 19–28 mm (range 4–60 mm) treated with endoscopic mucosal resection and adjuvant APC as required and followed for up for 13–71 months (range 4–151 months). Eradication was achieved in 86% of cases, and residual adenoma was often successfully treated with APC. Complications occurred in 9% and included 10 episodes of bleeding and one fatal perforation [58–61]. **Figure 27.10** shows an APC-induced duodenal perforation. Although adjuvant APC may minimize bleeding and recurrence, pancreatitis has been reported after APC in the duodenum [59,62].

Patients with FAP have 5–12% risk of small-bowel and periampullary cancer, and adenomatous polyps progress in size, number, and degree of cancer risk over time [63,64]. In a series of 14 FAP patients with 51 gastric or duodenal polyps, with a mean diameter of 10 mm (range 10–30 mm), a total of 18 procedures with endoscopic mucosal resection and APC or bipolar ablation were done. With a mean follow-up period of 6 months (range 1–18 months), all of the polyps were completely ablated in the 10 patients who were evaluated. Two of the 14 patients (14%) had complications, including one case of severe hemorrhage and one of mild pancreatitis [65]. In 42 FAP patients who had undergone colectomy, a median of two therapeutic procedures (range 0–12 procedures) were performed in the distal ileum and pouch over 49 months (range 0–168 months), with no complications. Seven percent had progression to advanced neoplasia [66]. Figure 27.11 shows APC of multiple rectal stump polyps.

Endoscopic resection of ampullary adenomas is initially successful in 75–100% of patients, and prophylactic pancreatic stenting is generally preformed to minimize the risk of pancreatitis. Adenomas recur in up to 33% of patients and can receive repeat treatment with APC. The morbidity rate is 8–27% [64]. Adjuvant APC ablation may reduce the recurrence rate [67]. APC delivers electrothermal energy to the tissue intimately associated with the plastic pancreatic and bile duct stents, but does not damage the stents themselves, as they are not electrically conductive (**Fig. 27.12**). APC can also be used to ablate adenomatous extension into the ducts. Strictures, which generally respond to stenting, should be expected. Ampullary adenomas can also be ablated with APC as primary therapy after pancreatic and biliary stenting, with or without sphincterotomy (**Fig. 27.13**) [64].

Colorectal Polyps and Cancer

Large sessile and flat polyps may require piecemeal resection with multiple snare attempts. This is associated with increased morbidity, incomplete resection, and frequent recurrence. Adjunctive APC on the margins, base, and residual polyp tissue appears to reduce the recurrence and morbidity rates [68]. In a prospective series of patients with polyps larger than 15 mm, 20 participants believed to have undergone complete snare resection were randomly assigned into equal groups to receive APC at the margins and base of the polyps, or no further treatment (controls). Another 13 patients with gross residual polyps had no APC and did not undergo randomization. Colonoscopy was repeated after 3 and 12 months, and recurrences were observed in significantly fewer of the treated patients (one of 10) in comparison with the untreated patients (seven of 10; $P < 0.02$). In addition, recurrences were observed in six of 13 patients who had had macroscopically incomplete resections [56]. Polyps that are difficult to snare can be ablated using APC

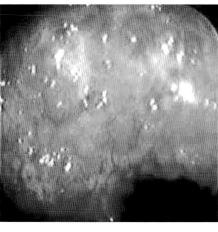 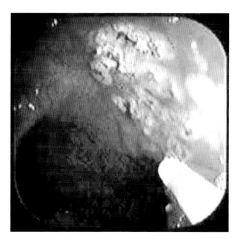 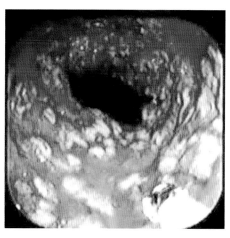

a, b
c

Fig. 27.11 a Multiple small rectal stump polyps in a patient with familial adenomatous polyposis (FAP) following subtotal colectomy and ileoproctostomy.

b APC with a 7-Fr lateral-firing probe in forced mode at 15 W and 1.2 L/min flow.
c The appearance after APC treatment of the multiple polyps.

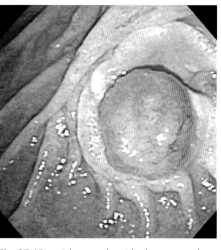 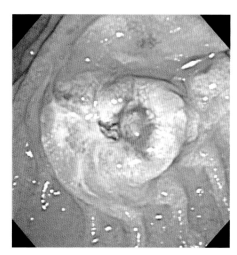 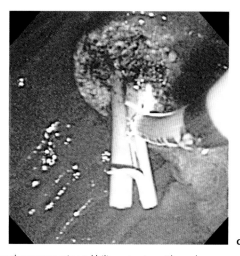

a, b
c

Fig. 27.12a A large polypoid adenoma at the ampulla of Vater.
b The same site after snare ampullectomy.
c Argon plasma coagulation is being applied via a 10-Fr axial-firing probe in forced mode at 20 W and 1.8 L/min flow. The argon plasma courses to the

tissue around and between the pancreatic and biliary stents, with no damage to the plastic.

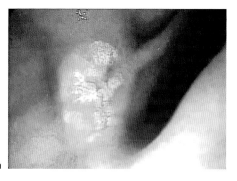 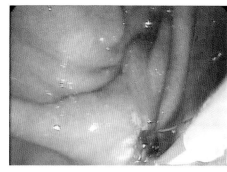

a
b

Fig. 27.13 a A flat ampullary adenoma with high-grade dysplasia, for ablation without resection.
b A biliary sphincterotomy was carried out to make space for pancreatic and bile duct stenting.
c Dual stents in place, with argon plasma coagulation being applied in pulsed mode with effect 1.
d The ampullary area 48 h later, with granulation tissue at the site of the ablated adenoma.

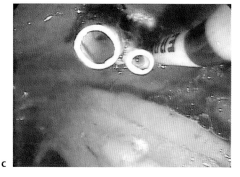 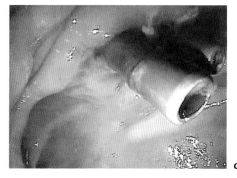

c
d

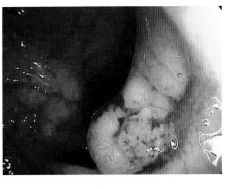

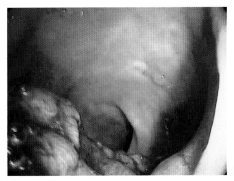

Fig. 27.14a A sessile colon polyp, mainly on the proximal margin of a fold.
b The appearance of the polyp after injection with saline and dilute methylene blue to lift the polyp distally and thicken the wall. A snare continually slipped over the polyp.
c APC with a 10-Fr probe in forced mode at 20 W and 1.4 L/min flow.
d The area after APC.

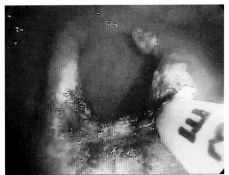

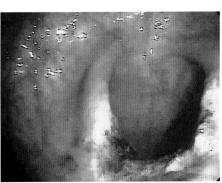

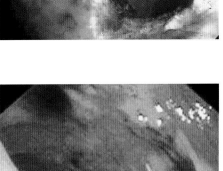

Fig. 27.15a Postpolypectomy bleeding in the sigmoid colon.
b The area after argon plasma coagulation in pulsed mode with effect 1, with hemostasis.

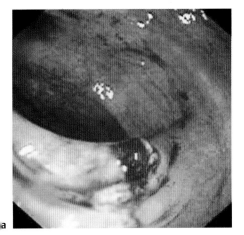

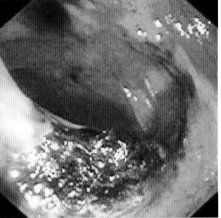

27

as the primary therapy (**Fig. 27.14**). APC is also useful for postpolypectomy bleeding, due to the limited depth of penetration (**Fig. 27.15**) [69,70]. It may be wise to inject saline before treatment. Palliative ablation of obstructing colon cancer was evaluated using pulsed and forced APC in 14 patients, in a series of 100 that also included patients with symptomatic esophageal and gastric tumors. Improvement in tumor-related symptoms occurred in more than 95% of the patients and recurrences developed in 6%, with no significant differences among the affected organs. The forced mode was associated with a shorter median treatment time [8]. **Figure 27.16** shows debulking of a colon cancer with APC.

Hemostasis

Vascular Lesions

Gastric antral vascular ectasia (GAVE), with or without portal hypertension, responds well to APC ablation. In six series including 135 patients with and without portal hypertension who underwent a mean of two sessions (range one to five sessions) and were followed for means of 15–30 months (range 1–61 months), success based on decreased transfusion requirements and increased hematocrit was achieved in 93% of cases, with morbidity including bleeding and stenosis in 5% [71–76]. There have been two series including 99 patients with arteriovenous malformations that were treated mostly with a single APC session. The patients were followed for means of 6–16 months (range 4–47 months). Success, as assessed by cessation of bleeding, was achieved in 83% of cases, and two cases were complicated by pneumoperitoneum [73,77]. **Figure 27.17** illustrates the use of APC to treat GAVE.

Another series included 100 patients with colorectal angiodysplasias who were treated with APC at 40–60 W, with a median follow-up period of 20 months (range 6–62 months). This resulted in cessation of bleeding and stabilization of hematocrit in 85% of cases, with no further transfusions in 90%. There were two complications (pneumoperitoneum and fever) [78]. Some authorities suggest using saline injection to thicken the wall for right colonic lesions, in an effort to prevent perforation [3,79]. **Figure 27.18** demonstrates APC of colonic angiodysplasias. There have been many

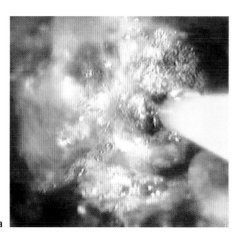

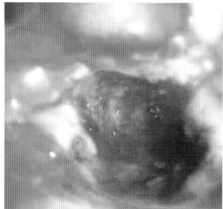

Fig. 27.16 a A near-obstructing dense sigmoid colon cancer being treated with prolonged static application of APC in forced mode at 60 W and 1.8 L/min flow.
b Successful restoration of the lumen after APC. The tissue will continue to slough for a few days, with a more pronounced effect.

V

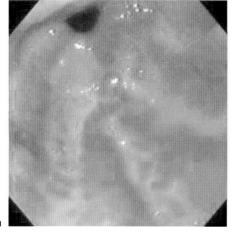

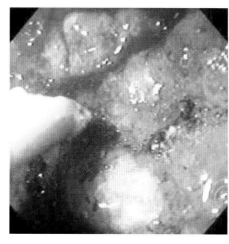

Fig. 27.17 a Gastric antral vascular ectasia (GAVE), showing the watermelon pattern.
b Argon plasma coagulation with pulsed mode effect 2.
c The appearance immediately after APC.
d Complete eradication of the vascular lesions 8 weeks later.

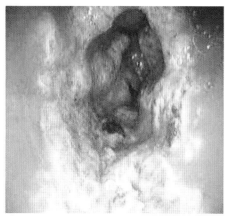

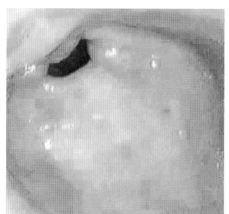

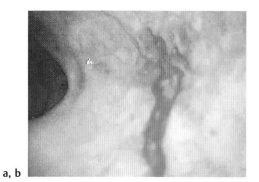

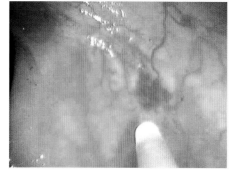

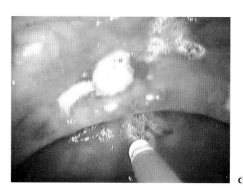

Fig. 27.18 a An oozing angiodysplastic lesion in the ascending colon.
b A 7-Fr lateral-firing APC probe in position.

c The appearance of the lesion after APC directed around and then to the center in precise mode.

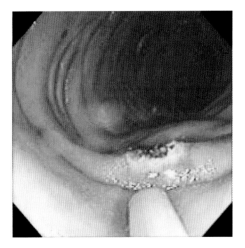

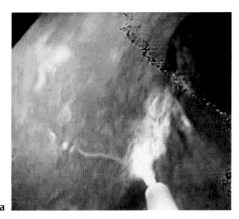

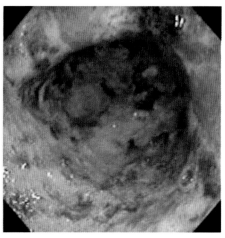

a
b

Fig. 27.19 Appearance after APC of a distal jejunal telangiectasia with a 7-Fr axial-firing probe in precise mode through an enteroscope.

Fig. 27.20 a Klippel–Trenaunay–Weber syndrome is characterized by massive visceral hemangiomas. APC coagulation is being applied to the affected sigmoid colon via a 7-Fr axial-firing probe in forced mode at 30 W and 1.8 L/min flow. The argon plasma is applied like spray paint to a wide area, with relatively deep penetration. Electronic interference with the video image is seen coursing from the 12-o'clock to 3-o'clock positions on the image.
b Following APC coagulation, there is relatively confluent and deep coagulation of the affected area. The intestinal bleeding abated after treatment.

other series reporting cases throughout the gastrointestinal tract, including lesions deep in the small bowel treated with balloon enteroscopy, with the treatment generally leading to excellent results [80]. **Figure 27.19** shows ACP of a jejunal telangiectasia. Other less common vascular lesions can also be treated with APC (**Fig. 27.20**).

Radiation proctitis is a syndrome that occurs as a result of radiation-induced neovascular telangiectasias that bleed. A total of 130 patients in four series including 25 or more patients each were treated with an approximate mean of three sessions (range one to eight sessions) at about 50 W, at intervals of about 3–5 weeks. Success—defined as improved bleeding and hematocrit, and reduced transfusions—was observed in 93 % of cases. There were nine complications (7 %), including three episodes of pain, three vagal events, and three intestinal explosions one of which required surgery. The explosions occurred in patients who had received enemas rather than full colonic preparation [81–84].

Dieulafoy lesions are submucosal arteries that erode through the mucosa in the absence of peptic ulcer and bleed. A retrospective series included 23 patients with bleeding from Dieulafoy lesions, of whom 39 % had severe comorbidities and 22 % had coagulopathies. Twenty of the lesions were in the upper tract, and 20 were actively bleeding at endoscopy. APC was applied at 40–60 W and three patients had an initial epinephrine injection, with hemostasis successfully achieved in all cases. During a mean follow-up period of 29 months, one case of recurrent hemorrhage was observed [85].

APC has been used to coagulate esophageal varices after ligation, to induce fibrosis and retard recurrence. There have been two randomized clinical trials comparing APC treatment with no APC treatment after ligation, including 90 patients who were followed for means of 16–18.5 months. Nonrecurrence of varices was seen more frequently in the APC group in both studies (100 % and 57 %, $P < 0.04$; 74 % and 50 %, $P < 0.05$). However, there were higher rates of post-treatment fever in the APC groups in both studies. This treatment should be considered investigational at present [86,87].

Peptic Ulcer Disease

There have been three randomized controlled trials of bleeding peptic ulcers, including a total of 326 patients assigned to APC or injection with epinephrine and polidocanol, APC or heat probe, and APC with epinephrine injection or heat probe with epinephrine injection. In each trial, the rates of hemostasis, rebleeding, transfusions, surgery, and mortality were similar between the groups [88–90]. A meta-analysis of the first two studies also showed similar outcomes [91].

Zenker's Diverticulum

Endoscopic treatment of Zenker's diverticulum can be carried out by passing a nasogastric tube and endoscopically incising along the impression from the tube with APC or other devices. APC has the advantage that it can control oozing or frank hemorrhage without the need to change instruments. Forty-one patients were treated with a mean of three sessions, with technical success in all. There was one perforation (2 %), which was treated conservatively, and seven cases of postprocedure fever (17 %). Recurrences were observed in five of 34 patients (15 %) followed for a mean of 16 months, and repeat treatment was successful in all cases [92]. In another series including 125 patients treated with a mean of 1.8 procedures, success was achieved in 100 %. Morbidity occurred in 24 (29 %) and included 17 episodes of subcutaneous emphysema, five of mediastinal emphysema, and two of bleeding. All were managed conservatively [93].

Stent Manipulation

Misplacement or migration of self-expanding metal stents may cause luminal obstruction and mucosal trauma and can complicate the placement of other stents. APC has been used to incise displaced stents for removal when they protrude into the lumen [94]. Incision usually occurs readily, but may leave long wires protruding into the lumen (**Fig. 27.21**), APC of ingrown and overgrown tissue in indwelling stents may facilitate removal. Eight covered and uncovered metal stents and four uncovered nitinol biliary stents implanted

27

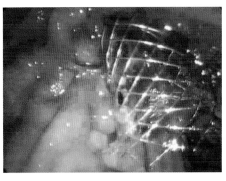
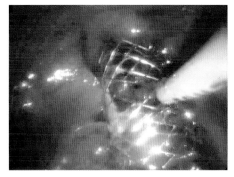
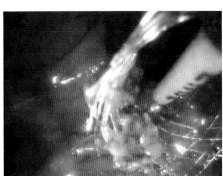
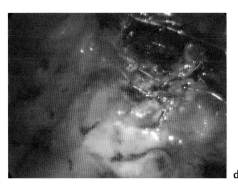

a

b

c

d

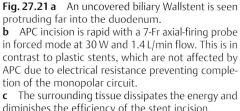

Fig. 27.21 a An uncovered biliary Wallstent is seen protruding far into the duodenum.
b APC incision is rapid with a 7-Fr axial-firing probe in forced mode at 30 W and 1.4 L/min flow. This is in contrast to plastic stents, which are not affected by APC due to electrical resistance preventing completion of the monopolar circuit.
c The surrounding tissue dissipates the energy and diminishes the efficiency of the stent incision.
d Post-incision changes in the stent architecture, with long individual wires protruding into the duodenum.

into swine were successfully incised with APC. There was mild superficial bile duct injury in two pigs [95]. In three series including 39 uncovered and covered stainless steel and nitinol stents (three esophageal, six duodenal, 27 biliary, and three colorectal), 38 (97%) were successfully manipulated with APC. Interventions included three fenestrations in duodenal stents to allow biliary cannulation, and cutting of malpositioned stents that were causing ulcers, bleeding pain, and/or obstruction, with relief of signs and symptoms in all cases. One covered duodenal stent could not be cut [95–98]. Careful technique with short bursts of the lowest possible energy to minimize thermal tissue energy is recommended.

References

1. Farin G, Grund KE. Technology of argon plasma coagulation with particular regard to endoscopic applications. Endosc Surg Allied Technol 1994;2:71–7.
2. Watson JP, Bennett MK, Griffin SM, Mattewson K. The tissue effect of argon plasma coagulation on esophageal and gastric mucosa. Gastrointest Endosc 2000;52:342–5.
3. Norton ID, Wang L, Levine SA, Burgart LJ, Hofmeister EK, Yacavone RF, et al. In vivo characterization of colonic thermal injury caused by argon plasma coagulation. Gastrointest Endosc 2002:55:631–6.
4. Goulet CJ, DiSario JA, Emerson L, Hilden K, Holubkov R, Fanc JC. In vivo evaluation of argon plasma coagulation in a porcine model. Gastrointest Endosc 2007;65:457–62.
5. American Society for Gastrointestinal Endoscopy Technology Committee. Mucosal ablation devices. Gastrointest Endosc 2008;68:1031–42.
6. Anonymous. APC in flexible endoscopy. Marietta, GA: Erbe USA, Inc., 2007.
7. Sumiyama K, Kaise M, Kato M, Saito S, Goda K, Odagi I, et al. New generation argon plasma coagulation in flexible endoscopy: ex vivo study and clinical experience. J Gastroenterol Hepatol 2006;21:1122–8.
8. Eickhoff A, Jakobs R, Schilling D, Hartmann D, Weickert U, Enderle MD, et al. Prospective nonrandomized comparison of two modes of argon beamer (APC) tumor desobstruction: effectiveness of the new pulsed APC versus forced APC. Endoscopy 2007;39:637–42.
9. Manner H, Enderle MD, Pech O, May A, Plum N, Riemann JF, et al. Second-generation argon plasma coagulation: two-center experience with 600 patients. J Gastroenterol Hepatol 2008;23:872–8.
10. Manner H, May A, Faerber M, Pech O, Plum N, Ell C. The tissue effect of second generation argon plasma coagulation (VIO APC) in comparison to

standard APC and Nd:YAG laser in vitro. Acta Gastroenterol Belg 2007;70:352–6.
11. Manner H, May A, Rabenstein T, Pech O, Nachbar L, Enderle MD, et al. Prospective evaluation of a new high-power argon plasma coagulation system (hp-APC) in therapeutic gastrointestinal endoscopy. Scand J Gastroenterol 2007;42:397–405.
12. Fujishiro M, Yahagi N, Nakamura M, Kakushima N, Kodashima S, Ono S, et al. Submucosal injection of normal saline may prevent tissue damage from argon plasma coagulation: an experimental study using resected porcine esophagus, stomach, and colon. Surg Laparosc Endosc Percutan Tech 2006;16:307–11.
13. Overholt BF, Wang KK, Burdick JS, Lightdale CJ, Kimmey M, Nava HR, et al. Five-year efficacy and safety of photodynamic therapy with Photofrin in Barrett's high–grade dysplasia. Gastrointest Endosc 2007;66:460–8.
14. Wang KK, Sampliner RE; Practice Parameters Committee of the American College of Gastroenterology. Updated guidelines 2008 for the diagnosis, surveillance and therapy of Barrett's esophagus. Am J Gastroenterol 2008;103:788–97.
15. Pech O, Behrens A, May A, Nachbar L, Gossner L, Rabenstein T, et al. Long-term results and risk factor analysis for recurrence after curative endoscopic therapy in 349 patients with high-grade intraepithelial neoplasia and mucosal adenocarcinoma in Barrett's esophagus. Gut 2008;57:1200–6.
16. Pouw RE, Sharma VK, Bergman JJ, Fleischer DE. Radiofrequency ablation for total Barrett's eradication: a description of the endoscopic technique, its clinical results and future prospects. Endoscopy 2008;40:1033–40.
17. Mörk H, Al-Taie O, Berlin F, Kraus MR, Scheurlen M. High recurrence rate of Barrett's epithelium during long-term follow-up after argon plasma coagulation. Scand J Gastroenterol 2007;42:23–7.
18. Ferraris R, Fracchia M, Foti M, Sidoli L, Taraglio S, Vigano L, et al. Barrett's oesophagus: long-term follow-up after complete ablation with argon plasma coagulation and the factors that determine its recurrence. Aliment Pharmacol Ther 2007;25:835–40.
19. Sharma P, Wani S, Weston AP, Bansal A, Hall M, Mathur S, et al. A randomized controlled trial of ablation of Barrett's oesophagus with multipolar electrocoagulation versus argon plasma coagulation in combination with acid suppression: long term results. Gut 2006;55:1233–9.
20. Manner H, May A, Miehlke S, Dertinger S, Wigginghaus B, Schimming W, et al. Ablation of nonneoplastic Barrett's mucosa using argon plasma coagulation with concomitant esomeprazole therapy (APBANEX): a prospective multicenter evaluation. Am J Gastroenterol 2006;101:1762–9.
21. Basu KK, Talwar V, de Caestecker JS. Effects of low-power argon plasma coagulation thermoablation of Barrett's epithelium on oesophageal motility. Eur J Gastroenterol Hepatol 2006;18:733–7.

22. Familiari L, Scaffidi M, Bonica M, Consolo P, Giacobbe G, Fichera D, et al. Endoscopic treatment of Barrett's epithelium with argon plasma coagulation. Long-term follow-up. Minerva Gastroenterol Dietol 2003;49: 63–70.

23. Ragunath K, Krasner N, Raman VS, Haqqani MT, Phillips CJ, Cheung I. Endoscopic ablation of dysplastic Barrett's oesophagus comparing argon plasma coagulation and photodynamic therapy: a randomized prospective trial assessing efficacy and cost-effectiveness. Scand J Gastroenterol 2005;40:750–8.

24. Pedrazzani C, Catalano F, Festini M, Zerman G, Tomezzoli A, Ruzzenente A, et al. Endoscopic ablation of Barrett's esophagus using high power setting argon plasma coagulation: a prospective study. World J Gastroenterol 2005;11:1872–5.

25. Madisch A, Miehlke S, Bayerdorffer E, Wiedemann B, Antos D, Sievert A, et al. Long-term follow-up after complete ablation of Barrett's esophagus with argon plasma coagulation. World J Gastroenterol 2005;11:1182–6.

26. Dulai GS, Jensen DM, Cortina G, Fontana L, Ippoliti A. Randomized trial of argon plasma coagulation vs. multipolar electrocoagulation for ablation of Barrett's esophagus. Gastrointest Endosc 2005;61:232–40.

27. Kelty CJ, Ackroyd R, Brown NJ, Stephenson TJ, Stoddard CJ, Reed MW. Endoscopic ablation of Barrett's oesophagus: a randomized-controlled trial of photodynamic therapy vs. argon plasma coagulation. Aliment Pharmacol Ther 2004;20:1289–96.

28. Attwood SE, Lewis CJ, Caplin S, Hemming K, Armstrong G. Argon beam plasma coagulation as therapy for high-grade dysplasia in Barrett's esophagus. Clin Gastroenterol Hepatol 2003;1:258–63.

29. Ackroyd R, Tam W, Schoeman M, Devitt PG, Watson DI. Prospective randomized controlled trial of argon plasma coagulation ablation vs. endoscopic surveillance of patients with Barrett's esophagus after antireflux surgery. Gastrointest Endosc 2004;59:1–7.

30. Kahaleh M, Van Laethem JL, Nagy N, Cremer M, Devière J. Long-term follow-up and factors predictive of recurrence in Barrett's esophagus treated by argon plasma coagulation and acid suppression. Endoscopy 2002;34:950–5.

31. Basu KK, Pick B, Bale R, West KP, de Caestecker JS. Efficacy and one year follow up of argon plasma coagulation therapy for ablation of Barrett's oesophagus: factors determining persistence and recurrence of Barrett's epithelium. Gut 2002;51:776–80.

32. Morris CD, Byrne JP, Armstrong GR, Attwood SE. Prevention of the neoplastic progression of Barrett's oesophagus by endoscopic argon beam plasma ablation. Br J Surg 2001;88:1357–62.

33. Tigges H, Fuchs KH, Maroske J, Fein M, Freys SM, Müller J, et al. Combination of endoscopic argon plasma coagulation and antireflux surgery for treatment of Barrett's esophagus. J Gastrointest Surg 2001;5:251–9.

34. Van Laethem JL, Jagodzinski R, Peny MO, Cremer M, Devière J. Argon plasma coagulation in the treatment of Barrett's high-grade dysplasia and in situ adenocarcinoma. Endoscopy 2001;33:257–61.

35. Pereira-Lima JC, Busnello JV, Saul C, Toneloto EB, Lopes CV, Rynkowski CB, et al. High power setting argon plasma coagulation for the eradication of Barrett's esophagus. Am J Gastroenterol 2000;95:1661–8.

36. Schulz H, Miehlke S, Antos D, Schentke KU, Vieth M, Stolte M, et al. Ablation of Barrett's epithelium by endoscopic argon plasma coagulation in combination with high-dose omeprazole. Gastrointest Endosc 2000; 51:659–63.

37. Van Laethem JL, Cremer M, Peny MO, Delhaye M, Devière J. Eradication of Barrett's mucosa with argon plasma coagulation and acid suppression: immediate and mid term results. Gut 1998;43:747–51.

38. Byrne JP, Armstrong GR, Attwood SE. Restoration of the normal squamous lining in Barrett's esophagus by argon beam plasma coagulation. Am J Gastroenterol 1998;93:1810–5.

39. Li YM, Li L, Yu CH, Liu YS, Cheng FX. A systematic review and meta-analysis of the treatment of Barrett's esophagus. Dig Dis Sci 2008;53: 2837–46.

40. Ell C, May A, Pech O, Gossner L, Guenter E, Behrens A, et al. Curative endoscopic resection of early esophageal adenocarcinomas (Barrett's cancer). Gastrointest Endosc 2007;65:3–10.

41. May A, Gossner L, Pech O, Müller H, Vieth M, Stolte M, et al. Intraepithelial high-grade neoplasia and early adenocarcinoma in short-segment Barrett's esophagus (SSBE): curative treatment using local endoscopic treatment techniques. Endoscopy 2002;34:604–10.

42. Ell C, May A, Gossner L, Pech O, Günter E, Mayer G, Henrich R, et al. Endoscopic mucosal resection of early cancer and high-grade dysplasia in Barrett's esophagus. Gastroenterology 2000;118:670–7.

43. Lopes CV, Hela M, Pesenti C, Bories E, Caillol F, Monges G, et al. Circumferential endoscopic resection of Barrett's esophagus with high-grade dysplasia or early adenocarcinoma. Surg Endosc 2007;21:820–4.

44. Peters FP, Kara MA, Rosmolen WD, Aalders MC, Ten Kate FJ, Bultje BC, et al. Endoscopic treatment of high-grade dysplasia and early stage cancer in Barrett's esophagus. Gastrointest Endosc 2005;61:506–14.

45. May A, Gossner L, Gunter E, Stolte M, Ell C. Local treatment of early cancer in short Barrett's esophagus by means of argon plasma coagulation: initial experience. Endoscopy 1999;31:497–500.

46. Eriksen JR. Palliation of non-resectable carcinoma of the cardia and esophagus by argon beam coagulation. Dan Med Bull 2002;49:346–9.

47. Heindorff H, Wojdemann M, Bisgaard T, Svendsen LB. Endoscopic palliation of inoperable cancer of the esophagus or cardia by argon electro-coagulation. Scand J Gastroenterol 1998;33:21–3.

48. Robertson GS, Thomas M, Jamieson J, Veitch PS, Dennison AR. Palliation of oesophageal carcinoma using the argon beam coagulator. Br J Surg 1996;83:1769–71.

49. Akhtar K, Byrne JP, Bancewicz J, Attwood SE. Argon beam plasma coagulation in the management of cancers of the esophagus and stomach. Surg Endosc 2000;14:1127–30.

50. Schumacher B, Lübke H, Frieling T, Haussinger D, Niederau C. Palliative treatment of malignant esophageal stenosis: experience with plastic versus metal stents. Hepatogastroenterology 1998;45:755–60.

51. Grund KE, Storek D, Becker HD. Highly flexible self-expanding meshed metal stents for palliation of malignant esophagogastric obstruction. Endoscopy 1995;27:486–94.

52. Dent J. Pathogenesis and classification of cancer around the gastroesophageal junction—not so different in Japan. Am J Gastroenterol 2006;101: 934–6.

53. Kitamura T, Tanabe S, Koizumi W, Mitomi H, Saigenji K. Argon plasma coagulation for early gastric cancer: technique and outcome. Gastrointest Endosc 2006;63:48–54.

54. Murakami M, Nishino K, Inoue A, Takaoka Y, Iwamasa K, Murakami B, et al. Argon plasma coagulation for the treatment of early gastric cancer. Hepatogastroenterology 2004;51:1658–61.

55. Sagawa T, Takayama T, Oku T, Hayashi T, Ota H, Okamoto T, et al. Argon plasma coagulation for successful treatment of early gastric cancer with intramucosal invasion. Gut 2003;52:334–9.

56. Brooker JC, Saunders BP, Shah SG, Thapar CJ, Suzuki N, Williams CB. Treatment with argon plasma coagulation reduces recurrence after piece-meal resection of large sessile colonic polyps: a randomized trial and recommendations. Gastrointest Endosc 2002;55:371–5.

57. Lienert A, Bagshaw PF. Treatment of duodenal adenomas with endoscopic argon plasma coagulation. ANZ J Surg 2007;77:371–3.

58. Alexander S, Bourke MJ, Williams SJ, Bailey A, Co J. EMR of large, sessile, sporadic nonampullary duodenal adenomas: technical aspects and long-term. Gastrointest Endosc 2009;69:66–73.

59. Lépilliez V, Chemaly M, Ponchon T, Napoleon B, Saurin JC. Endoscopic resection of sporadic duodenal adenomas: an efficient technique with a substantial risk of delayed bleeding. Endoscopy 2008;40:806–10.

60. Eswaran SL, Sanders M, Bernadino KP, Ansari A, Lawrence C, Stefan A, et al. Success and complications of endoscopic removal of giant duodenal and ampullary polyps: a comparative series. Gastrointest Endosc 2006;64: 925–32.

61. Apel D, Jakobs R, Spiethoff A, Riemann JF. Follow-up after endoscopic snare resection of duodenal adenomas. Endoscopy 2005;37:444–8.

62. Weigt J, Zimmermann LC, Mönkemüller K, Malfertheiner P. Acute pancreatitis after argon plasma coagulation of duodenal polyps in a patient with familial adenomatous polyposis. Endoscopy 2007;39(Suppl 1):E278.

63. Johnson JC, DiSario JA, Grady WM. Surveillance and treatment of periampullary and duodenal adenomas in familial adenomatous polyposis. Curr Treat Options Gastroenterol 2004;7:79–89.

64. Wong RF, DiSario JA. Approaches to endoscopic ampullectomy. Curr Opin Gastroenterol 2004;20:460–7.

65. DiSario J, Samowitz W, Burt R, Kuwada S. Endoscopic therapy of large gastroduodenal polyps in familial adenomatous polyposis [abstract]. Gastrointest Endosc 2002;55:AB138.

66. Gleeson FC, Papachristou GI, Riegert-Johnson DL, Boller AM, Gostout CJ. Progression to advanced neoplasia is infrequent in post colectomy familial adenomatous polyposis patients under endoscopic surveillance. Fam Cancer 2009;8:33–8.

67. Catalano MF, Linder JD, Chak A, Sivak MV Jr, Raijman I, Geenen JE, et al. Endoscopic management of adenoma of the major duodenal papilla. Gastrointest Endosc 2004;59:225–32.

68. Zlatanic J, Waye JD, Kim PS, Baiocco PJ, Gleim GW. Large sessile colonic adenomas: use of argon plasma coagulator to supplement piecemeal snare polypectomy. Gastrointest Endosc 1999;49:731–5.

27

69. Johanns W, Luis W, Janssen J, Kahl S, Greiner L. Argon plasma coagulation (APC) in gastroenterology: experimental and clinical experiences. Eur J Gastroenterol Hepatol 1997;9:581–7.

70. Wahab PJ, Mulder CJ, den HG, Thies JE. Argon plasma coagulation in flexible gastrointestinal endoscopy: pilot experiences. Endoscopy 1997;29:176–81.

71. Herrera S, Bordas JM, Llach J, Ginès A, Pellisé M, Fernández-Esparrach G, et al. The beneficial effects of argon plasma coagulation in the management of different types of gastric vascular ectasia lesions in patients admitted for GI hemorrhage. Gastrointest Endosc 2008;68:440–6.

72. Lecleire S, Ben-Soussan E, Antonietti M, Goria O, Riachi G, Lerebours E, et al. Bleeding gastric vascular ectasia treated by argon plasma coagulation: a comparison between patients with and without cirrhosis. Gastrointest Endosc 2008;67:219–25.

73. Kwan V, Bourke MJ, Williams SJ, Gillespie PE, Murray MA, Kaffes AJ, et al. Argon plasma coagulation in the management of symptomatic gastro-intestinal vascular lesions: experience in 100 consecutive patients with long-term follow-up. Am J Gastroenterol 2006;101:58–63.

74. Sebastian S, McLoughlin R, Qasim A, O'Morain CA, Buckley MJ. Endoscopic argon plasma coagulation for the treatment of gastric antral vascular ectasia (watermelon stomach): long-term results. Dig Liver Dis 2004;36:212–7.

75. Roman S, Saurin JC, Dumortier J, Perreira A, Bernard G, Ponchon T. Tolerance and efficacy of argon plasma coagulation for controlling bleeding in patients with typical and atypical manifestations of watermelon stomach. Endoscopy 2003;35:1024–8.

76. Probst A, Scheubel R, Wienbeck M. Treatment of watermelon stomach (GAVE syndrome) by means of endoscopic argon plasma coagulation (APC): long-term outcome. Z Gastroenterol 2001;39:447–52.

77. Rolachon A, Papillon E, Fournet J. Is argon plasma coagulation an efficient treatment for digestive system vascular malformation and radiation proctitis? Gastroenterol Clin Biol 2000;24:1205–10.

78. Olmos JA, Marcolongo M, Pogorelsky V, Herrera L, Tobal F, Dávolos JR. Long-term outcome of argon plasma ablation therapy for bleeding in 100 consecutive patients with colonic angiodysplasia. Dis Colon Rectum 2006;49:1507–16.

79. Suzuki N, Arebi N, Saunders BP. A novel method of treating colonic angiodysplasia. A novel method of treating colonic angiodysplasia. Gastrointest Endosc 2006;64:424–7.

80. May A, Nachbar L, Pohl J, Ell C. Endoscopic interventions in the small bowel using double balloon enteroscopy: feasibility and limitations. Am J Gastroenterol 2007;102:527–35.

81. Dees J, Meijssen MA, Kuipers EJ. Argon plasma coagulation for radiation proctitis. Scand J Gastroenterol Suppl 2006;(243):175–8.

82. Ben-Soussan E, Antonietti M, Savoye G, Herve S, Ducrotté P, Lerebours E. Argon plasma coagulation in the treatment of hemorrhagic radiation proctitis is efficient but requires a perfect colonic cleansing to be safe. Eur J Gastroenterol Hepatol 2004;16:1315–8.

83. Sebastian S, O'Connor H, O'Morain C, Buckley M. Argon plasma coagulation as first-line treatment for chronic radiation proctopathy. J Gastroenterol Hepatol 2004;19:1169–73.

84. Silva RA, Correia AJ, Dias LM, Viana HL, Viana RL. Argon plasma coagulation therapy for hemorrhagic radiation proctosigmoiditis. Gastrointest Endosc 1999;50:221–4.

85. Iacopini F, Petruzziello L, Marchese M, Larghi A, Spada C, Familiari P, et al. Hemostasis of Dieulafoy's lesions by argon plasma coagulation (with video). Gastrointest Endosc 2007;66:20–6.

86. Cipolletta L, Bianco MA, Rotondano G, Marmo R, Meucci C, Piscopo R. Argon plasma coagulation prevents variceal recurrence after band ligation of esophageal varices: preliminary results of a prospective randomized trial. Gastrointest Endosc 2002;56:467–71.

87. Nakamura S, Mitsunaga A, Murata Y, Suzuki S, Hayashi N. Endoscopic induction of mucosal fibrosis by argon plasma coagulation (APC) for esophageal varices: A prospective randomized trial of ligation plus APC vs. ligation alone. Endoscopy 2001;33:210–5.

88. Skok P, Krizman I, Skok M. Argon plasma coagulation versus injection sclerotherapy in peptic ulcer hemorrhage—a prospective, controlled study. Hepatogastroenterology 2004;51:165–70.

89. Cipolletta L, Bianco MA, Rotondano G, Piscopo R, Prisco A, Garofano ML. Prospective comparison of argon plasma coagulator and heater probe in the endoscopic treatment of major peptic ulcer bleeding. Gastrointest Endosc 1998;48:191–5.

90. Chau CH, Siu WT, Law BK, Tang CN, Kwok SY, Luk YW, et al. Randomized controlled trial comparing epinephrine injection plus heat probe coagulation versus epinephrine injection plus argon plasma coagulation for bleeding peptic ulcers. Gastrointest Endosc 2003;57:455–61.

91. Havanond C, Havanond P. Argon plasma coagulation therapy for acute non-variceal upper gastrointestinal bleeding. Cochrane Database Syst Rev 2005;(2):CD003791.

92. Rabenstein T, May A, Michel J, Manner H, Pech O, Gossner L, Ell C. Argon plasma coagulation for flexible endoscopic Zenker's diverticulotomy. Endoscopy 2007;39:141–5.

93. Mulder CJ. Zapping Zenker's diverticulum: gastroscopic treatment. Can J Gastroenterol 1999;13:405–7.

94. Chen YK, Jakribettuu V, Springer EW, Shah RJ, Penberthy J, Nash SR. Safety and efficacy of argon plasma coagulation trimming of malpositioned and migrated biliary metal stents: a controlled study in the porcine model. Am J Gastroenterol 2006;101:2025–30.

95. Topazian M, Baron TH. Endoscopic fenestration of duodenal stents using argon plasma to facilitate ERCP. Gastrointest Endosc 2009;69:166–9.

96. Christiaens P, Decock S, Buchel O, Bulté K, Moons V, D'Haens G, et al. Endoscopic trimming of metallic stents with the use of argon plasma. Gastrointest Endosc 2008;67:369–71.

97. Rerknimitr R, Naprasert P, Kongkam P, Kullavanijaya P. Trimming a metallic biliary stent using an argon plasma coagulator. Cardiovasc Intervent Radiol 2007;30:534–6.

98. Vanbiervliet G, Piche T, Caroli-Bosc FX, Dumas R, Peten EP, Huet PM, et al. Endoscopic argon plasma trimming of biliary and gastrointestinal metallic stents. Endoscopy 2005;37:434–8.

V

28 Polypectomy

Jerome D. Waye, Brian Saunders, Yasushi Sano, and Shinji Tanaka

Polypectomy with flexible instruments has been performed for the last 35 years. The removal of premalignant polyps has had an impact on the incidence, morbidity, and mortality of colorectal cancer [1,2]. The removal of colon polyps is one of the major landmarks of progress in gastroenterology during the past 50 years. The majority of colon polyps are relatively small—a feature that has made it possible to treat them successfully, and which has led to widespread use of the polypectomy technique throughout the world [3]. Most polyps are less than 1 cm in diameter, with only 20% being larger. All large polyps (greater than 35 mm) are adenomas, and they are usually located in the rectum or right colon. The majority of small polyps (less than 5 mm) in the rectum and distal sigmoid colon are non-neoplastic, but throughout the remainder of the colon, approximately 60–70% of small polyps are adenomas [4].

Fifty percent of patients with one adenoma will have another, and it is important to perform total colonoscopy to seek synchronous adenomas. No attempt should be made to remove large or difficult polyps during intubation, since larger unresectable polyps or a malignancy may be encountered further upstream, requiring surgery.

Principles of Colonoscopic Polypectomy

Heat Sealing of Blood Vessels

Safe polypectomy requires the ability to sever a polyp while achieving hemostasis and maintaining the integrity of the colon wall. A successful polypectomy depends on achieving a balance between the two forces employed whenever a larger polyp is transected with the wire snare. The two complementary forces involved are heat, which results in cauterization, and the shearing force exerted by tightening the wire loop. Both of these forces must be used simultaneously to result in a clean, bloodless polypectomy, without an excessive amount of burn to the colon wall. Heat alone will not sever a polyp, while guillotine force alone may cut through a polyp, but can result in immediate bleeding, as there is no capability for heat sealing of blood vessels. For this reason, some endoscopists perform final snare closure themselves, increasing the "squeeze" force applied to the snare to control the rate of transection through the polyp. An important point is that small, sessile polyps < 6 mm hardly ever have significant blood vessels in their base, and therefore "cold" techniques with biopsy forceps for tiny polyps < 2 mm in size and mini-snare "guillotine" for 2–5-mm polyps are the preferred polypectomy methods, as there is no danger of delayed, heat-related damage.

Type of Current

The type of current that should be used for polypectomy—whether coagulation or a blend of cutting and coagulation—is a point of some controversy. Both types of current can achieve tissue heating, but coagulation current produces a greater degree of hemostasis, while cutting current is designed to cause cell disruption, resulting in a risk of bleeding from the polypectomy site without adequate hemostasis. A clinical trial has shown that the use of blended current was associated with a greater incidence of immediate bleeding, whereas use of pure coagulation current was associated with a higher rate of delayed postpolypectomy bleeding [5]. Many endoscopists employ the Endocut mode (Erbe, Tubingen, Germany, providing pulsed cutting and coagulation current, when performing more advanced polypectomy techniques such as endoscopic mucosal resection (EMR).

Electrosurgical Unit

The power output of electrosurgical generator units is not standardized. There are no rules concerning the number of watt-seconds or joules used to separate broad or narrow attachments of polyps to the colon wall. In general, the dial settings should be medium to low, and the current may be either pure coagulation or blended. Pure cutting current is never used, because this type of energy output explodes cells without providing any hemostatic qualities. The delivery of energy may be continuous once polypectomy has commenced (there is no scientific justification for intermittent tapping of the foot switch), and the person who closes the snare should do so slowly (as opposed to rapid closure of the slide bar) after having been requested to begin tightening after current application. If transection does not occur within a reasonable period, the endoscopist should always reassess the volume of tissue that has been caught in the snare and whether it is safe to continue.

Coaptive Coagulation

Most polypectomies are performed without any blood loss. This is because the same principles are employed as in arresting bleeding in the upper gastrointestinal tract. During hemostasis of bleeding ulcers, the technique is to push hard on the hemostatic probe in order to tamponade the bleeding site. This coapts the walls of the bleeding vessel and stops the blood flow; only a small amount of heat is then needed to seal a coapted blood vessel in the absence of intravascular blood flow. Similarly, the tightened snare around the pedicle of a polyp effectively causes cessation of circulation in that polyp, enabling a relatively small amount of current to seal both the arteriole and vein. As there is no single large feeding blood vessel in a sessile polyp, it is difficult to achieve hemostasis as successfully as when a stalk is present.

Types of Polyp

There are two basic polyp configurations—pedunculated polyps, which are attached to the intestinal wall by a stalk, and sessile polyps, which arise directly from the wall without a pedicle. Pedunculated polyps may be attached by a short and thick or long and thin stalk. Sessile polyps may be attached to the colon wall in a variety of ways. Those that are less than 8 mm in diameter frequently have the shape of a split pea, with the base being the largest diameter of the polyp. Larger polyps can assume one of several configurations [6].

An internationally recognized classification system was agreed at a workshop of experts held in Paris and is known as the Paris classification [7]. This system describes polyps as pedunculated or flat and reclassifies "carpet adenomas" as laterally spreading tumors (LST), which may be granular or nongranular in appearance. Morphology appears to be important in determining the malignant potential of polyps; flat lesions that are depressed or flush with the mucosal surface and nongranular LSTs all have a significantly higher risk of containing high-grade dysplasia. The vast majority of polyps are sessile, with most pedunculated polyps being found in the left colon, where peristalsis is strong and tends to pull on polypoid protrusions, resulting in pedicle formation. Most sessile polyps have a broad base, and the largest are found in the rectum and right colon.

Chromoendoscopy

Polyps may be made more visible by chromoscopy, using surface staining during the examination or in the preparation phase [8]. The most commonly used dye is indigo carmine (0.1–0.5%) which highlights surface architecture, pooling in the innominate grooves and highlighting any mucosal depressions (**Fig. 28.1**). It is nontoxic at low doses and is generally preferred to methylene blue, which may cause DNA damage [9]. It is possible to have patients swallow a capsule of indigo carmine dye powder (100 mg) immediately after administration of a polyethylene glycol electrolyte lavage solution [10], but dye is usually applied directly onto the mucosal surface—either injected down the biopsy channel or sprayed over a wider surface area using a diffusion catheter. Tiny flat lesions can be detected during routine colonoscopic examination using dye, and this approach has become popular when examining high-risk patients such as those with polyposis syndromes and long-standing, extensive ulcerative colitis [11]. With magnification, it is usually possible to determine the histology of diminutive polyps visually according to well-established (crypt) pit patterns [12]. Without magnification, biopsy is always required to differentiate between hyperplastic and adenomatous lesions, although macroscopically hyperplastic polyps often have a characteristic pale and shiny appearance, with mucus clinging to their surface [13]. A trained endoscopist, using dye and a high-resolution endoscope, can achieve visual morphological distinction between these two groups of polyps in about 80–90% of cases [14,15].

Narrow-Band Imaging

White light is the standard illumination for endoscopy and is composed of an entire spectrum of wavelengths of visible light in the range of 400–800 nm. It was discovered that using extremely short wavelengths of light, in the 415-nm (blue) range, provides information on the capillaries and pit patterns of the superficial mucosa, while wavelengths of 540 nm (green) provide information on larger capillaries in the slightly deeper tissue. These wavelengths are quite narrow in comparison with the wavelengths of visible white light. The blue band of light is within the range of the hemoglobin absorption band and provides enhanced contrast of the capillary pattern in the superficial mucosal layer, allowing characterization of the vascular structures seen during endoscopy. Narrow-band imaging brings out the vascular architecture and is helpful for distinguishing between abnormal and normal mucosa. It can also differentiate hyperplastic, dysplastic, and malignant patterns in tissue [16]. Narrow-band imaging (NBI) is an innovative optical technology that has the potential to provide detailed characterization of a mucosal lesion on the basis of changes in the pattern and size of microvessels within tissue.

The NBI mode is present on many modern endoscopes and can be activated by pressing a button on the instrument's head. Other endoscopes provide a selection of narrow wavelengths that can be considered [17]. The NBI-enhanced superficial vascular patterns provide similar information to that obtained in chromoendoscopy, but without the need to spray dye onto the surface. NBI accentuates the vascular pattern, while chromoendoscopy accentuates the contours of a lesion and highlights the pit pattern of the colonic crypt but does not increase the visualization of vascular structures. In the NBI mode, meshed capillary vessels appear green-brown in color, while the surrounding normal colonic mucosa is yellow-orange (**Fig. 28.2**). Intestinal liquids, retained preparation fluid, and feces give a reddish color, while blood appears jet-black. Studies have reported that larger numbers of neoplastic lesions are seen with NBI in comparison with white-light endoscopy [18,19].

One study [16] has reported that lesions with invisible or faintly visible meshed capillary vessels on narrow-band imaging can be characterized as nonneoplastic, while lesions with clearly visible meshed capillary vessels are neoplastic. Hyperplastic polyps are seen as light brown lesions without a vascular network on narrow-band imaging, while adenomatous polyps appear to be dark brown, with a surface agglomeration of tiny blood vessels, known as the "meshed capillary" network. Using this scheme, it is possible to differentiate adenomas from hyperplastic polyps with accuracy, sensitivity, and specificity rates of 95.3%, 96.4%, and 92.3%, respectively. Narrow-band imaging is a useful and simple method for differentiating between neoplastic and nonneoplastic colorectal polyps.

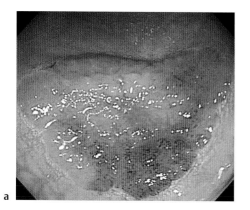 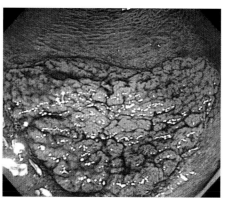

Fig. 28.1a, b Chromoendoscopy, showing the enhanced surface characteristics of a flat polyp.

a

b

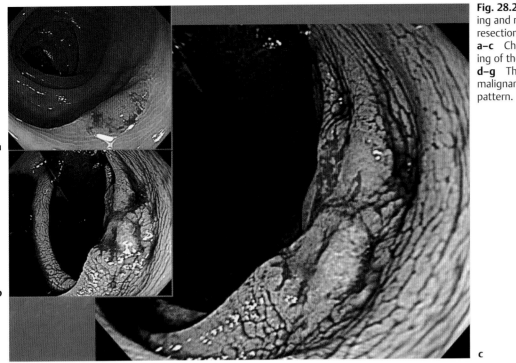

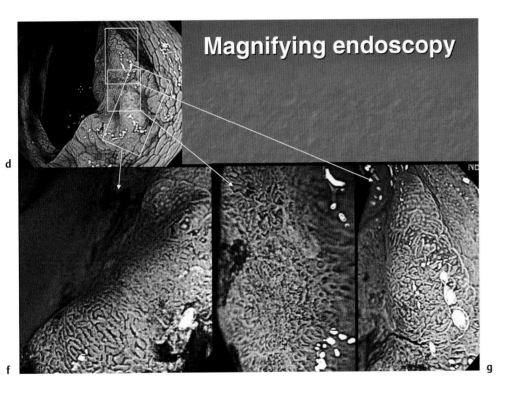

Fig. 28.2 Chromoendoscopy, narrow-band imaging and removal using endoscopic submucosal resection.
a–c Chromoendoscopy provides enhanced imaging of the surface characteristics of the lesion.
d–g The magnifying endoscopy images show malignant characteristics and a meshed capillary pattern.

Fig. 28.2h–p ▷

28

V

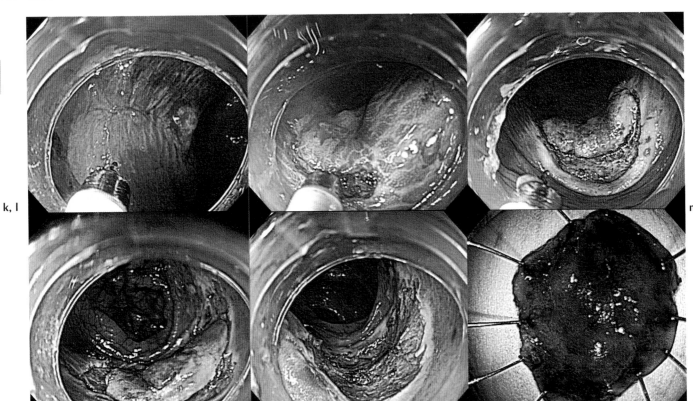

Fig. 28.2
h–j Magnifying endoscopy with various mucosal enhancement techniques: indigo carmine staining (**h**), crystal violet staining (**i**), and narrow-band imaging (**j**).

k–p Removal of the flat polyp with endoscopic submucosal dissection, resulting in curative treatment with a single large specimen.

Endoscopic Accessories

Electrosurgical Units

All of the available electrosurgical units are capable of producing continuous power output (cutting current), or an interrupted wave form (coagulation current). In most electrosurgical units, it is possible to combine the two wave forms with a setting termed "blended current." Most experts use pure coagulation current when removing stalked polyps and either coagulation or blended current for more sessile polyps—particularly in the right colon, when a quicker cut can reduce the risk of full-thickness diathermy injury. Once the electrosurgical unit has been adjusted to the optimal settings, there is no need to change the power output during polyp removal, regardless of whether the polyp base is large or small, or when switching between the polypectomy snare and the hot biopsy forceps.

Injector Needles

The injector needle is an important component of polypectomy equipment. It must be of sufficient length to traverse the colonoscope; the sheath should be strong enough to prevent buckling when pressure is applied to force it through several loops and convolutions of the scope when in the right colon. The needle should lock into position when extended, to prevent excess play of the needle when one is attempting to push it into the mucosa. In addition, the bevel of the needle is an important but often overlooked component, since a long bevel may pierce two or more layers and permit simultaneous injection into the submucosa while also spilling fluid into the peritoneal cavity. The distended bowel wall is relatively thin, with the total thickness varying from 1.5 to 2.5 mm [20]. Each layer (mucosa, submucosa, and muscularis propria) is about 0.5 mm thick, so the bevel has to be rather obtusely angled to allow precise submucosal injection. Even without a sharply angulated bevel, a needle with a smaller diameter is advantageous for delivering fluid into the submucosal layer without extravasation into the colon lumen. Generally, a 260-cm injector is used with a 25-G needle. More viscous solutions used for complex endoscopic resection require a slightly thicker 23-G needle.

Colonoscope

A single-channel colonoscope 168 cm long, with an accessory channel of 3.2 or 3.8 mm, is the instrument preferred for colonoscopy by all experts and most colonoscopists. The double-channel scopes are somewhat less flexible, can be difficult to pass through the entire colon, and are associated with more patient discomfort than the one-channel type. Variable-stiffness colonoscopes offer some advantage in terms of ease of insertion and now have standard-sized biopsy channels [21,22]. There are only a few occasions when there is a need to pass two accessory devices simultaneously through a colonoscope—such as grasping a polyp and lifting it while placing a snare [23–25]. This maneuver would appear to be relatively easy, but in practice it can be quite difficult, as the two accessories have to move together, rather than separately. It would be desirable to lift up the portion grasped by the forceps while seating the snare downward over the polyp, but such manipulation is not possible with current colonoscopes. Any attempt to use instruments passed through both channels requires that, before the polyp is grasped, the forceps must be passed through the open snare—but even when this has been accomplished, moving the scope tip to lift up the forceps and elevate the polyp also causes the snare to rise up.

Carbon Dioxide

Carbon dioxide colonic insufflation, once thought necessary to prevent spark-induced explosion [26], is now considered optional. Most endoscopists do not now use CO_2, and the major reason for using it is to speed up gas absorption during the examination, with a resultant decrease in postcolonoscopy cramps and distension [27].

Hot Biopsy Forceps

The hot biopsy forceps is an electrically insulated forceps through which electrical current flows in order to direct electrical energy around the tissue held within the jaws, allowing simultaneous cautery of a polyp base while a biopsy specimen is obtained. There has been a recent trend against the use of hot biopsy forceps, because of a perceived increased risk of excessive diathermy injury leading to the risk of delayed bleeding, particularly when the forceps is used in the right colon [28].

Heater Probe and BICAP

Two contact thermal devices, the heater probe and BICAP electrode, can control postpolypectomy arterial spurting, as well as lesser degrees of hemorrhage. When these devices are being used to stop colonic hemorrhage, the current delivery should be reduced by approximately 50% from the power used to treat upper intestinal hemorrhage. Multiple applications at this power setting appear to be safe in the colon. It is not wise to push with a great deal of force, as is recommended in the upper intestinal tract. The water jet from these probes is useful for precise localization of the bleeding site, allowing targeted application of the probe. Both of these probes require direct contact with the target tissue, and they can be applied directly end-on, laterally or tangentially to the tissue.

Argon Plasma Coagulator

The argon plasma coagulator delivers high-frequency current in a monopolar mode that does not require direct contact between the probe and tissue. When the distance from probe to tissue is optimal, the monopolar circuit is completed by the flow of electrons through the activated and ionized argon gas, which transmits the electrical ions from the probe electrode to the tissue. The ionized argon gas is known as argon plasma. Using a combination of voltage adjustment and motion of the probe tip, the extent of thermal penetration of tissue can be varied in a range from fractions of a millimeter up to 6 mm. In the colon, the power output setting depends on the system in use, and should usually be at 25–40 W, with a relatively low gas flow (0.8 L/min). The most recent instrument uses 25 W for intracolonic application. Uses in the large bowel include treatment of postpolypectomy bleeding and ablation of residual adenoma tissue after piecemeal resection [29–31] (**Fig. 28.3**). The delivery system for flexible endoscopy was developed in Germany (Erbe, Inc., Tübingen, Germany) [32,33].

Detachable Loop

There are two devices available for polypectomy, and both are underused: the detachable snare loop and clips [34]. The loop, used for additional hemostasis during or after polypectomy, is a nylon ligature that can be placed over a lesion (such as a pedunculated polyp) like a wire snare, and tightened with a one-way silicone-rubber stopper [35]. The stopper prevents opening of the loop once it has been closed (**Fig. 28.4**). The fully assembled mechanism, with an accompanying oversheath (to allow the soft nylon loop to pass through the instrument channel), has the same caliber as a snare. Once extruded from the end of the delivery system, the loop is maneuvered around the head of a polyp under direct vision. The tightened lasso is a self-retaining ligature; once deployed, the loop is separated from the insertion tube [35]. The loop is most often used for large polyps with a thick pedicle [36]. When an attempt is being made to encircle large polyps, the floppy nylon loop—which does not have the same tensile strength of a wire snare—may become caught in the bumpy nodularity of the polyp head, making it impossible to pass the loop completely over the polyp. If the loop becomes inadvertently enmeshed in the interstices of the polyp head, closure of the loop will result in tangential placement, interfering with snare positioning. If the head is encircled successfully, it is necessary for the loop to be placed on the pedicle far enough toward the colon wall to allow transection of the stalk above the

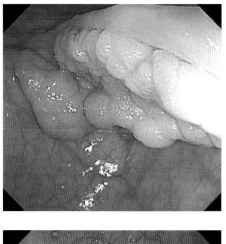

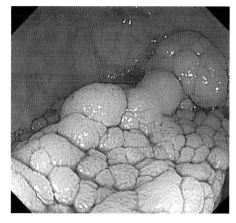

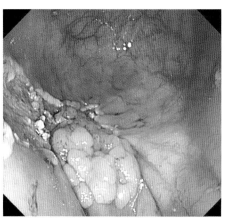

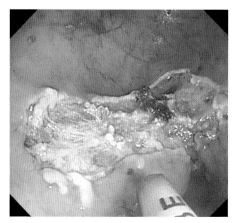

Fig. 28.3 Endoscopic mucosal resection and argon plasma coagulation.
a A flat polyp, seen with white-light endoscopy.
b The surface is enhanced with chromoendoscopy.
c Partial removal of the polyp with endoscopic mucosal resection.
d Treatment of the residual polyp fragment at the base, using the argon plasma coagulator. The probe can be seen in the foreground.

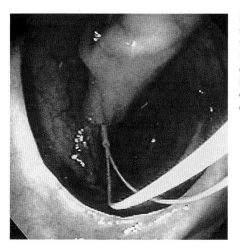

Fig. 28.4 A detachable snare has been placed at the base of a pedunculated polyp. The polyp can now be transected by placing the electrocautery snare above the detachable snare.

loop, with a sufficient margin to ensure safety if the polyp contains invasive cancer. After placement close to the bowel wall, polypectomy is carried out above the loop ligature. Transection of the pedicle close to the loop may cause the loop to slip off, with immediate bleeding as a complication. Placement prior to polyp removal may result in difficulty with snare placement because of the long "tail," which may overlay the site of snare application. As immediate postpolypectomy bleeding only occurs in about 1% of cases [37], an alternative use for this device is to place it on the resected stalk to ensure hemostasis after polypectomy—although tissue retraction may flatten the residual pedicle to the extent that the loop cannot be properly seated [38]. The loops spontaneously slough in 4–7 days, and endoscopy after detachment of the loops shows residual shallow ulcers. The loop and carrier device (HX-20) are manufac-

tured by Olympus, Inc.; the loop is available in two sizes, 2.5 cm and 4.0 cm.

Clips

Mucosal clips have been available for several years. These small tweezer-like devices are useful for temporary marking of lesions, to identify the distance reached by the colonoscope [39], and to mark the proximal and distal edges of tumors before expandable metal stents are placed. The clips can also be used for hemostasis [40]. Improvements in the application device have made it considerably easier to deploy clips, and the ability to rotate them allows more precise placement [41]. The clips are supplied in two different forms—one for hemostasis, and one for endoscopic mucosal marking. In practice, the two types of clip can be used interchangeably, and they are directly affixed to the bleeding site [42]. The clips are especially useful for bleeding from flat polypectomy sites. They have also been used successfully to stop arterial bleeding from the severed stalk of pedunculated polyps. It is theoretically possible to apply a clip to the base of a pedunculated polyp close to the bowel wall and to snare the polyp above the clip using standard snare techniques [43]. It is important that the wire snare should not touch the metal clip, as an aberrant current pathway can be activated, with potential burning of the colon wall. The clips spontaneously dislodge within a few days. The clips, when fully opened, are 9 or 11 mm in length and can be passed through a 2.8-mm accessory channel. A new clip design (Resolution; Boston Scientific, Natick, Massachusetts, USA) allows for reopening of the clip so that correct placement can be assessed before the clip is finally fired. Both loops and clips can be used prophylactically in patients with coagulation disorders, either spontaneous or iatrogenic (warfarin), when there is a risk of subsequent bleeding (**Fig. 28.5**).

Snares

Snares are available in a wide variety of shapes and sizes. The standard large snare is about 6 cm in length and 3 cm wide, and the small snare is 3 cm long and 1 cm wide. The technique is the same in all instances, whether the snare is oval, crescent-shaped, or hexagonal. The diameter of the wire is an important consideration, as thin snare wires will cut through a polyp faster than thick wires [44]. This variable needs to be taken into account when switching from one type of snare to another. A bipolar snare [45] is available, but this does not appear to provide any benefit in comparison with the standard monopolar electrocautery snare. Rotatable snares are available, but are considered unnecessary by most endoscopists.

Prepolypectomy Laboratory Testing

Routine testing for bleeding disorders before colonoscopic polypectomy is not necessary [46,47]. Any history of a bleeding disorder should be obtained, including any tendency to bleed excessively after lacerations, surgical procedures, or dental extraction. Patients do not need to be screened with a platelet count, prothrombin time, bleeding time, or clotting time.

Aspirin and Anticoagulants

Aspirin, at standard cardiac prophylactic doses (75–80 mg) with its known antiplatelet properties, has not been shown to be detrimental to hemostasis during polypectomy [48,49]. Combined antiplatelet therapy with clopidogrel and aspirin, however, is associated with a significant risk of bleeding, and generally polypectomy should be avoided. The colonoscopist should seek direct cardiology advice regarding the safety (or otherwise) of stopping clopidogrel in patients with drug-eluting coronary stents, because of the catastrophic risk of in-stent thrombosis. Diagnostic colonoscopy is relatively risk-free in patients who require continuous anticoagulation with warfarin, but polypectomy should be avoided because of the possibility of bleeding. When polyps are to be removed in patients receiving anticoagulation therapy who are at high risk for thrombotic episodes (such as those with prosthetic cardiac valves), anticoagulation must be maintained, and can be accomplished by injecting low-molecular-weight heparin, administered twice daily and discontinued at least 12 h before the procedure is performed. It can be continued after the procedure along with warfarin until therapeutic levels of anticoagulation are achieved. If intravenous heparin is used, a period of hospitalization is required [50]. The introduction of low-molecular-weight heparin has been reported to prevent deep vein thrombosis in orthopedic patients and provides an out-of-hospital option for short-term warfarin substitution, although it has not been studied for use in endoscopy [51].

Polypectomy Technique

Polyp Position

The industry standard for colonoscopes is for the suction/instrument channel to be situated at the 5-o'clock position in reference to the visual field. All accessories must enter the visual field in the lower right quadrant and progress toward the 11-o'clock position. This fixed reference point results in relatively easy snare capture of a polyp located in the right lower portion of the field, and occasionally those in the 5–11-o'clock axis, but makes it very difficult to ensnare a lesion that is not on that diagonal. Polypectomy will be easier if the

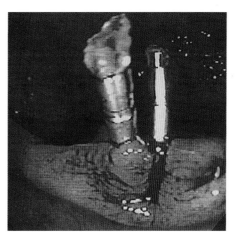

Fig. 28.5 Two clips have been placed on a polypectomy site due to slight bleeding and to ensure hemostasis, in a patient with factor XI deficiency.

instrument can be rotated to place the polyp in the right lower quadrant of the field of view.

Small Polyps

There are several ways of removing small polyps. A hot biopsy forceps provides a histologically identifiable tissue specimen, while electrocoagulation current ablates the polyp base in most instances [52]. In order to prevent deep thermal injury to the colon wall during use of the hot biopsy forceps, the polyp head, once grasped wholly or in part, should be tented away from the wall toward the colon lumen. As current is applied, a zone of white thermal injury will become visible on the stretched normal mucosa surrounding the polyp base. When this injury zone is 1–2 mm in size, the current should be discontinued and the specimen should be retrieved as with any biopsy technique. There is a high rate of residual adenoma when incomplete fulguration occurs [52–54]. Hot biopsy is only suitable for polyps < 6 mm in size, and as already mentioned, due to reported complications they are being employed less frequently than before [55]. Small polyps can also be removed with a wire snare. The mini-snare is suitable, as it is easier to manipulate it around the head of a polyp than the standard snare, since the standard snare requires that the full 6-cm length of wire be extended before the two wires are fully spread apart to form a loop. Small polyps in the range of 1–6 mm have small nutrient blood vessels and can safely be removed by "cheese-wiring" with the snare, in the absence of electric current. This technique is safe and results in minimal bleeding [56,57]. The defect after cold snare excision resembles a punch biopsy site, with a disk of missing mucosa. Streaming blood is only rarely seen afterward, but observation and flushing of the area always shows that it stops within 1–5 min.

Snare Catheter Placement

The most important step in polyp capture is to place the catheter tip at the precise site at which transection is desired once the open snare loop has been placed over the polyp [42]. If the polyp is pedunculated, the tip of the sheath should be advanced to the mid-portion of the stalk. If it is sessile, the sheath should be advanced to the line of visible demarcation between the adenoma and the colon wall. Closure of the loop will result in seating of the snare on the opposite side of the polyp, since the wire loop always concentrically closes toward the tip of the snare sheath, which is the fixed point in the polypectomy system. To ensure proper seating of the wire loop, it is important to look for and observe the tip of the wire loop as it is being withdrawn behind the polyp.

28

Pedunculated Polyps

It should be possible to remove a pedunculated polyp of any size with a single transection [6]. Attempts should be made to encircle the head of the polyp completely with the loop and to tighten it on the pedicle. This can usually be accomplished with any of the standard-sized commercially available polypectomy snares. If a pedunculated polyp is so large that the snare cannot be placed over the polyp head, piecemeal resection of the head can be carried out [58] until the residual portion of the polyp is small enough and adequately visualized to allow the pedicle to be encircled with the wire loop. An alternative approach has been reported to place several Endoclips on the pedicle and transect it with a needle-knife [59]. The polyp with a large broad base has an accompanying large vascular supply, and if the snare can be tightened on the pedicle, snare closure during application of electrocautery current should be considerably slower than usual in order to ensure coaptive coagulation of the blood vessels. When attempting such a polypectomy, prophylactic measures should be taken beforehand to control immediate post-polypectomy bleeding. These may include the ready availability of epinephrine for injection, clips, and a thermal modality such as a BICAP or heater probe.

Sessile Polyps

A polyp that has a wide attachment to the colon wall can be transected with one application of the wire snare, provided that it is located in the left colon and the base is less than 2 cm in diameter. In the right colon, where the wall is somewhat thinner, the endoscopist should consider piecemeal polypectomy or a submucosal injection technique for any polyp with a base larger than 1 cm. The heat produced by snare activation is localized to the area immediately around the wire loop, but also spreads toward the submucosa and serosa of the colon wall. The larger the polyp, the greater will be the volume of tissue captured within the wire loop, and a greater amount of thermal energy will be required to sever the polyp. This may cause a full-thickness burn in the colon wall, which can result in perforation of the bowel. It should be noted again that once the polyp and mucosa have been captured in the loop, the submucosal layers and muscularis propria are in total about 1 mm thick [20].

Endoscopic Mucosal Resection (EMR) and Submucosal Dissection (ESD)

Endoscopic submucosal dissection is a recently developed method of removing large flat superficial neoplastic lesions in the gastrointestinal tract. The initial technique is similar to endoscopic mucosal resection, in which fluid is injected under the polyp to elevate it from the colon wall. However, with endoscopic mucosal resection (EMR), small polyps can be removed with one application of the snare, but larger polyps require several snare applications for removal, with the possibility for heat to destroy residual portions of polyp after repeated piecemeal polypectomy. ESD, on the other hand, allows removal of large and flat lesions by incising the mucosa around the lesion and then dissecting with cautery in the submucosal plane to separate the polyp from the muscularis propria, with removal of the neoplasm in one large specimen (**Fig. 28.6**). This requires longer procedure times and a considerably greater level of skill [60] than EMR. Initial experience with this technique was obtained in the stomach, where the wall is thick, but the technique has been successfully applied in the colon as well [61,62]. The indications for ESD include polyps that cannot be resected in one piece with conventional EMR and those that require precise histo-

logical evaluation because of their significant malignant potential. This technique requires experience on the part of the operator and some special techniques [63]. A transparent hood is attached to the end of the endoscope, which maintains a distance from the tip of the endoscope and the target tissue, so that dissection can be carried out under direct vision in the submucosal plane. There is often a need for repeated fluid injections during ESD to ensure the expansion of the submucosal plane, which allows safe dissection and tends to prevent damage to the muscularis propria by the electrocautery knife. The electrosurgical tool can resemble a needle-knife, a slightly protruded tip of a snare, or a hook device. Characteristically, these devices are only protruded 1–2 mm from their sheath, so that deep damage does not occur. Standard electrosurgical units are used. Because of the length of time required for ESD, the fluid injected into the submucosa is usually a solution of higher viscosity, such as sodium hyaluronate [64–66], which tends to be absorbed at a slower rate than saline, the injection solution most often used for EMR. The en-bloc resection rate is high with ESD, and recurrences are unusual because of the wide margins of the specimen that are achieved during ESD. Bleeding occurs often, but can always be controlled with application of coagulation current by the dissection device or with coagulating (Coag-Grasper) forceps. Perforations do occur in approximately 5% of cases, but most can be treated non-surgically at the time of the ESD by applying clips [67].

Treatment of the Polyp Base after Removal

After a sessile polyp has been removed in piecemeal fashion, the base may be somewhat irregular, due to the several individual passes of the snare. If only ragged fragments of tissue are seen at the base, a repeat examination after 4–12 weeks may reveal that the polyp has completely disappeared, since the thermal energy delivered during polypectomy may slough the remnants. If visible adenoma is present, fulguration can be carried out with a variety of thermal devices, including the argon plasma coagulator, BICAP, heater probe, current applied to the barely extended snare wire, or a hot biopsy forceps [68]. Despite all attempts to remove large sessile polyps (over 3 cm in diameter) totally, even when the polyp appears to have been completely removed with the snare there is still a significant probability of finding residual or recurrent adenoma at the site of the original resection during the follow-up

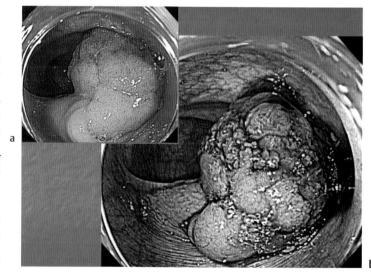

Fig. 28.6 Endoscopic submucosal dissection.
a, b A pseudopedunculated polyp seen with white-light endoscopy (**a**) and chromoendoscopy (**b**).

Fig. 28.3c–k ▷

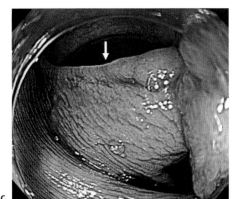

Fig. 28.6
c The thick pseudopedicle can be identified.
d–i The polyp is removed with endoscopic submucosal dissection, resulting in a clean base.
j, k The resected specimen in one large piece.

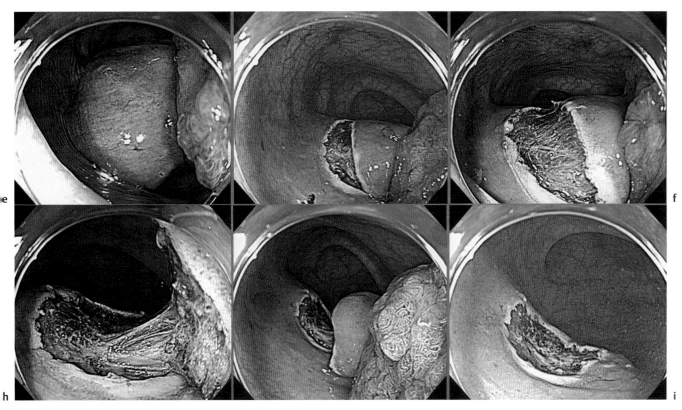

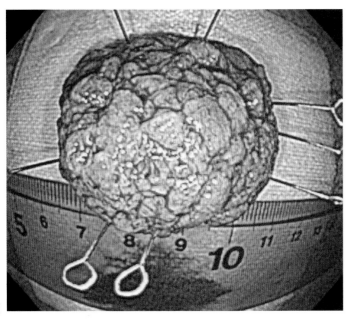

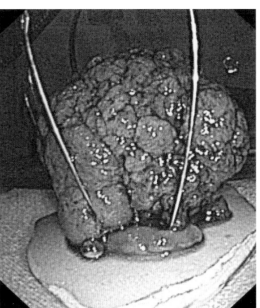

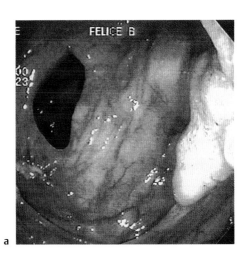
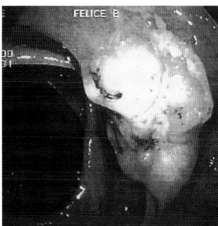
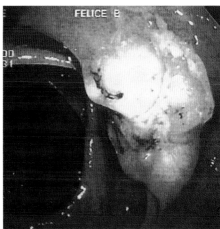
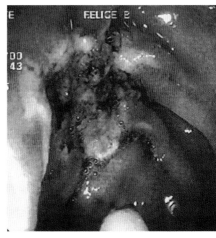

Fig. 28.7
a A flat polyp in the right colon.
b The polyp has been elevated by injecting saline. The translucent submucosa at the base of the elevated polyp should be noted.
c Fragments of polyp have been left at the site after piecemeal resection.
d Argon plasma coagulation of the residual polyp.

examination. If total polypectomy has not been achieved and there is visible residual adenoma at the polypectomy site, there is no possibility of subsequent total involution, and residual polyp will therefore be present at the follow-up examination. However, if visible residual adenoma is immediately treated with the argon plasma coagulator, the risk of residual adenoma falls to 50% [69] (**Fig. 28.7**). Most of these residual lesions can be resected endoscopically at the follow-up examination.

Methods for Safer Polypectomy

▥ Marking the Snare Handle

The endoscopic assistant who closes the snare around a large polyp feels resistance to closure when the slide bar is retracted to the point at which the wire loop is snug around the polyp. This resistance is perceived as a "spongy," resilient sensation, coupled with the inability to close the slide bar further. This closure sensation means that the wire loop has encircled an object and is tightly closed on it, and further retraction of the slide bar will result in guillotining of the polyp or the encircled tissue. If the polyp is very soft or very small, no closure sensation will be perceived, and in the absence of it, the slide bar may be effortlessly retracted and will inadvertently transect the encircled tissue, like a wire cutting through soft cheese. If it were possible for the assistant to know when to stop retracting the slide bar in the absence of any closure sensation, this type of inadvertent cheese-wiring of a polyp could be prevented. Knowledge of the exact point at which to stop slide bar retraction to prevent guillotining of a polyp can be readily obtained by a simple exercise.

This one-minute preparation requires that the slide bar should be retracted toward the thumb hole on the snare handle, stopping when the free tip of the wire loop (snare) is just even with the tip of the plastic sheath. Further closure of the slide bar would result in the snare tip fully entering the plastic sheath. The assistant should make a mark on the snare handle using the slide bar as a guide [6]. The mark can be made with a pencil or pen, forming a line across the handle where the edge of the slide bar crosses it. The mark must be on the thumb hole side of the slide bar crossing, not toward the plastic sheath.

Preventing inadvertent guillotining of a polyp. During snare closure, observing the line on the handle and stopping there, even without any closure sensation, will reassure the assistant that a polyp will not be sliced off unintentionally.

Estimating the tissue volume in the closed snare. The endoscopist may wish to know the approximate volume of tissue encircled by the snare. This is useful when an extremely large amount of tissue is captured. If the endoscopy assistant can inform the endoscopist that the volume of tissue within the closed loop is greater than expected for the estimated size of the polyp, then several interpretations of the estimate will be available for consideration—that the snare is seated across a wide area of the polyp (instead of at the narrow base); that the polyp base is too wide for a single transection; or that excess surrounding mucosa has also been included within the tightened loop. Using the mark on the handle as noted above, the amount of wire loop outside the sheath during snare closure can be estimated by the assistant, who can see the distance from the fully retracted slide bar (when spongy resistance is felt) to the previously

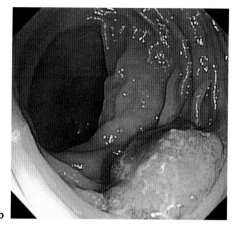
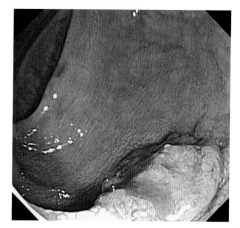
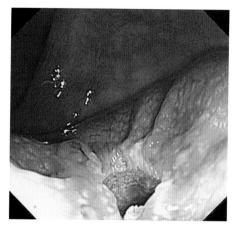

Fig. 28.8 Endoscopic mucosal resection.
a A sessile polyp.
b The appearance of the polyp following dye spraying.

c Total removal with one application of the snare after submucosal saline injection.

28

drawn mark. If a closure sensation has been noted and the slide bar is at the mark, then there is little likelihood of excess tissue being caught within the snare. If a closure sensation is perceived but the slide bar is not at the mark, the amount of tissue within the closed snare loop is directly proportional to the distance from the edge of the slide bar to the mark on the handle. If that distance is greater than 3 mm, there is a large volume of tissue within the loop. Knowing that a substantial volume of tissue has been captured, the endoscopist must reassess the situation and decide whether to remove the snare, to open and reposition the loop, or whether placement is appropriate (for instance, with snare lying tangentially across the polyp but acceptably positioned because piecemeal polypectomy will be necessary). Characteristically, larger portions of a polyp can be removed during the piecemeal technique than would ordinarily be resected by a single application of the wire loop around a single polyp. The decision as to whether large polyps should be removed piecemeal or with one transection is not necessarily related to the size of the polyp, but to the volume of tissue within the closed snare. Some large polyps may be soft and spongy, allowing a greater amount of slide bar retraction than is possible with a smaller but firmer polyp.

Submucosal Injection for Polypectomy

The submucosal injection technique can be used to remove sessile adenomas, whether small or large [70–73]. The total thickness of the colon wall is 1.5–2.5 mm, and thermal damage to deep layers of the colon frequently occurs [74]. Injection of fluid into the submucosa beneath the polyp increases the distance between the base of the polyp and the serosa. When current is then applied via a polypectomy snare, the lesion can be more safely removed, as there is a large submucosal "cushion" of fluid that reduces the likelihood of thermal injury to the serosal surface. The fluid, injected through a long and stiff sclerotherapy needle, may be saline (normal or hypertonic) [75], with or without methylene blue to enhance visualization, and with or without epinephrine [76]. Most endoscopists use normal saline only. Hypertonic solution and epinephrine are used to retain the fluid at the site for a longer period, but saline blebs last for 10–15 min, which is sufficient time to remove most polyps. There is a theoretical advantage to the injection of dilute epinephrine, to prevent bleeding at the time of polypectomy or to prevent delayed bleeding. However, the incidence of immediate bleeding is low (one in 100 procedures) [37], and the long-term effect of epinephrine injection is nil because its effect is measured in hours, not days.

The needle can be inserted into the submucosa just at the edge of a polyp, or if the polyp is large and flat, multiple injections may be given around the polyp or directly into the middle of the polyp. If a bleb does not form at the injection site when 1 mL of fluid has been given, the needle should be withdrawn, since the tip may have penetrated the wall and pierced the serosal surface. When the needle is in the right plane, continuous injection of saline will result in a bleb. A large localized fluid collection is the desired end point, with marked elevation of the polyp. When the tissues expand in response to fluid injection, the fluid is in the submucosal layer. The absence of a visible bleb does not indicate that a bleb is forming on the serosal surface, since the only location of areolar tissue in which fluid can collect is the submucosa. Neither the mucosa, the polyp, or the muscular layer will expand with fluid injection. If the needle placement is too superficial, the fluid will leak out from the beveled edge and spill into the lumen. This spilling is especially noticeable when a colored fluid is used, such as methylene blue or a carbon-based tattoo suspension. Several repeated needle placements and attempts at injection may be needed to locate the correct plane for elevating the polyp. One trick for finding the submucosal plane is to start injecting just before the mucosa is pierced, so that as soon as the needle hits the submucosal space, a bleb occurs. Approaching at 45° and using a slight "jabbing" action to pierce the mucosa can also help. The desired elevation of the polyp may require 3–4 mL of saline given in several places, although some authors use up to 30 mL of fluid [77]. Polyps up to 2 cm in diameter can be removed with one application of the snare (**Fig. 28.8**), but larger polyps may require several transections with a piecemeal technique [78]. It is permissible to remove a much larger piece using this technique than one would ordinarily resect when in the right colon without a cushion of fluid. The pieces should probably not be larger than 2 cm in diameter [77] (**Fig. 28.9**). With the fluid as protection against deep thermal tissue injury, it is even possible to fulgurate the base of the polyp resection site. The devices used for fulguration include a hot biopsy forceps, the tip of the snare, the argon plasma coagulator, or any other thermal device that delivers heat to the residual polyp site.

Volume of Injected Fluid

No specific volume of fluid is used when attempting submucosal injection polypectomy. Instead, the desired end point is reached when a large submucosal swelling is seen beneath the polyp and adjacent portions of the mucosa. When part of the polyp is hidden from view behind a fold, or is wrapped around a fold in clamshell

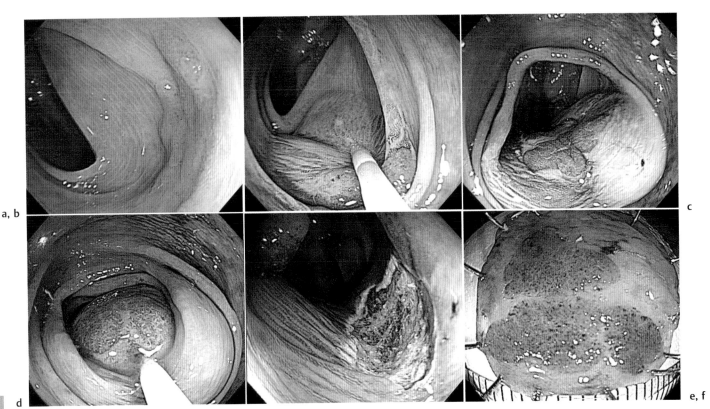

Fig. 28.9a–f Endoscopic mucosal resection, showing the injection technique and single-snare removal of a flat, sessile polyp.
a Laterally-spreading flat lesion (IIa) 15 mm in diameter in transverse colon.
b Injection of glycerol into submucosal layer at the oral side of lesion.
c View after injection.

d Snaring procedure.
e Ulcer after resection.
f Resected specimen should be flattened with pins like this to examine pathologic features.

fashion, injection of the part nearest to the colonoscope may elevate that portion—but may also result in an inability to see the rest of the polyp, as the mound of saline will block vision. This can be prevented. When the proximal edge of the polyp is hidden, an attempt should be made to pass the scope beyond the far edge of the polyp. While the tip is deflected toward the polyp, the injection should be made into the normal mucosa just at or near the edge of the polyp. Depending on the polyp size, several injections may be required to elevate the polyp so that snare placement is more readily accomplished. After the back portion of the polyp has been removed, saline can then be injected into the area closest to the scope to assist in completing the polypectomy.

Malignant Polyps

A colon cancer is a neoplasm that has invaded through the muscularis mucosa and into various levels of the submucosa; for more advanced cancers, the entire wall may be invaded with local or distant metastases [79]. A malignant colon polyp is a subcategory of colon cancer and has a more favorable outlook, as it can often be cured by endoscopic removal. "Malignant colon polyp" is the term used to describe the early stages of colon cancer, when neoplastic cells have invaded into the superficial submucosal tissues. Malignant colon polyps often appear visually to be benign, and the diagnosis of cancer within the polyp may only be found on histopathologic evaluation of the resected specimen. Some of the surface characteristics of a malignant polyp are: friability or spontaneous bleeding, concavity of the polyp head instead of a smooth convex contour, ulceration, or marked irregularity of the polyp. The difference between a polyp with high-grade dysplasia and a malignant polyp is that the malignant-appearing neoplastic cells in the polyp with high-grade dysplasia do not invade beyond the muscularis

mucosa. Since there are no lymphatic vessels superficial to the muscularis mucosa [80], a polyp with high-grade dysplasia is completely cured by polypectomy, because the tumor does not penetrate into the adjacent submucosa [81]. A polyp with high-grade dysplasia is not a malignant polyp and is cured by the polypectomy procedure. Once a polyp with high-grade dysplasia is removed colonoscopically, no special follow-up examinations are necessary.

One of the criteria for the ability to resect a sessile malignant polyp colonoscopically is the ability to lift the lesion with submucosal injection of saline. If the polyp fails to elevate (the nonlifting sign) when the injection is made into the right plane, this may be a sign of deep invasion of the tumor preventing elevation and separation of the lesion from deeper layers [82]. Kanao et al. [83], using narrow-band imaging, developed a classification of topographic appearances with which the endoscopist may be able to determine the depth of invasion of a malignant polyp with a fair degree of accuracy. In initial studies using chromoendoscopy with zoom colonoscopy, it was possible to see disruption of the pit pattern with advanced degrees of malignancy [84].

In pedunculated malignant polyps, the invasion of the carcinoma is into the submucosa of the polyp, whereas in sessile malignant polyps, the cancer invades into the submucosa of the colon wall. The decision as to whether to operate to remove that section of the colon in which the malignant polyp is located and any adjacent lymph nodes will depend on several factors. There are four factors that, if present in a malignant polyp, are associated with a very low rate of lymph-node metastasis, distant spread, or recurrent tumor. These four criteria are:

- The tumor is not poorly differentiated.
- The resection line is clear.
- There is no lymphatic or vascular invasion.
- The endoscopist feels that the entire tumor has been removed.

If all four of these "good" criteria are met, there is a low risk for residual cancer, lymphatic metastasis, or distant spread, varying from 0.3% to 1.5%, depending on whether the polyp was pedunculated or sessile [85,86]. However, it is important to know that even in the presence of any one of these four variables (the polyp is poorly differentiated, there is lymphatic or vascular invasion, the tumor extends to the margin of resection, or the endoscopist feels that the entire tumor was not removed), residual cancer, lymph-node spread, or distant metastases may be found in 8.5% of patients, not 100% [87]. Therefore, in the treatment algorithm for a malignant polyp, the assessment of whether the patient should have surgery will depend on the patient's risk of death associated with surgery relative to the risk of the patient's death due to recurrent/metastatic disease. If the patient is under 50 years of age, there is practically no risk of death from surgery, but as the patient's age increases, the risk of surgery also increases, and treatment options should be made on the basis of the risk of dying from the tumor in comparison with the risk of death from surgery. Comorbidities must also be taken into account in this assessment.

Removal of malignant colon polyps is often curative, even if performed in piecemeal fashion with endoscopic mucosal resection. However, if the lesion is large and multiple fragments of the polyp are removed, it may be difficult for the pathologist to determine whether the deep margin is involved or if the margin is free of tumor. In these circumstances, it is important to know whether the endoscopist felt that the entire tumor was removed, and if so, close follow-up of the moderate-risk or poor-risk patient may be the proper management. On the other hand, endoscopic submucosal dissection can result in a large single piece of tissue being sent for histopathologic examination, where the pathologist will readily be able to determine whether deep margins are involved [88].

If conservative management is selected, close follow-up should be performed with the first follow-up examination after 3 months. If nothing is found at the site, follow-up should be repeated after 1 year, and if there is no recurrence, the patient can revert to normal surveillance intervals.

Tumor Tracking

There is a theoretical possibility that injection through a malignant tumor might cause tracking of cancer cells into and even through the bowel wall. The risk of this happening is minimal, as experience gained from direct percutaneous needle aspiration of malignant tumors in other sites throughout the body suggests. In the latter instances, the risk of tumor tracking is one in 10 000 to one in 20 000 cases [89]. Parenthetically, it seems that any tumor capable of being elevated by a submucosal injection of fluid can be totally removed by endoscopic resection, even if invasive cancer is found on tissue examination. The ability to elevate a tumor indicates that there is only a limited degree of fixation to the submucosal layer, with the possibility of complete removal.

Air Aspiration

During the technique of sessile piecemeal polypectomy, with or without saline injection, an attempt should be made to place one edge of the wire snare at the edge of the adenoma or at the junction between the adenoma and the normal mucosal wall [46]. The other wire of the loop can then be sited over a portion of the polyp to encircle a large piece of tissue. Aspiration of air at this point will result in a decrease in the air-induced wall tension, resulting in a contracted segment of the wall. As the bowel diameter decreases, the footprint of the polyp will also decrease. Since the volume of the polyp does not change, as its base becomes smaller, the polyp will become taller, making it easier to ensnare.

The Tip of the Snare

As the snare is closed slowly, the endoscopist's attention should be directed toward the tip of the loop as it slides over the mucosal surface behind the polyp. It is often possible to see whether a portion of normal mucosa is being caught and dragged up into the loop along with the polyp, or whether the tip is sliding over the mucosa and engaging on the far margin of the polyp. This assessment is important, although in some cases in piecemeal polypectomy, the polyp itself may obscure direct vision.

Stopping at the Line

When complete visualization is not possible as the loop is being closed, the assistant should close until resistance is met, or, if there is no closure sensation, should stop at the marked line previously made on the handle of the snare. Once it is closed, the catheter sheath should be jiggled to and fro at the biopsy port while the colon walls around the polyp are observed. If extraneous portions of the mucosa have not been caught, the polyp will be seen to move independently of the surrounding colon walls as the sheath is jiggled. If the polyp and the surrounding wall move simultaneously, there is a strong probability that a portion of adjacent mucosa has been captured within the snare loop. Complete removal of the snare or partially opening the loop for repositioning is then advisable before electrocautery current is applied. Transection of a large fragment of inadvertently captured normal mucosa is not a desirable outcome of polypectomy, and may lead to perforation. If extra tissue is captured, there is no assurance that it will only consist of mucosa, for submucosa may also be entrapped, and when electrocautery current is applied, a deep burn may result.

Tent the Polyp away from the Base

After the wire is seated securely around the polyp, the sheath should be lifted slightly away from the wall, tenting it toward the lumen to separate the polyp from the submucosa [90]. This will limit the depth of thermal injury when current is applied, since the local zone of heating is less likely to damage the muscularis propria and serosa when the layers are being pulled away from each other. Tenting of the polyp can be accomplished by a variety of movements, with the success of any one being judged by its results. Often, a combination of efforts will be necessary—pushing the snare in or withdrawing it, elevation with the thumb on the up/down dial, or torque on the colonoscope shaft.

Piecemeal Polypectomy

During removal of a sessile polyp, the characteristic whitening at the site of wire placement when electrocautery current is applied often cannot be observed because the wire is embedded in the polyp. After a few seconds of current, the wire snare should be slowly closed until separation occurs. During piecemeal polypectomy, the next placement of the snare may be immediately adjacent to the first, with the edge of the wire being positioned in the denuded area just created by removal of the previous piece. In this fashion, multiple portions can be sequentially resected in an orderly fashion, with removal of each successive piece being facilitated by the previous one. Several applications may be required, with fragments being

28

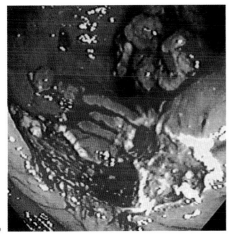
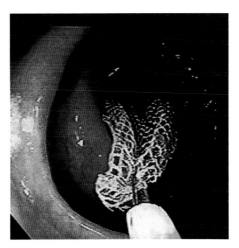
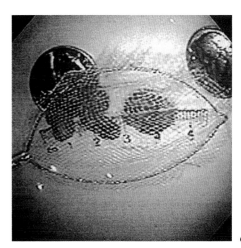

a, b

c

Fig. 28.10
a Multiple polyp fragments in the cecum after piecemeal polypectomy.
b The Roth basket is being deployed to collect all of the polyp fragments for retrieval.

c Multiple polyp fragments removed with the Roth basket.

removed until satisfactory polypectomy is achieved [91,92]. The polyp fragments can be removed by suction into a trap if they are small, or they can be retrieved using a Roth basket (**Fig. 28.10**) or (less effectively) with a Dormia basket or a tripod grasper. One or two fragments can be captured in a snare loop for removal.

Problems

Polyp Position

One of the most important factors in capturing a polyp is that it should be in the proper position relative to the tip of the colonoscope. One of the most frustrating problems encountered during polypectomy is that the polyp is in poor position. A polyp at the 5-o'clock position in the visual field is readily snared, since in colonoscopes the snare enters the field at this orientation. A polyp located between the 9-o'clock and 12-o'clock positions in the visual field is much more difficult to lasso than a polyp in the right lower quadrant, and those in the 3-o'clock or 8-o'clock position are impossible. An attempt should be made to bring all polyps into the 5-o'clock position to facilitate snare placement [46] (**Fig. 28.11**). This can usually be accomplished by rotating the scope to reposition its

face relative to the adenoma. Rotating the scope may be difficult during intubation, when the instrument shaft has loops and bends. Advantageous positioning may be best accomplished when the colonoscope shaft is straight, as a straight instrument transmits torque to the tip, whereas a loop in the shaft tends to absorb rotational motions applied to the scope. It is often difficult to capture a sigmoid polyp during intubation, when the obligatory sigmoid loop is present. It may not be possible to straighten the scope in the sigmoid, as rotation and loop withdrawal results in losing the scope's position. When there is a loop in the scope, the dial controls may no longer work effectively to turn the instrument tip, as the cables that transmit motion are maximally stretched by the loop. These two negative aspects—inability to torque effectively and loss of the cable-controlled tip deflection—combine to create an extremely difficult situation when attempts are made to maneuver the snare into position around a polyp. Maneuvering can be made considerably easier by passing the scope far beyond the polyp, even as far as the cecum (thus visualizing the rest of the colon) and then attempting capture during the withdrawal phase of the examination. As the scope is withdrawn, the loops are removed and a polyp that proved difficult to position during intubation may be quite easily ensnared, as both torque and tip deflection are responsive when the shaft is straight.

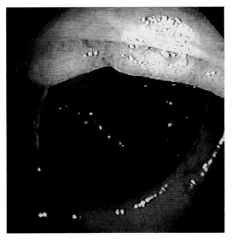
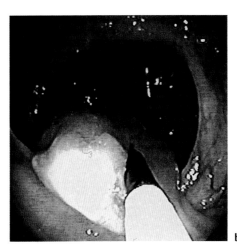

a

b

Fig. 28.11
a A polyp located opposite the ileocecal valve. The polyp is in a difficult location for removal, in the 11–2-o'clock portion of the field.
b The instrument has been rotated to place the polyp in the bottom half of the field. It should be noted that the notch of the ileocecal valve is now at the 12-o'clock position. Saline is being injected proximal to the polyp to elevate it toward the colonoscope.

When to Remove Polyps

There is no contraindication to removing a polyp during intubation and then continuing the examination to the cecum, despite the probability that the scope will rub against the polypectomy site. In general, if a small polyp of any size (< 5 mm) is seen during intubation, it should be removed, since it may be extremely difficult to find it during withdrawal of the colonoscope. If the polyp is of medium size and is in good position, it should be removed, but if it is not in good position it will be readily seen and removed on withdrawal. Small polyps that are transected during intubation should be collected in a polyp trap. The best trap is a multicompartment trap. Sessile polyps requiring piecemeal resection, or pedunculated polyps larger than 1 cm in diameter, should not be removed during the insertion phase, since there may be larger, more significant lesions proximally that could affect the decision for polypectomy. It is possible to spend a considerable amount of time and effort on removing a large hepatic flexure polyp and then to find an undetected carcinoma in the cecum that would require surgical resection including the polypectomy site.

Positional Changes and Abdominal Pressure

As noted previously, it is usually easier to position polyps properly for removal after total colonoscopy has been continued as far as the cecum. As the instrument straightens out with the shaft being pulled out of the colon, clockwise or counterclockwise torque combined with dial-control manipulation can result in unimpeded rotation of the colonoscope tip, so that a polyp encountered at the 10-o'clock position (which may be difficult to ensnare) can be moved to the 5-o'clock position even if it is located in the ascending colon. Additional techniques when trying to move a polyp into a more favorable position include changing the patient's position or applying abdominal pressure. Polyps partially hidden behind folds may come more prominently into view as the patient's position is altered. Polyps submerged in a pool of fluid can be rotated into a drier field by turning the patient so that fluid flows away from the base. Generally, optimal visualization of a polyp in the ascending colon or hepatic flexure is achieved with the patient in the left lateral position, whilst polyps in the transverse colon are best seen with the patient supine. Changing to the right lateral position often augments views of a polyp at the splenic flexure or descending colon.

Rotatable Snares

Rotatable snares are considered unnecessary by most endoscopists. With the wire loop extended, the combination of torque on the shaft and rotation of the dial controls affords much the same effect as snare wire rotation.

Mini-Snares

Some polyps may be extremely difficult to remove, whether they are large or small. There is no substitute for skill and experience in colonoscopy when dealing with a difficult polyp, since operators with special training and those who have excellent control of the instrument will readily be able to remove polyps that others might consider inaccessible. All of the tricks of instrument handling will be helpful in trying to make a polyp more accessible when difficulty is encountered. Sometimes even a small polyp can be difficult—such as those located deep between two intrahaustral folds or in an area distorted by diverticula, where the lumen is narrow and tip manipulation is almost nonexistent. The standard regular-sized polypectomy snare may not be able to capture a small polyp in a difficult and tight location in which there is insufficient space for the wire loop to open wide enough to be placed over the polyp. A problem with the standard snare is that it has to be completely extended to its full length of 6 cm in order for the loop to expand completely. During colonoscopy, it is often found that the wire loop can only be extended a few centimeters beyond the scope, due to a tight bend or because the tip of the loop impacts on an adjacent wall of the colon. When the snare loop cannot be fully extended, the two partially open parallel wires may not spread far enough apart to allow the polyp to be captured. In these conditions, a mini-snare 3 cm in length and 1.0 cm in width [46,93] is extremely valuable. This snare will open fully when extended only 3 cm beyond the sheath, making it useful in areas in which there are multiple bends (such as in a sigmoid narrowed with diverticulosis), or when polyps are located in the depth between intrahaustral folds. Since the vast majority of colon polyps are less than 1.0 cm in diameter, they are within the limits of this mini-snare.

Gastroscope for Better Tip Deflection

Even after total colonoscopy has been performed and the colonoscope has been straightened, there may still be difficulty in capturing a polyp in the sigmoid colon, due to narrowing caused by diverticula and thickened hypertrophic folds. Two techniques may allow easier endoscopic polypectomy. The first is to use a mini-snare as described above, which allows full extension of the snare within a short segment of the bowel. The second is to use a narrow-caliber scope to intubate the colon [94–96]. A pediatric colonoscope is useful, but these are not generally available. It has been shown that a standard upper intestinal gastroscope can be used effectively [88]. The main attributes of the gastroscope are that it has a tighter bending radius at the tip than a colonoscope does, and that the tip beyond the bending portion is shorter. These characteristics frequently allow easy snare positioning in locations in which the colonoscope is both cumbersome and difficult. There is a growing awareness among endoscopists that gastroscopes can be used easily and readily in the colon to intubate difficult and narrowed segments; to pass through strictures; and to make previously inaccessible polyps more readily manageable. The upper intestinal endoscope can be useful even in the rectum, where it may not be possible to snare a polyp on the proximal surface of one of the rectal valves. In this circumstance, the bending section of the colonoscope may be too long to allow a tight turn, whereas a gastroscope, with its greater tip deflection capability and shorter "nose" (or straight portion beyond the bending section), may allow easy visualization and removal of polyps.

New Colonoscopes

Instruments with variable stiffness have been designed by Olympus [21]. Rotating a knob on the control section varies the flexibility of the shaft of these colonoscopes from very soft to twice the firmness of a standard instrument. A pediatric model with a narrow tip deflection radius of the tip and a short bending section is an ideal all-around instrument for colonoscopy.

The Third-Eye Retroscope

Small lesions behind semilunar folds can represent "blind spots" that may be overlooked even with the most careful inspection. Endoscopists who allocate extra time to observe behind the colon

28

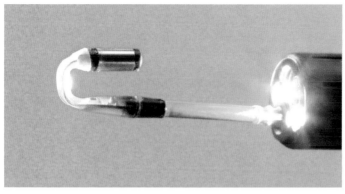

Fig. 28.12 The third-eye retroscope in position, with the lens directed toward the colonoscope to view the lumen behind the standard scope.

folds will reduce the overall incidence of missed polyps or other lesions. However, small polyps are often missed during colonoscopy [97]. In order to allow visualization of the proximal aspect of folds during antegrade inspection of the colon, a device called a "third-eye retroscope" (Avantis Medical Systems, Sunnyvale, California, USA) can be inserted through the instrument channel of a standard colonoscope. It extends beyond the tip of the colonoscope, carrying its own light source and imaging chip. As the "third eye" emerges

from the endoscope, it automatically flexes 180° to look at the face of the colonoscope (**Fig. 28.12**), and when positioned several centimeters away, it visualizes the inferior aspect of the colonic folds while the colonoscope image is shown simultaneously on an adjacent portion of the monitor (**Fig. 28.13**). With this additional visual perspective, the endoscopist can detect lesions that might be missed with the forward-viewing (antegrade image) colonoscope. In a pilot study [98], there was an 11.8% increase in the diagnostic yield of polyps found during routine colonoscopic examination using the third-eye retroscope. This auxiliary imaging device allows visualization behind folds of the colon to identify polyps that would otherwise have been overlooked with straight forward-viewing colonoscopy (**Fig. 28.14**).

■ Clamshell Polyps

In large sessile polyps wrapped around a fold in a "clamshell" fashion, it is usually possible to remove the distal portion readily, but resection of the proximal portion on the far side of the fold may be considerably more difficult. This type of polyp is often located in the right colon and should be removed in piecemeal fashion. With endoscopic mucosal resection or endoscopic submucosal dissection, there is a requirement for rotation of the colonoscope to place the polyp at the 5–6-o'clock position. During EMR, although it would be ideal to resect the total polyp in one session, it may only be possible

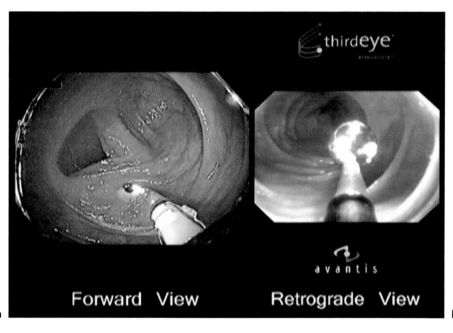

a

b

Fig. 28.13
a The third-eye retroscope has been extended beyond the colonoscope and is seen through the colonoscope.
b The colonoscope is seen by the third-eye retroscope.

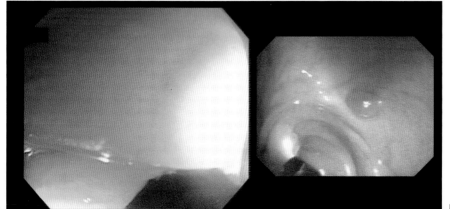

a

b

Fig. 28.14
a The bright light from the integrated light-emitting diode (LED) source in the third-eye retroscope can be seen through the colonic folds in this forward view from the colonoscope.
b The third-eye retroscope shows a polyp on the proximal side of the fold, which was not seen with the colonoscope.

V

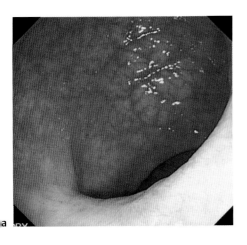
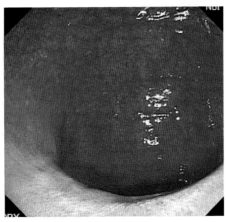

Fig. 28.15 Follow-up after polypectomy.
a The polypectomy scar at 6 o'clock on white-light endoscopy.
b The polypectomy scar seen with narrow-band imaging, demonstrating the absence of any adenoma, with restoration of mucosal patterns at the site of the polypectomy.

to remove the portion nearest to the scope, with some of the polyp on the far side of the fold being left for an interval resection. Subsequent scarring may flatten the polypectomy site, bringing the residual polyp into a favorable location for subsequent polypectomy. If the decision is taken to attempt total polypectomy during the first session, the stiffness of the plastic snare catheter can be used as a probe. After endoscopic transection of the portion closest to the scope, and with the loop extended, the tip of the catheter can be positioned on the ridge of the fold in the polypectomy site where a portion of the polyp has just been removed. Using a combination of torque and rotation of the large control knob, downward pressure on the ridge at the site of the polypectomy divot will often depress it sufficiently so that a portion of the residual adenoma will extend into the loop, allowing capture under direct vision. This maneuver is not dangerous. Several repeated snare applications and transections of this type will usually result in complete polypectomy. The tip of the instrument must be close to the polypectomy site for this technique to be effective, since the plastic polypectomy sheath becomes quite flexible when it is extended more than a few centimeters beyond the colonoscope. With its tip barely protruded, the sheath is stiff and will depress a fold when torque or tip deflection is applied to the colonoscope shaft. Pushing on a fresh polypectomy site in this manner is not associated with any adverse results. Injecting fluid into the submucosa, as described above, may help in attempting polypectomy, particularly aiming the initial injection proximal to the polyp to lift it towards the endoscope.

Retroversion

An alternative technique for removing a polyp located on the far side of a fold is to perform a U-turn maneuver. With standard instruments, this can only be accomplished in the cecum, ascending colon, and transverse colon. It is difficult, although not impossible, to resect a polyp in a U-turn mode, because the tip deflection responses are opposite to those usually expected. The third-eye retroscope permits visualization of the inferior portions of colon folds, but does not allow polypectomy.

Follow-Up Interval

All polypectomy fragments must be retrieved and sent to the pathologist to determine whether the polyp is malignant. If histopathological investigation shows that the resected specimen is benign, there is no rush for total removal of the polyp, and several months can safely elapse before the polypectomy is completed (**Fig. 28.15**). Even if some of the polyp is intentionally left behind, the interval between piecemeal polypectomies should range from 2–6 months

to allow healing to take place. There is no medical necessity for a short-interval (2–4 weeks) follow-up examination, and it is probably unwise to subject the patient to repeated preparation, with the colon being distended with air, shortly after the integrity of the wall has been compromised by a polypectomy.

Polyp Size

The size of the polyp is an obvious reason for difficulty with endoscopic resection. Most polyps are less than 1 cm in diameter, a size that should be well within the resection capability of any trained colonoscopist. Twenty percent of polyps are larger than 10 mm in diameter, and only 1% are over 35 mm in size. When polyps in the left colon grow to become larger than 1 cm in diameter, it is common for peristalsis to pull on the lesion, forming a tubular pedicle from the surrounding mucosa. A polyp of the same size in the right colon has a tendency to remain sessile, with a broad-based attachment.

Bleeding during Polypectomy

If bleeding obscures vision during piecemeal polypectomy, the blood can be dispersed by squirting water through the biopsy channel or by an integral water jet. Mild bleeding can be controlled by continuing piecemeal polypectomy, with cautery of the next segment heat-sealing the bleeding vessels at the previously cut edge. A BICAP, heater probe, or argon plasma coagulator may be useful to stop more severe bleeding, or a 1 : 10 000 solution of epinephrine can be injected into the bleeding site to promote hemostasis. A standard variceal sclerotherapy needle is used in injection therapy. A new and highly effective device is the Coag-Grasper from Olympus. This device has short, serrated metal jaws that can be used to grasp and coagulate visible vessels or bleeding points. Soft coagulation mode is used, and the grasped tissue is retracted away from the bowel wall before short 1–2-s bursts of diathermy are applied. The Coag-Grasper can be used to routinely coagulate submucosal vessels visible after endoscopic resection, and has proved valuable in cauterizing bleeding and destroying blood vessels at the base following endoscopic submucosal dissection.

Polyps Too Difficult to Remove

Flat Polyps

In spite of the knowledge and skill of modern endoscopists, not all colon polyps can be successfully removed with a colonoscope. Among these are lesions that extend over many centimeters, or that are circumferential. Such lesions are best referred for laparoscopic surgery or transendoscopic microsurgery (TEMS) if in the rectum. Ultimately, ease of endoscopic access and lifting characteristics are also key factors in determining suitability for endoscopic resection. Japanese endoscopists have pioneered the technique of endoscopic submucosal dissection (ESD) to remove very large, sessile and flat colorectal polyps [99]. This involves en-bloc dissection using a viscous, longer-lasting injection solution such as hyaluronate, with a diathermy knife to make a circumferential incision and perform submucosal dissection. In Western countries, if endoscopic resection is considered feasible, then piecemeal EMR, which is quick and relatively safe, remains the preferred technique [100].

Extremely Difficult Colonoscopy

If passage to the right colon has been arduous and prolonged and a large sessile polyp has been identified that has a broad attachment that would require several attempts at piecemeal polypectomy, the wisest approach may be to suggest surgical resection, so as to avoid the need for repeated difficult colonoscopies with repeated difficult polypectomies. The risk–benefit ratio depends on the location of the polyp; the right colon is somewhat thinner than the left, increasing the risk of colonoscopic removal. Occasionally, polyps arise from within the appendix orifice and extend around the cecal pole. These lesions are impossible to resect completely endoscopically and will require surgery.

Location of Lesions

At a time when laparoscopic surgical colonic resection is becoming as well accepted as primary colonoscopic treatment, the need for precise location of lesions is even more urgent, since the laparoscopist is not able to palpate the colon between the fingers during exploratory laparotomy [101]. For the laparoscopist, it is of great importance to have an easily visible marker that can be seen through the telescopic lens of the laparoscope. It is not acceptable for the endoscopist to state that a lesion is "in the transverse colon"; a more specific location is needed in order to avoid a subsequent open procedure to find the lesion.

Endoscopic Follow-Up

Precise location of the tip position during colonoscopy is equally important when there is a need to relocate a lesion or an area of the colon at a later time. It may be desirable to know the precise site at which a polyp was removed in piecemeal fashion, so that the area can be readily identified at the next follow-up colonoscopy—particularly if the polyp is on the back of a fold or just around a difficult bend in the colon.

Healing of Polypectomy Site

Even in circumstances in which an open laparotomy is to be performed, site identification becomes necessary when a specific portion of the large bowel requires resection and the lesion may not be readily apparent by visual or palpatory exploration. After endoscopic removal of a malignant adenoma, the site may heal completely in 8 weeks, and a locator mark may help both the surgeon and the pathologist to identify the site from which the lesion was removed.

Invalidity of Shaft Measurement

Localization by measuring the centimeters of the instrument introduced into the rectum is an extremely poor method of tip localization [102]. During introduction of the instrument, when looping is common, it is possible to advance the full length of a long colonoscope (180 cm) into the rectum, yet the tip may still be at the junction of the sigmoid and descending colon [103]. By repositioning the instrument, removing loops, and straightening it, it can be possible to reach the cecum in the same patient with a total inserted length of only 60 cm of the instrument. The actual number of centimeters inserted may bear no relationship to the actual tip location within the colon [104].

Endoscopic Landmarks

Landmarks are notoriously imprecise for exact localization of areas between the rectum and cecum. Even the most experienced colonoscopists may err in their estimate of tip location [101,103,105]. Indeed, in a large tortuous sigmoid colon, it may be difficult to localize a lesion to even the middle or upper sigmoid colon. Similarly, a lesion estimated by the endoscopist as being near the splenic flexure may be under the diaphragm; could be either proximal or distal to the flexure; or it might even be actually located at the junction between the sigmoid and descending colon. Precise location may be impossible because of tortuosity and multiple bends in that area of the colon. The only invariable localizing landmarks are when a lesion is located within 15 cm of the anus, since there is no doubt that it is close to or in the rectum, and when a lesion is near the endoscopically identified ileocecal valve which can be easily found by the surgeon. In the latter case, the problem is associated with the endoscopist's ability to recognize beyond doubt that the cecum has indeed been reached.

Clips

Clips can be inserted through the colonoscope and placed on the mucosa in any location. These will assist with radiographic or ultrasonographic location of the marked segment. However, clips tend to fall off after an average of approximately 10 days [106], with some falling off earlier and others continuing to be attached for longer intervals. Although it has been suggested that clips may be a helpful marker for surgical localization, it has been found that the clip devices are rather small to be palpated easily. In addition, the surgeon cannot be sure that a palpable clip has not spontaneously detached just prior to surgery and is actually at some distance from its original position during endoscopy. If a surgeon palpates a clip in the sigmoid colon and resects that segment, it is possible that the clip was actually placed at a location near the splenic flexure, and became detached and migrated distally. A report on eight patients in whom clips were placed during colonoscopy before laparoscopy stated that intraoperative ultrasound readily located the marked areas for surgical resection [107].

Intraoperative Colonoscopy

It is possible to locate the site of a tumor or a resected polypectomy site by carrying out intraoperative colonoscopy [108–110]. This technique has been avoided by most endoscopists, due to the need to perform an endoscopic examination in the operating room, with all the constraints of positioning the patient, handling the scope, and trying to use maneuvers such as torque and straightening techniques with the abdomen open. The amount of air insufflated for colonoscopy can create problems with surgical techniques once the endoscopist has completed the necessary localization. Because the site of a polypectomy may heal within a few weeks, there is a possibility that a polypectomy site may not be seen during intraoperative endoscopy.

▪ Marker Injections into the Colon Wall

The ideal method for lesion localization is to have an easily identifiable marker that will immediately attract the attention of the surgeon or endoscopist [105]. This can be achieved by injecting dye solutions. An experimental study has shown that of eight different dyes injected into the colon wall in experimental animals, only two persisted for more than 24 h [111]. These were indocyanine green and India ink. The indocyanine green was visible up to 7 days after injection, and it is known that India ink is a permanent marker that persists for the life of the patient, due to submucosal injection of carbon particles. Other dyes—such as methylene blue, indigo carmine, toluidine blue, sulfan blue, and hematoxylin and eosin— were all absorbed within 24 h, leaving no residual staining at the injection site. Indocyanine green is approved by the Food and Drug Administration (FDA) in the United States for human use, but India ink has not been so approved.

Indocyanine green is not associated with any significant tissue reaction and is relatively nontoxic, but ulceration of the injection sites has been reported in an animal model [111,112]. Clinical experience with indocyanine green tattoo in 12 patients demonstrated that the dye was easily visualized on the serosal surface of the colon at surgery within 36 h following injection [113] and may remain visible for up to 7 days [111]. In an animal model, the dye was not visible after 1 day [112]. The problem with a marker that has such a relatively short period of persistence is that the decision on whether to operate after removal of a malignant polyp may take a few weeks, with slide reviews and multiple consultations being required. An injection marking made at the time of polypectomy will have disappeared, while the site itself will become more difficult to locate with the passage of time.

India ink. Most experience with the dye injection technique has been gathered with India ink being used as a permanent marker [114,115]. The stain lasts for at least 10 years, with no reduction in intensity after that length of time. A permanent marker may be worthwhile for several reasons. A lesion that requires surgery may be injected, but surgery may be postponed for several weeks for clinical reasons—after which time a vital dye such as indocyanine green will have been absorbed, leaving the surgeon with no visible evidence of the injection site. Sometimes it is desirable to mark the site of a resected polyp for subsequent endoscopic localization, when it is anticipated that the area will be difficult to find on a follow-up examination, especially when the lesion is located around a fold or behind a haustral septum. A stain with a permanent marker such as India ink will immediately draw attention to the site, allowing more accurate and complete assessment. For the surgeon, a locator stain is an invaluable aid in the effort to seek and resect the area of the bowel containing the site of the lesion. When the lesion is relatively small, such as a flat cancer or a malignant polyp previously endoscopically resected that requires surgical resection, the site may not be evident from the serosal surface and may not even be palpable. If the area to be resected is in a redundant sigmoid colon or near the splenic flexure, it may be impossible to locate either visually or by palpation. Occasionally, even large lesions may not be palpable by the surgeon if they are soft and compressible [109]. As mentioned above, visible marking can assist with precise

surgical intervention for laparoscopy-assisted colon resections, or clips may be detected by an ultrasound probe.

Complications have been reported with India ink injection, but clinical symptoms resulting from the injection are relatively rare [116,117]. Tissue inflammation has been reported in an animal model [112]. The complications may in part be related to the wide variety of organic and inorganic compounds contained in the ink solution, such as carriers, stabilizers, binders, and fungicides [118]. It is possible that the toxic properties of India ink may be partially improved by substantial dilution of the ink. Ink diluted to 1 : 100 with saline produces as dark a spectrophotometric pattern as undiluted India ink, and in clinical tests, the tattoo made with 1 : 100 diluted India ink has been found to be readily visible by the endoscopist and by the surgeon. A small-volume injection (0.5 mL) may increase the safety of the procedure [112,119,120]. India ink is black drawing ink made with carbon particles. Permanent fountain pen ink is not an acceptable substitute. India ink is available from any stationery store, although it is supplied for medical uses in nonsterile form as a stain to enhance the diagnosis of cryptococcosis in the cerebrospinal fluid. The India ink may be sterilized in an autoclave after dilution, or it can be rendered bacteriologically sterile by passing the diluted solution through a 0.22-μm Millipore filter interposed between the syringe containing the dilute solution of India ink and the injection needle [121]. A standard sclerotherapy needle is used, long enough to traverse the accessory channel of a 168-cm colonoscope, and stiff enough for the plastic sheath not to crinkle up as it is being forced through the biopsy port when the tip of the instrument is deep in the colon and the colonoscope shaft has several convolutions and loops. Ideally, the needle should enter the mucosa at an angle in order to allow injections into the submucosa, rather than having the needle piercing the bowel wall. The edges of intrahaustral folds should be targeted. If a submucosal bleb is not immediately seen during an injection, the needle should be pulled back slightly, since it may have penetrated the full thickness of the wall and the ink may be squirting into the peritoneal cavity. An intracavity injection is not a clinical problem [113,122], but it may scatter black carbon particles around the abdominal cavity, which may be somewhat disconcerting for the surgeon. Since the colonoscopist cannot know which portion of the bowel is the superior aspect, multiple injections should be made circumferentially in the wall around a lesion to prevent a single injection site from being located in a "sanctuary" site, hidden from the eyes of the surgeon as the abdomen is opened with the patient lying supine [123]. Each injection should be of sufficient volume to raise a bluish bleb within the mucosa at the injection site. The injection volume may vary from 0.1 to 0.5 mL. If injections are made a few centimeters from the lesion, the surgeon should be informed whether the injections are proximal or distal to the site. With the 1 : 100 dilution of India ink, endoscopic visualization is still possible if some of the ink spills into the lumen, whereas with the more concentrated solutions, the endoscopic picture becomes totally black when ink covers the bowel walls [122]. Most endoscopists who use India ink to mark colonic lesions do not prescribe antibiotics before it is used, although it has been suggested that prophylactic antibiotics should be given before injections of indocyanine green [113]. India ink is indeed a permanent marker, with endoscopic visualization of the tattoo site being possible without any diminution in color in every case on follow-up examinations up to an interval of 10 years after the initial injection (Fig. 26.**12**). Several reports have attested to the safety as well as the efficacy of this technique [116,124,125].

An improved surgical marker. A pure, sterile, and dilute solution of carbon particles in suspension is now available and has received FDA approval for short-term surgical marking. The solution is prepackaged in syringes and is ready for use without any preparation.

28

Complications

The major complications that occur with therapeutic endoscopy are perforation of the bowel, bleeding, and postpolypectomy syndrome. The combined incidence of significant hemorrhage and perforation in therapeutic colonoscopy may range between 0.36% [126] and 1.7% [127,128].

▦ Perforation

Perforation occurs in 0.04–2.1% of colonoscopic polypectomies and is due to mechanical slicing across the wall with the wire snare or thermal necrosis of the wall that leads to perforation within a few hours after the polypectomy [129] (**Fig. 28.16**). The presence of free air after colonoscopy does not in and of itself mandate a surgical exploration if the clinical presentation is completely benign [130,131]. The literature states that a patient who has no signs or symptoms of perforation after endoscopy, with intraperitoneal or retroperitoneal air being the only sign of perforation, should be treated with antibiotics, nil by mouth, and careful observation [132]. It is possible that a small leak may spontaneously seal and not require surgical intervention. A condition termed "benign pneumoperitoneum" after colonoscopy has been described, in which it is thought that air may leak through a diverticulum. This was discovered in one out of 100 consecutive postcolonoscopy flat abdominal radiographs. The patient was completely asymptomatic and was treated conservatively, and the pneumoperitoneum resolved. The amount of free air seen on radiography or computed tomography may bear little relationship to the clinical picture. If the perforation occurs directly after polypectomy and is relatively small, an attempt can be made to close the defect with endoscopic clips. Multiple clips can be applied, and if good apposition of the muscle wall is achieved and there has been no contamination of the peritoneal cavity, then a good outcome can be expected, although with close patient observation and antibiotic coverage. On the other hand, if a large perforation is seen, with clear visualization of the peritoneal cavity or the serosal side of other organs, etc., then immediate surgical exploration is necessary (**Fig. 28.17**). There is no justification for waiting until symptoms develop, since they certainly will if there is a large through-and-through perforation. Whenever there is visible evidence of fat protruding through a hole in the colon, this is also evidence of a free perforation and mandates surgical exploration. Between the two extremes of the asymptomatic patient and the patient in whom there is an obvious large hole in the bowel wall, there is a subset of patients who have a high probability of perforation and who may or may not have free air, but who have localized peritonitis, without any signs of generalized peritonitis. These patients may have localized and rebound tenderness, leukocytosis, and a low-grade fever. Treatment with intravenous fluids, nil by mouth, and antibiotics will often allow the symptoms of acute inflammation to resolve [133,134]. If watchful waiting is the choice, then the patient must be closely monitored in the hospital setting by the gastroenterologist and a surgeon. If the situation deteriorates and it is deemed that the signs or symptoms of inflammation are spreading, then surgery should be performed. In these circumstances, a water-soluble contrast enema may be worthwhile in an attempt to identify the perforation site; this may be especially valuable in patients who have had multiple polyps removed, leading to doubt regarding the exact perforation site. Laparoscopic treatment of iatrogenic colon perforations has been successfully accomplished [135] and this may be a useful first-line surgical approach to the problem. If a small perforation occurring during polypectomy is recognized immediately, it may respond to transcolonoscopic clip application with closure of the hole [136].

▦ Postpolypectomy Coagulation Syndrome (Serositis, Transmural Burn, Postpolypectomy Syndrome)

This syndrome is known by several names, and is the result of a transmural burn causing irritation of the serosa, with a localized inflammatory response. This reaction to electrocautery current causes symptoms similar to those of any other intra-abdominal localized inflammatory response [137], such as appendicitis or diverticulitis. The difference is that an illness such as appendicitis is a response to an infectious process causing inflammation, whereas a transmural burn is a result of thermal injury to the colon wall. The postpolypectomy inflammatory response may cause localized pain, tenderness, guarding, and rigidity. There may or may not be fever, tachycardia, and leukocytosis. This syndrome occurs after 1% of colonoscopic polypectomies [37], and the symptoms begin 6 h to 5 days after polypectomy (average 2.3 days). As with all other syndromes in medicine, there are several grades of severity, with some patients having spontaneous discomfort with deep tender-

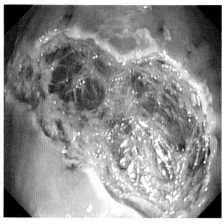

Fig. 28.16 The base of a polypectomy site following endoscopic submucosal resection. The bluish color is due to the indigo carmine that was added to the injection solution. The stellate pattern represents edema in the submucosal interstitial layer.

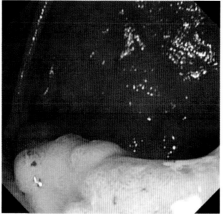
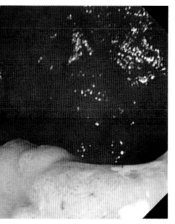

a

b

Fig. 28.17 Colon perforation.
a A flat polyp was present in the ascending colon.
b After an attempt at endoscopic submucosal resection, a through-and-through perforation was seen at the base of the polypectomy site. The bluish color is due to the indigo carmine that was added to the injection solution. This type of perforation cannot be closed with Endoclips, and the patient required surgical intervention.

ness on palpation, while others may have a full-blown inflammatory response with fever. Most patients with this syndrome have a mild ache or tenderness in the area overlying the polypectomy site. About 20% of patients will have more severe symptoms, such as guarding, rigidity, and fever, and should be treated with intravenous fluids and close observation in the hospital. All symptoms usually resolve in 2–5 days. The major differential diagnosis of the post-polypectomy coagulation syndrome involves perforation of the bowel [131]. Surgeons frequently consider this symptom complex as a "mini-perforation," although the major distinguishing characteristic between a free perforation and the postpolypectomy coagulation syndrome is that the latter does not show radiographic evidence of free air in the peritoneal cavity. Whenever the endoscopist is concerned about the integrity of the colon wall, a radiograph should be taken. If free air is seen under the diaphragm, the diagnosis is a perforation, and treatment decisions should be made in conjunction with surgical consultation. The worst outcome in this syndrome is a through-and-through burn of the wall, with rapidly developing necrosis and free perforation. The patient may have early evidence of localized peritonitis, which becomes increasingly severe, and when the necrotic wall perforates, air and bowel contents enter the abdominal cavity. There is no question that surgery is necessary at this time and should be performed urgently. In a recent prospective series of 777 polypectomies, this occurred in two patients (0.3 %) 1–9 days after polypectomy [37].

Postpolypectomy Hemorrhage

This is the most common complication after polypectomy [138]. In a series of colonoscopic resections of large sessile polyps, 2.3% of patients required blood transfusions [139]. The severity of the bleeding ranges from arterial pumping to a slight ooze. Whatever the severity, an attempt should be made to ensure hemostasis. Approximately 1.5% of patients will have bleeding immediately after the polyp is resected, and the hemorrhage should be controlled at that time.

Immediate bleeding. Most bleeding that occurs immediately after resection can be controlled by the endoscopist [37]. This may require several techniques performed in sequence. If a pedunculated polyp bleeds after transection, the hemorrhage can be stopped by regrasping the pedicle with a snare and applying pressure to it to stop the blood flow, initiating the hemostatic clotting cascade. Repeat transection of the pedicle can be performed, but this is not the preferred approach, since there may be too little of the pedicle remaining to allow it to be regrasped if repeated hemorrhage ensues. Most often, holding a snare around a bleeding pedicle tightly for 5 min will result in hemostasis. If bleeding starts again when the snare is loosened after 5 min, a second application of pressure for 5 min will always result in cessation of bleeding. A detachable loop (see the section on endoscopic accessories, above) may be useful, since it can often be applied after transection. Several techniques may be needed to control bleeding after removal of sessile polyps, but a flexible injector needle is the single most useful tool. Bleeding can often be controlled by injecting a 1 : 10,000 solution of epinephrine; several milliliters may be required. The desired effect is a large bleb at the bleeding site. Multiple injections can be made around the bleeding site. The heater probe, BICAP electrode, or argon plasma coagulator are helpful adjuncts to the hemostatic armamentarium. The hot biopsy forceps and more recently the Coag-Grasper can be used as cautery probes by directly applying diathermy current. Repeated light touching of the tissue with the activated hot biopsy forceps results in better fulguration than continuous pressure, since the latter may cause heating of tissue without hemostasis, whereas creating a spark gap results in a better

coagulum. Alternatively, Endoclips can be applied to the site of bleeding; it has been reported that these are easily deployed and successful [140].

Delayed bleeding occurs in approximately 2% of patients who have polyps removed [37]. If the patient comes to the hospital with active bleeding, as assessed by frequent bloody bowel movements, colonoscopy should be performed immediately [138]. Blood is a good cathartic, and usually cleans residual stool out of the colon. Even if the lesion is on the right side, patients can usually undergo endoscopy with adequate visualization of the site, allowing treatment to be delivered. However, if the frequency of bowel movements seems to be decreasing, this is the best clinical sign that bleeding has slowed or stopped, and emergency colonoscopy need not be carried out. If the patient begins to bleed again during observation, urgent endoscopic examination should be performed. An electrolyte preparation may provide an easier colonoscopy [141], but is not an absolute necessity when there is ongoing bleeding. A report of intraoperative colonoscopy for localization of acute severe lower gastrointestinal bleeding has demonstrated the effectiveness of intraoperative on-table irrigation via a catheter placed in the cecum [142]. Angiography may be beneficial when there is severe bleeding, with a vasopressin infusion causing hemostasis [143]. A band ligation device can be attached to the tip of a colonoscope to achieve hemostasis [144,145]. The ligator is a modification of the standard apparatus used to band esophageal varices. Delayed hemorrhage may occur at an average of 1 week after polypectomy, but it may also be seen from a few hours to 12 days later [37].

Hot Biopsy Forceps

This technique has to be used in a specific fashion to reduce the incidence of complications [146]. Under no circumstances should the hot biopsy forceps be pushed toward the colon wall when current is applied, since this will tend to push away the areolar tissue in the submucosa and decrease the distance between the mucosal surface, where the burn is occurring, and the serosal surface. Coaptation of the two layers may lead to a full-thickness burn effect, and even subsequent perforation of the wall. In a retrospective survey, hemorrhage after use of the hot biopsy forceps technique was reported as occurring in 0.41% of cases, and perforation in 0.05% [55]. A prospective series failed to detect any excess risk for either complication with the hot biopsy forceps [129], but the alternative technique of cold snaring appears to be associated with a negligible incidence of bleeding [56].

Results

Colon cancer is preceded by a benign precursor phase, which is the adenomatous polyp. There is no primary prevention for colon cancer, and colonoscopy with polypectomy is the only method for secondary prevention of colon cancer. Specifically, prevention of colon cancer is achieved by removing polyps before they have malignant degeneration. The vast majority of polyps throughout the colon can be removed with endoscopic techniques. Modern colonoscopes can inspect every portion of the colon, and with training and experience, the use of multiple polypectomy techniques will result in clean and bloodless polyp removal with a minimum of complications. The best results are achieved when the operator and assistant work together as a dedicated team with experience in removing colon polyps. It makes little difference whether the colonoscopic suite is large and modern, or small and cramped. The type of colonoscope used does not play a great part in achieving safe polypectomy, nor does the type of electrosurgical generator or the shape or brand of the snare wires used. The critical factors are the

28

capability of the endoscopist and the interaction between the endoscopist and the gastrointestinal endoscopy assistant. A good team ensures high-quality performance in endoscopic polypectomy. Not all polyps can be removed by all endoscopists. It is necessary to assess one's own operative skills continually, and if the proposed polypectomy has a high risk of complications, or if the endoscopist is concerned that the lesion is too large or cannot be approached in a safe manner, the procedure should not be performed. As in all forms of medical treatment, the patient's safety must be foremost at all times.

Checklist of Practice Points

- Teamwork is essential during colonoscopic polypectomy.
- A clean colon is mandatory.
- The history should include any abnormal bleeding tendency.
- Most polyps can be removed by colonoscopic polypectomy.
- A mark on the snare handle serves two purposes: to estimate the volume of polyp captured and to identify the point beyond which further closure will guillotine a polyp.
- Torque the colonoscope to place the polyp at the 5-o'clock position in the visual field before attempting snare placement.
- Have a full view of the polyp and surrounding areas. This may require torquing the instrument, further air insufflation, abdominal pressure, or moving the patient's position.
- Polyps with a base larger than 1.5 cm in the right colon should have a submucosal injection of fluid before polypectomy.
- During transection, closure of the handle should be slow and steady, while the operator provides continuous power application by standing on the foot switch.
- Postpolypectomy bleeding can be controlled with a variety of techniques, including epinephrine injection, heater probe, BICAP, hot biopsy forceps, Coag-Grasper, argon plasma coagulator, application of a detachable snare, or the use of clips.
- Lesions suspicious for malignancy, flat lesions, or those in a position that may be difficult to locate again later, should be marked with a permanent surgical marker (injection of a carbon particle-based suspension) to facilitate future localization either by the surgeon or at follow-up colonoscopies.

References

1. Winawer SJ, Zauber AG, Ho MN, O'Brien MJ, Gottlieb LS, Sternberg SS, et al. Prevention of colorectal cancer by colonoscopic polypectomy. N Engl J Med 1993;329:1977–81.
2. Rex DK. Colonoscopy. Gastrointest Endosc Clin N Am 2000;10:135–60.
3. Tolliver KA, Rex DK. Colonoscopic polypectomy. Gastroenterol Clin N Am 2008;37:229–51.
4. Waye JD, Lewis BS, Frankel A, Geller SA. Small colon polyps. Am J Gastroenterol 1988;83:120–2.
5. Van Gossum A, Cozzoli A, Adler M, Taton G, Cremer M. Colonoscopic snare polypectomy: analysis of 1485 resections comparing two types of current. Gastrointest Endosc 1992;38:472–5.
6. Geenen JE, Fleischer D, Waye JD. Techniques in therapeutic endoscopy. 2nd ed. New York: Gower Medical; 1992.
7. The Paris endoscopic classification of superficial neoplastic lesions: esophagus, stomach, and colon: November 30 to December 1, 2002. Gastrointest Endosc 2003;58(6 Suppl):S3–43.
8. Mitooka H, Fujimori T, Ohno S, Morimoto S, Nakashima T, Ohmoto A, et al. New methods, new materials: chromoscopy of the colon using indigo carmine dye with electrolyte lavage solution. Gastrointest Endosc 1992;38:373–4.
9. Sturmey RG, Wild CP, Hardie LJ. Removal of red light minimizes methylene blue-stimulated DNA damage in oesophageal cells: implications for chromoendoscopy. Mutagenesis 2009;24:253–8.
10. Mitooka H, Fujimori T, Maeda S, Nagasako K. Minute flat depressed neoplastic lesions of the colon detected by contrast chromoscopy using an indigo carmine capsule. Gastrointest Endosc 1995;41:453–9.
11. Rutter MD, Saunders BP, Schofield G, Forbes A, Price AB, Talbot IC. Pancolonic indigo carmine dye spraying for the detection of dysplasia in ulcerative colitis. Gut 2004;53:256–60.
12. Su MY, Ho YP, Chen PC, Chiu CT, Wu CS, Hsu cm, et al. Magnifying endoscopy with indigo carmine contrast for differential diagnosis of neoplastic and nonneoplastic colonic polyps. Dig Dis Sci 2004;49:1123–7.
13. Rex DK, Rahmani EY. New endoscopic finding associated with hyperplastic polyps. Gastrointest Endosc 1999;50:704–6.
14. Fleischer DE. Chromoendoscopy and magnification endoscopy in the colon. Gastrointest Endosc 1999;49:S45–9.
15. Apel D, Jakobs R, Schilling D, Weickert U, Teichmann J, Bohrer MH, et al. Accuracy of high-resolution chromoendoscopy in prediction of histologic findings in diminutive lesions of the rectosigmoid. Gastrointest Endosc 2006;63:824–8.
16. Rastogi A, Bansal A, Wani S, Callahan P, McGregor DH, Cherian R, et al. Narrow band imaging colonoscopy—a pilot feasibility study for the detection of polyps and correlation of surface patterns with polyp histologic diagnosis. Gastrointest Endosc 2008;67:280–6.
17. Pohl J, May A, Rabenstein T, Pech O, Ell C. Computed virtual chromoendoscopy: a new tool for enhancing tissue surface structures. Endoscopy 2007;39:80–3.
18. Inoue T, Murano M, Murano N, Kuramoto T, Kawakami K, Abe Y, et al. Comparative study of conventional colonoscopy and pan-colonic narrow-band imaging system in the detection of neoplastic colonic polyps: a randomized, controlled trial. J Gastroenterol 2008;43:45–50.
19. Uraoka T, Saito Y, Matsuda T, Sano Y, Ikehara H, Mashimo Y, et al. Detectability of colorectal neoplastic lesions using a narrow-band imaging system: a pilot study. J Gastroenterol Hepatol 2008;23:1810–5.
20. Tsuga K, Haruma K, Fujimura J, Hata J, Tani H, Tanaka S, et al. Evaluation of the colorectal wall in normal subjects and patients with ulcerative colitis using and ultrasonic catheter probe. Gastrointest Endosc 1998;48:477–84.
21. Brooker JC, Saunders BP, Shah SG, Williams CB. A new variable stiffness colonoscope makes colonoscopy easier randomised controlled trial. Gut 2000;46:801–5.
22. Othman MO, Bradley AG, Choudhary A, Hoffman RM, Roy PK. Variable stiffness colonoscope versus regular adult colonoscope: meta-analysis of randomized controlled trials. Endoscopy 2009;41:17–24.
23. Valentine JF. Double-channel endoscopic polypectomy technique for the removal of large pedunculated polyps. Gastrointest Endosc 1998;48:314–6.
24. Akahoshi K, Kojima H, Fujimaru T, Kondo A, Kubo S, Furuno T, et al. Grasping forceps assisted endoscopic resection of large pedunculated GI polypoid lesions. Gastrointest Endosc 1999;50:95–8.
25. Kawamoto K, Yamada Y, Furukawa N, Utsunomiya T, Haraguchi Y, Mizuguchi M, et al. Endoscopic submucosal tumorectomy for gastrointestinal submucosal tumors restricted to the submucosa: a new form of endoscopic minimal surgery. Gastrointest Endosc 1997;46:311–7.
26. Bigard MA, Gaucher P, Lassalle C. Fatal colonic explosion during colonoscopic polypectomy. Gastroenterology 1979;77:1307–10.
27. Stevenson GW, Wilson JA, Wilkinson J, Norman G, Goodacre RL. Pain following colonoscopy: elimination with carbon dioxide. Gastrointest Endosc 1992;38:564–7.
28. Singh N, Harrison M, Rex DK. A survey of colonoscopic polypectomy practices among clinical gastroenterologists. Gastrointest Endosc 2004;60:414–8.
29. Waye JD. New methods of polypectomy. Gastrointest Endosc Clin N Am 1997;7:413–22.
30. Johanns W, Luis W, Janssen J, Kahl S, Greiner L. Argon plasma coagulation (APC) in gastroenterology: experimental and clinical experiences. Eur J Gastroenterol Hepatol 1997;9:581–7.
31. Farin G, Grund KE. Technology of argon plasma coagulation with particular regard to endoscopic applications. Endosc Surg Allied Technol 1994;2:71–7.
32. Grund KE, Storek D, Farin G. Endoscopic argon plasma coagulation (APC): first clinical experiences in flexible endoscopy. Endosc Surg Allied Technol 1994;2:42–6.
33. Johanns W, Luis W, Janssen J, Kahl S, Greiner L. [Endoscopic argon gas coagulation—initial clinical experiences]. Z Gastroenterol 1993;31:675–9. German.
34. Carpenter S, Petersen BT, Chuttani R, Croffie J, DiSario J, Liu J, et al. Polypectomy devices. Gastrointest Endosc 2007;65:741–9.

35. Rey JF, Marek TA. Endoloop in the prevention of the post-polypectomy bleeding: preliminary results. Gastrointest Endosc 1997;46:387–9.

36. Katsinelos P, Kountouras J, Paroutoglou G, Beltsis A, Chatzimavroudis G, Zavos C, et al. Endoloop-assisted polypectomy for large pedunculated colorectal polyps. Surg Endosc 2006;20:1257–61.

37. Waye JD, Lewis BS, Yessayan S. Colonoscopy: a prospective report of complications. J Clin Gastroenterol 1992;15:347–51.

38. Matsushita M, Hajiro K, Takakuwa H, Kusumi F, Maruo T, Ohana M, et al. Ineffective use of a detachable snare for colonoscopic polypectomy of large polyps. Gastrointest Endosc 1998;47:496–9.

39. Ellis KK, Fennerty MB. Marking and identifying colon lesions: tattoos, clips, and radiology in imaging the colon. Gastrointest Endosc Clin N Am 1997;7:401–11.

40. Nagasu N, DiPalma JA. Bleeding ulcer: inject or clip? Am J Gastroenterol 1998;93:1998.

41. Hachisu T, Yamada H, Satoh S, Kouzu T. Endoscopic clipping with a new rotatable clip-device and a long clip. Dig Endosc 1996;8:127–33.

42. Uno Y, Satoh K, Tuji K, Wada T, Fukuda S, Saito H, et al. Endoscopic ligation by means of clip and detachable snare for management of colonoscopic postpolypectomy hemorrhage. Gastrointest Endosc 1999;49:113–5.

43. Iida Y, Miura S, Munemoto Y, Kasahara Y, Asada Y, Toya D, et al. Endoscopic resection of large colorectal polyps using a clipping method. Dis Colon Rectum 1994;37:179–80.

44. Cohen LB, Waye JD. Treatment of colonic polyps: practical considerations. Clin Gastroenterol 1986;15:359–76.

45. McNally DO, DeAngelis SA, Rison DR, Sudduth RH. Bipolar polypectomy device for removal of colon polyps. Gastrointest Endosc 1994;40:489–91.

46. Waye JD. Endoscopic treatment of adenomas. World J Surg 1991;15:14–9.

47. American Society for Gastrointestinal Endoscopy. ASGE guidelines: guideline on the management of anticoagulation and antiplatelet therapy for endoscopic procedures. Gastrointest Endosc 1998;48:672–5.

48. Kadakia SC, Angueira CE, Ward JA, Moore M. Gastrointestinal endoscopy in patients taking antiplatelet agents and anticoagulants: survey of ASGE members. Gastrointest Endosc 1996;44:309–16.

49. Friedland S, Soetikno R. Colonoscopy with polypectomy in anticoagulated patients. Gastrointest Endosc 2006;64:98–100.

50. Waye JD. Colonoscopy "my way": preparation, anticoagulants, antibiotic sedation. Can J Gastroenterol 1999;13:473–6.

51. Rutgeerts P, Wang TH, Llorens PS, Zuccaro G Jr. Gastrointestinal endoscopy and the patient with a risk of bleeding disorder. Gastrointest Endosc 1999;49:134–6.

52. Vanagunas A, Jacob P, Vakil N. Adequacy of "hot biopsy" for the treatment of diminutive polyps: a prospective randomized trial. Am J Gastroenterol 1989;84:383–5.

53. Peluso F, Goldner F. Follow-up of hot biopsy forceps treatment of diminutive colonic polyps. Gastrointest Endosc 1991;37:604–6.

54. Woods A, Sanowski RA, Wadas DD, Manne RK, Friess SW. Eradication of diminutive polyps: a prospective evaluation of bipolar coagulation versus conventional biopsy removal. Gastrointest Endosc 1989;35:536–40.

55. Wadas DD, Sanowski RA. Complications of the hot biopsy forceps technique. Gastrointest Endosc 1988;34:32–7.

56. Tappero G, Gaia E, DeGiuli P, Martini S, Gubetta L, Emanuelli G. Cold snare excision of small colorectal polyps. Gastrointest Endosc 1992;38:310–3.

57. Uno Y, Obara K, Zheng P, Miura S, Odagiri A, Sakamoto J, et al. Cold snare excision is a safe method for diminutive colorectal polyps. Tohoku J Exp Med 1997;183:243–9.

58. Waye JD. Techniques of polypectomy: hot biopsy forceps and snare polypectomy. Am J Gastroenterol 1987;82:615–8.

59. Cipoletta L, Bianco MA, Rotondano G, Catalano M, Prisco A, De Simone T. Endoclip-assisted resection of large pedunculated colon polyps. Gastrointest Endosc 1999;50:405–6.

60. Fujishiro M, Yahagi N, Nakamura M, Kakushima N, Kodashima S, Ono S, et al. Successful outcomes of a novel endoscopic treatment for GI tumors: endoscopic submucosal dissection with a mixture of high-molecular-weight hyaluronic acid, glycerin, and sugar. Gastrointest Endosc 2006; 63:243–249.

61. Yahagi N, Fujishiro M, Imagawa A. Endoscopic submucosal dissection for the reliable en bloc resection of colorectal mucosal tumors. Dig Endosc 2004;16:S89–92.

62. Yamamoto H, Kawata H, Sunada K, Sasaki A, Nakazawa K, Miyata T, et al. Successful en-bloc resection of large superficial tumors in the stomach and colon using sodium hyaluronate and small-caliber-tip transparent hood. Endoscopy 2003;35:690–4.

63. Tanaka S, Oka S, Kaneko I, Hirata M, Mouri R, Kanao H, et al. Endoscopic submucosal dissection for colorectal neoplasia: possibility of standardization. Gastrointest Endosc 2007;66:100–7.

64. Yamamoto H, Yube T, Isoda N, Sato Y, Sekine Y, Higashizawa T, et al. A novel method of endoscopic mucosal resection using sodium hyaluronate. Gastrointest Endosc 1999;50:251–6.

65. Fujishiro M, Yahagi N, Kashimura K, Mizushima Y, Oka M, Matsuura T, et al. Different mixtures of sodium hyaluronate and their ability to create submucosal fluid cushions for endoscopic mucosal resection. Endoscopy 2004;36:584–9.

66. Hirasaki S, Kozu T, Yamamoto H, Sano Y, Yahagi N, Oyama T, et al. Usefulness and safety of 0.4% sodium hyaluronate solution as a submucosal fluid "cushion" for endoscopic resection of colorectal mucosal neoplasms: a prospective multi-center open-label trial. BMC Gastroenterol 2009;9:1.

67. Taku K, Sano Y, Fu KI, Saito Y, Matsuda T, Uraoka T, et al Iatrogenic perforation associated with therapeutic colonoscopy: a multicenter study in Japan. J Gastroenterol Hepatol 2007;22:1409–14.

68. Walsh RM, Ackroyd FW, Shelito PC. Endoscopic resection of large sessile colorectal polyps. Gastrointest Endosc 1992;38:303–9.

69. Zlatanic J, Waye JD, Kim PS, Baiocco PJ, Gleim GW. Large sessile colonic adenomas: use of argon plasma coagulator to supplement piecemeal snare polypectomy. Gastrointest Endosc 1999;49:731–5.

70. Karita M, Tada M, Okita K, Kodama T. Endoscopic therapy for early colon cancer: the strip biopsy resection technique. Gastrointest Endosc 1991;37:128–32.

71. Karita M, Tada M, Okita K. The successive strip biopsy partial resection technique for large early gastric and colon cancers. Gastrointest Endosc 1992;38:174–8.

72. Karita M, Cantero D, Okita K. Endoscopic diagnosis and resection treatment for flat adenoma with severe dysplasia. Am J Gastroenterol 1993;88: 1421–3.

73. Waye JD. Advanced polypectomy. Gastrointest Endosc Clin N Am 2005;15:733–56.

74. Tsuga K, Haruma K, Fujimura J, Hata J, Tani H, Tanaka S, et al. Evaluation of the colorectal wall in normal subjects and patients with ulcerative colitis using an ultrasonic catheter probe. Gastrointest Endosc 1998;48:477–84.

75. Uchikawa H, Hirao M, Yamagutio M. Endoscopic mucosal resection combined with local injection of hypertonic saline epinephrine solution for early colorectal cancers and other tumors. Gastroenterol Endosc 1992;34: 1871–8.

76. Shirai M, Nakamura T, Matsuura A, Ito Y, Kobayashi S. Safer colonoscopic polypectomy with local submucosal injection of hypertonic saline–epinephrine solution. Am J Gastroenterol 1994;89:334–8.

77. Kanamori T, Itoh M, Yokoyama Y, Tsuchida K. Injection-incision-assisted snare resection of large sessile colorectal polyps. Gastrointest Endosc 1996;43:189–93.

78. Waye JD. Saline injection colonoscopic polypectomy [editorial]. Am J Gastroenterol 1994;89:305–6.

79. Cooper HS. Surgical pathology of endoscopically removed malignant polyps of the colon and rectum. Am J Surg Pathol 1983;7:613–23.

80. Fenoglio cm, Kaye GI, Lane N. Distribution of human colonic lymphatics in normal, hyperplastic, and adenomatous tissue. Its relationship to metastasis from small carcinomas in pedunculated adenomas. Gastroenterology 1973;64:51–66.

81. Eckardt VF, Fuchs M, Kanzler G, Remmele W, Stienen U. Follow-up of patients with colonic polyps containing severe atypia and invasive carcinoma. Cancer 1988;61:2552–7.

82. Ishiguro A, Uno Y, Ishiguro Y, Munakata A, Morita T. Correlation of lifting versus non-lifting and microscopic depth of invasion in early colorectal cancer. Gastrointest Endosc 1999;50:329–33.

83. Kanao H, Tanaka S, Oka S, Hirata M, Yoshida S, Chayama K. Narrow-band imaging magnification predicts the histology and invasion depth of colorectal tumors. Gastrointest Endosc 2009;69:631–6.

84. Katagiri A, Fu KI, Sano Y, Ikematsu H, Horimatsu T, Kaneko K, et al. Narrow band imaging with magnifying colonoscopy as diagnostic tool for predicting histology of early colorectal neoplasia. Aliment Pharmacol Ther 2008;27:1269–74.

85. Bond JH. Malignant colorectal polyps. Curr Treat Options Gastroenterol 1999;2:34–7.

86. Cranley JP, Petras RE, Carey WD, Paradis K, Sivak MV. When is endoscopic polypectomy adequate therapy for colonic polyps containing invasive carcinoma? Gastroenterology 1986;91:419–27.

87. Coverlizza S, Risio M, Ferrari A, Fenoglio-Presier cm, Rossini FP. Colorectal adenomas containing invasive carcinoma. Pathologic assessment of lymph node metastatic potential. Cancer 1989;64:1937–47.

88. Fujimori T, Fujii S, Saito N, Sugihara K. Pathological diagnosis of early colorectal carcinoma and its clinical implications. Digestion 2009;79: 40–51.

28

89. Schiano TD, Pfister D, Harrison L, Shike M. Neoplastic seeding as a complication of percutaneous endoscopic gastrostomy. Am J Gastroenterol 1994;89:131–3.

90. Waye JD. Polyps large and small [editorial]. Gastrointest Endosc 1992;38:391–2.

91. Nivatvongs S, Snover DC, Fang DT. Piecemeal snare excision of large sessile colon and rectal polyps: is it adequate? Gastrointest Endosc 1984;30:18–20.

92. Christie JP. Colonoscopic removal of sessile colonic lesions. Dis Colon Rectum 1978;21:12–4.

93. McAfee JH, Katon RM. Tiny snares prove safe and effective for removal of diminutive colorectal polyps. Gastrointest Endosc 1994;40:301–3.

94. Bat L, Williams CB. Usefulness of pediatric colonoscopes in adult colonoscopy. Gastrointest Endosc 1989;35:329–32.

95. Rogers BH. The use of small caliber endoscopes in selected cases increases the success rate of colonoscopy. Gastrointest Endosc 1989;35:352.

96. Kozarek RA, Botoman VA, Patterson DJ. Prospective evaluation of a small caliber upper endoscope for colonoscopy after unsuccessful standard examination. Gastrointest Endosc 1989;35:333–5.

97. Heresbach D, Barrioz T, Lapalus MG, Coumaros D, Bauret P, Potier P, et al. Miss rate for colorectal neoplastic polyps: a prospective multicenter study of back-to-back video colonoscopies. Endoscopy 2008;40:284–90.

98. Triadafilopoulos G, Watts HD, Higgins J, Van Dam J. A novel retrograde-viewing auxiliary imaging device (third eye retroscope) improves the detection of simulated polyps in anatomic models of the colon. Gastrointest Endosc 2007;65:139–44.

99. Fujishiro M, Yahagi N, Kakushima N, Kodashima S, Muraki Y, Ono S, et al. Outcomes of endoscopic submucosal dissection for colorectal epithelial neoplasms in 200 consecutive cases. Clin Gastroenterol Hepatol 2007;5:678–83.

100. Arebi N, Swain D, Suzuki N, Fraser C, Price A, Saunders BP. Endoscopic mucosal resection of 161 cases of large sessile or flat colorectal polyps. Scand J Gastroenterol 2007;42:859–66.

101. Hancock JH, Talbot RW. Accuracy of colonoscopy in localization of colorectal cancer. Int J Colorectal Dis 1995;10:140–1.

102. Dunaway MT, Webb WR, Rodning CB. Intraluminal measurement of distance in the colorectal region employing rigid and flexible endoscopes. Surg Endosc 1988;2:81–3.

103. Waye JD. Colonoscopy without fluoroscopy [editorial]. Gastrointest Endosc 1990;36:72–3.

104. Frager DH, Frager JD, Wolf EL, Beneventano TC. Problems in the colonoscopic localization of tumors: continued value of the barium enema. Gastrointest Radiol 1987;12:343–6.

105. Hilliard G, Ramming K, Thompson J Jr, Passaro E Jr. The elusive colonic malignancy: a need for definitive preoperative localization. Am Surg 1990;56:742–4.

106. Tabibian N, Michaletz PA, Schwartz JT, Heiser MC, Dixon WB, Smith JL, et al. Use of endoscopically placed clip can avoid diagnostic errors in colonoscopy. Gastrointest Endosc 1988;34:262–4.

107. Montorsi M, Opocher E, Santambrogio R, Bianchi P, Faranda C, Arcidiacono P, et al. Original technique for small colorectal tumor localization during laparoscopic surgery. Dis Colon Rectum 1999;42:819–22.

108. Forde KA, Cohen JL. Intraoperative colonoscopy. Ann Surg 1988;207:231–3.

109. Richter RM, Littman L, Levowitz BS. Intraoperative fiberoptic colonoscopy: localization of nonpalpable colonic lesions. Arch Surg 1973;106:228.

110. Sakanoue Y, Nakao K, Shoji Y, Yanagi H, Kusunoki M, Utsunomiya J. Intraoperative colonoscopy. Surg Endosc 1993;7:84–7.

111. Hammond DC, Lane FR, Welk RA, Madura MJ, Borreson DK, Passinault WJ. Endoscopic tattooing of the colon: an experimental study. Am Surg 1989;55:457–61.

112. Price N, Gottfried MR, Clary E, Lawson DC, Baillie J, Mergener K, et al. Safety and efficacy of India ink and indocyanine green as colonic tattooing agents. Gastrointest Endosc 2000;51:438–42.

113. Hammond DC, Lane FR, Mackeigan JM, Passinault WJ. Endoscopic tattooing of the colon: clinical experience. Am Surg 1993;59:205–10.

114. Ponsky JL, King JF. Endoscopic marking of colon lesions. Gastrointest Endosc 1975;22:42–3.

115. Cohen LB, Waye JD. Colonoscopic polypectomy of polyps with adenocarcinoma: when is it curative? In: Barkin JS, editor. Difficult decisions in digestive diseases. Chicago: Year Book Medical; 1989. p. 528–35.

116. Nizam R, Siddiqi N, Landas SK, Kaplan DS, Holtzapple PG. Colonic tattooing with India ink: benefits, risks, and alternatives. Am J Gastroenterol 1996;91:1804–8.

117. Gopal DV, Morava-Protzner I, Miller HAB, Hemphill DJ. Idiopathic inflammatory bowel disease associated with colonic tattooing with India ink preparation. Gastrointest Endosc 1999;49:636–9.

118. Lightdale CJ. India ink colonic tattoo: blots on the record [editorial]. Gastrointest Endosc 1991;37:68–71.

119. Poulard JB, Shatz B, Kodner I. Preoperative tattooing of polypectomy site. Endoscopy 1985;17:84–5.

120. Shatz BA. Small volume india ink injections [letter]. Gastrointest Endosc 1991;37:649–50.

121. Salomon P, Berner JS, Waye JD. Endoscopic India ink injection: a method for preparation, sterilization, and administration. Gastrointest Endosc 1993;39:803–5.

122. Shatz BA, Thavorides V. Colonic tattoo for follow-up of endoscopic sessile polypectomy. Gastrointest Endosc 1991;37:59–60.

123. Hyman N, Waye JD. Endoscopic four quadrant tattoo for the identification of colonic lesions at surgery. Gastrointest Endosc 1991;37:56–8.

124. Shatz BA, Weinstock LB, Swanson PE, Thyssen EP. Long-term safety of India ink tattoos in the colon. Gastrointest Endosc 1997;45:153–6.

125. McArthur CS, Roayaie S, Waye JD. Safety of preoperation endoscopic tattoo with India ink for identification of colonic lesions. Surg Endosc 1999;13:397–400.

126. Nahas SC, Alves PR, Borba MR, Nahas CS, Sobrado CW Jr, Araujo SE, et al. Polypectomies: colonic endoscopic resections. Arq Gastroenterol 1999;36:133–8.

127. Habr-Gama A, Waye JD. Complications and hazards of gastrointestinal endoscopy. World J Surg 1989;13:193–201.

128. Rankin GB. Indications, contraindications and complications of colonoscopy. In: Sivak MV Jr, editor. Gastroenterologic endoscopy. Philadelphia: Saunders; 1987. p. 868–80.

129. Shinya H. Complications: prevention and management. In: Shinya H, editor. Colonoscopy: diagnostic and treatment of colonic diseases. New York: Igaku-Shoin, 1982; p. 199–208.

130. Kavin H, Sinicrope F, Esker AH. Management of perforation of the colon at colonoscopy. Am J Gastroenterol 1992;87:161–7.

131. Waye JD, Kahn O, Auerbach ME. Complications of colonoscopy and flexible sigmoidoscopy. Gastrointest Endosc Clin N Am 1996;6:343–77.

132. Carpio G, Albu E, Gumbs MA, Gerst PH. Management of colonic perforation after colonoscopy: report of three cases. Dis Colon Rectum 1989;32:624–6.

133. Christie JP, Marrazzo J. "Mini-perforation" of the colon: not all postpolypectomy perforations require laparotomy. Dis Colon Rectum 1991;34:132–5.

134. Hall C, Dorricott NJ, Donovan IA, Neoptolemos JP. Colon perforation during colonoscopy: surgical versus conservative management. Br J Surg 1991;78:542–4.

135. Wullstein C, Koppen M, Gross E. Laparoscopic treatment of colonic perforations related to colonoscopy. Surg Endosc 1999;13:484–7.

136. Yoshikane H, Hidano H, Sakakibara A, Ayakawa T, Mori S, Kawashima H, et al. Endoscopic repair by clipping of iatrogenic colonic perforation. Gastrointest Endosc 1997;46:464–6.

137. Waye JD. The postpolypectomy coagulation syndrome. Gastrointest Endosc 1981;27:184.

138. Jensen DM, Machicado GA. Diagnosis and treatment of severe hematochezia. Gastroenterology 1988;95:1569–74.

139. Rex DK, Lewis BS, Waye JD. Colonoscopy and endoscopic therapy for delayed postpolypectomy hemorrhage. Gastrointest Endosc 1992;38:127–9.

140. Parra-Blanco A, Kaminaga N, Kojima T, Endo Y, Uragami N, Okawa N, et al. Hemoclipping for postpolypectomy and postbiopsy colonic bleeding. Gastrointest Endosc 2000;51:37–41.

141. Nivatvongs S. Complications in colonoscopic polypectomy: lessons to learn from an experience with 1576 polyps. Am Surg 1988;54:61–3.

142. Cussons PD, Berry AR. Comparison of the use of emergency mesenteric angiography and intraoperative colonoscopy with antegrade colonic irrigation in massive rectal hemorrhage. J R Coll Surg Edinb 1989;34:91–3.

143. Carlyle DR, Goldstein HM. Angiographic management of bleeding following transcolonoscopic polypectomy. Am J Dig Dis 1975;20:1196–9.

144. Slivka A, Parsons WG, Carr-Locke DL. Endoscopic band ligation for treatment of post-polypectomy hemorrhage: case report. Gastrointest Endosc 1994;40:230–2.

145. Smith RE, Doull J. Treatment of colonic post-polypectomy bleeding site by endoscopic band ligation. Gastrointest Endosc 1994;40:499–503.

146. Williams CB. Diathermy-biopsy: a technique for the endoscopic management of small polyps. Endoscopy 1973;5:215.

V

29 Dilation Techniques

Shabana F. Pasha and David E. Fleischer

Introduction

Esophageal dilation is a therapeutic procedure, often performed in conjunction with endoscopy, for the management of dysphagia secondary to structural or neuromuscular disorders of the esophagus. The technique of dilation has significantly evolved since its conception in the 17th century in the Algerian city of Bejaïa by Girolamo Fabricius (Hieronymus ab Aquapendente, 1537–1619), the Italian anatomist and embryologist, who used wax candles as rigid dilators [1]. (The city of Bejaïa, known in French as Bougie, was well known for its wax trade.) Bougienage as a method of stricture dilation was first reported by Hildreth in 1821 [2].

Modern dilation techniques involve the use of flexible bougie and balloon dilators. These have largely replaced the older Eder–Puestow and Hurst dilators, which were associated with a high rate of complications. Esophageal dilation allows successful management of the majority of patients with dysphagia, resulting in improved quality of life, and often obviates the need for invasive surgical procedures. However, as there is a significantly higher risk of complications when the procedure is carried out by inexperienced endoscopists, it is important that it should only be performed by endoscopists who are familiar with the nuances of the different dilators and dilation techniques. This chapter describes the techniques of esophageal dilation and outlines the management of common disorders that require dilation.

Predilation Evaluation

A thorough diagnostic evaluation before esophageal dilation is important for several reasons. It allows a precise diagnosis of the underlying etiology of dysphagia, whether secondary to a structural or motility disorder, as well as accurate determination of the length and complexity of strictures, if present. These factors, in turn, influence decisions regarding the type of dilator used and the technique employed for dilation. Predilation evaluation also facilitates recognition of the presence of diverticula, hiatal hernias, esophageal tortuosity, and other confounding factors that may increase the risk of complications related to the procedure [3]. The evaluation should include a detailed history, which may lead to an accurate diagnosis in up to 80 % of patients [4]. Additional diagnostic testing with esophagography, esophagogastroduodenoscopy (EGD), and/or esophageal motility studies should be considered, depending on the clinical presentation. Video fluoroscopy may be useful when a more proximal disorder involving the hypopharynx or cervical esophagus is suspected, and to test for swallowing with different consistencies. EGD has the advantage that biopsies can be taken, and it allows direct visualization of the esophagus. In addition, a retroflexed view on EGD allows diagnosis of lesions at the gastric cardia, which may be missed on barium esophagography. In most instances, endoscopic evaluation and dilation are performed together.

The diameter of an esophageal stricture can be estimated based on the degree of resistance to passage of the endoscope. As the standard EGD scope is 9 mm in diameter, subtle narrowing of the esophagus may be missed on endoscopy. A mild stricture is defined as a narrowing that allows passage of the endoscope with only minimal resistance, while moderate to severe strictures offer increasing resistance [5]. The caliber of a stricture can also be determined by comparing the luminal diameter to the size of an open biopsy forceps, which measures about 8 mm. Radiologically, the luminal diameter can be measured by the maximum-sized barium tablet that can pass through [6].

On the basis of the structural characteristics, an esophageal stricture can be categorized as simple or complex. A short (< 2 cm), straight stricture that allows passage of the endoscope with minimal to mild resistance is termed a simple stricture. A complex stricture is typically elongated (> 2 cm), angulated, or irregular, with a very narrow luminal diameter [7].

Indications and Contraindications

The main indications for esophageal dilation are classified as structural or mechanical obstruction, motility or neuromuscular disorders, and empiric dilation when the procedure is performed in the absence of an obvious underlying disorder (**Table 29.1**).

Esophageal dilation is absolutely contraindicated in the setting of a recent perforation. Relative contraindications to the procedure include bleeding diathesis, severe cardiopulmonary comorbidities, large thoracic aortic aneurysms, and all contraindications to standard upper endoscopy [8].

Table 29.1 Indications for esophageal dilation

Structural disorders
Benign
• Peptic stricture
• Schatzki ring
• Radiation-induced stricture
• Caustic stricture
• Pill-induced stricture
• Eosinophilic esophagitis
• Crohn's disease
• Postoperative stricture (anastomotic)
• Sclerotherapy-induced stricture
• Extrinsic compression
• Photodynamic therapy–induced stricture
Malignant
• Adenocarcinoma
• Squamous cell carcinoma
• Pseudoachalasia (infiltrative neoplasm at esophagogastric junction)
• Metastases
Motility disorders
Achalasia
Pseudoachalasia
Diffuse esophageal spasm
Empiric dilation

Preparation

Patients should be advised to fast for 4–6 h before the procedure in order to avoid any risk of aspiration. In addition, a clear liquid diet for at least 24 h before fasting should be advised to patients with achalasia, esophageal diverticula, or tight strictures, who are prone to esophageal stasis of food and oropharyngeal secretions [9]. The use of a large-bore nasogastric tube to remove retained esophageal contents may further reduce the risk of aspiration.

Esophageal dilation can result in significant bleeding in patients who are taking anticoagulants. The American Society for Gastrointestinal Endoscopy (ASGE) recommends that anticoagulants be withheld in all patients before esophageal dilation. In patients who are at low risk for thromboembolic events, oral anticoagulation should be suspended 5 days beforehand and can be reinitiated after completion of the procedure. Heparin as bridging therapy is recommended in patients who are at high risk for thromboembolic events on discontinuing oral anticoagulation [10].

The risk of bacteremia following esophageal dilation is estimated to be 12–22 %, and is predominantly due to Streptococcus viridans, a commensal of the upper gastrointestinal tract [69–71]. Bacteremia may be more common after dilation of malignant as compared to benign strictures, and has also been reported to be higher with passage of multiple dilators [72]. However, despite the high incidence of bacteremia, clinically significant infections, including endocarditis, are rare [73]. The AHA (American Heart Association) recommends antibiotic prophylaxis for all high risk patients (prosthetic valve, prior endocarditis, systemic-pulmonary shunt, synthetic vascular graft less than a year old, and complex cyanotic congenital heart disease), and optional prophylaxis for those with moderate risk cardiac conditions. For those patients, who have established infections of the gastrointestinal tract, which may be related to enterococci, the AHA has suggested that it may be reasonable that the antibiotic regimen includes an agent active against enterococci [74]. The ASGE no longer recommends antibiotic prophylaxis prior to endoscopic procedures, including esophageal dilation, solely to prevent infectious endocarditis, or infection of synthetic vascular grafts or nonvalvular cardiovascular devices (Grade 1C+). However, for patients with any high risk cardiac condition, undergoing a procedure in which the infecting flora may be enterococci, an antibiotic that covers these bacteria should be included in the antibiotic regimen (ampicillin, penicillin, or vancomycin) [75].

Types of Dilator

Esophageal dilators include weighted push-type dilators (Hurst and Maloney), polyvinyl wire-guided dilators (Savary–Gilliard and American Bard), balloon dilators (wire-guided and through the scope), and the newly introduced optical dilators.

Bougies were the first devices used for esophageal dilation. The older weighted bougie dilators were designed with blunted ends that contained either lead or mercury. Due to their toxicity, these metals have been replaced by tungsten in modern dilators. The push-type dilators currently available are Maloney dilators (Maloney Medovations, Inc., Germantown, Wisconsin, USA) (**Fig. 29.1**), which have largely replaced the older Hurst dilators and range in size from 4 to 20 mm (12–60 Fr) in diameter. These dilators can be passed into the esophagus either blindly or under fluoroscopic guidance. Due to their softer and pliable texture, they have the advantage of causing less pharyngeal and esophageal trauma in comparison with the polyvinyl dilators. The Maloney dilator has a more tapered tip in comparison with the Hurst dilator, with resultant improvement in safety due to a decrease in the shear force exerted during passage through the esophagus. In addition to their safety and ease of dilation, Maloney dilators can be reused several times and are the least expensive of all the dilators currently available. Push dilators can be used without sedation and are therefore commonly employed for self-dilation in patients requiring multiple dilation procedures. Their main disadvantage is their tendency to bend and buckle above narrow, complicated strictures, resulting in perforation [12].

Polyvinyl dilators are based on an earlier concept developed by Puestow, employing a steel guide wire passed through the stricture and a series of metal olives passed over the wire. Modern wire-guided dilators include the Savary–Gilliard (Wilson-Cook, Winston-Salem, North Carolina, USA) and American dilators (Bard Inc., Billerica, Massachusetts, USA), which range in size from 1 to 20 mm

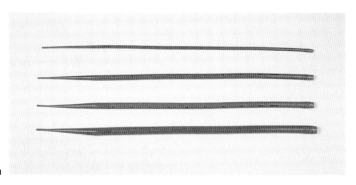

a

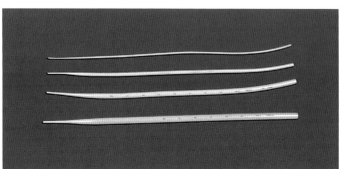

c

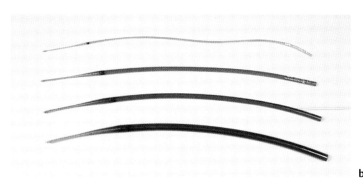

b

Fig. 29.1 Examples of bougie dilators.
a Maloney dilators (12–60 Fr).
b Savary–Gilliard dilators (3–60 Fr).
c American dilators (3–60 Fr)

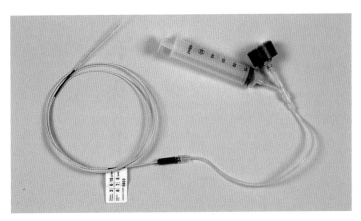

Fig. 29.2 Example of a Microvasive balloon dilator.

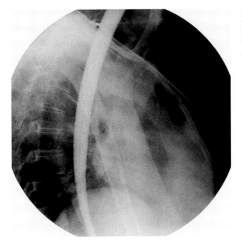

Fig. 29.3 Fluoroscopic image of wire-guided bougie dilation with an American dilator.

(3–60 Fr) in diameter. These dilators have a tapered and more rigid tip than the weighted push-type dilators, as well as a central hollow core to accommodate a guide wire. The Savary–Gillard dilators are marked with a radiopaque band at the level of their maximum diameter, which allows radiographic visualization during fluoroscopy. In comparison with the Savary dilators, American dilators have a shorter-tapered tip and are impregnated with barium throughout the body, allowing better visualization during fluoroscopy and thus a decreased risk of perforation. Polyvinyl dilators used under fluoroscopic guidance may be preferable to blind passage of push-type dilators for dilation of complicated strictures and in the presence of associated structural abnormalities of the esophagus. These dilators are also reusable, similar to push-type dilators.

Polyethylene balloon dilators (Microvasive/Boston Scientific Corporation, Watertown, Massachusetts, USA) (**Fig. 29.2**) include single-diameter and controlled radial expansion (CRE) models and can be used over a guide wire (over the wire, OTW) or passed through the scope (TTS). CRE balloons are designed to expand to increasing diameters with higher inflation pressures, and are therefore useful for sequential dilations with a single passage of the dilator. The balloon can be inflated with air, water, or radiopaque contrast. The size of the balloon dilator and the technique used (OTW or TTS) depend on the underlying esophageal disorder and the endoscopist's preference. Larger balloons (30–40 mm) are available for pneumatic dilation in patients with achalasia, while smaller ones (12–20 mm) are used in patients with mechanical strictures and other neuromuscular disorders. OTW balloon dilators, which allow a 0.035″ guide wire in the central lumen, are typically used under fluoroscopic guidance for dilation of tight strictures and achalasia. TTS dilators can be passed through the working channel of the scope and are being increasingly used due to their reported safety and the advantage of dilation under direct visualization, without the need for fluoroscopy [13].

The InScope Optical Dilator (InScope, Ethicon Endo-Surgery Inc., Cincinnati, Ohio, USA) is an over-the-scope dilator that combines the ease of use of a bougie dilator with the safety and convenience of a CRE balloon dilator. This is a single-use disposable instrument, made from a transparent flexible polymer that mounts over the endoscope, thereby allowing dilation under direct visualization. The dilator has three segments separated by markings to facilitate sequential dilation with a single passage of the endoscope. The dilator also allows passage of a guide wire for dilation of high-risk strictures in the cervical esophagus or hypopharynx [14].

All of these dilators have their own unique advantages and disadvantages, and none has been established as superior to the others [5,12,15,16]. Bougie dilators provide tactile feedback, which allows the endoscopist to estimate the amount of resistance offered to passage of the dilator and hence avoid overdilation and perforation. This tactile sensation is best perceived with the weighted push-type dilators, less with wire-guided polyvinyl dilators, and is absent with balloon dilators. Wire-guided polyvinyl dilators and balloon dilators have the advantage of allowing dilation under fluoroscopy (**Fig. 29.3**), and avoiding complications related to the blind passage of push-type dilators [12,17]. In addition, balloon and optical dilators can be used under direct visualization with the endoscope, with the additional advantage of sequential dilations with a single passage of the dilator. However, these dilators are less cost-effective than bougie dilators, as they are not reusable.

Physiology of Esophageal Dilation

Dilation is achieved by circumferential stretching or splitting of the mucosa and circular muscle of the esophagus. The bougie and balloon dilators differ in their underlying mechanism of action. Bougie dilators exert both radial and axial forces along the entire length of the stricture during forward passage through the esophagus. The amount of radial force generated depends on several factors, including the angle of taper, the surface friction of the dilator, the caliber of the dilator relative to the diameter of the stricture, and the intrinsic characteristics of the stricture [18]. As the radial dilation force is inversely proportional to the axial force generated, a bougie with a shallower taper has less shear force, with a corresponding mechanical advantage [6].

In contrast to bougie dilators, balloon dilators exert only radial force along the length of the stricture. This circumferential pressure exerted by the balloon is known as hoop stress and is a product of the diameter and pressure within the balloon. During dilation, the opposing static force of the stricture creates an hourglass-shaped waist in the balloon. The dilating force of a balloon dilator is inversely proportional to the diameter of the waist. A larger-sized balloon dilator thus exerts more radial force on a stricture and requires less pressure for dilation than a smaller balloon. On the same principle, a larger balloon has the disadvantage of a higher risk of perforation in comparison with a smaller balloon. The surface area of the stricture also influences the dilation force, with more effective dilation of longer strictures in comparison with shorter ones [6].

Dilation Techniques

An esophageal luminal diameter of 12 mm or less results in dysphagia, and symptomatic improvement usually requires dilation up to at least 15 mm [19]. The method of dilation employed is individualized on the basis of the underlying etiology of the dysphagia, the duration of symptoms, the severity and complexity of the strictures, and the physician's preference and expertise.

29

It is important to ensure that all necessary equipment is available in the endoscopy suite before the dilation procedure is started. The availability of a pediatric or ultrathin scope in addition to the standard EGD scope and fluoroscopy may be necessary when a tight stricture is suspected. It should also be ensured that medications and accessories, including steroid injections, biopsy forceps, or a needle-knife papillotome, are available in case adjunctive treatment is anticipated.

Blind passage of Maloney dilators can be performed with the patient in either the left lateral or upright position. The patient's head should be flexed to decrease the angle between the oropharynx and hypopharynx and facilitate passage of the dilator. The potential for the dilator to enter perpendicular to the hypopharynx, with resultant injury to the posterior pharyngeal wall, may be further reduced by removal of the mouthpiece and exertion of downward pressure on the tongue using the index and middle fingers. The dilator is lubricated generously and the shaft is grasped using the thumb and medial three fingers of the right hand, which allows better tactile feedback in comparison with a closed hand grip [3]. The dilator is slowly passed into the esophagus with clockwise and counterclockwise rotations until the widest diameter is distal to the stricture, as determined by the markings on the dilator. The dilator is then withdrawn in a single slow movement.

Wire-guided bougie dilation involves passage of a guide wire under direct visualization at endoscopy or fluoroscopy until the distal tip of the wire is positioned in the antrum. This distance is usually about 60 cm from the incisors in patients without prior esophagogastric surgery.

The endoscope is advanced through the stricture into the stomach if feasible, with placement of the guide wire under direct visualization, or positioned at the proximal margin of the stricture, followed by placement of the guide wire under fluoroscopic visualization. The dilator is then passed over the guide wire, lubricated, and advanced into the esophagus with a single smooth movement until its maximal diameter is beyond the narrowed area. It is important for the assistant to exert slight wire retraction, at the same time ensuring that the wire is not displaced from its original position. The dilator is then withdrawn slowly, in approximately 10-cm segments, with simultaneous advancement of the guide wire in a one-to-one method that ensures that the tip of the guide wire remains in place in the distal stomach. After passage of the last dilator, both the dilator and guide wire are withdrawn together.

With the technique of through-the-scope (TTS) balloon dilation, the endoscope is advanced to the proximal margin of the stricture. The catheter, with the balloon dilator, is then passed through the channel of the endoscope and advanced beyond the stricture. The length of the balloon is determined on the basis of the radiographic estimate of the length of the stricture. The balloon is inflated under direct visualization and maintained at the inflation pressure for 30 s or until there is a sudden drop in the manometric reading. Obliteration of the waist of the balloon at the proximal margin of the stricture indicates successful dilation. When over-the-wire (OTW) balloon dilation is employed, the guide wire is passed beyond the stricture into the antrum under fluoroscopic guidance, as described with polyvinyl dilators. The balloon dilator is passed over the guide wire and centered within the stricture, as indicated by radiopaque markers located at the center and ends of the balloon. Dilation is then performed to the desired diameter.

Dilation of Peptic Strictures

Peptic strictures are usually dilated by sequential passage of push dilators, bougies, or balloons. The size of the initial dilator should be approximately equal to, and no more than 1–2 mm larger than, the estimated diameter of the stricture [20]. Although there are data

suggesting that passage of a single large dilator with a diameter >15 mm, or incremental dilations with larger-diameter dilators, may be safe in uncomplicated peptic strictures, this is based on uncontrolled studies [21]. According to Boyce's "rule of threes," no more than three dilators of consecutively increasing size should be passed during a dilation session, after moderate resistance is encountered. Observation of this rule may reduce the risk of over-dilation and perforation [22]. Simple peptic strictures can also be dilated effectively using wire-guided or balloon dilators [5,16]. Administration of effective acid-suppressive medications has reduced the frequency of peptic strictures and the need for dilation.

Pneumatic Dilation for Achalasia

The objective of pneumatic dilation is to reduce lower esophageal sphincter pressure by forceful disruption of the circular muscle of the esophagus. Dilation is performed under fluoroscopic guidance, using polyethylene pneumatic balloon dilators (Microvasive Rigi-flex) passed over a guide wire. The presence of radiopaque markers on the center and ends of the balloon help confirm appropriate placement during dilation. The dilators are available in three sizes (30, 35, and 40 mm). Initial dilation is performed using the 30-mm balloon, with larger-caliber balloons reserved for patients who need additional dilation. The balloon is centered in the stricture and inflated until the waist is obliterated, after which the pressure is maintained for approximately a minute. The use of both high- and low-compliance balloons has been found to be equally effective in pneumatic dilation [23]. In addition, for subsequent dilations, the use of 30-mm diameter balloons inflated for shorter durations of up to 15 s appears to be as effective as larger-diameter balloons inflated for 1 min [24,25].

The reported efficacy of pneumatic dilation for achalasia is in the range of 58–95 % [26–28]. Lower response rates are seen in younger patients, males, and patients with a shorter duration of symptoms [29–31]. In addition, patients who have a poor response to initial dilation or experience rapid recurrence of symptoms have a lesser likelihood of response to additional dilations [32].

The reported risk of perforation is 3–5 %, and patients can present with delayed perforation not detected on immediate postprocedural imaging [33,34]. An esophagogram with water-soluble contrast (Gastrografin) should be obtained after the procedure before oral food intake is resumed [35]. Most cases of perforation can be managed conservatively, and only a minority require surgical intervention [36].

Dilation of Schatzki Rings

Dilation of a simple Schatzki ring may ideally be performed with a single large-caliber (≥20 mm) push-type dilator, which has a reported immediate response rate of almost 100 %. Alternatively, some endoscopists begin dilation with a medium-sized dilator (e.g., 12 mm). Contrary to the earlier view that there was a long-term response to a single dilation, studies have shown that dysphagia recurs in up to 90 % of patients during a 5-year follow-up period [37,38]. Alternative or adjunctive therapeutic options for dilation include rupture of the ring with four-quadrant biopsies or incision of the ring with a needle-knife papillotome [39,40].

Dilation of Caustic or Corrosive Strictures

Caustic strictures tend to be fibrotic, more extensive than other benign strictures, and may be noncircumferential. Due to the high risk of perforation in the acute setting, it is often recommended that

V

dilation be delayed for at least 3–6 weeks after the injury [41,42]. However, early bougienage has been shown to be safe in some studies, with early resolution of strictures in these patients [43].

Dilation of chronic corrosive strictures should be performed cautiously over several sessions (generally five or more), every 2–3 weeks, with gradual increments in the dilator size. In order to reduce the risk of perforation, the size of the initial dilator used should be equivalent to or one size less than the last dilator used at the previous session. The use of intralesional corticosteroids (e.g., triamcinolone) as an adjunct to dilation may lead to earlier resolution of strictures, in addition to increasing the interval between dilations [44]. Patients with severe strictures not amenable to antegrade dilation may respond to dilation using a retrograde or rendezvous technique [45]. Temporary placement of self-expanding plastic stents may also be effective in managing refractory strictures [46].

Dilation of Malignant Strictures

Malignant strictures should be dilated using wire-guided bougie or balloon dilators under fluoroscopic guidance, due to the complexity of these strictures and the risk of perforation, creation of false passages, and tracheo-esophageal fistulas with blind dilation techniques [47,48]. Although dilation improves dysphagia in up to 90 % of patients, the symptomatic relief is usually short-lived, and additional endoscopic treatment with stent placement, endoscopic mucosal resection, or photodynamic or thermal therapy may be necessary in the management of inoperable patients [48]. When endoscopic stent placement is planned, dilation may be performed in the same session or in two sessions to facilitate gradual stretching of the stricture and obtain an accurate measure of the stricture for appropriate-sized stent placement [49].

Self-Bougienage

Self-bougienage can be carried out by patients who need multiple and frequent dilations for benign esophageal strictures. The patients in whom this option is contemplated should be motivated and not fearful of performing the dilation. It is important for the patient to receive information about the anatomy of the upper gastrointestinal tract and the technique and complications of the procedure. The initial dilation sessions should be performed under the supervision of a gastroenterologist in order to familiarize the patient with the correct technique and overcome any apprehensions. It is important for patients to understand that they can contact the physician or nurse at any time, with an emphasis on the fact that support is always available to them. A single Maloney dilator is usually used (e. g., 14, 15, or 16 mm), and it is marked at two points: 20 cm from the tapered end and 10 cm beyond the estimated distal end of the stricture.

There are variations in the method used for self-dilation, but the procedure is usually performed as follows. The patient is in the sitting position. The dilator is lubricated with water, and using the left hand, the tapered end is introduced over the tongue into the oropharynx. When the tip of the dilator reaches the upper esophageal sphincter, the patient swallows, while the dilator is advanced using the right hand. When the patient visualizes the first marking at 20 cm, it indicates that the dilator is in the esophagus. The end of the dilator is then raised with the right hand above the head, which allows the tungsten to migrate to the tapered end. The dilator is then slowly pushed with the right hand into the esophagus, with the left hand being used to guide the direction of passage. Passage of the maximal diameter of the dilator beyond the stricture is confirmed when the second marking is seen at the level of the incisors. The dilator is then slowly withdrawn [49].

Refractory and High-Grade Strictures

Intralesional corticosteroid injection therapy has been reported to be beneficial in the management of refractory esophageal strictures, with an increase in the maximum postdilation diameter, a decrease in the number of dilation sessions, and an increase in the interval between dilations [44,49]. The underlying mechanism of action involves an inhibition of matrix protein genes, resulting in a decrease in the production of collagen and fibrous tissue. There are no standard guidelines regarding the dosage or concentration of the steroids injected. Triamcinolone acetonide is commonly used, with 0.2–0.5-mL aliquots injected into four quadrants of the stricture using a 23-gauge sclerotherapy needle. Although this is not common practice, reports have suggested that endoscopic ultrasound may be useful for accurate injection of intralesional steroids into the thickest portion of the stricture [50].

Expandable metal stents have been routinely used in the palliative management of malignant esophageal strictures. However, these stents have not been successful in the management of refractory benign strictures and have resulted in complications, including ingrowth of granulation tissue, migration, and perforation [51]. Recent reports have suggested advantages with self-expanding coated retrievable plastic stents (Polyflex, Boston Scientific, Natick, Massachusetts, USA), although their use has not been uniformly beneficial [46,52,53]. Biodegradable stents (InStent, Inc., Eden Prairie, Minnesota, USA) have also been used in the management of benign strictures, but these are no longer available for clinical use [54].

Retrograde dilation is employed for high-grade esophageal strictures with near-complete or complete luminal occlusion, which usually occur after radiotherapy for head and neck cancer. As the name suggests, the technique involves passage of the dilator into the stricture by a retrograde approach through the esophagogastric junction. A pediatric or ultrathin scope is introduced into the stomach through a mature gastrostomy tract. In some instances, the gastrostomy tract may require dilation before introduction of the scope. The endoscope is advanced into the esophagus to the distal margin of the stricture, in a cephalad direction via the esophagogastric junction. Using a rendezvous procedure, a second endoscopist simultaneously advances a separate endoscope via the oropharynx to the proximal margin of the stricture [55]. If the dilation can be carried out without a rendezvous, fluoroscopic guidance is used with insertion of a guide wire. Dilation is then performed using polyvinyl or balloon dilators passed in a retrograde manner [56]. After an adequate luminal diameter has been achieved, antegrade dilation can be performed.

Complications

The main complications related to esophageal dilation include aspiration, bleeding, perforation, and bacteremia with associated endocarditis.

The rate of esophageal perforation depends on many factors, including the endoscopist's level of experience, the etiology and complexity of the stricture, the type of dilator used, and the technique employed for dilation. Although radiographic evidence of contrast extravasation on barium esophagography may be seen in up to 12 % of patients after dilation, the reported rate of clinically significant perforations is about 0.1–2.0 % [12,57]. Among endoscopists who have performed fewer than 500 diagnostic EGDs, the perforation rate is reported to be four times higher than among more experienced endoscopists [58]. The underlying etiology may also play a role, with a greater risk for perforation in malignant strictures, peptic strictures with concomitant severe esophagitis, radiation-

29

induced strictures, caustic strictures, and eosinophilic esophagitis [59–62].

The clinical presentation after a perforation depends on the site and severity of perforation and the timing of presentation. Perforation usually occurs at the site of dilation and may be intracervical, intrathoracic, or intra-abdominal. It usually occurs proximal to the stricture with bougie dilators, or at the level of the stricture with balloon dilators. Perforation may rarely occur at a distant site as a result of kinking of the guide wire. Perforation of the cervical esophagus should be suspected in patients with symptoms of neck pain or tenderness, hoarseness, or dysphonia. The presence of subcutaneous emphysema helps confirm the complication. Patients with intrathoracic perforation often present with pleuritic chest or upper back pain. Additional symptoms include odynophagia, dysphagia, dyspnea, hematemesis, and rarely cardiac tamponade. The presence of mediastinal emphysema can demonstrated by the Hamman sign, described as a "crunching noise" on auscultation of the chest. An esophagogram with water-soluble contrast can help identify the site of perforation. Stable patients with minimal contrast extravasation on esophagography can be managed conservatively with antibiotics, analgesics, nil per os, and parenteral nutrition [63]. Surgery for closure of the leak may be necessary in patients who present late or have evidence of free perforation on esophagography [64]. Stents can be placed in patients who are poor candidates for surgery and in those with malignant strictures [65].

Although esophageal dilation has the highest rate of bacteremia among all endoscopic procedures, the risk of endocarditis is very rare [66,67]. Factors associated with bacteremia include bougie dilation, multiple dilations at a single session, and dilation of high-grade or malignant strictures [68]. Antibiotic prophylaxis is recommended for all high-risk cardiac patients (those with prosthetic valves, prior endocarditis, systemic–pulmonary shunt, synthetic vascular graft less than a year old, and complex cyanotic congenital heart disease) [11].

Aspiration, hemorrhage, bronchospasm, and arrhythmias are other complications that may occur with esophageal dilation [10, 50].

Conclusions

Esophageal dilation is a therapeutic procedure that offers the benefits of temporary or permanent relief of dysphagia, with an improved quality of life and avoidance of surgery. Thorough evaluation of the patient before the procedure and performance of dilation by an experienced endoscopist are essential to minimize the related risks. Multiple dilators are currently available for use, with none being established as superior to the others. The type of dilator and the dilation technique should be individualized on the basis of the underlying disorder and the endoscopist's preference. Adjunctive procedures may be beneficial for strictures that fail to respond to standard dilation techniques.

References

1. Kelly HD. Origins of oesophagology. Proc R Soc Med 1969;62:781–6.
2. Hildreth CT. Stricture of the esophagus. N Engl J Med Surg 1821;10:235.
3. Boyce HW. Dilation of difficult benign esophageal strictures. Am J Gastroenterol 2005;100:744–5.
4. Castell DO, Donner MW. Evaluation of dysphagia: a careful history is crucial. Dysphagia 1987;2:65–71.
5. Scolapio JS, Pasha TM, Gostout CJ, Mahoney DW, Zinsmeister AR, Ott BJ, et al. A randomized prospective study comparing rigid to balloon dilators for benign esophageal strictures and rings. Gastrointest Endosc 1999;50: 13–7.
6. Dryden GW, McClave SA. Methods of treating dysphagia caused by benign esophageal strictures. Tech Gastrointest Endosc 2001;3:135–43.
7. Lew RJ, Kochman ML. A review of endoscopic methods of esophageal dilation. J Clin Gastroenterol 2002;35:117–26.
8. [No authors listed.] Esophageal dilation. American Society for Gastrointestinal Endoscopy. Gastrointest Endosc 1998;48:702–4.
9. Devitta RJ, Reynolds JC. Esophageal dilation techniques. Pract Gastroenterol 2002;16:46–57.
10. Eisen GM, Baron TH, Dominitz JA, Faigel DO, Goldstein JL, Johanson JF, et al. Guideline on the management of anticoagulation and antiplatelet therapy for endoscopic procedures. Gastrointest Endosc 2002;55:775–9.
11. Hirota WK, Petersen K, Baron TH, Goldstein JL, Jacobson BC, Leighton JA, et al. Guidelines for antibiotic prophylaxis for GI endoscopy. Gastrointest Endosc 2003;58:475–82.
12. Hernandez LV, Jacobson JW, Harris MS. Comparison among the perforation rates of Maloney, balloon and Savary dilation of esophageal strictures. Gastrointest Endosc 2000;51:460–2.
13. Lindor KD, Ott BJ, Hughes RW Jr. Balloon dilation of upper digestive tract strictures. Gastroenterology 1985;89:545–8.
14. Jones MP, Bratten JR, McClave SA. The optical dilator: a clear over-the-scope bougie with sequential dilating segments. Gastrointest Endosc 2006;63:840–5.
15. Cox JG, Winter RK, Maslin SC, Dakkak M, Jones R, Buckton GK, et al. Balloon or bougie for dilatation of benign esophageal stricture? Dig Dis Sci 1994;39:776–81.
16. Saeed ZA, Winchester CB, Ferro PS, Michaletz PA, Schwartz JT, Graham DY. Prospective randomized comparison of polyvinyl bougies and through-the-scope balloons for dilation of peptic strictures of the esophagus. Gastrointest Endosc 1995;41:189–95.
17. McClave SA, Wright RA, Brady PG. Prospective randomized study of Maloney esophageal dilation: blinded versus fluoroscopic guidance. Gastrointest Endosc 1990;36:372–5.
18. Abele JE. The physics of esophageal dilation. Hepatogastroenterology 1992;39:486–9.
19. Schatzki R, Gary JE. Dysphagia due to a diaphragm-like localized narrowing in the lower esophagus (lower esophageal ring). Am J Roentgenol Radium Ther Nucl Med 1953;70:911–22.
20. Nostrant TT. Esophageal dilatation. Dig Dis Sci 1995;13:337–55.
21. Kozarek RA, Patterson DJ, Ball TJ, Gelfand MG, Jiranek GE, Bredfeldt JE, et al. Esophageal dilation can be done safely using selective fluoroscopy and single dilating sessions. J Clin Gastroenterol 1995;20:184–8.
22. Tulman AB, Boyce AB. Complications of esophageal dilation and guidelines for their prevention. Gastrointest Endosc 1981;27:229–34.
23. Muehldorfer SM, Hahn EG, Ell C. High- and low-compliance balloon dilators in patients with achalasia: a randomized prospective comparative trial. Gastrointest Endosc 1996;44:398–403.
24. Khan AA, Shah SW, Alam A, Butt AK, Shafqat F, Castell DO. Pneumatic balloon dilation in achalasia: a prospective comparison of balloon distention time. Am J Gastroenterol 1998;93:1064–7.
25. Gideon RM, Castell DO, Yarze J. Prospective randomized comparison of pneumatic dilation technique in patients with idiopathic achalasia. Dig Dis Sci 1999;44:1853–7.
26. West RL, Hirsch DP, Bartelsman JF, de Borst J, Ferwerda G, Tytgat GN, et al. Long term results of pneumatic dilation in achalasia followed for more than 5 years. Am J Gastroenterol 2002;97:1346–51.
27. Vaezi MF, Richter JE, Wilcox CM, Schroeder PL, Birgisson S, Slaughter RL, et al. Botulinum toxin versus pneumatic balloon dilatation for achalasia: a randomised trial. Gut 1999;44:231–9.
28. Bansal R, Nostrant TT, Scheiman JM, Koshy S, Barnett JL, Elta GH, et al. Intrasphincteric botulinum toxin versus pneumatic balloon dilation for treatment of primary achalasia. J Clin Gastroenterol 2003;36:209–14.
29. Clouse RE, Abramson BK, Todorczuk JR. Achalasia in the elderly. Effects of aging on clinical presentation and outcome. Dig Dis Sci 1991;36:225–8.
30. Ghoshal UC, Kumar S, Saraswat VA, Aggarwal R, Misra A, Choudhuri G. Long-term follow-up after pneumatic dilation for achalasia cardia: factors associated with treatment failure and recurrence. Am J Gastroenterol 2004;99:2304–10.
31. Farhoomand K, Connor JT, Richter JE, Achkar E, Vaezi MF. Predictors of outcome of pneumatic dilation in achalasia. Clin Gastroenterol Hepatol 2004;2:389–94.
32. Parkman HP, Reynolds JC, Ouyang A, Rosato EF, Eisenberg JM, Cohen S. Pneumatic dilatation or esophagomyotomy treatment for idiopathic achalasia: clinical outcomes and cost analysis. Dig Dis Sci 1993;38:75–85.
33. Vaezi MF, Richter JE. Current therapies for achalasia: comparison and efficacy. Journal of Clinical Gastroenterology 1998;27:21–35.

34. Reynolds JC, Parkman HP. Achalasia. Gastroenterol Clin North Am 1989; 18:223–55.

35. Ott DJ, Richter JE, Wu WC, Chen YM, Castell DO, Gelfand DW. Radiographic evaluation of esophagus immediately after pneumatic dilatation for achalasia. Dig Dis Sci 1987;32:962–7.

36. Swedlund A, Traube M, Siskind BN, McCallum RW. Nonsurgical management of esophageal perforation from pneumatic dilatation in achalasia. Dig Dis Sci 1989;34:379–84.

37. Groskreutz JL, Kim CH. Schatzki's ring: long-term results following dilation. Gastrointest Endosc 1990;36:479–81.

38. Eckardt FE, Kanzler G, Willems D. Single dilation of symptomatic Schatzki rings. A prospective evaluation of its effectiveness. Dig Dis Sci 1992;37: 577–82.

39. Chotiprasidhi P, Minocha A. Effectiveness of single dilation with Maloney dilator versus endoscopic rupture of Schatzki's ring using biopsy forceps. Dig Dis Sci 2000;45:281–84.

40. Burdick JS, Venu RP, Hogan WJ. Cutting the defiant lower esophageal ring. Gastrointest Endosc 1993;39:616–19.

41. Katzka DA. Caustic injury to the esophagus. Curr Treat Options Gastroenterol 2001;4:59–66.

42. Keh SM, Onyekwelu N, McManus K, McGuigan J. Corrosive injury to upper gastrointestinal tract: still a major surgical dilemma. World J Gastroenterol 2006;12:5223–8.

43. Tiryaki T, Livanelioglu Z, Atayurt H. Early bougienage for relief of stricture formation following caustic esophageal burns. Pediatr Surg Int 2005;21: 78–80.

44. Lee M, Kubik CM, Polhamus CD, Brady CE 3 rd, Kadakia SC. Preliminary experience with endoscopic intralesional steroid injection therapy for refractory upper gastrointestinal strictures. Gastrointest Endosc 1995;41: 598–601.

45. Vimalraj V, Rajendran S, Jyotibasu D, Balachandar TG, Kannan D, Jeswanth S, et al. Role of retrograde dilatation in the management of pharyngoesophageal corrosive strictures. Dis Esophagus 2007;20:328–32.

46. Evrard S, Le Moine O, Lazaraki G, Dormann A, El Nakadi I, Devière J. Self-expanding plastic stents for benign esophageal lesions. Gastrointest Endosc 2004;60:894–900.

47. Dua KS. New approach to malignant strictures of the esophagus. Curr Gastroenterol Rep 2003;5:198–205.

48. Tietjen TG, Pasricha PJ, Kalloo AN. Management of malignant esophageal stricture with esophageal dilation and esophageal stents. Gastrointest Endosc Clin N Am 1994;4:851–62.

49. Fleischer DE. Esophageal dilation [slides]. 2nd ed. New York: Gower Medical, 1992. (Slide atlas of therapeutic endoscopy, unit 2.)

50. Bhutani MS, Usman N, Shenoy V, Qarqash A, Singh A, Barde CJ, et al. Endoscopic ultrasound miniprobe-guided steroid injection for treatment of refractory esophageal strictures. Endoscopy 1997;29:757–9.

51. Ackroyd R, Watson DI, Devitt PG, Jamieson GG. Expandable metallic stents should not be used in the treatment of benign esophageal strictures. J Gastroenterol Hepatol 2001;16:484–7.

52. Song HY, Jung HY, Park SI, Kim SB, Lee DH, Kang SG, et al. Covered retrievable expandable nitinol stents in patients with benign esophageal strictures: initial experience. Radiology 2000;217:551–7.

53. Triester SL, Fleischer DE, Sharma VK. Failure of self-expanding plastic stents in treatment of refractory benign esophageal strictures. Endoscopy 2006;38:533–7.

54. Fry SW, Fleischer DE. Management of a refractory benign esophageal stricture with a new biodegradable stent. Gastrointest Endosc 1997;45: 179–82.

55. Bueno R, Swanson SJ, Jaklitsch MT, Lukanich JM, Mentzer SJ, Sugarbaker DJ. Combined antegrade and retrograde dilation: a new endoscopic technique in the management of complex esophageal obstruction. Gastrointest Endosc 2001;54:368–72.

56. Steele NP, Tokayer A, Smith RV. Retrograde endoscopic balloon dilation of chemotherapy and radiation-induced esophageal stenosis under direct visualization. Am J Otolaryngol Head Neck Med Surg 2007;28:98–102.

57. Kang SG, Song HY, Lim MK, Yoon HK, Goo DE, Sung KB. Esophageal rupture during balloon dilation of strictures of benign or malignant causes: prevalence and clinical importance. Radiology 1998;209:741–6.

58. Quine MA, Bell GD, McCloy RF, Matthews HR. Prospective audit of perforation rates following upper gastrointestinal endoscopy in two regions of England. Br J Surg 1995;82:530–3.

59. Van Dam J, Rice TW, Catalano MF, Kirby T, Sivak MV Jr. High-grade malignant stricture is predictive of esophageal tumor stage. Risks of endosonographic evaluation. Cancer 1993;71:2910–7.

60. Swaroop VS, Desai DC, Mohandas KM, Dhir V, Dave UR, Gulla RI, et al. Dilation of esophageal strictures induced by radiation therapy for cancer of the esophagus. Gastrointest Endosc 1994;40:311–5.

61. Broor SL, Raju GS, Bose PP, Lahoti D, Ramesh GN, Kumar A, et al. Long term results of endoscopic dilatation for corrosive oesophageal strictures. Gut 1993;34:1498–501.

62. Shafi MA, Eisen GE, Al Kawas FH. Increased risk of esophageal perforation with dilation in patients with multiple esophageal webs (feline esophagus): a case–control study [abstract]. Gastrointest Endosc 1997;45: AB56.

63. Williamson, WA, Ellis, FH. Esophageal perforation. In: Taylor MB, Gollan JL, Steer MJL, Wolfe MM, editors. Gastrointestinal emergencies. Baltimore: Williams & Wilkins; 1997. p. 31–47.

64. Bladergroen MR, Lowe JE, Postlethwait RW. Diagnosis and recommended management of esophageal perforation and rupture. Ann Thorac Surg 1986;42:235–9.

65. Ferguson MK. Esophageal perforation and caustic injury: management of perforated esophageal cancer. Dis Esophagus 1997;10:90–4.

66. Botoman VA, Surawicz CM. Bacteremia with gastrointestinal endoscopic procedures. Gastrointest Endosc 1986;32:342–6.

67. Niv Y, Bat L, Motro M. Bacterial endocarditis after Hurst bougienage in a patient with a benign esophageal stricture and mitral valve prolapse. Gastrointest Endosc 1985;31:265–7.

68. Nelson DB, Sanderson SJ, Azar MM. Bacteremia with esophageal dilation. Gastrointest Endosc 1998;48:563–7.

69. Zuccaro G Jr, Richter JE, Rice TW, et al. Viridans streptococcal bacteremia after esophageal stricture dilation. Gastrointestinal Endoscopy 1998;48:568–73

70. Nelson DB, Sanderson SJ, Azar MM. Bacteremia with esophageal dilation. Gastrointestinal Endoscopy 1998;48:563–7

71. Hirota WK, Wortmann GW, Maydonovitch CL, et al. The effect of oral decontamination after esophageal dilation: a prospective trial. Gastrointestinal Endoscopy 1999;50:475–9

72. Nelson DB, Sanderson SJ, Azar MM. Bacteremia with esophageal dilation. Gastrointestinal Endoscopy 1998;48:563–7

73. Banerjee S, Shen B, Baron TH, et al. ASGE Standards of Practice Committee. Antibiotic prophylaxis for GI endoscopy. Gastrointestinal Endoscopy 2008; 67:791–8

74. Wilson W, Taubert KA,Gewitz M, et al. Prevention of infective endocarditis: guidelines from the American Heart Association: a guideline from the American Heart Association Rheumatic Fever, Endocarditis, and Kawasaki Disease Committee, Council on Cardiovasculart Disease in the Young,and the Council on Clinical Cardiology, Council on Cardiovascular Surgery and Anesthesia, the the Quality of Care and Outcomes Research Interdisciplinary Working Group. Circulation 2007;116:1736–54

75. Banerjee S, Shen B, Baron TH, et al. ASGE Standards of Practice Committee. Antibiotic prophylaxis for GI endoscopy. Gastrointestinal Endoscopy 2008; 67:791–8

29

30 Endoscopic Resection, Ablation, and Dissection

Hiroyuki Ono, Stefan Seewald, and Nib Soehendra

Introduction: the History of Endoscopic Treatment

Endoscopic treatment for early gastrointestinal tumors is now common throughout the world. In Japan, the increased use of this form of treatment resulted from improved early detection of cancer due to widely available physical examinations and advances in endoscopic instruments—from gastrocameras to electronic scopes. In terms of the resulting quality of life, endoscopic treatment is clearly superior to open and laparoscopic surgery for early gastrointestinal tumor. In this chapter, the term "endoscopic mucosal resection" (EMR) is used refer to endoscopic resection, while "endoscopic submucosal dissection" (ESD) refers to endoscopic dissection.

The history of endoscopic treatment for cancer is outlined in **Table 30.1**. Rosenberg et al. performed polypectomy as the first endoscopic treatment in 1955, using a rigid scope in patients with rectal and sigmoid polyps [1]. The development of techniques for polypectomy was followed by the introduction of laser treatment. Polypectomy can only be used for pedunculated polyps, and laser treatment does not provide tissue for histological evaluation of the tumor depth and type, so that the treatment outcome may be unclear. The current method of EMR for endoscopic resection of sessile colonic polyps was first developed by Deyhle et al. [2]. In this method, saline is injected into the submucosa to swell the lesion and facilitate its removal with a snare. Takekoshi et al. developed a method in which the polyp is held and lifted up with two snares before removal [3], but the strip biopsy technique described by Tada et al. is more commonly used in Japan [4]. In Europe and the United States, where fewer cases of early gastric cancer are treated in comparison with Japan, the method of endoscopic mucosal resection using a transparent plastic cap (EMR-C), developed by Inoue et al., is commonly used due to its ease and usefulness [5,6]. EMR is also used to treat superficial esophageal cancer. Soehendra et al. described a simple suction technique in which a lesion can be easily removed using a snare alone [7].

These EMR methods are not capable of being used to remove large lesions (≥ 2 cm) or lesions that have an ulcer scar as a single fragment, and such lesions are therefore often removed in multiple fragments. With lesions in the esophagus and large intestine, the resection margin is clear, and recurrences resulting from residual neoplastic tissue are rare even when the lesions are removed in multiple fragments. There are therefore no clinical problems with EMR in such cases. In contrast, gastric cancer lesions often have a vague margin, and removing them in multiple fragments is associated with a risk of recurrence. In Japan, most EMR procedures for early gastric cancer used to be performed using strip biopsy or EMR-C. However, local recurrences are sometimes observed following resection in multiple fragments (**Table 30.2**) [8]. One-piece resection is also preferable, as it is often difficult to reconstruct the entire lesion from multiple-fragment specimens, and local recurrences can often be attributed to inappropriate assessment of the multiple fragments of a resected specimen. New endoscopic resection techniques were therefore needed to replace conventional EMR and allow en bloc resection of large and difficult lesions (≥ 20 mm or with ulceration).

In 1983, Hirao et al. described a method of endoscopic resection using a hypertonic saline–epinephrine (ERHSE) injection, in which the mucosa is dissected with a needle-knife and removed by snaring

Table 30.2 Recurrence rate in resected specimens [8]

	n	Complete resection (n = 292) (%)	NE (n = 81) (%)	Incomplete resection (n = 47) (%)	Recurrence rate (n = 21) (%)
1 piece	244	81	10	9	2
2 pieces	134	61	28	11	6
3 pieces	24	46	33	21	26
4 or more	18	17	55	28	24

NE, not evaluable.

Table 30.1 History of endoscopic treatment for early gastrointestinal lesions

Date	Procedure	Technique	First author, ref.
1955	Polypectomy with a rigid scope (colon)	Saline injection	Rosenberg [1]
1973	Polypectomy for sessile polyps (colon)	Saline injection and snaring	Deyhle [2]
1980	Double-snare polypectomy (stomach)	Grasping and snaring	Takekoshi [3]
1983	Development of electronic scope system		
1983	Endoscopic resection with hypertonic saline–epinephrine (ERHSE) solution (stomach)	Injection, precutting, and snaring	Hirao [9]
1984	Strip biopsy (stomach)	Injection, grasping, and snaring	Tada [4]
	Endoscopic mucosal resection (EMR) (esophagus)	Injection, snaring using an overtube	Makuuchi [6]
1990	Endoscopic mucosal resection using a transparent plastic cap (EMR-C) (esophagus)	Injection, snaring with a cap	Inoue [5]
1996	Endoscopic submucosal dissection (ESD) using insulated-tip (IT) knife (stomach)	Injection, precutting mucosa, and dissecting submucosa	Hosokawa, Ono [9, 10]
1997	Simple suction technique	Snaring	Soehendra [7]

[9]. However, this method is associated with a high risk of perforation due to the use of the needle-knife and is not applicable to large lesions because of the need for snaring. The ERHSE technique has therefore been limited to a small number of institutions.

Further changes in operating techniques and in the design of accessory equipment followed. Hosokawa and Yoshida [10] and Ono et al. [11] developed a specialized endoscopic knife, known as the insulated-tip (IT) diathermic knife, which consists of a needle-knife tipped with a ceramic ball [10,11]. This can be used to cut the submucosa safely and remove a lesion completely. This and several other knives were developed in Japan [12,13] for use in ESD.

Diagnosis and Indications

EMR/ESD for gastrointestinal cancer is generally carried out as a local treatment and is limited to cancer associated with a low risk of metastasis to the lymph nodes—i. e., early-stage cancer. The procedures involved include diagnosis of lesions using endoscopy, radiography, and endoscopic ultrasonography before resection; collection of a resected specimen for histopathology; and complete resection of lesions when possible, with avoidance of side effects such as burning.

▥ Pathology

The standards for histological diagnosis of gastric cancer differ in Japan and the West [14], with mucosal cancer often being diagnosed as dysplasia in the West, but as cancer in Japan. However, attempts to achieve a consensus on histological criteria are gradually reducing these differences [15]. The extent of resection of EMR/ESD specimens is evaluated carefully both endoscopically and histopathologically in slices at intervals of 2 mm [16]. After resection in multiple fragments, this evaluation is based on completely reconstructed specimens. Submucosal massive invasion and/or vessel involvement are indicators of a high risk of positive nodes or distant metastasis, and surgical intervention is strongly recommended in such cases. Invasion on the lateral margin is classified into the following three groups on the basis of endoscopic and histopathological evidence:

- Complete resection: when the lateral margin is clear endoscopically and pathologically (minimal probability of local recurrence).
- Incomplete resection: when the tumor has definitely invaded as far as the lateral margin endoscopically and pathologically (high probability of local recurrence).
- Not evaluable: when the tumor has been removed endoscopically, but its lateral margin cannot be evaluated pathologically due to burning (caused by diathermic treatment) or mechanical damage, or when reconstruction is difficult due to multiple-fragment resection.

▥ New Diagnostic Technologies

Recent technological developments (described in detail in other chapters) such as chromoendoscopy, magnifying endoscopy, and imaging-enhanced endoscopy have led to new diagnostic approaches. These methods use narrow band-imaging (NBI) [17], Fujinon Intelligent Color Enhancement (FICE) [18], and autofluorescence imaging (AFI) [19]. The diagnostic mechanisms in NBI and FICE depend on the difference in the penetration depth of light of different wavelengths, which can be used to assess capillaries on the mucosal surface and fine mucosal patterns. In AFI, the tissue is irradiated with excitation light at 390–470 nm to detect autofluor-

escence emitted from fluorescent substrates such as collagen and with light at 540–560 nm, which is absorbed by hemoglobin in blood. This makes it possible to distinguish between neoplastic lesions and normal mucosa, as they can be highlighted in different colors (**Fig. 30.1**).

▥ Esophageal Cancer

In Europe and the United States, adenocarcinoma accounts for more than 50% of esophageal cancers and for about 70% of such cases among white males. The primary site for adenocarcinoma is the lower esophagus, which is also the site of 70% or more of all esophageal cancers. In contrast, in Japan, squamous cell carcinoma (SCC) accounts for 90% or more of esophageal cancers. SCC often occurs in the mid-esophagus, and more than 60% of esophageal cancers develop in the upper and mid-esophagus, resulting in different treatments, surgical approaches, and outcomes. In Japan, screening tests for the upper gastrointestinal tract have been developed to detect gastric cancer, and this has led to more than 20% of cases of esophageal cancer being detected at stage I. Fewer stage I cases are found in Europe and the United States, and consequently fewer patients are treated with EMR/ESD there.

Early esophageal cancer lesions show a slight concavity or an irregular surface, but are often difficult to detect using regular endoscopy. As smoking and drinking are risk factors for squamous cell carcinoma, a 1–3% potassium iodine solution is used in high-risk patients to facilitate diagnosis; normal mucosa containing glycogen-rich granules stains a dense dark brown, whereas carcinoma and dysplasia show little staining [20]. The rate of detection of esophageal adenocarcinoma can be increased using NBI and magnifying endoscopy in obese patients and those with reflux esophagitis. The standard application of endoscopic therapy is for lesions within the mucosal layer and up to two-thirds of the whole esophageal circumference, in which resection does not cause stenosis after resection. In such cases, the risk of lymph-node metastasis is less than 5%. However, metastases occur in approximately 40% of patients with submucosal cancer, with a subsequent requirement for chemoradiotherapy and surgical treatment.

▥ Gastric Cancer

The term "early gastric cancer" (EGC) refers to T1 tumors, in which invasion is confined to the mucosa or submucosa regardless of the presence of regional lymph-node metastasis. The macroscopic types and endoscopic findings are shown in **Fig. 30.2**. EGC is classified into these types, or as "type IIa + IIc" or "IIc + III" for complex types [21]. The aim of the Japanese classification is to provide a common language for the clinical and pathological description of gastric cancer and thereby to contribute to improved treatment and diagnosis. More than 50% of gastric cancers in Japan [22], but less than 5% in the West [23], are early lesions, suggesting that these cancers may be missed in the West. Both knowledge and technique are important in detecting EGC. Since most early gastric cancers are not symptomatic, searches based on symptoms are not usually performed. In Japan, mass screening using the barium meal approach was initiated 40 years ago, and the proportion of cases of EGC among patients with gastric cancer has increased.

Experience with EGC has shown that preparation before gastroscopy is very important. Pronase, a proteolytic enzyme solution, and simethicone are first administered to remove mucus and bubbles, respectively. During gastroscopy, retention of air and the use of Buscopan as an antispasmodic agent are important for maintaining a good view of the whole stomach. Chromoendoscopy using indigo

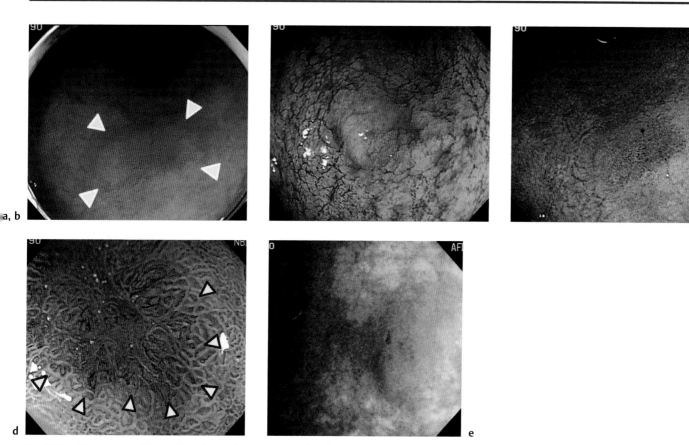

Fig. 30.1 A lesion in a patient with early gastric cancer located in the lesser curvature of the mid-region of the stomach.

a Examination of the lesion (yellow arrows) with a normal optical scope. The lesion was a generally flat elevated polyp with a diameter of 10 mm and a central part that was slightly red and recessed. The lesion was diagnosed as a grade 0 IIa + IIc early gastric cancer and intramucosal cancer.

b Chromoendoscopic image after spraying with indigo carmine.

c On narrow-band imaging (NBI), the recessed part of the lesion appears as a brownish area.

d NBI image combined with magnifying endoscopy. The arrow line indicates the margin between normal mucosa and the cancer. The normal glandular structure is lost, and abnormal blood vessels with a large diameter are present in the lesion. Using NBI with magnifying endoscopy improved the diagnostic accuracy for the lesion margin.

e A relatively unclear autofluorescence image (AFI), showing the surrounding normal mucosa in green and the lesion in magenta.

30

carmine dye is useful to accentuate any lesions present, and NBI with magnifying endoscopy and AFI are also helpful (**Fig. 30.1**).

The standard indications for endoscopic treatment proposed by the Japanese Gastric Cancer Association [24] include:

- Differentiated adenocarcinoma
- Intramucosal cancer
- Lesion ≤ 20 mm in size
- No ulceration

Lesions that meet all of these criteria are considered to have a negligible risk of lymph-node metastasis. However, these criteria also take into account the technical difficulty that a lesion that is 2 cm or larger in size cannot be removed in a single fragment using EMR. This technical problem has been solved by ESD, and clinical trials are in progress to cover the following wider range of indications:

- Differentiated adenocarcinoma
- Intramucosal cancer
- Lesions of any size but with no ulceration, or lesions ≤ 30 mm with ulceration.

We have shown that lesions that meet these criteria have a negligible risk of lymph-node metastasis [25].

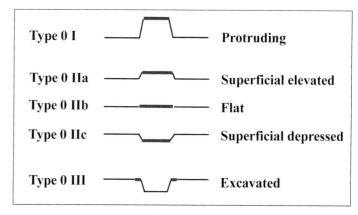

Fig. 30.2 Macroscopic types of early gastric cancer.

Colonic Cancer

Polypectomy has been carried out for early colonic cancer on the basis of the adenoma–carcinoma sequence proposed by Morson et al. [26]. The indications have not been fully established. Neoplastic lesions < 5 mm in diameter have been found to harbor intramucosal cancer and submucosal cancer in 1–2 % and 0.1–0.2 % of cases, respectively. These are extremely low incidences, indicating that pedunculated and elevated adenomas with a diameter of 6 mm or more should be resected at present. Widespread colonoscopy screening and the development of a high-resolution electronic endoscope have shown that superficial flat or depressed-type tumors are relatively common [27], but these tumors are difficult to remove completely using polypectomy and are treated with EMR.

The criteria for EMR are a tumor with almost no risk of lymph-node metastasis and a tumor with a size and site that allow complete resection. A large tumor that cannot be completely dissected can be removed in pieces [28]. Relapses after incomplete piecemeal resection are frequently observed with tumors in the ascending colon and cecum, laterally spreading tumors, and tumors 2–3 cm or more in diameter. Such tumors can therefore only be treated using ESD in a few institutions, due to technical difficulties. Approaches with low invasiveness, including laparoscopic surgery, are used where possible, but if any of the following risk factors for metastasis is found in histopathological tests, radical surgery is required [29]:

● Positive vertical (surgical) margin
● Submucosal invasion of 1000 µm or more in depth
● Positive lymphatic and vascular invasion
● Poorly differentiated adenocarcinoma

Treatment Procedures

▦ Principles

EMR/ESD has few aftereffects and allows patients to maintain a better quality of life in comparison with open and laparoscopic surgery. Endoscopic surgery should therefore be chosen whenever possible, although it must be borne in mind that this is a local treatment that has to be performed in accordance with the indications. Endoscopic surgery in patients in whom the procedure is not indicated should be carried out only in the context of clinical trials, and informed consent should be obtained after the risks and benefits of the procedure have been fully explained to the patient. Treatment can also be performed using laser ablation, argon plasma coagulation (APC), and photodynamic therapy, but these all result in tissue destruction, which prevents the collection of samples for postoperative histopathological assessment. In patients with an incomplete preoperative diagnosis, EMR/ESD may be the best approach for obtaining adequate specimens for histologic examination. This allows the extent of cancer invasion, the presence of

lymphatic and vascular invasion, and the histological type to be established postoperatively, with subsequent decision-making regarding the need for further surgical resection.

▦ Endoscopic Mucosal Resection

EMR techniques for esophageal and gastric lesions can be broadly divided into two methods: strip biopsy using a double-channel endoscope, in which a polyp is held and pulled with forceps and removed by a snare; and EMR-C, in which the polyp is lifted up by suction and removed with a snare. In the large intestine, pedunculated polyps are removed by polypectomy, whereas sessile polyps are removed using a snare following submucosal injection.

Strip biopsy consists of the following steps (**Fig. 30.3**):
● A mark is made around the polyp with a needle-knife (**Fig. 30.3 a**).
● A saline–epinephrine solution (diluted 1 : 500 000–1 : 1 000 000) is injected into the submucosa to raise the lesion (**Fig. 30.3 b**).
● The polyp is lifted with grasping forceps, and the polyp and surrounding tissue are caught with a snare (**Fig. 30.3 c**).
● Resection is performed using high-frequency current, preferably coagulating current (**Fig. 30.3 d**).
● The lesion is collected (**Fig. 30.3 e**).

EMR-C consists of the following steps (**Fig. 30.4**):
● A mark is made around the polyp with a needle-knife.
● A transparent plastic cap is placed on the tip of the endoscope, and a saline–epinephrine solution (diluted 1 : 500 000–1 : 1 000 000) is injected into the submucosa to raise the lesion (**Fig. 30.4 a**). Local injection into the distal part of the lesion then makes the lesion rise forward.
● A small-diameter snare is fixed onto the rim of the cap (the prelooping process) and the lesion is sucked completely inside the cap (**Fig. 30.4 b**).
● The snare is pulled, and the injected saline prevents the muscle layer from catching (**Fig. 30.4 c**).
● The snare contents are resected using high-frequency current (**Fig. 30.4 d**).

In patients with Barrett's esophagus, it is difficult to distinguish cancer endoscopically from high-grade or low-grade intraepithelial neoplasia (HGIN and LGIN, respectively). The current guidelines of the American College of Gastroenterology recommend a surveillance protocol based on histological diagnosis [30]. A patient with LGIN on biopsy should have repeat endoscopy for confirmation and then surveillance endoscopy annually until no further dysplasia is observed. For those with HGIN on biopsy, endoscopy should be repeated to search for cancer. For multifocal HGIN, surgery or photodynamic therapy have been recommended. In recent years, patients with a low risk of lymph-node metastasis (HGIN, intramucosal cancer) are increasingly being treated with EMR [31].

For extensive EMR of Barrett's esophagus containing premalignant and early malignant lesions, and for early intramucosal SCC (m1–2) in the esophagus, EMR using a modified multiple-band ligator (with the ligate-and-cut technique) is increasingly being used in Western countries. This technique facilitates multiple mucosal resections in the esophagus without the need to withdraw the endoscope. Submucosal injection is not required [32]. The targeted mucosa is sucked into the barrel, and the rubber band is deployed in the same manner as in variceal ligation by creating a pseudopolyp. The pseudopolyp is then immediately resected using pure coagulating current. The second ligation is performed by suctioning the adjacent mucosa with a bit overlapping to ensure that no Barrett's remnant remains (**Fig. 30.5**).

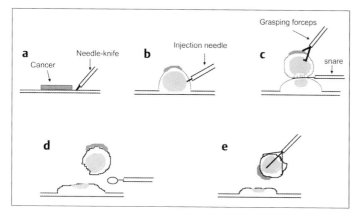

Fig. 30.3 Steps in strip biopsy.
a A mark is made around the polyp with a needle-knife.
b Saline–epinephrine solution is injected into the submucosa to raise the lesion.
c The polyp is lifted with grasping forceps. The polyp and surrounding tissue are caught with a snare.
d Resection is performed using a high-frequency current preferably coagulating current.
e The lesion is collected.

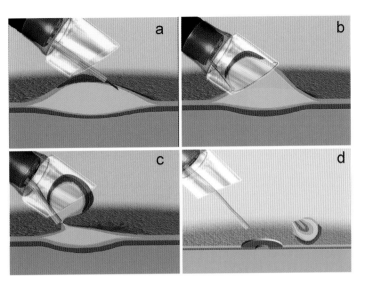

Fig. 30.4 Steps in endoscopic mucosal resection using a transparent plastic cap (EMR-C).
a A transparent plastic cap is placed on the tip of the endoscope and a saline–epinephrine solution is injected into the submucosa to raise the lesion.
b A small-diameter snare is fixed onto the rim of the cap, and the lesion is sucked completely inside the cap.
c The snare is pulled, and the injected saline prevents the muscle layer from catching.
d The snare contents are resected using high-frequency current.

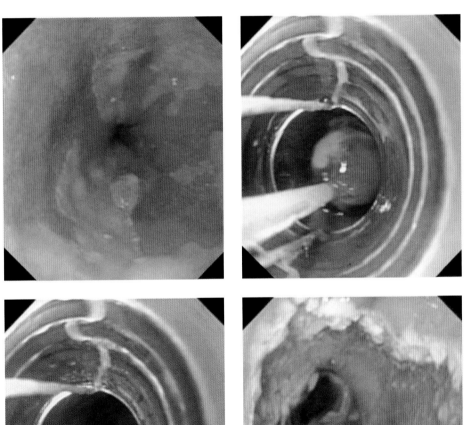

Fig. 30.5 Endoscopic images of complete endoscopic mucosal resection of a 4-cm long segment of Barrett's esophagus using a modified multiple-band ligator kit (Duette; Cook Medical, Bloomington, Indiana, USA).
a Barrett's esophagus with a nodule confirmed histologically as intramucosal cancer.
b Suctioning and ligating the tumor-bearing mucosa to create a pseudopolyp.
c Resection of the pseudopolyp.
d Sequential ligation and cutting continues until the entire Barrett's mucosa has been resected.

30

Table 30.3 Rates of margin-free and one-piece resection

	< 20 mm	20–30 mm	> 30 mm	Total
ESD with IT knife	87 % (686/785)	91 % (187/206)	83 % (146/176)	87 % (1019/1167)
EMR by strip-off biopsy	45 % (172/386)	24 % (8/34)	0 % (0/10)	42 % (180/430)

EMR, endoscopic mucosal resection ESD, endoscopic submucosal dissection; IT, insulated-tip.

Barrett's mucosa without dysplasia can be eradicated using radiofrequency ablation [33]. Recently, good results have been reported with circumferential and focal ablation of persistent dysplasia following endoscopic resection for intraepithelial neoplasia in Barrett's esophagus [33,34].

Endoscopic Submucosal Dissection

Endoscopic mucosal resection is a valuable technique, but it is technically difficult to achieve complete removal of large lesions (≥ 2 cm) and those with ulcer scars. The rates of margin-free and one-piece resection for EMR and ESD in patients with gastric cancer are shown relative to tumor diameter in **Table 30.3** [8]. The EMR rate is only 50 % even for tumors up to 2 cm in diameter, and the relapse rates after resection in multiple fragments are high (**Table 30.2**), with subsequent surgical resection often being required. To solve these problems, the technique of ESD was developed to allow removal of lesions as single fragments, to minimize the local recurrence rate, and to increase the percentage of negative margins (**Table 30.3**). ESD was initially applied as a method of treatment for early gastric cancer, and it is now also used in early esophageal cancer. EMR is still the major method for early cancer in the large intestine, but the use of ESD to treat large, sessile lesions such as laterally spreading tumors has been increasing.

The ESD protocol is shown in **Fig. 30.6**. In principle, the site surrounding a lesion margin is circumferentially dissected with a high-frequency knife, and subsequently the submucosa is removed in order to ablate the entire lesion. The high-frequency knife is safer than a needle-knife and has been a breakthrough in ESD. In 1996, we developed a specialized endoscopic knife, the insulated-tip (IT) diathermy knife, which is a needle-knife with a ceramic ball at the tip (**Fig. 30.7 a**) [10,11]. An insulated small ceramic sphere connected to the tip of the high-frequency needle-knife allows safe and easy incision and separation of the mucosal and submucosal layers. Following this invention, several other endoscopic knives [13,35] have been developed in Japan (**Fig. 30.7 c, d**). Rösch et al. performed ESD using an IT knife and reported complete removal of only 25 % of the tumor [36], which indicates the difficulty of the ESD technique and the need for sufficient training in order to obtain good outcomes. It has been recognized that the IT knife has three technical drawbacks: firstly, it is not easy to cut a lesion while looking downward; secondly, lateral cutting performance is relatively poor; and thirdly, the ceramic tip may become stuck to the cutting edge of the mucosa, as it is made of insulating material. To address these issues, we have developed an improved IT knife, the IT knife-2 (IT-2) (**Fig. 30.7 b**). Its superiority in comparison with the original IT knife, particularly in shortening the operating time, has been reported [37].

Case Presentation

Step 1: preparation and pretreatment. With the exception of sedation, pretreatment procedures are similar to those in regular endoscopy. Diazepam (10 mg) and pethidine hydrochloride (35 mg) are injected intravenously immediately before initiation of ESD. Diazepam and midazolam are then administered intravenously as required. In Europe, propofol is widely used for conscious sedation. Oxygen saturation with pulse oximetry (SpO_2) electrocardiography,

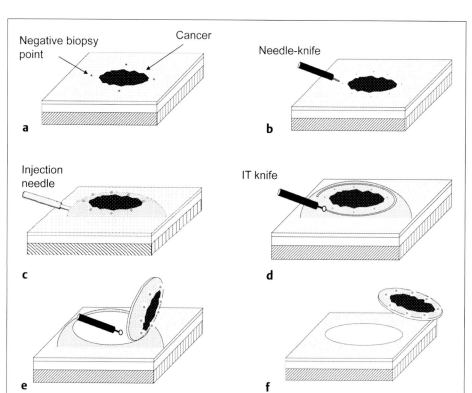

Fig. 30.6 Scheme for endoscopic submucosal dissection (ESD) using an insulated-tip (IT) knife.
a Before ESD, negative biopsies were taken outside the lesion to confirm the cancer margin.
b Circumferential marking using the needle-knife (or an argon plasma coagulation probe).
c Injection of 4 % hyaluronic acid solution into the submucosal layer.
d Circumferential incision of the mucosal layer using an IT knife-2.
e Dissection of the submucosal layer.
f Retrieving the tumor.

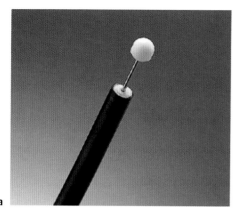
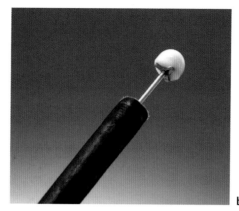
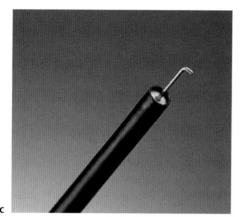
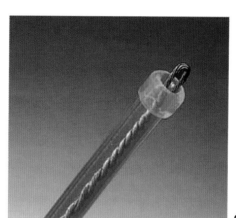

Fig. 30.7 Knives used for endoscopic submucosal dissection.
a Original model insulated-tip (IT) knife.
b IT knife-2.
c Hook knife.
d Flex knife.

and blood pressure should be monitored, as drug administration may reduce blood pressure and cause respiratory depression.

Step 2: marking (Fig. 30.8 a, b). The lesion was a stage IIa early gastric cancer, 2 cm in diameter, in the lesser curvature beneath the cardia. An area approximately 5 mm outside the lesion margin is marked with a dot at intervals of several millimeters. For specimen arrangement, it is useful to place a mark to identify the direction of the resected specimen (on the proximal or distal side).

Step 3: local injection (Fig. 30.8 c). For local injection before circumferential dissection, a needle is inserted slightly outside the mark to ensure that adequate swelling of the mucosa is obtained. Saline or a 4% sodium hyaluronate solution containing epinephrine at 0.5 mg/100 mL and a moderate amount of indigo carmine is injected. Epinephrine should be reduced or should not be used in patients with hypertension or ischemic heart disease.

Step 4: precutting and circumferential mucosal dissection (Fig. 30.8 d). A precut of 1–2 mm for insertion of the IT knife is made using the cutting edge of a needle-knife. Care needs to be taken to avoid perforation, as the edge of the needle-knife is not insulated. The precut is made at the distal margin of the lesion. For a large lesion or one in a difficult site, several additional precuts make it easier to dissect the lesion. The edge of the IT knife is inserted into the precut and the mucosa is dissected circumferentially about 2–3 mm outside the mark in dissection mode (VIO, dry cut 50 W, effect 4; Erbe, Germany). The IT knife is used to press down and dissect the mucosa from back to front and slightly downward in the vertical direction.

Step 5: submucosal dissection and removal (Fig. 30.8 e, f). Following circumferential dissection, a local injection is given again to swell the entire lesion. The submucosa is identified by blue staining with indigo carmine and then dissected and removed with the knife in the end-cut mode (ICC 200; Erbe, effect 3, 80 W) or swift coagulation mode (VIO, effect 4, 100 W). With an image of the line of the stomach wall being borne in mind, the IT knife is run parallel to the stomach wall to remove the submucosal tissue while giving sufficient tension to the submucosa when handling the endoscope and IT knife. Since the operation site is covered with the removed mucosa, the mucosa is lifted with a disposable attachment placed on the tip of the endoscope (Olympus Corporation, Japan) to maintain vision with the scope and provide countertraction.

Step 6: specimen collection and hemostasis. The resected specimen is collected with grasping forceps and then examined histopathologically (**Fig. 30.8 g**). If there is hemorrhage, coagulation (soft mode, 80 W, ICC 200; or swift coagulation, VIO, Erbe) with hemostatic forceps should be carried out. Bleeding makes the scope view extremely narrow and leads to complications such as perforation. Even slight bleeding should therefore be completely arrested. After removal and collection of the specimen, the endoscope is inserted again for hemostasis.

Step 7: postoperative care. A proton-pump inhibitor should be administered orally or by injection on and after the day ESD is performed. Food should be started on postoperative day 2.

Some physicians prefer to use needle-type knives, which are not insulated, such as a hook knife (**Fig. 30.7 c**) or flex knife (**Fig. 30.7 d**), and others. These knives can cut the submucosa steadily under direct vision. However, it sometimes takes longer to complete the procedure, as the cutting length is short in comparison with the IT knife. **Figure 30.9** illustrates the hook knife technique.

Complications

Complications of gastrointestinal ESD can occur intraoperatively and postoperatively. Hemorrhage, perforation, and sequelae associated with perforation may occur intraoperatively. The sequelae can be classified into conditions induced by air leakage outside the gastrointestinal tract and those due to infection. Gastric perforation is associated with pneumoperitoneum and peritonitis; esophageal

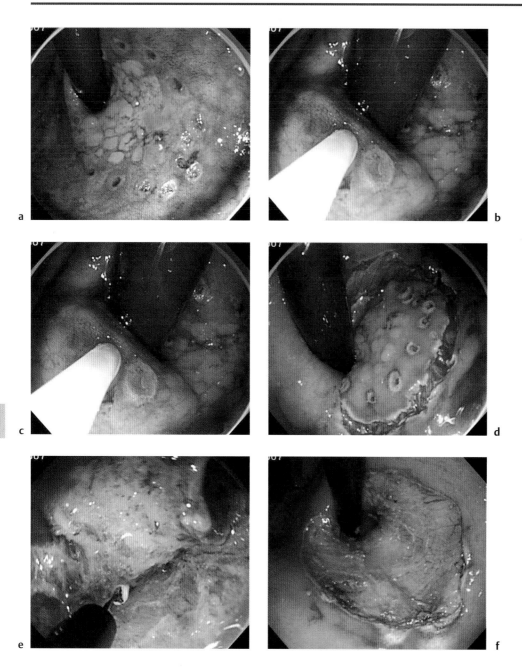

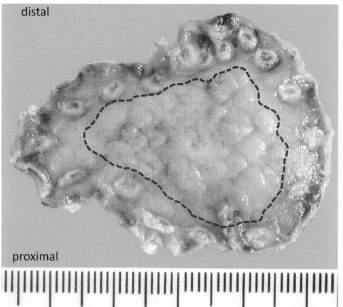

Fig. 30.8 An endoscopic submucosal dissection (ESD) procedure.
a A type IIa early gastric cancer, 2 cm in size, is located at the lesser curvature, just below the cardia.
b Circumferential marking using an argon plasma coagulation probe.
c Injection of 4 % hyaluronic acid solution into the submucosal layer.
d Circumferential incision of the mucosal layer using an IT knife-2.
e Dissection of the submucosal layer.
f The ESD ulcer after retrieval of the tumor.
g Histological examination of the specimen revealed intramucosal cancer and lymphatic and vascular invasion (dotted red line), with the horizontal and vertical margins free from cancer. The specimen measured 51 × 35 mm and the lesion 29 × 21 mm.

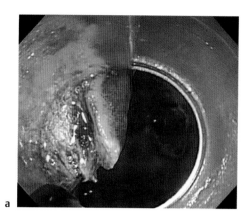 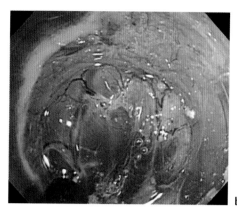

Fig. 30.9 a Dissecting submucosa with a hook knife. The tip of the hook is moving in the direction of the lumen.
b Precutting coagulation of the vessel. The tip of the hook is inserted under the vessel and coagulation is carried out as it moves in the direction of the lumen.

perforation with mediastinal and subcutaneous emphysema, pneumothorax, and mediastinitis; and large-intestinal perforation with pneumoperitoneum, retroperitoneal emphysema, and peritonitis. Other intraoperative complications include changes in cardiorespiratory dynamics (hypotension, arrhythmia, hypoxemia) and Mallory–Weiss syndrome. Postoperative complications include secondary hemorrhage and delayed perforation, which both occur within a few days after EMR/ESD and are considered to be early postoperative complications; and gastrointestinal stenosis (obstruction), which can occur more than 1 week after surgery as a late postoperative complication. Aspiration pneumonia, fever, and pain may also occur postoperatively.

Hemorrhage

Conventional EMR causes almost no intraoperative hemorrhage, whereas the ESD procedure may cause hemorrhage. The incidence has not been fully defined, but Oda et al. reported that Hb decreased by ≥ 2 g/dL on the day after gastric ESD in 7 % of patients (63 of 945) [38]. Intraoperative hemorrhage in gastric ESD often occurs in lesions from the cardia to the anterior/posterior wall of the lesser curvature in the upper part of the gastric body and in lesions with ulcer scars, indicating that particular care is required when ESD is carried out for such lesions. In the esophagus and large intestine, hemorrhage is less of a concern as a complication of ESD. However, bleeding makes the scope view extremely narrow and causes complications including perforation, incomplete resection, and prolonged treatment time. It is therefore important to prevent and treat bleeding using hemostatic forceps and surgical clips. It is also important to maintain vision with the scope using attachments such as a water jet, and to handle the knife under direct vision whenever possible.

Perforation

The incidence of intraoperative gastric perforation is higher in ESD (1–4 %) than in EMR (0.2 %). The usual treatment is closure with clips, and the safety of this approach has been confirmed [39], indicating the value of conservative treatment whenever possible. After perforation occurs, a nasogastric tube should be inserted to drain the gastric contents. Perforation induces pneumoperitoneum due to air leakage into the peritoneal cavity. A small air leak may not cause a serious problem, but a large leak may induce deteriorating respiratory status and lead to shock. In a patient with severe pneumoperitoneum or changes in vital signs, the air should be released by abdominal puncture.

Esophageal perforation is an extremely serious complication that is often associated with mediastinal and subcutaneous emphysema

and pneumothorax, and can result in mediastinitis and mediastinal abscess. The esophageal wall is thin and the external membrane is fragile, and this can allow air leaks due to an exposed muscle layer, in the absence of obvious perforation. In esophageal ESD, it is therefore important to remove the lesion with the submucosa intact in order to limit exposure of the muscle layer and prevent perforation and mediastinal emphysema.

Large-intestinal perforation is also a serious complication in ESD. The wall of the large intestine is thin and its tertiary structure is more complicated (due to the haustra) than that of the stomach and esophagus. Care therefore needs to be taken when performing ESD for a lesion crossing a haustrum. The incidence of ESD-induced perforation in the large intestine has been reported to range from 2 % to 6 %. Leakage of fecal fluid into the peritoneal cavity due to perforation may cause diffuse peritonitis, and this fluid should always be vacuumed away in EMR/ESD. Fecal fluid around a perforated site should be immediately vacuumed, and the site should be closed with clips. Antibiotics should then be administered and the patient should be fasted, with neither food nor beverages allowed. Oral intake should be started carefully several days later, with close observation of clinical symptoms and inflammatory reactions.

Stenosis

In narrow areas such as the esophagus and the gastric cardia and pylorus, wide (circumferential) EMR/ESD may induce stenosis associated with ulcer scar healing. It has been reported that stenosis in the esophagus and gastric pylorus is frequently induced by dissection of 75 % or more of the perimeter, and it may occur with dissection of only half the perimeter. Stenosis can be treated with balloon dilation, but a long stenosis in the esophagus and gastric antrum is a severe condition. It is therefore very important to prevent stenosis by avoiding unnecessary mucosal dissection. In treating a lesion in which stenosis is anticipated, minimum resection of nontumorous mucosa and maintenance of normal mucosa can contribute to preventing or reducing stenosis. Treatment is very difficult once an ulcer scar has become stiff and stenosis has developed, and bougie treatment should be performed after wide and circumferential resection. Stenosis often occurs 10–20 days after ESD, and bougie treatment may therefore be performed about 7 days after ESD.

Ablation

Ablation methods include laser therapy, photodynamic therapy (PDT), and argon plasma coagulation (APC), which were the major treatment methods for early gastrointestinal cancer until the emergence of EMR and ESD. However, these methods destroy tissue and

30

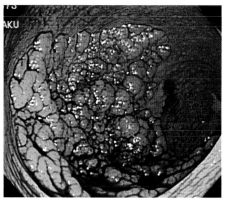
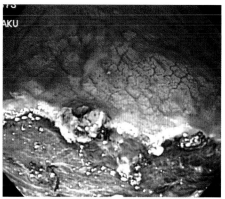
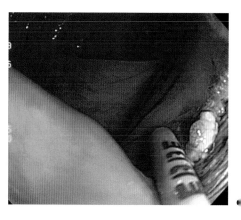

a, b

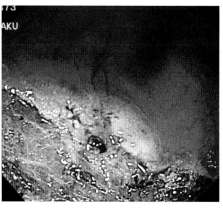
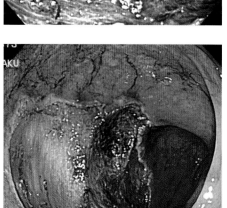

d

e

Fig. 30.10 a A laterally spreading tumor in the rectum (60 mm in size).
b A tiny residual tumor.
c, d After argon plasma coagulation, the tumor is no longer visible.
e The ulcer after endoscopic mucosal resection.

do not allow postoperative histopathological examination, unlike EMR and ESD. In the United States, high-grade dysplasia in Barrett's esophagus has been treated using PDT [40], and relapse after EMR and ESD is sometimes treated with APC. Recently, balloon-based radiofrequency ablation has been used to ablate Barrett's esophagus without dysplasia. This technique is much easier to apply, and the complication rate is lower in comparison with PTD and APC [32]. For further details, see Chapters 26, 27, and 32.

Case Presentation

Figure 30.10 illustrates a case in which a laterally spreading tumor with a diameter of 6 cm was found in the rectum (**Fig. 30.10 a**) and removed using EMR. A slight residual tumor was observed around the margin (**Fig. 30.10 b**) and was ablated with APC, resulting in disappearance of the tumor (**Fig. 30.10 c–e**).

Conclusions

EMR and ESD provide resected specimens that can be examined histopathologically. In cases in which the preoperative diagnosis is found to be incorrect and there is a risk of lymph-node metastasis, the treatment strategy can be changed. Despite technical difficulties, the use of ESD has been increasing in Japan, as it is applicable to large lesions and those with an ulcer scar. ESD is also becoming more common in Europe and the United States for the treatment of intramucosal gastric cancers. The method is likely to become increasingly useful as better devices and techniques are developed.

Acknowledgments

The authors are indebted to Dr. Inoue and Dr. Oyama for permission to use **Fig. 30.3** and **Fig. 30.9**, respectively.

References

1. Rosenberg N. Submucosal saline wheal as safety factor in fulguration of rectal and sigmoidal polyps. Arch Surg 1955;70:120–2.
2. Deyhle P, Largiader F, Jenny S, Fumagalli I. A method for endoscopic electroresection of sessile colonic polyps. Endoscopy 1973;5:38–40.
3. Takekoshi T, Baba Y, Ota H, Kato Y, Yanagisawa A, Takagi K, et al. Endoscopic resection of early gastric carcinoma: results of a retrospective analysis of 308 cases. Endoscopy 1994;26:352–8.
4. Tada M, Murakami A, Karita M, Yanai H, Okita K. Endoscopic resection of early gastric cancer. Endoscopy 1993;25:445–50.
5. Inoue H, Endo M. Endoscopic esophageal mucosal resection using a transparent tube. Surg Endosc 1990;4:198–201.
6. Makuuchi H, Machimura T, Sugihara T. Endoscopic diagnosis and treatment of mucosal cancer of the esophagus [in Japanese]. Endosc Dig 1990;2:447–52.
7. Soehendra N, Binmoeller KF, Bohnacker S, Seitz U, Brand B, Thonke F, et al. Endoscopic snare mucosectomy in the esophagus without any additional equipment: a simple technique for resection of flat early cancer. Endoscopy 1997;29:380–3.
8. Ono H. Early gastric cancer: diagnosis, pathology, treatment techniques and treatment outcomes. Eur J Gastroenterol Hepatol 2006;18:863–6.
9. Hirao M, Masuda K, Asanuma T, Naka H, Noda K, Matsuura K, et al. Endoscopic resection of early gastric cancer and other tumors with local injection of hypertonic saline–epinephrine. Gastrointest Endosc 1988;34:264–9.
10. Hosokawa K, Yoshida S. Recent advances in endoscopic mucosal resection for early gastric cancer [in Japanese with English abstract]. Jpn J Cancer Chemother 1998;25:476–83.
11. Ono H, Kondo H, Gotoda T, Shirao K, Yamaguchi H, Saito D, et al. Endoscopic mucosal resection for treatment of early gastric cancer. Gut 2001;48:225–9.

V

12. Oyama T, Kikuchi Y. Aggressive endoscopic mucosal resection in the upper GI tract: hook knife EMR method. Min Invas Ther Allied Technol 2002;11:291–5.

13. Yahagi N, Fujishiro M, Kakushima N, Kobayashi K, Hashimoto T, Oka M, et al. Endoscopic submucosal dissection for early gastric cancer using the tip of an electro-surgical snare (thin type). Dig Endosc 2004;16:34–8.

14. Schlemper RJ, Itabashi M, Kato Y, Lewin KJ, Riddell RH, Shimoda T, et al. Differences in diagnostic criteria for gastric carcinoma between Japanese and Western pathologists. Lancet 1997;348:1725–9.

15. Schlemper RJ, Riddell RH, Kato Y, Borchard F, Cooper HS, Dawsey SM, et al. The Vienna classification of gastrointestinal epithelial neoplasia. Gut 2000;47:251–5.

16. Japanese Gastric Cancer Association. Japanese classification of gastric carcinoma. 2nd English edition. Gastric Cancer 1998;1:10–24.

17. Sano Y, Muto M, Tajiri H, Ohtsu A, Yoshida S. Optical/digital chromoendoscopy during colonoscopy using narrow-band imaging system. Dig Endosc 2005;17(Suppl):S 60–5.

18. Osawa H, Yoshizawa M, Yamamoto H, Kita H, Satoh K, Ohnishi H, et al. Optimal band imaging system can facilitate detection of changes in depressed-type early gastric cancer. Gastrointest Endosc 2008;67:226–34.

19. Haringsma J, Tytgat GN, Yano H, Iishi H, Tatsuta M, Ogihara T, et al. Autofluorescence endoscopy: feasibility of detection of GI neoplasms unapparent to white light endoscopy with an evolving technology, Gastrointest Endosc 2001;53:642–50.

20. Endo M, Takeshita K, Yoshida M. How can we diagnose the early stage of esophageal cancer? Endoscopic diagnosis. Endoscopy 1986;18:11–8.

21. [No authors listed.] The Paris endoscopic classification of superficial neoplastic lesions: esophagus, stomach, and colon: November 30 to December 1, 2002. Gastrointest Endosc 2003;58(6 Suppl):S 3–43.

22. Shimizu S, Tada M, Kawai K. Early gastric cancer: its surveillance and natural course. Endoscopy 1995;27:27–31.

23. Ballantyne KC, Morris DL, Jones JA, Gregson RH, Hardcastle JD. Accuracy of identification of early gastric cancer. Br J Surg 1987;74:618–9.

24. Japanese Gastric Cancer Association. JGCA gastric cancer treatment guidelines. 2nd ed. Tokyo: Kanehara, 2004.

25. Gotoda T, Yanagisawa A, Sasako M, Ono H, Nakanishi Y, Shimoda T, et al. Incidence of lymph node metastasis from early gastric cancer: estimation with a large number of cases at two large centers. Gastric Cancer 2000;3:219–25.

26. Morson BC, Dawson IMP. The polyp–cancer sequence. In: Morson BC, Dawson IMP. Gastrointestinal pathology. Oxford: Blackwell Scientific; 1972. p. 542–7.

27. Kudo S. Early colorectal cancer: detection of depressed types of colorectal carcinoma. Tokyo: Igaku-Shoin, 1996.

28. Nivatvongs S, Snover DC, Fang DT. Piecemeal snare excision of large sessile colon and rectal polyps: is it adequate? Gastrointest Endosc 1984;30:18–20.

29. Kitajima K, Fujimori T, Fujii S, Takeda J, Ohkura Y, Kawamata H, et al. Correlations between lymph node metastasis and depth of submucosal invasion in submucosal invasive colorectal carcinoma: a Japanese collaborative study. J Gastroenterol 2004;39:534–43.

30. Sampliner RE. Updated guidelines for the diagnosis, surveillance, and therapy of Barrett's esophagus. Am J Gastroenterol 2002;97:1888–95.

31. Seewald S, Ang TL, Soehendra N. Endoscopic mucosal resection of Barrett's oesophagus containing dysplasia or intramucosal cancer. Postgrad Med J 2007;83:367–72.

32. Soehendra N, Seewald S, Groth S, Omar S, Seitz U, Zhong Y, et al. Use of modified multiband ligator facilitates circumferential EMR in Barrett's esophagus (with video). Gastrointest Endosc 2006;63:847–52.

33. Sharma VK, Wang KK, Overholt BF, Lightdale CJ, Fennerty MB, Dean PJ, et al. Balloon-based circumferential endoscopic radiofrequency ablation of Barrett's esophagus: 1-year follow-up of 100 patients (with video). Gastrointest Endosc 2007;65:185–95.

34. Gondrie JJ, Pouw RE, Sondermeijer CMT, Peters FP, Curvers WL, Rosmolen WD, et al. Stepwise circumferential and focal ablation of Barrett's esophagus with high-grade dysplasia: results of the first prospective series of 11 patients. Endoscopy 2008;40:359–69.

35. Oyama T, Kikuchi Y. Aggressive endoscopic mucosal resection in the upper GI tract: hook knife EMR method. Min Invas Ther Allied Technol 2002;11:291–5.

36. Rösch T, Sarbia M, Schumacher B, Deinert K, Frimberger E, Toermer T, et al. Attempted endoscopic en bloc resection of mucosal and submucosal tumors using insulated-tip knives: a pilot series. Endoscopy 2004;36:788–801.

37. Ono H, Hasuike N, Inui T, Takizawa K, Ikehara H, Yamaguchi Y, et al. Usefulness of a novel electrosurgical knife, the insulation-tipped diathermic knife-2, for endoscopic submucosal dissection of early gastric cancer. Gastric Cancer 2008;11:47–52.

38. Oda I, Gotoda T, Hamanaka H, Eguchi T, Saito Y, Matsuda T, et al. Endoscopic submucosal dissection for early gastric cancer technical feasibility, operation time and complications from a large consecutive series. Dig Endosc 2005;17:54–8.

39. Minami S, Gotoda T, Ono H, Oda I, Hamanaka H. Complete endoscopic closure of gastric perforation induced by endoscopic resection of early gastric cancer using endoclips can prevent surgery (with video). Gastrointest Endosc 2006;63:596–601.

40. Overholt BF, Lightdale CJ, Wang KK, Canto MI, Burdick S, Haggitt RC, et al. Photodynamic therapy with porfimer sodium for ablation of high-grade dysplasia in Barrett's esophagus: international, partially blinded, randomized phase III trial. Gastrointest Endosc 2005;62:488–98.

30

31 Clipping and Suturing

Keiichi Ikeda and Paul Swain

Introduction

Endoscopic clipping devices enable endoscopists to achieve tissue approximation during gastrointestinal endoscopy and have been used for hemostasis of gastrointestinal bleeding, to mark the location of tumors for stenting or surgery, to attach pH measurement capsules, and to close mucosal defects or perforations. Endoscopic submucosal dissection (ESD) was developed to allow en bloc resection of early gastrointestinal cancer [1], but the procedure is associated with a higher risk of perforation than the standard endoscopic mucosal resection (EMR) technique. Endoscopic clipping is still useful for such perforations [2], although a more secure device for approximating tissue when iatrogenic perforations of this type occur would be desirable.

Several companies have been actively conducting research during the last 10 years to develop endoscopically controlled suturing devices. Endoscopic plication treatment for gastroesophageal reflux disease (GERD) an attractive indication for such devices, and the advent of a new approach to endoscopic therapy, natural orifice transluminal endoscopic surgery (NOTES), has accelerated the development of various types of endoscopic suturing device. This chapter outlines the features of several types of device for endoscopic clipping and suturing, along with relevant applications for them.

Endoscopic Clipping

An endoscopic clipping device capable of being passed through the accessory channel was first developed in 1975 by Hayashi et al. [3], and the design was modified by Hachisu et al. [4–6]. Endoscopic clipping is now an essential technique in the field of gastrointestinal endoscopy and has a wide range of clinical applications, including endoscopic treatment for gastrointestinal hemorrhage. In contrast to laser, diathermy, and injection therapy, the mechanical method of hemostasis has clear theoretical advantages. With an expanding range of indications, clips are now used to close perforations and fistulas, to secure catheters and stents, to attach pH telemetry devices, and as markers to guide endoscopic, surgical, and radiological therapy.

Several endoscopic clip designs are currently commercially available, and each type may have advantages for various specific uses.

EZ Clip and QuickClip (Olympus Medical Systems, Tokyo, Japan). The reusable EZ Clip and preloaded disposable QuickClip are stainless-steel devices, 1.2 mm wide, available in several lengths (short, standard, and long), with opening angles of 90° or 135° (**Fig. 31.1 a**). Each clip is housed in a color-coded cartridge (**Fig. 31.1 b**), and in comparison with earlier types of device they are easy to load (**Fig. 31.1 c**). The preloaded single-use QuickClip avoids the need for clip loading.

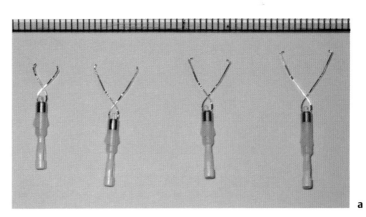

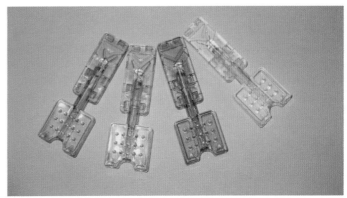

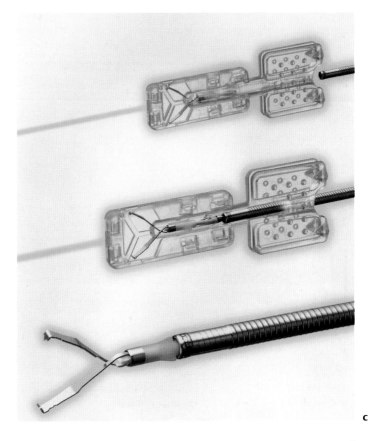

Fig. 31.1 a Different types of QuickClip (Olympus Medical Systems, Tokyo, Japan).
b The QuickClip color-coded cartridge.
c Quick, single-action loading with the QuickClip.

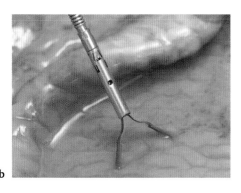
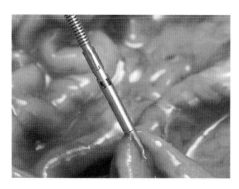
a, b
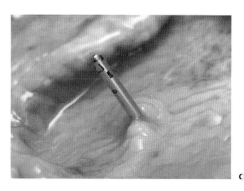
c

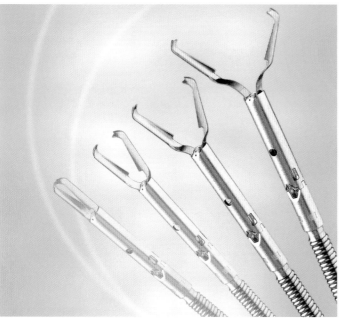
d

Fig. 31.2 a–d The Resolution Clip (Boston Scientific Corporation, Natick, Massachusetts, USA).

than other commercially available clips. In a porcine model, Shin et al. compared the duration of attachment in all of the commercially available clips [7]. The study showed that the Resolution Clip is retained longest at the site of application (more than 4–5 weeks).

TriClip (Cook Medical, Inc., Bloomington, Indiana, USA). In the new TriClip device, the aim is to overcome problems by using a three-pronged design, coupled with an ergonomic handling device to enhance orientation and performance (**Fig. 31.3**) [8]. With the three arms, it is more likely that one arm will be on each side of the vessel when the clip is closed.

MultiClips (InScope, Inc., Cincinnati, Ohio, USA). Another clip device that is close to commercial launch in the United States is the MultiClip Applier from InScope, Inc. (a division of Ethicon Endo-Surgery). The MultiClip is a single-use device with four premounted two-pronged clips. The clips can also be rotated, closed, reopened, and repositioned for optimal application. Raju et al. evaluated the feasibility and outcome of endoluminal closure of a small perforation of the colon with this device in a porcine model [9]. The study showed that endoluminal closure of a 2-cm colon perforation with clips was successful in preventing peritonitis and adhesions, and it was accomplished quickly with the new device. Clip closure at 1-cm intervals was sufficient for successful closure of a 2-cm colon perforation.

Endoscopic Suturing

The development of endoscopically controlled suturing devices may enable endoscopists and surgeons to perform a range of surgical procedures without the need to make external incisions. During flexible endoscopy, the problems involved in sewing are different from those experienced at open surgery or laparoscopy. It is not easy to manipulate a needle holder and exert sufficient force to drive a curved needle through tissue in such a way that it returns to the lumen and to be caught again and pulled, along with the thread, through the tissue. It is also difficult to manipulate two graspers practically for suturing, even with a double-channeled endoscope, as they tend to move coaxially to each other. Flexible endoscopy usually only allows access to one side of the tissue.

EndoCinch (Bard, Inc., Murray Hill, New Jersey, USA). The Endo-Cinch was the first effective flexible endoscopic suturing device. It was first used in patients in the United Kingdom in 1994 and was approved by the Food and Drugs Administration (FDA) in 1998 [10–12]. It has been used in at least 5000 patients, mostly for treating GERD [13]. The device works by sucking a fold of tissue into a cavity. The cavity size is selected to allow the stitch to penetrate the deep muscle and serosal surface of human stomach tissue. The hollow needle is then pushed through the sucked fold of tissue, and a "tilt stitch," consisting of a metal tag with a long attached length of nylon thread, is pushed through the hollow needle and caught in the device's reception chamber. The suction is then released, allowing the tissue through which the stitch has been placed to fall out of the device. The endoscope is then withdrawn, retaining

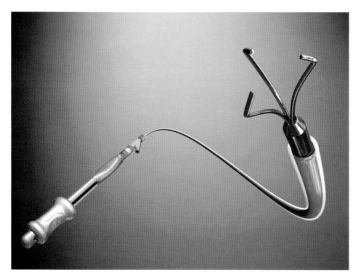

Fig. 31.3 The TriClip (Cook Medical, Inc., Bloomington, Indiana, USA).

Resolution Clip (Boston Scientific Corporation, Natick, Massachusetts, USA). A unique feature of the Resolution Clip is that it can be reopened and repositioned up to five times after closing, as long as the device has not been fired (**Fig. 31.2**). This feature allows precise positioning of the clips. The Resolution Clip also has longer arms

the thread and thus pulling the thread through the tissue. The thread and tilt stitch are released from the device outside the mouth, so that the thread passes from the mouth through the gastric tissue and back up to the mouth again. The nylon thread and metal tag can be reloaded onto the machine and further stitches can be placed in selected areas to form a continuous suture.

Plicator (NDO Surgical, Inc., Mansfield, Massachusetts, USA). Other suturing devices have been developed specifically for reflux treatment. The Plicator is an unusual suturing device designed to place two tags through a fold of tissue [14]. The tags are attached to a single thread, which passes through a pledget to spread the load over the tissue. When attached, the threads are fairly loose; it was found that separation reduced the frequency of displacement. There is a corkscrew, which is driven into the deep muscle and is designed to retract the tissue into the jaws of the device so that the stitches are placed deeply. This device has received FDA approval and has been used in more than 200 patients [15].

Tissue Apposition System (TAS; Ethicon Endo-Surgery, Inc., Cincinnati, Ohio, USA) (**Fig. 31.4**). A new and comparatively simple suturing method has recently been developed [16,17]. This uses a flexible hollow needle to deliver a threaded tag through tissue. It can be used to place stitches to any desired depth and to sew into the submucosa or deep muscle. Thread-locking methods and thread cutting can be accomplished in a single action. This method has some advantages over the others described above. All of the suturing components can be passed through the 2.8-mm accessory channel of a flexible endoscope, and an overtube is not required. The view is not obscured in any way by other components of the suturing process. The device can be used much more quickly than other flexible endoscopic suturing methods and should also be low in cost thanks to its simplicity.

This suturing method can also be used with endoscopic ultrasound guidance, allowing sutures to be placed in structures in or beyond the wall of the gastrointestinal tract with precision and safety. Using endoscopic ultrasound with this method, a posterior gastropexy has been carried out, with the cardia being sutured to the median arcuate ligament (the posterior attachment of the diaphragm, more than 1 cm thick and is easily identifiable above the celiac axis) to increase lower esophageal sphincter pressure [18]. In another example, ultrasound guidance was used when placing stitches into lymph nodes adjacent to the stomach in order to mark them and then follow the thread using a transgastric incision to remove the tagged lymph node [19]. This experimental approach might allow less invasive assessment of sentinel nodes and could improve staging and perhaps therapy for early gastric cancer. This suturing method has also been used through a flexible endoscope for a variety of endosurgical applications. It has also been used to close incisions made following full-thickness gastric resection [20,21] and to perform anastomoses, including a transgastric sutured gastrojejunostomy [22] and sutured biliary anastomosis [23], and to close transgastric incisions for NOTES procedures [24]. It has already been used in a few patients to close a perforated duodenal ulcer and a leaking gastroenterostomy [25].

Brace Bar (Olympus Medical Systems, Tokyo, Japan). A prototype double T-bar suturing device has been developed by Olympus [26]. It consists of a puncture needle and a suture unit. The suture unit has two metal tags at the distal end of a bifurcated nylon thread. The proximal end of the bifurcated thread has a stopper that can be moved forward to cinch the tags. The two metal tags are housed inside the tip of the needle in tandem (**Fig. 31.5**). The puncture needle's operating handle has mechanisms for delivering each tag and pushing the stopper forward to cinch the bifurcated thread. Using this newly developed bifurcated double T-bar suturing device, a suture can be completed consecutively through an accessory channel without the need to withdraw the device.

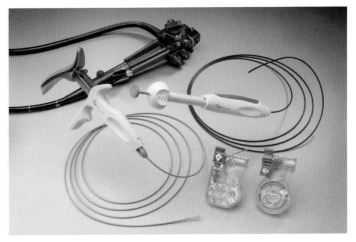

Fig. 31.4 Components of the Tissue Apposition System (TAS; Ethicon Endo-Surgery, Inc., Cincinnati, Ohio, USA).

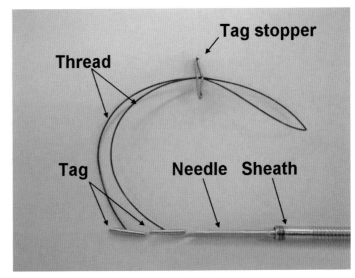

Fig. 31.5 A suture unit and the tip of the Brace Bar (Olympus Medical Systems, Tokyo, Japan).

Spiderman (Ethicon Endo-Surgery, Inc., Cincinnati, Ohio, USA). This suturing device uses a curved needle that forms approximately two-thirds of a circle. It is housed in a curved receptacle attached at the front of a flexible endoscope, which has an empty cavity occupying about one-third of the circle. Tissue can either be sucked into this cavity or positioned without suction in the curved receptacle, and the curved needle can be advanced through the tissue using a ratchet action. The needle is caught on the far side of the receptacle and can advance to the proximal side. The device can then be repositioned for the next stitch. This suturing device can place a running stitch in tissue.

EagleClaw (Olympus Medical Systems, Tokyo, Japan). Another complex flexible endoscopic suturing machine with an unusual action is the EagleClaw [27]. This was the first endoscopic device that attempted to solve the difficulties of sewing using a curved needle (**Fig. 31.6**). Most surgical stitches, of course, whether placed at open surgery or laparoscopy, are delivered using a curved needle. The proximal end of the thread is passed through a thread lock, which is tightened using a pushing catheter passed through a channel in the device once the two stitches have been placed. This device has not yet been used in patients, but several procedures have been performed with it in a porcine model, including endoscopic gastrojejunostomy, endoscopic plication for bleeding peptic ulcers, and endoscopic closure of colon perforations [28–31].

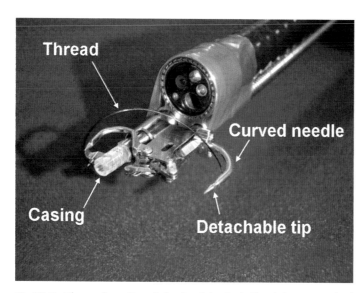

Fig. 31.6 The configuration of the tip of the EagleClaw (Olympus Medical Systems, Tokyo, Japan).

g-Prox (USGI Medical, Inc., San Clemente, California, USA). The USGI g-Prox can be passed in its narrowest configuration through the 6-mm accessory channel. The instrument is 5.5 mm in diameter and the toothed jaws are 25 mm long, providing a large, secure bite for manipulating tissue. Closing the jaws allows a needle to be advanced through the tissue at a 90° angle, enabling full visualization as the needle is passed through the tissue. A pair of self-expanding polyester mesh baskets is preloaded into the system; these act as tissue anchors to hold the grasped layer or layers of tissue. The first basket is deployed through the hollow needle and the needle is then retracted, leaving the basket on one side of the tissue. This distal basket is connected via a suture to another basket, which can be released on the proximal side of the tissue. The two baskets are strung onto a length of suture, with a terminal suture knot and a one-way cinch. The anchors are advanced towards each other and locked at the desired distance. The baskets then act on the tissue to form a plate-like configuration, tending to cinch the tissues together into a fold with the central connection between the baskets passing through the serosal surface. Additional anchors can be loaded into the g-Prox without the need to withdraw or reposition the instrument. This device has already been used in patients, in combination with the USGI TransPort multiple-lumen operating system, for gastric closure during NOTES procedures [32,33].

Future Prospects

Considerable activity is currently taking place in this field, with numerous patents being filed for flexible endoscopic suturing devices. This flowering of interest is due to the increasing numbers of procedures suitable for flexible endoscopic suturing. The advent of NOTES has led to the development and use of endoscopically sutured closure methods, as well as other intraperitoneal suturing applications. The expansion of endoscopic mucosal resection techniques and endoscopic submucosal dissection has also led to interest in endoscopic full-thickness resection with subsequent closure, as well as interest in closure of inadvertent perforations during large or deep tissue resections.

Bariatric surgery is another driving factor behind the development of endoscopic suturing methods. Bariatric surgery can be currently divided into gastric restriction procedures (the Lap-Band procedure is currently favored for this) and operations intended to lead to malabsorption, usually combined with gastric restriction—

for example, gastric bypass. There is considerable interest in developing less invasive methods that might mimic these procedures. An endoscopically sutured method of performing gastric restriction would be valuable. Less invasive methods for forming anastomoses using sutures placed via flexible endoscopes—e.g., for gastrojejunostomy or enteroenteral anastomoses—might reduce the invasiveness of current bypass procedures.

A number of other new developments have also been taking place. Internal electrode attachment for gastric pacing, duodenal ulcer closure, suturing of bleeding vessels, pyloroplasty, Heller myotomy, gastropexy, hiatus hernia repair, stent fixation, and lymphadenectomy are examples that have attracted recent interest. Reflux is rather out of fashion at present as a target for less invasive suturing devices, as is Nissen fundoplication. Although it seems clear from sham-controlled trials and physiological data that pathological reflux and the resulting symptoms are reduced in the majority of endoscopically treated patients, there is still a need for improvement. It seems clear that more stitches, and stitches that will hold their position permanently, are needed if the clinical results are to improve. Suturing devices need to be developed to improve the results. There have been no recent improvements in drug therapy for reflux, and many patients are dissatisfied with having to take long-term medication.

Conclusions

Progress in the field of gastrointestinal endoscopy has expanded the range of indications for it, and endoscopic clip applications have played an important role here. In addition, the advent of NOTES as a new approach to endoscopic surgery has led to the development of suturing devices for flexible endoscopy and multitasking platforms for NOTES procedures. There is a particular need for cheap, simple, and multipurpose suturing methods that can be used for most applications. Such devices are now in the advanced stages of development and early clinical use. The variety of new technologies being developed can be expected to contribute to further progress in the fields of gastrointestinal endoscopy and laparoscopic surgery.

■ Disclosures

Paul Swain acts as a consultant for Ethicon Endo-Surgery, USGI, and was an inventor of the Bard EndoCinch. Keiichi Ikeda acts as a consultant for the Olympus Medical Systems Corporation.

References

1. Miyamoto S, Muto M, Hamamoto Y, Boku N, Ohtsu A, Baba S, et al. A new technique for endoscopic mucosal resection with an insulated-tip electrosurgical knife improves the completeness of resection of intramucosal gastric neoplasms. Gastrointest Endosc 2002;55:576–81.
2. Minami S, Gotoda T, Ono H, Oda I, Hamanaka H. Complete endoscopic closure of gastric perforation induced by endoscopic resection of early gastric cancer using Endoclips can prevent surgery (with video). Gastrointest Endosc 2006;63:596–601.
3. Hayashi T, Yonezawa M, Kawabara T. [The study on staunch clip for the treatment by endoscopy]. Gastroenterol Endosc 1975;17:92–101. Japanese.
4. Hachisu T. Evaluation of endoscopic hemostasis using an improved clipping apparatus. Surg Endosc 1988;2:13–7.
5. Hachisu T, Miyazaki S, Hamaguchi K. Endoscopic clip-marking of lesions using the newly developed HX-3 L clip. Surg Endosc 1989;3:142–7.
6. Hachisu T, Yamada H, Satoh S. Endoscopic clipping with a new rotatable clip-device and a long clip. Dig Endosc 1996;8:127–33.
7. Shin EJ, Ko CW, Magno P, Giday SA, Clarke JO, Buscaglia JM, et al. Comparative study of endoscopic clips: duration of attachment at the site of clip application. Gastrointest Endosc 2007;66:757–61.

8. Chan CY, Yau KK, Siu WT, Wong KH, Luk YW, Tai TY, et al. Endoscopic hemostasis by using the TriClip for peptic ulcer hemorrhage: a pilot study. Gastrointest Endosc 2008;67:35–9.

9. Raju GS, Ahmed I, Xiao SY, Brining D, Poussard A, Tarcin O, et al. Controlled trial of immediate endoluminal closure of colon perforations in a porcine model by use of a novel clip device (with videos). Gastrointest Endosc 2006;64:989–97.

10. Kadirkamanathan SS, Evans DF, Gong F, Yazaki E, Scott M, Swain CP. Antireflux operations at flexible endoscopy using endoluminal stitching techniques: an experimental study. Gastrointest Endosc 1996;44:133–43.

11. Swain P, Park PO, Mills T. Bard EndoCinch: the device, the technique, and pre-clinical studies. Gastrointest Endosc Clin N Am 2003;13:75–88.

12. Filipi CJ, Lehman GA, Rothstein RI, Raijman I, Stiegmann GV, Waring JP, et al. Transoral, flexible endoscopic suturing for treatment of GERD: a multi-center trial. Gastrointest Endosc 2001;53:416–22.

13. Rothstein RI, Filipi CJ. Endoscopic suturing for gastroesophageal reflux disease: clinical outcome with the Bard EndoCinch. Gastrointest Endosc Clin N Am 2003;13:89–101.

14. Chuttani R, Kozarek R, Critchlow J, Lo S, Pleskow D, Brandwein S, et al. A novel endoscopic full-thickness plicator for treatment of GERD: an animal model study. Gastrointest Endosc 2002;56:116–22.

15. Chuttani R. Endoscopic full-thickness plication: the device, technique, pre-clinical and early clinical experience. Gastrointest Endosc Clin N Am 2003;13:109–16.

16. Fritscher-Ravens A, Mosse CA, Mills TN, Mukherjee D, Park PO, Swain P. A through-the-scope device for suturing and tissue approximation under endoscopic ultrasound control. Gastrointest Endosc 2002;56:737–42.

17. Swain P, Park PO. Endoscopic suturing. Best Pract Res Clin Gastroenterol 2004;18:37–47.

18. Fritscher-Ravens A, Mosse CA, Mukherjee D, Yazaki E, Park PO, Mills T, et al. Transgastric gastropexy and hiatal hernia repair for GERD under EUS control: a porcine model. Gastrointest Endosc 2004;59:89–95.

19. Fritscher-Ravens A, Mosse CA, Ikeda K, Swain P. Endoscopic transgastric lymphadenectomy by using EUS for selection and guidance. Gastrointest Endosc 2006;63:302–6.

20. Ikeda K, Fritscher-Ravens A, Mosse CA, Mills T, Tajiri H, Swain CP. Endoscopic full-thickness resection with sutured closure in a porcine model. Gastrointest Endosc 2005;62:122–9.

21. Ikeda K, Mosse CA, Park PO, Fritscher-Ravens A, Bergström M, Mills T, et al. Endoscopic full-thickness resection: circumferential cutting method. Gastrointest Endosc 2006;64:82–9.

22. Bergström M, Ikeda K, Swain P, Park PO. Transgastric anastomosis by using flexible endoscopy in a porcine model (with video). Gastrointest Endosc 2006;63:307–12.

23. Park PO, Bergström M, Ikeda K, Fritscher-Ravens A, Swain P. Experimental studies of transgastric gallbladder surgery: cholecystectomy and chole-cystogastric anastomosis (videos). Gastrointest Endosc 2005;61:601–6.

24. Sclabas GM, Swain P, Swanstrom LL. Endoluminal methods for gastro-stomy closure in natural orifice transenteric surgery (NOTES). Surg Innov 2006;13:23–30.

25. Bergström M, Swain P, Park PO. Early clinical experience with a new flexible endoscopic suturing method for natural orifice transluminal endoscopic surgery and intraluminal endosurgery (with videos). Gastro-intest Endosc 2008;67:528–33.

26. Ikeda K, Tajiri H. Evaluation of bifurcated double T-bar suturing device for effective closure of gastric perforation in ex vivo porcine models, aimed at clinical application of NOTES [abstract]. Gastrointest Endosc 2008;67:AB116.

27. Hu B, Chung SC, Sun LC, Lau JY, Kawashima K, Yamamoto T, et al. Endo-scopic suturing without extracorporeal knots: a laboratory study. Gastro-intest Endosc 2005;62:230–3.

28. Kantsevoy SV, Jagannath SB, Niiyama H, Chung SS, Cotton PB, Gostout CJ, et al. Endoscopic gastrojejunostomy with survival in a porcine model. Gastrointest Endosc 2005;62:287–92.

29. Chiu PW, Hu B, Lau JY, Sun LC, Sung JJ, Chung SS. Endoscopic plication of massively bleeding peptic ulcer by using the Eagle Claw VII device: a feasibility study in a porcine model. Gastrointest Endosc 2006;63:681–5.

30. Hu B, Chung SC, Sun LC, Kawashima K, Yamamoto T, Cotton PB, et al. Eagle Claw II: A novel endosuture device that uses a curved needle for major arterial bleeding: a bench study. Gastrointest Endosc 2005;62:266–70.

31. Pham BV, Raju GS, Ahmed I, Brining D, Chung S, Cotton P, et al. Immediate endoscopic closure of colon perforation by using a prototype endoscopic suturing device: feasibility and outcome in a porcine model (with video). Gastrointest Endosc 2006;64:113–9.

32. Swanstrom LL, Whiteford M, Khajanchee Y. Developing essential tools to enable transgastric surgery. Surg Endosc 2008;22:600–4.

33. Swanstrom LL, Kozarek R, Pasricha PJ, Gross S, Birkett D, Park PO, et al. Development of a new access device for transgastric surgery. J Gastro-intest Surg 2005;9:1129–36.

31

32 Photodynamic Therapy

Rami J. Badreddine and Kenneth K. Wang

Introduction

The most important clinical feature of photodynamic therapy (PDT) is its ease of clinical application. It requires the least degree of endoscopic skill to apply effectively in the gastrointestinal tract, since the endoscopist's primary role is to produce mucosal destruction. The second great strength of this form of treatment is that it is possible to perform PDT almost anywhere within the hollow viscera.

The earliest forms of photodynamic therapy probably date back to the ancient Egyptians, who found that pitch (tar) could be applied to psoriatic skin lesions, but that sunlight was needed to truly heal the lesions. Modern PDT was carried out experimentally in a wide variety of tumors during the 1960s, with only modest success in advanced tumors. However, clinical PDT was first found to truly benefit patients with early endobronchial lung cancer in the early 1980s [1]. Since these early successes, PDT has become more widely used in the gastrointestinal tract and has been standardized for treatment of patients with esophageal cancer, Barrett's esophagus, and cholangiocarcinoma. In comparison with pulmonary therapy, PDT in the gastrointestinal tract has the advantage that it does not requiring a "clean-up" procedure after treatment, as the debris is usually excreted or absorbed by the gastrointestinal tract.

PDT has moved from being a palliative procedure to become a curative method of treating superficial cancers. Specialized instruments have been developed that allow treatment of different types of gastrointestinal lesion. Newer flexible fibers are being developed to allow easier passage through endoscopes.

Principles of PDT

PDT uses the principle of the photochemical interaction of light with a photosensitizing drug, leading to tumor necrosis [2]. Three elements are thus required for PDT: oxygen, light, and a photosensitizing drug. The photosensitizer agent absorbs energy from light and transfers it to oxygen, creating singlet oxygen that produces tissue damage (**Figs. 32.1, 32.2**). The energy transfer allows the energized photosensitizer to diffuse into the tissue much further than singlet oxygen, which only has a half-life of nanoseconds to milliseconds in tissue. The degree of tissue damage depends on the wavelength and amount of the exciting light, the type and concentration of the photosensitizer, and the oxygen concentration in the tissue [3]. The advantage of this system is that all of these parameters can be manipulated to control the delivery of treatment. Real-time monitoring of therapeutic efficacy is possible by measuring the photosensitizer concentration, which decreases with treatment as a result of photobleaching or destruction of the photosensitizer due to photoradiation.

Photosensitizers

Several photosensitizing drugs can be modified to produce photosensitizers that are tissue-specific [4]. The only photosensitizers available in the United States are porfimer sodium (Photofrin II; Axcan Pharma, Montreal, Quebec, Canada) and aminolevulinic acid

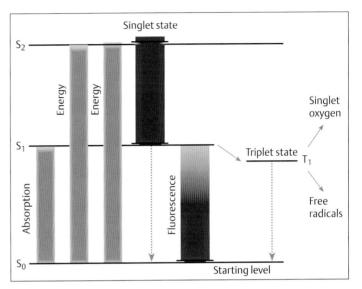

Fig. 32.1 Processes involved in activation by laser light.

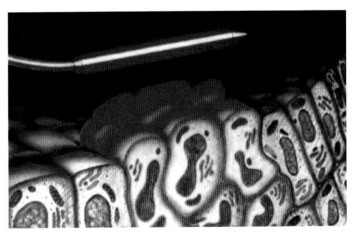

Fig. 32.2 The mechanism of photodynamic action.

(ALA, Levulan; DUSA Pharmaceuticals, Wilmington, Massachusetts). Porfimer sodium has Food and Drug Administration (FDA) approval, whereas ALA has only been approved by the FDA as a topical formulation.

Porfimer sodium (Photofrin) is a derivative of porphyrin consisting of trimers and tetramers of porphyrin rings. These rings are bound through an acetylation reaction and have a central space created by four pyrrole rings and a nitrogen atom. The nitrogen atom faces inward and coordinates metals to form nearly planar 1 : 1 ligand–metal complexes. It is thought that when these compounds are administered, they migrate preferentially to areas with leaky vasculature such as those found around tumors. Once there, they can infiltrate into the interstitial space and bind to tumor tissues. This is considered to be the basis for the selectivity of the drug for

Table 32. 1 Porfimer sodium versus aminolevulinic acid (ALA)

Aminolevulinic acid	Porfimer sodium
Oral route	Intravenous route
FDA orphan drug	FDA-approved
Photosensitivity risk for 1–2 weeks	Photosensitivity risk for up to 8 weeks
Depth of penetration < 2 mm	Penetration > 2 mm

FDA, Food and Drug Administration.

neoplastic lesions. This selectivity is at most two to three times greater in tumor tissue than in normal tissues. Sodium porfimer is given intravenously at a dose of 2 mg/kg, typically 48 h before photoradiation treatment.

The kinetics of the drug are complex. It can remain bound to tissues for over a month after administration, particularly in cutaneous tissue, which is the reason for the prolonged photosensitivity observed after administration. The drug is actually best activated in the blue–green light region, but this is not used as an activating light wavelength because of the decreased depth of penetration with light at this wavelength. Red light (630 nm) is used, although its absorption by porfimer sodium is at least 10 times lower due to the increased depth of penetration. In clinical practice, the absorption problem is overcome by administering very large doses of light.

Side effects of porfimer sodium administration are rare except in cases of allergy. Cutaneous sensitivity persists for 30–90 days. Photobleaching of the drug is needed in order to eliminate the drug from the skin completely, so that careful exposure to sunlight is needed. Complete protection from sunlight (in areas of skin protected by clothing) followed by large amounts of sunlight exposure, as may occur during vacations in tropical countries, can lead to skin reactions many months after administration of the drug. Cutaneous reactions can be treated with antihistamines, as the initial cutaneous reaction is histamine-mediated.

The other agent available for PDT in the United States is 5-ALA. This is a prodrug that has to be converted to the active photosensitizer, protoporphyrin IX, in cellular mitochondria [5]. It is used in dermatology as a topical treatment for actinic keratosis, as it produces less scar formation than other treatments. For gastrointestinal applications, it is usually administered orally. **Table 32.1** summarizes the main differences between porfimer sodium and ALA. ALA is selective for the mucosa and produces much less deep injury than porfimer sodium. ALA is a less efficient photosensitizer than porfimer sodium, so that much larger dosages of light are needed. Protoporphyrin IX has a similar absorption peak to that of porfimer sodium, at 605 nm. ALA has several side effects, including elevated values in liver function tests and even jaundice when it is administered in large dosages. Nausea is not uncommon after ingestion and split dosages are often used, as they are better tolerated.

PDT Light Sources for Gastrointestinal Applications

To enhance the delivery of light to large surface areas through fiberoptics, laser-based light is typically used in gastroenterology. Both the optical properties of the tissue and the light wavelength dictate the depth of penetration of the light used. Longer wavelengths of visible light, for example, have a deeper tissue penetration than light with shorter wavelengths. There is a large rise in penetration that occurs between 600 and 680 nm, which plateaus between 700 and 800 nm. For this reason, red light is the preferred form for PDT.

Many laser sources have been used in PDT. These include dye lasers (Coherent Lambda Plus, Santa Clara, California, USA; or Laserscope Model 630, San Jose, California, USA), which use one source of laser energy (an argon gas laser) to produce red light from a dye (Kiton red). These dyes deteriorate over time and have to be exchanged in order to maintain power output. These laser systems also have very large power requirements. More recent laser sources that have been used include a solid-state diode laser (Diomed 630PDT; Cambridge, United Kingdom), which can operate with standard power outlets and can be air-cooled. This diode system can supply a power of 2 W using a wavelength of 630 nm. The latter wavelength is thus chosen when PDT is performed, as it can activate porphyrin compounds.

It is worth noting that the rate at which light is delivered is also important, since higher rates produce thermal effects, causing coagulation and reducing the light penetration. In addition, high light fluence rates can produce increased photobleaching and eliminate the photosensitizer without producing singlet oxygen. To avoid this, light is typically delivered at a rate lower than 150 mW/cm^2. The thermal effect is thought to increase tissue injury and is used by some investigators in addition to the photodynamic effect for a more beneficial outcome [6].

Light Dosimetry and Application Systems

It is essential to apply treatment homogeneously when performing PDT. For this to happen, serious consideration must be given to optical properties and the location and size of a tumor so that necrosis occurs in all regions of the lesion. Analytical light dosimetry modeling helps estimate the ideal light dosage required for PDT to be successful.

Fluence is the amount of light delivered to a tumor and is measured in joules per square centimeter (J/cm^2). The fluence used depends on the type and concentration of the PDT agent, the light wavelength used, and the intrinsic photosensitivity of the tumor. When porfimer sodium is used, a dose of 2 mg/kg is given intravenously 48 h before PDT. Photoradiation is then performed using light at a wavelength of 630 nm. There are three methods of applying photoradiation in the gastrointestinal tract: cylindrical surface (CS), cylindrical insertion (CI), and front surface (FS).

CS is a line source centered within a cylindrical lumen, whereas CI is a line source embedded in the tumor tissue. CI is typically used for bulky tumors with protruding nodules [7]. When the tumor is small and discrete, FS is used, consisting of a uniform irradiance incident beam. FS is typically used in pulmonary applications. Most photoradiation in the gastrointestinal tract uses a cylindrical surface light source (CS) (**Fig. 32.3**). To deliver the light homogenously, different balloon applicators have been developed for use in the esophagus [8,9] (**Fig. 32.4**). However, these balloon applicators are no longer commercially available at present, as they have not been found to enhance therapy clinically. Formulas are used to calculate the depth of tissue necrosis and treatment time. The treatment time (in seconds) could be computed, for example, by dividing the desired energy density (fluence) in J/cm^2 by the measured power density (irradiance) in W/cm^2. Most clinical trials on PDT with light at a 630-nm wavelength have produced tumor necrosis to a depth of 5 mm, and rarely as deep as 10 mm.

Clinical Applications and Complications of PDT in the Gastrointestinal Tract

PDT has been used in the treatment of malignant and premalignant lesions throughout the gastrointestinal tract—esophageal cancer and Barrett's esophagus, gastric cancer, cholangiocarcinoma, pancreatic cancer, and colon cancer. Although the treatment of each of these cancers is associated with specific complications, which will be discussed below, cutaneous phototoxicity from the photosensitizer is a possible complication whenever PDT is performed.

Photosensitivity

Cutaneous phototoxicity includes edema, pruritus, blistering, large-scale erythema, bullae, and urticarial lesions. Photofrin can produce cutaneous phototoxicity within hours after intravenous administration of the drug. This occurred in 19% of patients treated by PDT for esophageal carcinoma in a multicenter study using Photofrin [10]. The risk of developing these complications is significantly reduced if light exposure precautions are undertaken. It is essential to warn patients that because of the half-life of the medication, photosensitivity may persist for 4–8 weeks. If the patient is suddenly exposed to large amounts of light, as may occur on vacations in tropical countries, the duration of photosensitivity may be even more prolonged. Strict light-protective measures are usually discussed with patients. These include wearing appropriate clothing that does not allow light to pass. It is essential to cover all the skin, including the scalp, back of the neck, face, nose, ears, and hands. The patient needs to understand that sunscreen use blocks ultraviolet light, while the drug is actually activated by visible light, which is not affected by sunscreen. Patients can be recommended to wear wide-brimmed hats to provide additional protection. Preparation of the home and working environment is also crucial to provide protection against possible phototoxicity. This includes draping windows that cannot be avoided, using light-proof coverings. Televisions, computer monitors, and regular house lighting are not dangerous. Patients will need a companion who can drive them during sunlight hours. We ask our patients to observe full protection for 4 weeks, after which they can gradually reexpose a limited area of skin to sunlight. If they can do this without cutaneous phototoxicity, sun exposure is gradually increased. If phototoxicity develops, on the other hand, then we ask them to delay any further sun exposure until they are able to successfully expose a small portion of the skin to sunlight.

Treatment of cutaneous photosensitivity is usually conservative. This includes elimination of further sun exposure, diphenhydramine and acetaminophen orally, and appropriate dressings. Topical or oral antibiotics are rarely needed. The endoscopist needs to discuss potential phototoxicity and the appropriate management with the patient in detail. Extreme caution must also be taken during intravenous administration of the drug, as extravasation can result in long-term photosensitivity in the affected area.

PDT in the Esophagus

Esophageal adenocarcinoma is the most common type of esophageal cancer seen in the United States and western Europe. Barrett's esophagus is a well-known risk factor for esophageal adenocarcinoma and is believed to be found in 6–12% of patients undergoing endoscopy for gastroesophageal reflux disease (GERD) and in 1% of all patients undergoing endoscopy. Traditionally, treatment for high-grade dysplasia (HGD) and cancer in patients with Barrett's

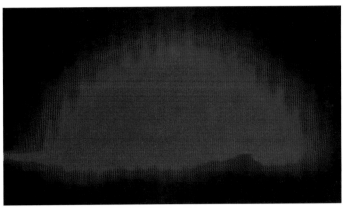

Fig. 32.3 A cylindrical diffuser applicator for perpendicular irradiation in the gastrointestinal tract (Rare Earth Medical, Inc., West Yarmouth, Massachusetts, USA).

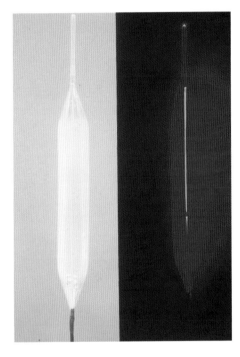

Fig. 32.4 A centering balloon applicator, which can be positioned through the endoscope under direct vision for surface illumination (TTC PDT Balloon, Wilson-Cook, Germany).

esophagus has been surgical. However, more recent ablative treatments, including PDT, have proved to be very effective.

A cylindrical-tipped fiber is most commonly used in PDT for Barrett's esophagus. It is essential to choose the length of the diffuser tip to match the length of the lesion being treated. Although the tissue effects of PDT in the esophagus are delayed, visible evidence of mucosal damage usually develops several hours after photoradiation. The treatment parameters for HGD in Barrett's esophagus using porfimer sodium include: red light (630 nm) at a power of 400 mW/cm fiber for a total energy of 200 J/cm fiber. If ALA is used, a wavelength of 635 nm is required, as ALA is activated at this wavelength. Preliminary data, mostly based on case series, supported the use of PDT in the treatment of HGD and early-stage intramucosal carcinoma in patients with Barrett's esophagus (**Figs. 32.5–32.10**). More recently, larger trials have confirmed this [11–14]. On the basis of the current data, PDT can eliminate HGD in 88–100% of cases (**Figs. 32.11–32.13**). There are also strong data showing that the rate of carcinoma declines after ablation of HGD in Barrett's esophagus using PDT [15]. Recently, Overholt et al. reviewed the 5-year efficacy and safety rates with Photofrin PDT in the treatment of Barrett's esophagus with HGD [16]. In this multi-

32

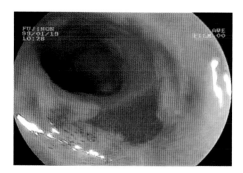

Fig. 32.5 Macroscopically unclear high-grade dysplasia in Barrett's esophagus.

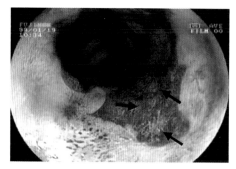

Fig. 32.6 Multifocal high-grade dysplasia in Barrett's esophagus after vital staining with methylene blue. Arrows: unstained areas or areas with heterogeneous staining, with biopsy-confirmed high-grade dysplasia.

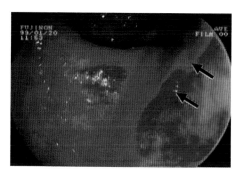

Fig. 32.7 Barrett's esophagus with early mucosal cancer type IIa (arrows).

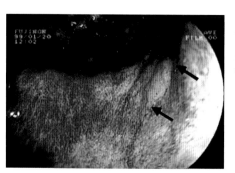

Fig. 32.8 Barrett's esophagus with early mucosal cancer type IIa (arrows) after methylene blue staining.

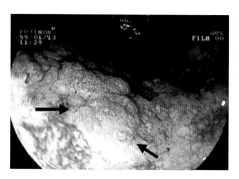

Fig. 32.9 Identification of a type IIa early Barrett's cancer (arrows) after indigo carmine application.

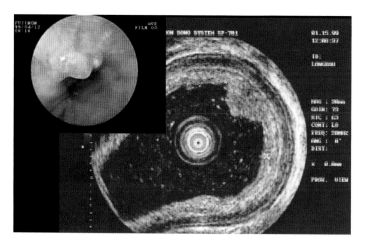

Fig. 32.10 Early Barrett's cancer type I, strictly confined to the mucosa, as demonstrated by high-resolution endoscopic ultrasound (20 MHz).

center, prospective randomized study, patients with Barrett's esophagus and HGD were either treated with omeprazole alone or PDT and omeprazole. The main outcome measure was the rate of HGD ablation after 5 years, with a secondary outcome of rates of cancer progression in both groups. After 5 years, PDT plus omeprazole was significantly more effective than omeprazole alone in eliminating HGD (77% vs. 39%; $P < 0.0001$). Progression to cancer was also significantly lower in the PDT group (15% vs. 29%; $P = 0.027$). **Table 32.2** summarizes landmark studies on PDT in Barrett's esophagus [17–19].

PDT complications specific to the esophagus include: chest pain and odynophagia, nausea, vomiting, and esophageal strictures leading to dysphagia. Problems with odynophagia and nausea are usually transient. We advise all patients on the importance of maintaining food and hydration and provide them with antiemetic suppositories and narcotic patches for symptomatic control. We ask patients to avoid all nonsteroidal anti-inflammatory drugs for at least 2 weeks; acetaminophen is allowed for pain control.

A more troublesome complication is stricture formation. Esophageal strictures typically develop within 2–3 weeks of PDT and present with the development of progressive dysphagia for solid food. This occurs in 27–34% of treated patients [20,21]. Strictures occur despite the use of centering balloons, and they are not prevented by pretreatment with systemic steroids [22]. Prasad et al. at the Mayo Clinic investigated predictive factors for stricture formation after PDT for HGD [23]. Twenty-seven percent of 131 patients developed strictures. Risk factors for the development of strictures after PDT included a history of esophageal stricture, performance of endoscopic mucosal resection (EMR) before PDT, and more than one PDT application in one treatment session. The use of centering balloons was not associated with a statistically significant reduction in the risk of stricture formation [23]. Recurrent dilations are needed in a few patients with recurrent strictures. It is important to continue surveillance for dysplasia in patients with Barrett's esophagus after PDT, since although the risk is small, there have been reports of buried or hidden Barrett's mucosa underlying neosquamous epithelium (**Figs. 32.14–32.16**).

V

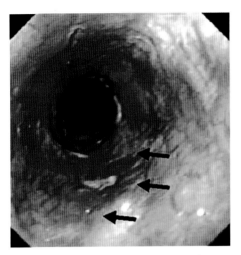

Fig. 32.11 High-grade dysplasia (arrows) in a long-segment Barrett's esophagus before photodynamic therapy.

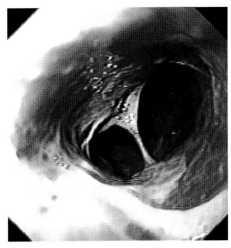

Fig. 32.12 Fibrinoid necrosis 24 h after photodynamic therapy with 5-aminolevulinic acid.

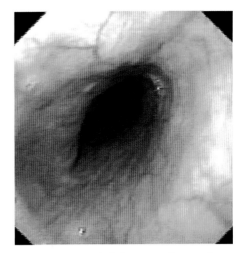

Fig. 32.13 Reepithelialization with normal squamous mucosa after 1 year of acid-suppressant treatment with proton-pump inhibitors. Biopsy confirmed there was no dysplasia.

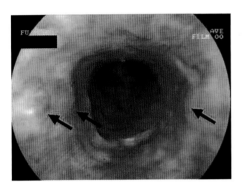

Fig. 32.14 Multifocal early squamous-cell cancer (arrows) in the upper third of the esophagus.

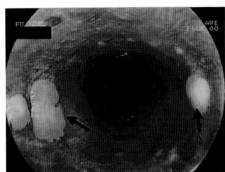

Fig. 32.15 Multifocal early squamous-cell cancer (arrows) after staining with Lugol's solution.

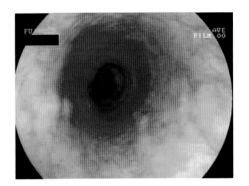

Fig. 32.16 Complete remission after photodynamic therapy with 5-aminolevulinic acid: the esophagus is macroscopically and microscopically tumor-free 18 months after the treatment.

Table 32.2 Landmark trials of photodynamic therapy in patients with Barrett's esophagus

First author	Year	Patients (n)	Drug	Adjuvant therapy	HGD elimination (%)	Follow-up (months)
Barr [17]	1996	5	ALA	No	100	44
Gossner [9]	1999	10	ALA	No	100	5.4
Overholt [11]	1999	73	Photofrin	Yes	88	19
Wang [18]	1999	26	HpD	No	88	24
Krishnadath [14]	2000	56	Photofrin	No	100	46
Panjehpour [22]	2000	43	Photofrin	Yes	96	12
Schnell [13]	2001	208	Photofrin	No	80	6
Javaid [12]	2002	4	Temoporfin	No	100	27
Overholt [16]	2007	208	Photofrin	Yes	77	60

ALA: aminolevulinic acid; HGD, high-grade dysplasia; HpD: hematoporphyrin derivative.

PDT in the Stomach

Gastric cancer is still one of the most common cancers throughout the world, with an incidence of 870 000 cases and 650 000 deaths per year [24]. Approximately 50% of patients have advanced incurable disease at presentation, and most of those who undergo resection will have recurrences.

PDT for gastric carcinoma is not as widely used in the United States as it is in Japan [25]. The most effective form of treatment has been resection. Patients who are not candidates for surgery may benefit from PDT as a palliative treatment [26]. PDT can control hemorrhage and relieve obstruction in these patients. More recent trials have found that PDT is also beneficial for early gastric cancer (**Figs. 32.17, 32.18**). It appears to be superior to other modalities, including thermal laser, particularly when the depth of invasion is not beyond the submucosa and when the margins of the lesions are unclear [27,28]. There have been no large trials of PDT in gastric cancer, and the response rates in the different series using PDT for this indication have ranged from 55% to 100%, with minor complications including phototoxicity and local pain.

32

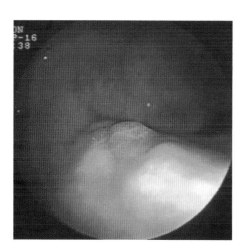

Fig. 32.17 Early gastric cancer, type II a + c.

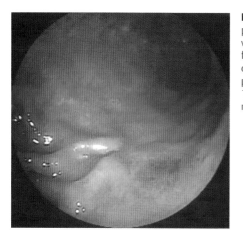

Fig. 32.18 A scar after photodynamic therapy with temoporfin at the former tumor site. Biopsy confirmed that the patient was tumor-free 12 months after treatment.

PDT in the Colon

In the United States, colorectal cancer ranks second to lung cancer as a cause of cancer deaths. Approximately 150 000 new cases are diagnosed each year, 107 000 of which are colon and the remainder rectal cancers [29]. Approximately 35% of patients with this type of cancer are not candidates for aggressive surgical therapy due to distant metastases, local invasion, poor functional status, or because they decline surgery.

Few studies have been performed describing the use of PDT in colorectal cancer. Barr et al. reported a study including 10 patients with colorectal carcinoma treated with PDT [30]. Hematoporphyrin derivative was used as the photosensitizer drug. Light doses of 50 J/cm^2 were used, with a diffusing fiber placed in the tumor. The response was relatively poor in patients who had bulky tumors. This and other studies have shown that PDT appears to be most effective in smaller colorectal tumors or smaller areas that need to be sterilized after surgery, making PDT a possible adjuvant treatment. This was described in a randomized trial using porfimer sodium PDT after surgical resection for rectosigmoid tumors [31]. The results did not show any improvement in the rate of local recurrence or survival, and further research in this area is therefore required. Complications reported in various trials included bleeding and photosensitization leading to sunburn.

PDT in the Pancreas

Pancreatic cancer is the second most frequent cause of gastrointestinal-related death after colorectal cancer. Because of the late presentation, only 15–20% of the patients are deemed resectable at the time of diagnosis. Even after surgery, the median survival is 12–18 months and the 5-year survival rate is less than 20% [32,33]. PDT was first used to treat pancreatic cancer in the early 1980s [34]. It is an attractive treatment option for pancreatic cancer, as the photosensitizer has poor uptake in normal pancreatic cells, allowing some selectivity. In 2002, Bown et al. reported their experience in treating 16 patients with inoperable, biopsy or cytology proven pancreatic adenocarcinoma [35]. Ampullary cancers and possible cholangiocarcinomas were excluded. They used temoporfin (mTHPC) as a photosensitizer. This drug has a much greater depth of penetration than porfimer sodium and is a more efficient photosensitizer. The approach taken was transcutaneous transabdominal PDT via needles placed under computed-tomographic or ultrasound guidance deep in the tumor. PDT fibers were then passed through the needles and PDT was applied using laser light at 652 nm. There were no treatment-related mortalities, and the median survival time after PDT was 9.5 months. Seven of 16 patients (44%) were alive 1 year after treatment. Complications included bleeding (in two patients) and duodenal obstruction (in three patients). These results are promising, but more data and randomized trials are needed before PDT can be regarded as a potential treatment for pancreatic cancer.

PDT in the Biliary Tree

Cholangiocarcinoma accounts for 3% of gastrointestinal malignancies, with a prevalence of 0.01–0.046% in autopsy studies [36]. This tumor has a very poor prognosis, with an average 5-year survival rate of less than 10%. Surgery is the only curative option, but even then few patients have tumor-free resection margins.

Photodynamic therapy is becoming more widely used in the treatment of unresectable cholangiocarcinoma. Earlier uncontrolled trials showed a palliation benefit and an extended survival period in patients with advanced bile duct cancer who were treated with PDT [37]. These and other results prompted randomized controlled trials, which showed a survival benefit in these patients in comparison with stenting alone [38,39]. Reported side effects include cholangitis, cholecystitis, photosensitivity, and biloma.

Patients receive intravenous antibiotics before the procedure. Endoscopic retrograde cholangiography (ERCP) is performed to define the proximal and distal extent of the intraductal tumor. The tumor length is determined by using the endoscope diameter as a reference. The cylindrical diffusing fiber used for PDT in esophageal carcinoma (Fibers Direct, Andover, Massachusetts, USA) is usually 1.0–2.5 cm long. The fiber is preloaded into a double-lumen catheter (Howell Introducer-1; Cook Endoscopy, Winston-Salem, North Carolina, USA). This is done to protect the photoradiation fiber, which is stiff and subject to fracture. The tip of the catheter contains a metal marker. The tip of the catheter is cut just below the marker to allow the fiber to pass. The preloaded catheter is passed over a 0.035-inch guide wire positioned in the biliary tree. Use of the elevator should be avoided in order prevent fiber fracture. Angled 0.035-inch Terumo guide wires (Angled Glidewire; Boston Scientific, Natick, Massachusetts, USA) are used to access the right and left hepatic ducts as needed. For passage of the PDT catheter, the wires are exchanged for a standard long ERCP guide wire (X-Wire; ConMed, Utica, New York, USA).

Photoradiation is carried out using a laser (Lambda Plus, Coherent, Palo Alto, California, USA, or Diomed, Diomed, Inc., Andover, Massachusetts, USA) that produces 630-nm light with a power output of 180 J/cm^2 of light fluence at the mucosal surface. Tumor segments are treated sequentially in a proximal-to-distal fashion. After PDT is performed, either 10-Fr or 11.5-Fr plastic biliary stents are inserted to ensure adequate decompression and bile drainage. All ducts that are accessed and injected are drained, unless there is associated parenchymal atrophy. Patients usually receive prophylactic oral antibiotics for 1 week after the procedure.

■ Contraindications to PDT

There are relatively few contraindications to PDT. Apart from the usual contraindications for anesthesia or endoscopy, the following are worth mentioning:

- Any known previous allergic reaction or hypersensitivity to porphyrins
- Known porphyria
- Impaired renal function
- Impaired liver function
- Low blood counts (whole blood cell count < 2.5 × 10^9/L, platelets < 50 × 10^9/L, INR > 1.5 times upper limit of normal)

Conclusion

PDT is emerging as an effective treatment for many types of gastrointestinal cancer. Ablation of premalignant conditions such as dysplasia in Barrett's esophagus using PDT has been extensively studied, with very good long-term results, and further research will undoubtedly lead to the method being used to treat other types of gastrointestinal cancer in the future as well. The main side effects of PDT are photosensitivity and stricture formation, which make it unattractive to some practitioners. However, the development of newer photosensitizers and newer flexible fibers may overcome these limitations. With the advent of newer imaging techniques, the more flexible fibers will be able to reach previously inaccessible regions in the gastrointestinal tract. As the technical difficulties and cost of PDT decrease, the indications for the procedure will certainly expand. In the future, PDT may be incorporated into treatment protocols for gastrointestinal cancer as an adjuvant or neoadjuvant treatment.

References

1. Hayata Y, Kato H, Konaka C, Ono J, Takizawa N. Hematoporphyrin derivative and laser photoradiation in the treatment of lung cancer. Chest 1982;81:269–77.
2. Dougherty TJ, Gomer CJ, Henderson BW, Jori G, Kessel D, Korbelik M, et al. Photodynamic therapy. J Natl Cancer Inst 1998;90:889–905.
3. Boyle RW, Dolphin D. Structure and biodistribution relationships of photodynamic sensitizers. Photochem Photobiol 1996;64:469–85.
4. Kessel D, Poretz RD. Sites of photodamage induced by photodynamic therapy with a chlorin e6 triacetoxymethyl ester (CAME). Photochem Photobiol 2000;71:94–6.
5. Ackroyd R, Brown N, Vernon D, Roberts D, Stephenson T, Marcus S, et al. 5-Aminolevulinic acid photosensitization of dysplastic Barrett's esophagus: a pharmacokinetic study. Photochem Photobiol 1999;70:656–62.
6. Moore JV, West CM, Whitehurst C. The biology of photodynamic therapy. Phys Med Biol 1997;42:913–35.
7. Beyer W. Systems for light application and dosimetry in photodynamic therapy. J Photochem Photobiol B 1996;36:153–6.
8. Overholt BF, DeNovo RC, Panjehpour M, Petersen MG. A centering balloon for photodynamic therapy of esophageal cancer tested in a canine model. Gastrointest Endosc 1993;39:782–7.
9. Gossner L, May A, Sroka R, Ell C. A new long-range through-the-scope balloon applicator for photodynamic therapy in the esophagus and cardia. Endoscopy 1999;31:370–6.
10. Lightdale CJ, Heier SK, Marcon NE, McCaughan JS Jr, Gerdes H, Overholt BF, et al. Photodynamic therapy with porfimer sodium versus thermal ablation therapy with Nd:YAG laser for palliation of esophageal cancer: a multicenter randomized trial. Gastrointest Endosc 1995;42:507–12.
11. Overholt BF, Panjehpour M, Haydek JM. Photodynamic therapy for Barrett's esophagus: follow-up in 100 patients. Gastrointest Endosc 1999;49: 1–7.
12. Javaid B, Watt P, Krasner N. Photodynamic therapy (PDT) for oesophageal dysplasia and early carcinoma with mTHPC (m-tetrahydroxyphenyl chlorin): a preliminary study. Lasers Med Sci 2002;17:51–6.
13. Schnell TG, Sontag SJ, Chejfec G, Aranha G, Metz A, O'Connell S, et al. Long-term nonsurgical management of Barrett's esophagus with high-grade dysplasia. Gastroenterology 2001;120:1607–19.
14. Krishnadath KK, Wang KK, Taniguchi K, Sebo TJ, Buttar NS, Anderson MA, et al. Persistent genetic abnormalities in Barrett's esophagus after photodynamic therapy. Gastroenterology 2000;119:624–30.
15. Overholt BF, Lightdale CJ, Wang KK, Canto MI, Burdick S, Haggitt RC, et al. Photodynamic therapy with porfimer sodium for ablation of high-grade dysplasia in Barrett's esophagus: international, partially blinded, randomized phase III trial. Gastrointest Endosc 2005;62:488–98.
16. Overholt BF, Wang KK, Burdick JS, Lightdale CJ, Kimmey M, Nava HR, et al. Five-year efficacy and safety of photodynamic therapy with Photofrin in Barrett's high-grade dysplasia. Gastrointest Endosc 2007;66:460–8.
17. Barr H, Shepherd NA, Dix A, Roberts DJ, Tan WC, Krasner N. Eradication of high-grade dysplasia in columnar-lined (Barrett's) oesophagus by photodynamic therapy with endogenously generated protoporphyrin IX. Lancet 1996;348:584–5.
18. Wang KK. Current status of photodynamic therapy of Barrett's esophagus. Gastrointest Endosc 1999;49(3 Pt 2):S20–3.
19. Wang KK, Nijhawan PK. Complications of photodynamic therapy in gastrointestinal disease. Gastrointest Endosc Clin N Am 2000;10:487–95.
20. Wang KK, Kim JY. Photodynamic therapy in Barrett's esophagus. Gastrointest Endosc Clin N Am 2003;13:483–9, vii.
21. Wolfsen HC, Hemminger LL, Wallace MB, Devault KR. Clinical experience of patients undergoing photodynamic therapy for Barrett's dysplasia or cancer. Aliment Pharmacol Ther 2004;20:1125–31.
22. Panjehpour M, Overholt BF, Haydek JM, Lee SG. Results of photodynamic therapy for ablation of dysplasia and early cancer in Barrett's esophagus and effect of oral steroids on stricture formation. Am J Gastroenterol 2000;95:2177–84.
23. Prasad GA, Wang KK, Buttar NS, Wongkeesong LM, Lutzke LS, Borkenhagen LS. Predictors of stricture formation after photodynamic therapy for high-grade dysplasia in Barrett's esophagus. Gastrointest Endosc 2007; 65:60–6.
24. Lau M, Le A, El-Serag HB. Noncardia gastric adenocarcinoma remains an important and deadly cancer in the United States: secular trends in incidence and survival. Am J Gastroenterol 2006;101:2485–92.
25. Tajiri H, Daikuzono N, Joffe SN, Oguro Y. Photoradiation therapy in early gastrointestinal cancer. Gastrointest Endosc 1987;33:88–90.
26. Spinelli P, Mancini A, Dal Fante M. Endoscopic treatment of gastrointestinal tumors: indications and results of laser photocoagulation and photodynamic therapy. Semin Surg Oncol 1995;11:307–18.
27. Nakamura H, Yanai H, Nishikawa J, Okamoto T, Hirano A, Higaki M, et al. Experience with photodynamic therapy (endoscopic laser therapy) for the treatment of early gastric cancer. Hepatogastroenterology 2001;48: 1599–603.
28. Mimura S, Ito Y, Nagayo T, Ichii M, Kato H, Sakai H, et al. Cooperative clinical trial of photodynamic therapy with photofrin II and excimer dye laser for early gastric cancer. Lasers Surg Med 1996;19:168–72.
29. Jemal A, Siegel R, Ward E, Murray T, Xu J, Smigal C, et al. Cancer statistics, 2006. CA Cancer J Clin 2006;56:106–30.
30. Barr H, Krasner N, Boulos PB, Chatlani P, Bown SG. Photodynamic therapy for colorectal cancer: a quantitative pilot study. Br J Surg 1990;77:93–6.
31. Allardice JT, Abulafi AM, Grahn MF, Williams NS. Adjuvant intraoperative photodynamic therapy for colorectal carcinoma: a clinical study. Surg Oncol 1994;3:1–10.
32. Yeo CJ, Cameron JL, Lillemoe KD, Sitzmann JV, Hruban RH, Goodman SN, et al. Pancreaticoduodenectomy for cancer of the head of the pancreas. 201 patients. Ann Surg 1995;221:721–3.
33. Nitecki SS, Sarr MG, Colby TV, van Heerden JA. Long-term survival after resection for ductal adenocarcinoma of the pancreas. Is it really improving? Ann Surg 1995;221:59–66.
34. Ayaru L, Bown SG, Pereira SP. Photodynamic therapy for pancreatic and biliary tract carcinoma. Int J Gastrointest Cancer 2005;35:1–13.
35. Bown SG, Rogowska AZ, Whitelaw DE, Lees WR, Lovat LB, Ripley P, et al. Photodynamic therapy for cancer of the pancreas. Gut 2002;50:549–57.

32

36. Vauthey JN, Blumgart LH. Recent advances in the management of cholangiocarcinomas. Semin Liver Dis 1994;14:109–14.
37. Berr F, Wiedmann M, Tannapfel A, Halm U, Kohlhaw KR, Schmidt F, et al. Photodynamic therapy for advanced bile duct cancer: evidence for improved palliation and extended survival. Hepatology 2000;31:291–8.
38. Ortner ME, Caca K, Berr F, Liebetruth J, Mansmann U, Huster D, et al. Successful photodynamic therapy for nonresectable cholangiocarcinoma: a randomized prospective study. Gastroenterology 2003;125:1355–63.
39. Zoepf T, Jakobs R, Arnold JC, Apel D, Riemann JF. Palliation of nonresectable bile duct cancer: improved survival after photodynamic therapy. Am J Gastroenterol 2005;100:2426–30.

V

33 Endoscopic Treatment for GERD

Byung Moo Yoo, George Triadafilopoulos, and Glen A. Lehman

Introduction

Gastroesophageal reflux disease (GERD) affects millions of people throughout the world, significantly impairing their quality of life and causing persistent and/or recurrent symptoms. The management of GERD has gained increasing attention during the past two decades due to the high prevalence of the disease in Western societies, a better understanding of its pathophysiology, the availability of powerful new antisecretory drug therapies, and the advent of minimally invasive surgery and various innovative incisionless endoscopic therapies [1]. Surgery has been proposed as an alternative, and good results have been reported in some surgical studies. However, recent studies have suggested that many patients require continued medical therapy after surgery [2]. Thus, minimally invasive endoscopic antireflux therapies—preferably those with the potential to correct the underlying cause of the disorder—would be quite appealing. The general reasons for considering endoscopic therapy for GERD are listed in **Table 33.1** [3].

From a pathophysiologic point of view, endoscopic therapies should prevent reflux in the following ways: 1, they should alter the compliance of the cardia and prevent lower esophageal sphincter (LES) shortening/relaxation; 2, they should increase the baseline LES tone; or 3, they should increase the intra-abdominal LES length [4]. Thus far, most endoscopic GERD therapy studies have been restricted to patients with typical GERD symptoms, abnormal GERD health-related quality of life (GERD-HRQL) scores, and patients who are not receiving proton-pump inhibitors (PPIs), are near-normal on therapy, and have an abnormal total reflux time with pH < 4. Patients with esophageal motor disorders, erosive esophagitis above Los Angeles grade II, including Barrett's esophagus, prior esophagogastric surgery, and those with fixed hiatal hernia (> 3 cm) have been excluded. Techniques for which clinical data have been published fall into four general categories: radiofrequency ablation, injection/implantation, plication devices, and miscellaneous others (**Table 33.2**).

Radiofrequency Ablation

The possibility of radiofrequency (RF) energy being used for GERD therapy was explored after successful treatment of snoring and sleep apnea by shrinking hypopharyngeal structures [4].

The Stretta device (Curon Medical, Inc., Sunnyvale, California, USA) consists of a flexible, handheld, disposable 20-Fr catheter and a distal balloon (max. 3 cm) with four externally attached 5.5-mm NiTi (nitinol) needle electrodes that deliver computer-regulated radiofrequency energy to the gastroesophageal junction zone at approximately 56 separate sites (**Fig. 33.1**). Inflation of the balloon deploys the four electrodes circumferentially in the esophageal wall to make deep, intramuscular thermal lesions (**Fig. 33.2**). The procedure time is about 40–60 min.

Stretta delivers thermal energy in a controlled manner with constant mucosal and muscular temperature monitoring and automated modulation of RF power output. With time, such thermal injury causes shrinkage and a cellular response in the submucosal tissue surrounding the puncture sites, decreasing the frequency of

Table 33.1 Reasons for considering endoscopic therapies for gastroesophageal reflux disease (GERD)

GERD refractory to medical therapy
• Persistent heartburn despite escalating proton-pump inhibitor (PPI) dose
• Residual regurgitation without heartburn while on PPI therapy
PPI intolerance ($\approx 2\%$ of users)
Desire to stop drug therapy (concern about long-term effects)
Concern about side effects of surgical fundoplication (e.g., dysphagia, gas bloating)
Symptomatic GERD after fundoplication

Table 33.2 Endoscopic therapy for gastroesophageal reflux disease

Radiofrequency energy
• Stretta device (Curon Medical, Sunnyvale, California, USA)
Injection/implantation
• Enteryx (Boston Scientific, Natick, Massachusetts, USA)
• Gatekeeper (Medtronic, Minneapolis, Minnesota, USA)
• Plexiglas (polymethylmethacrylate, PMMA)
Endoscopic plication devices
• EndoCinch (C.R. Bard, Inc., Murray Hill, New Jersey, USA)
• NDO Plicator (NDO Surgical, Mansfield, Massachusetts, USA)
• EsophyX (EndoGastric Solutions, Redmond, Washington, USA)
• Medigus SRS endoscopic stapling system (Medigus Ltd., Tel Aviv, Israel)
• Syntheon ARD plicator (Syntheon LLC, Miami, Florida, USA)
Others

transient LES relaxations (tLESRs) by 50% and leading to reduced acid reflux due to a less compliant gastroesophageal junction [5].

Table 33.3 lists selected series and results from published trials on the Stretta device [6–13]. In a multicenter open-label trial with a 12-month follow-up period, significant improvement in heartburn, GERD, and satisfaction scores was observed. PPIs were discontinued in 30% of the patients and reduced in 58%, while acid exposure as measured with pH monitoring improved significantly from 10.2% to 6.4% [6]. In a randomized sham-controlled study, daily heartburn symptoms and GERD-HRQL were found to be significantly improved at 6 and 12 months. However, there were no significant differences in daily medication use or in esophageal acid exposure at 6 months [9].

Most Stretta series have reported its efficacy for patients who respond to PPI treatment, although one study reported outcomes for patients in whom double-dose PPI therapy had failed, who almost certainly were truly refractory patients or had a hypersensitive esophagus [14]. In such series, PPIs could only be stopped in 6.25% of the patients, with the dose reduced in 56%.

In addition, most series have reported outcomes after a single treatment session. Ayman et al. have presented a preliminary report on a randomized controlled trial in which single-session Stretta was superior to a sham procedure, while two Stretta sessions were statistically superior to sham and single-session Stretta [12]. Un-

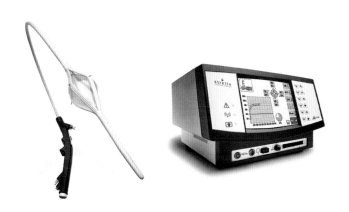
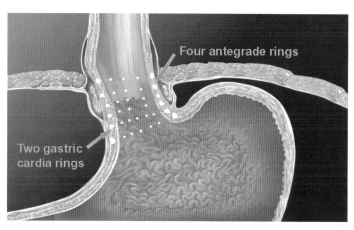

Fig. 33.1 a The Stretta catheter and control module (Curon Medical Inc., Sunnyvale, California, USA). **b** Distribution of cautery sites with the Stretta device in the distal esophagus and cardia.

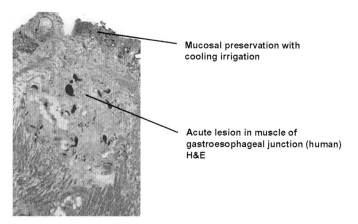

Fig. 33.2 Human gastroesophageal junction treated with Stretta just prior to esophagectomy. This hematoxylin–eosin stain of the cardia demonstrates a well-defined lesion in the muscle and a narrow needle tract through the mucosa. The mucosa is preserved via the delivery of chilled irrigation through the catheter during radiofrequency ablation.

fortunately, two cases of worsening gastroparesis were reported in the double Stretta group.

During the initial, learning curve phase with the Stretta procedure, serious complications such as aspiration pneumonia, esophageal perforation, and death occurred. Subsequently, the number of complications was reduced by the addition of a guide wire and a

reduction in the total number of ablations delivered per session. Nevertheless, despite its moderate overall efficacy and relative safety, worldwide sales and third-party reimbursement did not support continuous manufacturing, and the device is no longer commercially available.

Injection/Implantation

This technique is attractive because of its relative simplicity and similarity to other techniques familiar to endoscopists, such as variceal sclerosis. Historically, dermatologists and plastic surgeons have used a number of "filler" materials successfully. Years ago, bovine dermal collagen implants into the LES for the treatment of GERD had shown modest efficacy, but lacked durability [15]. Although Enteryx was the first nonbiodegradable agent to undergo large-series trials and marketing, other injection/implantation approaches have also been introduced in human trials.

Enteryx

Enteryx (Boston Scientific, Natick, Massachusetts, USA) consists of a biocompatible polymer—8 % weight by volume (w/v) ethylene-vinyl alcohol (EVOH) copolymer—with a radiopaque contrast agent (30 % w/v tantalum powder) dissolved in an organic liquid carrier (dimethyl sulfoxide, DMSO) [16]. As it is not biodegradable and has no

Table 33.3 Summary of selected publications on endoscopic treatment for gastrointestinal reflux disease (GERD) with Stretta

First author (ref.)	Study design			% off PPIs	Heartburn score	GERD-HRQL	Time pH <4 (%)		Follow-up (months)
	Type	Patients (n)	Follow-up (months)				Before	After	
Triadafilopoulos [6]	OL, MC	118	12	30	+ *	+ *	10.2	6.4*	6
Wolfsen [7]	OL, MC	558	8	51	+ *	NA	NA	NA	NA
Tam [8]	OL, SC	20	12	65	+ *	+ *	10.6	6.8*	6
Corley [9]	RCT, SC	35/29	6/6	45/39	+ §	+ §	9.5/9.5	9.9/10.7	6/6
Cipolletta [10]	OL, SC	32	12	56	+ *	+ *	11.7	8.4	18
Reymunde [11]	OL, SC	83	48	89 #	+ *	+ *	NA	NA	NA
Mavrelis [12]	OL, SC	32	30	66 #	NA	+ *	NA	NA	NA
Noar [13]	OL, SC	109	48	75 #	+ *	+ *	NA	NA	NA

*GERD-HRQL, Gastroesophageal Reflux Disease Health-Related Quality of Life (score); MC, multicenter; NA, not available; OL, open-labeled; RCT, randomized controlled trial, SC, single center. +, Improved; * significant difference (P < 0.05); § significant difference in comparison with sham treatment ; # including patients with reduced usage of medication.*

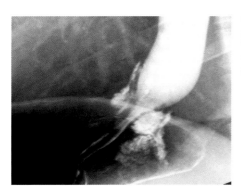

Fig. 33.3 A barium swallow after Enteryx injection. The intramural radiopaque material should be noted.

antigenic properties, Enteryx has been used to embolize arteriovenous malformations [17]. After contact with tissues or body fluids, the solvent, DMSO, rapidly diffuses, resulting in precipitation of the polymer (EVOH) to a spongy mass. Neither migration through vessels or lymphatics nor shrinkage after injection has been observed or reported. Enteryx is injected deep into the wall beneath the LES under fluoroscopic monitoring, forming a globular mass or a ring to augment LES pressure and decrease the frequency of tLESRs (**Fig. 33.3**). Although the exact mechanism of the Enteryx effect in humans remains to be fully characterized, fibrous encapsulation and scarring may functionally lengthen and narrow the LES.

Table 33.4 shows selected series and results from the Enteryx trials [18–20]. In a pilot study, LES pressure had increased in 86% of patients at 1 month, and the increase was sustained at a median follow-up of 6 months [16]. There was also a sustained reduction in heartburn scores at 1 month and at the final follow-up. Devière et al. published a randomized sham-controlled multicenter trial in which, after 3 months, 81% of the Enteryx-treated group had a ≥50% reduction in PPI use, in comparison with 53% of the sham group [18]. In this trial, a higher proportion of the Enteryx group (68%) than the sham group (41%) completely ceased PPI use. Improvement by >50% in GERD-HRQL heartburn scores was achieved in 67% of the Enteryx group, versus 22% of the sham group [18]. At 3 months after implantation of Enteryx, the mean estimated residual implant volume was 67%, while no residual implant could be detected in two patients.

Several thousand patients have been treated with Enteryx since it was approved for use in the United States in 2003. Common adverse events after Enteryx included retrosternal pain, transient dysphagia, and fever. Although infrequent, serious adverse events were also reported, including pericarditis, embolization to the kidney, and mediastinitis [21–24]. Due to such complications, the

manufacturer initiated a voluntary recall of Enteryx and the procedure is no longer available.

Gatekeeper Reflux Repair System

Gatekeeper (Medtronic, Minneapolis, Minnesota, USA) is a hydrated prosthesis that is implanted into the submucosa of the cardia/LES. It consists of a specially designed 16-mm overtube assembly, a prosthesis delivery system with a diameter of 2.4 mm (1-mm diameter needle, dilator, and 2.4-mm diameter sheath), a push-rod assembly, and 1 × 15 mm prostheses. With the overtube positioned at the LES level, hydrogel bioprostheses can be inserted into the submucosa of the distal esophagus. The prostheses are made from an inert polyacrylonitrile-based hydrogen (Hypan) that becomes hydrated by body water and expands to a cylinder-shaped soft, pliable cushion 6 × 15 mm in size. Following an initial positive pilot study, an international multicenter sham-controlled study was conducted, but unfortunately, after randomization of nearly 100 patients, the active treatment arm was not superior to sham and the study and further marketing were terminated [25,26]. Evaluation of this or similar devices with different size, shape, and number or sites of therapy would be of interest.

Plexiglas

Plexiglas (polymethylmethacrylate) is a gelatinous suspension of microspheres implanted at the LES. It was first used for dental prostheses. With improvements in manufacturing methods, it has been successfully used in plastic surgery for skin defects and wrinkles. As with other injected materials, the needle is inserted into the submucosal layer 1–2 cm above the Z-line, and the implant is injected. In a pilot study in humans, the mean symptom severity score and esophageal acid exposure were significantly improved. Complete discontinuation of medical treatment occurred in 70% of patients (seven of 10), and there were no serious complications [27]. The product has not yet been approved by the Food and Drug Administration (FDA) in the United States.

Endoscopic Plication Devices

In 1986, Swain and Mills designed an endoscopic sewing device that was used through the biopsy channel [28]. Many other endoscopic suturing or plication devices have followed, with all of which the

Table 33.4 Summary of selected publications on endoscopic treatment of gastroesophageal reflux disease with Enteryx

First author (ref.)	Study design			% off PPIs	Heartburn score	GERD-HRQL	Time pH <4 (%)		
	Type	Patients (n)	Follow-up (months)				Before	After	Follow-up (months)
Johnson [19]	OL, MC	85	12	88	+ *	+ *	11.3	8.0*	12
Cohen [20]	OL, MC	144	24	68	+ *	+ *	10.0	6.4*	12
Devière [18] (active/sham)	RCT, MC	32/32	3/3	68/41 §	NA	+/– § #	13.3/14.0	11.2/NA	6/NA ¶

GERD-HRQL, Gastroesophageal Reflux Disease Health-Related Quality of Life (score); NA, not available; OL, open-labeled; MC, multicenter; RCT, randomized controlled trial.
+ Improved; – did not improve; * significant difference (P < 0.05), § significant difference compared with sham; # GERD-HRQL and heartburn score; ¶ prolonged pH-metry was not consistently performed at the same follow-up visit.

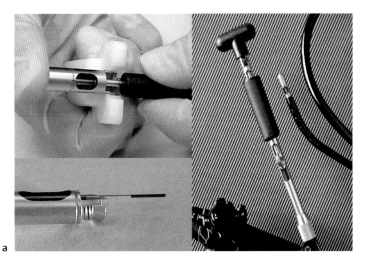

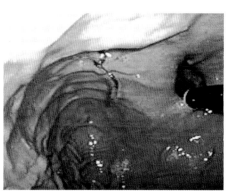

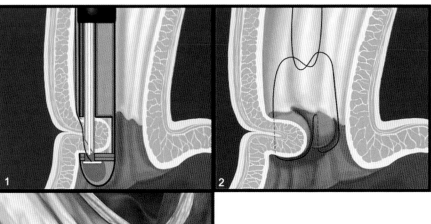

Fig. 33.4 a The EndoCinch device (C.R. Bard, Inc., Murray Hill, New Jersey, USA).
b The technique of endoscopic gastric plication with the EndoCinch. 1, suction of tissue just beneath the Z-line and needle with a preloaded suture advanced; 2, cinching/cutting catheter advanced to the tissue; 3, final appearance of the plication in the cardia.
c A failed EndoCinch procedure after 6 months. The patulous cardia and residual sutures remote from the cardia should be noted.

aim is to cinch the gastroesophageal junction and mechanically prevent backflow of gastric contents into the esophagus.

■ EndoCinch

EndoCinch (C.R. Bard, Inc., Murray Hill, New Jersey, USA) was the first suture placement device to be approved and marketed in the United States for the treatment of GERD (**Fig. 33.4 a**) [28]. The technique uses an endoscopic sewing device to create pleats through a series of sutures passed through adjoining folds at the cardia (**Fig. 33.4 b**). Although the exact working mechanism remains uncertain, this treatment is designed to "tighten" the cardia component of the LES and impose a barrier to acid reflux.

A substantial number of clinical trials on EndoCinch treatment have been published (**Table 33.5**) [29–36]. In a pivotal study, symptoms (heartburn severity and frequency, regurgitation) and 24-h intraesophageal pH monitoring scores were significantly improved at 6 months, irrespective of the plication configuration (linear or circumferential) [29]. In another prospective multicenter open-la-

bel trial, heartburn, regurgitation, and PPI use were significantly improved at 12 months [32]. In a randomized, sham-controlled trial, EndoCinch reduced acid-suppressive drug use and improved GERD symptoms and GERD-HRQL at 3 and 12 months in comparison with a sham procedure [35]. However, the reduction in esophageal acid exposure recorded on pH monitoring was no greater after Endo-Cinch than after a sham procedure [35].

Although the short-term results with EndoCinch have yielded promising results, more recent long-term results have been disappointing. In one study of 70 patients, treatment was considered to have failed in 80% after 18 months [34]. In the randomized sham-controlled trial, at 3 months, the percentage of patients who had reduced drug use by ≥50% was greater in the active treatment group than in the sham group. Although the active treatment effects on PPI use persisted after 6 and 12 months of open-label follow-up, 29% of patients received repeat treatment with PPIs in this period [35]. Overall, the performance of the EndoCinch procedure appears to be modest to poor in the intermediate to long-term follow-up results [32,34]. These results were likely related to the endoscopic observation that the intact plications were seen in only 10–17% of

Table 33.5 Summary of selected publications on endoscopic treatment of gastroesophageal reflux disease with EndoCinch

First author (ref.)	Study design			% off PPIs	Heartburn score	GERD-HRQL	Time pH < 4 (%)		
	Type	Patients (n)	Follow-up (months)				Before	After	Follow-up (months)
Filipi [29]	OL, MC	64	6	62	+ *	+ *	9.6	8.5*	6
Mahmood [30]	OL, SC	26	12	64	+ *	+ *	11.1	9.3*	3
Abou-Rebyeh [31]	OL, SC	38	12	20	NA	NA	15.4	8.7*	2
Chen [32]	OL, MC	85	24	41	+ *	NA	9.4	5.8*	3–6
Arts [33]	OL, SC	20	12	30	+ *	NA	17.0	8.1*	3
Schiefke [34]	OL, SC	70	18	6	+ *	NA	9.1	8.6	12
Schwartz [35] (active/ sham)	RCT, SC	20/20	3/3	40/5	+/– (§§)	+/– (§§)	9.5/9.6	6.8/7.7	3/3
Liao [36]	OL, SC	21	24	81/48 (1/24 mo)	+ *	+ *	8.4	4.6*	3

GERD-HRQL, Gastroesophageal Reflux Disease Health-Related Quality of Life (score); MC, multicenter; NA, not available; OL, open-labeled; RCT, randomized controlled trial; SC, single center. + Improved; – did not improve; * significant difference (P < 0.05), § significant difference in comparison with sham.

patients, while complete loss of plication sutures was noted in 6–74% of patients (**Fig. 33.4 c**) [31,34]. Such lack of durability is probably related to the superficial (mucosa or submucosal) location of the sutures, and it is anticipated that next-generation devices will suction a larger and deeper bite of tissue.

The EndoCinch procedure is usually well tolerated and relatively low-risk. Minor complications such as minimal bleeding and pharyngeal pain are common, but infrequent serious complications such as esophageal perforation and bleeding requiring transfusion have been reported [37]. In order to prevent perforation, all stitches and plications should be placed below the squamocolumnar junction. Plications on the lesser curvature of the cardia may be more likely to bleed.

NDO Plicator

The NDO Plicator (NDO Surgical, Mansfield, Massachusetts, USA) (**Fig. 33.5 a**) is an endoscopic full-thickness plication device designed to place a serosa-to-serosa pleat near the gastroesophageal junction under direct retroflexed endoscopic visualization [38]. The NDO Plicator, approved in the United States for the endoscopic treatment of GERD, differs from the EndoCinch device in that it creates a large transmural plication just distal to the gastroesophageal junction, using two grasping arms attached to an overtube device. The plicator was designed to apply a full-thickness pledget-reinforced U stitch near the gastroesophageal junction with serosa-to-serosa apposition, restoring the antireflux barrier (**Fig. 33.5 b**).

Table 33.6 lists selected series and results from NDO Plicator trials [38–42]. In a randomized, sham-controlled study, GERD-HRQL scores, complete cessation of PPI therapy, and esophageal acid exposure times were significantly improved in comparison with the sham group at 3 months [40]. A multicenter study further confirmed the efficacy and safety of the device; there were no perforations, while the treated patients had fewer GERD symptoms, less PPI use, and shorter esophageal acid exposure times at 6 months [38]. After a 5-year follow-up period in 33 of 64 evaluable patients, 67% remained off daily PPI therapy and GERD-HRQL scores continued to show significant improvement [42].

The NDO Plicator is relatively safe. There have been no deaths in the reported series, while common adverse events have included mild chest, epigastric, or abdominal pain, radiating shoulder pain, and postprocedural nausea and vomiting. In the sham-controlled study, radiating shoulder pain and abdominal pain were signifi-

cantly higher in the treated group than in the sham group [40]. Other infrequent events have included dyspnea, pneumothorax, and gastric perforation [38]. Rarely, intractable postplication pain has required the plication suture to be removed [40].

Despite its overall moderate short-term and long-term efficacy and relative safety, worldwide sales and third-party reimbursement did not support continuous manufacturing and marketing, and the device is no longer commercially available.

EsophyX

The EsophyX transoral incisionless fundoplication (TIF) procedure (EndoGastric Solutions, Inc., Redmond, Washington, USA) is based on the principle of surgical repair of the antireflux barrier, similar to laparoscopic fundoplication. The goal of TIF is to create an omega-shaped gastroesophageal valve (3–5 cm long) with 200–310° of circumferential wrap. This is accomplished using multiple T-fasteners that pleat the fundus to the esophageal wall, acting like an interrupted suture line and in turn restoring the angle of His, reducing the hiatal hernia, if present, and creating serosa-to-serosa fusions (**Fig. 33.6**). The procedure is performed by two operators, with the patient under general anesthesia, and takes 60–120 min.

Table 33.7 shows selected series and results from the EsophyX trials [43–45]. In an early study of 17 patients to assess the feasibility of EsophyX for the treatment of GERD, a transoral incisionless fundoplication was successfully completed in all cases without serious complications [44]. After 12 months, the GERD-HRQL scores were significantly improved in 67% of the patients, while 82% of patients were satisfied or very satisfied with the outcome of the procedure. PPI use was completely discontinued in 82% of the patients; 63% of the patients had normal esophageal acid exposure. In 81% of the patients, the newly created valve appeared endoscopically snug at 12 months, and hiatal hernia continued to be reduced in 62% of the patients [44]. In a prospective multicenter trial, the GERD-HRQL score improved significantly in 68% of the patients at 12 months. Cessation of daily PPI use was feasible in 85% of patients, while esophageal acid exposure time was significantly reduced or normalized in 61% of patients. The mean LES resting pressure was also increased significantly in 53% of patients. Endoscopy revealed that the mean length of the reconstructed valve was 2.5 cm and had a mean circumference of 180° (range 0–280° range). Most of the valves were Hill grade I or II. Sliding hiatal hernias, present in 36% of patients at 12 months, were reduced in size 60% of cases, and this was associated with reduced esophagitis in 57% of patients. Overall,

33

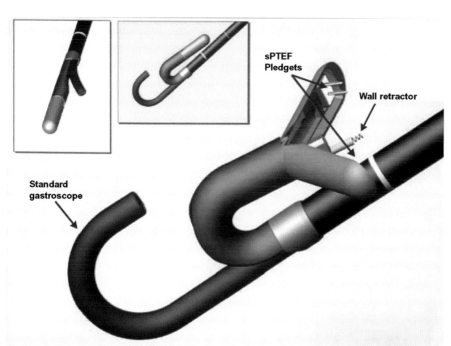

Fig. 33.5 a NDO Plicator (NDO surgical, Mansfield, Massachusetts, USA).
b The full-thickness plication technique with the NDO Plicator. 1, the plicator and gastroscope retroflexed to the gastroesophageal junction; 2, the arms are opened and the tissue retractor is advanced to the serosa; 3, the gastric wall is retracted; 4, the arms are closed and a single pre-tied implant is deployed; 5, the resulting full-thickness plication.

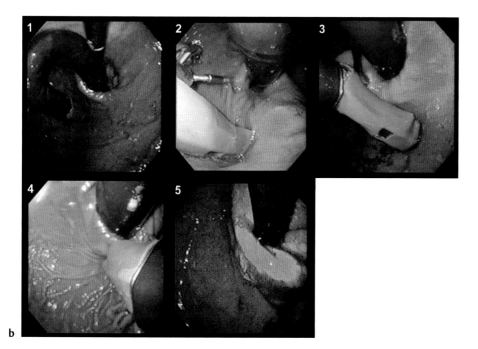

Table 33.6 Summary of selected publications on endoscopic treatment of gastroesophageal reflux disease with the NDO Plicator

First author (ref.)	Study design			% off PPIs	Heartburn score	GERD-HRQL	Time pH <4 (%)		
	Type	Patients (n)	Follow-up (months)				Before	After	Follow-up (months)
Pleskow [38]	OL, MC	64	6	74	NA	+ *	10	8*	6
Pleskow [39]	OL, MC	57	12	68	NA	+ *	10	8	6
Rothstein [40] (active/sham)	RCT, MC	72/72	3/3	57/25 §	–	+/– §	10/9	7/10*	3/3
Renteln [41]	OL, MC	41	6	59	+ *	+ *	11	9*	6
Pleskow [42]	OL, MC	33	60	67	NA	+ *	NA	NA	NA

GERD-HRQL, Gastroesophageal Reflux Disease Health-Related Quality of Life (score); MC, multicenter; NA, not available; OL, open-labeled; RCT, randomized controlled trial.
+ Improved; – did not improve; * significant difference (P< 0.05), § significant difference in comparison with sham.

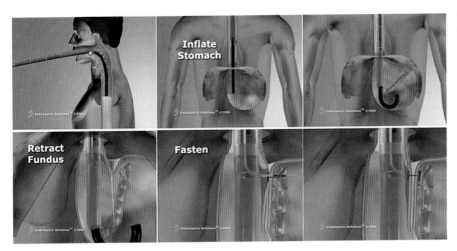

Fig. 33.6 The technique of transoral incisionless fundoplication (TIF) with the EsophyX device.

Table 33.7 Summary of selected publications on endoscopic treatment of gastroesophageal reflux disease with EsophyX

First author (ref.)	Study design			% off PPIs	Heartburn score	GERD-HRQL	Time pH <4 (%)		
	Type	Patients (n)	Follow-up (months)				Before	After	Follow-up (months)
Bergman [43]	OL, SC	8	2	50 §	NA	NA	NA	NA	NA
Cadière [44]	OL, SC	17	12	82	NA	+ *	NA	4.7	12
Cadière [45]	OL, MC	86	12	68	+ *	+ *	10	7*	12

GERD-HRQL, Gastroesophageal Reflux Disease Health-Related Quality of Life (score); OL, open-labeled; MC, multicenter; NA, not available; SC, single center.
+ Improved; * significant difference (P < 0.05); § including patients with reduced usage of medication.

33

56 % of the patients were considered to be "cured" of their GERD on the basis of the clinically significant reduction in heartburn and complete cessation of PPI use, accompanied by normalization or significant reduction of esophageal acid exposure in 80 %.

The reported adverse events have been few, mild, and transient. In more than 700 TIF procedures that have been performed to date throughout the world, two cases of esophageal perforation and three cases of bleeding have been reported during insertion of the device [45]. Shoulder pain, which has been reported in up to 18 % of cases, results from indirect or direct irritation of the phrenic nerve [46]. Larger series with long-term follow-up are awaited.

Medigus SRS Endoscopic Stapling System

The Medigus SRS endoscopic stapling system (Medigus, Tel Aviv, Israel) (**Fig. 33.7 a**) is used to staple the fundus of the stomach to the esophagus in two or three locations, 2–4 cm above the gastroesophageal junction. The stapled fundus covers part of the circumference of the distal esophagus, on its left and anterior sides (**Fig. 33.7 b**). The partial wrap created is intended to restore the angle of His and to create a flap valve similar to the valve created with a surgical partial anterior fundoplication.

In ex vivo experiments, a configuration with two staples 90° apart at the coronal angle, 2.5–3.0 cm from the gastroesophageal junction, was found to effectively prevent esophageal reflux at a gastric pressure exceeding 40 mmHg. In a pilot study, 13 of 14 patients (93 %) with a grade 1 gastroesophageal flap valve (GEFV) had GERD-HRQL scores that had improved by > 50 % 6 weeks after

the procedure in comparison with the baseline values. A grade 1 GEFV was always achieved with three staple sets, but succeeded in only 63 % of the cases with two staples and was not possible with a single staple set. Thirteen of the fourteen patients (93 %) with grade 1 GEFV were able to discontinue daily PPI therapy, and nine were able to stop all GERD medications. The 24-h acid exposure decreased from a median of 15 % at baseline to 6 % (P < 0.002). One patient developed benign pneumoperitoneum, which resolved spontaneously within 2 days. The efficacy of the Medigus endoscopic stapling system appears to depend on the creation of a grade 1 GEFV. An international multicenter trial is underway.

Syntheon ARD Plicator

This full-thickness plicator places a single titanium implant into the gastric cardia. It establishes a serosa-to-serosa apposition and alters the anatomy of the proximal stomach in a similar way to the NDO device. However, the important distinction is that the Syntheon Antireflux Device (ARD; Syntheon LLC, Miami, Florida, USA) and the endoscope are passed independently of each other. Preliminary results are available from a multicenter clinical trial including 57 patients [47]. The GERD-HRQL scores had improved at 6 months. Sixty-three percent of the patients were off all antisecretory therapy. There was a median decrease of 27 % in the 24-h esophageal acid exposure time. Despite the overall moderate efficacy and relative safety of the procedure, the FDA withheld approval.

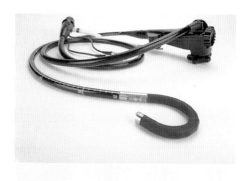

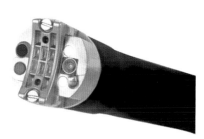

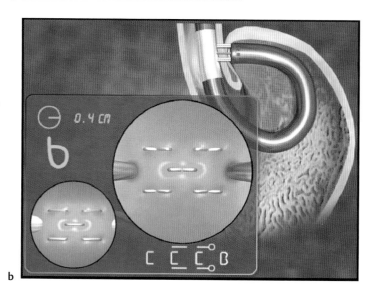

Fig. 33.7 a The SRS endoscopic stapling system (Medigus, Tel Aviv, Israel).
b The technique of endoscopic stapling with the SRS endoscopic stapling system.

Anti-Obesity Technique

Some similar endoscopic techniques have been used in efforts to manage obesity. The EndoCinch (C.R. Bard, Murray Hill, New Jersey, USA) endoscopic suturing device, the Transoral Gastroplasty (TOGA) system (Satiety Inc., Palo Alto, California, USA), and the Eagle Claw (Olympus, Tokyo, Japan) have been used or developed to manage obesity. These devices place the suture line near the cardia, which creates a small compartment in the upper part of the stomach (similar to vertical banding gastroplasty). In 64 patients included an open-label uncontrolled study with the EndoCinch suturing system, the mean body mass index (BMI) decreased significantly at 12 months ($39.9 \pm 5 \, \text{kg/m}^2$ versus $30.6 \pm 5 \, \text{kg/m}^2$; $P < 0.001$) and the percentage of excess weight loss (% EWL) was 21.1 ± 6, 39.6 ± 11, and 58.1 ± 20 at 1, 3, and 12 months, respectively [48]. In multicenter study with the TOGA system including 21 patients, the patients lost an average 8.0 kg at 1 month, 11.1 kg at 3 months, and 12 kg at 6 months after treatment (% EWL 16.2%, 22.6%, and 24.4%, respectively) [49]. Additional studies with sham controls and longer follow-up periods are awaited.

Miscellaneous

Many other endoscopic devices and techniques are currently undergoing study. These include submucosal magnets, mucosectomy with resultant scarring, mucosectomy and suture apposition of mucosectomy sites, and other injectable agents. Preliminary results are awaited.

Conclusions

Endoscopic treatment for GERD is continuing to evolve. All current and future techniques strive to maintain a balance between technical difficulty, efficacy, safety, and cost-effectiveness. Conceptually, a technically simple, "5-minute" safe procedure with only 50% efficacy might be widely acceptable, particularly if it could be repeated easily. Alternatively, procedures with higher costs and risks need to have greater efficacy in order to be accepted. No procedure will be widely utilized and hence remain viable unless reimbursement is easily achieved. Some of the techniques described above are no longer available; however, some may become available after modification or refinancing of the manufacturing companies. Even if they are not reintroduced, there are lessons to be learned from the data. Continuing further developments in this area of endoscopic research are likely to have a major impact on future algorithms for GERD treatment.

References

1. DiBaise JK. And then there were three—endotherapy for gastroesophageal reflux disease. Am J Gastroenterol 2003;98:1909–12.
2. Vakil N, Shaw M, Kirby R. Clinical effectiveness of laparoscopic fundoplication in a U.S. community. Am J Med 2003;114:1–5.
3. Triadafilopoulos G. GERD: the potential for endoscopic intervention. Dig Dis 2004;22:181–8.
4. Iqbal A, Salinas V, Filipi CJ. Endoscopic therapies of gastroesophageal reflux disease. World J Gastroenterol 2006;12:2641–55.
5. Gustavson K. The contraction of collagen, particularly hydrothermal shrinkage and crosslinking reactions. New York: Academic Press; 1956.
6. Triadafilopoulos G, DiBaise JK, Nostrant TT, Stollman NH, Anderson PK, Wolfe MM, et al. The Stretta procedure for the treatment of GERD: 6 and 12 month follow-up of the U.S. open label trial. Gastrointest Endosc 2002;55:149–56.
7. Wolfsen HC, Richards WO. The Stretta procedure for the treatment of GERD: a registry of 558 patients. J Laparoendosc Adv Surg Tech A 2002;12:395–402.
8. Tam WC, Schoeman MN, Zhang Q, Dent J, Rigda R, Utley D, et al. Delivery of radiofrequency energy to the lower oesophageal sphincter and gastric cardia inhibits transient lower oesophageal sphincter relaxations and gastro-oesophageal reflux in patients with reflux disease. Gut 2003;52:479–85.
9. Corley DA, Katz P, Wo JM, Stefan A, Patti M, Rothstein R, et al. Improvement of gastroesophageal reflux symptoms after radiofrequency energy: a randomized, sham-controlled trial. Gastroenterology 2003;125:668–76.
10. Cipolletta L, Rotondano G, Dughera L, Repici A, Bianco MA, De Angelis C, et al. Delivery of radiofrequency energy to the gastroesophageal junction (Stretta procedure) for the treatment of gastroesophageal reflux disease. Surg Endosc 2005;19:849–53.
11. Reymunde A, Santiago N. Long-term results of radiofrequency energy delivery for the treatment of GERD: sustained improvements in symptoms, quality of life, and drug use at 4-year follow-up. Gastrointest Endosc 2007;65:361–6.
12. Ayman M, Aziz A, Sadek A, Mattat S, McNulty G, Lehman GA. A prospective randomized trial of sham, single Stretta and double Stretta for the treatment of gastroesophageal reflux disease (GERD) [abstract]. Gastrointest Endosc 2007;65:AB144.
13. Noar MD, Lotfi S. Radiofrequency correction of GERD (Stretta) results in significant, long term 4-year improvement in symptoms, quality of life and medication use in the medically refractory GERD patient [abstract]. Gastrointest Endosc 2006;63:AB134.
14. Mavrelis P, Ayman M, Aziz A, Rearick C, Richards L, McNulty G, et al. Longer term clinical outcomes after radiofrequency therapy for refractory gastroesophageal reflux disease (GERD). Pract Gastroenterol 2007;31:73–80.
15. O'Connor KW, Lehman GA. Endoscopic placement of collagen at the lower esophageal sphincter to inhibit gastroesophageal reflux: a pilot study of 10 medically intractable patients. Gastrointest Endosc 1988;34:106–12.
16. Devière J, Pastorelli A, Louis H, de Maertelaer V, Lehman G, Cicala M, et al. Endoscopic implantation of a biopolymer in the lower esophageal sphincter for gastroesophageal reflux: a pilot study. Gastrointest Endosc 2002;55:335–41.
17. Terada T, Nakamura Y, Nakai K, Tsuura M, Nishiguchi T, Hayashi S, et al. Embolization of arteriovenous malformations with peripheral aneurysms using ethylene vinyl alcohol copolymer. Report of three cases. J Neurosurg 1991;75:655–60.
18. Devière J, Costamagna G, Neuhaus H, Voderholzer W, Louis H, Tringali A, et al. Nonresorbable copolymer implantation for gastroesophageal reflux disease: a randomized sham-controlled multicenter trial. Gastroenterology 2005;128:532–40.
19. Johnson DA, Ganz R, Aisenberg J, Cohen LB, Devière J, Foley TR, et al. Endoscopic implantation of Enteryx for treatment of GERD: 12-month results of a prospective, multicenter trial. Am J Gastroenterol 2003;98:1921–30.
20. Cohen LB, Johnson DA, Ganz RA, Aisenberg J, Devière J, Foley TR, et al. Enteryx implantation for GERD: expanded multicenter trial results and interim postapproval follow-up to 24 months. Gastrointest Endosc 2005;61:650–8.
21. U.S. Food and Drug Administration. Enteryx™ procedure kit – P020 006. Summary of safety and effectiveness data. Silver Spring, MD: U.S. Food and Drug Administration, 2003. Available from: http://www.fda.gov/cdrh/pdf2/p020 006.html.
22. Tintillier M, Chaput A, Kirch L, Martinet JP, Pochet JM, Cuvelier C. Esophageal abscess complicating endoscopic treatment of refractory gastroesophageal reflux disease by Enteryx injection: a first case report. Am J Gastroenterol 2004;99:1856–8.
23. Noh KW, Loeb DS, Stockland A, Achem SR. Pneumomediastinum following Enteryx injection for the treatment of gastroesophageal reflux disease. Am J Gastroenterol 2005;100:723–6.
24. Wong RF, Davis TV, Peterson KA. Complications involving the mediastinum after injection of Enteryx for GERD. Gastrointest Endosc 2005;61:753–6.
25. Fockens P, Bruno MJ, Gabbrielli A, Odegaard S, Hatlebakk J, Allescher HD, et al. Endoscopic augmentation of the lower esophageal sphincter for the treatment of gastroesophageal reflux disease: multicenter study of the Gatekeeper Reflux Repair System. Endoscopy 2004;36(8):682–9.
26. Fockens P. Gatekeeper Reflux Repair System: technique, pre-clinical, and clinical experience. Gastrointest Endosc Clin N Am 2003;13:179–89.
27. Feretis C, Benakis P, Dimopoulos C, Dailianas A, Filalithis P, Stamou KM, et al. Endoscopic implantation of Plexiglas (PMMA) microspheres for the treatment of GERD. Gastrointest Endosc 2001;53(4):423–6.
28. Swain CP, Mills TN. An endoscopic sewing machine. Gastrointest Endosc 1986;32:36–8.
29. Filipi CJ, Lehman GA, Rothstein RI, Raijman I, Stiegmann GV, Waring JP, et al. Transoral, flexible endoscopic suturing for treatment of GERD: a multicenter trial. Gastrointest Endosc 2001;53:416–22.
30. Mahmood Z, McMahon BP, Arfin Q, Byrne PJ, Reynolds JV, Murphy EM, et al. EndoCinch therapy for gastro-oesophageal reflux disease: a one year prospective follow up. Gut 2003;52:34–9.
31. Abou-Rebyeh H, Hoepffner N, Rösch T, Osmanoglou E, Haneke JH, Hintze RE, et al. Long-term failure of endoscopic suturing in the treatment of gastroesophageal reflux: a prospective follow-up study. Endoscopy 2005;37:213–6.
32. Chen YK, Raijman I, Ben-Menachem T, Starpoli AA, Liu J, Pazwash H, et al. Long-term outcomes of endoluminal gastroplication: a U.S. multicenter trial. Gastrointest Endosc 2005;61:659–67.
33. Arts J, Lerut T, Rutgeerts P, Sifrim D, Janssens J, Tack J. A one-year follow-up study of endoluminal gastroplication (EndoCinch) in GERD patients refractory to proton pump inhibitor therapy. Dig Dis Sci 2005;50:351–6.
34. Schiefke I, Zabel-Langhennig A, Neumann S, Feisthammel J, Moessner J, Caca K. Long term failure of endoscopic gastroplication (EndoCinch). Gut 2005;54:752–8.
35. Schwartz MP, Wellink H, Gooszen HG, Conchillo JM, Samsom M, Smout AJ. Endoscopic gastroplication for the treatment of gastro-oesophageal reflux disease: a randomised, sham-controlled trial. Gut 2007;56:20–8.
36. Liao CC, Lee CL, Lin BR, Bai CH, Hsieh YH, Wu CH, et al. Endoluminal gastroplication for the treatment of gastroesophageal reflux disease: a 2-year prospective pilot study from Taiwan. J Gastroenterol Hepatol 2008;23:398–405.
37. Tuebergen D, Rijcken E, Senninger N. Esophageal perforation as a complication of EndoCinch endoluminal gastroplication. Endoscopy 2004;36:663–5.
38. Pleskow D, Rothstein R, Lo S, Hawes R, Kozarek R, Haber G, et al. Endoscopic full-thickness plication for the treatment of GERD: a multicenter trial. Gastrointest Endosc 2004;59(2):163–71.
39. Pleskow D, Rothstein R, Lo S, Hawes R, Kozarek R, Haber G, et al. Endoscopic full-thickness plication for the treatment of GERD: 12-month follow-up for the North American open-label trial. Gastrointest Endosc 2005;61:643–9.
40. Rothstein R, Filipi C, Caca K, Pruitt R, Mergener K, Torquati A, et al. Endoscopic full-thickness plication for the treatment of gastroesophageal reflux disease: A randomized, sham-controlled trial. Gastroenterology 2006;131:704–12.
41. von Renteln D, Brey U, Riecken B, Caca K. Endoscopic full-thickness plication (Plicator) with two serially placed implants improves esophagitis and reduces PPI use and esophageal acid exposure. Endoscopy 2008;40:173–8.
42. Pleskow D, Rothstein R, Kozarek R, Haber G, Gostout C, Lo S, et al. Endoscopic full-thickness plication for the treatment of GERD: Five-year long-term multicenter results. Surg Endosc 2008;22:326–32.

43. Bergman S, Mikami DJ, Hazey JW, Roland JC, Dettorre R, Melvin WS. Endoluminal fundoplication with EsophyX: the initial North American experience. Surg Innov 2008;15:166–70.

44. Cadière GB, Rajan A, Germay O, Himpens J. Endoluminal fundoplication by a transoral device for the treatment of GERD: A feasibility study. Surg Endosc 2008;22:333–42.

45. Cadière GB, Buset M, Muls V, Rajan A, Rösch T, Eckardt AJ, et al. Antireflux transoral incisionless fundoplication using EsophyX: 12-month results of a prospective multicenter study. World J Surg 2008;32:1676–88.

46. Wynyard M, Kletschka HD. The crural branches of the phrenic nerves. Their surgical significance. Minn Med 1966;49:1821–4.

47. Ramage JI, Rothstein RI, Edmundowicz SA. Endoscopically placed titanium plicator for GERD: pivotal phase—preliminary 6-month results [abstract]. Gastrointest Endosc 2006;63:AB126.

48. Fogel R, De Fogel J, Bonilla Y, De La Fuente R. Clinical experience of transoral suturing for an endoluminal vertical gastroplasty: 1-year follow-up in 64 patients. Gastrointest Endosc 2008;68:51–8.

49. Devière J, Ojeda Valdes G, Cuevas Herrera L, Closset J, Le Moine O, Eisendrath P, et al. Safety, feasibility and weight loss after transoral gastroplasty: First human multicenter study. Surg Endosc 2008;22: 589–98.

V

34 Endoscopic Papillotomy and Endoscopic Sphincterotomy

Christian Prinz and Meinhard Classen

Introduction

The treatment of biliary stones is little more than a century old—a few years after Langenbuch carried out the first cholecystectomy, at the end of the 19th century, McBurney introduced surgical sphincterotomy. The first endoscopic papillotomies of the main duodenal papilla were carried out in June 1973 in Germany [1], and shortly afterward in Japan [2]. The procedure was soon taken up by endoscopic centers in the United States [3,4], in 1980 by An Rong in China, and in other countries as well. Endoscopic papillotomy (EPT) is now an established therapeutic procedure for various disorders of the main papilla, biliary tract, and pancreas. The procedure widens the abnormally narrow opening of the biliary and pancreatic ducts, and also facilitates access to the ductal systems, making it possible to obtain tissue samples using fluoroscopically guided biopsies and allowing endoscopic treatments such as biliary decompression using a nasobiliary tube or endoprosthesis, balloon dilation of ductal stenoses, and local photodynamic therapy for unresectable tumors. Stones in the bile duct and in the pancreatic duct can be extracted using Dormia baskets or balloon catheters. Mechanical and hydraulic methods, as well as different types of laser and extracorporeal shock-wave lithotripsy, are used to fragment and reduce the size of stones so that they can be extracted using the above methods.

Indications (Table 34.1)

Endoscopic retrograde cholangiopancreatography (ERCP) was used exclusively for diagnosis between 1970 and 1973, but the range of indications for ERCP has narrowed with the development of magnetic resonance cholangiopancreatography (MRCP). During the last 27 years, there has been a continuing increase in the number of therapeutic procedures carried out at our own and many other centers, and these now account for 60% or more of the indications for ERCP. Another shift in the indications for EPT has been away from stone treatment and toward the endoscopic management of bile duct tumors by biliary stenting. Obtaining endoscopic access to the pancreatic duct system to treat sequelae of pancreatitis such as strictures, stones, and pseudocysts, and also to treat tumors, is now an established procedure.

The range of indications has broadened and now includes virtually all causes of obstruction in the biliary system, as well as organic and functional dyskinesia of the sphincter of Oddi and occlusion of pancreatic ducts in certain situations—such as stone near the papilla, pancreas divisum, pseudocysts, and tumors. **Figures 34.1–34.3** illustrate some indications for and techniques of papillotomy.

Main Duodenal Papilla and Minor Papilla

The motility disorder of the sphincter of Oddi known as sphincter of Oddi dysfunction (SOD) [5] is characterized by recurrent pain, suspected to be caused by a structural or functional pancreatic and/or biliary sphincter abnormality, with or without clinical evidence of any abnormality of the pancreas or liver, or of biliary function.

Table 34.1 Indications for endoscopic papillotomy

Main duodenal papilla and minor papilla
Sphincter of Oddi dysfunction (SOD)
Postoperative strictures
Adenoma: sporadic, or familial adenomatous polyposis
Carcinoma
Bile ducts
Choledocholithiasis
Cholangitis: septic, suppurative, acute obstructive
"Sump syndrome"
Tumor metastases
Leakage: external, internal
Biliary strictures, postoperative (cholecystectomy, liver transplantation)
Worms: *Ascaris lumbricoides, Echinococcus cysticus*
Occluded stents
Primary sclerosing cholangitis
AIDS cholangiopathy
Pancreatic disorders
Pancreatitis: acute biliary; chronic, with ductal stones/obstruction
Pseudocyst
Tumor
Pancreas divisum
Enhancement of diagnostic measures

Sphincter of Oddi manometry (SOM) may reveal hypertension of the biliary sphincter, pancreatic sphincter, or both (>40 mmHg). However, SOM—particularly of the pancreatic sphincter—may lead to complications in up to 40% of cases and is a procedure that should only be used by very experienced examiners.

In benign papillary stenoses that are either spontaneous or postoperative, EPT with or without stenting is the treatment of choice. Juxtapapillary adenoma and carcinoma have been treated using EPT or endoscopic papillectomy (also known as ampullectomy) when obstruction of the ductal systems occurs. The large samples that can be removed by snare excision improve the histological detection of cancerous areas within an adenoma [6].

Bile Ducts

Stones in the common bile duct are an indication for EPT and stone extraction (**Fig. 34.1**). In the first few years after EPT was introduced, it was generally held that the loss of sphincter function after EPT (**Fig. 34.2**) in patients under 50 years of age might have deleterious consequences. This is regarded today as an overprotective approach. There is now more than 35 years' experience with the technique since the introduction of EPT, and negative long-term effects due to the loss of the barrier function or due to a shift in the composition of bile do not appear to have any clinical significance [7–9]. The Asian form of biliary ductal stones is different from the Western one, as the

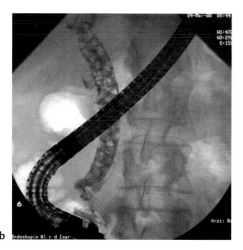
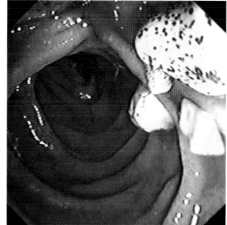
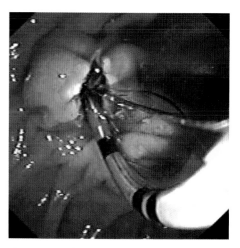

a, b

Fig. 34.1
a Choledocholithiasis.
b Extracted stones in the duodenum.

Fig. 34.2 Endoscopic papillotomy.

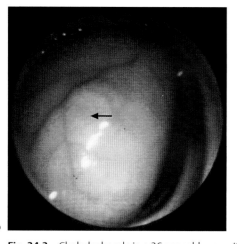
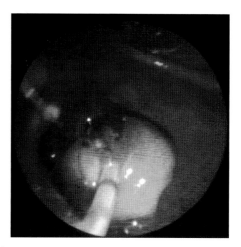
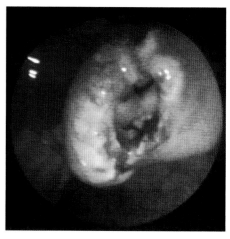

a, b

c

Fig. 34.3 Choledochocele in a 36-year-old man with recurrent pancreatitis.
a The choledochocele is seen bulging into the duodenal orifice (arrow).
b The tip of the papillotome has been positioned in the orifice, and stones are visible leaving the sac.

c View of the common bile duct immediately after papillotomy. The opening of the main pancreatic duct is covered with debris.

stones usually lodge in the intrahepatic branches of the biliary tree in the Asian type.

The presence or absence of the gallbladder is not relevant when the indication for EPT is urgent decompression of the bile duct in patients with acute suppurative and septic cholangitis. In these cases, removal of the stone obstructing the hepatic or common bile duct is of the greatest clinical importance, and it substantially improves the patient's condition if the procedure is not performed too late [10,11].

Choledochocele (**Fig. 34.3**) is a rarely occurring anomaly of the common bile duct. The distal sac-like dilation of the common bile duct bulges into the duodenum. EPT is the method of choice in type III patients (in Todani's classification) [12].

Acute obstructive cholangitis (also known as suppurative or septic cholangitis) is a life-threatening condition and an emergency indication for EPT and EPT-associated methods of stone removal and/or drainage by nasobiliary tube or biliary endoprosthesis [10,11]. **Figure 34.4** shows what is known as a balloon papilla, with the procedure indicated by obstruction at the distal end by a stone. The most common causes of the obstruction are stones, tumors, postoperative strictures, occlusion of biliary stents, and parasites. The endoscopic treatment methods are chosen accord-

ingly. Urgent endoscopic drainage is mandatory, in combination with resuscitation and antibiotic treatment if necessary. Antibiotic treatment alone, without biliary drainage, does not resolve this dangerous situation [13]. Early intervention is needed in patients with already existing or developing septicemia, and they should be treated within 8 h of admission [14]. The presence or absence of the gallbladder is of no relevance in these patients.

A condition known as the "sump syndrome" occurs after side-to-side choledochoduodenostomy or choledochojejunostomy procedures, when the distal portion of the common bile duct becomes a "sump" in which bile, vegetable material, and debris accumulate, or in which parasites can be found. **Figures 34.4 d** and **34.5–34.7** illustrate these conditions. Obstruction of the anastomosis, cholestasis, and cholangitis may occur. EPT and removal of the foreign material through the papilla of Vater have been carried out successfully [15].

Tumors obstructing the common bile duct are rarely benign; malignant tumors originate from the biliary duct epithelium, the pancreatic head, lymph nodes, and liver metastases (**Figs. 34.8–34.10**). Endoscopic therapy allows drainage of the bile and can therefore be used for therapeutic or palliative purposes, as in photodynamic therapy for bile duct cancer.

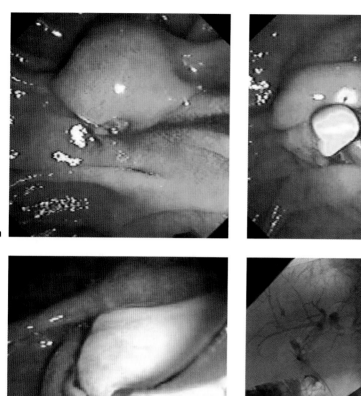

a

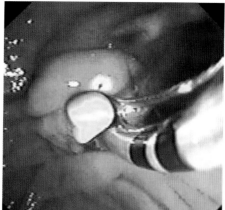

b

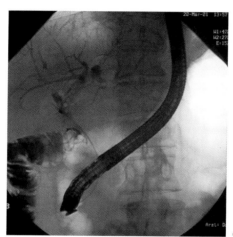

c

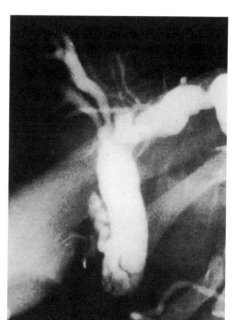

d

Fig. 34.4
a Balloon dilation of the papilla.
b Mobilization of the stone.
c Putrid bile.
d Sump syndrome after hepaticojejunostomy.

34

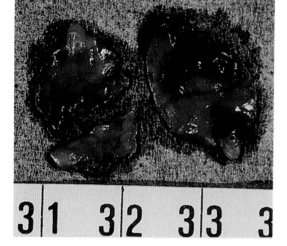

Fig. 34.5 *Fasciola hepatica* extracted from the bile duct after endoscopic papillotomy.

Fig. 34.6 Biliary fascioliasis in the prepapillary common bile duct.

External and internal leakage of the bile or cystic duct have been treated successfully using EPT (**Fig. 34.11**), with or without ductal stenting [16]. The number of patients undergoing this procedure appears to be increasing along with the growing use of laparoscopic methods of removing the gallbladder. Biliary strictures, which occur in about 0.5 % of cases after laparoscopic cholecystectomy

(**Fig. 34.12**), have become a generally accepted indication for endoscopic treatment with balloon dilation and stenting. EPT and endoscopic removal of postoperative blood clots or parasites—e. g., *Ascaris lumbricoides, Echinococcus cysticus, Fasciola hepatica,* and others [17,18]—are frequently carried out in areas of the world in which these parasites are endemic.

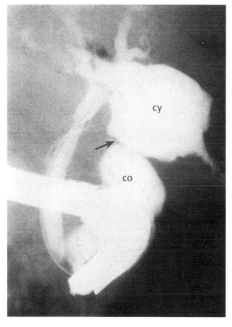

Fig. 34.7 Hepatic echinococcosis, with formation of a cyst (cy) at the hilum of the liver. The cyst is in communication (arrow) with the colon (co).

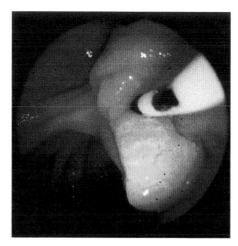

Fig. 34.8 Papillary adenoma.

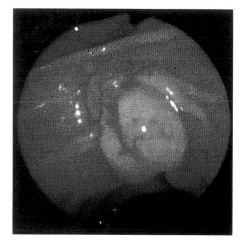

Fig. 34.9 Carcinoid originating from the papilla.

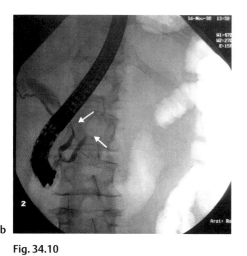

a, b

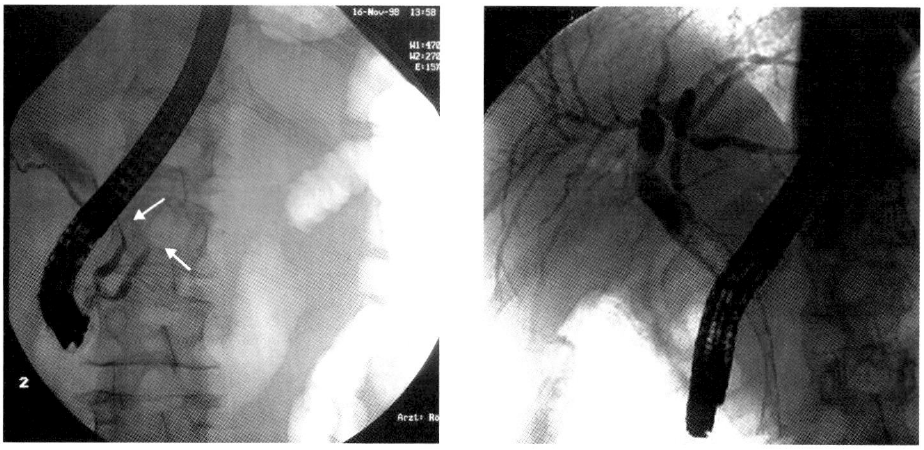

Fig. 34.10
a Double duct sign: pancreatic cancer obstructing the biliary tract.
b Use of a metal stent to bridge a biliary stricture caused by pancreatic cancer.

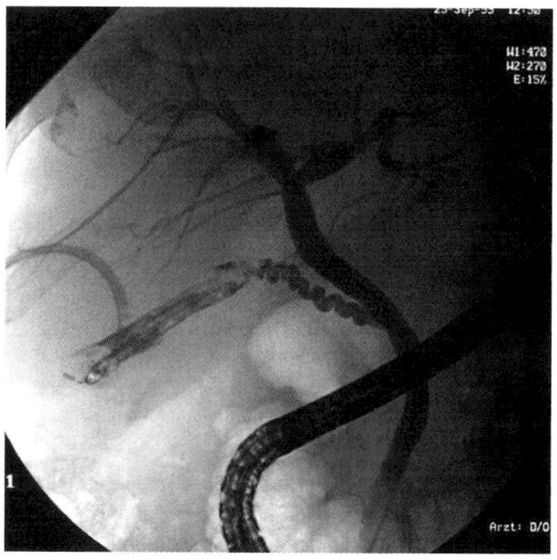

Fig. 34.11 Cystic stump insufficiency.

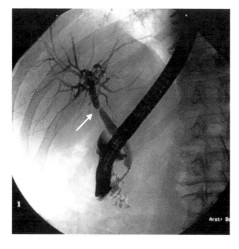

Fig. 34.12 Postsurgical biliary stricture.

Primary sclerosing cholangitis and acquired immune deficiency syndrome (AIDS) cholangiopathy may be indications for EPT and stenting when strictures dominate the clinical picture (**Fig. 34.13**).

▓ Pancreas

Acute pancreatitis and biliary obstruction, microlithiasis. EPT is indicated in acute pancreatitis when biliary ductal stones or strictures are present. However, microlithiasis in the distal bile duct—a condition that can be detected by computed tomography (CT) or endoscopic ultrasonography—appears to occur not infrequently, in some 30 % of cases [10]. The indication for EPT, or even ERCP, in seriously ill patients with acute pancreatitis has been challenged by some, and the procedure should only be carried out when symptoms or signs of cholestasis and especially cholangitis are present [19–23].

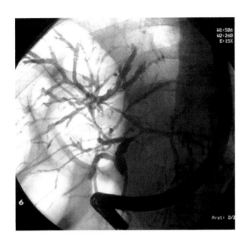

Fig. 34.13 Primary sclerosing cholangitis.

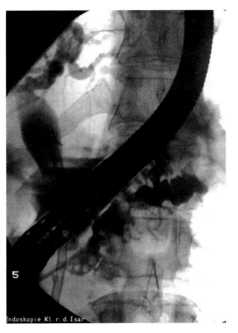

Fig. 34.14 Chronic obstructive pancreatitis.

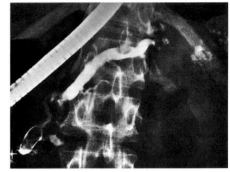

Fig. 34.15 Pancreatolithiasis with strictures and dilation of the duct.

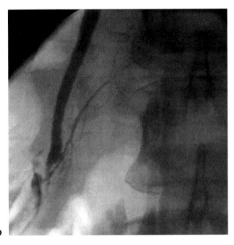

Fig. 34.16 Pancreas divisum.
a Ventral duct.

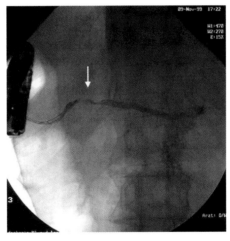

b Dorsal duct with proximal stenosis.
c Stenting of the dorsal duct.

34

Chronic pancreatitis. The rationale in endoscopic therapy for chronic pancreatitis is to treat the papillary stenosis or a dominant stricture of the pancreatic duct (**Figs. 34.14, 34.15**), or to break up the obstructing stones in parts of the ductal system near the papilla of Vater. Some larger-diameter stones can only be extracted after destruction using a laser lithotriptor or extracorporeal shock-wave lithotripsy.

In some patients with chronic calcifying pancreatitis, access to the main pancreatic duct is easier through the minor papilla and Santorini duct than through the major duodenal papilla, because of stones or strictures obstructing the main pancreatic duct.

Pseudocysts bulging into the stomach or duodenal wall can be evacuated by introducing a stent, after endoscopic ultrasonography (EUS) and determination of a suitable puncture site. Pseudocysts connected with the pancreatic duct can be treated after EPT using a transpapillary stent or a nasocystic tube. A tumor of the pancreatic head may infiltrate and obstruct the common bile duct or the papilla of Vater (**Fig. 34.10 b**).

It has been assumed that in patients with pancreas divisum and accompanying pancreatitis, the minor papilla is anatomically and functionally incapable of passing pancreatic juice from the main portion of the pancreatic parenchyma. However, some authors do not share this assumption [24]. Cannulation of the minor papilla can be accomplished in approximately 90% of patients with pancreas divisum, and demonstrates pathological findings in 20–70% of cases. Whether pancreatitis is caused by this anatomical variant in these patients is still a matter of debate [25]. EPT of the minor papilla and stenting of the Santorini duct have been carried out in patients with symptomatic pancreas divisum, as well as in those with recurrent episodes of acute pancreatitis and in others with chronic pancreatitis [26] (**Fig. 34.16**).

Admission, Premedication, and Instruments

▥ Circumstances of Admission (In-Patient or Outpatient)

Endoscopic papillotomy is an invasive procedure. The patient, and relatives when appropriate, must therefore be informed beforehand concerning the aim and nature of the procedure, its risks and potential complications, and the possible alternatives using endoscopic treatment. In the past, EPT was always carried out on an in-patient basis. Several authors have suggested that patients can be discharged following the procedure after a few hours of observation in the recovery room [27]. However, a policy of overnight hospitalization has been shown to produce a better outcome overall [28].

▥ Preparation (see also Chapter 6)

The methods of preparation and sedation are broadly similar to those used for diagnostic ERCP. There are no data to support routine preprocedural testing in patients undergoing elective gastrointestinal procedures. Endoscopists should pursue preprocedural testing selectively, based on the patient's medical history and physical examination [29]. The legal implications differ in various countries. In some countries, a coagulation profile should be obtained, and any coagulopathy should be corrected beforehand. We assess prothrombin time and partial thromboplastin time to check plasma coagulation; platelet count and bleeding time are required to detect platelet dysfunction (associated with prior acetylsalicylic acid or nonsteroidal anti-inflammatory drug intake; see also the section on prevention below). There is considerable variability in individual thrombocyte responses to aspirin. It has been shown that persons with low acetylsalicylic acid esterase activity have a greater prolongation time than those who metabolize the drug quickly [30]. Cardiopulmonary status should be assessed as for a surgical intervention. Patients who are unfit for surgery can generally be treated, but close monitoring of blood pressure, pulse rate, and oxygen saturation are required. Sedative drugs such as propofol may only be administered by anesthesiologists in some countries, while in others this restriction does not apply. When this drug is used in severely ill patients (American Society of Anesthesiologists grade III

or higher), an additional doctor experienced in resuscitation and in the use of the relevant equipment should be at hand [31].

The endoscopist should work in close cooperation with an experienced abdominal surgeon, as serious complications may occur during or after the procedure.

Although hemorrhage is a recognized and potentially life-threatening complication of EPT, units of cross-matched blood are only rarely needed before the procedure. It is doubtful whether using endoscopic Doppler ultrasonography to locate the retroduodenal artery in the wall of the duodenum, as well as any branches of the vessel in the region of the papilla, can be helpful in preventing life-threatening hemorrhage during EPT.

Views in the literature diverge concerning whether prophylactic antibiotic treatment should be given in all patients before EPT. In its guidelines, the European Society of Gastrointestinal Endoscopy (ESGE) recommends prophylactic antibiotic administration for all therapeutic ERCP-related interventions [32].

High-level disinfection of endoscopes and all accessories is even more important for endoscopic procedures in the bile and pancreatic ducts than in other procedures. The patient should be in a fasting state.

▥ Instruments

Endoscopes, papillotomes, and high-frequency electrosurgical generator. All duodenoscopes with lateral viewing systems are suitable for EPT. Considerable technical improvements have been made, which have been particularly important for implanting the endoprosthesis. The improvements include replacement of the viewing fiber bundle with a charge-coupled device (CCD) chip; an increase in the viewing angle; improvements in the range and tightness of the deflection angle of the instrument tip; and an increase in the diameter of the instrumentation channel.

With some modifications, the Demling–Classen papillotome (the pull type) is now in general use (**Figs. 34.17, 34.18**) [33]. The tip of the catheter, which does not have a wire attached, serves as pathfinder during cannulation of the bile duct. Needle-knife papillotomes are useful for precutting sphincterotomy. Several types of needle-knife are produced by Olympus and the instruments are undergoing continuous further development. Most needle-knives consist of an outer plastic sheath (1.85 mm) and an inner stainless-steel wire, and they have a length of 3 mm projecting from the plastic sheath. The needle-knife can be used to puncture the roof the duodenal papilla (fistulotomy) or to make an incision in it.

The modified Erlangen-type precutting papillotome has several theoretical advantages over the needle-knife: firstly, the risk of injury to the pancreatic orifice and pancreatic duct may be lower, since these structures are protected by the convex Teflon catheter, and a small leading tip of 1 mm ensures that the cutting wire is only in contact with tissue cranial to the wire. Secondly, the incision can be better controlled, since the tip of the instrument functions as a stabilizing fulcrum.

In push-type papillotomes, including what is known as the "shark-fin" variant, the wire is pushed out to form a bow. Push-type papillotomes are only used rarely, as the direction of the incision produced with this device is less predictable (**Fig. 34.19**).

All papillotome catheters should have a side port to allow injection of contrast material, and a guide wire to serve as a pathfinder. A type known as a "safety sphincterotome," which has a guide wire with a tapered tip, a metal marker, a long nose, and an insulated cutting wire, has been proposed (**Fig. 34.20**) [34]. Several other developments for carrying out EPT in patients who have undergone Billroth II surgery have been presented, including one device that has the advantage of using a shape-memory plastic material for the catheter, ensuring that the sigmoid shape of the

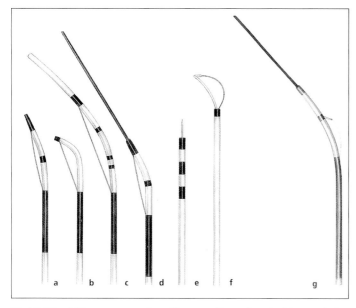

Fig. 34.17 Different types of papillotome. (Reproduced with permission from Soehendra et al., *Praxis der therapeutischen Endoskopie,* Stuttgart: Thieme, 1997.)

V

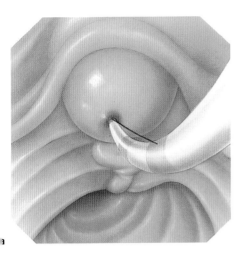

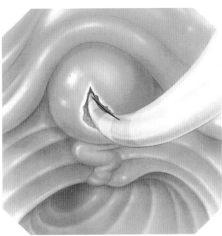

b

Fig. 34.18
a Introducing the papillotome into the duct.
b Carrying out the papillotomy. (Reproduced with permission from Soehendra et al., *Praxis der therapeutischen Endoskopie*, Stuttgart: Thieme, 1997.)

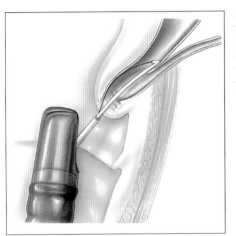

Fig. 34.19 The push-type papillotome. (Reproduced with permission from Soehendra et al., *Praxis der therapeutischen Endoskopie*, Stuttgart: Thieme, 1997.)

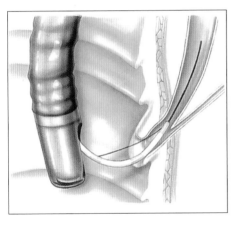

Fig. 34.20 The safety sphincterotome. (Reproduced with permission from Soehendra et al., *Praxis der therapeutischen Endoskopie*, Stuttgart: Thieme, 1997.)

allowing coagulation at tissue temperatures of approximately 70 °C. During EPT, the cutting and coagulation mode is automatically controlled, and the examiner should therefore stay on the pedal while cutting instead of repeatedly pushing the button. Modern devices with a rapid-start function have an electronic safety facility that provides initial high-power current for a short time (a fraction of a second) to ensure an electrosurgical incision no matter what level of electric resistance is encountered.

Accessories or additional instruments. Guide wires are indispensable as pathfinders during cannulation of the intended duct, as well as for passing ductal obstructions caused by strictures, stones, and tumors. The guide wire should avoid the need for repeated filling of the pancreatic duct with contrast material and should reduce the risk of local tissue damage. The diameter of a suitable guide wire for the papillotome is 0.89 mm (0.35 inches). Guide wires with a hydrophilic coating (Terumo type) are needed to pass various types of tumor. A properly insulated guide wire must be used if the papillotomy is to be performed with the wire in place [36]. Double-lumen papillotomes have two insulated channels that make it possible to maintain deep cannulation with the guide wire during EPT (**Fig. 34.21**), without the risk of current being conducted through the guide wire. These papillotomes are larger and less flexible, and the data available indicate that the use of the single-lumen papillotome together with a guide wire insulated with plastic coating is safe and effective [37].

Multipurpose guide wires are used during ERCP, to facilitate cannulation and access through strictures, and also for exchanging interventional devices. The efficacy and cost-effectiveness of these guide wires in comparison with single-use wires is being studied.

Conventional Dormia baskets of various sizes, or balloon tubes, are needed for removal of stones from the common bile duct and pancreatic duct. Drainage from the ductal systems can be ensured using a nasobiliary tube (which also allows the bile or pancreatic juice to be studied) (**Fig. 34.22**) and using various endoprostheses (stents) made of various types of plastic material or of a metal mesh (see Chapter 36). Mechanical lithotripsy within the ducts has been carried out using heavy-duty baskets that capture and pulverize the stone, gradually reducing its size (**Fig. 34.23**) [38]. Dormia-type baskets can also be used to hold the stone in a constant location so that electrohydraulic forces can destroy the stone, but not the wall [39]. Modern "smart" lasers, with tissue-detection systems, automatically switch off when the stone is out of the laser's focus [40,41]. Use of this type of laser could become the method of choice, as the procedure can be monitored using endoscopy or fluoroscopy. Extracorporeal shock-wave lithotripsy is still used by some for large stones several centimeters in diameter that are difficult to reach endoscopically [40–46].

wire is retained after it has been passed through the instrument channel. An instrument known as the "baby papillotome" has been described for primary cannulation and papillotomy, and this also allows precutting [35].

Disposable sphincterotomes serve to reduce infectious complications, but at considerable cost. When there is adequate sterilization of disposable sphincterotomes, there is no increase in the infection rate. When reusable papillotomes are reprocessed in vitro, functional integrity is maintained for a mean of five to ten uses. These instruments may allow significant cost savings. However, the medicolegal implications still need to be clarified.

A modern high-frequency electrosurgical generator with cutting and coagulation modes is adequate for EPT. The device delivers currents at a frequency above 350 kHz. In the cutting mode, tension is maintained, while in the coagulation mode, tension is reduced,

34

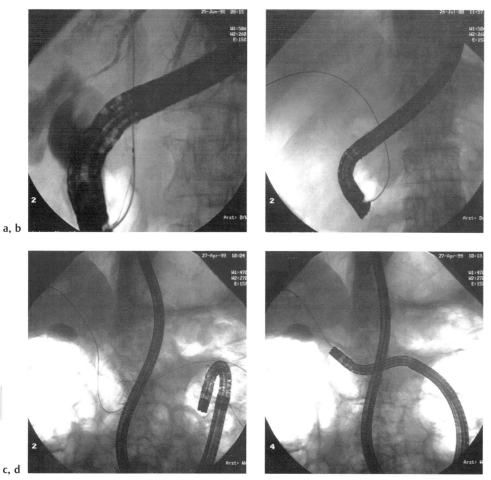

a, b

c, d

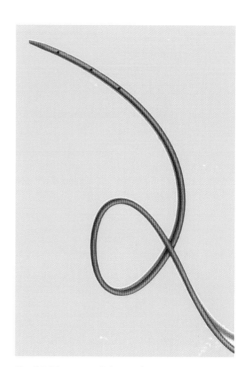

Fig. 34.21 a–d Different methods of carrying out papillotomy using guide wires.
a Wire-guided insertion of a papillotome.
b The papillotome is being inserted over a guide wire that has been placed via the percutaneous transhepatic approach (rendezvous technique).
c Positioning of an endoscope over a percutaneously inserted guide wire in a patient with Billroth II anatomy.
d The instrument is successfully guided to the papilla.

Fig. 34.22 A nasobiliary tube.

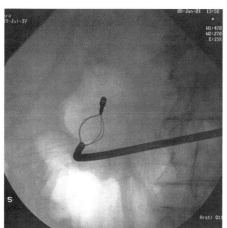

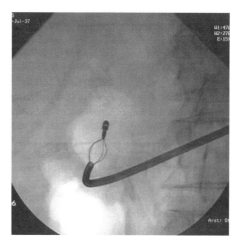

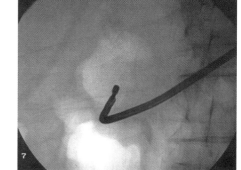

a, b

c

Fig. 34.23 a–c Various stages of mechanical lithotripsy.
a The stone has been trapped in the basket.

b Disintegration of the stone.
c The basket has been closed, and the stone is in fragments.

Methods of Endoscopic Papillotomy

Biliary Papillotomy

The technique of endoscopic papillotomy has remained virtually unchanged since the first reports were published in 1973. After endoscopic retrograde ductography, the standard papillotome is introduced, with its position at the papilla and within the duct being monitored endoscopically and fluoroscopically. If there is any doubt as to whether the papillotome has been positioned in the intended duct, a small amount of contrast medium can be instilled through the papillotome for confirmation, or a suitable guide wire can be introduced (**Figs. 34.21 a, b; 34.24, 34.25**). Guide wires with a hydrophilic coating are particularly helpful in stenosis of the terminal bile duct. The roof of the papilla should "ride" up and down on the cutting wire of the papillotome when tension is applied to the wire, as this ensures that the cut will correspond to the course of the bile duct and that the tension on the wire is not excessive. It should be checked that about one-third to half of the length of the tensed cutting wire can be seen outside the papilla. This ensures that the cutting procedure will be controlled and that cutting will proceed in increments. If the papillotome is introduced too deeply into the duct, the cut cannot be controlled, and a rapid incision of excessive length may occur, with the attendant risk of perforation or hemorrhage, or both. The common error is to have too much wire inside the duct and the papilla, and to apply too much bowing tension. In this situation, cutting will not occur promptly, and there is a tendency to increase the current settings and tension on the wire. This may result in cutting through an already coagulated area at high speed (an effect known as the "zipper cut"), with the associated risk of significant bleeding. The adequacy of the incision depends on the individual anatomical situation. In general, the incision will be about 10–15 mm when the appearance of the papilla is normal. Short pulses of current incise the papilla as far as it enters the duodenal wall. In general, this point can be seen endoscopically, as the dilated common bile duct produces a bulge in the duodenal wall all the way down to the papillary orifice, defining the course of the bile duct endoscopically. However, if the papilla is small and flat and the bile duct is not dilated, it may be difficult to determine the length to which the cut can be made safely. Here, the relationship between the bile duct and duodenal wall as observed fluoroscopically is of importance in judging the length of the incision. If the duct

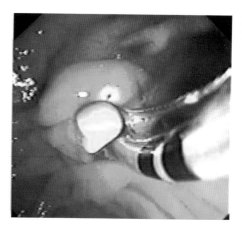

Fig. 34.24 Endoscopic papillotomy.

lies close to the duodenal wall and is dilated, a relatively long incision can be made safely. If the duct is not dilated for the most part, and fluoroscopy indicates a course distant from the duodenal wall, then it is safe to reduce the length of the incision. In difficult situations after initial failure of duct cannulation, interrupting the procedure and repeating endoscopic retrograde cholangiography (ERC) and EPT later on should be considered in patients in whom the indication is not urgent. A repeat intervention by the same endoscopist yielded a considerable increase (87.5%) in the success rate [47]. In addition, switching to a more experienced endoscopist, if available, should also be considered.

Precut Papillotomy

The precut papillotome (or modified Demling–Classen papillotome) described above basically has the same architecture as the standard papillotome, but with a short cutting wire that may extend to the tip of the cannula (**Fig. 34.26**). Its use is indicated when the standard papillotome cannot be selectively introduced into the desired duct to a sufficient depth. The precut papillotome is introduced into the papillary orifice, and the cautery wire is tensed in an 11-o'clock to 12-o'clock direction, approximating the direction of the ampulla of Vater. When the roof of the ampulla is incised as far as possible, the bile-stained mucosa can be seen. The precut papillotome can then be exchanged for the standard papillotome, with which selective

34

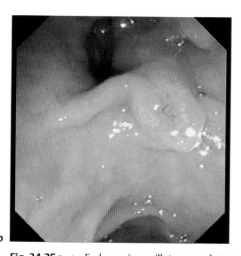
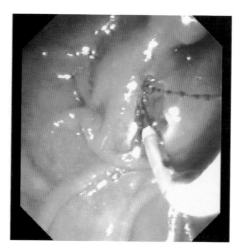
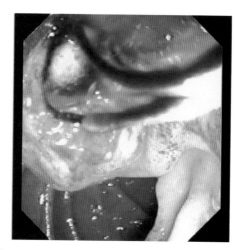

Fig. 34.25 a–c Endoscopic papillotomy and stone extraction.
a Papilla of Vater adjacent to a duodenal diverticulum.
b Insertion of the papillotome, cutting through the wire using HF-currents.
c Extraction of the stone using Dormia basket.

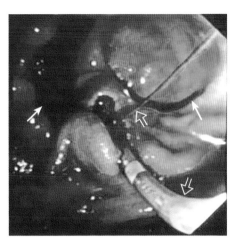

Fig. 34.26 Precut papillotomy alongside a ridge between juxtapapillary diverticula (thin arrow: diverticulum; thick arrows: papillotome).

plications [48–53]. Needle-knives are more problematic when the biliary ostium is not opened and instead a second lumen is generated, leading to perforation and false cannulations into the retroperitoneum. The major disadvantage of this method is thus a higher rate of complications, including bleeding, perforation, and pancreatitis, especially in the hands of inexperienced examiners. Kasmin et al. [54] assessed the safety and efficacy of needle-knife sphincterotomy in 72 patients in whom bile duct cannulation had been unsuccessful using standard procedures. An overall success rate of 93 % was reported by these experienced authors. Complications including pancreatitis, bleeding, and perforation occurred in eight of the 72 patients (11.1 %). The efficacy and safety of needle-knife fistulotomy and needle-knife precut papillotomy was further evaluated in a prospective randomized trial [55]. The first group included 74 patients who underwent needle-knife fistulotomy avoiding the papillary orifice, while a second group included 79 patients who underwent needle-knife precut papillotomy starting from the papillary orifice. Bile duct cannulation was successful in approximately 90 % of cases in both groups, and the overall complication rate was 13.1 %. In patients receiving needle-knife precut papillotomy, post-ERCP pancreatitis was observed in six of the 79 patients (7.6 %). In contrast to these results, Freeman [56] reported higher complication rates (24.3 %) using needle-knife precut sphincterotomy techniques in a series of 111 patients. The high rates of pancreatitis and bleeding might therefore prevent younger investigators from using the technique.

cannulation of the desired duct is usually successful. There may be instability in the papillotome's position within the papilla that impairs the direction and the depth of cutting. In this case, the application of a needle-knife may be preferable.

Needle-Knife Papillotomy (Figs. 34.27–34.29)

The needle-knife precut papillotomy technique has been used for difficult cannulation of the biliary tract since the 1980s. Needle-knife papillotomy is highly successful when performed by expert endoscopists, but is associated with an increased potential for com-

Needle-knife precutting technique. Most experts start the precutting sphincterotomy from the papillary orifice and extend the incision in short movements, with the action of the elevator causing a to-and-fro motion of the needle-knife; or by withdrawing the endo-

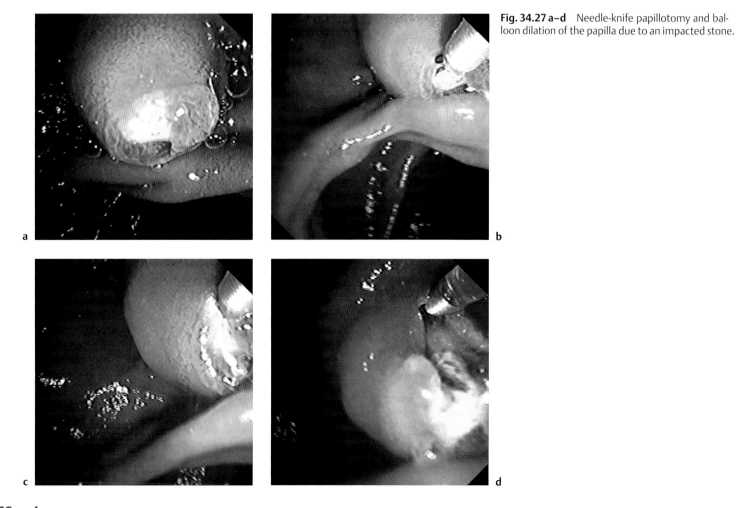

a

b

c

d

Fig. 34.27 a–d Needle-knife papillotomy and balloon dilation of the papilla due to an impacted stone.

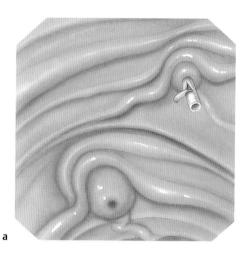
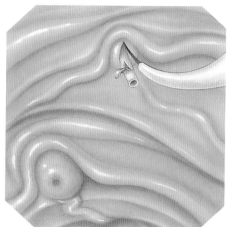

Fig. 34.28 a, b Needle-knife papillotomy over a stent in the minor papilla. (Reproduced with permission from Soehendra et al., *Praxis der therapeutischen Endoskopie,* Stuttgart: Thieme, 1997.)

a

b

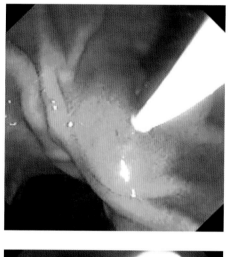
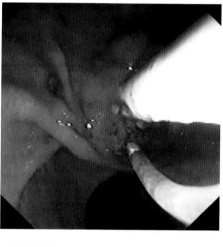

Fig. 34.29 a–d Needle-knife papillotomy over a stent in a patient with Billroth II anatomy.

a

b

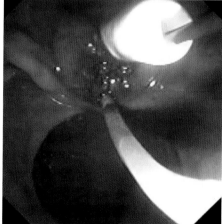
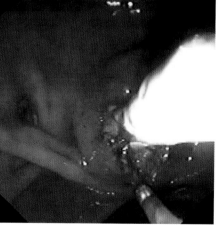

c

d

34

scope, making the needle-knife move progressively up the papilla (**Fig. 34.29**).

The needle-knife is initially lifted with the elevator and placed in contact with the bulging papilla approximately 5 mm from the orifice. The needle-knife is cut onto the papilla by dropping the elevator, and sometimes by gentle downward angulation of the endoscope. Starting the needle-knife sphincterotomy in either an upward or downward direction, as a rule, the incision should be made in the 11-o'clock to 12-o'clock direction from the orifice of the papilla, corresponding to the direction of the common bile duct. The exception to this rule (11-o'clock to 12-o'clock) is in patients with

post–Billroth II subtotal gastrectomy, who have the papilla in a "reversed" or "upside down" position. In these cases, the needle-knife should be placed at the six-o'clock position at the papillary orifice, and the incision should be made in a caudad direction. After the repeated to-and-fro motions of the needle-knife, with minimal pressure and using short bursts of current, seepage of bile may be seen, showing that entrance into the common bile duct has been achieved. Gentle probing with a blunt ERCP catheter can be used to enter the common bile duct, progressing to cholangiography or sphincterotomy as indicated.

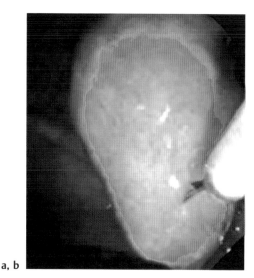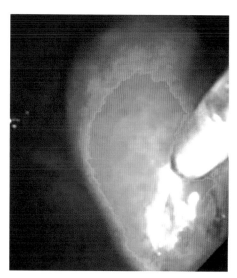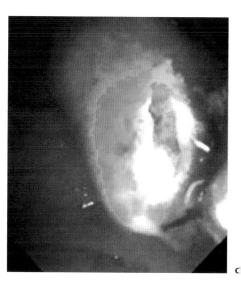

a, b

c

Fig. 34.30 a–c Fistulotomy using a needle-knife papillotome.

If free access to the common bile duct is not successfully obtained, a repeat examination can be arranged 4–7 days later, at which time the biliary orifice is usually evident and easily cannulated. In the case of a small papilla, periampullary diverticula, papillary stenosis, or extrinsic compression of the duodenum around the papilla—when needle-knife sphincterotomy may be technically difficult—injection of 1–2 mL of normal saline into the papillary tissue at the 12-o'clock position 1–2 mm above the superior margin of the papillary orifice makes the papilla clearly bulge into the duodenal lumen.

Fistulotomy, Papillectomy (Ampullectomy)

Endoscopic fistulotomy (choledochoduodenostomy) is another endoscopic technique for puncturing and incision of the common bile duct. This technique is appropriate when the orifice of the main papilla is obstructed. In these cases, the distal bile duct produces a prominent bulging of the duodenal wall that can be seen endoscopically proximal to the papilla (**Fig. 34.30**). The prominence of this intramural common bile duct (CBD) segment is usually the result of dilation of the distal bile duct proximal to the obstruction. In addition, it is advisable to inject contrast medium into the bile duct to demonstrate dilation and to establish the proximity of the bile duct to the wall of the duodenum. When these prerequisites have been met, the intramural segment is simply punctured using an electrosurgical device such as a needle-knife. It may be possible to complete the cutting procedure with a standard papillotome. As with the precut techniques, endoscopic fistulotomy should be performed only by the most experienced endoscopists.

Transpancreatic Sphincter Precutting Approach

A standard Olympus papillotome (Olympus Europe Ltd., Hamburg, Germany) is used to carry out the precut procedure using pure cutting current, with an Erbe electrosurgical generator and the cut mode set at step 3 (Erbe Elektromedizin Ltd., Tübingen, Germany). The cut is directed toward the 12-o'clock position to allow an approach to the bile duct over a length of 5–8 mm. To make this technique possible, the scope may also be pushed into a deeper position, with the small wheel allowing right lateral movement being used. Careful attention is given to performing the sphincterotomy incision directed toward the bile duct, through the septum

between the bile duct and the pancreatic duct, avoiding an incision into the deeper region of the papilla. The bile duct is then selectively cannulated once the ostium can be detected due to the secretion of bile. This technique was initially described by Goff [57] and subsequently validated in several studies in comparison with needle-knife precutting.

Several other studies have now validated the success of this precutting technique guided by placement of a wire in the pancreatic duct. The success and complication rates with the technique were initially investigated in 51 patients [58]. Contrast extravasation was observed in only one of the 51 patients. The overall complication rate with the technique was thus 2%, and there were no patients with post-ERCP pancreatitis. Akashi et al. [58] studied a total of 172 patients who underwent a pancreatic precut along the midline, above the papillary elevation, using either the common channel or the pancreatic duct in the ampulla of Vater for guidance. This technique did not use a guide wire. The septum between the pancreatic duct and the bile duct was removed, and separate openings to the pancreatic and bile ducts were created, followed by complete biliary sphincterotomy. Using this technique, biliary cannulation was successful in 95% of cases. Mild complications occurred in 10%. Similar results were observed in the study by Kahaleh et al. [59]. The authors reported immediate biliary access after pancreatic precutting in 85% of cases. Complications, including bleeding (2.3%), pancreatitis (8%), and retroperitoneal perforation (1.7%), occurred in 12% of the patients.

As there is still a substantial complication rate with the pancreatic precut, further improvement of the technique is needed. When using a pancreatic duct stent to guide difficult common bile duct cannulation, Goldberg et al. [60] reported a 97.4% success rate with bile duct cannulation (38 of 39 patients). Procedure-related pancreatitis occurred in two of the 39 patients (5.1%). Placement of a pancreatic stent during the wire-guided precut thus appears technically feasible, and a meta-analysis of prophylactic stent placement showed that this additional stent placement reduced the rate of pancreatitis [61]. Further studies to evaluate the benefit of prophylactic pancreatic stent placement after transpancreatic precut sphincterotomy are currently being conducted at our institution.

In the most recent prospective studies, pancreatic precut techniques were found to be extremely safe for cannulating the bile duct [62]. In this study, Weber et al. investigated 108 patients in whom bile duct access was difficult for various reasons. In contrast to the above study, an overall complication rate of 11.1% was observed. Successful bile duct cannulation using wire-guided transpancreatic

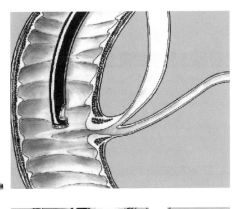 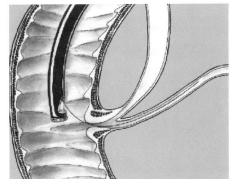

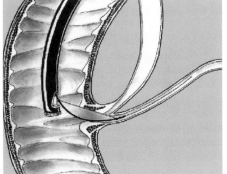 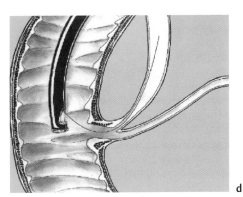

Fig. 34.31 a–d The pancreatic precut technique.
a Duodenoscope positioned in front of the papilla of Vater.
b Soft guide wire in main pancreatic duct.
c Incision of the papilla in 12 o'clock direction.
d Ostium of the CBD is now opened. Guide wire is introduced into the biliary system.

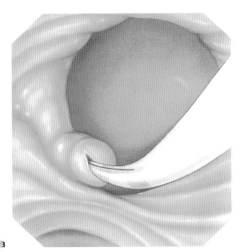 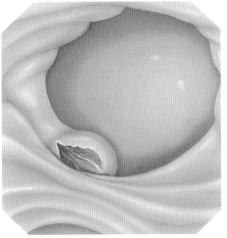

Fig. 34.32 a, b Papillotomy in a papilla positioned within a diverticulum.

sphincterotomy was achieved in 95.4 % of the patients. Placement of a soft guide wire in the pancreatic duct allowed orientation regarding the correct placement of the papillotome. When the papillotome was being introduced, precuts were performed in the direction of the presumed bile duct. This made the ostium of the bile duct visible, allowing precise control of the introduction of the catheter (**Fig. 34.31**). These data indicate that transpancreatic precut sphincterotomy is highly successful (95.4 %), with only a moderate rate of complications such as mild pancreatitis (5.6 %) and bleeding (5.6 %).

Minor Papilla Papillotomy

Papillotomy of the minor papilla is required in patients with symptomatic pancreas divisum. A catheter with a tapered tip is needed to cannulate the minute orifice. A stent with a diameter of 5–7 Fr can then be positioned as a guide for the subsequent needle-knife incision in a 9–11-o'clock direction. The stent can be removed a few days later.

Juxtapapillary Diverticula

Juxtapapillary diverticula are not associated with an increased risk of perforation in EPT. Occasionally, the papilla is entirely positioned within a diverticulum, and cannulation may be difficult or impossible. Even if the papillotome is placed in the bile duct, in some cases the distorted anatomy makes it difficult to control the incision (**Fig. 34.32**). If the papilla is at the distal margin of a shallow diverticulum, a ridge-like structure may bisect the diverticulum from proximal to distal and terminate at the papilla. This is usually the bile duct. EPT may be easier in this case, as the bile duct is clearly visible and the duct is close to the duodenal lumen. Selective biliary cannulation is often difficult when there is a juxtapapillary diverticulum, especially when the papilla is within the diverticulum (**Fig. 34.33**). Another technique can be used in which the papilla is kept out of the diverticulum by placing a pancreatic duct stent and needle-knife sphincterotomy is then carried out to obtain biliary access. Biliary entry was immediately successful at a second attempt in five of eight patients in whom the initial biliary cannulation had

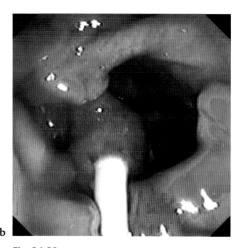
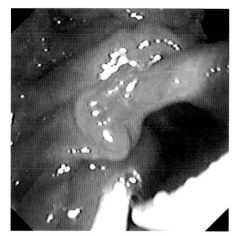
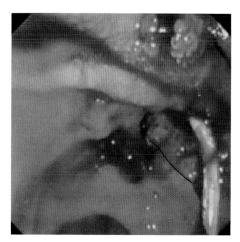

a, b

Fig. 34.33
a A percutaneously inserted biliary drain in a papilla located within a diverticulum.
b Needle-knife papillotomy over the stent.

Fig. 34.34 Antegrade papillotomy in a patient with Billroth II anatomy. The papillotome is inserted percutaneously, and cutting is controlled endoscopically.

failed. There is continuing debate regarding the possible relationship between juxtapapillary diverticula and biliary pathology, particularly bile duct stones.

Billroth II Gastrectomy

The papilla of Vater is occasionally difficult to find in patients who have undergone a Billroth procedure. The type of anastomosis (retrocolic, antecolic, or Roux-en-Y) may prohibit entry into the different loops or make it impossible to locate the papilla. In addition, the inverted position of the endoscope in relation to the papilla of Vater and the intramural segment of the common bile duct makes papillotomy technically demanding. Even using an endoscope with a forward-viewing lens does not always solve this problem. Papillotomes with a sigmoid shape (reverse bow) have been designed for use in these patients. These devices are believed to reduce the risk of injury to the pancreas. Other specialized instruments and techniques include graduated endoscopes, various steerable catheters, specialized papillotomes, and antegrade sphincterotomy via percutaneous transhepatic cholangioscopy (**Fig. 34.34**) [63–66]. Some believe that the most important technical development is represented by duodenoscopes with short distal tips. Fluoroscopy allows quick identification of the loop that the endoscope has entered. Identifying the papilla of Vater is the first important step, but intubation of the standard papillotome is frequently aligned with the pancreatic duct.

The success rates of endoscopic papillotomy in patients with a prior Billroth II gastrectomy have been reported as ranging from 66 % to 97 %. Good success rates have definitely been achieved with endoscopic techniques alone, but some investigators recommend using the percutaneous approach not just as a second-line treatment, but as an initial step (see the section on the rendezvous technique below).

Rendezvous Technique

This procedure is used when the papilla can be reached with the endoscope, but it is not possible to intubate it. A guide wire is therefore introduced into the biliary system via the percutaneous transhepatic route and is advanced through the papilla into the small bowel with radiographic monitoring. The guide wire is then grasped using the endoscope, and the papillotome is positioned in

the papilla of Vater over the guide wire. This method also has the advantage that the position of the papillotome is secured by the wire, while access to the bile duct is still ensured [14] (see **Fig. 34.22**).

Complications of Endoscopic Papillotomy

Short-Term Complications

Definitions. The principal complications of EPT are pancreatitis, hemorrhage, cholangitis, and perforation (**Table 34.2**) [67]. Only case reports have so far appeared regarding additional complications such as subcutaneous emphysema, pneumothorax, and pneumopericardium. When cholecystitis occurs after EPT, it is often difficult to judge whether it is a genuine complication, or simply the natural course of the disease in the presence of gallstones.

Pancreatitis. Hyperamylasemia frequently occurs after endoscopic papillotomy. The term "post-EPT pancreatitis" is used to describe abdominal pain that persists for at least 24 h, with an accompanying rise in serum enzymes (amylase, lipase) to 2.5–5 times normal levels [56].

Milder, spontaneously resolving *secondary hemorrhage* is a frequent occurrence after incision of the papilla of Vater. This is not regarded as a complication, but may suggest a risk of later hemorrhage. However, when hematemesis and/or anal blood loss occurs, with a fall in the hemoglobin level by at least 2 g/dL, this does constitute severe bleeding that represents a complication (**Fig. 34.35**).

Table 34.2 Complications of endoscopic papillotomy (from Freeman et al. [67])

	All		Severe		Fatal	
	n	%	n	%	n	%
Bleeding	48	2.0	12	0.5	2	0.1
Acute pancreatitis	127	5.4	9	0.4	1	<0.1
Acute biliary sepsis	24	1.0	2	0.1	1	<0.1
Perforation	8	0.3	5	0.2	1	<0.1
Miscellaneous	25	1.1	8	0.3	5	0.2
Total complications	229	9.8	38	1.6		
Fatal complications					10	0.4

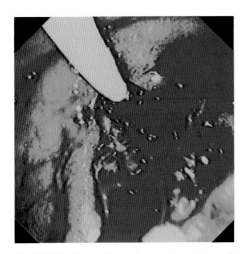

Fig. 34.35 Hemorrhage after endoscopic papillotomy.

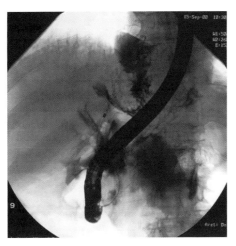

Fig. 34.36 Perforation after endoscopic papillotomy.

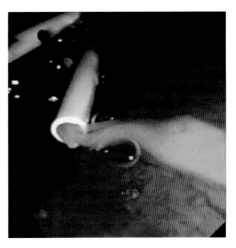

Fig. 34.37 Cholangitis after endoscopic papillotomy and stent insertion.

Perforations of the esophagus, stomach, and duodenum during passage of the endoscope are extremely rare, and usually require surgical treatment. Perforations of the duodenobiliary junction by the guide wire or papillotome can be recognized from the abnormal course of the guide wire as it passes the perforation site, or by cloudy contrast discharge into the retroperitoneum. In general, perforations of the ampulla or bile duct can be successfully treated using biliary drainage (stent, nasobiliary tube), parenteral nutrition, and antibiotic administration for a few days (**Fig. 34.36**).

Like the other complications, *cholangitis* can also occur after EPT at any grade of severity, including the septic form (**Fig. 34.37**). The causes include failure to remove an obstruction to drainage; the stent remaining wholly or partially in the bile duct; and the Dormia basket becoming detached and incapable of being removed from the common bile duct together with the stone that has been captured. Rarely, endoscopic instruments or accessories do not function correctly, so that the procedure has to be interrupted before the treatment goal has been achieved. In all cases, an attempt must be made to obtain effective drainage even when there is a persistent obstacle in the bile duct.

Rare complications of endoscopic gallstone therapy include gallstone ileus and perforation of the cystic duct. In older patients with comorbid conditions, disorders of other organs occasionally develop during the course of endoscopic treatment procedures—e. g., myocardial infarction or pulmonary embolism. There is no justification for a fatalistic view that these are events lying beyond the scope of endoscopic management.

Incision of the ampulla and biliary sphincter (Fig. 34.38).

Despite the increasing extension and expansion of the range of indications, the rate of complications has remained more or less constant, at approximately 10 %. Substantial variations in the distribution of the various complications are the result of the different techniques used—e. g., with the needle-knife—and of varying definitions of the type and severity of complications.

A very large American–Canadian multicenter study with a prospective design confirmed earlier retrospective observations and also identified risk factors for the occurrence of complications. In this study, by Freeman and colleagues [67], a total of 2347 patients were observed in detail before and after EPT. Complications occurred in 9.8 % of the cases, and 0.4 % of the patients died. Post-EPT pancreatitis was the most frequent complication, at 5.4 %, followed by hemorrhage at 2 %. Biliary sepsis (1 %) and perforation (0.3 %) were less important numerically.

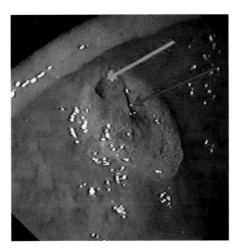

Fig. 34.38 Endoscopic papillotomy of both sphincters.

34

Risk factors. The most frequent ERCP-related complication is acute inflammation—i. e., pancreatitis—which is mild in the majority of patients and does not lead to a significantly extended hospital stay. The frequency of post-ERCP pancreatitis is similar in diagnostic and therapeutic procedures. Specific patient-related and technique-related characteristics that may increase the risk of post-ERCP complications can be identified. Several factors may be responsible for the pathogenesis of post-ERCP hyperamylasemia and pancreatitis, both technical and patient-related, acting independently or together [68–70]. Some technical factors are: frequent injection of contrast material into the pancreatic duct, especially when cannulation of the bile duct is difficult; the type of contrast medium used; injection under pressure, leading to complete acinar filling of the pancreas; the type of diathermy used; young female patients; pregnancy; and a history of previous pancreatitis [68,69]. Serum amylase levels higher than four to five times the upper limit of normal, together with pancreatic-type pain 24 h after ERCP strongly suggest the development of pancreatitis. If any of the predictive risk factors are found to coexist during a procedure, it is better either to abandon the procedure and try again later or, if the situation is urgent, to resort to an alternative technique such as precut or needle-knife papillotomy earlier [70].

Evangelou and his group stated that "Endoscopic papillotomy for stones by experts is safe, even in younger patients with normal ducts" [71]. In the study by Freeman et al. [67], some groups of patients were found to be at higher risk—adolescents, patients with

Table 34.3 Pancreatic sphincter hypertension is a significant risk factor for post-ERCP pancreatitis (from Patel et al. [72])

	PSH			No PSH		
	n	Σ	%	n	Σ	%
PEP after diagnostic ERCP	22	28	79	6	28	21
PEP after biliary EPT	13	16	81	3	16	19
PEP after subsequent ERCP/ manometric study	3	34*	8.5	2	9	22

* EPT/stenting failed in all cases.
EPT, endoscopic papillotomy; ERCP, endoscopic retrograde cholangiopancreatography; PEP, post-ERCP pancreatitis; PSH, pancreatic sphincter hypertension.

Table 34.4 Complication and mortality rates associated with needle-knife papillotomy in 691 patients who underwent endoscopic papillotomy for therapeutic indications at Nankai Hospital, Tianjin, China, between 1984 and 1999

Complication	Patients		Surgery required	Deaths
	n	%		
Bleeding	9	1.3	1	
Perforation	1	0.14	1	
Pancreatitis	15	2.1	2	1
Cholangitis	8	1.2	1	1
Acute cholecystitis	4	0.6	4	
Total	37		9	2

Complication rate 37/691 (5.35%); rate of surgery required 9/691 (1.3%); mortality rate 2/691 (0.29%).

Table 34.5 Frequency of use of the needle-knife papillotomy procedure and associated complication rates and mortality rates (after Huibregtse et al. [51])

First author, ref.	Frequency of use (%)	EPT		Needle-knife	
		Compli-cations (%)	Mor-tality (%)	Compli-cations (%)	Mor-tality (%)
Huibregtse 1986 [51]	19.2	2.1	0	2.6	0
Vaira 1989 [76]	< 1	6.9	0.6	–	0
Siegel 1989 [77]	–	–	–	6.7	0
Dowsett 1990 [52]	12.8	–	–	5.2	2
Tweedle 1991 [78]	4.2	7	0	12	0
Leung 1990 [53]	3.9	–	–	20	0
Booth 1990 [79]	9.7	9	0	16	1
Sherman 1991 [80]	15.4	7	0	6.2	0
Shakoor 1992 [81]	3.8	6	0.1	11	0
Martin 1992 [82]	–	–	–	6.3	0
Foutch 1995 [48]	11	9.7	0	5.7	0

EPT: endoscopic papillotomy.

a history of post-ERCP pancreatitis, and patients in whom sphincter of Oddi dysfunction (SOD) was the indication for EPT. An investigation conducted by Cotton's group confirmed that pancreatic sphincter hypertension is a significant risk factor for the development of post-ERCP pancreatitis (**Table 34.3**) [72]. Freeman et al. [67] also showed that the examination technique is an important factor; the more difficult the cannulation was, the more frequent the complications were. Another important point was the examiner's level of personal experience. Endoscopists with small case numbers (less than 50 EPTs per year) had a higher complication rate (not unexpectedly) than colleagues practicing the technique frequently.

Risk factors for the occurrence of bleeding during or after EPT are coagulation disorders, the presence of cholangitis, and anticoagulation therapy within 3 days before the EPT procedure. Mild bleeding during EPT also increases the probability of later hemorrhage. Another prospective study identified additional risk factors for hemorrhage during and after EPT, including coagulopathy, long incisions (> 5 mm), and admission to the intensive-care unit (comorbidity?) [72–75].

Higher complication rates when the needle-knife is used are observed in patients with SOD (8.6%) in comparison with patients who undergo needle-knife papillotomy for other indications (3.3%) (**Tables 34.4, 34.5**) [48,51–53,76–84]. The high morbidity rate in the series reported by Leung et al. [53] undoubtedly resulted from the fact that the needle-knife was always used when sphincterotomy with the standard papillotome had been unsuccessful. In the study by Freeman [56], use of the precut technique to obtain access to the bile duct was also identified as a specific risk factor. Complications are particularly to be feared when access to the bile duct or pancreatic duct has to be achieved forcibly in order to establish a diagnosis with EPT (**Table 34.6**).

Follow-up examinations. Some physicians consider that a plain radiograph of the right upper abdomen with the patient in the supine position should always be carried out as a routine procedure after needle-knife sphincterotomy. Others have proposed short-term follow-up with anteroposterior and oblique radiography, as well as regular clinical examinations of the patient for symptoms and physical evidence of perforation. If the needle-knife is used only by experienced endoscopists whose personal complication rates are low, these recommendations may not be necessary in all cases.

Prevention. There are also differences of opinion regarding the need for coagulation testing before standard sphincterotomy [30]. To prevent the coagulation effect during papillotomy, the use of pure cutting current has been proposed [84]. However, Gorelick and colleagues [85] have shown that hemorrhage after the use of cutting current can be significantly reduced by using mixed current during the papillotomy, without this leading to a higher rate of post-EPT pancreatitis. As was mentioned above, patients in whom the duodenobiliary junction is perforated by the guide wire or papillotome can usually be adequately treated with biliary drainage, intravenous nutrition, and antibiotics. Demands for routine prophylactic administration of antibiotics to prevent microbial inflammation of the pancreaticobiliary ductal system have not been generally accepted if there is no suspicion or evidence of cholangitis, cholecystitis, pancreatic pseudocysts, or similar conditions. However, the ESGE guideline contrary to this should be noted.

These substantial method-related problems have of course given rise to repeated quests for methods that might be capable of reducing the complication rate. In particular, a large number of agents and drugs to prevent post-ERCP and post-EPT pancreatitis have been investigated, although as yet without any marked success. Prophylactic administration of gabexate, somatostatin, and heparin has been studied [86–89]. Another interesting approach to reducing the rate of pancreatitis involves insertion of a stent into the pancreatic duct before carrying out EPT of the biliary system. Interesting initial results have been presented in particular for high-risk patients with sphincter of Oddi dysfunction [90]. A report that injection of botulinum toxin into the residual pancreatic sphincter after EPT may reduce the risk of pancreatitis has as yet only been presented in abstract form [91].

Pancreatic sphincterotomy. *Major duodenal papilla.* It was only after EPT of the biliary sphincter had become a widely used technique that pancreatic sphincterotomy was also attempted—mainly for the treatment of stones, dominant strictures, and leaks [92]. It was

V

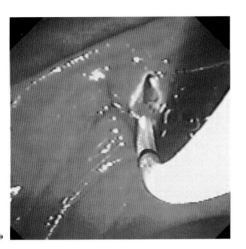
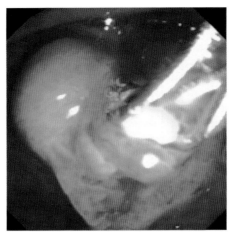
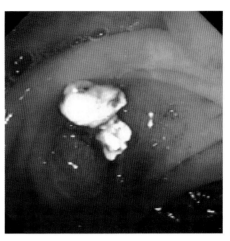

Fig. 34.39
a Endoscopic papillotomy of the pancreatic sphincter.

b Stone extraction from the pancreatic duct.

c Pancreatic duct stones.

Table 34.6 Complication rate and mortality rate associated with needle-knife papillotomy in 466 patients in whom diagnostic endoscopic retrograde cholangiopancreatography was intended (data from at Nankai Hospital, Tianjin, China, between 1984 and 1999)

Complication	Patients		Surgery required	Deaths (n)
	n	%		
Bleeding	6	1.2		
Perforation	1	0.2	1	
Pancreatitis	2	0.4	1	1
Cholangitis	0		0	
Acute cholecystitis	2	0.4	2	
Total	11		4	1

Complication rate 11/466 (2.36 %); rate of surgery required 4/466 (0.86 %); mortality rate 1/466 (0.21 %).

found that the risks, particularly for the occurrence of postintervention pancreatitis, did not differ significantly from those with biliary sphincterotomy. In a review of 349 patients, Desilets and colleagues observed short-term complications in only 5 % of the cases. Pancreatitis, hemorrhage, and perforation were also observed with this technique, as in biliary EPT (**Fig. 34.39**). During a follow-up period of 34 months (median), repeat interventions were required in 10 % of the cases (recurrent stenosis and expansion of the EPT), and there was no method-related mortality [93]. Introducing a stent into the pancreatic duct, either to serve as a "pathfinder" for EPT or to ensure drainage after EPT, appears to reduce the risk of pancreatitis. An interesting study on pancreatic sphincterotomy conducted by Cotton's group has reported a lower complication rate when the needle-knife papillotome was used, in comparison with the bow papillotome. The study also confirms the preventive effect of temporary stenting on the development of post-EPT pancreatitis, particularly after needle-knife EPT [94]. However, it must be admitted that the indication for the procedure and the success of endoscopic treatment are still matters of controversy, particularly in relation to chronic pancreatitis [95].

Papillotomy of the minor duodenal papilla. The most frequent anatomical variant in the pancreatic duct system is a fusion anomaly of the dorsal and ventral pancreatic duct primordia [96]. In this condition, the majority of the pancreas drains via the small minor papilla. The pancreatitis frequently observed with this variant is usually attributed to the drainage disorder caused by the disparity—although again, this interpretation is not undisputed [96]. Complications of EPT of the minor papilla in pancreas divisum include acute pancreatitis (13–70 %) and recurrent pain [27,97,98]. The use of stents reduces the risk of developing pancreatitis from 80 % in untreated patients to 10 % over a follow-up period of nearly 3 years [99] (**Fig. 34.28**). An endoscopic intervention with papillotomy and stent placement is by far the most effective form of treatment in the group of patients with recurrent acute episodes of pancreatitis (acute relapsing pancreatitis). Positive long-term results, with complete freedom from pain, are achieved in around 50 % of the cases [100]. The risks are similar to those with EPT at the major papilla, and also do not appear to be substantially different in terms of the numerical distribution [101]. Treatment of these complications is mainly conservative.

Long-Term Complications

The principal long-term complication after papillotomy is recurrent stenosis of the papilla of Vater, of the biliary or pancreatic sphincter (**Fig. 34.40**). This may encourage the development of recurrent stones, particularly in the bile duct, and cholangitis and pancreatitis may be caused. The frequency of cholangitis as a long-term complication after EPT varies considerably, with reports ranging from 1 % to 24 % [102,103].

In addition to papillary stenosis, bile duct strictures and intra-ampullary duodenal diverticula, the diameter of the bile duct also plays a role in the formation of recurrent stones. Bile duct dilation of more than 13 mm [104] or 22 mm [105] represents a risk factor for recurrent stones. An issue that has not been fully resolved is that of gallbladder in situ after EPT [106–108]. A general recommendation to remove the calculous gallbladder after EPT cannot be given. The occurrence of "biliary symptoms," with corresponding laboratory and ultrasound findings of cholecystitis, represents an indication for cholecystectomy.

Finally, some mention should be made of the issue of whether the risk of developing cholangiocellular carcinoma increases after EPT. The investigations carried out so far have not provided any conclusive evidence of this. However, the study by Hakamada et al. [109] should be noted—although it included patients who had undergone surgical sphincteroplasty a median of 18 years previously. The authors found that 7.4 % of the patients had cholangiocellular carcinoma; this topic will therefore continue to require attention.

34

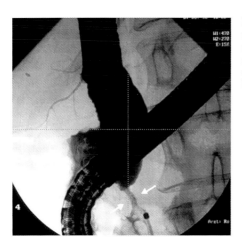

Fig. 34.40 Recurrent stenosis after endoscopic papillotomy (arrows), with prestenotic dilation of the common bile duct.

Table 34.7 Endoscopic papillotomy after Billroth II gastrectomy (after Huibregtse et al. [51])

First author, ref.	Frequency of use (%)	Complications (%)	Mortality (%)	Success (%)
Safrany 1980 [123]	–	4.3	0	66
Osnes 1986 [64]	34	4.2		92
Ricci 1989 [122]	51	4.7	0	89
Costamagna 1994 [124]	61	5.9	0	97
Meenan 1996 [125]	48	5.8	0*	95

Results and Outcome

Technical Success

EPT of the biliary sphincter. Even in the initial period after the method was introduced, success rates higher than 90% were reported. Currently, success rates approaching 100% are being reached (**Fig. 34.41**) [29,76,80,107,108,110–120]. The success rate with EPT here depends quite decisively on the examiner's experience, skill, and choice of equipment [121,122]. Even in this difficult situation, however, some research groups have achieved success rates of 90% (**Table 34.7**) [51,52,64,122–127]. After total gastrectomy and Roux-en-Y anastomosis, the papilla of Vater cannot be safely reached via the transduodenal route. Although a success rate of 33%

has been reported [127], this is an exception. The same also applies to biliodigestive anastomoses with the jejunum, and particularly to patients who have undergone a Whipple's procedure. In all of these cases, percutaneous transhepatic access to the bile duct system is a valuable alternative.

EPT of the pancreatic sphincter. Technically, sphincterotomy of the pancreatic duct does not differ substantially from that of the bile duct (apart from a slight alteration in the direction of the incision). Papillotomy of the minor papilla is more difficult, although the success rates are around 90% here as well, often with the use of a needle-knife (needle-knife EPT) [128]. The introduction of a stent before the EPT procedure provides better control of the direction of the incision, on the one hand, and reduces the risk of post-EPT pancreatitis on the other.

Effects of EPT. After successful EPT, the biliary sphincter is usually left in a nonfunctional condition [129], and the duodenal contents and pancreatic juice can flow into the bile duct. Increasing bacterial colonization develops, which may be of significance for the development of recurrent stones in the bile duct [130] but is otherwise of no clinical significance. The duodenobiliary reflux that can be observed radiographically is also without negative sequelae [8], provided there is no drainage disorder. Amylase measurements of the bile duct contents—which are initially increased after EPT—return to the pre-EPT values by 1 year after the procedure [131]. After EPT, the contractility of the gallbladder and nucleation time increase, and the cholesterol saturation time decreases [106,131,132].

It is currently assumed that EPT does not affect the risk of carcinoma in the bile duct region [8]. However, after surgical sphincteroplasty (median follow-up period 18 years), an increase in the frequency of cholangiocellular carcinoma has been observed [109].

EPT in Individual Indications

Although it was only the technical success of the intervention that used to be evaluated, today it is the course of the disease or functional disorder as affected by EPT that is assessed. This approach to the long-term results also includes the patient's assessment of the success of the procedure in relation to his or her symptoms and quality of life (the outcome). However, outcome research is still in its youth in the field of gastrointestinal endoscopy, and only very few studies meet the relevant criteria.

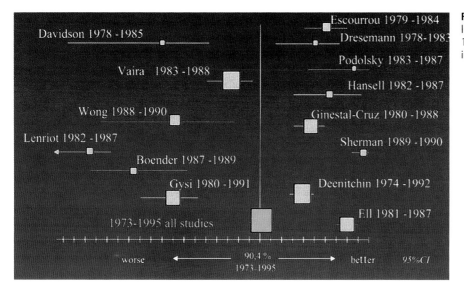

Fig. 34.41 Endoscopic papillotomy and choledocholithiasis: comparative success rates in the period 1973–1975 reported in a meta-analysis [138]. The bars indicate 95% confidence intervals.

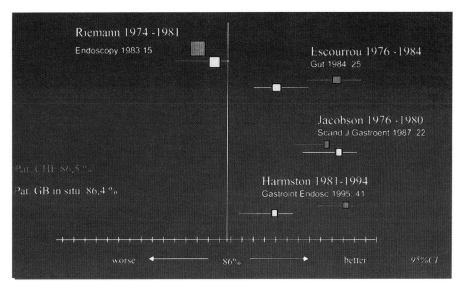

Fig. 34.42 Endoscopic papillotomy and choledocholithiasis: long-term results reported in a meta-analysis [138]. The bars indicate 95 % confidence intervals. The white squares indicate patients with gallbladder in situ (success rate 86.4 %) and the pink squares show those undergoing cholecystectomy (success rate 86.5 %).

Choledocholithiasis. Ever since its introduction, EPT has always been the method most frequently used in the treatment of choledocholithiasis. It provides access to the bile ducts, allowing removal of the stones in 90 % of cases using a simple Dormia basket or balloon [133,134]. If "difficult" stones are encountered—i. e., when the position of the stone (e. g., far proximal in the intrahepatic bile ducts or proximal to stenoses) or its size mean that it cannot be removed using the above techniques—then resort can be made to various technical innovations. In mechanical lithotripsy, even stones with a diameter of more than 20 mm can be successfully treated in nearly 80 % of cases [135,136]. Pulsed-dye lasers with stone recognition systems ("intelligent lasers") achieve fragmentation rates of 100 %, and are significantly superior to extracorporeal shock-wave lithotripsy (ESWL) [50]. ESWL can now be replaced by other, simpler, methods in all but a very few cases [50].

The long-term results with EPT after successful management of bile duct stones are good in both adults and children [137,138]. In a large meta-analysis including 10,335 patients, the results of EPT for choledocholithiasis were found to have improved significantly, probably due to the use of intraductal fragmentation of bile duct stones and combined use of EPT with percutaneous techniques. However, the complication rates have remained more or less constant [139]. The meta-analysis also showed that in around 90 % of the patients, no recurrent stones developed and there was continuing freedom from symptoms (**Fig. 34.42**) [116,140,141]. The risk factors for the development of recurrent stones were already mentioned above [139,142].

ERCP followed by cholecystectomy: therapeutic splitting. A combination of endoscopic stone treatment of the common bile ducts and laparoscopic cholecystectomy is today preferred by 80 % of surgeons, according to a study conducted in Europe [143–145]. There have been studies comparing preoperative endoscopic clearance of the CBD plus laparoscopic cholecystectomy with laparoscopic removal of the gallbladder and stones from the ducts [146,147]. The technically demanding technique of choledochoscopy and stone removal during laparoscopic cholecystectomy may in the future come into competition with the joint endoscopic–laparoscopic approach. However, it is already practiced in some centers [134,145]. In the presence of stones in the gallbladder and bile duct, cholecystectomy and choledochotomy can be discussed with the surgeon concerned on the basis of the individual case. In this situation, the mildness of the endoscopic procedure—although it may require several sessions in some cases—needs to be weighed up against the shorter hospitalization period after surgical treatment. Endo-

Table 34.8 Outcome of endoscopic papillotomy in high-risk patients with acute cholangitis in a meta-analysis [138]. There was a significant difference between the high-risk and low-risk patient groups (**P<0.5**)

	Success rate (%)	Complication rate (%)	Mortality rate (%)
Groups with >50 % high-risk patients *	87.7	10.7	3.7
Groups with <50 % high-risk patients †	73.8	11.9	7.2

* Boender et al. 1995 [13], Lam 1984 [147], Leung et al. 1989 [148], Himal 1991 [149], Lai et al. 1992 [150].
† Gogel et al. 1987 [11], Davidson et al. 1988 [107].

34

scopic treatment for choledocholithiasis in the context of laparoscopic cholecystectomy is already being practiced at some centers [134,145].

Cholangitis and biliary pancreatitis. EPT with removal of the stones and maintenance or restoration of bile drainage is the treatment of choice for the main complications of choledocholithiasis, cholangitis, and biliary pancreatitis. Particularly in the case of cholangitis, EPT—carried out as early as possible with stone removal and stent placement if appropriate—is now an undisputed and successful technique that has driven the surgical alternative into the background (**Table 34.8**) [11,13,107,138,139,147–152]. Risk factors for ERCP are age above 75, liver cirrhosis, kidney malfunction, and thrombocytopenia.

Biliary pancreatitis is defined as acute pancreatitis, detection of gallstones, and elevation of liver transaminases. ERC with EPT is also the treatment of choice in biliary pancreatitis when cholestasis with cholangitis is found, while absence of cholestasis is an unfavorable parameter. In a synopsis of three controlled studies [19–21], in addition to numerous uncontrolled reports [22], biliary EPT is regarded as a reasonable procedure that should be performed as soon as possible when septic cholangitis is present (**Table 34.9**) [20–23].

Sphincter of Oddi dysfunction (see also Chapters 45 and 52). Fifty percent of patients with acute relapsing pancreatitis have a form of SOD that responds well to EPT (**Table 34.10**) [5,18,152–157]. Numerous patients with pancreatic SOD become free of symptoms even after EPT of the biliary sphincter alone [18]. In biliary sphincter of Oddi dysfunction, EPT is all the more successful the more definite

Table 34.9 Three controlled studies [20–22] and an uncontrolled study [23]. Endoscopic papillotomy is indicated in patients with biliary pancreatitis and cholestasis

First author, ref.	Patients (n)	Time to ERC	Severe pancreatitis	ERC success rate	Gallstones
Neoptolemos 1988 [22]	121	72 h	44 %	88 %	85 %
Fan 1993 [20]	195	24 h	42 %	90 %	65 %
Fölsch 1997 [21]	238	72 h*	14 %	96 %	46 %
Nowak 1998 [23]	280	24 h	n.a.	n.a.	n.a.
Sharma (pooled)	834	Analysis of above	30 %	92 %	61 %

ERC, endoscopic retrograde cholangiography.

Table 34.10 Sphincter of Oddi dysfunction: long-term outcome of biliary endoscopic papillotomy correlated with abnormal biliary and pancreatic sphincter pressures (after Eversman et al. [157])

	Baseline sphincter pressure		
Biliary sphincter	Elevated	Elevated	Normal
Pancreatic sphincter	Normal	Elevated	Elevated
Patients (n)	37	62	33
Repeat intervention	16 % *	29 % †	39 % ‡

* vs. †, $P < 0.05$; * vs. ‡, $P < 0.05$.

the diagnosis is, or the more marked the changes it causes. In patients with type I biliary SOD, characterized by increased cholestasis parameters, delayed biliary drainage, and a dilated bile duct, the success rates are 80–95 %. The results with EPT in the type II and III groups of patients are markedly poorer, and probably differ due to the heterogeneity of the underlying disorders.

Brush cytology and biopsy during ERCP. Tissue collection during endoscopic retrograde cholangiography (ERC) is widely performed to provide a definitive diagnosis in patients with indeterminate strictures. To obtain tissue, brush cytology and/or forceps biopsy are routinely performed with wire-guided brushes and with forceps of different sizes, with branches usually 3–4 mm wide. Several studies have reported that brush cytology and/or forceps biopsy are sensitive in the diagnosis of malignant biliary strictures [158,159]. Pugliese et al. [160] reported that both brush cytology and forceps biopsy are sensitive in patients with malignant bile duct strictures. The 36 patients included in the study had a wide range of diagnoses, including pancreatic cancer (n = 12), cholangiocarcinoma (n = 10), intra-ampullary carcinoma (n = 9), metastatic cancer (n = 3), and malignant islet cell tumor (n = 2). Cytological and histological investigation was positive in 19 of the 36 patients (53 %). Ponchon et al. [161] also investigated a heterogeneous patient group with malignant bile duct stenoses. In this series, 27 of the 73 patients had cholangiocarcinomas, although the stricture locations were not stated. Cytology was positive for malignant bile duct stenosis in 12 of 25 patients (48 %), and biopsy was positive for the condition in seven of 16 (44 %) patients. In a study by our own group [162], brush cytology and forceps biopsy were carried out in patients with hilar cholangiocarcinoma treated in our department from 1995 to 2005. The location of the biliary strictures was classified relative to the confluence of the hepatic ducts as described by Bismuth. The Bismuth stage was classified using ERC at the time of the primary diagnosis. In this series, the sensitivity of transpapillary brush cytology was 24.4 % relative to the number of cytological samples and 33.9 % relative to the number of patients, whereas the sensitivity of forceps biopsy was 32.1 % relative to the number of tissue samples and 44.8 % relative to the number of patients. Combined cytology and biopsy increased the sensitivity only slightly to 33.3 % and 46.4 %, respectively. Overall, the sensitivity for detecting cancer

only averages around 50 %, and new approaches to improve detection are currently being investigated.

Stent insertion. After favorable experience with endoscopic treatment of stenotic bile duct tumors, which has largely replaced palliative surgery [163–168], the indication for endoscopic stent placement is increasingly being extended to benign changes as well. Strictures can be caused by chronic inflammatory or cicatricial changes in the bile ducts and papilla of Vater—such as papillary stenosis due to adenomyosis, passage of stones, or surgical dilation—as well as by primary sclerosing cholangitis (PSC) (**Fig. 34.43**). In PSC, the often characteristic strictures of the small and smallest intrahepatic branches cannot be reached with stent therapy, although good treatment of distal stenoses, particularly of the common bile duct and papilla of Vater, is possible. It should always also be borne in mind that recognition and treatment of malignant transformation in PSC should not be delayed, depriving the patient of the option of timely transplantation. Choledochoceles and choledochal cysts can be treated using EPT with a good success rate (approximately 80 %) if they are located in the intraduodenal part of the CBD. In the early forms, the symptoms of cholestasis, cholangitis, and pancreatitis resolve very quickly after the procedure. Long-term complications of choledochal cysts include recurrent stenoses of the papilla, which are easily treated, and strictures of the hepatic duct.

Postoperative bile duct lesions. The advent of laparoscopic cholecystectomy, with its associated increase in iatrogenic bile duct lesions—above all among novices to the method—led to a parallel increase in endoscopic therapy. In postoperative bile duct strictures, usually occurring at the level of the cystic duct outlet, rigorous stent treatment, potentially with several simultaneous stents positioned for at least 1 year, is successful (i. e., with persistent dilation and freedom from symptoms without any need for further intervention) in up to 60 % or more of cases [169–173].

Another increasingly important indication for stent treatment is anastomotic stenosis after liver transplantation. Biliary complications, mainly consisting of strictures, are observed in 10–35 % of cases after transplantation. Endoscopic intervention is regarded as the treatment of choice [174,175]. In cases of postoperative biliary leakage, the results of papillotomy with placement of a nasobiliary drain or stent are even more satisfactory. The success rates reach 100 %, and it is particularly notable that successful treatment is long-lasting [176–178]. In the large series reported by Haber's group, only three of 100 patients with large postoperative bile duct leaks required surgery (two patients with clips across the CBD, one with an incomplete cholecystectomy) [176].

ERCP and chronic pancreatitis. Biliary stenoses in the context of chronic pancreatitis respond to stent treatment at best only in the initial period. The long-term results are disappointing. Only about 30 % of the patients treated can manage after stent therapy without further bile duct treatment [179,180]. It is not yet clear whether

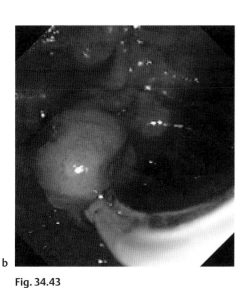
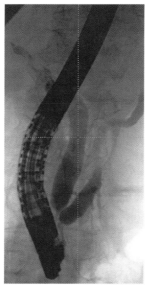
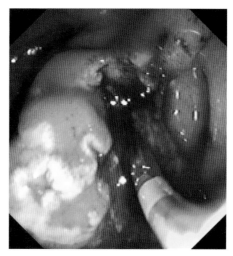

Fig. 34.43
a An enlarged papilla.
b Papillary stenosis causing obstruction of the biliary duct as well as the pancreatic duct.

c Sphincterotomy.

surgical treatment, either with duodenum-preserving pancreatic head resection or with biliodigestive anastomosis alone, should be used with this type of stenosis. Studies conducted by our own research group have led to the conclusion that the long-term results with endoscopic treatment are inferior to those with surgery [181]. However, selected patients may well be able to receive successful long-term stent treatment, although regular stent exchanges are necessary. The use of the currently available types of metal stent for this type of benign condition should be regarded with considerable reservation, as these stents are virtually impossible to remove and can therefore lead to local problems, or make later interventions difficult or entirely impossible.

Several reviews in the literature suggest that most physicians consider pancreatic duct stenting to be a safe and effective treatment in advance of surgical procedures for patients with chronic abdominal pain [179]. The primary goal of endoscopic stent placement is to relieve pain. The multicenter study by Rösch et al. [180], a major study in this field, focused on pain relief during stent therapy in patients with chronic pancreatitis. In an intention-to-treat analysis, approximately 67 % were successfully treated. Similarly, Morgan et al. [181] investigated a total of 25 patients and assessed pain relief. Fourteen patients had a single stent placed, with a mean duration of 93 days and a range of 10–975 days. Eleven patients had sequential stents placed (after relapses), with a mean duration of 173 days and a range of 47–349 days.

To evaluate the clinical benefits of endoscopic intervention with subsequent stent therapy, we prospectively investigated a total of 19 consecutive patients with symptomatic chronic pancreatitis [182]. The pain situation was evaluated before stent therapy, during stent therapy, and over a 2-year follow-up period after stent extraction. Initially, sphincterotomy was performed in each patient to facilitate ductal access and minimize potential papillary trauma due to stent placement or stone extraction. In chronic pancreatitis, pancreatic sphincterotomy for ductal access followed by tube drainage is reported to have short-term morbidity rates of less than 1 %. We used a short-term stenting protocol to avoid long-term stricture development. The mean duration of stenting was 5.6 months. It should be mentioned that a recent study has also emphasized the benefits of surgery in this indication; our experience, however, is that most patients favor endoscopy at the onset of these clinical problems [183].

Alternatives to EPT

Balloon dilation of the papilla. As discussed above, the risks of EPT also depend on the endoscopist's level of experience and the technical facilities at his or her disposal. Although endoscopic papillotomy led to a reduction in the level of risk associated with surgical procedures in the biliary and pancreatic system, which were the only methods available previously, seeking alternatives that might be capable of reducing the risks and complication rates even further is nevertheless a valuable and justified approach. Current possibilities might include balloon dilation of the papilla of Vater, as proposed by Staritz et al. [65]. In a randomized study, Bergman and colleagues [184] showed that balloon dilation (sphincteroclasia) is as successful as EPT in choledocholithiasis. The increase in the rate of pancreatitis that had been feared was not observed. However, in an editorial [185], the same authors point out that sphincteroclasia can at present only be regarded as an important supplement to EPT for use in difficult situations. This is because balloon dilation of the papilla only allows smaller stones to be extracted, and in 9 % of the cases Bergman and colleagues also had to use EPT for dilation to be able to extract medium-sized and larger stones. Tanaka et al. reported similar complication rates and success rates (90 %), but pointed out that any endoscopist who carries out balloon dilation of the papilla must also be in a position to switch to EPT in case of failure [186]. Recently, Lee et al. combined EPT with dilation using an 18-mm balloon to remove multiple larger stones [187].

Wehrmann and colleagues [188] have developed an interesting alternative or supplementary procedure after primary EPT. Endoscopic injection of botulinum toxin into the papilla led to a marked improvement of the symptoms in some 50 % of the patients affected. In addition, patients who responded well to botulinum toxin injection also appear to derive particular benefit from EPT, so that this form of injection therapy might possibly be of predictive value for treatment planning.

Double-balloon endoscopy has also recently made it possible to reach the papilla or biliary anastomosis using a retrograde approach [189–191]. Papillotomy, dilation and stent insertion through the long scopes has been reported. Currently, it remains to be investigated whether this procedure is superior to percutaneous transhepatic biliary drainage.

34

References

1. Classen M, Demling L. Endoskopische Sphinkterotomie der Papilla Vateri und Steinextraktion aus dem Ductus choledochus. Dtsch Med Wochenschr 1974;99:496–7.
2. Kawai K, Akaska Y, Murakami K, Tada M, Kohli Y, Nakajima M. Endoscopic sphincterotomy of the ampulla of Vater. Gastrointest Endosc 1974;20:148–51.
3. Geenen JE. Endoscopic papillotomy. In: Demling L, Classen M, editors. Endoscopic sphincterotomy of the papilla of Vater. Stuttgart: Thieme; 1978. p. 81–2.
4. Zimmon DS, Falkenstein DB, Kessler RE. Endoscopic papillotomy for choledocholithiasis. N Engl J Med 1975;293:1181–2.
5. Geenen JE, Nash JA. The role of sphincter of Oddi manometry and biliary microscopy in evaluating idiopathic recurrent pancreatitis. Endoscopy 1998;30:237–41.
6. Huibregtse K, Tytgat GNJ. Carcinoma of the ampulla of Vater: the endoscopic approach. Endoscopy 1988;20:223–6.
7. Cotton PB, Geenen JE, Sherman S, Cunningham JT, Howell DA, Carr-Locke DL, et al. Endoscopic sphincterotomy for stones by experts is safe, even in younger patients with normal ducts. Ann Surg 1998;227:201–4.
8. Frimberger E. Long-term sequelae of endoscopic papillotomy. Endoscopy 1998;30(Suppl 2):A221–7.
9. Tarnasky PR, Tagge EP, Hebra A, Othersen B, Adams DB, Cunningham JT, et al. Minimally invasive therapy for choledocholithiasis in children. Gastrointest Endosc 1998;47:189–92.
10. Classen M, Sandschin W, Born P. 25 years' experience with ERCP and endoscopic papillotomy (EPT) [abstract]. Endoscopy 1997;29:E6.
11. Gogel HK, Runyon BA, Volpicelli NA, Palmer RC. Acute suppurative obstructive cholangitis due to stones: treatment by urgent endoscopic sphincterotomy. Gastrointest Endosc 1987;33:210–3.
12. Venu RP, Geenen JE, Hogan WJ, Dodds WJ, Wilson SW, Stewart ET. Role of endoscopic retrograde cholangiopancreatography in the diagnosis and treatment of choledochocele. Gastroenterology 1984;87:1144–9.
13. Boender J, Nix GAJJ, de Ridder MAJ, Dees J, Schütte HE, van Buuren HR, et al. Endoscopic sphincterotomy and biliary drainage in patients with common bile duct stones. Am J Gastroenterol 1995;90:233–8.
14. Classen M, Born P. Endoscopic sphincterotomy. In: Tytgat GNJ, Classen M, Waye JD, Nakazawa S, editors. Practice of therapeutic endoscopy. 3 rd ed. Philadelphia: Saunders; 2000. p. 129–46.
15. Baker AR, Neoptolemos JP, Carr-Locke DL, Fossard DP. Sump syndrome following choledochoduodenostomy and its endoscopic treatment. Br J Surg 1985;72:433–5.
16. Del Olmo L, Merono E, Moreira VF, Garcia T, Garcia-Plaza A. Successful treatment of postoperative external biliary fistulas by endoscopic sphincterotomy. Gastrointest Endosc 1988;34:307–9.
17. El Sheikh Mohamed AR, al Karawi MA, Yasawy MI. Modern techniques in the diagnosis and treatment of gastrointestinal and biliary tree parasites. Hepatogastroenterology 1991;38:180–8.
18. Al Karawi MA, El Sheikh Mohamed AR, Sultan Khurro M, Neuhaus H. Bedeutung der Endoskopie in der Diagnostik und Therapie gastrointestinaler und biliarer Parasiten. Internist 1988;29:807–14.
19. Sharma VK, Howden CW. Metaanalysis of randomized controlled trials of endoscopic retrograde cholangiography and endoscopic sphincterotomy for the treatment of acute biliary pancreatitis. Am J Gastroenterol 1999;94:3211–4.
20. Fan ST, Lai ECS, Mok FPT, Lo CM, Zheng SS, Wong J. Early treatment of acute biliary pancreatitis by endoscopic papillotomy. N Engl J Med 1993;328:228–32.
21. Fölsch UR, Nitsche R, Lüdtke R, Hilgers RA, Creutzfeldt W. Early ERCP and papillotomy compared with conservative treatment for acute biliary pancreatitis. The German Study Group on Acute Biliary Pancreatitis. N Engl J Med 1997;336:237–42.
22. Neoptolemos JP, Carr-Locke DL, London NJ, Bailey IA, James D, Fossard DP. Controlled trial of urgent endoscopic retrograde cholangiopancreatography and endoscopic sphincterotomy versus conservative treatment for acute pancreatitis due to gallstones. Lancet 1988;ii:979–83.
23. Nowak A, Nowakowska-Dulawa E, Marek TA, Rybicka J. Final results of the prospective randomized controlled study on endoscopic sphincterotomy versus conventional management in acute biliary pancreatitis [abstract]. Gastroenterology 1998;108:A380.
24. Cotton PB. Pancreas divisum: curiosity or culprit? Gastroenterology 1985;89:1431–5.
25. Bernard JP, Sahel J, Giovannini M, Sarles H. Pancreas divisum is a probable cause of acute pancreatitis: a report of 137 cases. Pancreas 1990;5:248–54.
26. Lehman GA, Sherman S, Nisi R, Hawes RH. Pancreas divisum: results of minor papilla sphincterotomy. Gastrointest Endosc 1993;39:1–8.
27. Mehta SN, Pavone E, Barkun AN. Outpatient therapeutic ERCP: a series of 262 consecutive cases. Gastrointest Endosc 1996;44:443–9.
28. Howell DA, Oringer JA, Ku PM. Overnight hospitalization following endoscopic sphincterotomy produces a higher quality outcome [abstract]. Gastrointest Endosc 1999;49:AB217.
29. ASGE Standards of Practice Committee, Levy MJ, Anderson MA, Baron TH, Banerjee S, Dominitz JA, et al. Position statement on routine laboratory testing before endoscopic procedures. Gastrointest Endosc 2008;68:827–32.
30. Seymour RA, Williams FM, Oxley A, Ward A, Fearns M, Brighan K, et al. A comparative study of the effects of aspirin and paracetamol (acetaminophen) on platelet aggregation and bleeding time. Eur J Clin Pharmacol 1984;26:567–71.
31. Riphaus A, Wehrmann T, Weber B, Arnold J, Beilenhoff U, Bitter H, et al. [S 3-guidelines—sedation in gastrointestinal endoscopy]. Z Gastroenterol 2008;46:1298–330. German.
32. Rey JR, Axon A, Budzynska A, Kruse A, Nowak A. Guidelines of the European Society of Gastrointestinal Endoscopy (ESGE): antibiotic prophylaxis for gastrointestinal endoscopy. Endoscopy 1998;30:318–24.
33. Soehendra N, Binmoeller KF, Seifert H, Schreiber HW. Praxis der therapeutischen Endoskopie. Stuttgart: Thieme; 1997.
34. Martin DF, England R, Martin O. The safety sphincterotome: the device, the technique, and preliminary results. Endoscopy 1998;30:375–8.
35. Seiffert H, Schmitt T, Dietrich CF, Caspary JW, Wehrmann T. Endoscopic sphincterotomy with a newly developed baby papillotome: a prospective randomized study [abstract]. Gastrointest Endosc 1999;49:AB131.
36. Johlin FC, Tucker RD, Ferguson S. The effect of guidewires during electrosurgical sphincterotomy. Gastrointest Endosc 1992;38:536–40.
37. Schoenfeld PS, Jones DM, Lawson JM. Conducted current on guidewires in single lumen papillotomes. Gastrointest Endosc 1991;37:344–6.
38. Riemann JF, Seuberth K, Demling L. Clinical application of a new mechanical lithotriptor for smashing common bile duct stones. Endoscopy 1982;14:226–30.
39. Riemann JF, Seuberth K, Demling L. Mechanical lithotripsy through the intact papilla of Vater. Endoscopy 1983;15:111–3.
40. Bonnel DH, Liguory CE, Cornud FE, Lefebvre JFP. Common bile duct and intrahepatic stones: results of transhepatic electrohydraulic lithotripsy in 50 patients. Radiology 1991;180:345–8.
41. Classen M, Hagenmüller F, Knyrim K, Frimberger E. Giant bile duct stones: nonsurgical treatment. Endoscopy 1988;20:21–6.
42. Martin EC, Wolff M, Neff RA, Casarella WJ. Use of the electrohydraulic lithotriptor in the biliary tree in dogs. Radiology 1981;139:215–7.
43. Tanaka M, Yoshimoto H, Ikeda S, Matsumoto S, Guo RX. Two approaches for electrohydraulic lithotripsy in the common bile duct. Surgery 1985;98:313–8.
44. Neuhaus H. Fragmentation of pancreatic stones by extracorporeal shockwave lithotripsy. Endoscopy 1991;23:161–5.
45. Neuhaus H, Hoffmann W, Zillinger C, Classen M. Laser lithotripsy of difficult bile duct stones under direct visual control. Gut 1993;34:415–21.
46. Neuhaus H, Zillinger C, Born P, Ott R, Allescher H, Rösch T, et al. Randomized study of intracorporeal laser lithotripsy versus extracorporeal shockwave lithotripsy for difficult bile duct stones. Gastrointest Endosc 1998;47:327–34.
47. Ramirez FC, Dennert B, Sanowski RA. Success of repeat ERCP by the same endoscopist. Gastrointest Endosc 1999;49:58–61.
48. Foutch PG. A prospective assessment of results for needle-knife papillotomy and standard endoscopic sphincterotomy. Gastrointest Endosc 1995;41:25–32.
49. Fuji T, Amano H, Ohmura R, Akiyama T, Aibe T, Takemoto T. Endoscopic pancreatic sphincterotomy: technique and evaluation. Endoscopy 1989;21:27–30.
50. Rabenstein T, Ruppert T, Schneider HT, Hahn EG, Ell C. Benefits and risks of needle-knife papillotomy. Gastrointestinal Endosc 1997;46:207–11.
51. Huibregtse K, Katon RM, Tytgat GN. Precut papillotomy via fine-needle knife papillotome: a safe and effective technique. Gastrointestinal Endosc 1986;32:403–5.
52. Dowsett JF, Polydorou AA, Vaira D, D'Anna LM, Ashraf M, Croker J, et al. Needle knife papillotomy: how safe and how effective? Gut 1990;31:905–8.
53. Leung JWC, Banez VP, Chung SCS. Precut (needle knife) papillotomy for impacted common bile duct stones at the ampulla. Am J Gastroenterol 1990;85:991–3.

54. Kasmin FE, Cohen D, Batra S, Cohen SA, Siegel JH. Needle-knife sphincterotomy in a tertiary referral center: efficacy and complications. Gastrointest Endosc 1996;44:48–53.

55. Mavrogiannis C, Liatsos C, Romanos A, Petoumenos C, Nakos A, Karvountzis G. Needle-knife fistulotomy versus needle-knife precut papillotomy for the treatment of common bile duct stones. Gastrointest Endosc 1999; 50:334–9.

56. Freeman M. Complications of endoscopic biliary sphincterotomy: a review. Endoscopy 1997;29:288–97.

57. Goff JS. Common bile duct pre-cut sphincterotomy: transpancreatic sphincter approach. Gastrointest Endosc 1995;41:502–5.

58. Akashi R, Kiyozumi T, Jinnouchi K, Yoshida M, Adachi Y, Sagara K. Pancreatic sphincter pre-cutting to gain selective access to the common bile duct: a series of 172 patients. Endoscopy 2004;36:405–10.

59. Kahaleh M, Tokar J, Mullick T, Bickston SJ, Yeaton P. Prospective evaluation of pancreatic sphincterotomy as a precut technique for biliary cannulation. Clin Gastroenterol Hepatol 2004;2:971–7.

60. Goldberg E, Titus M, Haluszka O, Darwin P. Pancreatic-duct stent placement facilitates difficult common bile duct cannulation. Gastrointest Endosc 2005;62:592–6.

61. Singh P, Das A, Isenberg G, Wong RC, Sivak MV Jr, Agrawal D, et al. Does prophylactic pancreatic stent placement reduce the risk of post-ERCP acute pancreatitis? A meta-analysis of controlled trials. Gastrointest Endosc 2004;60:544–50.

62. Weber A, Roesch T, Pointner S, Born P, Neu B, Meining A, et al. Transpancreatic precut sphincterotomy for cannulation of inaccessible common bile duct: a safe and successful technique. Pancreas 2008;36:187–9.

63. Osnes M, Myren J. Endoscopic retrograde cholangiopancreatography (ERCP) in patients with Billroth II gastrectomies. Endoscopy 1975;7:227–32.

64. Osnes M, Rosseland AR, Aabakken L. Endoscopic retrograde cholangiography and endoscopic papillotomy in patients with a previous Billroth II resection. Gut 1986;27:1193–8.

65. Staritz M, Baas U, Ewe K, Meyer zum Büschenfelde KH. ERCP using a special catheter with external steering: a reliable aid in typical ERCP problems. Endoscopy 1985;17:26–8.

66. Wurbs D, Dammermann R, Osenberg FW, Classen M. Descending sphincterotomy of the papilla of Vater through the T-drain under endoscopic view: variants of endoscopic papillotomy (EPT). Endoscopy 1978;10: 199–203.

67. Freeman ML, Nelson DB, Sherman S, Haber GB, Herman ME, Dorsher PJ, et al. Complications of endoscopic biliary sphincterotomy. N Engl J Med 1996;335:909–18.

68. Vandervoort J, Soetikno RM, Tham TC, Woong RC, Ferrari AP, Mentes H, et al. Risk factors for complications after performance of ERCP. Gastrointest Endosc 2002;56:652–6.

69. Mehta SN, Pavone E, Barkun JS, Bouchard S, Barkun AN. Predictors of post-ERCP complications in patients with suspected choledocholithiasis. Endoscopy 1998;30:457–63.

70. Christoforidis E, Goulimaris I, Kanellos I, Tsalis K, Demetriades C, Betsis D. Post-ERCP pancreatitis and hyperamylasemia: patient-related and operative risk factors. Endoscopy 2002;34:286–92.

71. Evangelou H, Eng D, Bosco JJ, Hanson BL, Hoffman BJ, Rahaman SM, et al. Endoscopic sphincterotomy for stones by experts is safe, even in younger patients with normal ducts. Ann Surg 1998;227:201–4.

72. Patel R, Hawes RH, Nelles SE, Cunningham JT, Payne KM, Cotton PB. Pancreatic sphincter hypertension is a significant risk factor for post-ERCP pancreatitis [abstract]. Gastrointest Endosc 1999;49:653.

73. Rabenstein T, Hoepfner L, Roggenbuch S, Framke B, Martus P, Hochberger J, et al. Hemorrhage after EPT: risk factors and endoscopic management: final results of a prospective study [abstract]. Gastrointest Endosc 2000; 51:4619.

74. Rabenstein T, Schneider HAT, Hahn EG, Ell C. 25 years of endoscopic sphincterotomy in Erlangen: assessment of the experience in 3498 patients. Endoscopy 1998;30:A194–201.

75. Rabenstein T, Ruppert T, Schneider HT, Hahn EG, Ell C. Benefits and risks of needle-knife papillotomy. Gastrointest Endosc 1997;46:207–11.

76. Vaira D, D'Anna L, Ainley C, Dowsett J, Williams S, Baillie J, et al. Endoscopic sphincterotomy in 1000 consecutive patients. Lancet 1989;2: 431–4.

77. Siegel JH, Ben-Zvi JS, Pullano W. The needle knife: a valuable tool in diagnosis and therapeutic ERCP. Gastrointest Endosc 1989;35:499–503.

78. Tweedle DE, Martin DF. Needle knife papillotomy for endoscopic sphincterotomy and cholangiography. Gastrointest Endosc 1991;37:518–21.

79. Booth FV, Doerr RJ, Khalafi RS, Luchette FA, Flint LM Jr. Surgical management of complications of endoscopic sphincterotomy with precut papillotomy. Am J Surg 1990;159:132–5.

80. Sherman S, Ruffolo TA, Hawes RH, Lehman GA. Complications of endoscopic sphincterotomy: a prospective series with emphasis on the increased risk associated with sphincter of Oddi dysfunction and nondilated bile ducts. Gastroenterology 1991;101:1068–75.

81. Shakoor T, Geenen JE. Pre-cut papillotomy. Gastrointest Endosc 1992;38: 623–7.

82. Martin DF, Tweedle DE. Risks of precut papillotomy and the management of patients with duodenal perforation. Am J Surg 1992;163:273–4.

83. Cotton PB. Precut papillotomy: a risky technique, for experts only. Gastrointest Endosc 1989;35:578–9.

84. Elta GH, Barnett JL, Wille RT, Brown KA, Chey WD, Scheiman JM. Pure cut electrocautery current for sphincterotomy causes less post-procedure pancreatitis than blended current. Gastrointest Endosc 1998;47:149–53.

85. Gorelick AB, Cannon ME, Barnett JL, Chey WD, Scheiman JM. Sphincterotomy outcome with two different electrocautery currents [abstract]. Gastrointest Endosc 1999;49(Part 2):AB179.

86. Andriulli A, Leandr G, Niro G, Mangia A, Festa V, Gambassi G, et al. Pharmacologic treatment can prevent pancreatic injury after ERCP: a meta-analysis. Gastrointest Endosc 2000;51:1–7.

87. Bordas JM, Toledo-Pimentel V, Llach J, Elena M, Mondelo F, Gines A, et al. Effects of bolus somatostatin in preventing pancreatitis after endoscopic pancreatography: results of a randomized study. Gastrointest Endosc 1998;47:230–4.

88. Cavallini G, Titobello A, Frulloni L, Masci E, Mariani A, Di Francesco V, et al. Gabexate for the prevention of pancreatic damage related to endoscopic retrograde cholangiopancreatography. N Engl J Med 1996;335:919–23.

89. Rabenstein T, Ell C, Franke B, Schneider HF, Hahn EG. Kann eine niedrigdosierte Antikoagulation das Risiko einer akuten Pankreatitis nach endoskopischer Sphinkterotomie (EST) senken? Z Gastroenterol 1998;36:721.

90. Tarnasky PR, Palesch YY, Cunningham JT, Mauldin PD, Cotton PB, Hawes RH. Pancreatic stenting prevents pancreatitis after biliary sphincterotomy in patients with sphincter of Oddi dysfunction. Gastroenterology 1998;115:1518–24.

91. Gorelick AB, Barnett JL, Chey WD, Elta GH. A novel method to reduce post-ERCP pancreatitis in patients with sphincter of Oddi dysfunction: botulinum toxin injection in the residual pancreatic sphincter [abstract]. Gastrointest Endosc 2000;51(Part 2):AB239.

92. Kozarek RA, Ball TJ, Patterson DJ, Brandabur JJ, Traverso LW, Raltz S. Endoscopic pancreatic duct sphincterotomy: indications, technique and analysis of results. Gastrointest Endosc 1994;40:592–8.

93. Desilets DJ, Howell DA, Elton E, Dy RM, Hanson BL. Endoscopic pancreatic sphincterotomy: long-term follow-up [abstract]. Gastrointest Endosc 2000;51(Part 2):AB180.

94. Patel R, Hawes RH, Cunningham JT, Payne KM, Cotton PB. Pancreatitis after pancreatic sphincterotomy: bow papillotome vs. needle-knife [abstract]. Gastrointest Endosc 1999;49:652.

95. Riemann JF, Jakobs R. Pankreasgang-Stenting bei chronischer Pankreatitis: Kontroversen. Z Gastroenterol 2000;38:365–6.

96. Boerma D, Huibregtse K, Gulik TM, Rauws EAJ, Obertop H, Gouma DJ. Long-term outcome of endoscopic stent placement for chronic pancreatitis associated with pancreas divisum. Endoscopy 2000;32:452–6.

97. Cohen SA, Kasmin FE, Siegel JH. Minor papilla sphincterotomy in pancreas divisum. Gastrointest Endosc 1994;40:117–8.

98. Galdermans D, Michielsen P, Pelckmans P, Cremer M, van Maercke Y. Postendoscopic sphincterotomy stenosis. Endoscopy 1989;21:237–9.

99. Lans JI, Geenen JE, Johanson JF, Hogan WJ. Endoscopic therapy in patients with pancreas divisum and acute pancreatitis: a prospective, randomized, controlled clinical trial. Gastrointest Endosc 1992;38:430–4.

100. Catalano MF, Sial SH, Geenen JE, Hogan WJ. Minor papilla stent therapy in patients with symptomatic pancreas divisum: indications, efficacy and long-term outcome [abstract]. Gastrointest Endosc 2000;51(Part 2): AB203.

101. Kozarek RA, Ball TJ, Patterson DJ. Endoscopic approach to pancreatic duct calculi and obstructive pancreatitis. Am J Gastroenterol 1992;87:600–3.

102. Bergman JJGHM, van der Mey S, Rauws EAJ, Tijssen JGP, Gouma DJ, Tytgat GNJ, et al. Long-term follow-up after endoscopic sphincterotomy for bile duct stones in patients younger than 60 years of age. Gastrointest Endosc 1996;44:643–9.

103. Gregg JA, De Girolami P, Carr-Locke DL. Effects of sphincteroplasty and endoscopic sphincterotomy on the bacteriologic characteristics of the common bile duct. Am J Surg 1985;149:668–71.

34

104. Kim DI, Kim MH, Lee SK. The risk factors for the recurrence of primary common bile duct stones after endoscopic biliary sphincterotomy [abstract]. Gastrointest Endosc 2000;51:4639.

105. Costamagna G, Tringali A, Mutignani M. Endoscopic sphincterotomy for common bile duct stones: long-term follow-up and risk analysis for recurrence [abstract]. Gastrointest Endosc 2000;51:4633.

106. Caroli-Bosc FX, Montet JC, Salmon L, Demarquay JF, Dumas R, Montet AM, et al. Effect of endoscopic sphincterotomy on bile lithogenicity in patients with gallbladder in situ. Endoscopy 1999;31:437–41.

107. Davidson BR, Neoptolemos JP, Carr-Locke DL. Endoscopic sphincterotomy for common bile duct calculi in patients with gallbladder in situ considered unfit for surgery. Gut 1988;29:114–20.

108. Dresemann G, Kautz G, Bunte H. Long-term results of endoscopic sphincterotomy in patients with gallbladder in situ. Dtsch Med Wochenschr 1988;113:500–5.

109. Hakamada K, Sasaki M, Endoh M, Itoh T, Morita T, Konn M. Late development of bile duct cancer after sphincteroplasty: a ten- to twenty-two-year follow-up study. Surgery 1998;121:488–92.

110. Tanaka M, Konomi H, Matsunaga H, Yokohata K, Utsonomiya N, Takeda T. Endoscopic sphincterotomy for common bile duct stones: impact of recent technical advances. J Hepatobiliary Pancreat Surg 1997;4:16–9.

111. Wong PY, Lane MR, Hamilton I. Endoscopic management of bile duct stones at Auckland Hospital in 1988 and 1989. N Z Med J 1991;104:403–5.

112. Lenriot JP, Le-Neel JC, Hay JM, Jaeck D, Millat B, Fagniez PL. Retrograde cholangiopancreatography and endoscopic sphincterotomy for biliary lithiasis: prospective evaluation in surgical circle. Gastroenterol Clin Biol 1993;17:244–50.

113. Boender J, Nix GA, de Ridder MAJ, van Blankenstein M, Schutte HE, Dees J, et al. Endoscopic papillotomy for common bile duct stones: factors influencing the complication rate. Endoscopy 1994;26:209–16.

114. Gysi B, Schmassmann A, Scheurer U, Halter F. 12 years of endoscopic stone removal. Schweiz Med Wochenschr 1993;123:1115–7.

115. Escourrou J, Cordova JA, Lazorthes F, Frexinos J, Ribet A. Early and late complications after endoscopic sphincterotomy for biliary lithiasis with and without the gallbladder "in situ." Gut 1984;25:598–602.

116. Hansell DT, Millar MA, Murray WR, Gray GR, Gillespie G. Endoscopic sphincterotomy for bile duct stones in patients with intact gall bladders. Br J Surg 1989;76:856–58.

117. Ginestal-Cruz A, Grima N, Correia AP, Duarte V, Correia JP. Endoscopic sphincterotomy in choledocholithiasis: analysis of an experience of 530 interventions. Acta Med Port 1990;3:133–40.

118. Deenitchin GP, Konomi H, Kimura H, Ogawa Y, Naritomi G, Chijiiwa K, et al. Reappraisal of safety of endoscopic sphincterotomy for common bile duct stones in the elderly. Am J Surg 1995;170:51–4.

119. Ell C, Rabenstein T, Ruppert T, Forster P, Hahn EG, Demling L. 20 years of endoscopic papillotomy: analysis of 2752 patients in Erlangen Hospital. Dtsch Med Wochenschr 1995;120:163–7.

120. Kim MH, Lee SK, Lee MH, Myung SJ, Yoo BM, Seo DW, et al. Endoscopic retrograde cholangiopancreatography and needle-knife sphincterotomy in patients with Billroth II gastrectomy: a comparative study of the forward-viewing endoscope and the side-viewing duodenoscope. Endoscopy 1997;29:82–5.

121. Van Buuren HR, Boender J, Nix GA, van Blankenstein M. Needle-knife sphincterotomy guided by a biliary endoprosthesis in Billroth II gastrectomy patients. Endoscopy 1995;27:229–32.

122. Ricci E, Bertoni G, Conigliaro R, Contini S, Mortilla MG, Bedogni G. Endoscopic sphincterotomy in Billroth II patients: an improved method using a diathermic needle as sphincterotome and a nasobiliary drain as guide. Gastrointest Endosc 1989;35:47–50.

123. Safrany L, Neuhaus B, Portocarrero G, Krause S. Endoscopic sphincterotomy in patients with Billroth II gastrectomy. Endoscopy 1980;12:16–22.

124. Costamagna G, Mutignani M, Perri V, Gabrielli A, Locicero P, Crucitti F. Diagnostic and therapeutic ERCP in patients with Billroth II gastrectomy. Acta Gastroenterol Belg 1994;57:155–62.

125. Meenan J, Rauws EA, Huibregtse K. Benign biliary strictures and sclerosing cholangitis. Gastrointest Endosc Clin N Am 1996;6:127–38.

126. Hintze RE, Adler A, Veltzke W, Abou-Rebyeh H. Endoscopic access to the papilla of Vater for endoscopic retrograde cholangiopancreatography in patients with Billroth II or Roux-en-Y gastrojejunostomy. Endoscopy 1997;29:69–73.

127. Siegel JH, Ben-Zvi JS, Pullano W, Cooperman A. Effectiveness of endoscopic drainage for pancreas divisum: endoscopic and surgical results in 31 patients. Endoscopy 1990;22:129–33.

128. Bergman JJGHM, van Berkel AM, Groen AK, Schoeman MN, Offerhaus J, Tytgat GNJ, et al. Biliary manometry, bacterial characteristics, bile com-

129. Tanaka M, Takahata S, Konomi H, Matsunaga H, Yokohata K, Takeda T, et al. Long-term consequence of endoscopic sphincterotomy for bile duct stones. Gastrointest Endosc 1998;48:465–9.

130. Sugiyama M, Atomi Y. Does endoscopic sphincterotomy cause prolonged pancreaticobiliary reflux? Am J Gastroenterol 1999;94:795–8.

131. Sharma BC, Agarwal DK, Baijal SS, Negi TS, Choudhuri G, Saraswat VA. Effect of endoscopic sphincterotomy on gallbladder bile lithogenicity and motility. Gut 1998;42:288–92.

132. Lehman GA. Endoscopic therapy and lithotripsy: are these effective options? Bethesda, MD: American Gastroenterological Association; 1996 (AGA Postgraduate Course Digestive Diseases Week Supplement).

133. Wurbs DF, Sivak MV. Calculus disease of the bile ducts. In: Sivak MV, editor. Gastroenterologic endoscopy. Philadelphia: Saunders; 2000. p. 923–47.

134. Nakajima M, Yasuda K, Cho E, Mukai H, Ashihara T, Hirano S. Endoscopic sphincterotomy and mechanical basket lithotripsy for management of difficult common bile duct stones. J Hepatobiliary Pancreat Surg 1997;4:5–10.

135. Schneider MU, Matek W, Bauer R, Domschke W. Mechanical lithotripsy of bile duct stones in 209 patients. Effect Tech Adv Endosc 1988;20:248–53.

136. Catalano MF, Nayor R, Geenen JE. ERCP for CBD stones in children: presentation, efficacy and long-term outcome [abstract]. Gastrointest Endosc 1999;49:191.

137. Catalano MF, Khan FN, Sial SH, Geenen JE. Long-term outcome of biliary and pancreatic endoscopic sphincterotomy in adolescents [abstract]. Gastrointest Endosc 2000;51:3567.

138. Classen M, Sandschin W, Born P, Kassem AM. 20 years' experience in the endoscopic therapy of acute biliary cholangitis: a meta-analysis [abstract]. Endoscopy 1997;29:E52.

139. Jacobsen O, Matzen P. Long-term follow-up study of patients after endoscopic sphincterotomy for choledocholithiasis. Scand J Gastroenterol 1987;22:903–6.

140. Harmston GE, DiSario JA, Bjorkman DJ. Endoscopic therapy for common bile duct stones (CBD): long-term outcomes [abstract]. Gastrointest Endosc 1995;41:AB399.

141. Vlodov J, Abdullah M, Lapin S. Cholecystectomy should follow sphincterotomy in patients with choledocholithiasis: a meta-analysis [abstract]. Digestive Diseases Week Abstracts 2000:287.

142. Cotton PB, Williams CB. Practical gastrointestinal endoscopy. 3rd ed. Cambridge, MA: Blackwell Scientific, 1990.

143. Neoptolemos JP, Carr-Locke DI, Fossard DP. A prospective randomised study of preoperative endoscopic sphincterotomy versus surgery alone on common bile duct stones. Br Med J 1987;294:470–4.

144. Neubrand M, Sackmann M, Caspary WF, Feussner H, Schild H, Lauchart W, et al. Leitlinien der Deutschen Gesellschaft für Verdauungs- und Stoffwechselkrankheiten zur Behandlung von Gallensteinen. Z Gastroenterol 2000;38:449–68.

145. Rhodes M, Sussman L, Cohen L, Lewis MP. Randomised trial of laparoscopic exploration of common bile duct versus postoperative endoscopic retrograde cholangiography for common bile duct stones. Lancet 1998; 351:159–61.

146. Suc B, Escat J, Cherqui D, Fourtanier G, Hay JM, Fingerhut A, et al. Surgery vs. endoscopy as primary treatment in symptomatic patients with suspected common bile duct stones: a multicenter randomized trial. French Associations for Surgical Research. Arch Surg 1998;133:702–8.

147. Lam SK. A study of endoscopic sphincterotomy in recurrent pyogenic cholangitis. Br J Surg 1984;71:262–6.

148. Leung JW, Chung SC, Sung JJ, Banez VP, Li AK. Urgent endoscopic drainage for acute suppurative cholangitis. Lancet 1989;i:1307–9.

149. Himal HS. The role of endoscopic papillotomy in ascending cholangitis. Am Surg 1991;57:241–4.

150. Lai ECS, Mok FPT, Tan ESY, Lo CM, Fan ST, You KT, et al. Endoscopic biliary drainage for severe acute cholangitis. N Engl J Med 1992;326:1582–6.

151. Tarnasky PR, Cotton PB. Early ERCP and papillotomy for acute biliary pancreatitis. N Engl J Med 1997;336:1835.

152. Kaw M, Verma R, Brodmerkel GJ Jr. ERCP, biliary analysis, sphincter of Oddi manometry (SOM) in idiopathic pancreatitis (IP) in response to endoscopic sphincterotomy (ES) [abstract]. Am J Gastroenterol 1996;91: 1935A.

153. Coyle W, Tarnasky P, Knapple W. Evaluation of unexplained acute pancreatitis using ERCP, sphincter of Oddi manometry (SOM) and endoscopic ultrasound [abstract]. Gastrointest Endosc 1996;43:378A.

154. Botoman VA, Kozarek RA, Novell LA, Patterson DJ, Ball TJ, Wechter DG, et al. Long-term outcome after endoscopic sphincterotomy in patients with

position and histological changes fifteen to seventeen years after endoscopic sphincterotomy. Gastrointest Endosc 1997;45:400–5.

biliary colic and suspected sphincter of Oddi dysfunction. Gastrointest Endosc 1994;40:165–70.

155. Geenen JE, Hogan WJ, Dodds WJ, Toouli J, Venu RP. The efficacy of endoscopic sphincterotomy after cholecystectomy in patients with sphincter-of-Oddi dysfunction. N Engl J Med 1989;320:82–7.

156. Gill M, Freeman ML, Cars OW. Long-term outcome of endoscopic sphincter of Oddi dysfunction [abstract]. Gastrointest Endosc 2000:51:AB137.

157. Eversman D, Fogel E, Phillips S, Sherman S, Lehman G. Sphincter of Oddi dysfunction (SOD): long-term outcome of biliary sphincterotomy (BES) correlated with abnormal biliary and pancreatic sphincters [abstract]. Gastrointest Endosc 1999;49:116.

158. Jailwala J, Fogel EL, Sherman S, Gottlieb K, Flueckiger J, Bucksot LG, et al. Triple-tissue sampling at ERCP in malignant biliary obstruction. Gastrointest Endosc 2000;51:383–90.

159. Mansfield JC, Griffin SM, Wadehra V, Matthewson KA. A prospective evaluation of cytology from biliary strictures. Gut 1997;49:671–7.

160. Pugliese V, Conio M, Nicolò G, Saccomanno S, Gatteschi B. Endoscopic retrograde forceps biopsy and brush cytology of biliary strictures: a prospective study. Gastrointest Endosc 1995;42:520–6.

161. Ponchon T, Gagnon P, Berger F, Labadie M, Liaras A, Chavaillon A, et al. Value of endobiliary brush cytology and biopsies for the diagnosis of malignant bile duct stenosis: results of a prospective study. Gastrointest Endosc 1995;42:565–72.

162. Weber A, von Weyhern C, Fend F, Schneider J, Neu B, Meining A, et al. Endoscopic transpapillary brush cytology and forceps biopsy in patients with hilar cholangiocarcinoma. World J Gastroenterol 2008;14:1097–101.

163. Born P, Rösch T, Brühl K, Sandschin W, Weigert N, Ott R, et al. Long-term outcome in patients with advanced hilar bile duct tumors undergoing palliative endoscopic or percutaneous drainage. Z Gastroenterol 2000;38:483–9.

164. Chang WH, Kortan P, Haber GB. Outcome in patients with bifurcation tumors who undergo unilateral versus bilateral hepatic duct drainage. Gastrointest Endosc 1998;47:354–62.

165. Dowsett JF, Polydorou A, Vaira D. Endoscopic stenting for malignant biliary obstruction: how good really? A review of 641 consecutive patients [abstract]. Gut 1988;29:1458A.

166. Huibregtse K. Endoscopic biliary and pancreatic drainage. New York: Thieme; 1988.

167. Nayar R, Catalano MF, Geenen JE. Experience with choledochal cysts of the biliary tract in an adult population at a large GI referral center [abstract]. Gastrointest Endosc 1999;49:499.

168. Bergman JJGHM, van den Brink GR, Rauws EAJ, deWit L, Obertop H, Huibregtse K, et al. Treatment of bile duct lesions after laparoscopic cholecystectomy. Gut 1996;38:141–7.

169. Born P, Rösch T, Brühl K, Sandschin W, Allescher HD, Frimberger E, et al. Long-term results of endoscopic and percutaneous transhepatic treatment of benign biliary strictures. Endoscopy 1999;31:725–31.

170. Coene PPLO, Tytgat GNJ, Huibregtse K. Endoscopic stenting for postoperative biliary strictures. Gastrointest Endosc 1992;38:12–8.

171. Davids PHP, Tanka AKF, Rauws EAJ, van Gulik TM, van Leeuwen DJ. Benign biliary strictures: surgery or endoscopy? Ann Surg 1994;217:237–43.

172. Rizk RS, McVicar JP, Emond MJ, Rohrmann CA Jr, Kowdley KV, Perkins J, et al. Endoscopic management of biliary strictures in liver transplant recipients: effect on patient and graft survival. Gastrointest Endosc 1998;47:128–35.

173. Rossi AF, Grosso C, Zanasi G, Gambitta P, Bini M, De Carlis L, et al. Long-term efficacy of endoscopic stenting in patients with stricture of the biliary anastomosis after orthotopic liver transplantation. Endoscopy 1998;30:360–6.

174. Born P, Brühl K, Rösch T, Ungeheuer A, Neuhaus H, Classen M. Long-term follow-up of endoscopic therapy in patients with post-surgical leakage. Hepatogastroenterology 1996;43:477–82.

175. Ryan ME, Geenen JE, Lehman GA, Aliperti G, Freeman ML, Silverman WB, et al. Endoscopic intervention for biliary leaks after laparoscopic cholecystectomy: a multicenter review. Gastrointest Endosc 1998;47:261–6.

176. Sandha GS, Bourke MJ, Haber GB. Endoscopic therapy in 207 bile leaks: validation of a treatment strategy [abstract]. Gastrointest Endosc 2000; 51:4670.

177. Born P, Rösch T, Brühl K, Ulm K, Sandschin W, Frimberger E, et al. Long-term results of endoscopic treatment of biliary duct obstruction due to pancreatic disease. Hepatogastroenterology 1998;45:833–9.

178. Smits ME, Rauws EAJ, van Gulik TM, Gouma DJ, Tytgat GNJ, Huibregtse K. Long-term results of endoscopic stenting and surgical drainage for biliary stricture due to chronic pancreatitis. Br J Surg 1996;83:764–8.

179. Cremer M, Devière J, Delhaye M, Baize M, Vandermeeren A. Stenting in severe chronic pancreatitis: results of medium-term follow-up in seventy-six patients. Endoscopy 1991;23:171–6.

180. Rösch T, Daniel S, Scholz M, Huibregtse K, Smits M, Schneider T, et al. Endoscopic treatment of chronic pancreatitis: a multicenter study of 1000 patients with long-term follow-up. Endoscopy 2002;34:765–71.

181. Morgan DE, Smith JK, Hawkins K, Wilcox CM. Endoscopic stent therapy in advanced chronic pancreatitis: relationships between ductal changes, clinical response, and stent patency. Am J Gastroenterol 2003;98:821–6.

182. Weber A, Schneider J, Neu B, Meining A, Born P, Schmid RM, et al. Endoscopic stent therapy for patients with chronic pancreatitis: results from a prospective follow-up study. Pancreas 2007;34:287–94.

183. Cahen DL, Gouma DJ, Nio Y, Rauws EA, Boermeester MA, Busch OR, et al. Endoscopic versus surgical drainage of the pancreatic duct in chronic pancreatitis. N Engl J Med 2007;356:676–84.

184. Bergman JJGHM, Rauws EAJ, Fockens P, van Berkel AM, Bossuyt PMM, Tijssen JGP, et al. Randomised trial of endoscopic balloon dilatation versus endoscopic sphincterotomy for removal of bile duct stones. Lancet 1997;349:1124–9.

185. Bergman JJ, Huibregtse K. What is the current status of endoscopic balloon dilation for stone removal? Endoscopy 1998;30:43–5.

186. Tanaka S, Sawayama T, Yoshioka T. Endoscopic papillary balloon dilation and endoscopic sphincterotomy for bile duct stones: long-term outcomes in a prospective randomized controlled trial. Gastrointest Endosc 2004;59:614–8.

187. Lee DK, Lee BJ. EST, EPBD and EPLBD (cut, stretch, or both?). In: Niwa H, Tajiri H, Nakajima M, editors. New challenges in gastrointestinal endoscopy. New York: Springer, 2008. p. 385–97.

188. Wehrmann T, Seifert H, Seipp M, Lembcke B, Caspary WF. Endoscopic injection of botulinum toxin for biliary sphincter of Oddi dysfunction. Endoscopy 1998;30:702–7.

189. Chu YC, Yang CC, Yeh YH, Chen CH, Yueh SK. Double-balloon enteroscopy application in biliary tract disease—its therapeutic and diagnostic functions. Gastrointest Endosc 2008;68:585–91.

190. Maaser C, Lenze F, Bokemeyer M, Ullerich H, Domagk D, Bruewer M, et al. Double balloon enteroscopy: a useful tool for diagnostic and therapeutic procedures in the pancreaticobiliary system. Am J Gastroenterol 2008;103:894–900.

191. Chu YC, Su SJ, Yang CC, Yeh YH, Chen CH, Yueh SK. ERCP plus papillotomy by use of double-balloon enteroscopy after Billroth II gastrectomy [abstract]. Gastrointest Endosc 2007;66:1234.

34

35 Gastrointestinal Stenting

Todd H. Baron and Richard A. Kozarek

Introduction

Endoscopic palliation of luminal obstruction can be achieved with the use of gastrointestinal stents. Although rigid esophageal stents were initially used for palliation of dysphagia, self-expanding stents composed of metal or plastic materials are now almost exclusively used. Self-expanding plastic and fully covered self-expanding metal stents have been used to treat benign esophageal conditions. Self-expanding metal stents are used for palliation of malignant gastroduodenal and colonic obstruction and can be deployed as far distally from the mouth or as far proximally from the anus as can be reached with long endoscopes passed either orally or rectally. This chapter reviews the use of stents in the gastrointestinal tract.

Basic Principles

Self-expanding metal stents (SEMS) are composed of a variety of metal alloys with varying shapes and sizes, depending on the individual manufacturer and organ of placement [1]. SEMS are preloaded in a collapsed (constrained) position, mounted on a small-diameter delivery catheter. A central lumen within the delivery system allows for passage over a guide wire. Once the guide wire has been advanced beyond the site of pathology, the predeployed stent is passed over the guide wire and positioned across the stricture. The constraint system is released or withdrawn, which results in subsequent radial expansion of the stent and of the stenosed lumen (if present) during deployment (**Fig. 35.1**). The radial expansile forces and degree of shortening differ between stent types [2]. SEMS may also have a covering membrane (covered or coated stents) to close fistulas and prevent tumor ingrowth through the mesh wall (which leads to recurrent obstruction).

The uncovered portion of SEMS becomes deeply incorporated into both the tumor and the surrounding tissue [3,4]. This prevents migration. Covering of the SEMS prevents embedding and promotes stent migration; fully covered metal stents do not embed and can be removed. Partially covered stents are therefore most commonly used in malignant conditions.

Esophageal Stenting

In the early 1990s, SEMS were introduced for palliation of malignant dysphagia [5]. More recently, a self-expanding plastic stent (SEPS) has been used for the treatment of benign esophageal disease, including esophageal fistulas, stenoses, and anastomotic leaks. Stent placement is a frequently used method for palliation of malignant dysphagia. Before 1990, endoscopically placed rigid plastic stents with fixed internal and external diameters were used. SEMS are now used almost exclusively and have advantages over conventional plastic tubes [6]. The predeployment diameter of the SEMS delivery system is 5–10 mm, requiring minimal or no dilation before placement. After placement, SEMS gradually expand, decreasing the risk of stent-related placement complications in comparison with plastic stents. A larger luminal diameter is achieved, with a significant improvement in swallowing in comparison with plastic prosthetic

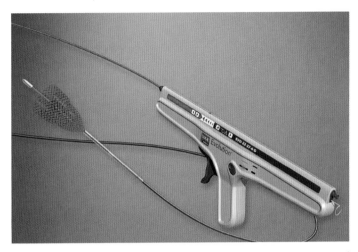

Fig. 35.1 View of a commercially available self-expanding metal stent and delivery system (with pistol release). The stent is partially deployed.

tubes [7]. However, delayed complications may be as frequent or greater [8,9].

SEMS from various manufacturers differ in design, luminal diameter, radial expansile force, and degree of shortening. All SEMS have a covering to prevent tumor ingrowth and to close fistulas [10]. Covered SEMS are more likely to migrate than uncovered SEMS, especially when deployed in the region of the distal esophagus and cardia [10,11]. Several esophageal SEMS are available (**Table 35.1**; **Fig. 35.2**) [12]. Data from several studies suggest there are minor differences in the efficacy and complication rates between most SEMS [13–17].

▪ Placement of Esophageal SEMS

Placement of stents is usually performed on an outpatient basis using fluoroscopic assistance, although placement using endoscopic visualization alone is also performed [18,19]. If a contrast esophagram has been obtained, it provides information about the stricture and about the presence of fistulas (**Fig. 35.3**). In addition to fluoroscopic markers on the stent, other fluoroscopic markers can be used to indicate the location of the stricture and assist in placement. Usually, the proximal and distal margins of the stricture are identified endoscopically and corresponding radiopaque markers are used. Markers can be external (applied to the skin) or internal (using tissue clips or intramucosal injection of a radiopaque contrast agent). External markers become inaccurate if the patient is rotated [20]. Predilation of the stricture to a diameter of 10–12 mm allows passage of a standard upper endoscope and complete assessment of the stricture length and location. However, aggressive stricture dilation increases the risk of perforation. Alternatively, injection of water-soluble contrast under fluoroscopic guidance or passage of a small-caliber (pediatric) endoscope can be used to assess the stricture, avoiding the need for dilation. A guide wire is placed across the stricture (preferably a stiff guide wire) into the stomach or duodenum, and the endoscope is withdrawn. Dilation may be required for

Table 35.1 Currently available types of covered metal esophageal stent

	Ultraflex	Wallflex	Z-stent*	Evolution	Alimaxx	Flamingo Wallstent	Choo stent	Dostent*	Hanarostent	Niti-S†	Bonastent	FerX-ELLA (Boubella A and E)	SX-ELLA (Flexella and HV)*
Stent material	Nickel titanium (nitinol)	Nickel titanium (nitinol)	Stainless steel	Nickel titanium (nitinol)	Nitinol	Cobalt-based alloy	Nitinol	Nitinol	Nitinol	Nitinol	Nitinol	Stainless steel	Nitinol
Delivery system diameter (Fr)	16	16	28	24	21	18	28	18		16	15		
Covering	Partial	Partial	Partial	Partial	Full	Full	Full	Full	Full	Full	Full	Full and partial	Fully covered
Design	Mesh	Mesh	Zigzag	Mesh		Mesh	Zigzag	Mesh	Mesh	Mesh	Mesh	Zigzag	Braided
Radial force	+	++	++	+++		+++	++					++++	
Length (cm)	10, 12, 15	10, 12, 15	6, 8, 10, 12, 14	8, 10, 12.5, 15	7, 12, 15	12, 14	8, 11, 14, 17			6, 9, 12, 15	9, 12, 15	Multiple, 4–16	Multiple, 8.5–15
Lumen diameter: flanges (mm)	23, 28	23, 28	21, 25	25	Proximal 27, 23 Distal 25, 21	24, 30							25
Lumen diameter: shaft (mm)	18, 23	18, 23	18, 22	20	18, 22	16, 20	18			16, 18, 20	20, 22		20
Release system	Proximal/distal	Distal	Distal	Distal	Distal	Distal	Distal	Distal	Distal	Proximal/distal	Distal	Distal	Distal
Flexibility	+++	+++	+	+++	++	++	+			++			
Degree of shortening	30–40%	30–40%	0–10%		0%	20–30%	0–10%					Minimal	
FDA approved	Yes	Yes	Yes	Yes	Yes	No	No	No	No	No	No	No	No
Manufacturer	Boston Scientific, Natick, MA, USA	Boston Scientific, Natick, MA, USA	Cook Medical, Winston-Salem, NC, USA	Cook Medical, Winston-Salem, NC, USA	Alveolus, Charlotte, NC, USA	Boston Scientific, Natick, MA, USA	MI Tech, Seoul, South Korea	MI Tech, Seoul, South Korea	MI Tech, Seoul, South Korea	Taewong Medical, Seoul, South Korea	Standard Sci-Tech, Seoul, Korea	ELLA-CS, Hradec Králové, Czech Republic	ELLA-CS, Hradec Králové, Czech Republic

* Available only with antireflux valve.
† Available with antireflux valve.

passage of stents with larger predeployment delivery systems. The preloaded stent is then advanced over the wire. The stent is then deployed using fluoroscopy, or endoscopically by reintroducing the endoscope alongside the predeployed stent, or both (**Fig. 35.4**). After deployment, one should avoid passing the endoscope through the stent if resistance is encountered, in order to prevent dislodgment. Repositioning the stent after deployment from distal to proximal is much easier than from proximal to distal and can be achieved by pulling on the upper rim of the stent, or on a string that is attached to the inside of the proximal flange of some stents and causes the radial diameter of the stent to decrease [21]. The Z-stent can be withdrawn using a string attached to the end of the stent and attached to the delivery system. After correct positioning has been confirmed, the string is cut at the end of the procedure, just before removal of the delivery system. When the stent is placed across the gastroesophageal junction (GEJ), care must be taken not to place an excessive amount of distal stent into the stomach, to prevent impaction against the greater curvature of the stomach [5].

Efficacy and Complications

The technical success rate for placement of esophageal SEMS is close to 100%. Failure may occur if the lumen cannot be traversed with a guide wire. Improvement in dysphagia occurs in most patients and may be sustained [12]. Procedure-related complication rates have remained stable, with complications such as perforation, aspiration pneumonia, and pain occurring in approximately 10% of patients [20]. Complications are described in detail elsewhere [20] and may be classified as intraprocedural and postprocedural (immediate or delayed) (**Table 35.2**). Delayed complications include bleeding, fistula formation, gastroesophageal reflux, stent migration, food bolus obstruction, and tumor overgrowth at either end of the stent. These complications occur in up to 35–45% of patients [12,20].

SEMS placed across the GEJ have higher complication rates in comparison with stents placed in the mid-esophagus [21,22]. Larger-diameter stents prevent migration when placed across the GEJ [15,23]. When the stent crosses the GEJ, proton-pump inhibitors (PPIs) should be administered and the patient should be counseled about raising the head of the bed in order to prevent reflux symptoms at night and reduce the risk of aspiration. Stents with an antireflux mechanism have been developed, but studies have shown mixed results with these in relation to reflux symptoms [24–30].

Placing SEMS after previous radiotherapy and/or chemotherapy may be associated with an increase in major stent-related complications [31–35]. On the other hand, concurrent radiotherapy and chemotherapy may not be associated with such risks [36].

Most outcome data following stent placement are derived from studies of palliative treatment for intrinsic lesions in patients with esophageal cancer. Significant improvement in dysphagia can also be achieved in patients with extrinsic causes of dysphagia [37]. In addition, nearly all prospective studies of self-expanding stents exclude patients with cervical strictures, and it has been suggested that the stricture should be a distance of 2 cm below the upper esophageal sphincter before a stent is placed. However, there are several small studies showing that stents can be placed very proximally in the esophagus and allow effective palliation [38,39]. However, there may be less improvement in dysphagia following stent placement for very proximal strictures, and the rate of foreign-body sensation may be greater. Smaller-diameter stents and those with a shorter proximal flange [40], if available, are preferable for very proximal strictures in order to minimize the foreign-body sensation.

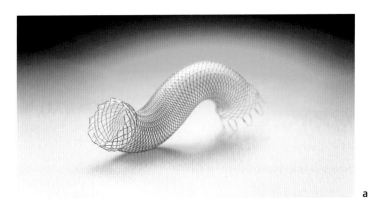

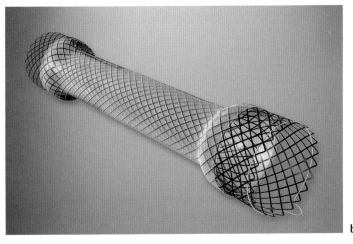

Fig. 35.2 Two commercially available self-expanding esophageal stents in their fully deployed state.
a Wallflex (Boston Scientific).
b Evolution (Cook Medical).

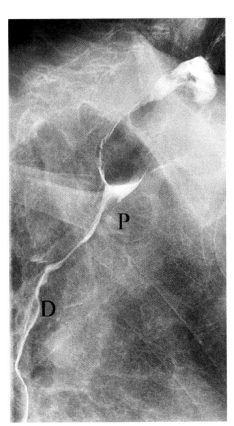

Fig. 35.3 A barium esophagram showing a malignant stricture in the proximal esophagus. No fistula is seen. This information facilitates stent placement without passage of the endoscope across the lesion. D: distal; P: proximal.

35

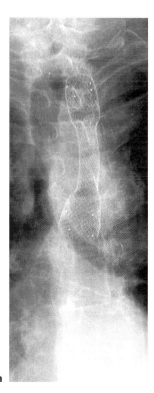

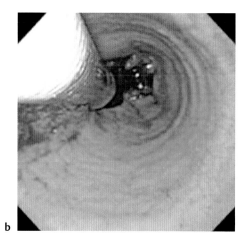

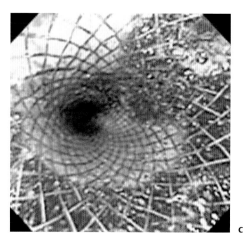

Fig. 35.4 Palliation of esophageal obstruction (same patient as in **Fig. 35.3**).
a The fluoroscopic view immediately after placement of a partially covered self-expanding metal stent.
b The endoscopic view when the endoscope is passed alongside the stent during deployment.
c The endoscopic view immediately after placement.

Table 35.2 Complications of self-expanding metal esophageal stents

Early complications
Perforation
Chest pain
Bleeding (mild)
Airway obstruction
Aspiration
Late complications
Perforation
Tracheoesophageal fistula   Obstruction: tumor ingrowth, overgrowth, tissue hyperplasia
Food impaction   Reflux with aspiration, esophagitis
Bleeding (often massive)
Migration

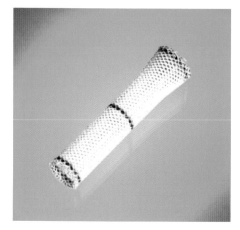

Fig. 35.5 A Polyflex self-expanding plastic stent (Boston Scientific).

Self-Expanding Plastic Stents

The Polyflex stent (Boston Scientific, Natick, Massachusetts, USA) can easily be removed, as no embedding occurs. It is the only available nonmetallic self-expanding stent and is composed of polyester mesh completely covered in silicone (**Fig. 35.5**). The largest available Polyflex flares to 25 mm at the proximal end. The expanded mid-body diameter ranges from 16 to 21 mm. Disadvantages are that the stent needs to be loaded onto the delivery device before placement and that the diameter of the delivery system is large and relatively inflexible [12].

The Polyflex stent has been shown to be safe and effective for the palliation of malignant dysphagia, with no inducement of tissue hyperplasia or tumor ingrowth [41,42]. Stent migration occurs in up to 25 % [43]. In the only randomized trial comparing the Polyflex stent with a partially covered SEMS for palliation of malignant dysphagia, equivalent results for palliation were achieved, but late stent migration was more frequent with the Polyflex stent [44].

Biodegradable Stents

Biodegradable stents have the potential to allow treatment of benign disease without the need for additional procedures to remove them. One such stent is the SX-ELLA (ELLA-CS, Hradec Králové, Czech Republic), designed for the treatment of benign strictures and of achalasia refractory to other therapies. Stent integrity is maintained for up to 6–8 weeks, with complete degradation by 12 weeks. Unfortunately, acid reflux accelerates degradation. As yet, there are no data on the outcome following placement of these stents.

Treatment of Malignant Esophageal Fistula

Progressive esophageal carcinoma, primary lung cancer, and radiotherapy for malignancy can produce a fistula between the esophagus and the respiratory tract [45]. In addition, pressure necrosis at the proximal edge of a previously placed SEMS can cause a fistula. Retrospective and prospective series [46–52] have shown that complete sealing of fistulas occurs using covered SEMS in more than 90 % of patients.

Placement of Self-Expanding Stents for Benign Disease

The indications for placement of self-expanding stents in patients with benign disease include closure of leaks and perforations, as well as the treatment of benign refractory esophageal strictures. Although the use of partially covered self-expanding metal stents has been described for the treatment of benign esophageal strictures [53], tissue embedding in the uncovered portion can make removal of the stent difficult. Nonmalignant perforations of the esophagus may occur as a result of endoscopic therapy (dilation, tumor resection) and spontaneously (Boerhaave syndrome). Esophageal leaks after esophageal surgery, as well as perforations, can be successfully closed with Polyflex stent placement [54–58]. The stents are retrieved endoscopically after closure. In the absence of a stricture, a large-diameter Polyflex stent may migrate less frequently, although in the studies mentioned above, stent migration was observed in 17–30 % of patients. Refractory strictures have been successfully treated with Polyflex stents [59,60], although with relatively high complication rates [61–63]. Completely covered SEMS are potentially removable [64,65] and can be used to treat leaks and strictures, followed by removal, although there are few data on their use [65–67].

Malignant Gastric Outlet Obstruction

Malignant gastric outlet obstruction produces postprandial abdominal pain, early satiety, vomiting, and intolerance of oral intake. SEMS placement for malignant gastric outlet obstruction was first described in 1992 [68]. Since then, there have been many publications describing the efficacy of SEMS for palliating gastric outlet obstruction. In a systematic review of 32 case series, including 10 prospective series, the efficacy of SEMS for gastroduodenal malignancies was reported [69]. The majority of malignancies included were gastric and pancreatic in origin. In all, 606 patients underwent attempted stent placement. Technical success, defined as successful stent placement and deployment, was achieved in 589 (97 %). Technical failure was attributed to severe obstruction, difficult anatomy, malpositioning, and one failed delivery. Clinical success, defined as relief of symptoms and improved oral intake, occurred in 89 % of the technical successes. Clinical failures were due to early stent migration (20 %) and disease progression (61 %), as well as procedural complications (15 %) such as malpositioned stents or partially expanded stents. Severe complications included bleeding (1 %). There were no procedure-related deaths. Nonsevere complications occurred in 27 % of attempted stent placements. The most commonly reported nonsevere complication was stent occlusion (17 %), primarily due to tumor growth or obstruction away from the stent. Migration occurred in 5 % of patients and was generally managed with additional stent placement. Pain was reported in 2 % of the patients. Evidence of biliary obstruction after stent placement was noted in 1 %. The mean survival was 12.1 weeks.

Surgical gastroenterostomy has been compared to endoscopic SEMS for palliation of unresectable malignant antropyloric stenosis [70]. In a small, randomized prospective trial including 18 patients, stent placement was successful in 100 %. The mean time to oral intake was 6.3 days for surgical patients and 2.1 days for stent treatment ($P < 0.0001$). The median period of hospital stay was longer in the surgical group at 10 days, in comparison with 3.1 days in the stent group. The mean procedure time was twice as long in compar-

ison with the endoscopy group. One major complication each occurred in the stent and surgery groups—stent dislocation and postoperative hemorrhage, respectively. No differences in the morbidity or mortality rates were seen.

Other retrospective studies have shown similar results. The time to ingestion of both liquids and a light-consistency diet, as well as the postprocedural length of the hospital stay, are significantly shorter in the endoscopic stent group in comparison with surgical groups. Postprocedural and procedural costs are higher in the gastrojejunostomy groups [71]. Indeed, in a systematic review [72], endoscopic placement of SEMS was the preferred strategy over open or laparoscopic gastrojejunostomy for palliation of malignant gastric outlet obstruction in patients with a short life expectancy, on the basis of effectiveness, fewer complications, reduced costs, and earlier resumption of oral intake.

Gastroduodenal and Small-Bowel Self-Expanding Stents

Several stents are available for gastroduodenal placement (**Table 35.3**). These stents pass directly through the working channel of the endoscope (through the scope, TTS). Non-TTS stent placement is difficult, but possible. Optimal endoscopic stent placement may be impaired by the presence of retained gastric contents. Placing the patient in the left lateral decubitus position prevents aspiration, but often results in a suboptimal fluoroscopic image. Placing the patient in the prone or supine position is preferable for fluoroscopic visualization, but if the latter position is chosen, the patient should be carefully monitored and suctioning should be carried out and any gastric contents removed if possible as soon as the stomach is entered. In addition, one may consider endotracheal intubation to prevent aspiration. Before gastroduodenal stent placement is undertaken, it is important to assess the status of the biliary tree first, since placement of a self-expanding stent across the papilla may make subsequent endoscopic access to the papilla difficult, if not impossible. In addition, in patients with proximal duodenal strictures, the stent may not need to cross the papilla to achieve palliation. Thus, a stent should be chosen that is sufficient to cross the lesion, but not excessively long so as to prevent access to the papilla. Large-caliber therapeutic-channel endoscopes (with a working channel ≥ 3.8 mm) are needed for placement of TTS stents, and thus it is frequently not possible to pass the endoscope across the stricture; this is not necessary to achieve placement, and aggressive dilation of the stricture should be avoided in order to prevent perforation. The stricture is traversed using biliary endoscopic techniques and accessories, with fluoroscopic guidance. Sphincterotomes are also useful, as they can be bowed to change the direction of orientation, especially those that can be rotated. In addition, changing from a forward-viewing endoscope to a side-viewing endoscope may improve access to the lumen of the stricture. Once the stricture has been traversed with the guide wire and catheter, contrast can be injected to define the length of the stricture (**Fig. 35.6 a**). The stent chosen should be about 4 cm longer than the measured stricture.

Gastroduodenal stents foreshorten up to 40 % during deployment, and all deploy from the distal end. In order to prevent malpositioning of the stent, it is therefore important to maintain the endoscope in a position about 3–4 cm proximal from the proximal end of the stricture, while continuously monitoring the proximal end. The stent will appear to move away from the tip of the endoscope as it is delivered and while it expands and shortens. The endoscopist almost always needs to pull back on the delivery system during deployment in order to maintain the proper position.

For strictures in the second duodenum, there is some debate about whether or not the proximal end of the stent should remain

Table 35.3 Self-expanding duodenal and colonic stents

	Materials	Deployed diameters	Deployed lengths (cm)	Features
Boston Scientific				
Ultraflex Precision Colonic	Nitinol	25 mm (proximal flare 30 mm)	5.7, 8.7, 11.7	Not TTS; non-reconstrainable; 23 % foreshortening
Wallstent Enteral	Elgiloy (cobalt–chromium–nickel)	20 mm, 22 mm	6, 9	TTS delivery; reconstrainable; 39–49 % foreshortening during expansion
Wallflex Enteral Duodenal	Nitinol	22 mm body, 27 mm proximal flare	6, 9, 12	TTS delivery; reconstrainable; 30–38 % foreshortening during expansion
Wallflex Enteral Colonic	Nitinol	25 mm body, 30 mm proximal flare	6, 9, 12	TTS delivery; reconstrainable; 30–38 % foreshortening during expansion
		22 mm body, 27 mm proximal flare		
Cook Endoscopy				
Colonic Z-stent	Stainless steel	25 mm	4, 6, 8,10,12	Non-TTS; no foreshortening
Evolution Duodenal Stent	Nitinol	22 mm (proximal and distal flares 27 mm)	6, 9, 12	TTS delivery; reconstrainable; 45 % foreshortening during expansion
Evolution Colonic Stent	Nitinol	25 mm (proximal and distal flares 30 mm)	6, 8, 10	TTS delivery; reconstrainable; 45 % foreshortening during expansion
MI Tech				
Hanarostent, colorectal	Nitinol	22 mm	8, 11, 14	TTS delivery, partially reconstrainable
Hanarostent, pyloroduodenal	Nitinol	18 mm		TTS delivery (uncovered), reconstrainable
	Uncovered		8, 11, 14	
	Partially covered		6, 9, 11, 13	
Taewong Medical				
Colorectal	Nitinol	20, 22, 24 mm (proximal and distal flares 28 and 30 mm)	6, 8, 10, 12	Non-TTS delivery, reconstrainable
	Uncovered			
	Covered			
	Double-layer			
Pyloric	Nitinol	18, 20 (proximal and distal flares 24 and 28 mm)	6, 8, 10, 12	TTS delivery
	Uncovered			
	Covered			
ELLA-CS				
SX-ELLA, pyloroduodenal	Nitinol	20, 22, 25	8, 9, 11, 13.5	TTS delivery
	Uncovered			
SX-ELLA, colorectal	Nitinol	22, 25, 30	7.5, 8, 9, 11, 13.5	TTS delivery
	Uncovered			
	Covered			

TTS, through the scope.

in the proximal duodenum or in the gastric antrum (**Fig. 35.6 b**), because of the potential difference in the functional result. When the proximal end remains in the duodenum, stent-induced perforation has been reported with stents that have sharp ends [73]. However, newer stents with rounded edges may reduce this complication.

Colonic Obstruction

The mortality rate associated with acute colonic obstruction is high, and colonic obstruction due to malignancy is the number one cause of emergency large-bowel surgery [74].

SEMS are placed for several indications in patients with obstructive colorectal malignancies [75]. Stents can be used for temporary decompression before resection of operable colonic tumors, allowing a one-stage bowel resection. Advantages of preoperative stent placement include laparoscopic resection of the stent and tumor [76], as well as the ability to perform an elective preoperative

colonoscopy to exclude synchronous lesions [77]. Secondly, stents can be used for palliation of inoperable obstructive colorectal malignancies. Extrinsic compression causing obstruction from pelvic malignancies and lymphadenopathy can also be treated palliatively with stents. Finally, a covered stent can be placed in the rectum to seal fistulas to the vagina and bladder [78].

Sebastian et al. [79] published a comprehensive report on the efficacy and safety of SEMS for malignant colorectal obstruction based on studies published from 1990 to 2003. No randomized trials were identified. Fifty-four case series including 1198 patients were included in this pooled analysis; 791 of the patients had undergone stent placement for palliation. In the remaining patients, stenting was performed as a bridge to surgery. Of the patients treated palliatively, technical success in stent placement was achieved in 93 % and clinical success was achieved in 91 % (cumulative rates). Perforations, predominantly in the rectosigmoid region, occurred in 3.8 % of the patients, 64 % of whom required emergency surgery. In 17.7 % of the perforations, predilation was thought to be a causative factor. The use of laser therapy in the present setting was also considered

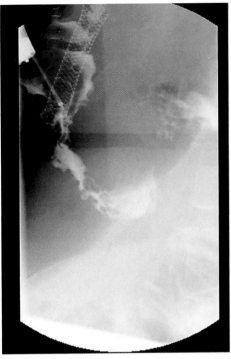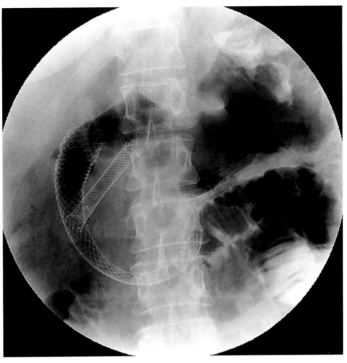

b

Fig. 35.6 Palliation of duodenal obstruction due to pancreatic cancer. **a** Injection of contrast through a biliary catheter outlines the stricture in the duodenum. An indwelling biliary self-expanding stent is already in place.

b Radiograph taken immediately after deployment of the duodenal self-expanding metal stent. The proximal end is in the gastric antrum.

to have contributed to perforation in a few cases. Perforations were attributed to balloon dilation, stent wires, and guide wires. Migration after technically successful stent placement occurred in 11.8 % of cases, two-thirds of which occurred within the first week. Most migrations were distal (94.7 %). Fifteen percent of the palliative stents migrated, in comparison with only 3.9 % of the stents used as a bridge to surgery. The cumulative procedure-related mortality rate for all stent placements was 0.58 %. The majority of these deaths were among patients receiving palliative therapy. Recurrent obstruction was noted in 7.3 % of patients after a median of 24 weeks. Recurrent obstruction was due to tumor ingrowth in most cases. Other causes of obstruction, including fecal impaction, mucosal prolapse, tumor overgrowth, and peritoneal seeding occurred less frequently. Laser, argon plasma coagulation, stent replacement, and surgery were among the methods used to treat recurrent obstruction. For stents placed in the left colon, there are few or no data for comparisons between stent types, although one study suggested that there may be differences [80]. It is important to note that stent placement in the right colon is also effective [81]. Complications of gastroduodenal/colonic (enteral) SEMS are listed in **Table 35.4**.

Placement of SEMS in patients with benign disease is limited by the fact that uncovered stents are incapable of being removed, while partially covered stents almost always migrate. In patients with benign conditions and a need for preoperative decompression, there are no concerns regarding long-term complications of uncovered stents due to lack of removability, since the stent is removed at the time of surgery. There is an emerging literature on preoperative SEMS placement for benign disease [82].

Table 35.4 Complications of enteral stents

Perforation: immediate/delayed
Obstruction: tumor ingrowth, overgrowth, and tissue hyperplasia
Bleeding
Migration
Tenesmus, incontinence, and pain (distal rectal stent placement only)

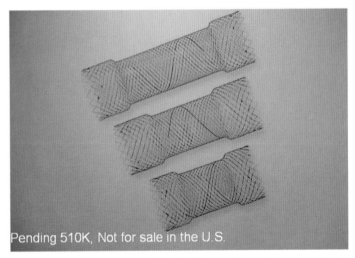

Pending 510K, Not for sale in the U.S.

Fig. 35.7 Examples of fully deployed self-expanding colonic stents (Evolution, Cook Medical).

Stent Types

Several types of self-expanding metal stent are available for colonic use (**Table 35.3**; **Fig. 35.7**). It is important to realize that some of these are non-TTS, while others are TTS. In addition, the degree of stent shortening after placement varies greatly. Placement of SEMS

in the rectum and distal sigmoid using non-TTS stents is analogous to esophageal stent placement, as described previously. TTS stent placement is necessary to treat more proximal obstruction and is analogous to the techniques described above for gastroduodenal stent placement.

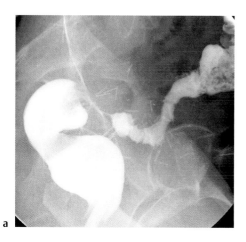
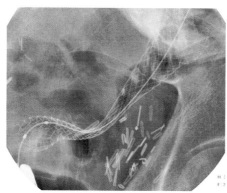

Fig. 35.8   Palliative stent placement for recurrent sigmoid cancer.
a   A retrograde contrast study showing a tight stricture.
b   The radiographic view immediately after successful stent deployment. The waist in the mid-portion corresponds to the obstructing lesion.

Patient Preparation

Adequate endoscopic visualization is essential to allow optimal stent placement. Complete bowel preparation is usually not necessary in patients with complete colonic obstruction, as feces are evacuated below the obstruction. Enema preparation is usually adequate. Similarly, in patients with distal sigmoid and rectal obstruction, stool can easily be evacuated with enema preparation. Standard colonoscopy preparation is administered in patients with subtotal obstruction located more proximally.

Although a radiographic retrograde contrast study is not essential, it makes it possible to assess the anatomy and the length of stricture and avoids the need for passage of the endoscope beyond the lesion to determine the length and characteristics (**Fig. 35.8 a**).

Placement Techniques

The traditional left lateral decubitus position is frequently not optimal for interpreting fluoroscopic images; rotating the patient into the supine position is often preferable.

Endoscopic placement alone is possible. This is best reserved for patients with incomplete obstruction, since a small-caliber endoscope can usually be passed across the stricture. A guide wire can be placed and a non-TTS approach taken for stent deployment, since SEMS will not pass through such endoscopes and the endoscope has to be removed before stent placement. Alternatively, a larger-diameter endoscope can be used, but cautious dilation is needed (12–15 mm) to pass the endoscope beyond the lesion. Once the endoscope is passed across the stricture, a guide wire is passed. In non-TTS stents, the endoscope is withdrawn and the length of the stricture is measured. The endoscope is then positioned distal to the lesion.

Combined endoscopic and fluoroscopic placement avoids the need for passage of the endoscope across the lesion and is analogous to the approach described for gastroduodenal stent placement. The endoscope is inserted to the lesion. Water-soluble contrast is used to outline the stricture, either by injecting through the working channel of the endoscope using a large syringe or by using a biliary catheter. A biliary stone balloon catheter is inflated to a diameter of 15–18 mm to provide pressure for injection across the stricture. A guide wire is passed through the catheter lumen under fluoroscopic guidance. The stricture is measured, and the stent is deployed as described previously while the deployment is monitored endoscopically and fluoroscopically (**Fig. 35.8 b**).

If overlapping stents are required, it is essential to have an overlap of at least 2 cm after deployment, since with further expansion after placement the stents may shorten and separate. Because of the angulations within the colon—at the rectosigmoid, sigmoid–descending colon junction, and hepatic flexures—the ends of the stent may be oriented toward the wall rather than toward the lumen, preventing adequate passage of fecal material. It may therefore be preferable to use a longer stent than anticipated in order to ensure that the ends are directed toward the lumen. Very distal rectal lesions may require the stent to be deployed close to the dentate line. This leaves less room for error (similar to very proximal esophageal lesions), and it may not be possible to allow for 2 cm or more of stent below the tumor. When a choice between a smaller-diameter or larger-diameter stent is available, the smaller diameter may be more appropriate for lesions in the right colon, as the stool is still liquefied and it is hypothetically possible that delayed perforations may be less likely with a smaller stent. Conversely, for lesions in the left colon, a larger-diameter stent should be used to potentially prevent solid stool impaction within the stent lumen.

Conclusions

Endoscopic placement of self-expanding stents allows palliation of malignant and nonmalignant luminal obstruction. Stent placement is the frequently the only endoscopic management option that restores luminal continuity in patients with malignant gastroduodenal and colonic obstruction. In the colon, stents can be used to restore luminal patency both preoperatively and for palliation in order to avoid colostomy.

References

1. Baron TH. Expandable gastrointestinal stents. Gastroenterology 2007; 133:1407–11.
2. Chan AC, Shin FG, Lam YH, Ng EK, Sung JJ, Lau JY, et al. A comparison study on physical properties of self-expandable esophageal metal stents. Gastrointest Endosc 1999;49:462–5.
3. Silvis SE, Sievert CE Jr, Vennes JA, Abeyta BK, Brennecke LH. Comparison of covered versus uncovered wire mesh stents in the canine biliary tract. Gastrointest Endosc 1994;40:17–21.
4. Bethge N, Sommer A, Gross U, von Kleist D, Vakil N. Human tissue responses to metal stents implanted in vivo for the palliation of malignant stenoses. Gastrointest Endosc 1996;43:596–602.
5. Siersema PD, Marcon N, Vakil N. Metal stents for tumors of the distal esophagus and gastric cardia. Endoscopy 2003;35:79–85.
6. Knyrim K, Wagner HJ, Bethge N Keymling M, Vakil N. A controlled trial of an expansile metal stent for palliation of esophageal obstruction due to inoperable cancer. N Engl J Med 1993;329:1302–7.

7. Roseveare CD, Patel P, Simmonds N, Goggin PM, Kimble J, Shepherd HA. Metal stents improve dysphagia, nutrition and survival in malignant oesophageal stenosis: a randomized controlled trial comparing modified Gianturco Z-stents with plastic Atkinson tubes. Eur J Gastroenterol Hepatol 1998;10:653–7.

8. Kozarek RA, Ball TJ, Brandabur JJ, Patterson DJ, Low D, Hill L, et al. Expandable versus conventional esophageal prostheses: easier insertion may not preclude subsequent stent-related problems. Gastrointest Endosc 1996;43:204–8.

9. Eickhoff A, Knoll M, Jakobs R, Weickert U, Hartmann D, Schilling D, et al. Self-expanding metal stents versus plastic prostheses in the palliation of malignant dysphagia: long-term outcome of 153 consecutive patients. J Clin Gastroenterol 2005;39:877–85.

10. Vakil N, Morris AI, Marcon N, Segalin A, Peracchia A, Bethge N, et al. A prospective, randomized, controlled trial of covered expandable metal stents in the palliation of malignant esophageal obstruction at the gastro-esophageal junction. Am J Gastroenterol 2001;96:1791–6.

11. Saranovic DJ, Djuric-Stefanovic A, Ivanovic A, Masulovic D, Pesko P. Fluoroscopically guided insertion of self-expandable metal esophageal stents for palliative treatment of patients with malignant stenosis of esophagus and cardia: comparison of uncovered and covered stent types. Dis Esophagus 2005;18:230–8.

12. Siersema PD. New developments in palliative therapy. Best Pract Res Clin Gastroenterol 2006;20:959–78.

13. May A, Hahn EG, Ell C. Self-expanding metal stents for palliation of malignant obstruction in the upper gastrointestinal tract. Comparative assessment of three stent types implemented in 96 implantations. J Clin Gastroenterol 1996;22:261–6.

14. Schmassmann A, Meyenberger C, Knuchel J, Binek J, Lammer F, Kleiner B, et al. Self-expanding metal stents in malignant esophageal obstruction: a comparison between two stent types. Am J Gastroenterol 1997;92:400–6.

15. Siersema PD, Hop WC, van Blankenstein M, van Tilburg AJ, Bac DJ, Homs MY, et al. A comparison of 3 types of covered metal stents for the palliation of patients with dysphagia caused by esophagogastric carcinoma: a prospective, randomized study. Gastrointest Endosc 2001;54:145–53.

16. Sabharwal T, Hamady MS, Chui S, Atkinson S, Mason R, Adam A. A randomized prospective comparison of the Flamingo Wallstent and Ultraflex stent for palliation of dysphagia associated with lower third oesophageal carcinoma. Gut 2003;52:922–6.

17. Verschuur EM, Homs MY, Steyerberg EW, Haringsma J, Wahab PJ, Kuipers EJ, et al. A new esophageal stent design (Niti-S stent) for the prevention of migration: a prospective study in 42 patients. Gastrointest Endosc 2006;63:134–40.

18. Rathore OI, Coss A, Patchett SE, Mulcahy HE. Direct-vision stenting: the way forward for malignant oesophageal obstruction. Endoscopy 2006;38:382–4.

19. Martin DF. Endoscopy is superfluous during insertion of expandable metal stents in esophageal tumors. Gastrointest Endosc 1997;46:98–9.

20. Baron TH. Minimizing endoscopic complications: endoluminal stents. Gastrointest Endosc Clin N Am 2007;17:83–104.

21. Baron TH. Expandable metal stents for the treatment of cancerous obstruction of the gastrointestinal tract. N Engl J Med 2001;344:1681–7.

22. Spinelli P, Cerrai FG, Ciuffi M, Ignomirelli O, Meroni E, Pizzetti P. Endoscopic stent placement for cancer of the lower esophagus and gastric cardia. Gastrointest Endosc 1994;40:455–7.

23. Verschuur EM, Steyerberg EW, Kuipers EJ, Siersema PD. Effect of stent size on complications and recurrent dysphagia in patients with esophageal or gastric cardia cancer. Gastrointest Endosc 2007;65:592–601.

24. Dua KS, Kozarek R, Kim J, Evans J, Medda BK, Lang I, et al. Self-expanding metal esophageal stent with anti-reflux mechanism. Gastrointest Endosc 2001;53:603–13.

25. Laasch HU, Marriott A, Wilbraham L, Tunnah S, England RE, Martin DF. Effectiveness of open versus antireflux stents for palliation of distal esophageal carcinoma and prevention of symptomatic gastroesophageal reflux. Radiology 2002;225:359–65.

26. Do YS, Choo SW, Suh SW, Kang WK, Rhee PL, Kim K, et al. Malignant esophagogastric junction obstruction: palliative treatment with an antireflux valve stent. J Vasc Interv Radiol 2001;12:647–51.

27. Homs MY, Wahab PJ, Kuipers EJ, Steyerberg EW, Grool TA, Haringsma J, et al. Esophageal stents with antireflux valve for tumors of the distal esophagus and gastric cardia: a randomized trial. Gastrointest Endosc 2004;60:695–702.

28. Wenger U, Johnsson E, Arnelo U, Lundell L, Lagergren J. An antireflux stent versus conventional stents for palliation of distal esophageal or cardia cancer: a randomized clinical study. Surg Endosc 2006;20:1675–80.

29. Schoppmeyer K, Golsong J, Schiefke I, Mössner J, Caca K. Antireflux stents for palliation of malignant esophagocardial stenosis. Dis Esophagus 2007;20:89–93.

30. Shim CS, Jung IS, Cheon YK, Ryu CB, Hong SJ, Kim JO, et al. Management of malignant stricture of the esophagogastric junction with a newly designed self-expanding metal stent with an antireflux mechanism. Endoscopy 2005;37:335–9.

31. Kinsman KJ, DeGregorio BT, Katon RM, Morrison K, Saxon RR, Keller FS, et al. Prior radiation and chemotherapy increase the risk of life-threatening complications after insertion of metallic stents for esophagogastric malignancy. Gastrointest Endosc 1996;43:196–203.

32. Siersema PD, Hop WC, Dees J, Tilanus HW, van Blankenstein M. Coated self-expanding metal stents versus latex prostheses for esophagogastric cancer with special reference to prior radiation and chemotherapy: a controlled, prospective study. Gastrointest Endosc 1998:47:113–20.

33. Bartelsman JF, Bruno MJ, Jensema AJ, Haringsma J, Reeders JW, Tytgat GN. Palliation of patients with esophagogastric neoplasms by insertion of a covered expandable modified Gianturco-Z endoprosthesis: experiences in 153 patients. Gastrointest Endosc 2000;51:134–8.

34. Homs MY, Hansen BE, van Blankenstein M, Haringsma J, Kuipers EJ, Siersema PD. Prior radiation and/or chemotherapy has no effect on the outcome of metal stent placement for esophagogastric carcinoma. Eur J Gastroenterol Hepatol 2004;16:163–70.

35. Lecleire S, Di Fiore F, Ben-Soussan E, Antonietti M, Hellot MF, Paillot B, et al. Prior chemoradiotherapy is associated with a higher life-threatening complication rate after palliative insertion of metal stents in patients with oesophageal cancer. Aliment Pharmacol Ther 2006;23(12):1693–702.

36. Ludwig D, Dehne A, Burmester E, Wiedemann GJ, Stange EF. Treatment of unresectable carcinoma of the esophagus or the gastroesophageal junction by mesh stents with or without radiochemotherapy. Int J Oncol 1998;13:583–8.

37. Bethge N, Sommer A, Vakil N. Palliation of malignant esophageal obstruction due to intrinsic and extrinsic lesions with expandable metal stents. Am J Gastroenterol 1998;93:1829–32.

38. Eleftheriadis E, Kotzampassi K. Endoprosthesis implantation at the pharyngo-esophageal level: problems, limitations and challenges. World J Gastroenterol 2006;12:2103–8.

39. Macdonald S, Edwards RD, Moss JG. Patient tolerance of cervical esophageal metallic stents. J Vasc Interv Radiol 2000;11:891–8.

40. Shim CS, Jung IS, Bhandari S, Ryu CB, Hong SJ, Kim JO, et al. Management of malignant strictures of the cervical esophagus with a newly-designed self-expanding metal stent. Endoscopy 2004;36(6):554–7.

41. Dormann AJ, Eisendrath P, Wigginghaus B, Huchzermeyer H, Devière J. Palliation of esophageal carcinoma with a new self-expanding plastic stent. Endoscopy 2003;35(3):207–211.

42. Szegedi L, Gal I, Kosa I, Kiss GG. Palliative treatment of esophageal carcinoma with self-expanding plastic stents: a report on 69 cases. Eur J Gastroenterol Hepatol 2006;18(11):1197–201.

43. Costamagna G, Shah SK, Tringali A, Mutignani M, Perri V, Riccioni ME. Prospective evaluation of a new self-expanding plastic stent for inoperable esophageal strictures. Surg Endosc 2003;17:891–5.

44. Conio M, Repici A, Battaglia G, De Pretis G, Ghezzo L, Bittinger M, et al. A randomized prospective comparison of self-expandable plastic stents and partially covered self-expandable metal stents in the palliation of malignant esophageal dysphagia. Am J Gastroenterol 2007;102:2667–77.

45. Yoruk Y. Esophageal stent placement for the palliation of dysphagia in lung cancer. Thorac Cardiovasc Surg 2007;55:196–8.

46. Do YS, Song HY, Lee BH, Byun HS, Kim KH, Chin SY, et al. Esophagorespiratory fistula associated with esophageal cancer: treatment with a Gianturco stent tube. Radiology 1993;187:673–7.

47. Bethge N, Sommer A, Vakil N. Treatment of esophageal fistulas with a new polyurethane-covered, self-expanding mesh stent: a prospective study. Am J Gastroenterol 1995;90:2143–6.

48. Kozarek RA, Raltz S, Brugge WR, Schapiro RH, Waxman I, Boyce HW, et al. Prospective multicenter trial of esophageal Z-stent placement for malignant dysphagia and tracheoesophageal fistula. Gastrointest Endosc 1996;44:562–7.

49. Low DE, Kozarek RA. Comparison of conventional and wire mesh expandable prostheses and surgical bypass in patients with malignant esophagorespiratory fistulas. Ann Thorac Surg 1998;65:919–23.

50. May A, Ell C. Palliative treatment of malignant esophagorespiratory fistulas with Gianturco-Z stents. A prospective clinical trial and review of the literature on covered metal stents. Am J Gastroenterol 1998;93:532–5.

35

51. Raijman I, Siddique I, Ajani J, Lynch P. Palliation of malignant dysphagia and fistulae with coated expandable metal stents: experience with 101 patients. Gastrointest Endosc 1998;48:172–9.

52. Dumonceau JM, Cremer M, Lalmand B, Devière J. Esophageal fistula sealing: choice of stent, practical management, and cost. Gastrointest Endosc 1999;49:70–8.

53. Low DE, Kozarek RA. Removal of esophageal expandable metal stents: description of technique and review of potential applications. Surg Endosc 2003;17:990–6.

54. Siersema PD, Homs MY, Haringsma J, Tilanus HW, Kuipers EJ. Use of large-diameter metallic stents to seal traumatic nonmalignant perforations of the esophagus. Gastrointest Endosc 2003;58:356–61.

55. Hünerbein M, Stroszcynski C, Moesta KT, Schlag PM. Treatment of thoracic anastomotic leaks after esophagectomy with self-expanding plastic stents. Ann Surg 2004;240:801–7.

56. Gelbmann CM, Ratiu NL, Rath HC, Rogler G, Lock G, Schölmerich J, et al. Use of self-expandable plastic stents for the treatment of esophageal perforations and symptomatic anastomotic leaks. Endoscopy 2004;36:695–9.

57. Schubert D, Scheidbach H, Kuhn R, Wex C, Weiss G, Eder F, et al. Endoscopic treatment of thoracic esophageal anastomotic leaks by using silicone-covered, self-expanding polyester stents. Gastrointest Endosc 2005;61:891–6.

58. Freeman RK, Ascioti AJ, Wozniak TC. Postoperative esophageal leak management with the Polyflex esophageal stent. J Thorac Cardiovasc Surg 2007;133:333–8.

59. Repici A, Conio M, De Angelis C, Battaglia E, Musso A, Pellicano R, et al. Temporary placement of an expandable polyester silicone-covered stent for treatment of refractory benign esophageal strictures. Gastrointest Endosc 2004;60:513–9.

60. Evrard S, Le Moine O, Lazaraki G, Dormann A, El Nakadi I, Devière J. Self-expanding plastic stents for benign esophageal lesions. Gastrointest Endosc 2004;60:894–900.

61. Dua KS, Vleggaar FP, Santharam R, Siersema PD. Removable self-expanding plastic esophageal stent as a continuous, non-permanent dilator in treating refractory benign esophageal strictures: a prospective two-center study. Am J Gastroenterol 2008;103:2988–94.

62. Triester SL, Fleischer DE, Sharma VK. Failure of self-expanding plastic stents in treatment of refractory benign esophageal strictures. Endoscopy 2006;38:533–7.

63. Holm AN, De La Mora Levy JG, Gostout CJ, Topazian MD, Baron TH. Self-expanding plastic stents in treatment of benign esophageal conditions. Gastrointest Endosc 2008;67:20–5.

64. Baron TH, Burgart LJ, Pochron NL. An internally covered (lined) self-expanding metal esophageal stent: tissue response in a porcine model. Gastrointest Endosc 2006;64:263–7.

65. Song HY, Park SI, Do YS, Yoon HK, Sung KB, Sohn KH, et al. Expandable metallic stent placement in patients with benign esophageal strictures: results of long-term follow-up. Radiology 1997;203:131–6.

66. Fiorini A, Fleischer D, Valero J, Israeli E, Wengrower D, Goldin E. Self-expandable metal coil stents in the treatment of benign esophageal strictures refractory to conventional therapy: a case series. Gastrointest Endosc 2000;52:259–62.

67. Song HY, Jung HY, Park SI, Kim SB, Lee DH, Kang SG, et al. Covered retrievable expandable nitinol stents in patients with benign esophageal strictures: initial experience. Radiology 2000;217:551–7.

68. Truong S, Bohndorf V, Geller H, Schupelick V, Gunther RW. Self-expanding metal stents for palliation of malignant gastric outlet obstruction. Endoscopy 1992;24:433–5.

69. Dormann A, Meisner S, Verin N, Wenk Lang A. Self-expanding metal stents for gastroduodenal malignancies: systematic review of their clinical effectiveness. Endoscopy 2004;36:543–50.

70. Fiori E, Lamazza A, Volpino P, Burza A, Paparelli C, Cavallaro G, et al. Palliative management of malignant antro-pyloric strictures. Gastroenterostomy vs. endoscopic stenting. A randomized prospective trial. Anticancer Res 2004;24:269–71.

71. Mittal A, Windsor J, Woodfield J, Casey P, Lane M. Matched study of three methods for palliation of malignant pyloroduodenal obstruction. Br J Surg 2004;91:205–9.

72. Jeurnink SM, van Eijck CH, Steyerberg EW, Kuipers EJ, Siersema PD. Stent versus gastrojejunostomy for the palliation of gastric outlet obstruction: a systematic review. BMC Gastroenterol 2007;7:18.

73. Small AJ, Petersen BT, Baron TH. Closure of a duodenal stent-induced perforation by endoscopic stent removal and covered self-expandable metal stent placement (with video). Gastrointest Endosc 2007;66: 1063–5.

74. Baron TH. Benign and malignant colorectal strictures. In: Waye JD, Rex DK, Williams CB, editors. Colonoscopy: principles and practice. Maldon, MA: Blackwell; 2003. p.611–23.

75. Baron TH, Rey JF, Spinelli P. Expandable metal stent placement for malignant colorectal obstruction. Endoscopy 2002;34:823–30.

76. Stipa F, Pigazzi A, Bascone B, Cimitan A, Villotti G, Burza A, et al. Management of obstructive colorectal cancer with endoscopic stenting followed by single-stage surgery: open or laparoscopic resection? Surg Endosc 2008;22:1477–81.

77. Vitale MA, Villotti G, d'Alba L, Frontespezi S, Iacopini F, Iacopini G. Pre-operative colonoscopy after self-expandable metallic stent placement in patients with acute neoplastic colon obstruction. Gastrointest Endosc 2006;63:814–9.

78. Repici A, Reggio D, Saracco G, Marchesa P, De Angelis C, Barletti C, et al. Self-expanding covered esophageal ultraflex stent for palliation of malignant colorectal anastomotic obstruction complicated by multiple fistulas. Gastrointest Endosc 2000;51:346–8.

79. Sebastian S, Johnston S, Geoghegan T, Torreggiani W, Buckley M. Pooled analysis of the efficacy and safety of self-expanding metal stenting in malignant colorectal obstruction. Am J Gastroenterol 2004;99:2051–7.

80. Small AJ, Baron TH. Comparison of Wallstent and Ultraflex stents for palliation of malignant left-sided colon obstruction: a retrospective, case-matched analysis. Gastrointest Endosc 2008;67:478–88.

81. Repici A, Adler DG, Gibbs CM, Malesci A, Preatoni P, Baron TH. Stenting of the proximal colon in patients with malignant large bowel obstruction: techniques and outcomes. Gastrointest Endosc 2007;66:940–4.

82. Small AJ, Young-Fadok TM, Baron TH. Expandable metal stent placement for benign colorectal obstruction: outcomes for 23 cases. Surg Endosc 2008;22:454–62.

36 Biliary and Pancreatic Stenting

Guido Costamagna, Pietro Familiari, and Andrea Tringali

Introduction

Endoscopic biliopancreatic stent placement is a well-established technique. The procedure has a universally recognized role in the management of malignant biliary obstruction and treatment of selected patients with benign biliopancreatic disorders. The range of benign diseases amenable to endoscopic stenting has expanded in recent years and currently includes chronic pancreatitis, postoperative biliary injuries, pancreatic fistulas and ascites, primary sclerosing cholangitis, large biliary stones, pancreatic pseudocysts, and cholecystitis.

This chapter reviews the most recent data available on stent types and characteristics, the technique of stent insertion and self-expanding metal stent deployment, the clinical indications for stent insertion, the management of complications, and possible future applications for biliopancreatic stents.

Types of Stent

Plastic Stents

Plastic stents were the first endoprostheses used in the management of biliary strictures. The first biliary stent placement was reported in the late 1970s by Soehendra and Reynders-Frederix [1,2]. At that time, endoscopic single-pigtail plastic stents were made by the endoscopist when clinically required, using the cut end of an angiographic catheter.

A variety of plastic stents are now available, and they differ in size, shape, and polymer composition. Research is currently focusing on improving the patency period and performance of stents by modifying the design (with side holes, anchoring flaps, and systems for preventing duodenobiliary reflux) and materials.

Shape and size. Plastic stents can be divided into two main types—pigtail stents and straight stents. Pigtail stents were the first stents to be created. They are available in different lengths and diameters, varying from 5 Fr to 10 Fr. They are usually tapered at one end to make it easier to negotiate tight strictures. Stents can have "pigtails" either at one end (the single-pigtail stent) or at both ends (the double-pigtail stent). The pigtails are straightened over a guide wire for insertion and resume their shape after the wire has been withdrawn. The pigtail provides excellent anchorage and prevents migration of the stent. However, these stents have a small inner caliber and have been used relatively infrequently, in selected cases, since the development of new anchoring systems (**Fig. 36.1a**).

Straight stents are currently the standard design used for biliary and pancreatic indications. Straight stents for endoscopic application are available with different lengths (5–8 cm), diameters (3.0–11.5 Fr) and shapes. The choice of stent depends on the patient's anatomy, the clinical indication, and the physician's preference. Most straight stents are slightly bent to conform to the anatomy of the biliary or pancreatic ducts. They may have side holes to improve the flow of bile or pancreatic juice, and they are provided with side flaps for anchoring.

The most common plastic endoprosthesis used for biliary stenting is the Cotton–Leung or "Amsterdam" stent. It is made of polyethylene, slightly bent approximately halfway up the stent length and is tapered at the proximal end to make it easier to negotiate tight strictures. It has two flaps (at the proximal and distal end) to prevent stent migration and three side holes (one close to the proximal end and two at the level of the two anchoring flaps) (**Fig. 36.1b**).

The Cotton–Huibregtse biliary stent is similar to the "Amsterdam" stent with regard to materials, side holes, and anchoring system, but it is bent at the distal (duodenal) end (**Fig. 36.1b**).

The Soehendra–Tannenbaum stent is substantially different. It was developed in order to overcome the problem of early occlusion of the standard Amsterdam-type stents [3] (**Fig. 36.1c**). Soehendra–Tannenbaum stents are made of Teflon, which has a lower coefficient of friction in comparison with polyethylene. There are no side holes, but there are four anchoring flaps at each end, cut into the thickness of the stent wall. Theoretically, this polymer and shape should help prevent protein adsorption and sludge accumulation in the stent lumen. The absence of side holes limits turbulence of the bile flow through the stent, which may play a role in stent occlusion [4–7]. However, clinical trials have not demonstrated that Soehendra–Tannenbaum stents have improved patency in comparison with Cotton–Leung stents [8–13].

The choice of stent length depends on the distance between the proximal end of the stricture and the papilla of Vater. Ideally, the proximal flap of a deployed stent should extend no more than 1 cm above the upper level of the stricture, while the distal flap should be at the level of the native papilla. Other factors may influence stent length and performance. In a C-shaped, curved common bile duct, a stent may impact onto the bile duct wall and malfunction. On the other hand, with a stent that is too long there is a risk of downward migration and impaction into the opposite duodenal wall.

The diameter of biliary stents varies from 7 Fr to 11.5 Fr. Large-bore stents (> 8.5 Fr in diameter) are too large to be inserted through the accessory channel of standard diagnostic or pediatric duodenoscopes. Clinical studies have shown that the larger the diameter, the longer the patency [14,15]. However, it may be impossible or very difficult to place large-bore stents when there is a tight biliary stricture or when placement of multiple stents is indicated (e.g., hilar strictures). In addition, the placement of 11.5-Fr stents does not significantly improve clinical outcomes [16], and most endoscopists usually prefer to place 10-Fr stents.

Pancreatic stents are similar to biliary stents. They are manufactured using the same polymers and can be anchored with pigtails or side flaps. In contrast to biliary stents, pancreatic stents usually have multiple side holes, at approximately 1-cm intervals, to allow drainage of the pancreatic duct side branches. In most cases, the standard Amsterdam stent, with a couple of side holes added using a scalpel blade, can be used instead of specially designed pancreatic stents.

Specially designed pancreatic plastic stents are produced by the major stent manufacturers, and include the Geenen stent, the Johlin pancreatic wedge stent, the Cremer pancreatic stent, the Zimmon (single-pigtail) pancreatic stent (with or without anchoring flap) and many others (**Figs. 36.2, 36.3**).

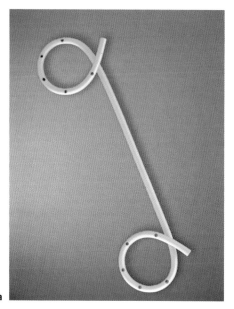

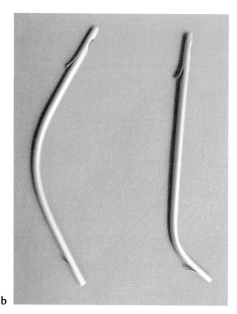

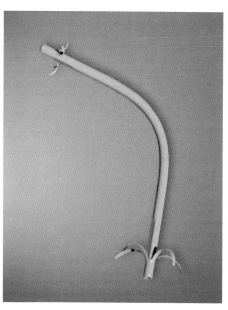

a

b

c

Fig. 36.1 Different types of plastic biliary stent.
a A double-pigtail stent, made of polyethylene, with multiple side holes on both the proximal and distal anchoring pigtails. This type of stent is used only in situations in which excellent anchorage is necessary (e.g., for drainage of pancreatic fluid collections, transpapillary endoscopic gallbladder drainage, and unretrievable common bile duct stones).

b Two different straight stents. *Left:* a standard "Amsterdam" (or Cotton–Leung) polyethylene stent; *right,* a Cotton–Huibregtse polyethylene stent. These stents both have proximal and distal anchoring flaps and three side holes.
c A Soehendra–Tannenbaum stent. This stent is made of Teflon, with no side holes, and has four anchoring flaps at each end.

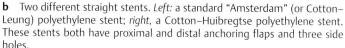

Fig. 36.2 A Geenen pancreatic stent. This stent was specifically designed for pancreatic applications. It is made of polyethylene and has multiple side holes and four flaps to prevent upward or downward migration after placement. Depending on the clinical indication, various diameters are available for pancreatic stents, usually ranging from 3 Fr to 11.5 Fr.

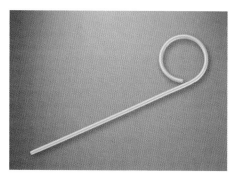

Fig. 36.3 A single-pigtail pancreatic stent, without anchoring flaps. The absence of proximal anchoring flaps allows spontaneous stent migration a few days after placement. The distal pigtail (at the duodenal end) prevents trauma and impaction into the duodenal wall. In selected cases, this stent (with a diameter of 5–7 Fr) is placed after endoscopic sphincterotomy to prevent post-ERCP pancreatitis.

The diameter of stents for pancreatic use usually ranges from 5 Fr to 11.5 Fr. Following preliminary mechanical or pneumatic dilation, most pancreatic strictures can be traversed with a 7-Fr stent. Like biliary stents, pancreatic stents may occlude over time. Pancreatic stent obstruction is mainly caused by deposits of proteins and calcium carbonate crystals; as with biliary stents, the larger the diameter, the longer the patency period [17–19].

Pancreatic duct stents may induce changes in the main pancreatic duct similar to the findings in chronic pancreatitis in patients with normal or slightly abnormal pancreatic ducts. These include ductal irregularity, narrowing, and side-branch changes. These ductal changes do not resolve completely immediately after stent removal and may persist or progress despite stent removal [20–25]. The relationship between ductal changes and stent size is still a matter of controversy. Some studies have shown no correlation between stent-induced changes and stent size [23]. Other authors have reported that ductal changes are less predominant when small-caliber (3-Fr) pancreatic stents are used [20]. However, very small-caliber stents occlude early and currently do not provide an effective endoscopic treatment for chronic pancreatitis. Their role is currently limited to the prevention of pancreatitis following endoscopic retrograde cholangiopancreatography (ERCP).

Materials. Three different polymers are used for biliary and pancreatic stents—polyethylene, Teflon, and polyurethane. In the early 1980s, homemade stents were in widespread use. Polyethylene was chosen because it becomes soft and malleable at a relatively low temperature (87 °C), and it can be easily shaped and molded using boiling water and subsequently fixed by immersing it in cold water. Polyethylene is softer than Teflon and makes it much easier to cut side holes and anchoring flaps [26]. Given the variety of stents commercially available, many endoscopists prefer to modify the shape and curvature of the stents personally in order to adapt them to the curvature of the duct, or to shorten the stents, or to make additional flaps or side holes. For these reasons, most plastic stents used for biliary and pancreatic indications are currently also made of polyethylene.

The coefficient of friction of the polymer used to make the stent is one of the factors that influence the process of stent occlusion [5,27,28]. Electron microscopy has shown that the inner surface of polytetrafluoroethylene (Teflon) or polyurethane stents is smoother than that of polyethylene stents and has a lower coefficient of friction [29,30]. However, clinical studies have not demonstrated that Teflon or polyurethane stents have longer patency in comparison with standard polyethylene stents [8–13,31,32].

V

During the last 10 years, a variety of other polymers have been investigated in efforts to prolong the patency of biliary stents. These new polymers include polyamidoamine cross-linked to polyurethane chains [33], hydromer-coated polyurethane [34], and perfluoro-aloxy combined with polyamide elastomer [35]. Despite promising preliminary studies, none of these materials has been shown to have definite advantages in terms of longer patency in comparison with standard polyethylene stents in clinical practice.

Self-Expanding Metal Stents

Self-expanding metal stents (SEMS) for endoscopic use were developed in the early 1990s to improve the quality and the durability of biliary drainage. These stents are inserted into the bile duct in a compressed state and after deployment expand to a diameter of up to 10 mm. Even in the first comparative studies, SEMS were shown to have a longer patency period than plastic stents [36–39]. The use of SEMS can therefore reduce or even avoid the need for periodic stent exchange. However, the high cost of these devices has limited their use in clinical practice.

A variety of different SEMS are currently available. The features and characteristics of the ideal SEMS are: good fluoroscopic visibility, adequate radial force, excellent flexibility, small-caliber introducer, intuitive and easy deployment, limited shortening after deployment, stability during removal, and compatibility with magnetic resonance imaging (MRI). There is as yet no ideal SEMS, and the choice of device should therefore be made on an individualized basis according to clinical need.

SEMS also become occluded over time, and most of them are not designed to allow removal [40,41]. In patients with benign biliary strictures, SEMS should therefore only be used in exceptional clinical situations [42].

The major biomedical manufacturers have focused on improving stent performance and are currently supporting clinical research to improve the overall quality of SEMS, reduce the occlusion rate, and assess the removability of SEMS and their efficacy in the management of benign strictures.

Materials. A stainless-steel alloy was initially used to manufacture biliary SEMS. However, the stainless-steel alloy SEMS were poorly flexible and reduced the quality of magnetic resonance images. SEMS are currently manufactured from two different materials—Elgiloy (a cobalt–chromium–nickel alloy) and nitinol. Elgiloy SEMS provide excellent visibility on fluoroscopy and have a high radial force. Elgiloy is malleable and can be reduced to very thin wires, preserving elasticity and flexibility. However, Elgiloy SEMS are usually stiff, with poor flexibility, and in cases of C-curved bile ducts, the risk of impacting on the bile duct wall after deployment increases with time. In contrast to stainless-steel alloy SEMS (now only available for extrabiliary applications), Elgiloy SEMS are compatible with MRI. Patients undergoing MRI do not have any additional hazards or risks, and Elgiloy endoprostheses do not have an adverse effect on the image quality (**Fig. 36.4**).

Nitinol SEMS are usually less radiopaque than Elgiloy SEMS. Most nitinol SEMS compensate for the poor fluoroscopic visibility using gold, silver, or platinum radiopaque markers. Nitinol has at least two unique properties—the shape-memory effect and superelasticity. Thermal shape-memory enables nitinol implants to be compressed for insertion into small-caliber delivery systems; they resume their original shape after deployment in situ at body temperature. Superelasticity is highly advantageous for applications in which flexibility, constancy of applied stress, and large expansion or deformation ratios are required. Because of this property, nitinol stents are more flexible than stainless-steel or Elgiloy SEMS. Nitinol is less reactive with epithelium than stainless steel and should theoret-

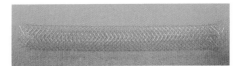

Fig. 36.4 An Elgiloy (cobalt–chromium–nickel alloy) uncovered self-expanding metal stent (Wallstent; Boston Scientific, Natick, Massachusetts, USA). This stent has a woven braided mesh and barbed sharp ends. It provides excellent visibility on fluoroscopy and outstanding radial force, but it has little flexibility, so that it may impact into the bile duct wall in patients with curved bile ducts. A partly covered version of this stent is also available.

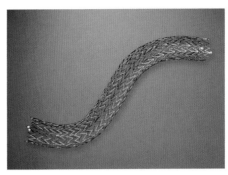

Fig. 36.5 An uncovered nitinol self-expanding metal stent (Zilver, Cook Endoscopy). This stent is laser-cut from a nitinol tube. The special zigzag design provides excellent flexibility and the stent does not become shorter after deployment. The shape-memory nitinol alloy allows good expansion of the stent after deployment. Nitinol is poorly visible on fluoroscopy, and gold radiopaque markers therefore have been added to the stent.

36

ically be associated with a longer patency period (although this has been never demonstrated in clinical practice). In addition, nitinol is not ferromagnetic and nitinol SEMS are MRI-compatible.

Mesh type and design. The overall characteristics of a SEMS depend on the stent mesh design. The SEMS used in the biliary tract can be divided into two types—those made with a woven, braided mesh and those made from a single nitinol wire cut with a spiral zigzag design. Most SEMS available for biliary use are made with a woven braided mesh (Elgiloy or nitinol). A braided mesh combines good flexibility and radial force with resistance to longitudinal traction (very important if there is a need to remove the stent) [43]. Adjustments of the mesh size might improve performance; theoretically, the thinner the mesh, the more flexible the stent. Another important characteristic that may affect the overall performance of a SEMS is the design of the stent edges. A soft, rounded and flexible end may reduce epithelial reactivity and thus the risk of tissue overgrowth, although it may also facilitate migration. By contrast, ends that are flared or barbed, or both, may prevent stent migration but can induce tissue overgrowth [44]. Currently available braided mesh stents are available in two versions—uncovered, or covered with a stent coating to prevent tumor ingrowth.

SEMS with a spiral zigzag design are laser-cut from a single nitinol tube. This special SEMS design provides excellent flexibility associated with good radial force. In addition, these SEMS can be compressed into a very small-caliber introducer and do not become shorter after deployment, allowing perfect SEMS positioning across the stricture. Unfortunately, the special mesh design does not allow them to be moved or removed after deployment. The thin nitinol wire tends to break if it is pulled with a foreign-body forceps or snare. In addition, most stents with a spiral zig-zag mesh are only available uncovered, and they can therefore become occluded by tumor ingrowth (**Fig. 36.5**).

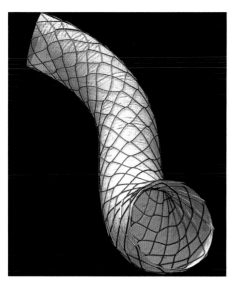

Fig. 36.6 A fully covered nitinol self-expanding metal stent made with a woven braided mesh (Niti-S; Taewoong Medical, Seoul, South Korea). The particular mesh design in this stent provides excellent flexibility and good radial force. A plastic covering is inserted between the inner and the outer mesh in order to enhance flexibility and prevent stent migration. Different versions of this stent are available, including partly covered, uncovered, and fully covered devices.

Uncovered versus polymer-coated SEMS. Tissue ingrowth (hyperplasia or neoplasia) through the mesh of a SEMS is one of the main causes of SEMS malfunction [40,41,45–50]. SEMS with a plastic polymer covering were therefore developed in recent years, and most stent manufacturers now have both covered and uncovered biliary SEMS on their product lists. The currently available covered SEMS may be fully covered or partly covered (with uncovered ends, to minimize migration) (**Figs. 36.6, 36.7**).

The results of clinical trials comparing covered and uncovered SEMS for palliative treatment of jaundice and cholangitis are controversial. Covered SEMS may occlude with time, but their patency period is significantly longer than with uncovered SEMS. However, increased SEMS migration rates and SEMS-related cholecystitis rates have been observed with covered SEMS [46–49]. Placement of covered SEMS in patients with hilar strictures requires careful evaluation. A covered SEMS with the proximal end placed above the biliary bifurcation may occlude one of the main hepatic ducts or other secondary sectorial or segmental ducts, leading to biliary obstruction and cholangitis.

As some reports have demonstrated that the removal of covered SEMS is feasible and completely safe, research is currently focusing on the possible role of covered SEMS in patients with benign disease, with an emphasis on postoperative biliary strictures and biliary strictures related to chronic pancreatitis [43,51–58].

Stenting Technique

Positioning of Plastic Stents

Biliary stents (either plastic or metal) can be positioned with or without a prior sphincterotomy. The technique of endoscopic plastic stent placement is now well-established. The procedure begins with guide-wire cannulation of the selected duct. Various guide wires can be used for this purpose. Straight-tipped or angle-tipped fully hydrophilic guide wires are very useful for very tight strictures, but hybrid guide wires with a hydrophilic tip and coil wire shaft can be used for routine application. Pigtail and 5-Fr or 7-Fr straight stents can be inserted into the biliary or pancreatic duct directly over the guide wire and advanced with a stent pusher.

By contrast, placement of large-bore straight stents requires a different approach. A 5-Fr or 6-Fr guiding catheter (for an 8.5-Fr or 10–11.5-Fr stent, respectively) is advanced over the guide wire beyond the stricture. The guiding catheter should lie well above the stricture, preferably in a major intrahepatic duct [59]. The large-bore stent is then loaded over the guiding catheter and pushed with the stent pusher (**Fig. 36.8**).

This three-accessory system was simplified into an all-in-one stent set that combines the guiding catheter, stent, and pusher [60]. There is considerable friction in this system, and the inner catheter tends to move upward with the pusher movements. Continuous fluoroscopic monitoring of the correct positioning of guide wire and guiding catheter in the intrahepatic ducts is therefore required. The assistant should help with stent insertion by applying moderate traction on the inner catheter against the pusher catheter. This is particularly important with very tight common bile duct strictures and hilar strictures.

During stent insertion, the tip of the endoscope should be very close to the papilla in order to avoid any bowing in the catheter and to push the stent along the axis of the common bile duct. The stent is pushed in through the combined action of the endoscope's elevator, of the tip of the endoscope (angled up), and the stent pusher. With tight strictures, a fourth movement sometimes helps increase the efficacy of the pushing action. The stent should be locked with the elevator in the full up position and pushed in by pulling back on the

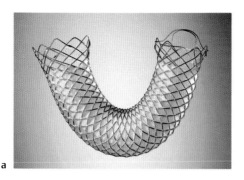

a

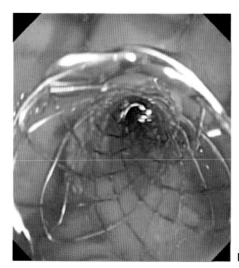

b

Fig. 36.7 A partly covered nitinol self-expanding metal stent (WallFlex; Boston Scientific, Natick, Massachusetts, USA).
a This stent is made of a nitinol woven and braided mesh. The nontraumatic, flared, uncovered ends prevent stent migration after deployment. The distal end is provided with a loop to make stent removal easier if necessary. This stent is very flexible and has excellent visibility on fluoroscopy and good radial force.
b An endoscopic image of a biliary WallFlex immediately after deployment.

V

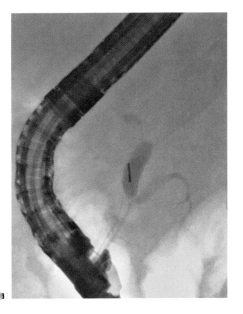

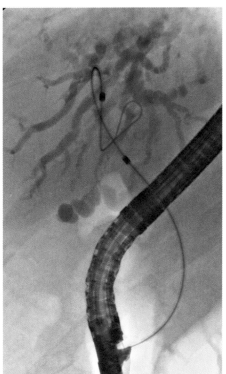

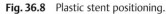

Fig. 36.8 Plastic stent positioning.
a Endoscopic retrograde cholangiopancreatography shows a distal common bile duct stricture due to pancreatic cancer.
b A guide wire has been maneuvered into position to traverse the stricture.
c A guiding catheter is pushed over the guide wire, through the stricture. Guiding catheters for plastic stent insertion are usually provided with radiopaque markers to allow measurement of the length of the stricture.
d An Amsterdam-type plastic stent is being pushed over the guiding catheter across the stricture, using a stent pusher. The stent is eventually released by withdrawing the guiding catheter and the guide wire.

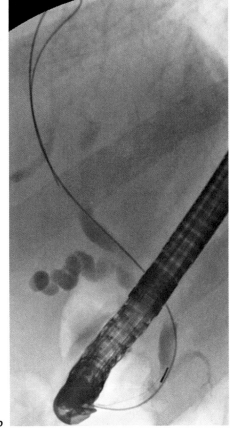

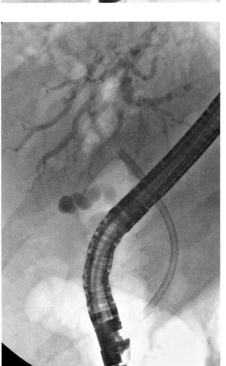

c

d

36

endoscope shaft to force the stent inward. This maneuver is particularly useful in hilar strictures.

Once the proximal end of the stent is above the stricture and the distal end is 1 cm from the papilla, the stent can be released by pulling out the inner guiding catheter completely.

Metal Stent Deployment

Deploying a SEMS is an easy maneuver. However, SEMS are expensive, and once they have been completely deployed, it is difficult to adjust the stent position. SEMS deployment therefore requires special attention on the part of the endoscopist and the assistant.

The procedure can usually be carried out without any previous stricture dilation. SEMS introducers have a diameter varying from 6 Fr to 11.5 Fr, like the standard plastic stents. In the delivery system, the SEMS are constrained between an inner catheter (which allows passage of the guide wire) and an outer sheath. The delivery system is advanced over the guide wire and positioned across the stricture. As some SEMS become significantly shorter after deployment, the appropriate SEMS length should be carefully evaluated on preliminary cholangiography by using appropriately graduated catheters [59]. SEMS is usually left extending about 5–10 mm beyond the papilla into the duodenum. There is no evidence that placing the SEMS completely inside the duct prolongs patency, but subsequent endoscopic intervention may be more difficult if the stent malfunc-

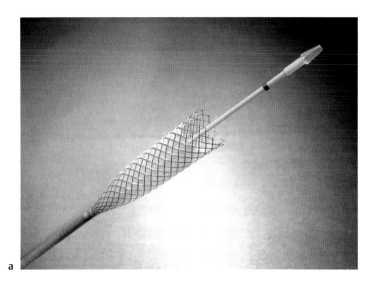

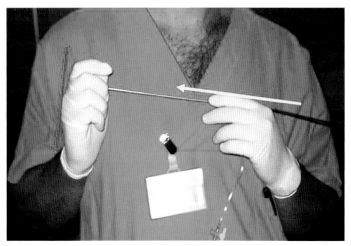

Fig. 36.9   Deployment of a self-expanding metal stent (SEMS).
a   SEMS are supplied compressed into a small-caliber (7.5–11.5 Fr) delivery system, between an inner catheter that allows guide wire passage and an outer transparent sheath. The delivery system usually has radiopaque markers. Part of the covered biliary Wallstent seen here is still compressed inside the delivery system.
b   The assistant releases the stent by sliding the outer sheath (yellow arrow) back over the inner catheter, which is firmly held with the other hand (red line).

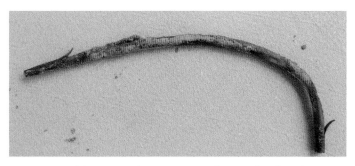

Fig. 36.10   A biliary stent that was removed 4 months after placement. Diffuse crystallized sludge deposits are visible (light orange) on the outer surface of the stent.

tions. Once the delivery system is in position, the SEMS is released by carefully pulling back the outer sheath. This maneuver must be continuously monitored by fluoroscopy to allow minor adjustments of the SEMS position before final release. If necessary, a SEMS can be reinserted into the delivery system before it has been totally deployed (e.g., in case of erroneous placement or inappropriate SEMS

length). In this case, the outer sheath is gently pushed in and advanced over the SEMS until it is completely constrained. After the necessary adjustments, the SEMS can be deployed. After deployment, the delivery system is withdrawn through the expanded SEMS (**Fig. 36.9**).

Management of Malfunctioning Stents

Sooner or later, all biliary and pancreatic stents malfunction or become occluded. Stent occlusion is usually clinically significant and leads to recurrent signs of biliary and pancreatic obstruction, including jaundice, cholangitis, abdominal pain, pancreatitis, and infections (hepatic abscesses and pancreatic abscesses). Prompt intervention is always required if there is suspected stent malfunction, in order to prevent deteriorating clinical conditions and more severe complications.

▦ Plastic Stents

The mean patency period with biliary plastic stents is approximately 100 days, varying depending on the number of stents placed, their diameter, and the level of the obstruction [4,44,61–63]. Plastic stents may malfunction for various reasons. They may impact into the bile duct wall, leading to poor bile drainage, especially in patients with C-curved bile ducts or when inappropriately long stents are used [44]. They can migrate upward or downward and impact into the duodenal wall [44]. However, the most frequent cause of plastic stent occlusion is stent clogging. The mechanism leading to stent clogging is not completely understood. In vitro studies have demonstrated that the development of a biofilm of bacteria and proteinaceous material on the inner surface of the plastic stent may be the initial event [27,28,30,64–68]. Bacterial enzymes may promote bilirubin deconjugation and precipitation of biliary salts and calcium bilirubinate inside the plastic stent. Clinical research has focused on finding ways of prolonging stent patency [3,4,6,8–10,26, 27,31,33–35,69–77]. However, the polymer type, stent shape, and administration of antibiotics and biliary salts have unfortunately not been found to prolong stent patency significantly in clinical practice (**Fig. 36.10**).

Pancreatic stents occlude over time in the same way as their biliary counterparts. The biochemical events that promote pancreatic stent obstruction are similar to those that cause biliary stent clogging, and include bacterial adhesion to a protein matrix and precipitation of calcium carbonate [17–19] (**Fig. 36.11**). In comparison with biliary stents, pancreatic stent obstruction is slower, and when the stent becomes occluded it may be clinically silent for months (stent exchange is required after a mean of 6–12 months). The low incidence of pancreatic pain and pancreatitis may be partly explained by the nature of the disease leading to pancreatic stent placement, which in most patients is chronic pancreatitis. Chronic pancreatitis causes gradual fibrosis and atrophy of the pancreas, with less frequent pain attacks.

When biliary and pancreatic stents malfunction, they can be easily removed and replaced with a new plastic or metal stent. When the stents are still visible beyond the papilla of Vater, removing them is easy and does not require special instructions. Stents can be grasped with a foreign-body forceps or snare and removed through the accessory channel of the endoscope, or by removing the endoscope from the patient's mouth. When the stent has migrated above the papilla of Vater, extracting it may be more complicated. Stents can be removed using a foreign-body forceps, a Dormia basket, or a snare, which can be opened inside the biliary or pancreatic duct [78–82] (**Fig. 36.12**).

V

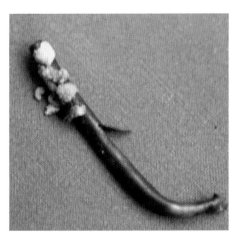

Fig. 36.11 An occluded pancreatic stent, 6 months after placement. There is proteinaceous material and calcium carbonate soiling at the proximal end of the stent.

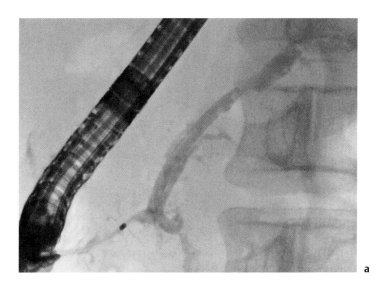

a

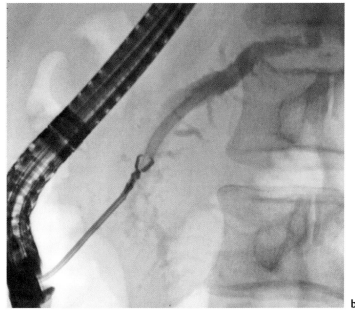

b

A special accessory has been developed for over-the-wire stent exchange—the Soehendra stent retriever [83]. The device consists of a flexible metal catheter with a threaded tip. After cannulation of the migrated stent using a guide wire, the Soehendra stent retriever is advanced over the wire and its tip is screwed into the stent by rotating the device clockwise. When the stent has been completely engaged, it can be removed through the endoscope's accessory channel, leaving the wire in place ready for implantation of a new stent. A variety of different techniques and tricks for removing migrated plastic stents have been described in the literature, and these can be used in specific situations (**Fig. 36.13**).

Following retrieval of a plastic stent, a new plastic stent can be immediately inserted through the stricture. However, in some clinical situations, plastic stents may become easily occluded due to the presence of pus, thick sludge, or clots. In this situation, placing a SEMS may be more appropriate, regardless of the patient's life expectancy [84,85].

SEMS

The mean patency period for SEMS is approximately 7 months. The reported occlusion rates show wide variations, between 10% and 65%, depending on the patient and the characteristics of the SEMS used. However, most patients undergoing SEMS placement for tumor palliation die without recurrent symptoms of biliary obstruction [45,46,48,49,51,86–92].

Covered and uncovered SEMS are likely to become occluded for different reasons, and the management of malfunctioning covered and uncovered SEMS is therefore also different [40,41,50,93,94]. The main reason for occlusion of uncovered SEMS is ingrowth. If the patient survives long enough, a neoplasm sooner or later grows through the mesh of an uncovered SEMS until it becomes completely occluded. The easiest way to treat patients with an obstructed uncovered SEMS is to place a new stent inside the occluded one [40,41,50,93,94]. The choice between a plastic stent or a new SEMS should be weighed up in accordance with the quality of the bile above the stricture (sludge, clots, and pus will lead to early plastic stent occlusion) and the patient's presumed life expectancy (**Fig. 36.14**).

Covered SEMS are more likely to become occluded due to sludge and debris or neoplastic overgrowth [47,49]. Mechanical cleaning (with a Dormia basket or an extraction balloon) may be the first-line approach for the management of covered SEMS occluded by stones or sludge. In this case, the treatment only takes a short time and is relatively inexpensive. Placement of a nasobiliary drain for a couple of days and continuous bile duct perfusion with saline solution may also be helpful (**Fig. 36.15**). Over time, a neoplasm may grow through the mesh of the uncovered end of a covered SEMS or above

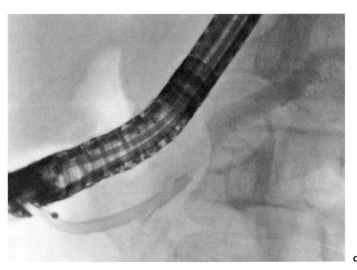

c

Fig. 36.12 Removal of a migrated pancreatic stent.
a Endoscopic retrograde cholangiopancreatography shows a pancreatic stent that has completely migrated inside the pancreatic duct.
b The stent is grasped with a foreign-body forceps that has been introduced into the pancreatic duct.
c The stent is being removed through the endoscope's accessory channel.

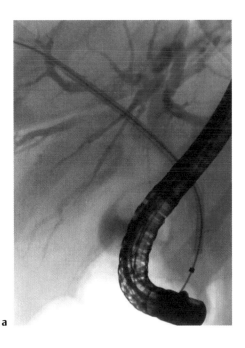

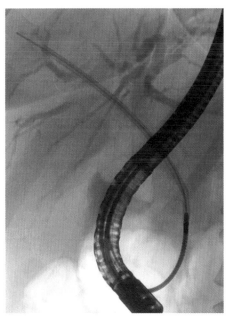

Fig. 36.13 Over-the-wire removal of a migrated biliary stent.
a A biliary stent has migrated proximally above the papilla of Vater. A guide wire has been inserted into the stent lumen using a catheter.
b A Soehendra stent retriever is advanced over the wire up to the distal end of the stent. The stent retriever tip is screwed into the stent by rotating the whole device clockwise. When the stent has been completely engaged, it can be removed through the endoscope's accessory channel.

a

b

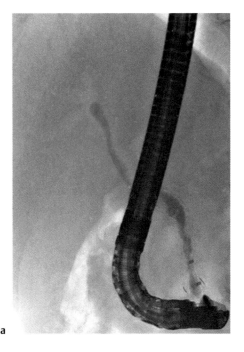

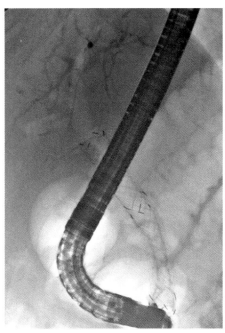

Fig. 36.14 Management of occluded self-expanding metal stents.
a Endoscopic retrograde cholangiopancreatography shows an uncovered stent occluded by neoplastic ingrowth and overgrowth.
b Insertion of a new self-expanding metal stent inside the occluded one. The massive pneumobilia at the end of the procedure should be noted.

a

b

the SEMS, contributing to malfunction [47,49]. As with ingrowth, placement of a new stent inside the occluded SEMS is probably the best way of treating overgrowth [40,41,50,93,94]. Although it happens less frequently than with uncovered SEMS, ingrowth can also affect the patency of covered SEMS if the integrity of the coating material is not sufficiently long-lasting [95].

Covered SEMS may migrate and in some cases impact into the duodenal wall [46–49,88,96]. SEMS migration may be facilitated by palliative chemoradiotherapy. The management of patients with migrated stents should be evaluated on a case-to-case basis. SEMS that impact into the duodenal wall should be removed (whenever possible) or trimmed using argon plasma coagulation [97–100] in order to avoid more severe complications, including duodenal perforation and bleeding (**Fig. 36.16**).

With a C-curved bile duct, a SEMS may impact into the medial bile duct wall, leading to obstruction. Theoretically, this complication is more likely to occur with Elgiloy SEMS, which are stiffer and

have a tendency to straighten after deployment. Placement of a longer SEMS inside the previous one may solve this problem.

When SEMS have been inserted for palliation of hilar strictures, they may occlude side branches or the contralateral hepatic duct. This complication is more likely to occur with covered SEMS, but can also be a consequence of ingrowth or overgrowth. Endoscopic management of patients with hilar strictures and occluded SEMS can be very difficult, with a greater likelihood of failure. The rescue approach is percutaneous cholangiography with external biliary drainage.

Although most SEMS are not designed to be extracted, it has been demonstrated that removing them is feasible and safe in selected cases [43,52,53]. Proposed indications for stent removal are as follows: 1, distal migration with impaction against the duodenal wall opposite the papilla, or stent malfunction resulting from an inappropriately long distal end lying in the duodenum; 2, impaction of the proximal end of the stent into the bile duct wall; 3, disease

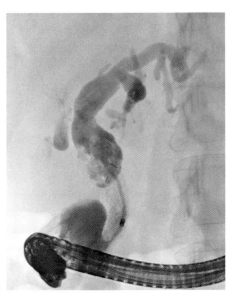

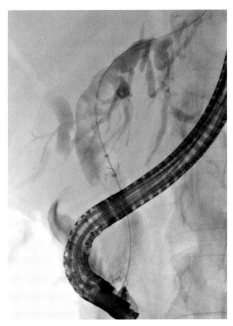

Fig. 36.15 Management of occluded self-expanding metal stents.

a A covered self-expanding metal stent completely occluded by debris and biliary sludge. The intrahepatic biliary ducts are dilated.

b Mechanical cleaning of the stent using an extraction balloon.

c Pneumobilia at the end of the procedure.

d A nasobiliary drain was placed at the end of the procedure. Cholangiography after 3 days showed complete cleaning of the bile duct and stent and a good flow of contrast medium into the duodenum.

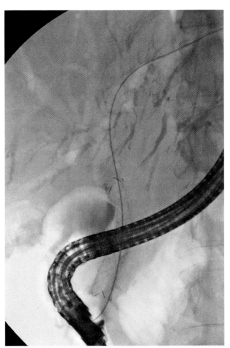

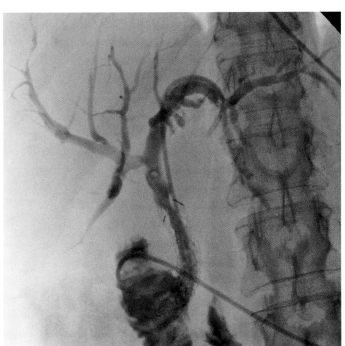

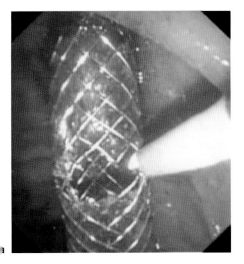

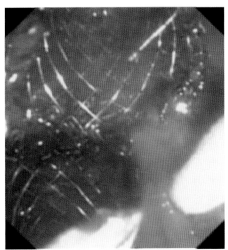

Fig. 36.16 Trimming of self-expanding metal stents.

a A covered stainless-steel metal stent has been deployed with the distal end protruding excessively into the duodenum and impacting into the duodenal wall. The stent is shortened using argon plasma coagulation (70–90 W, 1–2 L/min).

b The self-expanding metal stent has been completely trimmed.

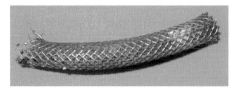

Fig. 36.17 A new partly covered Wallstent that was removed after 2 years. The plastic covering is still intact.

progression, tissue ingrowth, or overgrowth, necessitating an increased number of SEMS; and 4, inappropriate length of the stent, causing occlusion of intrahepatic ducts. Removal of covered SEMS is not a particularly demanding procedure if the covering has successfully prevented ingrowth (**Figs. 36.17, 36.18**). Removing uncovered SEMS affected by severe ingrowth is more likely to be unsuccessful. Recently, completely covered SEMS specifically designed to be removable in case of malfunction have been developed [101].

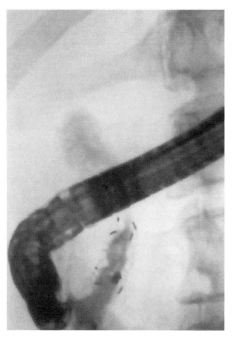

a

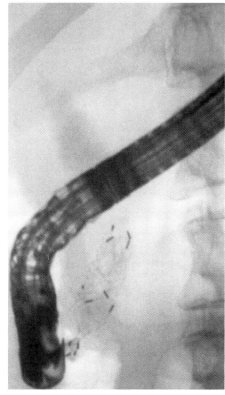

b

Fig. 36.18 Endoscopic removal of self-expanding metal stents.
a Endoscopic retrograde cholangiopancreatography shows partial distal migration of a covered self-expanding metal stent.
b, c The stent is captured with a polypectomy snare and removed through the endoscope's accessory channel.
d A new biliary self-expanding metal stent was placed at the end of the procedure.

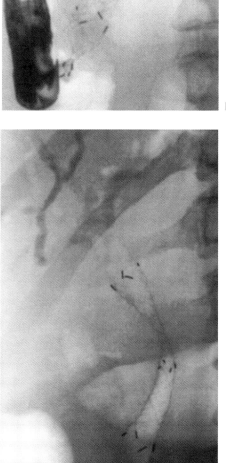

c

d

Biliary Stenting

Malignant Strictures

Endoscopic placement of stents is the gold standard for palliative treatment of malignant biliary strictures. Stenting improves the patient's quality of life, is less invasive than surgical or percutaneous drainage, and is well accepted by patients [102].

Common bile duct strictures. Most malignant common bile duct strictures are due to pancreatic cancer. Less frequently, they are caused by lymph-node metastases or primary distal cholangiocarcinoma. Stenting for malignant common bile duct strictures has an extremely high success rate (**Fig. 36.19**).

The choice of stent type for malignant biliary stricture stenting is a matter of debate. In comparison with plastic stents, SEMS have longer patency periods and require fewer days of hospitalization, less use of antibiotics, and fewer ERCPs and transabdominal ultrasound examinations, with a lower overall cost. It is now generally accepted that SEMS placement is the appropriate palliative procedure for patients without distant metastases and an expected survival period of at least 4–6 months at the initial stent placement. A metal stent would be cost-effective if future interventions were to cost more than $1820 [103,104]. Patients in whom resection is possible can also benefit from SEMS, as it provides a longer patency period and ensures the continuity of neoadjuvant chemoradiotherapy. It has recently been demonstrated that surgical resection is possible with a SEMS in place [105].

Hilar strictures. Stenting in malignant hilar biliary strictures is a challenge for the endoscopist, as it is technically difficult and the results are unsatisfactory due to the high incidence of infectious complications. The number of stents required to drain complex hilar strictures is still under debate. Injection of contrast above hilar strictures and subsequent partial drainage, leaving opacified and undrained biliary ducts, was the cause of the high incidence of cholangitis reported in early studies [106,107]. Magnetic resonance cholangiography (MRC), providing a detailed map of the intrahepatic ducts above a malignant hilar stricture, can guide the endoscopist for drainage of selected and dilated intrahepatic ducts (**Fig. 36.20**).

Plastic stents 12 or 15 cm long are usually needed for hilar strictures. A complete sphincterotomy is suggested if multiple stenting is planned. Inserting multiple plastic stents in the presence of an undilated common bile duct below the stricture and a tight hilar stricture is technically difficult and can fail. Unilateral plastic stent insertion using MRC as a "road map," with drainage only of opacified intrahepatic biliary ducts [108], reduces the incidence of infectious complications and ensures resolution of jaundice, provided that a large enough portion of the liver is affected. This technique also results in an easier and shorter procedure.

36

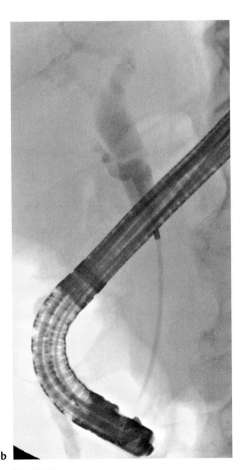
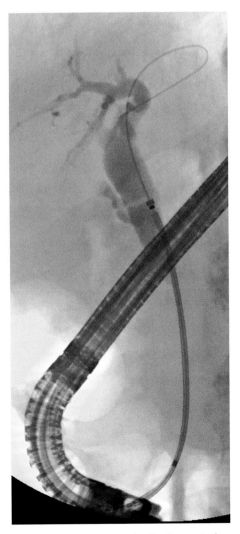
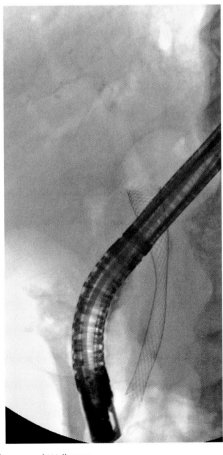

b

c

Fig. 36.19
a A malignant common bile duct stricture secondary to pancreatic cancer.
b Deployment of a partly covered Wallstent.
c The Wallstent is released; pneumobilia is present.

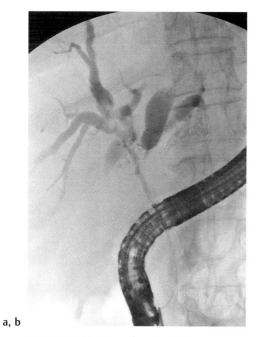 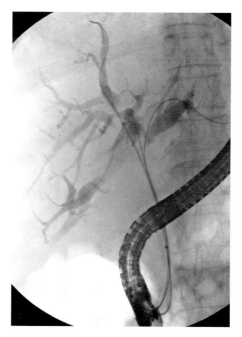

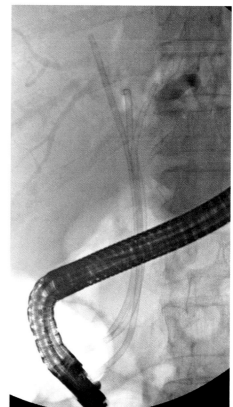

a, b

Fig. 36.20 Stenting of proximal biliary strictures.
a Endoscopic retrograde cholangiopancreatography shows a Bismuth–Corlette type III malignant hilar stricture.
b Three guide wires are positioned in the ducts above the stricture.
c Insertion of three plastic stents, with complete drainage of all the opacified ducts.

c

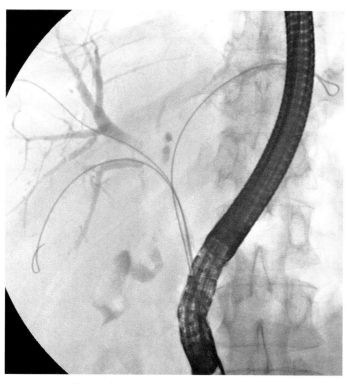

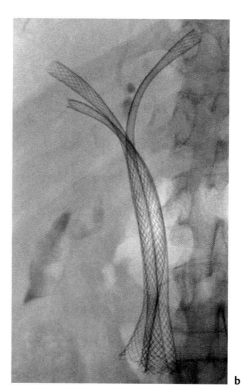

a

b

Fig. 36.21 Self-expanding metal stents for proximal biliary strictures.
a A Bismuth–Corlette type III malignant hilar stricture, with three guide wires positioned over the stricture.

b Insertion of three uncovered Wallstents, in a patient with inoperable hilar cholangiocarcinoma.

In comparison with plastic stents, SEMS are associated with better short-term outcomes, independently of the Bismuth classification [109]. Inserting multiple SEMS for unresectable hilar strictures is very expensive and technically difficult, and later management of clogged SEMS can be very challenging (**Fig. 36.21**). Uncovered SEMS are preferable to ensure drainage of lateral bile ducts. Unilateral MRC-targeted and computed tomography–targeted drainage of hilar strictures using a single SEMS has shown satisfactory results [110,111]. Endoscopic drainage is recommended as the first-line procedure for palliative treatment of jaundice in patients with inoperable Klatskin tumor of Bismuth–Corlette types II and III, while the percutaneous approach is preferable in type IV [112,113].

Benign Indications

Plastic biliary stenting represents the standard treatment for benign biliary strictures, as the stents are removable and surgery is always still possible if endoscopic treatment fails. There may be a role for SEMS treatment for benign biliary strictures in selected cases (biliary strictures in chronic pancreatitis), but this is not accepted as a standard treatment due to the poor results and the scarcity of data in the literature.

Postoperative biliary strictures. Postoperative biliary strictures following cholecystectomy are the most common benign biliary strictures. Postoperative biliary strictures benefit from an "aggressive" endoscopic approach, with the insertion of an increasing number of plastic stents at 3-monthly stent exchange intervals until there is complete morphologic disappearance of the stricture, independent of the duration of the treatment [114,115]. This treatment reduced the stricture recurrence rate during the long-term follow-up in comparison with the standard approach (placement of two 10-Fr stents with 3-monthly exchanges for a period of 1 year) [116] (**Fig. 36.22**). Anastomotic strictures following liver transplantation can also benefit from this aggressive approach [117] (**Fig. 36.23**). In patients with benign disease, a complete sphincterotomy is necessary before multiple placement of plastic stents, to allow stent insertion. It has been proposed that SEMS should be used to dilate benign biliary strictures, but the results have generally been poor, with high medium and long-term morbidity rates [55,118–120].

Primary sclerosing cholangitis. Dominant strictures of the extrahepatic bile ducts occur in 15–20% of patients with primary sclerosing cholangitis. These strictures are well diagnosed with MRC and can be treated endoscopically using pneumatic dilation or stenting [121,122]. Short-term stenting (2 weeks) with a single 10-Fr plastic stent is suggested for patients with primary sclerosing cholangitis; longer periods of stenting increase the risk of cholangitis. In patients with primary sclerosing cholangitis, endoscopic treatment of dominant biliary strictures provides drainage of the bile ducts and relief from obstructions, with acceptable procedure-related complications and higher than expected 3-year and 4-year survival rates [123]. In recent years, many experts have preferred balloon dilation alone to stenting in primary sclerosing cholangitis [124].

Chronic pancreatitis and biliary stricture. Patients with biliary strictures secondary to chronic pancreatitis presenting with cholangitis, jaundice, or persistent cholestasis may benefit from endoscopic plastic stenting (**Fig. 36.24**).

Common bile duct strictures occurring in the course of chronic pancreatitis may be reversible (due to pancreatic edema or compression from a pseudocyst) or nonreversible (due to pancreatic fibrosis). Biliary strictures disappear in about one-third of the patients who undergo single plastic stenting for 3–6 months. An aggressive approach with multiple simultaneous side-by-side stents to obtain calibration of the biliary stricture appears to be superior to single stent placement, providing good long-term benefit [125,126]. If the stricture does not disappear after 1 year of plastic stenting, the patient should undergo surgical hepaticojejunostomy, which is the definitive treatment option [127]. Importantly, the presence of an endoprosthesis does not compromise the potential for surgical treatment.

36

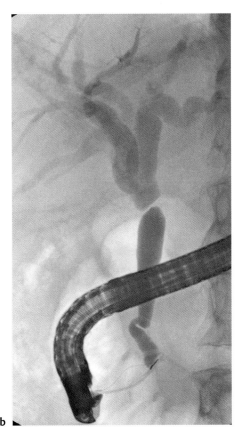
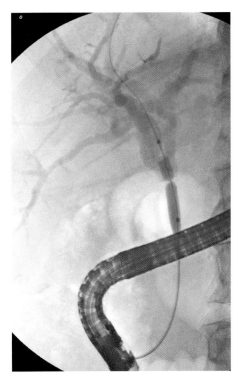
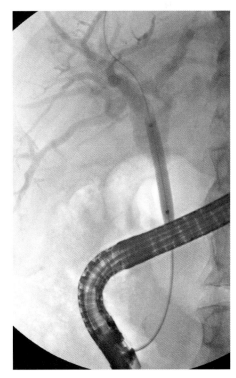

b

c

Fig. 36.22 Endoscopic management of postoperative biliary strictures.
a Endoscopic retrograde cholangiopancreatography shows a Bismuth type II benign biliary stricture following open cholecystectomy.

b Dilation of the stricture. The waist on the balloon should be noted.
c The balloon is fully expanded.

Fig. 36.22d–h ▷

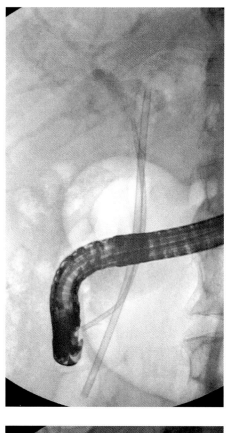

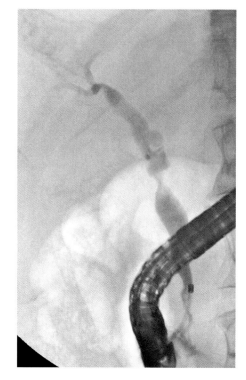

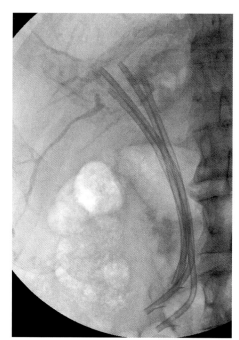

d

e,

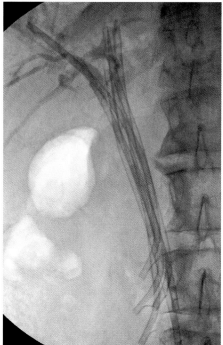

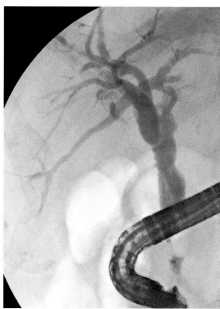

g

h

Fig. 36.22d–h
d   Insertion of two plastic stents.
e, f   Three months later, after removal of the stents, the stricture diameter has improved, and four large-bore plastic stents are inserted.
g   After a further 3 months, six plastic stents were placed.
h   The cholangiogram at the end of the treatment shows complete resolution of the stricture.

Patients with unrelenting strictures after plastic stenting who are unfit for surgery, or those who decline surgery, can be offered SEMS placement. The results with uncovered [54,128] and partly covered SEMS [129] are similar, with stent occlusion/dysfunction in almost half of the cases after a mean follow-up of 2–4 years. Sphincterotomy is suggested before plastic or metal stenting in these patients.

A new option for refractory chronic pancreatitis–related biliary strictures is dilation using temporary placement of fully covered removable SEMS. A recent study reported unsatisfactory results due to failure to remove fully covered SEMS in one-third of the cases

[101]. Future evaluation of removable SEMS and improvement in the materials and shape design is expected.

Bile duct leaks. Healing of biliary leaks (iatrogenic and post-traumatic) is achieved by reducing the pressure gradient between the biliary tree and the duodenum using endoscopic sphincterotomy and/or stenting, and/or nasobiliary catheter insertion. All of these treatments are effective [130,131]. Biliary stenting appears to be the most widely accepted technique for treating biliary leaks, as the sphincter of Oddi remains intact and the procedure is associated

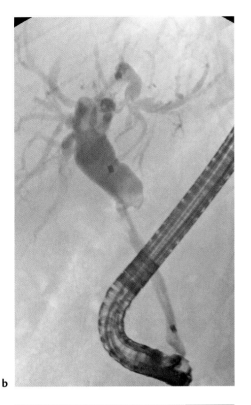

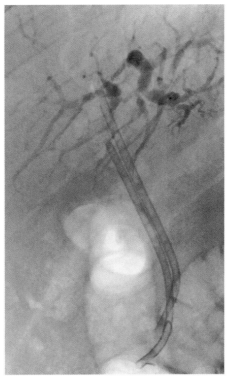

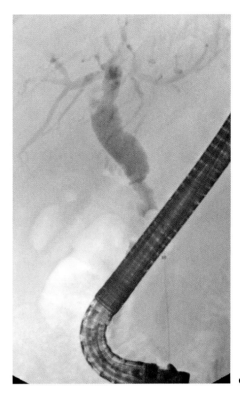

b

c

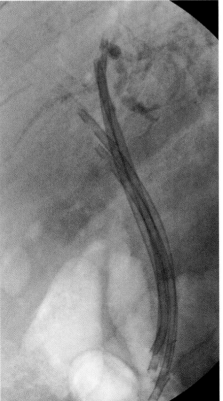

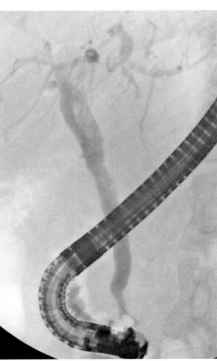

d

e

Fig. 36.23 Endoscopic dilation of an anastomotic biliary stricture after liver transplantation.
a The anastomotic biliary stricture following liver transplantation.
b Insertion of two large-bore plastic stents.
c, d Three months later, after removal of the stents, the stricture has improved, and four plastic stents are placed.
e The final cholangiogram showing complete stricture resolution after a further 3 months.

36

with less discomfort for the patient than a nasobiliary catheter. The disadvantage of internal stenting is the need for repeat endoscopy for stent removal 4–8 weeks after initial placement. Long, large-diameter (10 Fr or larger), leak-traversing plastic stents are preferred [132], although in a recent study no advantage was observed for 10-Fr stents in comparison with 7-Fr stents [133]. Temporary placement of partly covered SEMS for biliary leaks not responding to conventional endoscopic stenting was recently described, with a high success rate and with no problems in removing the SEMS after 3 months [56]. This approach can be regarded as a rescue therapy in referral centers.

Biliary stones. In patients with large, unretrievable stones, plastic stents can be placed to drain the bile duct and prevent cholangitis before further attempts at removal with or without previous intracorporeal or extracorporeal lithotripsy. It has been reported that the

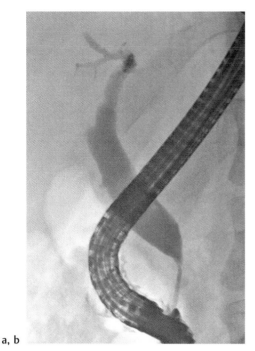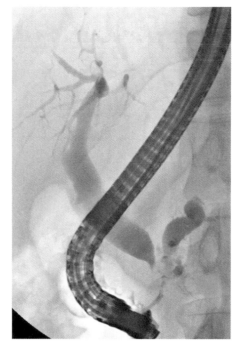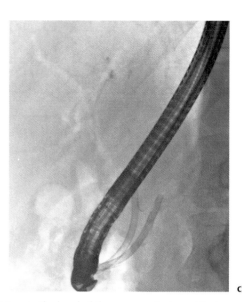

a, b
c

Fig. 36.24 Biliary stricture secondary to chronic pancreatitis.
a Endoscopic retrograde cholangiopancreatography shows a benign biliary stricture secondary to chronic pancreatitis.

b A pancreatic duct stricture in the head of the pancreas is also evident.
c Insertion of biliary and pancreatic plastic stents.

V

presence of a stent, through continuous grinding of the stone and along with administration of ursodeoxycholic acid, can make the stone smaller in 70% of cases, facilitating subsequent removal [134,135]. Definitive stenting for unretrievable bile duct stones is indicated in elderly and high-risk patients, with good immediate results in relieving biliary obstruction and maintaining bile duct patency [136]. Due to the high incidence of recurrent cholangitis and related mortality, permanent biliary stenting should preferably be restricted to patients who are unfit for elective treatment at a later stage and who have a short life expectancy [137].

Cholecystitis. Retrograde cannulation of the cystic duct with hydrophilic guide wires and insertion of a 7-Fr double-pigtail plastic stent or nasocholecystic drainage have been used in high-risk patients and those with neoplasia as a "bridge to surgery" or as a definitive treatment for acute cholecystitis. Successful retrograde drainage of the gallbladder is reported in over 70% of cases, with a favorable clinical outcome in over 85% of the patients [138,139]. Retrograde drainage of the gallbladder in cases of acute cholecystitis represents an alternative to percutaneous drainage, particularly in patients with ascites, coagulopathy, and those who are receiving anticoagulants or antiplatelet drugs.

Pancreatic Stenting

Chronic Pancreatitis

In patients with chronic pancreatitis, pancreatic stenting plays a major role for drainage of the main pancreatic duct obstructed by strictures and/or stones, and for drainage of pancreatic pseudocysts.

Pancreatic duct strictures. Symptomatic patients with a single pancreatic duct stricture located in the head of the pancreas are the best candidates for pancreatic stenting. In cases of tight main pancreatic duct strictures that cannot be traversed with a 5-Fr or 6-Fr guiding catheter, dilation before stent insertion becomes mandatory in or-

der to insert large-bore (8.5–11.5 Fr) stents, which provide a longer patency period (**Fig. 36.25**). Pain relief is achieved after single pancreatic stenting in chronic pancreatitis in more than 75% of the cases [140,141].

Main pancreatic duct stricture relapse after stent removal is reported in 38% of cases [140]. Calibration of a single pancreatic duct stricture in the head of the pancreas with multiple stents is a promising approach, with stricture resolution in 95% of cases and 84% of the patients free of pain after a mean follow-up period of 3 years [142]. The mean pancreatic stent patency period is 6–12 months. "On-demand" stent exchange instead of prophylactic substitution every 3 months is the preferred strategy [143], as the length of the clinical effect of a pancreatic stent is rather unpredictable. Removal of temporary, fully covered pancreatic SEMS was feasible 3 months after placement, but the incidence of stricture recurrence after stent removal was over 50% [144]. These results come from a pilot study, and the use of SEMS in the pancreatic duct is currently far from representing clinical practice.

Pancreatic stones. Calcified pancreatic stones can become impacted in the ductal wall or above a stricture, making extraction impossible without prior fragmentation using extracorporeal shock-wave lithotripsy (ESWL). Following ESWL, pancreatic stenting is frequently required due to a concomitant stricture of the main pancreatic duct [145]. Complete removal of pancreatic stone fragments is important, as they can occlude the stent. If ESWL is not available, drainage of the main pancreatic duct can be obtained by inserting a plastic stent alongside the stone. Stent insertion alongside a pancreatic stone fails in half of the cases, can require aggressive mechanical dilation, and insertion of a pancreatic stent larger than 7 Fr is rare. As an alternative to ESWL when there are pancreatic stones above a stricture, inserting an uncovered SEMS and removing it after 4–7 days allowed stricture dilation, eventually leading to stone extraction, in four cases [146]. This represents an unusual indication for SEMS and ESWL is still the gold standard treatment for pancreatic stones.

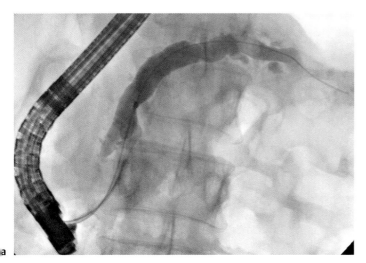
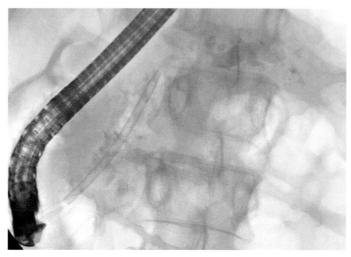

Fig. 36.25 Pancreatic duct obstruction due to chronic pancreatitis.
a Pancreatic stones are extracted with a Dormia basket.

b Insertion of a pancreatic stent, with complete drainage of contrast.

Pseudocysts. The indications for drainage of pancreatic pseudocysts are mainly symptom-driven (pain, fever, vomiting, and jaundice due to gastrointestinal or biliary compression), and drainage should also be considered when cysts are becoming larger [147]. Endoscopic management of pancreatic pseudocysts consists of two approaches—transmural and transpapillary.

Transmural drainage involves establishing a communication between the pseudocyst and the lumen of the stomach (cystogastrostomy) or duodenum (cystoduodenostomy). This approach is possible only when there is evidence of clear bulging of the pseudocyst into the gastric or duodenal wall. Endoscopic ultrasonography has expanded the endoscopic options, making it possible to drain nonbulging pancreatic pseudocysts [148,149]. After puncture, one or more transmural large-bore plastic stents are inserted into the cyst from the stomach or the duodenum in order to maintain the fistula, and usually one or two nasocystic drainage tubes are inserted to flush the cyst, especially if it is infected. The use of double-pigtail plastic stents reduces the risk of stent migration and complications in comparison with straight stents [127].

Transpapillary endoscopic drainage with plastic stents is preferred in the presence of small (< 6 cm) and solitary pseudocysts communicating with the main pancreatic duct and distant from the stomach and duodenum. When these pseudocysts are associated with pancreatic stones or strictures occluding the main pancreatic duct, relieving the obstruction by stent insertion is important in order to avoid later recurrence of the pseudocysts. Relief of symptoms after endoscopic treatment of pancreatic pseudocysts is reported in over 88% of cases, and this result is sustained after a minimum follow-up of 6 months [150,151].

Other Pancreatic Indications

Pancreatic duct leaks. Pancreatic duct leaks usually occur after acute pancreatitis, surgery, or trauma. Endoscopic interventions are reserved for fistulas that do not respond to conservative treatment.

The aim of endoscopic treatment is to traverse the ductal defect by placing a stent or a nasopancreatic drain across the leak point, whenever possible. As an alternative, an attempt can be made to reduce pancreatic duct pressure by performing a pancreatic sphincterotomy or by placing a pancreatic stent downstream from the leak. The pancreatic stent diameter should be adjusted in accordance with pancreatic duct diameter; 7-Fr and 8.5-Fr plastic stents are most commonly used. Pancreatic sphincterotomy appears to be important in order to avoid recurrent fistula due to an increase in ductal pressure after the stent is removed. Transpapillary stenting is effective in obtaining healing of pancreatic duct leaks in approximately two-thirds of cases [152–154].

Pancreas divisum. There is no consensus regarding the appropriate endoscopic treatment for acute recurrent pancreatitis associated with pancreas divisum. Endoscopic papillotomy of the minor papilla appears to lead to clinical improvement in most cases [155]. A short 5-Fr pancreatic stent can be inserted before needle-knife sphincterotomy of the minor papilla in order to identify the landmarks for the appropriate depth and height of incision; a stent without an internal flange can facilitate spontaneous migration, avoiding the need for a repeated ERCP for removal of the stent. To avoid minor papilla sphincterotomy, dorsal duct stenting (5 Fr or 7 Fr) in patients with acute recurrent pancreatitis and pancreas divisum has also been used, with good clinical results 2 years after stent removal [155]. Pancreatic stenting also resulted in effective symptom relief in patients with chronic pancreatitis and pancreas divisum [156].

Obstructive pancreatic-type pain. If pancreatic pain in patients with pancreatic cancer is related to meals (known as "obstructive" pain), the patients may benefit from pancreatic stenting. Stent insertion may fail due to tumor necrosis at the level of the stricture. When plastic stenting (7–10 Fr) is successful, approximately 60% of patients treated for "obstructive" pain become symptom-free, and a further 20–25% have a significant reduction in the analgesic drug dosage required [157–159].

Future Developments in Biliopancreatic Stenting

Current research is focusing on efforts to prolong the patency of biliary and pancreatic stents. Over many years, stent manufacturers have attempted to modify the polymer used and the shape of plastic stents, but without achieving any significant improvements in patency rates. At the same time, the development of plastic-coated SEMS did not completely solve the problem of SEMS occlusion. At present, the most interesting and promising advances in biliary stents are drug-eluting stents and bioabsorbable stents, a recently developed stent with an anti-duodenobiliary reflux valve, and the "wing stent"—a stent without a central lumen that has been designed to drain fluid around itself, along multiple grooved wings.

36

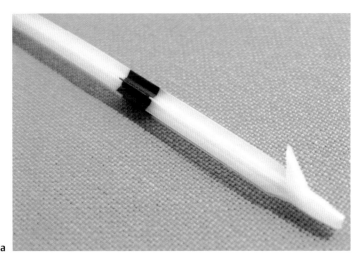

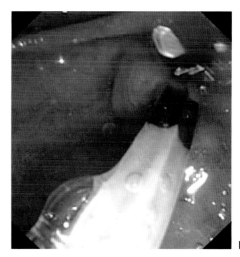

Fig. 36.26 The "wing" stent, a pancreatic stent without the central lumen. **a** Close-up view of this recently developed stent for biliary and pancreatic applications. This polyurethane stent has a star-shaped cross-section, with several wings radiating outward from the center. Bile and pancreatic juice flows along the "wings." **b** Endoscopic view of a 10-Fr "wing" stent placed in the pancreatic duct.

Drug-eluting stents. Drug-eluting stents are used in clinical practice for coronary strictures with good results and no apparent systemic toxicity. Similar stents impregnated with chemotherapeutic agents could be of value in the management of cholangiocarcinoma. Only a few published experiences with stents coated with carboplatin and paclitaxel are available [160,161]. The results of the pilot studies are promising, and future research on drug-eluting stents for biliopancreatic endoscopy is expected.

Bioabsorbable stents. Bioabsorbable biliary and pancreatic stents could have a role in the treatment of benign strictures. Although removable SEMS have recently been developed [101], their actual efficacy in the management of benign strictures needs to be further evaluated [42]. Theoretically, abrupt dilation of the scar of a benign stricture might induce further inflammation and eventually lead to a recurrent stricture. Eventually, every SEMS will occlude, and this would limit the role of SEMS for biliary strictures related to chronic pancreatitis and other permanent benign strictures (which are better managed using surgery). However, bioabsorbable stents could partly solve the problems related to the placement of large-bore expandable metal stents in benign strictures. To date, only a few published reports on experience in animals are available, with promising results in the treatment of benign biliary and pancreatic disorders [162–165].

Stents with an anti-duodenobiliary reflux valve and "wing" stents. Duodenobiliary reflux may play a role in the clogging of plastic stents that have been placed across the papilla of Vater. A special Soehendra–Tannenbaum plastic stent with an attached 4-cm windsock-shaped tubular valve made of expanded polytetrafluoroethylene material was tested in a clinical trial on a few patients. A preliminary in vitro evaluation showed that the newly developed antireflux biliary stent was effective in reducing duodenobiliary reflux without interfering with antegrade flow. In a prospective clinical evaluation, this new stent remained patent for a longer period (mean 145 days) in comparison with a standard stent [166]. However, further trials are needed in order to confirm the impact of reducing duodenobiliary reflux on the stent patency rate.

In the standard stents, bile and pancreatic juice flow is ensured by a central lumen. Over time, stents may become occluded due to deposits of bacteria, proteinaceous material, or sludge [27,28,30,64–68]. To overcome this problem, a new "winged" stent (a polyurethane stent with a star-shaped cross-section, with several wings radiating outward from the center and with no central lumen

except for a small central channel allowing the passage of a guide wire) has recently been developed, and it is currently available on the market [21,167] (**Fig. 36.26**).

Preliminary data have shown that in the short term, the new wing stent is likely to be at least as effective as standard Amsterdam stents in relieving signs of biliary obstruction [167]. In an animal study, a 5-Fr pancreatic wing stent was reported to cause less injury to the pancreatic duct than a standard 5-Fr pancreatic stent [21]. Although the preliminary results are promising, whether this type of stent will prove to be better than its conventional counterpart in clinical practice remains to be established.

Conclusions

Drainage of biliopancreatic ducts by ERCP and stenting can today be achieved in almost all cases. New materials have been developed during the last 10 years, but a perfect, clog-free biliary and pancreatic stent is as yet still not available. SEMS perform better than plastic stents in malignant strictures but, despite expanding indications, their cost is still too high for them to come into widespread use. The development of covered SEMS significantly improved the overall performance of metal stents, and ongoing research is investigating their possible role in the management of benign diseases. Some case reports and case series using SEMS in various benign biliopancreatic diseases have been published during the last 2–3 years. However, it will only be possible to assess the role of covered and removable SEMS in patients with benign biliopancreatic disease conclusively through prospective multicenter controlled clinical trials. SEMS are today indicated only for malignant biliary strictures, and plastic stents are approved for benign biliopancreatic strictures.

References

1. Soehendra N, Reynders-Frederix V. Palliative bile duct drainage—a new endoscopic method of introducing a transpapillary drain. Endoscopy 1980;12:8–11.
2. Soehendra N, Reynders-Frederix V. [Palliative biliary duct drainage. A new method for endoscopic introduction of a new drain]. Dtsch Med Wochenschr 1979;104:206–7. German.
3. Seitz U, Vadeyar H, Soehendra N. Prolonged patency with a new-design Teflon biliary prosthesis. Endoscopy 1994;26:478–82.
4. Libby ED, Leung JW. Prevention of biliary stent clogging: a clinical review. Am J Gastroenterol 1996;91:1301–8.

5. Libby ED, Leung JW. Ultrasmooth plastic to prevent stent clogging. Gastrointest Endosc 1994;40:386–7.

6. Binmoeller KF, Seitz U, Seifert H, Thonke F, Sikka S, Soehendra N. The Tannenbaum stent: a new plastic biliary stent without side holes. Am J Gastroenterol 1995;90:1764–8.

7. Coene PP, Groen AK, Cheng J, Out MM, Tytgat GN, Huibregtse K. Clogging of biliary endoprostheses: a new perspective. Gut 1990;31:913–7.

8. Catalano MF, Geenen JE, Lehman GA, Siegel JH, Jacob L, McKinley MJ, et al. "Tannenbaum" Teflon stents versus traditional polyethylene stents for treatment of malignant biliary stricture. Gastrointest Endosc 2002; 55:354–8.

9. van Berkel AM, Boland C, Redekop WK, Bergman JJ, Groen AK, Tytgat GN, et al. A prospective randomized trial of Teflon versus polyethylene stents for distal malignant biliary obstruction. Endoscopy 1998;30:681–6.

10. Terruzzi V, Comin U, De Grazia F, Toti GL, Zambelli A, Beretta S, et al. Prospective randomized trial comparing Tannenbaum Teflon and standard polyethylene stents in distal malignant biliary stenosis. Gastrointest Endosc 2000;51:23–7.

11. Schilling D, Rink G, Arnold JC, Benz C, Adamek HE, Jakobs R, et al. Prospective, randomized, single-center trial comparing 3 different 10F plastic stents in malignant mid and distal bile duct strictures. Gastrointest Endosc 2003;58:54–8.

12. England RE, Martin DF, Morris J, Sheridan MB, Frost R, Freeman A, et al. A prospective randomised multicentre trial comparing 10 Fr Teflon Tannenbaum stents with 10 Fr polyethylene Cotton–Leung stents in patients with malignant common duct strictures. Gut 2000;46:395–400.

13. Barkun AN. A prospective randomised multicentre trial comparing 10F Teflon Tannenbaum stents with 10F polyethylene Cotton–Leung stents in patients with malignant common duct strictures. Gastrointest Endosc 2001;53:399–401.

14. Pedersen FM. Endoscopic management of malignant biliary obstruction. Is stent size of 10 French gauge better than 7 French gauge? Scand J Gastroenterol 1993;28:185–9.

15. Speer AG, Cotton PB, MacRae KD. Endoscopic management of malignant biliary obstruction: stents of 10 French gauge are preferable to stents of 8 French gauge. Gastrointest Endosc 1988;34:412–7.

16. Kadakia SC, Starnes E. Comparison of 10 French gauge stent with 11.5 French gauge stent in patients with biliary tract diseases. Gastrointest Endosc 1992;38:454–9.

17. Devière J. Why do pancreatic stents become occluded? Gastrointest Endosc 2005;61:867–8.

18. Smits ME, Groen AK, Mok KS, van Marle J, Tytgat GN, Huibregtse K. Analysis of occluded pancreatic stents and juices in patients with chronic pancreatitis. Gastrointest Endosc 1997;45:52–8.

19. Provansal-Cheylan M, Bernard JP, Mariani A, Soehendra N, Cremer M, Sahel J, et al. Occluded pancreatic endoprostheses—analysis of the clogging material. Endoscopy 1989;21:63–9.

20. Lawrence C, Cotton PB, Romagnuolo J, Payne KM, Rawls E, Hawes RH. Small prophylactic pancreatic duct stents: an assessment of spontaneous passage and stent-induced ductal abnormalities. Endoscopy 2007;39:1082–5.

21. Raju GS, Gomez G, Xiao SY, Ahmed I, Brining D, Bhutani MS, et al. Effect of a novel pancreatic stent design on short-term pancreatic injury in a canine model. Endoscopy 2006;38:260–5.

22. Sherman S, Hawes RH, Savides TJ, Gress FG, Ikenberry SO, Smith MT, et al. Stent-induced pancreatic ductal and parenchymal changes: correlation of endoscopic ultrasound with ERCP. Gastrointest Endosc 1996;44:276–82.

23. Smith MT, Sherman S, Ikenberry SO, Hawes RH, Lehman GA. Alterations in pancreatic ductal morphology following polyethylene pancreatic stent therapy. Gastrointest Endosc 1996;44:268–75.

24. Sherman S, Alvarez C, Robert M, Ashley SW, Reber HA, Lehman GA. Polyethylene pancreatic duct stent-induced changes in the normal dog pancreas. Gastrointest Endosc 1993;39:658–64.

25. Kozarek RA. Pancreatic stents can induce ductal changes consistent with chronic pancreatitis. Gastrointest Endosc 1990;36:93–5.

26. Leung JW, Del FG, Cotton PB. Endoscopic biliary prostheses: a comparison of materials. Gastrointest Endosc 1985;31:93–5.

27. Yu JL, Andersson R, Ljungh A. Protein adsorption and bacterial adhesion to biliary stent materials. J Surg Res 1996;62:69–73.

28. McAllister EW, Carey LC, Brady PG, Heller R, Kovacs SG. The role of polymeric surface smoothness of biliary stents in bacterial adherence, biofilm deposition, and stent occlusion. Gastrointest Endosc 1993;39:422–5.

29. van Berkel AM, van MJ, Groen AK, Bruno MJ. Mechanisms of biliary stent clogging: confocal laser scanning and scanning electron microscopy. Endoscopy 2005;37:729–34.

30. van Berkel AM, van MJ, van VH, Groen AK, Huibregtse K. A scanning electron microscopic study of biliary stent materials. Gastrointest Endosc 2000;511:19–22.

31. van Berkel AM, Bruno MJ, Bergman JJ, van Deventer SJ, Tytgat GN, Huibregtse K. A prospective randomized study of hydrophilic polymer-coated polyurethane versus polyethylene stents in distal malignant biliary obstruction. Endoscopy 2003;35:478–82.

32. Landoni N, Wengrower D, Chopita N, Goldin E. [Randomized prospective study to compare the efficiency between standard plastic and polyurethane stents in biliary tract malignant obstruction]. Acta Gastroenterol Latinoam 2000;30:501–4.

33. Cetta F, Rappuoli R, Montalto G, Baldi C, Gori M, Cetta D, et al. New biliary endoprosthesis less liable to block in biliary infections: description and in vitro studies. Eur J Surg 1999;165:782–5.

34. Costamagna G, Mutignani M, Rotondano G, Cipolletta L, Ghezzo L, Foco A, et al. Hydrophilic hydromer-coated polyurethane stents versus uncoated stents in malignant biliary obstruction: a randomized trial. Gastrointest Endosc 2000;51:8–11.

35. Tringali A, Mutignani M, Perri V, Zuccalà G, Cipolletta L, Bianco MA, et al. A prospective, randomized multicenter trial comparing DoubleLayer and polyethylene stents for malignant distal common bile duct strictures. Endoscopy 2003;(35):992–7.

36. Huibregtse K. Plastic or expandable biliary endoprostheses? Scand J Gastroenterol Suppl 1993;200:3–7.

37. Schmassmann A, von GE, Knuchel J, Scheurer U, Fehr HF, Halter F. Wallstents versus plastic stents in malignant biliary obstruction: effects of stent patency of the first and second stent on patient compliance and survival. Am J Gastroenterol 1996;91:654–9.

38. Yeoh KG, Zimmerman MJ, Cunningham JT, Cotton PB. Comparative costs of metal versus plastic biliary stent strategies for malignant obstructive jaundice by decision analysis. Gastrointest Endosc 1999;49:466–71.

39. Kaassis M, Boyer J, Dumas R, Ponchon T, Coumaros D, Delcenserie R, et al. Plastic or metal stents for malignant stricture of the common bile duct? Results of a randomized prospective study. Gastrointest Endosc 2003; 57:178–82.

40. Bueno JT, Gerdes H, Kurtz RC. Endoscopic management of occluded biliary Wallstents: a cancer center experience. Gastrointest Endosc 2003;58:879–84.

41. Tham TC, Carr-Locke DL, Vandervoort J, Wong RC, Lichtenstein DR, Van Dam J, et al. Management of occluded biliary Wallstents. Gut 1998;42:703–7.

42. Costamagna G. Covered self-expanding metal stents in benign biliary strictures: not yet a "new paradigm" but a promising alternative. Gastrointest Endosc 2008;67:455–7.

43. Familiari P, Bulajic M, Mutignani M, Lee LS, Spera G, Spada C, et al. Endoscopic removal of malfunctioning biliary self-expandable metallic stents. Gastrointest Endosc 2005;62:903–10.

44. Raijman I. Biliary and pancreatic stents. Gastrointest Endosc Clin N Am 2003;13:561–92, vii–viii.

45. Born P, Neuhaus H, Rösch T, Ott R, Allescher H, Frimberger E, et al. Initial experience with a new, partially covered Wallstent for malignant biliary obstruction. Endoscopy 1996;28:699–702.

46. Isayama H, Komatsu Y, Tsujino T, Sasahira N, Hirano K, Toda N, et al. A prospective randomised study of "covered" versus "uncovered" diamond stents for the management of distal malignant biliary obstruction. Gut 2004;53:729–34.

47. Fumex F, Coumaros D, Napoleon B, Barthet M, Laugier R, Yzet T, et al. Similar performance but higher cholecystitis rate with covered biliary stents: results from a prospective multicenter evaluation. Endoscopy 2006;38:787–92.

48. Park do H, Kim MH, Choi JS, Lee SS, Seo DW, Kim JH, et al. Covered versus uncovered Wallstent for malignant extrahepatic biliary obstruction: a cohort comparative analysis. Clin Gastroenterol Hepatol 2006;4:790–6.

49. Yoon WJ, Lee JK, Lee KH, Lee WJ, Ryu JK, Kim YT, et al. A comparison of covered and uncovered Wallstents for the management of distal malignant biliary obstruction. Gastrointest Endosc 2006;63:996–1000.

50. Rogart JN, Boghos A, Rossi F, Al-Hashem H, Siddiqui UD, Jamidar P, et al. Analysis of endoscopic management of occluded metal biliary stents at a single tertiary care center. Gastrointest Endosc 2008;68:676–82.

51. O'Brien SM, Hatfield AR, Craig PI, Williams SP. A 5-year follow-up of self-expanding metal stents in the endoscopic management of patients with benign bile duct strictures. Eur J Gastroenterol Hepatol 1998;10:141–5.

52. Shin HP, Kim MH, Jung SW, Kim JC, Choi EK, Han J, et al. Endoscopic removal of biliary self-expandable metallic stents: a prospective study. Endoscopy 2006;38:1250–5.

36

53. Kahaleh M, Tokar J, Le T, Yeaton P. Removal of self-expandable metallic Wallstents. Gastrointest Endosc 2004;60:640–4.

54. van Berkel AM, Cahen DL, van Westerloo DJ, Rauws EA, Huibregtse K, Bruno MJ. Self-expanding metal stents in benign biliary strictures due to chronic pancreatitis. Endoscopy 2004;36:381–4.

55. Kahaleh M, Behm B, Clarke BW, Brock A, Shami VM, De La Rue SA, et al. Temporary placement of covered self-expandable metal stents in benign biliary strictures: a new paradigm? (with video). Gastrointest Endosc 2008;67:446–54.

56. Kahaleh M, Sundaram V, Condron SL, De La Rue SA, Hall JD, Tokar J, et al. Temporary placement of covered self-expandable metallic stents in patients with biliary leak: midterm evaluation of a pilot study. Gastrointest Endosc 2007;66:52–9.

57. Eickhoff A, Jakobs R, Leonhardt A, Eickhoff JC, Riemann JF. Self-expandable metal mesh stents for common bile duct stenosis in chronic pancreatitis: retrospective evaluation of long-term follow-up and clinical outcome pilot study. Z Gastroenterol 2003;41:649–54.

58. Kahl S, Zimmermann S, Glasbrenner B, Pross M, Schulz HU, McNamara D, et al. Treatment of benign biliary strictures in chronic pancreatitis by self-expandable metal stents. Dig Dis 2002;20:199–203.

59. Dumonceau JM, Devière J, Delhaye M, Baize M, Minet M, Cremer M. A guiding catheter to facilitate accurate stent length determination. Gastrointest Endosc 1998;48:203–6.

60. Lawrie BW, Pugh S, Watura R. Bile duct stenting: a comparison of the One-Action Stent introduction system with the conventional delivery system. Endoscopy 1996;28:299–301.

61. Matsuda Y, Shimakura K, Akamatsu T. Factors affecting the patency of stents in malignant biliary obstructive disease: univariate and multivariate analysis. Am J Gastroenterol 1991;86:843–9.

62. Frakes JT, Johanson JF, Stake JJ. Optimal timing for stent replacement in malignant biliary tract obstruction. Gastrointest Endosc 1993;39:164–7.

63. Donelli G, Guaglianone E, Di RR, Fiocca F, Basoli A. Plastic biliary stent occlusion: factors involved and possible preventive approaches. Clin Med Res 2007;5:53–60.

64. Speer AG, Cotton PB, Rode J, Seddon AM, Neal CR, Holton J, et al. Biliary stent blockage with bacterial biofilm. A light and electron microscopy study. Ann Intern Med 1988;108:546–53.

65. Hoffman BJ, Cunningham JT, Marsh WH, O'Brien JJ, Watson J. An in vitro comparison of biofilm formation on various biliary stent materials. Gastrointest Endosc 1994;40:581–3.

66. Maillot N, Aucher P, Robert S, Richer JP, Bon D, Moesch C, et al. Polyethylene stent blockage: a porcine model. Gastrointest Endosc 2000;51:12–8.

67. Weickert U, Venzke T, Konig J, Janssen J, Remberger K, Greiner L. Why do bilioduodenal plastic stents become occluded? A clinical and pathological investigation on 100 consecutive patients. Endoscopy 2001;33:786–90.

68. Swidsinski A, Schlien P, Pernthaler A, Gottschalk U, Bärlehner E, Decker G, et al. Bacterial biofilm within diseased pancreatic and biliary tracts. Gut 2005;54:388–95.

69. Barrioz T, Ingrand P, Besson I, de Ledinghen V, Silvain C, Beauchant M. Randomised trial of prevention of biliary stent occlusion by ursodeoxycholic acid plus norfloxacin. Lancet 1994;344:581–2.

70. Ghosh S, Palmer KR. Prevention of biliary stent occlusion using cyclical antibiotics and ursodeoxycholic acid. Gut 1994;35:1757–9.

71. Sung JJ, Chung SC, Tsui CP, Co AL, Li AK. Omitting side-holes in biliary stents does not improve drainage of the obstructed biliary system: a prospective randomized trial. Gastrointest Endosc 1994;40:321–5.

72. Luman W, Ghosh S, Palmer KR. A combination of ciprofloxacin and Rowachol does not prevent biliary stent occlusion. Gastrointest Endosc 1999;49:316–21.

73. Sung JJ, Sollano JD, Lai CW, Ismael A, Yung MY, Tumala I, et al. Long-term ciprofloxacin treatment for the prevention of biliary stent blockage: a prospective randomized study. Am J Gastroenterol 1999;94:3197–201.

74. De Lédinghen V, Person B, Legoux JL, Le Sidaner A, Desaint B, Greef M, et al. Prevention of biliary stent occlusion by ursodeoxycholic acid plus norfloxacin: a multicenter randomized trial. Dig Dis Sci 2000;45:145–50.

75. Faigel DO. Preventing biliary stent occlusion. Gastrointest Endosc 2000;51:104–7.

76. Halm U, Schiefke I, Fleig WE, Mossner J, Keim V. Ofloxacin and ursodeoxycholic acid versus ursodeoxycholic acid alone to prevent occlusion of biliary stents: a prospective, randomized trial. Endoscopy 2001;33:491–4.

77. Seitz U, Block A, Schaefer AC, Wienhold U, Bohnacker S, Siebert K, et al. Biliary stent clogging solved by nanotechnology? In vitro study of inorganic-organic sol-gel coatings for Teflon stents. Gastroenterology 2007;133:65–71.

78. Goh PM, Sim EK, Isaac JR. Endoscopic extraction of a proximally migrated Amsterdam-type biliary endoprosthesis. Gastrointest Endosc 1990;36:539–40.

79. Eppel MN, Duden K, McCown R. Biopsy forceps removal of proximally migrated biliary stent. Gastrointest Endosc 1992;38:730.

80. Chaurasia OP, Rauws EA, Fockens P, Huibregtse K. Endoscopic techniques for retrieval of proximally migrated biliary stents: the Amsterdam experience. Gastrointest Endosc 1999;50:780–5.

81. Vandervoort J, Carr-Locke DL, Tham TC, Wong RC. A new technique to retrieve an intrabiliary stent: a case report. Gastrointest Endosc 1999;49:800–3.

82. Rerknimitr R, Phuangsombat W, Naprasert P. Endoscopic removal of proximally migrated pancreatic stent by a grasping tripod. Endoscopy 2007;39(Suppl 1):E42.

83. Soehendra N, Maydeo A, Eckmann B, Bruckner M, Nam VC, Grimm H. A new technique for replacing an obstructed biliary endoprosthesis. Endoscopy 1990;22:271–2.

84. Moparty B, Carr-Locke DL. Metal or plastic stent for malignant biliary obstruction: what's got the most bang for your buck? Eur J Gastroenterol Hepatol 2007;19:1041–2.

85. Weber A, Mittermeyer T, Wagenpfeil S, Schmid RM, Prinz C. Self-expanding metal stents versus polyethylene stents for palliative treatment in patients with advanced pancreatic cancer. Pancreas 2009;38:e7–e12.

86. Chen JH, Sun CK, Liao CS, Chua CS. Self-expandable metallic stents for malignant biliary obstruction: efficacy on proximal and distal tumors. World J Gastroenterol 2006;12:119–22.

87. Hoepffner N, Foerster EC, Hogemann B, Domschke W. Long-term experience in Wallstent therapy for malignant choledochal stenosis. Endoscopy 1994;26:597–602.

88. Kahaleh M, Tokar J, Conaway MR, Brock A, Le T, Adams RB, et al. Efficacy and complications of covered Wallstents in malignant distal biliary obstruction. Gastrointest Endosc 2005;61:528–33.

89. Kawamoto H, Ishida E, Okamoto Y, Okada H, Sakaguchi K, Nakagawa M, et al. Evaluation of covered metallic stents in malignant biliary stenosis—prominent effectiveness in gallbladder carcinoma. Hepatogastroenterology 2005;52:1351–6.

90. Nakai Y, Isayama H, Komatsu Y, Tsujino T, Toda N, Sasahira N, et al. Efficacy and safety of the covered Wallstent in patients with distal malignant biliary obstruction. Gastrointest Endosc 2005;62:742–8.

91. Shah RJ, Howell DA, Desilets DJ, Sheth SG, Parsons WG, Okolo P 3rd, et al. Multicenter randomized trial of the spiral Z-stent compared with the Wallstent for malignant biliary obstruction. Gastrointest Endosc 2003;57:830–6.

92. Shim CS, Lee YH, Cho YD, Bong HK, Kim JO, Cho JY, et al. Preliminary results of a new covered biliary metal stent for malignant biliary obstruction. Endoscopy 1998;30:345–50.

93. Menon K, Barkun A. Management of occluded biliary Wallstents. Gastrointest Endosc 1999;49:403–5.

94. Togawa O, Kawabe T, Isayama H, Nakai Y, Sasaki T, Arizumi T, et al. Management of occluded uncovered metallic stents in patients with malignant distal biliary obstructions using covered metallic stents. J Clin Gastroenterol 2008;42:546–9.

95. Jaganmohan S, Raju GS. Tissue ingrowth in a fully covered self–expandable metallic stent (with videos). Gastrointest Endosc 2008;68:602–4.

96. Egan LJ, Baron TH. Endoscopic removal of an embedded biliary Wallstent by piecemeal extraction. Endoscopy 2000;32:492–4.

97. Vanbiervliet G, Piche T, Caroli-Bosc FX, Dumas R, Peten EP, Huet PM, et al. Endoscopic argon plasma trimming of biliary and gastrointestinal metallic stents. Endoscopy 2005;37:434–8.

98. Rerknimitr R, Naprasert P, Kongkam P, Kullavanijaya P. Trimming a metallic biliary stent using an argon plasma coagulator. Cardiovasc Intervent Radiol 2007;30:534–6.

99. Christiaens P, Decock S, Buchel O, Bulté K, Moons V, D'Haens G, et al. Endoscopic trimming of metallic stents with the use of argon plasma. Gastrointest Endosc 2008;67:369–71.

100. Chen YK, Jakribettuu V, Springer EW, Shah RJ, Penberthy J, Nash SR. Safety and efficacy of argon plasma coagulation trimming of malpositioned and migrated biliary metal stents: a controlled study in the porcine model. Am J Gastroenterol 2006;101:2025–30.

101. Cahen DL, Rauws EA, Gouma DJ, Fockens P, Bruno MJ. Removable fully covered self-expandable metal stents in the treatment of common bile duct strictures due to chronic pancreatitis: a case series. Endoscopy 2008;40:697–700.

102. Luman W, Cull A, Palmer KR. Quality of life in patients stented for malignant biliary obstructions. Eur J Gastroenterol Hepatol 1997;9:481–4.

103. Moss AC, Morris E, Leyden J, MacMathuna P. Do the benefits of metal stents justify the costs? A systematic review and meta-analysis of trials comparing endoscopic stents for malignant biliary obstruction. Eur J Gastroenterol Hepatol 2007;19:1119–24.

104. Somogyi L, Chuttani R, Croffie J, DiSario J, Liu J, Mishkin DS, et al. Biliary and pancreatic stents. Gastrointest Endosc 2006;63:910–9.

105. Kahaleh M, Brock A, Conaway MR, Shami VM, Dumonceau JM, Northup PG, et al. Covered self-expandable metal stents in pancreatic malignancy regardless of resectability: a new concept validated by a decision analysis. Endoscopy 2007;39:319–24.

106. Chang WH, Kortan P, Haber GB. Outcome in patients with bifurcation tumors who undergo unilateral versus bilateral hepatic duct drainage. Gastrointest Endosc 1998;47:354–62.

107. Devière J, Baize M, de TJ, Cremer M. Long-term follow-up of patients with hilar malignant stricture treated by endoscopic internal biliary drainage. Gastrointest Endosc 1988;34:95–101.

108. Hintze RE, bou-Rebyeh H, Adler A, Veltzke-Schlieker W, Felix R, Wiedenmann B. Magnetic resonance cholangiopancreatography-guided unilateral endoscopic stent placement for Klatskin tumors. Gastrointest Endosc 2001;53:40–6.

109. Perdue DG, Freeman ML, DiSario JA, Nelson DB, Fennerty MB, Lee JG, et al. Plastic versus self-expanding metallic stents for malignant hilar biliary obstruction: a prospective multicenter observational cohort study. J Clin Gastroenterol 2008;42:1040–6.

110. Freeman ML, Overby C. Selective MRCP and CT-targeted drainage of malignant hilar biliary obstruction with self-expanding metallic stents. Gastrointest Endosc 2003;58:41–9.

111. Singh V, Singh G, Verma GR, Singh K, Gulati M. Contrast-free unilateral endoscopic palliation in malignant hilar biliary obstruction: new method. J Gastroenterol Hepatol 2004;19:589–92.

112. Khan SA, Davidson BR, Goldin R, Pereira SP, Rosenberg WM, Taylor-Robinson SD, et al. Guidelines for the diagnosis and treatment of cholangiocarcinoma: consensus document. Gut 2002;51(Suppl 6):VI1–9.

113. Lee SH, Park JK, Yoon WJ, Lee JK, Ryu JK, Yoon YB, et al. Optimal biliary drainage for inoperable Klatskin's tumor based on Bismuth type. World J Gastroenterol 2007;13:3948–55.

114. Costamagna G, Pandolfi M, Mutignani M, Spada C, Perri V. Long-term results of endoscopic management of postoperative bile duct strictures with increasing numbers of stents. Gastrointest Endosc 2001;54:162–8.

115. Kuzela L, Oltman M, Sutka J, Hrcka R, Novotna T, Vavrecka A. Prospective follow-up of patients with bile duct strictures secondary to laparoscopic cholecystectomy, treated endoscopically with multiple stents. Hepatogastroenterology 2005;52:1357–61.

116. Bergman JJ, Burgemeister L, Bruno MJ, Rauws EA, Gouma DJ, Tytgat GN, et al. Long-term follow-up after biliary stent placement for postoperative bile duct stenosis. Gastrointest Endosc 2001;54:154–61.

117. Morelli J, Mulcahy HE, Willner IR, Cunningham JT, Draganov P. Long-term outcomes for patients with post-liver transplant anastomotic biliary strictures treated by endoscopic stent placement. Gastrointest Endosc 2003;58:374–9.

118. Dumonceau JM, Devière J, Delhaye M, Baize M, Cremer M. Plastic and metal stents for postoperative benign bile duct strictures: the best and the worst. Gastrointest Endosc 1998;47:8–17.

119. Siriwardana HP, Siriwardena AK. Systematic appraisal of the role of metallic endobiliary stents in the treatment of benign bile duct stricture. Ann Surg 2005;242:10–9.

120. Stainier L, Hubert C, Jouret M, Deprez P, Goffette P, Gigot JF. Self-expanding metallic stents in benign postoperative biliary strictures: a difficult surgical obstacle? Hepatogastroenterology 2007;54:999–1003.

121. Kaya M, Petersen BT, Angulo P, Baron TH, Andrews JC, Gostout CJ, et al. Balloon dilation compared to stenting of dominant strictures in primary sclerosing cholangitis. Am J Gastroenterol 2001;96:1059–66.

122. Ponsioen CY, Lam K, van Milligen de Wit AW, Huibregtse K, Tytgat GN. Four years experience with short term stenting in primary sclerosing cholangitis. Am J Gastroenterol 1999;94:2403–7.

123. Gluck M, Cantone NR, Brandabur JJ, Patterson DJ, Bredfeldt JE, Kozarek RA. A twenty-year experience with endoscopic therapy for symptomatic primary sclerosing cholangitis. J Clin Gastroenterol 2008;42:1032–9.

124. Johnson GK, Saeian K, Geenen JE. Primary sclerosing cholangitis treated by endoscopic biliary dilation: review and long-term follow-up evaluation. Curr Gastroenterol Rep 2006;8:147–55.

125. Catalano MF, Linder JD, George S, Alcocer E, Geenen JE. Treatment of symptomatic distal common bile duct stenosis secondary to chronic pancreatitis: comparison of single vs. multiple simultaneous stents. Gastrointest Endosc 2004;60:945–52.

126. Pozsar J, Sahin P, Laszlo F, Forro G, Topa L. Medium-term results of endoscopic treatment of common bile duct strictures in chronic calcifying pancreatitis with increasing numbers of stents. J Clin Gastroenterol 2004;38:118–23.

127. Cahen DL, van Berkel AM, Oskam D, Rauws EA, Weverling GJ, Huibregtse K, et al. Long-term results of endoscopic drainage of common bile duct strictures in chronic pancreatitis. Eur J Gastroenterol Hepatol 2005;17:103–8.

128. Devière J, Cremer M, Baize M, Love J, Sugai B, Vandermeeren A. Management of common bile duct stricture caused by chronic pancreatitis with metal mesh self expandable stents. Gut 1994;35:122–6.

129. Cantu P, Hookey LC, Morales A, Le MO, Devière J. The treatment of patients with symptomatic common bile duct stenosis secondary to chronic pancreatitis using partially covered metal stents: a pilot study. Endoscopy 2005;37:735–9.

130. Pinkas H, Brady PG. Biliary leaks after laparoscopic cholecystectomy: time to stent or time to drain. Hepatobiliary Pancreat Dis Int 2008;7:628–32.

131. Sandha GS, Bourke MJ, Haber GB, Kortan PP. Endoscopic therapy for bile leak based on a new classification: results in 207 patients. Gastrointest Endosc 2004;60:567–74.

132. Shah JN. Endoscopic treatment of bile leaks: current standards and recent innovations. Gastrointest Endosc 2007;65:1069–72.

133. Katsinelos P, Kountouras J, Paroutoglou G, Chatzimavroudis G, Germanidis G, Zavos C, et al. A comparative study of 10-Fr vs. 7-Fr straight plastic stents in the treatment of postcholecystectomy bile leak. Surg Endosc 2008;22:101–6.

134. Johnson GK, Geenen JE, Venu RP, Schmalz MJ, Hogan WJ. Treatment of non-extractable common bile duct stones with combination ursodeoxycholic acid plus endoprostheses. Gastrointest Endosc 1993;39:528–31.

135. Chan AC, Ng EK, Chung SC, Lai CW, Lau JY, Sung JJ, et al. Common bile duct stones become smaller after endoscopic biliary stenting. Endoscopy 1998;30:356–9.

136. Christoforidis E, Vasiliadis K, Blouhos K, Tsalis K, Tsorlini E, Tsachalis T, et al. Feasibility of therapeutic endoscopic retrograde cholangiopancreatography for bile duct stones in nonagenarians: a single unit audit. J Gastrointest Liver Dis 2008;17:427–32.

137. Bergman JJ, Rauws EA, Tijssen JG, Tytgat GN, Huibregtse K. Biliary endoprostheses in elderly patients with endoscopically irretrievable common bile duct stones: report on 117 patients. Gastrointest Endosc 1995;42:195–201.

138. Kjaer DW, Kruse A, Funch-Jensen P. Endoscopic gallbladder drainage of patients with acute cholecystitis. Endoscopy 2007;39:304–8.

139. Itoi T, Sofuni A, Itokawa F, Tsuchiya T, Kurihara T, Ishii K, et al. Endoscopic transpapillary gallbladder drainage in patients with acute cholecystitis in whom percutaneous transhepatic approach is contraindicated or anatomically impossible (with video). Gastrointest Endosc 2008;68:455–60.

140. Eleftherladis N, Dinu F, Delhaye M, Le Moine O, Baize M, Vandermeeren A, et al. Long-term outcome after pancreatic stenting in severe chronic pancreatitis. Endoscopy 2005;37:223–30.

141. Weber A, Schneider J, Neu B, Meining A, Born P, Schmid RM, et al. Endoscopic stent therapy for patients with chronic pancreatitis: results from a prospective follow-up study. Pancreas 2007;34:287–94.

142. Costamagna G, Bulajic M, Tringali A, Pandolfi M, Gabbrielli A, Spada C, et al. Multiple stenting of refractory pancreatic duct strictures in severe chronic pancreatitis: long-term results. Endoscopy 2006;38:254–9.

143. Delhaye M, Matos C, Devière J. Endoscopic technique for the management of pancreatitis and its complications. Best Pract Res Clin Gastroenterol 2004;18:155–81.

144. Sauer B, Talreja J, Ellen K, Ku J, Shami VM, Kahaleh M. Temporary placement of a fully covered self-expandable metal stent in the pancreatic duct for management of symptomatic refractory chronic pancreatitis: preliminary data (with videos). Gastrointest Endosc 2008;68:1173–8.

145. Sasahira N, Tada M, Isayama H, Hirano K, Nakai Y, Yamamoto N, et al. Outcomes after clearance of pancreatic stones with or without pancreatic stenting. J Gastroenterol 2007;42:63–9.

146. Yang XJ, Lin Y, Zeng X, Shi J, Chen YX, Shen JW, et al. A minimally invasive alternative for managing large pancreatic duct stones using a modified expandable metal mesh stent. Pancreatology 2008;9:111–5.

147. Jacobson BC, Baron TH, Adler DG, Davila RE, Egan J, Hirota WK, et al. ASGE guideline: The role of endoscopy in the diagnosis and the management of cystic lesions and inflammatory fluid collections of the pancreas. Gastrointest Endosc 2005;61:363–70.

148. Giovannini M, Pesenti C, Rolland AL, Moutardier V, Delpero JR. Endoscopic ultrasound-guided drainage of pancreatic pseudocysts or pancreatic abscesses using a therapeutic echo endoscope. Endoscopy 2001;33:473–7.

36

149. Sanchez Cortes E, Maalak A, Le Moine O, Baize M, Delhaye M, Matos C, et al. Endoscopic cystenterostomy of nonbulging pancreatic fluid collections. Gastrointest Endosc 2002;56:380–6.

150. Hookey LC, Debroux S, Delhaye M, Arvanitakis M, Le MO, Devière J. Endoscopic drainage of pancreatic-fluid collections in 116 patients: a comparison of etiologies, drainage techniques, and outcomes. Gastrointest Endosc 2006;63:635–43.

151. Kahaleh M, Shami VM, Conaway MR, Tokar J, Rockoff T, De La Rue SA, et al. Endoscopic ultrasound drainage of pancreatic pseudocyst: a prospective comparison with conventional endoscopic drainage. Endoscopy 2006;38: 355–9.

152. Costamagna G, Mutignani M, Ingrosso M, Vamvakousis V, Alevras P, Manta R, et al. Endoscopic treatment of postsurgical external pancreatic fistulas. Endoscopy 2001;33:317–22.

153. Kim HS, Lee DK, Kim IW, Baik SK, Kwon SO, Park JW, et al. The role of endoscopic retrograde pancreatography in the treatment of traumatic pancreatic duct injury. Gastrointest Endosc 2001;54:49–55.

154. Brennan PM, Stefaniak T, Palmer KR, Parks RW. Endoscopic transpapillary stenting of pancreatic duct disruption. Dig Surg 2006;23:250–4.

155. Ertan A. Long-term results after endoscopic pancreatic stent placement without pancreatic papillotomy in acute recurrent pancreatitis due to pancreas divisum. Gastrointest Endosc 2000;52:9–14.

156. Vitale GC, Vitale M, Vitale DS, Binford JC, Hill B. Long-term follow-up of endoscopic stenting in patients with chronic pancreatitis secondary to pancreas divisum. Surg Endosc 2007;21:2199–202.

157. Wehrmann T, Riphaus A, Frenz MB, Martchenko K, Stergiou N. Endoscopic pancreatic duct stenting for relief of pancreatic cancer pain. Eur J Gastroenterol Hepatol 2005;17:1395–400.

158. Tham TC, Lichtenstein DR, Vandervoort J, Wong RC, Slivka A, Banks PA, et al. Pancreatic duct stents for "obstructive type" pain in pancreatic malignancy. Am J Gastroenterol 2000;95:956–60.

159. Costamagna G, Alevras P, Palladino F, Rainoldi F, Mutignani M, Morganti A. Endoscopic pancreatic stenting in pancreatic cancer. Can J Gastroenterol 1999;13:481–7.

160. Mezawa S, Homma H, Sato T, Doi T, Miyanishi K, Takada K, et al. A study of carboplatin-coated tube for the unresectable cholangiocarcinoma. Hepatology 2000;32:916–23.

161. Kalinowski M, Alfke H, Kleb B, Durfeld F, Joachim WH. Paclitaxel inhibits proliferation of cell lines responsible for metal stent obstruction: possible topical application in malignant bile duct obstructions. Invest Radiol 2002;37:399–404.

162. Ginsberg G, Cope C, Shah J, Martin T, Carty A, Habecker P, et al. In vivo evaluation of a new bioabsorbable self-expanding biliary stent. Gastrointest Endosc 2003;58:777–84.

163. Laukkarinen J, Nordback I, Mikkonen J, Karkkainen P, Sand J. A novel biodegradable biliary stent in the endoscopic treatment of cystic-duct leakage after cholecystectomy. Gastrointest Endosc 2007;65:1063–8.

164. Meng B, Wang J, Zhu N, Meng QY, Cui FZ, Xu YX. Study of biodegradable and self-expandable PLLA helical biliary stent in vivo and in vitro. J Mater Sci Mater Med 2006;17:611–7.

165. Laukkarinen J, Lamsa T, Nordback I, Mikkonen J, Sand J. A novel biodegradable pancreatic stent for human pancreatic applications: a preclinical safety study in a large animal model. Gastrointest Endosc 2008;67: 1106–12.

166. Dua KS, Reddy ND, Rao VG, Banerjee R, Medda B, Lang I. Impact of reducing duodenobiliary reflux on biliary stent patency: an in vitro evaluation and a prospective randomized clinical trial that used a biliary stent with an antireflux valve. Gastrointest Endosc 2007;65:819–28.

167. Raju GS, Sud R, Elfert AA, Enaba M, Kalloo A, Pasricha PJ. Biliary drainage by using stents without a central lumen: a pilot study. Gastrointest Endosc 2006;63:317–20.

V

37 Intestinal Decompression

Todd H. Baron and Faris M. Murad

Introduction

Endoscopic intestinal decompression is carried out to relieve distension due to a variety of causes that lead to luminal dilation in the stomach, small bowel, and colon. The settings in which bowel decompression is required range from benign to malignant and from functional to mechanical. A major consideration in the management of these patients is the short-term and long-term nature of the disease processes. Decompression is most often achieved using tubes passed into the gastrointestinal tract, and when placed endoscopically these are passed after placement of a guide wire. Expandable metal stents can also be used to achieve intestinal decompression, and are discussed in Chapter 35. The present chapter reviews methods of intestinal decompression other than the use of expandable stents.

Gastric and Small-Bowel Decompression

The various causes leading to a need for decompression of the stomach and small intestine are outlined in **Table 37.1**. Decompression not only improves symptoms of pain related to abdominal distension, but can also prevent vomiting and potential aspiration. The method of decompression selected depends on the etiology and also on the need for short-term or long-term decompression. Each of these topics is discussed separately below.

Short-Term Decompression

Any cause of gastric outlet distension or small-bowel obstruction or distension can usually be relieved by placing a nasogastric decompression tube. Almost always, these tubes can be placed at the bedside, without the need for endoscopy. However, endoscopy is required in some patients when failure to pass a nasogastric tube occurs due to anatomical difficulties in the nasal cavity, oropharynx, or esophagus. Endoscopic placement of nasogastric tubes can be performed using standard endoscopes passed transorally. After the endoscope is passed into the stomach, a guide wire is advanced through the channel and positioned in the antrum or duodenum. The endoscope is withdrawn, leaving the wire in place. The wire is then rerouted through the nose, and the tube is passed over the guide wire. It is important to realize that standard, commercially available nasogastric tubes do not have end holes to allow the wire to pass, as the tip is closed. Cutting the tip of the nasogastric tube allows for wire passage. Fluoroscopy is not usually necessary for endoscopic placement. Transnasal endoscopy using a small-caliber endoscope is a way to obviate transfer of the guide wire from the mouth to the nose. The nasogastric tube is then passed directly over the guide wire after the endoscope has been withdrawn from the nose.

Although most patients with small-intestinal obstruction can receive decompression treatment using a nasogastric tube, there are data suggesting that nasointestinal tube decompression is superior to gastric decompression. This can be achieved endoscopically using the transnasal technique, as described above [1,2]. The endo-

Table 37.1 Scenarios for gastric and small-intestinal decompression

Benign
Postoperative ileus
Acute pancreatitis
Gastroparesis
Small-bowel adhesions
Intestinal pseudo-obstruction
Peptic ulcer disease

Malignant
Gastric cancer
Gastric lymphoma
Pancreaticobiliary malignancies with duodenal invasion
Small intestinal cancer, localized
Diffuse peritoneal carcinomatosis

scope only needs to be passed into the duodenum. A guide wire is then advanced under fluoroscopy beyond the ligament of Treitz. After removal of the endoscope, the tube is advanced to the jejunum. Hydrophilic intestinal decompression tubes are available, such as the Super Denis Tube (Nippon Sherwood, Tokyo, Japan) and One-Step Ileus Tube (Sumitomo Bakelite, Tokyo, Japan), with a diameter of 16 Fr and a length of 300 cm. Although there are no data on the use of nasojejunal feeding tubes (typically 12 Fr in diameter) as decompression tubes, they should allow effective decompression and are readily available in most endoscopy units.

Long-Term Decompression

Long-term decompression of the stomach is required in the setting of chronic gastroparesis of any cause and in patients with peritoneal carcinomatosis. Patients with peritoneal carcinomatosis have diffuse obstruction that leads to intractable nausea and vomiting. In these situations, percutaneous endoscopic gastrostomy (PEG) placement is frequently the only alternative to nasogastric tube decompression, which with long-term use can cause pharyngeal and esophageal irritation, sinusitis, and a risk of mucosal necrosis and perforation. PEG tube placement allows for more suitable long-term decompression. Important technical considerations when placing PEG tubes for decompression are the size of the PEG tube, the presence and degree of ascites, and the relative inability to achieve transillumination and indentation due to omental caking. Larger PEG tubes (28 Fr) may allow better decompression and symptom relief in comparison with 20-Fr tubes.

Ascites is nearly always present in patients with peritoneal carcinomatosis. Minimal to moderate ascites, especially when limited to the pelvis or not seen anteriorly on abdominal imaging studies, is usually of no consequence. Large-volume ascites, presenting anteriorly between the stomach and abdominal wall on imaging studies, portends a risk of leakage and subsequent peritonitis. In this situation, large-volume paracentesis is required before PEG placement [3,4]. Serial imaging studies may be useful to assess the need for

Table 37.2 Scenarios for colonic decompression

Benign
Acute colonic pseudo-obstruction (Ogilvie syndrome)
Chronic pseudo-obstruction
Sigmoid volvulus
Diverticulitis with obstruction
Malignant
Primary or recurrent colorectal cancer
Pelvic malignancies
Metastatic disease

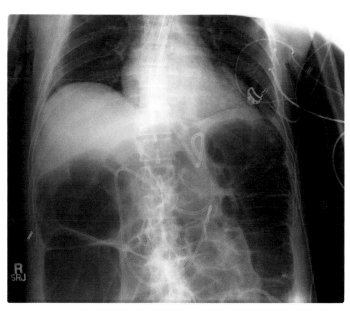

Fig. 37.1 A plain abdominal radiograph, showing acute colonic pseudo-obstruction in a patient hospitalized for spinal cord injury.

Table 37.3 Conservative management of acute colonic pseudo-obstruction

- Rule out mechanical obstruction
- Fasting
- Nasogastric tube placement
- Rectal tube and/or periodic rectal examination
- Regular changes in patient position
- Ambulation, if possible
- Reversal of precipitating factors
- Intravenous fluids and correction of electrolyte imbalance

repeat paracenteses until the PEG tract has matured. Gastropexy sutures can also secure the stomach to the abdominal wall [5].

In patients with gastroparesis, a small-bowel feeding tube is also necessary. The combination of decompression and feeding tubes limits the ability to decompress the stomach, as the feeding tube occupies part of the gastrostomy lumen. In these cases, the patient may benefit from placement of a direct percutaneous endoscopic jejunostomy (DPEJ) tube for feeding. This allows the entire lumen of the PEG tube to be used for gastric decompression.

Jejunostomy tubes can also be used for long-term gastric and small-bowel decompression. In patients with peritoneal carcinomatosis, the stomach is often encased by omental tumor, precluding the transillumination and indentation that are necessary for PEG placement. Jejunostomy placement may be feasible in these patients and may provide decompressive palliation. In addition, in patients with altered anatomy (e. g., after distal esophagectomy or

gastric resection), PEG placement may not be feasible, but direct percutaneous endoscopic jejunostomy placement is possible [6,7] and can be accomplished safely and with effective decompression [8].

Colonic Decompression

Severe colonic distension is a medical emergency, because of the potential for bowel ischemia, perforation, and sepsis with peritonitis if not rapidly and appropriately treated. There are a number of causes of colonic distension, some of which are functional, while others are mechanical (**Table 37.2**). The approach differs depending on this differentiation and on whether the need is for short-term or long-term decompression.

■ Functional Obstruction

Functional obstruction of the colon is most often due to acute colonic pseudo-obstruction (ACPO) (**Fig. 37.1**), also known as Ogilvie syndrome. This is an uncommon condition that presents as acute dilation of the colon. Patients with acute colonic pseudo-obstruction are often debilitated and receiving narcotic medications. This is an important clinical entity to recognize, as it carries a significant risk of perforation. Acute colonic pseudo-obstruction usually presents in patients who are already hospitalized with multiple medical problems. While it has well-recognized features, misdiagnosis can lead to increased morbidity and mortality. If it is diagnosed early and treated appropriately, resolution of the condition usually follows.

Clinical features of acute colonic pseudo-obstruction include abdominal pain as the most common presenting symptom. Patients are usually noted to have marked abdominal distension, which is tympanitic on percussion. Abdominal pain is typically mild, but if it is increasing or severe, then the development of ischemia and impending perforation must be considered. Bowel sounds will be present and high-pitched. Nausea and vomiting occur in 50–80 % of patients [9].

Acute colonic pseudo-obstruction should be considered in a patient with symptoms and signs of colonic obstruction when there is no apparent organic cause, especially in patients hospitalized for another condition. It is important to exclude conditions that may mimic acute colonic pseudo-obstruction such as volvulus, obstructing colonic neoplasms, and acute diverticulitis, since these conditions require different management.

Once acute colonic pseudo-obstruction has been diagnosed, the initial management is conservative (**Table 37.3**). These steps include nasogastric tube placement, rectal tube placement, changing the patient's position, ambulation (if possible), and administration of intravenous fluids with correction of electrolytes. If there is no resolution or improvement in symptoms after 24 h, intravenous neostigmine should be administered, as long as there are no contraindications to its use. Neostigmine should be administered slowly at a dose of 2.0 mg over 3–5 min. It is imperative that continuous electrocardiographic monitoring and blood pressure monitoring be performed during administration, to monitor for bradycardia, arrhythmias, and hypotension. If the patient has contraindications to neostigmine, then colonoscopic decompression should be attempted (**Fig. 37.2**). This algorithm should be repeated each day, with careful monitoring for perforation until resolution occurs.

Decompression is performed to relieve distension and prevent cecal ischemia and perforation. The risk of perforation increases when the cecal diameter reaches 12 cm and when the distension is prolonged for more than 6 days [10]. Management includes removal of precipitating factors and administration of neostigmine. Endoscopic decompression is indicated in patients who fail to re-

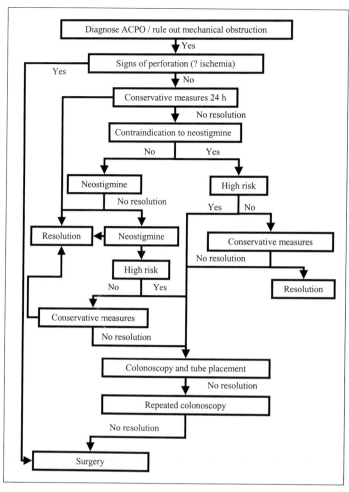

Fig. 37.2 Algorithm for the management of acute colonic pseudo-obstruction. "High risk" is present when the cecal diameter is larger than 12 cm, dilation is prolonged, or the patient is of advanced age.

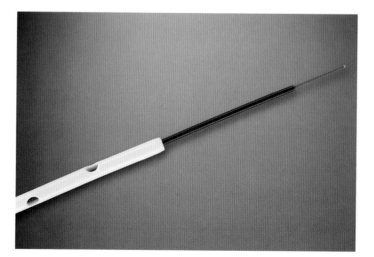

Fig. 37.3 View of a commercially available colonic decompression tube (Cook Endoscopy, Winston-Salem, North Carolina, USA).

spond to conservative management and who have contraindications to neostigmine or fail to respond to it. Decompression can be achieved by colonoscopy alone with air removal, although the recurrence rate is high [11]. No oral preparation is required before colonoscopy for acute colonic pseudo-obstruction. A large-channel therapeutic colonoscope allows more effective suctioning of air and liquid stool. Air insufflation should be kept to a minimum, with a

focus on aspirating stool and air. The goal is to reach the cecum without compromising the patient's safety. Placement of a colonic decompression tube for several days after colonoscopic decompression reduces the risk of recurrence. Commercially available colonic decompression tube kits are available (**Fig. 37.3**). The tube has an inner catheter that accepts a guide wire. The endoscope is passed as far proximally as possible, and a guide wire is positioned. If fluoroscopy is used, the guide wire can be advanced proximal to the endoscope. If fluoroscopy is not used, we prefer to pass the endoscope to the cecum and use a stiff Savary guide wire (Cook Endoscopy, Winston-Salem, North Carolina, USA). The endoscope is withdrawn, and the tube is passed over the wire. The wire and inner catheter are then removed (**Fig. 37.4**). The tube is placed to intermittent suction and irrigated with tap water several times per day. A plain abdominal film is obtained immediately after tube placement to assess the position and the extent of decompression (**Fig. 37.5**).

Patients who have recurrent acute colonic pseudo-obstruction, chronic intestinal pseudo-obstruction, and those with neurogenic bowel may require long-term, intermittent decompression. Colostomy tubes in these situations can be useful for large-bowel decompression and administration of laxative medications for bowel irrigation. This can be achieved by placing a percutaneous endoscopic colostomy (PEC) tube. The method used for PEC placement is similar to that with PEG placement. The colonoscope is advanced to the cecum and transillumination is used to identify it in the right lower quadrant. Digital indentation of the cecum or right colon confirms the correct position. After the abdominal wall has been prepared in the usual sterile fashion, a smaller-caliber needle available on all standard PEG trays is passed into the lumen of the large bowel. We prefer to grasp the needle tightly with a snare, to prevent the bowel moving away from the abdominal wall. A 19-gauge trocar is then passed alongside the smaller-caliber needle into the cecum. The smaller needle is released. The trocar is secured with the snare until the securing loop is passed through the trocar and grasped with the snare. The colonoscope and loop are then withdrawn from the colon. A gastrostomy tube is then secured to the loop and slowly pulled retrograde through the colon to exit the abdominal wall, as in the PEG pull method. The tube is then secured in place with external bolsters. This method allows the cecum to be affixed to the abdominal wall and reduces the chances of leakage and peritonitis developing. Several series have now been published describing percutaneous endoscopic cecostomy (PEC) tube placement in adults [12–16]. Most of the reports have used traditional PEG placement methods, although some authors have used fasteners to prevent intra-abdominal leakage of fecal contents at the time of placement [17]. Many of these patients present with significant large-bowel distension, and care has to be taken to minimize air insufflation during colonoscopy in order to reduce the risk of perforation. It must be emphasized that severe complications may arise after PEC placement, including peritonitis and sepsis [18].

Mechanical Obstruction

Primary colon cancer. Short-term and long-term relief of malignant obstruction from colorectal cancer can be achieved using self-expandable metal stents (SEMS) and is discussed in detail in Chapter 35. An alternative to SEMS placement for the short-term relief of obstruction and to allow preoperative decompression for obstructing left-sided colon cancer is the use of a specially designed large-bore decompression tube [19,20]. A colonoscope is advanced to the site of the tumor. Under fluoroscopic and endoscopic guidance, a large-diameter guide wire (0.052″) is passed across the point of obstruction. After the guide wire has been positioned, an overtube with an outer diameter of 20 mm is positioned in the left colon. A transanal drainage tube (7.3 mm, 22-Fr outer diameter, 120 cm long

37

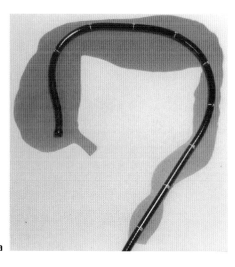
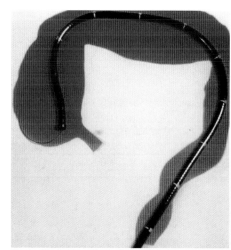

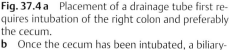

Fig. 37.4 a Placement of a drainage tube first requires intubation of the right colon and preferably the cecum.
b Once the cecum has been intubated, a biliary-type wire should be placed, which can be stiffened with a 6-Fr biliary stent pusher. The colonoscope is then slowly withdrawn with suction, and the wire position is maintained under fluoroscopic control.
c, d Once the colonoscope has been withdrawn, the drainage tube can be placed in a coaxial fashion over the wire under fluoroscopic control.

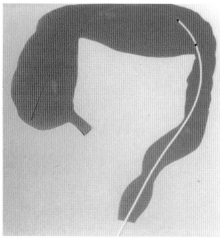
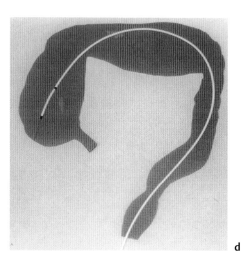

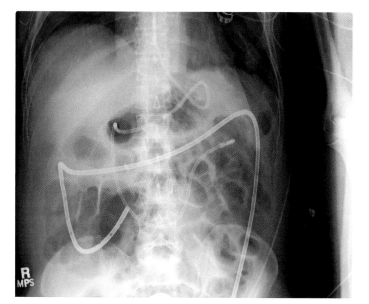

Fig. 37.5 A plain abdominal radiograph taken several hours after colonic decompression and tube placement (same patient as in **Fig. 37.1**). The endoscopic procedure was performed without fluoroscopy.

Dennis colon decompression tube; Nippon Sherwood, Tokyo, Japan) is passed over the wire and through the overtube and advanced beyond the tumor. A balloon at the tip of the decompression tube is insufflated with 30 mL of saline, and the overtube is withdrawn. Successful decompression using this technique has been reported in over 90 % of patients [20,21]. Following successful decompression, a one-stage operation or stent placement is subsequently performed. Other authors have described similar results using tube decompression without an overtube [22].

Colonic volvulus. Sigmoid and cecal volvuli have characteristic appearances on plain radiographs and can be confirmed by computed tomography. Endoscopic decompression can be achieved by passing across the area of torsion into the proximal bowel, and in some patients derotation is possible [23]. Placement of a colonic decompression tube may prevent immediate recurrence (**Fig. 37.6**). Patients who are candidates for surgery usually undergo an elective procedure, with either resection or sigmoidopexy to prevent recurrence. Poor surgical candidates with sigmoid volvulus can be treated by placement of one or two PEC tubes into the left colon [15,16].

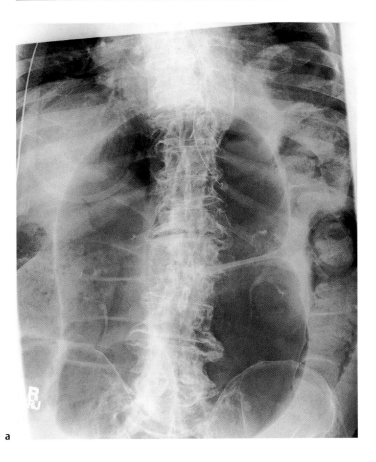

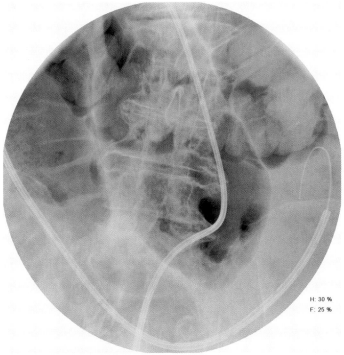

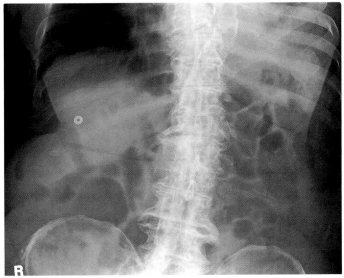

Fig. 37.6 Endoscopic management of sigmoid volvulus.
a A plain abdominal radiograph, showing typical findings of sigmoid volvulus.
b A plain radiograph taken at the time of endoscopic derotation and fluoroscopic placement of a colonic decompression tube in the descending colon.
c An abdominal radiograph taken after removal of the decompression tube, showing a sustained response.

References

1. Sato R, Watari J, Tanabe H, Fujiya M, Ueno N, Konno Y, et al. Transnasal ultrathin endoscopy for placement of a long intestinal tube in patients with intestinal obstruction. Gastrointest Endosc 2008;67:953–7.
2. Ishizuka M, Nagata H, Takagi K, Kubota K. Transnasal fine gastrointestinal fiberscope-guided long tube insertion for patients with small bowel obstruction. J Gastrointest Surg 2009;13:550–4.
3. Ryan JM, Hahn PF, Mueller PR. Performing radiologic gastrostomy or gastrojejunostomy in patients with malignant ascites. AJR Am J Roentgenol 1998;171:1003–6.
4. Lee MJ, Saini S, Brink JA, Morrison MC, Hahn PF, Mueller PR. Malignant small bowel obstruction and ascites: not a contraindication to percutaneous gastrostomy. Clin Radiol 1991;44:332–4.
5. Wejda BU, Deppe H, Huchzermeyer H, Dormann AJ. PEG placement in patients with ascites: a new approach. Gastrointest Endosc 2005;61: 178–80.
6. Rathore OI, Coss A, Patchett SE, Mulcahy HE. Direct-vision stenting: the way forward for malignant oesophageal obstruction. Endoscopy 2006; 38:382–4.
7. Martin DF. Endoscopy is superfluous during insertion of expandable metal stents in esophageal tumors. Gastrointest Endosc 1997;46:98–9.
8. Scheidbach H, Horbach T, Groitl H, Hohenberger W. Percutaneous endoscopic gastrostomy/jejunostomy (PEG/PEJ) for decompression in the upper gastrointestinal tract. Initial experience with palliative treatment of gastrointestinal obstruction in terminally ill patients with advanced carcinomas. Surg Endosc 1999;13:1103–5.
9. Vanek VW, Al-Salti M. Acute pseudo-obstruction of the colon (Ogilvie's syndrome): an analysis of 400 cases. Dis Colon Rectum 1986;29:203–10.
10. Saunders MD. Acute colonic pseudo-obstruction. Best Pract Res Clin Gastroenterol 2007;21:671–87.
11. Geller A, Petersen BT, Gostout CJ. Endoscopic decompression for acute colonic pseudo-obstruction. Gastrointest Endosc 1996;44:144–50.
12. Lynch CR, Jones RG, Hilden K, Wills JC, Fang JC. Percutaneous endoscopic cecostomy in adults: a case series. Gastrointest Endosc 2006;64:279–82.
13. Ramage JI Jr, Baron TH. Percutaneous endoscopic cecostomy: a case series. Gastrointest Endosc 2003;57:752–5.
14. Einwachter H, Hellerhoff P, Neu B, Prinz C, Schmid R, Meining A. Percutaneous endoscopic colostomy in a patient with chronic intestinal pseudo-obstruction and massive dilation of the colon. Endoscopy 2006;38:547.

15. Cowlam S, Watson C, Elltringham M, Bain I, Barrett P, Green S, et al. Percutaneous endoscopic colostomy of the left side of the colon. Gastrointest Endosc 2007;65:1007–14.
16. Baraza W, Brown S, McAlindon M, Hurlstone P. Prospective analysis of percutaneous endoscopic colostomy at a tertiary referral centre. Br J Surg 2007;94:1415–20.
17. Uno Y. Introducer method of percutaneous endoscopic cecostomy and antegrade continence enema by use of the Chait Trapdoor cecostomy catheter in patients with adult neurogenic bowel. Gastrointest Endosc 2006;63:666–73.
18. Bertolini D, De Saussure P, Chilcott M, Girardin M, Dumonceau JM. Severe delayed complication after percutaneous endoscopic colostomy for chronic intestinal pseudo-obstruction: a case report and review of the literature. World J Gastroenterol 2007;13:2255–7.
19. Horiuchi A, Maeyama H, Ochi Y, Morikawa A, Miyazawa K. Usefulness of Dennis Colorectal Tube in endoscopic decompression of acute, malignant colonic obstruction. Gastrointest Endosc 2001;54:229–32.
20. Horiuchi A, Nakayama Y, Tanaka N, Kajiyama M, Fujii H, Yokoyama T, et al. Acute colorectal obstruction treated by means of transanal drainage tube: effectiveness before surgery and stenting. Am J Gastroenterol 2005;100:2765–70.
21. Xu M, Zhong Y, Yao L, Xu J, Zhou P, Wang P, et al. Endoscopic decompression using a transanal drainage tube for acute obstruction of the rectum and left colon as a bridge to curative surgery. Colorectal Dis 2008 May 29 [Epub ahead of print].
22. Fischer A, Schrag HJ, Goos M, Obermaier R, Hopt UT, Baier PK. Transanal endoscopic tube decompression of acute colonic obstruction: experience with 51 cases. Surg Endosc 2008;22:683–8.
23. Renzulli P, Maurer CA, Netzer P, Büchler MW. Preoperative colonoscopic derotation is beneficial in acute colonic volvulus. Dig Surg 2002;19:223–9.

V

38 Approach to Gastrointestinal Foreign Bodies

Benjamin K. Poulose and Jeffrey L. Ponsky

The management of foreign bodies in the gastrointestinal tract has been a challenge to physicians and surgeons for centuries. The endoscopic removal of foreign objects was developed and described in the early part of the 20th century using open-lumen rigid endoscopes [1]. Early on after the introduction of flexible endoscopes, there was uncertainty whether removal of foreign objects could be effectively carried out with these instruments, due to their small operating channels. With enhanced experience and skill, the effectiveness of flexible endoscopes in the removal of foreign bodies has not only equaled that of rigid instruments, but also provided access to deeper reaches of the gastrointestinal tract [2].

Ingestion of foreign bodies is a common event and may occur by intention or accident (**Fig. 38.1**). Patients of all ages are affected. Although most ingested objects will traverse the alimentary tract without harm, a small number may cause significant harm and even death [3]. The optimal management of patients who have ingested foreign bodies requires knowledge of the nature of the foreign body in question, endoscopic skill, and ingenuity. In certain situations, a combined endoscopic and surgical approach may be warranted. Ex vivo practice with the endoscope, accessories, and an object similar to that ingested will greatly facilitate the actual extraction process.

Approach to the Patient with Foreign-body Ingestion

It is estimated that between 80 % and 93 % of ingested foreign bodies that reach the stomach ultimately pass through the gastrointestinal tract [4]. In general, objects wider than 2 cm or longer than 5 cm often do not pass into the duodenum [5]. Clinical observation and appropriate studies are warranted to assess for signs and symptoms of obstruction or perforation. Most swallowed foreign bodies that result in obstruction become lodged in the anatomic narrowings of the esophagus at the levels of the upper esophageal sphincter, aortic arch, left mainstem bronchus, or diaphragm. The overall probability of perforation is less than 1 %, but this percentage increases dramatically when only sharp or pointed objects are considered (15–35 %) [4]. Other factors, such as position of the object and techniques used for removal, can influence the probability of iatrogenic perforation during object retrieval. Once an object is in the small intestine, perforation or obstruction usually occur in the region of the terminal ileum or cecum [4].

The patient's age, mental status, and the nature of the ingested foreign body will dictate how the clinical situation is approached. Although many cases will easily lend themselves to endoscopic extraction under conscious sedation, young children, combative patients, and situations in which foreign-body extraction poses a potential threat of airway compromise should be managed with general anesthesia and endotracheal intubation.

The patient and his or her family are often extremely anxious regarding the ingestion, and time should be taken to provide reassurance and counseling regarding the events to follow. A careful history should be taken to define the interval between the ingestion and presentation, the nature of the ingested article, and any symptoms that have developed following ingestion. In addition, knowledge of prior surgical and endoscopic procedures can provide important information regarding anatomy and previous pathology in the gastrointestinal tract. Preexistent gastrointestinal symptoms may provide important information regarding the reason for food bolus ingestion.

Plain films of the neck and abdomen are valuable for assessing an ingested object (**Fig. 38.2**). Lateral as well as anteroposterior films are important for defining the location and orientation of the ingested object, and to look for evidence of perforation. The presence of air in the soft tissues of the neck may indicate a full-thickness injury to the pharynx or esophagus. Metallic objects will be clearly seen on plain radiographic examination. Nonmetallic objects such as bones, food boluses, or plastic may be more difficult or impossible to see on plain films. Computed tomography may help localize nonmetallic objects and assess the soft-tissue reaction to the foreign body, but can potentially delay needed endoscopic intervention unless it is readily available. In general, early endoscopy is the best diagnostic and therapeutic approach.

Food Bolus Impaction

Esophageal obstruction by a food bolus is the most common type of foreign-body ingestion seen in adults. This phenomenon is usually an acute and dramatic event, associated with dysphagia and great anxiety. The obstruction is often complete and may be associated with increased salivation, inability to swallow even liquids, and substernal pain. Meat is the most common offending food. The meat may impact at a point of esophageal narrowing, frequently a Schatzki ring or peptic stricture. With the increasing use of gastric restrictive procedures to treat morbid obesity, impaction can also occur above the point of restriction (**Fig. 38.3**). Esophageal carcinoma may also underlie such an event. Patients with a history of gastric restrictive operations for morbid obesity often present with food bolus impaction, due to the narrowing of the anastomotic or restrictive site. It is not unusual to obtain a history of similar less dramatic and transient obstructions preceding the current event. Although using the Heimlich maneuver may be very effective and even life-saving for dislodging and evacuating an impacted tracheal or esophageal food bolus, complications such as gastric or esophageal rupture have been reported [6]. The use of meat tenderizer was once thought to be an effective therapy for impaction of food, but this has since been shown to be ineffective and potentially dangerous [7]. Early endoscopy is a safe and highly effective method of removing impacted food and determining the etiology of impaction.

Endoscopy for the removal of an impacted food bolus is usually performed with topical pharyngeal anesthesia. A standard gastroscope is used, and an overtube may be useful to allow multiple passages of the instrument, as well as to protect the airway from debris as it is withdrawn [8]. Some have suggested that a food bolus may be gently pushed past the obstruction into the stomach. While this may be possible at times, the risk of perforation is real, and extraction is preferable. A variety of instruments are available to allow manipulation of the food bolus. These include polypectomy snares, wire baskets, and grasping forceps (**Figs. 38.4, 38.5**). The food bolus will often fragment during manipulation, requiring mul-

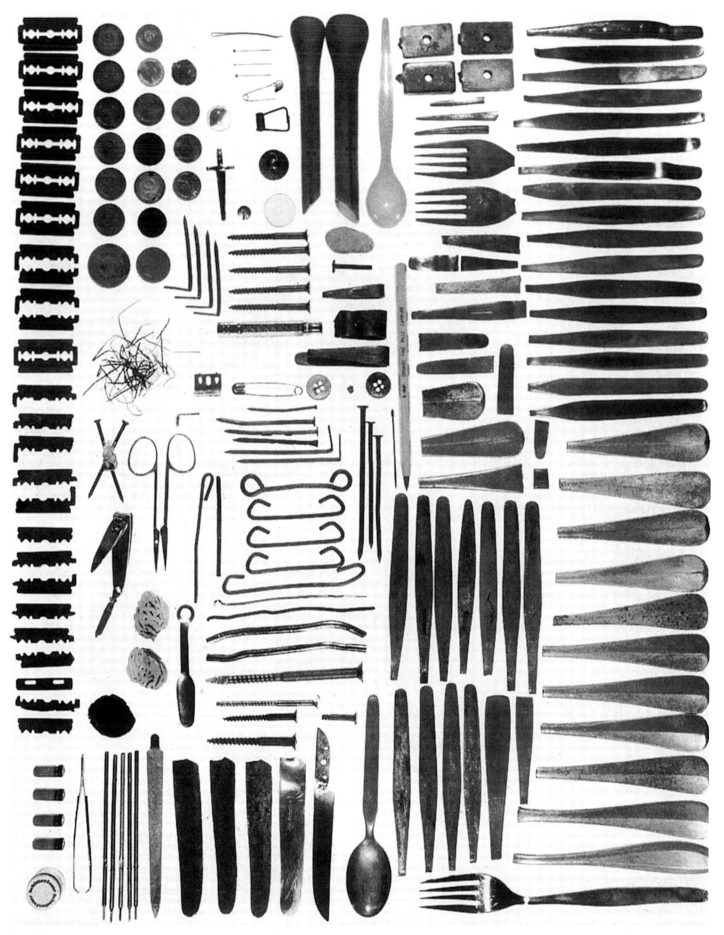

Fig. 38.1 Foreign bodies extracted endoscopically from the upper gastrointestinal tract—selected from a collection. Reproduced by kind permission of B. Manegold, Mannheim, Germany.

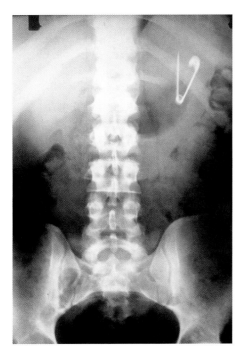

Fig. 38.2 A plain film of the abdomen should be obtained to ascertain the nature, number, and location of ingested foreign bodies.

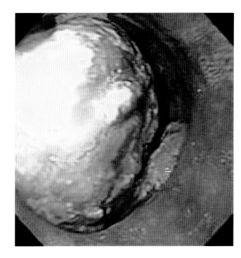

Fig. 38.3 Meat may impact above a stricture, in this case following previous gastric banding.

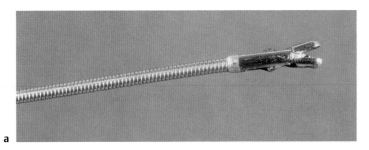

a

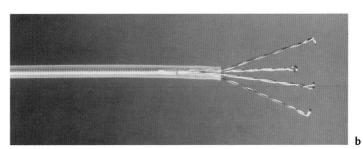

b

Fig. 38.4 a, b A variety of grasping forceps, toothed forceps, baskets, and snares are available for manipulating and holding foreign bodies.

tiple passages of the gastroscope. A very effective approach is to fit the tip of the endoscope with the cap used in esophageal variceal banding (**Fig. 38.6**). This allows the creation of a chamber at the tip of the scope into which the food bolus can be suctioned, and it frequently facilitates extraction of the bolus in one piece.

After removal of the impacted food, it is imperative to carry out a careful examination of the point of obstruction to discern what might have precipitated the event. Strictures or areas of possible tumor should be biopsied. Dilation can be performed after extraction of the foreign body, or scheduled soon after the acute event.

Coins

Children will frequently ingest coins. Most of these pass harmlessly through the gastrointestinal tract without incident, and reassurance and watchful waiting are warranted. The stools should be examined to note passage of the object, or periodic radiographs can be obtained. In some cases, however, problems may arise. A plain film of the neck and abdomen should be obtained as soon as possible after the ingestion. If the coin is located in the neck, it should prompt further action. Foreign bodies typically lodge at the cricopharyngeus

or the thoracic inlet. If the thin edge of the coin is seen on the anteroposterior film, it is most often lodged in the larynx or trachea. Prompt bronchoscopy should be performed to remove it and prevent airway compromise. When the broad face of the coin is noted on the anteroposterior film, the coin is most often in the esophagus (**Fig. 38.7**). Lateral neck films are useful for making this distinction. Early endoscopy is also indicated when a coin does not pass from the esophagus. It is important to repeat radiography just prior to starting the endoscopy, as the coin will often have passed spontaneously into the stomach, obviating the need for the procedure.

In rare cases, coins may linger in the stomach for more than a week. In such instances, they should be removed endoscopically. Rubber-tipped grasping forceps, alligator jaw forceps, or a standard polypectomy snare can be used to retrieve the coin (**Fig. 38.8**). Another accessory that is particularly useful in approaching foreign bodies is the Roth Net (U.S. Endoscopy, Mentor, Ohio, USA) (**Fig. 38.9**). This is a mesh bag covering the structure of a polypectomy snare. The foreign article can be entrapped in the bag, and the snare closed to capture it. This is particularly useful when the foreign body is difficult to grasp, or when there is a risk of losing the article into the airway.

38

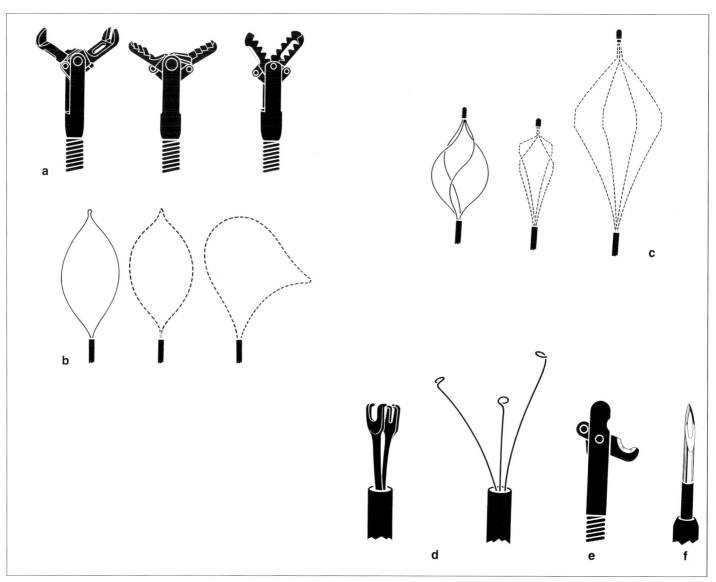

Fig. 38.5 Instruments for extracting foreign bodies in combination with endoscopes.
a Foreign-body forceps: hook-tipped forceps, alligator forceps for hard foreign bodies, alligator forceps for soft foreign bodies.
b Foreign-body loops: symmetrical and asymmetrical, made of monofilament or plaited wire.

c Dormia baskets, made of monofilament or plaited wire.
d Grasping instruments: two-armed for solid foreign bodies, three-armed for soft ones.
e Flexible scissors for cutting threads.
f Flexible and withdrawable puncture needle.

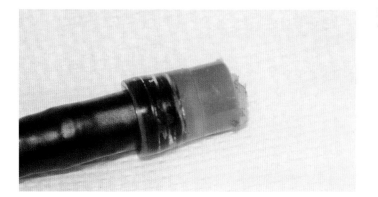

Fig. 38.6 The cap of a variceal ligating device can serve as a suction chamber and is very effective in removing impacted food boluses.

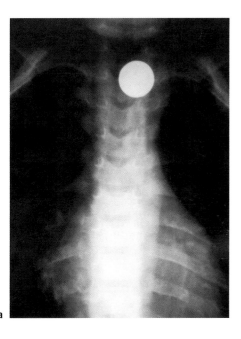

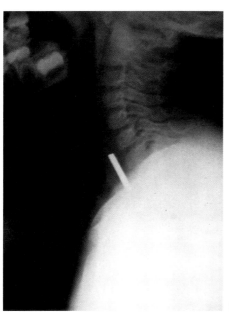

Fig. 38.7 a A plain film of the neck and chest reveals the flat face of an ingested coin, suggesting it is located in the esophagus rather than the trachea. **b** A lateral film shows that the coin is in the esophagus, posterior to the air-filled trachea.

a

b

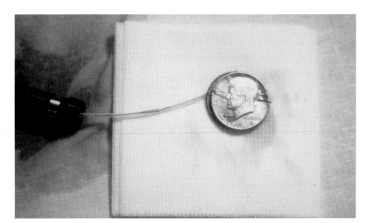

Fig. 38.8 Once in the stomach, coins can be captured with a snare.

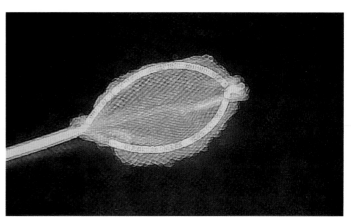

Fig. 38.9 The Roth Net (U.S. Endoscopy, Inc., Mentor, Ohio, USA) combines a mesh basket with a snare and is useful for retrieving and holding foreign bodies as well as preserving loss of the object in the airway.

Sharp Objects

Foreign bodies with sharp edges may pose a real risk of gastrointestinal tract injury. Perforation is the most common complication [9]. When possible, these objects should be endoscopically removed as soon after ingestion as possible. Plain radiographs may help identify the nature of the foreign body and its position (**Fig. 38.10**). Computed tomography greatly facilitates locating the foreign body and provides information regarding the surrounding soft tissues (**Fig. 38.11**). Evidence of compression necrosis (soft-tissue stranding with accompanying mural or extraluminal air) may assist in therapeutic decision-making. When the object or objects have passed the duodenum, it may be that observation is the best course. Despite the risk of perforation, most of these items will be surrounded with food materials and will pass safely through the gastrointestinal tract. However, when the object is observed in the esophagus, stomach, duodenum, or colon, endoscopic removal may reduce the incidence of complications.

The larger a sharp object, the more danger it poses. Needles, pins, tacks, and pieces of glass are commonly seen (**Fig. 38.12**). For secondary gain, some prisoners have been known to ingest safety pins

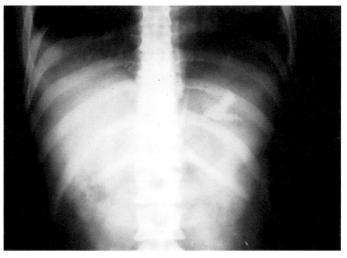

Fig. 38.10 Plain radiography can help identify the location and nature of the foreign body.

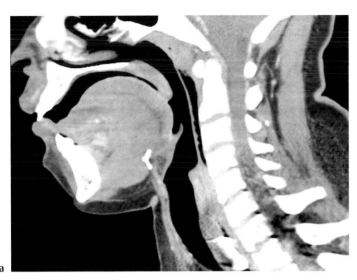

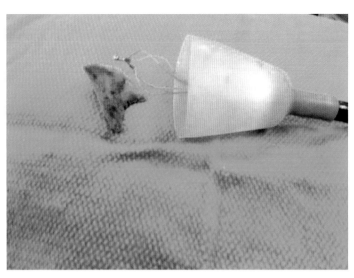

Fig. 38.11 a   A sagittal computed-tomographic image of an impacted foreign body in the lumen of the esophagus. There is evidence of soft-tissue inflammation and intraluminal air, suggestive of mucosal compromise.

b   The steak bone specimen after successful endoscopic extraction using a protective hood.

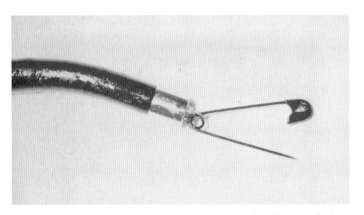

Fig. 38.12   A large safety pin that has been removed endoscopically from the duodenum.

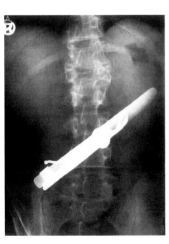

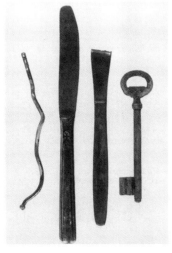

Fig. 38.13   A 28-year-old psychiatric patient who had had foreign bodies in his stomach for 14 days. The foreign bodies were extracted with the patient under general anesthesia.
a   Foreign bodies in situ.
b   After extraction.

or razors (**Fig. 38.13**). These may be wrapped in tape to facilitate swallowing. Once in the stomach, the tape is digested, and the sharp edges of the item become exposed. The use of an overtube may greatly enhance the safety of the removal process. The sharp article can be grasped with a foreign-body forceps or snare and withdrawn into the overtube for safe removal. When needles, pins, and nails are being removed, it is important to remember the axiom "a trailing point never perforates." A safety pin is grasped at the hinged end and pulled back with the point trailing (**Fig. 38.14**). A protective rubber hood has sometimes been attached to the tip of the endoscope to shield a sharp foreign body as it is pulled up the esophagus [10] (**Fig. 38.15**).

Irregularly shaped objects such as bones or soda can tops may prove particularly challenging and pose a significant threat of perforation. This is even more true if the object is impacted in the esophagus, where the luminal diameter is small (**Fig. 38.16**). If the sharp end or ends of an object in the stomach are oriented upward, it may be wise to advance the object into the stomach with the points trailing and then turn it round to facilitate extraction. Firmly impacted objects may be more safely approached surgically, or with a combined endoscopic and surgical procedure.

Batteries and Magnets

Batteries present the danger of obstruction and caustic ulceration in the gastrointestinal tract. They contain either metallic salts (mercuric oxide, silver oxide, zinc oxide, or lithium oxide) or alkali (sodium or potassium hydroxide) [11]. Button batteries—common in cameras, watches, and many modern electronic devices—are particularly prone to ingestion and are difficult to handle endoscopically [12,13]. If a battery is found to be out of reach of the endoscope, it may be followed closely through the gastrointestinal tract with serial radiographs. If it does not progress, surgery is indicated. When accessible, the battery should be removed endoscopically. Instruments useful for manipulating a battery may include a polypectomy snare, Dormia stone baskets, and the Roth net.

Ingested magnets pose a unique and potentially dangerous problem for patients. Usually observed in the pediatric population, magnets in the gastrointestinal tract can lead to pressure necrosis in the luminal wall due to attractive magnetic forces. Several reports of perforation resulting from this phenomenon warrant an aggressive

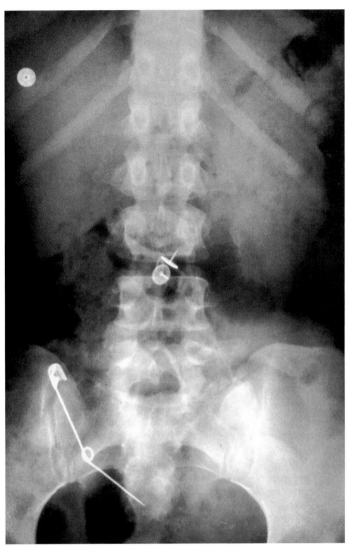

Fig. 38.14 When a sharp foreign body is grasped, it should be removed with the point trailing.

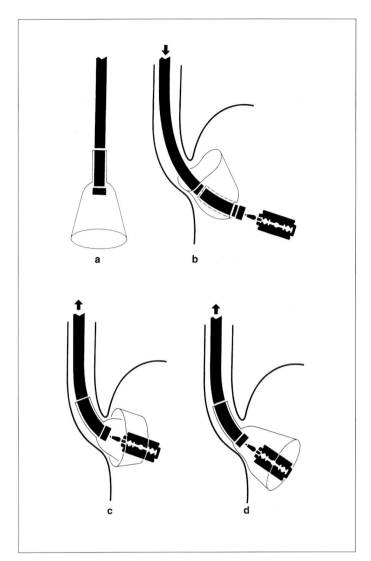

Fig. 38.15 Removing sharp-edged foreign bodies from the stomach.
a A flexible protective funnel mounted at the distal end of the endoscope.
b The funnel turns inside out when the instrument is introduced around the shaft.
c, d When the instrument has securely grasped the foreign body and the endoscope is withdrawn into the cardia, the funnel deploys over the object.

38

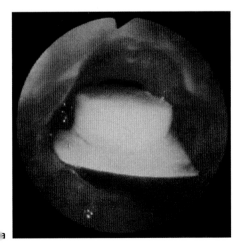

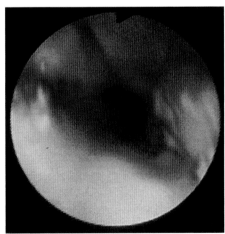

Fig. 38.16 A 75-year-old man who had swallowed a handful of morning tablets.
a One tablet had been swallowed along with its sharp-edged packaging.
b Longitudinal decubital ulcers in the esophagus ("tablet ulcers") were visible within a few hours after ingestion.

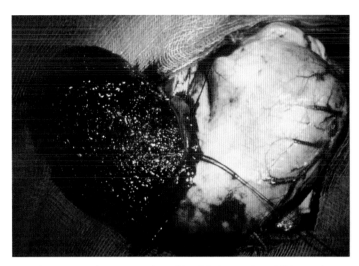

Fig. 38.17 Large bezoars, such as this trichobezoar in a child, may form a cast of the stomach and are often best removed surgically.

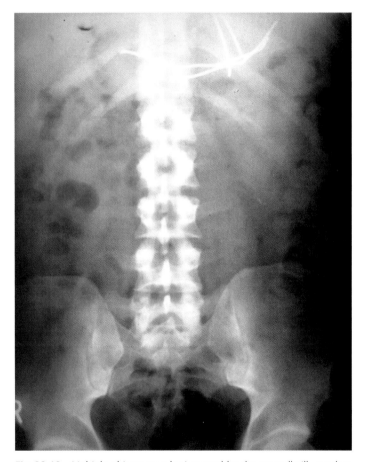

Fig. 38.18 Multiple objects may be ingested by the mentally ill, or when secondary gain is anticipated.

approach to removal, especially if more than one magnet is known to have been ingested [14,15]. Endoscopic removal techniques are similar to those described for battery retrieval.

Bezoars

Bezoars are concretions of foreign material that become fixed in the stomach and occasionally the duodenum. They may be of vegetable origin (phytobezoar), or consist of ingested hair (trichobezoar) [16].

Phytobezoars are particularly common in patients with delayed gastric emptying after previous partial gastrectomy and vagotomy. Patients will present with a chronic history of vomiting, dyspepsia, abdominal discomfort, or weight loss. A barium upper gastrointestinal series may allow diagnosis, but diagnostic endoscopy may be therapeutic as well as diagnostic.

Treatment of phytobezoars using enzymatic digestion has occasionally been effective. This has been particularly true with the use of cellulose, which will digest vegetable matter. Large bezoars may be fixed to the gastric wall and difficult to manipulate endoscopically. Use of an overtube allows multiple passages of the endoscope and protects the patient's airway as the procedure is conducted. Accessories such as snares and stone baskets are useful for fragmenting and removing large portions of the bezoar. Vigorous irritation with a device that provides a forceful jet stream will also be effective in some cases. Multiple sessions may be required to completely fragment and remove the bezoar. Some bezoars, particularly trichobezoars, may be so large and fixed as to form a cast of the stomach (**Fig. 38.17**). In such extreme cases, prompt surgical therapy may be most effective. After removal of a bezoar, it is important to try and prevent recurrent formation. This may require diet and behavioral modification, as well as prokinetic agents in some cases to enhance gastric emptying.

Unusual Foreign Bodies

In the management of foreign bodies, the endoscopist must expect the unexpected. A wide variety of unusual objects will be encountered, particularly in the mentally ill or in those seeking secondary gain. Frequently in such patients, a large number of objects will be ingested. These may include knives, forks, spoons, hairpins, tacks, safety pins, batteries, toothbrushes, and even bottles (**Fig. 38.18**). Dental bridges and chicken bones are not uncommonly swallowed, and may have potentially harmful sharp edges (**Fig. 38.19**).

Once again, preprocedural ex vivo practice with similar objects will prepare the endoscopist for the actual procedure and clarify which tools and methods will be most effective in the process [17] (**Fig. 38.20**). The use of an overtube may be extremely important for extracting sharp or multiple objects, and general anesthesia may be required in pediatric patients, the mentally impaired, recalcitrant patients, and in situations in which airway control is imperative.

Ingestion of latex condoms or balloons filled with drugs such as heroin or cocaine (body packing) is well known [18] (**Fig. 38.21**). The outlines of these vessels may be seen on plain abdominal films. Endoscopic extraction may be feasible in some cases, but can be hazardous, as rupture of the condom or balloon will release large amounts of the drug, and absorption will be toxic. Observation for spontaneous passage or surgical extraction may be preferable.

Rectal and Colonic Foreign Bodies

Foreign bodies in the rectum, often the result of sexual play, are frequently considered a subject of humor, but provide a very serious problem for the physician and patient. These foreign bodies may be large and irregularly shaped. Frequently they may be made of breakable substances such as glass, which may penetrate the rectal wall if broken. Sometimes the object may migrate upward into the sigmoid colon and can become impacted in the curves of the colon (**Fig. 38.22**). For these reasons, removal of rectal and colonic foreign bodies may be very challenging, if not dangerous. Good radiographs and possibly computed tomographic scans documenting the position of the foreign object and ruling out perforation should be obtained before any manipulation. The patient should most often be sedated, and general anesthesia will be employed in many cases.

V

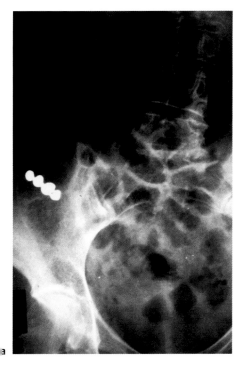

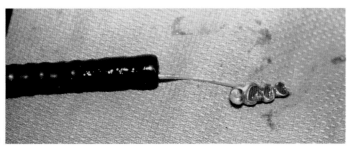

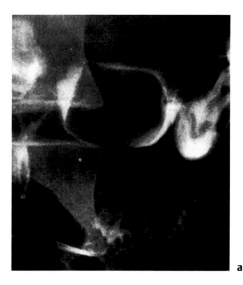

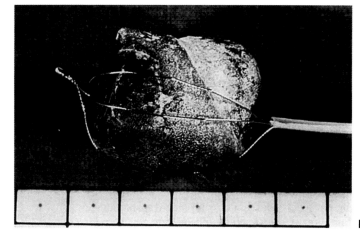

Fig. 38.19 a A plain film demonstrates a swallowed dental bridge that has come to rest in the cecum. Such items may pass spontaneously, but endoscopic removal may prevent the occasional perforation. If the object fails to pass within a few days, colonoscopic removal should be considered.
b Using a snare, the bridge is removed with a colonoscope.

Fig. 38.20 A 49-year-old woman with Bouveret syndrome (gastric outlet syndrome).
a Penetration of the gallstone from the gallbladder into the duodenal bulb, with complete stenosis of the gastric outlet.
b Endoscopic stone extraction.

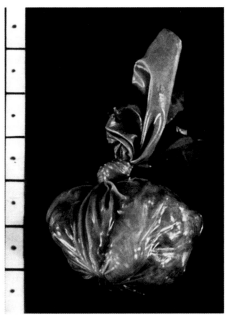

Fig. 38.21 A container with 5 g of heroin that was extracted endoscopically from the stomach of a body packer. The street value of the package was approximately $ 7500.

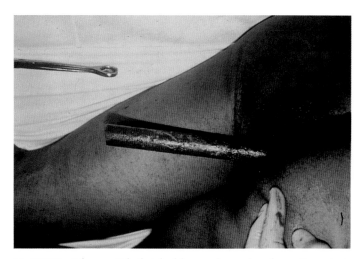

Fig. 38.22 A broomstick that had been advanced as far as the splenic flexure of the colon has been maneuvered distally with a combination of abdominal compression and manipulation through a large-diameter rigid sigmoidoscope.

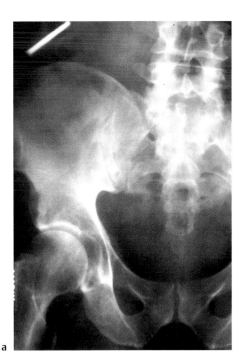

a

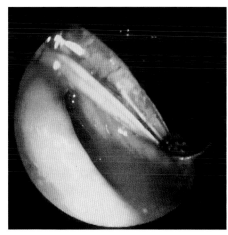

b

Fig. 38.23 a A thermometer swallowed by a patient had remained impacted in the ileum for several years. It is visualized endoscopically.
b The snared thermometer is removed with the colonoscope. Care must be taken not to grasp the glass object too tightly.

The flexible endoscope may be useful in identifying the object and assessing its location. Smaller and more proximal objects may be grasped and retrieved with snares or baskets (**Fig. 38.23**). When larger objects appear to be impacted or difficult to maneuver with a flexible endoscope, attempts at retrieval with larger-lumen rigid instruments are occasionally valuable. In some cases, laparoscopy or laparotomy may be required.

Surgically Assisted Endoscopic Foreign-Body Removal

The successful and safe management of recalcitrant ingested foreign bodies sometimes requires innovative techniques that combine endoscopic and surgical approaches. In general, indications for hybrid approaches include foreign bodies that cannot be safely retrieved endoscopically and require extraluminal manipulation to facilitate endoscopic removal, or localization of intraluminal objects. In the upper gastrointestinal tract, impacted foreign bodies or those that perforate can require gastrotomy or duodenotomy for removal [19]. A hybrid approach can limit the size of incursion into the lumen, provide a means of safe extraction, facilitate removal of peritoneal soilage, and test the integrity of luminal closure [5]. At times, the colon may be manipulated surgically to advance the foreign body distally until it can be grasped with an endoscope or emerges from the anus. When manipulation may result in danger to the patient, as with impacted condoms containing narcotics, open colotomy and extraction may be necessary. Often, surgical assistance can be provided via a laparoscopic approach. Successful hybrid removal of foreign bodies is highly dependent on the skills of the surgeon, endoscopist, nurses, and technical staff associated with both teams.

Conclusion

Foreign-body ingestion is a common, ubiquitous problem. While most objects will pass uneventfully through the gastrointestinal tract and exit without harm, sharp objects, items likely to obstruct or perforate, batteries, and items that fail to progress should be removed. Careful attention to airway protection, appropriate sedation, and the use of protective overtubes are vital aspects of this process. The endoscopist should also become familiar with the endoscopic manipulation of foreign objects by preprocedural ex vivo practice using similar items. A hybrid surgical–endoscopic approach or a purely surgical approach should be considered when objects appear to have perforated, are impacted, or present a toxic threat. In most cases, however, the endoscopic approach is highly effective and safe.

References

1. Jackson C, Jackson CL. Personal gastroscopy. JAMA 1935;104:269–75.
2. Sanowski RA, Harrison ME, Young MF, Berggreen PJ. Foreign body extraction. In: Sivak M, editor. Gastrointestinal endoscopy. 2nd ed. Philadelphia: Saunders; 2000. p. 801–12.
3. Devanesan J, Pisani A, Sharma P, Kazarian KK, Mersheimer WL. Metallic foreign bodies in the stomach. Arch Surg 1977;112:664–5.
4. Henderson CT, Engel J, Schlesinger P. Foreign body ingestion: review and suggested guidelines for management. Endoscopy 1987;19:68–71.
5. Iafrati MD, Fabry SC, Lee YM, Obrien JW, Schwaitzberg SD. A novel approach to the removal of sharp foreign bodies from the stomach using a combined endoscopic and laparoscopic technique. Gastrointestinal Endoscopy 1996;43:67–70.
6. Bintz M, Cogbill TH. Gastric rupture after the Heimlich maneuver. J Trauma 1996;40:159–60.
7. Holsinger JW, Fuson RL, Sealy WC. Esophageal perforation following meat impaction and papain ingestion. JAMA 1968;204:734–5.
8. Rogers BH, Kot C, Meiri S, Epstein M. An overtube for the flexible fiberoptic esophagogastroduodenoscope. Gastrointest Endosc 1982;28:256–7.
9. Oshima T, Shimizu I, Horie T. A case of penetration of the large intestinal wall by a toothpick. Dig Endosc 1999;11:350–2.
10. Bertoni G, Pacchione D, Sassatelli R, Ricci E, Mortilla MG, Gumina C. A new protector device for safe endoscopic removal of sharp gastroesophageal foreign bodies in infants. J Pediatr Gastroenterol Nutr 1993;16:393–6.
11. Litovitz TL. Battery ingestions: product accessibility and clinical course. Pediatrics 1985;75:469–76.
12. Litovitz TL. Button battery ingestions: a review of 56 cases. JAMA 1983;249:2495–500.
13. Webb WA. Management of foreign bodies of the upper gastrointestinal tract. Gastroenterology 1988;83:476–8.

V

14. Schierling S, Snyder SK, Custer M, Pohl JF, Easley D. Magnet ingestion. J Pediatr 2008;152:294.

15. Butterworth J, Feltis B, Butterworth J, Feltis B. Toy magnet ingestion in children: revising the algorithm. J Pediatr Surg 2007;42:e3–5.

16. Andrus CH, Ponsky JL. Bezoars: classification, pathophysiology, and treatment. Am J Gastroenterol 1988;83:476–8.

17. Ahmed A, Cummings SA. Novel endoscopic approach for removal of a rectal foreign body. Gastrointest Endosc 1999;50:872–4.

18. Suarez CA, Aranjo A, Lester JL 3 rd. Cocaine-condom ingestion: surgical treatment. JAMA 1977;238:1391–2.

19. Lanitis S, Filippakis G, Christophides T, Papaconstandinou T, Karaliotas C. Combined laparoscopic and endoscopic approach for the management of two ingested sewing needles: one migrated into the liver and one stuck in the duodenum. J Laparoendosc Adv Surg Tech A 2007;17:311–4.

38

39 Biliary Lithotripsy

Chan-Sup Shim

Introduction

Lithotripsy, a procedure that fragments stones, is used to reduce the size of large or difficult-to-remove stones to facilitate their removal or passage via the biliary ducts, or to dislodge impacted stones. Lithotripsy can be carried out using intracorporeal modalities, such as mechanical lithotripsy (ML), electrohydraulic lithotripsy (EHL), or laser lithotripsy (LL) during peroral access (via endoscopic retrograde cholangiopancreatography, ERCP) or percutaneous access (via percutaneous transhepatic cholangioscopy, PTC), or via extracorporeal shock-wave lithotripsy (ESWL). Approximately 80% of common bile duct stones can be removed endoscopically using standard basket or balloon extraction techniques. The addition of ML has improved success rates by a further 10%. Recent technological advances have led to breakthroughs in the endoscopic management of difficult stones, enabling endoscopists to successfully fragment and remove nearly 100% of bile duct stones.

Indications

Lithotripsy is used for stones in the intrahepatic and extrahepatic bile ducts that cannot be removed by conventional methods. Stone removal from the common bile duct (CBD) may be technically difficult, due to factors such as the size of the stone (> 2 cm), impaction of the stone in an undilated bile duct, stones above a bile duct stricture, or a narrowed retropancreatic portion of the distal CBD. In these circumstances, ML is commonly used. Shock-wave lithotripsy, including EHL or LL, should be reserved for stones in which ML fails. This may occur if the stone is too large to be captured in the basket, or if the basket is unable to open completely over an impacted stone or unfold around the stone. In other cases, stones lodged in the cystic duct at the junction with the CBD (Mirizzi syndrome) or intrahepatic stones may be inaccessible to basket extraction for anatomic reasons. Percutaneous access can be used when the papilla cannot be reached endoscopically following previous surgery, as with Billroth II resection or Roux-en-Y anastomosis procedures and biliodigestive anastomoses.

Equipment and Techniques

In most centers, side-viewing video endoscopes are available, with a large channel and special modifications to accommodate standard accessories. This obviates the need to change instruments when therapeutic procedures are required. Peroral cholangioscopy is now routine, with the use of an ultrathin endoscope inserted through a large-channel duodenoscope. The ultrathin endoscope allows direct visual examination of the biliary system and lithotripsy procedures. Percutaneous choledochoscopic lithotripsy is also possible using thin choledochoscopes inserted through percutaneous tracts.

Peroral Cholangioscopy

Equipment. Intraductal shock-wave lithotripsy without a stone–tissue recognition system can cause injury to the bile duct wall and should therefore be performed under cholangioscopic guidance. A mother–baby endoscope system is required for this procedure (**Fig. 39.1**). The baby scope (cholangioscope) is inserted through the working channel of the mother scope (duodenoscope). Two operators, or a single operator with an external cholangioscope fixation device, are needed in order to perform peroral cholangioscopy [1,2].

Commercially available cholangioscopes designed for passage through the working channel of a therapeutic duodenoscope (4.2-mm working channel) include the Olympus CHF-BP30 (non-video; Olympus Optical Co. Ltd., Tokyo, Japan), Pentax FCP9P (non-video; Pentax, Orangeburg, New York, USA), and Olympus CHF-B160/BP260/B260 (video scope). The scope diameters range from 2.6 to 3.4 mm, with a working channel of 1.2 mm. The Olympus video scope has a smaller tip deflection (70° up and down) than the nonvideo scope (160° up and 130° down). A new single-operator cholangioscopy system with four-way tip deflection and dedicated irrigation and biopsy channels (SpyGlass Direct Visualization System; Boston Scientific Corporation, Natick, Massachusetts, USA) has received Food and Drug Administration clearance and is currently under clinical investigation [2,3]. We have recently used an ultra-slim upper endoscope (Olympus GIF-260N or GIF-XP260N) for intraductal balloon-guided peroral cholangioscopy or overtube balloon-assisted direct peroral cholangioscopy as a new technique for lithotripsy [4,5].

Technical tip. Cholangioscopy-guided shock-wave lithotripsy requires two experienced endoscopists, one to operate each of the endoscopes. The endoscopist operating the mother scope is responsible for guiding the baby scope into the bile duct and directing it to the stone, and the endoscopist operating the baby scope fine-tunes the position of the shock-wave probe at the stone surface. A fluid medium is required around the stone for effective generation and conduction of shock waves with EHL, and is also helpful for flushing out stone debris after fragmentation. A nasobiliary catheter (**Fig. 39.1a**) should be inserted above the stone for irrigation with physiological saline, as the operating channel of the baby scope is too small to be useful for irrigation, especially with the lithotripsy probe in place. Continuous irrigation of the bile duct is frequently required because stone debris, sludge, or pus may obscure the cholangioscopic view.

Percutaneous Choledochoscopy

Equipment. Preliminary dilation of the percutaneous tract makes it possible to accommodate small-caliber choledochoscopes. Percutaneous choledochoscopes have an outer diameter of 3.0–6.0 mm and an instrumentation channel of 1.2–2.6 mm. Most choledochoscopes can be maneuvered bidirectionally (e.g., Olympus CHF-P2Q), providing tip deflection in four directions. For therapeutic choledochoscopic procedures such as stone fragmentation and extraction, a durable choledochoscope with a larger caliber would be better.

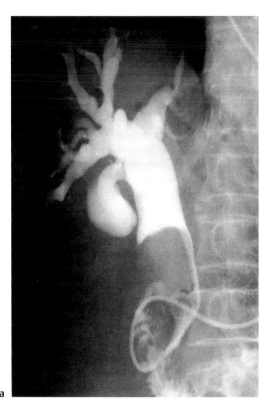

a

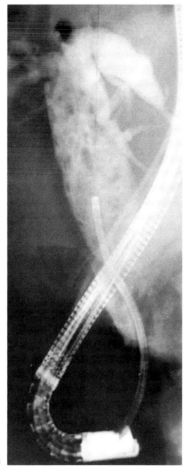

b

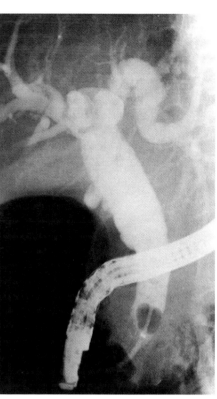

c

Fig. 39.1   Radiographic views of peroral cholangioscopic electrohydraulic lithotripsy (EHL) of a common bile duct (CBD) stone using the mother–baby scope unit.

a   A nasobiliary catheter is inserted above the stone for irrigation with physiological saline.

b   The cholangioscope has been inserted into the CBD and positioned for EHL. A large CBD stone is being fragmented using EHL.

c   After fragmentation, the fragmented stones are completely evacuated using a retrieval balloon.

Technical tip   The site of percutaneous access is variable. For intrahepatic stones, access depends on the location of the stones, and routes via the left and right hepatic duct are used when necessary. In the case of CBD lesions, either tract can be chosen. We prefer the left access route, as it is better tolerated by patients. In addition, the cutaneobiliary fistula can be established quickly and is more stable. For bilateral intrahepatic stones, a left intrahepatic duct approach is recommended, as it is easier to pass the choledochoscope from a left intrahepatic duct to a right intrahepatic duct or to the common duct. For right-sided access, a posterior rather than an anterior approach is preferable, to avoid the angulations of the anterior segment [6]. The choledochoscope is passed into the biliary system via a preexisting percutaneous tract; the procedure should not be performed at the initial percutaneous tract, due to the lack of a mature tract. After full dilation of the percutaneous tract to a diameter of between 12 and 18 Fr, 7–10 days are typically required for the sinus tract to mature [6].

Choledochoscopic examination can be performed after complete maturation of a sufficiently dilated percutaneous tract (**Fig. 39.2**).

We generally recommend waiting 3–4 weeks for the tract to mature and permit sequential dilation to a size of 12–14 Fr or larger [7,8]. When percutaneous choledochoscopic lithotomy with a basket and EHL are used to remove intrahepatic duct stones, fragments or small stones usually remain in the bile duct that are too small to be captured with a basket. Percutaneous transhepatic papillary balloon dilation (PTPBD) of the sphincter of Oddi (**Fig. 39.3**) and clearance of residual bile duct stones and stone fragments by pushing them through the papilla with the tip of choledochoscope is simple and effective in patients undergoing percutaneous choledochoscopic lithotomy [9]. PTPBD may be an acceptable alternative to percutaneous retrieval of stones and stone fragments, which reduces the number of times the choledochoscope has to be inserted and the time required to clear the bile ducts of stones.

Given its more invasive nature and the associated morbidity of PTC in comparison with ERCP, this approach should only be used for intraductal lithotripsy of stones that are inaccessible with a transpapillary retrograde approach.

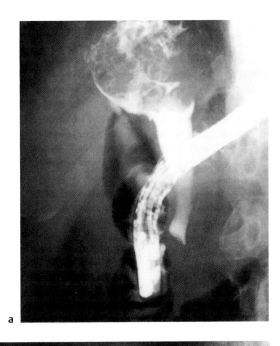
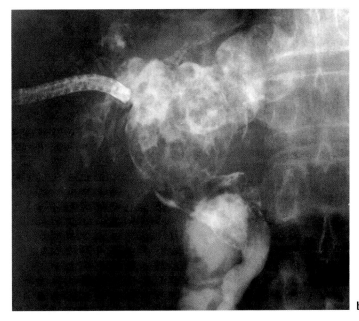

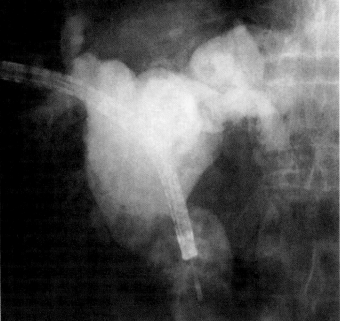
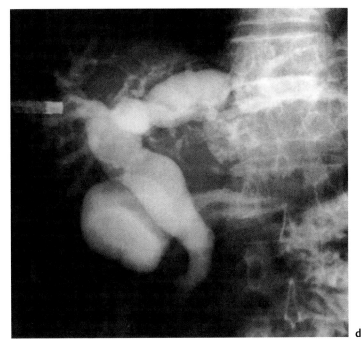

39

Fig. 39.2 Radiographic views of percutaneous choledochoscopic lithotripsy.
a Endoscopic retrograde cholangiopancreatography, showing conglomerated multiple intrahepatic stones.
b After complete maturation of a sufficiently dilated percutaneous tract, the choledochoscope is inserted into the intrahepatic bile duct.

c The electrohydraulic lithotripsy (EHL) probe is inserted through the choledochoscope and positioned.
d All the stones in the intrahepatic duct and common bile duct are completely evacuated.

Mechanical Lithotripsy (ML)

Equipment. ML is the simplest and typically the most cost-effective method of fragmenting stones in the bile duct. A mechanical lithotriptor consists of a wire basket, a metal sheath, and a handle that allows mechanical retraction of the basket into the metal sheath, directing a crushing force onto the stone. Two types of mechanical lithotriptor are in use, depending on whether lithotripsy is being carried out on an emergency or elective basis.

Some models can be passed through the endoscope, whereas others require removal of the endoscope before the metal sheath is positioned. The specifications of some recent commercially available mechanical lithotriptors are shown in **Table 39.1** [10].

- The LithoCrushV single-use mechanical lithotriptor (Olympus) is available in wire-guided and bullet-tip styles. The wire-guided version (Olympus BML-V437QR-30, V442QR-30) (**Fig. 39.4a**, **b**) uses a monorail construction with a guide-wire lumen at the distal end; this design makes it easier to exchange catheters and insert the basket into the papilla. It also facilitates a selective approach to the intrahepatic bile ducts or other target sites. The bullet-tip style (Olympus BML-V232QR-26/30, BML-V237QR-30, and BML-V242QR-30) (**Fig. 39.4c**) consists of a three-layer system, with a strong four-wire basket, a Teflon tube sheath, and an overlying metal coil sheath. This design effectively combines the benefits of the tube's outstanding insertion ability with the coil's remarkable torque performance. The set-up is designed to break

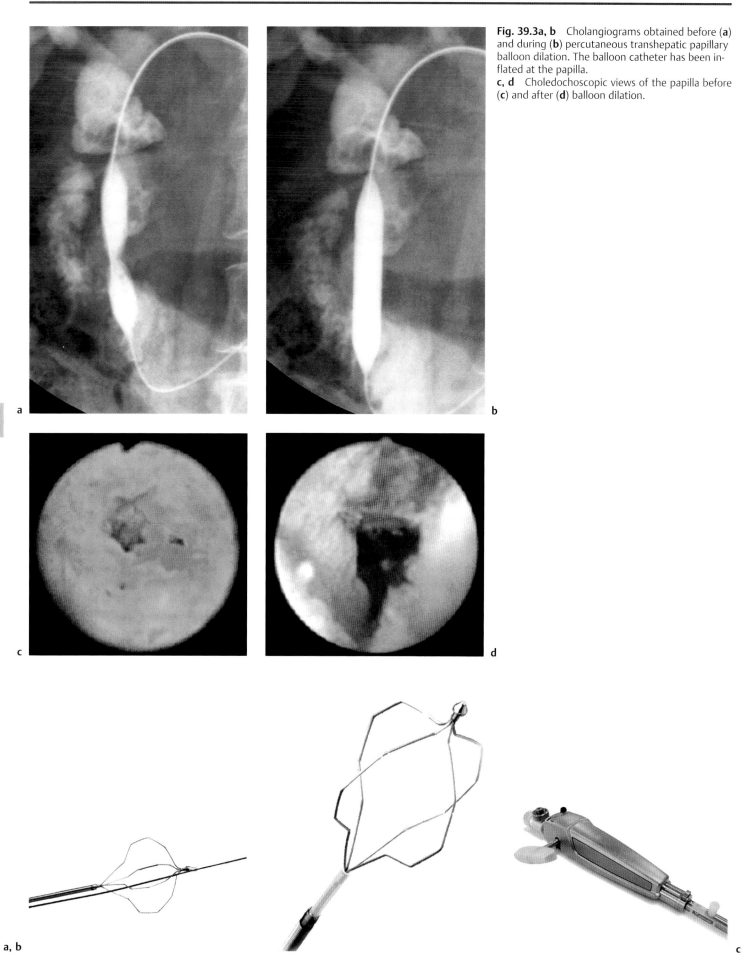

Fig. 39.3a, b Cholangiograms obtained before (**a**) and during (**b**) percutaneous transhepatic papillary balloon dilation. The balloon catheter has been inflated at the papilla.
c, d Choledochoscopic views of the papilla before (**c**) and after (**d**) balloon dilation.

Fig. 39.4 Olympus rotatable mechanical lithotriptors (LithoCrushV) are available in new wire-guided (**a**) and standard bullet-tip styles (**b**), with a new handle design (**c**).

Table 39.1 Mechanical lithotriptors

Device	Contrast injection capability	Working channel (mm)	Crush > 1 stone
Integrated			
Olympus			
• BML-V242QR-30	Yes	4.2	Yes
• BML-V237QR-30	Yes	3.7	Yes
• BML-V232QR-30	Yes	3.2	Yes
• BML-V232QR-26	Yes	3.2	Yes
• BML-V442QR-30 (w/GW)	Yes	4.2	Yes
• BML-V437QR-30 (w/GW)	Yes	3.7	Yes
Microvasive (Boston Scientific)			
• Trapezoid RX	Yes	3.2	Yes
Salvage			
Olympus			
• MAJ-441(compatible with basket)	No	Remove scope	No
• BML-110A-1	No	3.2–4.2	No
Cook Endoscopy			
• Conquest TTC lithotriptor cable (disposable)			
• TTCL-1 (sheath)	No	3.2	No
• TTCL-10 (sheath)	No	3.7	No
• Soehendra lithotriptor cable (reusable), SLC-2	No	Remove scope	No
• Soehendra lithotriptor handle (reusable), SLH-1	NA	NA	NA

NA, not available.

at the point of connection between the basket system and the crank handle. The handle is reusable and autoclavable.

- The Trapezoid RX Lithotripsy Compatible (Boston Scientific) (**Fig. 39.5**) is a single-piece disposable ML system with the basket, metal sheath, and crank handle all built into a single unit. Once it has been advanced through an endoscope and into the common bile duct, this device serves as a retrieval apparatus with crushing capability, and complete stone fragments can be removed. In the event that the biliary stone cannot be crushed, the Trapezoid RX has been designed for the basket's tip to disengage, minimizing the potential for stone entrapment in the basket. Four basket sizes (1.5, 2.0, 2.5, 3.0 cm) are available.
- The Soehendra lithotriptor (Cook Endoscopy, Winston-Salem, North Carolina, USA) consists of a 14-Fr metal sheath and a self-locking crank handle (**Fig. 39.6**). The lithotriptor can be used with large lithotripsy baskets or standard stone extraction baskets. Typically, lithotripsy baskets are four-wire hexagonal baskets with an average size of 2 × 3 cm or 3 × 5 cm (diameter × length).
- A hybrid variation of the above lithotriptor types consists of a thin-diameter 7.8-Fr coil sleeve that fits through the endoscope working channel and a cranking device (Medi-Globe Lithotriptor; Medi-Globe, Tempe, Arizona, USA) (**Fig. 39.7**). This lithotriptor is used in conjunction with a lithotripsy-compatible Dormia basket, which has a removable handle. The basket is used in the standard fashion for stone extraction; if lithotripsy is required, the basket handle and outer sheath are removed and replaced with the metal sleeve. The basket wires and sleeve are then secured to the cranking device for lithotripsy.

Technical tip. Integrated devices incorporate all components of the system and are designed for use through the operating channel of the duodenoscope. The system can be applied through the scope in anticipation of lithotripsy for large common duct or intrahepatic stones above a strictured/stenosed bile duct, and there is then no need to remove the duodenoscope. Once the stone is properly trapped in the basket (**Fig. 39.8**), the metal sheath is advanced up

39

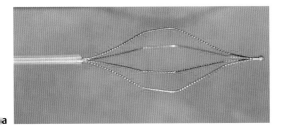
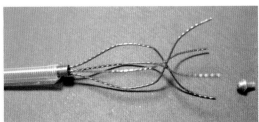

a

Fig. 39.5
a A single-piece disposable mechanical lithotripsy system (Trapezoid RX, Boston Scientific).
b The basket is designed in such a way that the basket tip can disengage, minimizing the potential for stone entrapment in the basket.

b

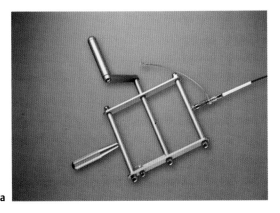
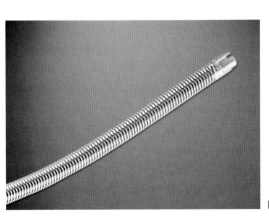

a

Fig. 39.6a, b A Soehendra emergency lithotriptor, consisting of a cranking device (**a**) and a flexible metal coil sheath (**b**).

b

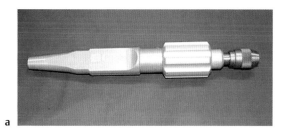

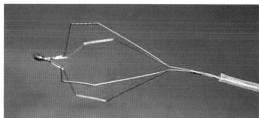

a

Fig. 39.7a, b The Medi-Globe mechanical lithotriptor, consisting of a flexible metal coil and cranking device (**a**). The lithotriptor can be used on an elective or emergency basis, and can also be used in conjunction with a lithotripsy-compatible Dormia basket (**b**).

b

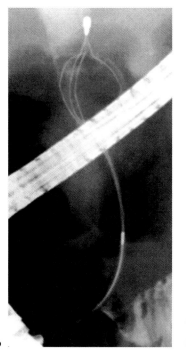

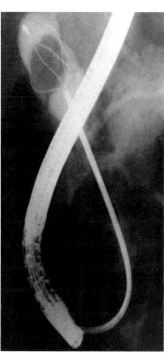

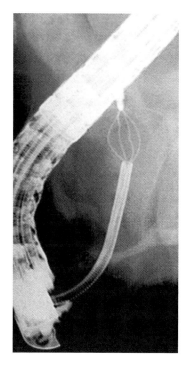

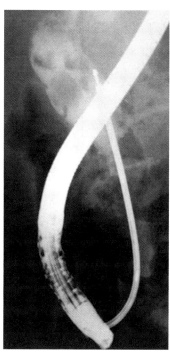

a, b

c

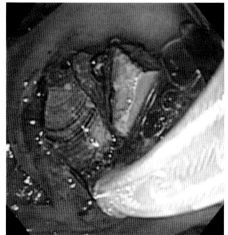

e

Fig. 39.8 Cholangiographic views showing mechanical lithotripsy using an endoscopic mechanical lithotriptor to treat a common duct stone.
a A large stone has been captured in the lithotriptor basket.
b The metal sheath is advanced up to the level of the stone.
c Mechanical lithotripsy is carried out by pulling the stone against the metal sleeve using a cranking device.
d The large stone is fragmented into multiple small pieces.
e The endoscopic view shows the multiple fragmented stones that have been removed with a Dormia basket.

to the level of the stone by adjusting the controls on the shaft of the lithotripsy basket. Tension is then applied to the wires by turning the control knob to crush the stone. The metal sheath is retracted into the channel of the duodenoscope, so that only the Teflon catheter and basket are used to cannulate the bile duct. The Teflon catheter is then pulled back using the opened basket to engage the stone. Trapping of the stone may be difficult, as a large stone may not leave sufficient space within the bile duct for basket manipulation. Shaking the basket often does not work. If necessary, the metal sheath is railroaded up the Teflon catheter to provide stiffness for manipulation of the basket. Gentle twisting of the scope will

transmit a rotational force to the basket to facilitate movement of the basket wires around the stone for stone engagement. Advancing the scope farther into the second part of the duodenum is sometimes helpful in straightening the axis of the basket and the bile duct to facilitate stone engagement.

Salvage devices consisting of just the metal sheath and the handle are used when a basket containing a stone becomes impacted in the duct during attempted stone extraction. Salvage devices are designed to be applied over a variety of stone-removal baskets, but not all baskets are lithotriptor-compatible. Basket designs must include failure points that break safely and allow basket re-

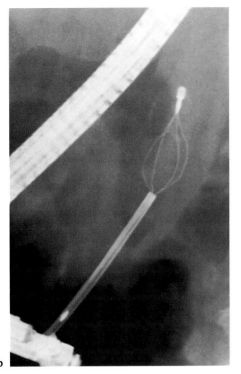
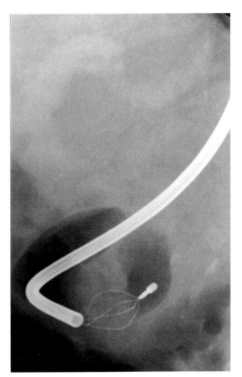
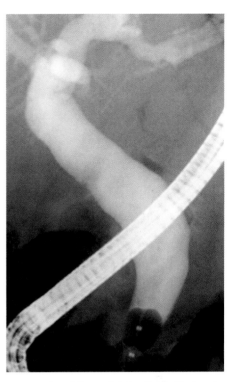

Fig. 39.9 Radiographs illustrating an emergency lithotripsy.
a A large stone has been engaged in a mechanical lithotripsy Dormia basket, but stone extraction has failed.

b The duodenoscope was removed, and the metal sheath of a Soehendra lithotriptor was inserted over the traction wire to the level of stone.
c The fragmented stones were completely evacuated.

39

moval from around the stone and the duct when the application of maximum force fails to achieve stone fragmentation. When lithotripsy is required, the basket handle is cut off, the metal lithotriptor sheath is passed over the plastic sheath and the wires of the impacted basket, and the lithotripsy handle is attached to the metal sheath and the basket wires. Under fluoroscopic guidance, rotation of the handle retracts the basket and the stone against the sheath, breaking the stone or the basket and allowing the basket to be removed (**Fig. 39.9**).

Shock-Wave Lithotripsy

Intracorporeal shock waves can be generated using either electrohydraulic or laser technology, which creates a plasma that rapidly expands and collapses at the surface of the stone. Vaporizing fluid with high-voltage sparks across a pair of electrodes produces shock waves.

Electrohydraulic Lithotripsy (EHL)

Equipment. An electrohydraulic shock-wave generator (Olympus LithoTron EL-27) set at an output of 2000 V can be used to generate shock waves of increasing frequency (with an intensity up to 500 mJ), which are applied as a continuous sequence of discharges. The lithotripsy probes are available in 3-Fr and 4.5-Fr sizes.

Technical tip. The 4.5-Fr probe, which fills the working channel of the baby scope, is usually used in conjunction with a nasobiliary catheter for saline irrigation. In the absence of a nasobiliary catheter, it is necessary to use the 3-Fr probe so as to be able to irrigate alongside the probe. When a charge is transmitted across the elec-

trodes at the tip of the probe, a spark is created. This induces expansion of the surrounding fluid and an oscillating spherical shock wave with a pressure sufficient to fragment the stone. Continuous irrigation with saline solution is required to provide a medium for the transmission of shock-wave energy to ensure visualization and to flush away debris. The procedure is usually performed under direct choledochoscopic guidance to avoid erroneous application of shock waves, which can cause ductal trauma and perforation. The probe is aimed directly at the stone and is optimally positioned ≥ 5 mm from the tip of the endoscope and 1–2 mm from the stone [11].

When direct cholangioscopic control is not available or is limited, EHL with a balloon catheter may be an alternative [11]. A balloon catheter can be used to center the EHL probe on the stone and to avoid contact with the bile duct wall (**Fig. 39.10**). The lumen of a standard extraction balloon catheter (Wilson-Cook Medical Inc., Winston-Salem, North Carolina, USA), with an 18-mm diameter balloon, is expanded to accommodate the 3-Fr EHL probe. The catheter is 6.8 Fr in diameter and 2 m long. The EHL probe, 3 m long and with a 3-Fr radiopaque tip (Olympus), is passed through the lumen of the modified balloon catheter. The balloon catheter is then inserted through the 3.2-mm accessory channel of a standard duodenoscope (Olympus JF-240). The balloon catheter with the EHL probe then is introduced into the bile duct. The tip of the balloon catheter is positioned near the stone and the balloon is expanded. The tip of the EHL probe is advanced a few millimeters beyond the radiopaque tip of the balloon catheter under fluoroscopic guidance to ensure that the EHL probe is positioned on the surface of the stone. Fluoroscopy is used to target the stone and to monitor fragmentation. Due to the risk of serious complications, however, balloon catheter EHL should be limited to cases in which the stones are not amenable to conventional endoscopic methods.

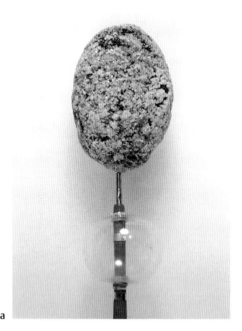

a

Laser Lithotripsy (LL)

Since the first report of successful retrograde laser-induced shock-wave lithotripsy of bile duct stones in 1986 [12], various solid-state laser and pulsed-dye laser systems have been developed and introduced for lithotripsy of bile duct stones [13]. The combination of a rhodamine 6G-dye laser with a stone–tissue detection system, which minimizes the risk of bile duct injury, allows the safe disintegration of bile duct stones without cholangioscopic guidance [14,15]. However, this system is expensive, bulky, requires a high voltage supply [15], and has limited fragmentation power. Recently, a new solid-state laser lithotriptor, the *fr*equency-*d*oubled *d*ouble-pulse neodymium:yttrium–aluminum–garnet laser system ("FREDDY"), was developed in Germany [16,17]. This system promises to combine the advantages of dye and solid-state lasers, such as reliability, effectiveness, and low price [17,18]. The FREDDY laser system uses wavelengths of 532 nm (20%) and 1064 nm (80%). The green light ignites a plasma at the stone surface, while the infrared laser energy boosts this plasma to form a rapidly collapsing bubble, which produces a strong shock wave that fragments the

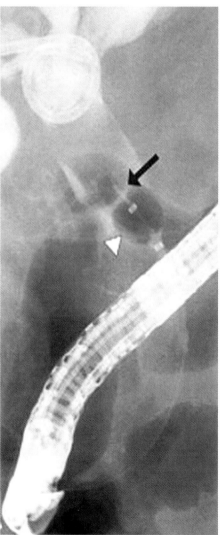

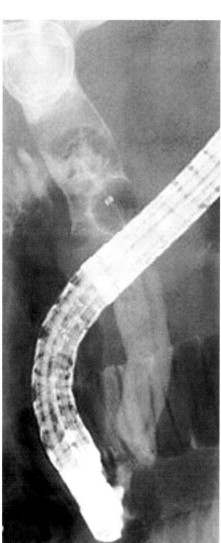

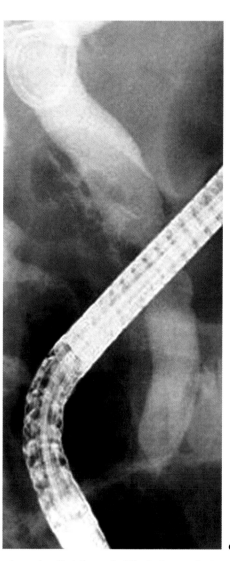

b, c

d

Fig. 39.10 Radiographs showing electrohydraulic lithotripsy using the balloon catheter.
a A bile-duct stone and balloon catheter with an electrohydraulic lithotripsy probe.
b The cholangiogram shows a stone impacted in the bile duct, with the metal tip of the electrohydraulic lithotripsy (EHL) probe (arrow) in contact

with the stone. The balloon (arrowhead) at the end of the balloon catheter has been inflated to position the probe properly.
c The cholangiogram during EHL, showing multiple stone fragments.
d The cholangiogram shows complete clearance of stones from the bile duct.

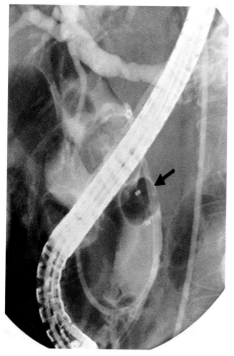 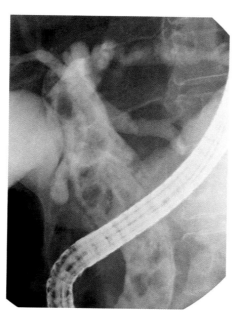 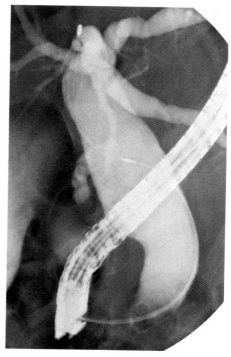

, b

c

Fig. 39.11 Radiographs illustrating laser lithotripsy (FREDDY) under fluoroscopic guidance with a balloon catheter.
a The cholangiogram shows multiple large common bile duct stones. The patient underwent two sessions of laser lithotripsy under fluoroscopic guidance with a balloon catheter (arrow).

b After one session of laser lithotripsy, the large stones are fragmented into smaller stones.
c The postprocedure cholangiogram shows complete clearance of the bile duct.

stones [16] (**Fig. 39.11**). The laser pulse duration is 1.2 ms at 160 mJ, with single or dual pulses at adjustable rates of 1, 3, 5, or 10 Hz with 110-volt alternating current, or 15 or 20 Hz with 220-volt electricity [10]. We use the following laser parameters for all patients: energy output, 120 mJ/pulse; pulse rate, 10 Hz; and maximum number of pulses per laser session, 3000. The laser beam is transmitted via a 0.73-mm diameter laser fiber. These fibers can be inserted through the ports of most choledochoscopes.

The FREDDY laser causes minimal or no ductal injury and has been used through the guide-wire port of a stone-extraction balloon to keep it in the center of the duct. To avoid damage to the working channel of the endoscope by the sharp laser fiber, the laser fiber was passed through the lumen of a standard balloon-tipped catheter (Escort II/Tri-Ex; Wilson-Cook). Correct apposition of the laser tip on the stone is assessed radiographically, and the transmission of the shock wave is monitored by listening to the typical "tick, tick" percussion sound using a stethoscope taped to the patient's upper abdomen.

FREDDY lithotripsy under percutaneous transhepatic choledochoscopy guidance (**Fig. 39.12**) appears to be the most effective treatment for intrahepatic bile duct stones. It is less likely to cause mucosal damage than EHL or ultrasound lithotripsy due to its stone–tissue recognition system. The fragmentation of stones under saline irrigation allows them to be spontaneously evacuated, without the tedious manipulation of baskets [19]. In our experience, however, when the stones are located above an acutely angulated bile duct, overcoming the angulation with the laser fiber is difficult, as the tip of the laser fiber is not flexible (**Table 39.2**).

Tex et al. [20] compared fragmentation and fiber burn-off for human gallstones using FREDDY rhodamine-6G and holmium: yttrium–aluminum–garnet (Ho:YAG) lasers. They suggested that with a higher laser energy than its prototype, the 150-mJ FREDDY is an inexpensive and promising laser system that produces fragmentation results significantly better than or equal to those of

Table 39.2 Advantages and disadvantages of laser lithotripsy

Advantages

- Thanks to the stone–tissue discrimination system (STDS), it is less likely than electrohydraulic lithotripsy to cause mucosal damage
- Fragmentation of stones under saline irrigation allows spontaneous evacuation of stones without tedious manipulation with basket forceps
- The STDS further increases safety when the tip of the fiber is difficult to visualize endoscopically during fragmentation, due to biliary sludge or location inside a stone

Disadvantages

- It is difficult and time-consuming to target stones using fluoroscopy, as the position of the radiolucent laser fiber inserted through a catheter is not visible. The tip of laser fiber is not fluoroscopically visible
- The laser fiber is fragile and may be inadvertently broken during procedures
- Hemobilia develops due to direct mechanical trauma to the bile duct mucosa by the sharp laser fiber tip

established laser systems, such as the rhodamine-6G and Ho:YAG lasers.

Extracorporeal Shock-Wave Lithotripsy (ESWL)

The reasons for the failure of conventional endoscopic therapy include impacted or extremely large stones, stones located intrahepatically or proximal to a bile duct stenosis, or previous surgery such as a Billroth II gastrojejunostomy preventing endoscopic access to the major papilla.

ESWL focuses high-pressure shock-wave energy at a designated target point, while minimizing energy exposure to adjacent tissues. Shock waves can be generated by an underwater spark gap (electrohydraulic), piezoelectric crystals, or electromagnetic membrane

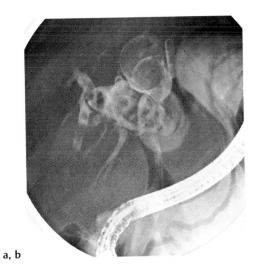
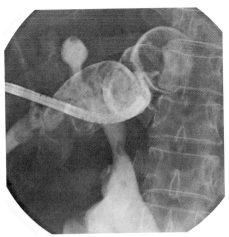
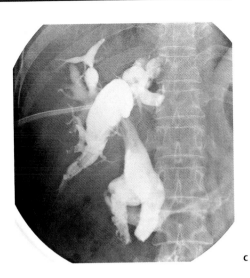

a, b

c

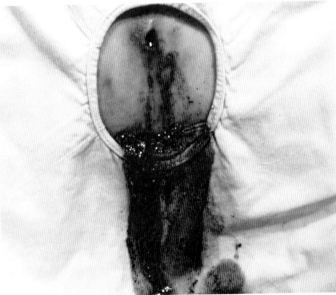

d

Fig. 39.12 Radiographs of percutaneous laser lithotripsy (FREDDY) of intrahepatic stones.
a Endoscopic retrograde cholangiopancreatography shows multiple intrahepatic stones.
b The intrahepatic duct stones were removed using percutaneous laser lithotripsy with percutaneous cholangioscopic guidance.
c The final cholangiogram after the sixth session of percutaneous transhepatic cholangioscopy and laser lithotripsy shows complete clearance of the intrahepatic bile duct stones.
d Flushing of the biliary tree with normal saline achieves clearance of the fine fragmented stone particles.

technologies. The energy can be focused by elliptical reflectors, fixation of piezoelectric crystals to an elliptical dish, or by acoustic lenses. Spark-gap lithotriptors are more powerful and may lead to better stone clearance rates. When shock waves reach the stone, cavitation occurs at the surface, and the changes in acoustic impedance release compressive and tensile forces, resulting in fragmentation.

When stones are located in the bile duct, a nasobiliary catheter is usually needed for contrast administration. The major drawback of ESWL is the time-consuming approach involved in the endoscopic retrograde cholangiography (ERC) steps, with the insertion of a nasobiliary catheter, one or more sessions of treatment, and finally fragment extraction using ERC. Common duct stones amenable to ESWL are localized using fluoroscopy or ultrasonography.

▥ Novel Application of Direct Cholangioscopy

Peroral cholangioscopy provides direct visualization of the bile duct and allows diagnostic procedures or therapeutic interventions. Currently, the "mother–baby" scope system that is available is not widely used, as it has several limitations. However, direct cholangioscopy using an ultraslim upper endoscope with a guide wire has been reported to be an easy way of conducting a direct visual examination of the biliary tree.

Direct peroral cholangioscopy (direct POC) using an ultraslim upper endoscope with an overtube balloon to maintain access and direct POC using an ultraslim endoscope with an intraductal balloon are also possible [4,5]. An endoscopic sphincterotomy or papillary balloon dilation with a large balloon is necessary before the ultraslim endoscope is introduced. The overtube (TS-13140; Fujinon Corporation, Saitama, Japan) for a double-balloon enteroscope is equipped with an ultraslim upper endoscope (Olympus GIF-260N). After the endoscope with the overtube has been advanced into the duodenal bulb, the overtube position is fixed by balloon inflation. The slim endoscope is then advanced directly into the bile duct through the ampulla of Vater. Using a balloon catheter to maintain access, an ultraslim upper endoscope (GIF-260N or GIF-XP260N; Olympus Medical Systems Corp., Tokyo, Japan) can be advanced over the balloon catheter directly into the bile duct through the ampulla of Vater (**Fig. 39.13**).

Wire-guided direct POC was performed successfully in five of 10 patients (50%). The success rate of intraductal balloon-guided direct POC was 93.3% (14 of 15 patients; $P < 0.05$). Overtube balloon-assisted direct POC was performed successfully in nine of 11 patients (81.8%). A forceps biopsy with direct visualization of the intraductal lesions and therapeutic interventions, including laser lithotripsy or EHL, were also successfully performed [21]. Intraductal balloon-guided direct peroral cholangioscopy appears to be a promising new procedure for direct visual examination of the bile ducts.

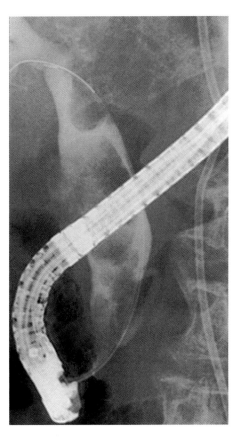

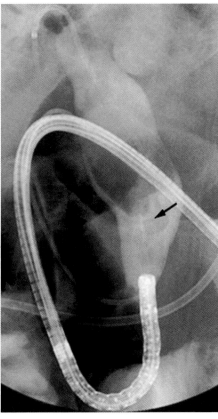

Fig. 39.13
a A 72-year-old man presented with retained common bile duct (CBD) stones.
b The patient underwent intraductal balloon-guided direct peroral cholangioscopy to fragment the stones using electrohydraulic lithotripsy (EHL). With a balloon catheter being used to maintain access, an ultraslim endoscope was advanced into the bile duct and lithotripsy was carried out.
c, d The endoscopic images shows the EHL probe (arrow) near the CBD stone (**c**) and fragmentation of the stones (**d**).

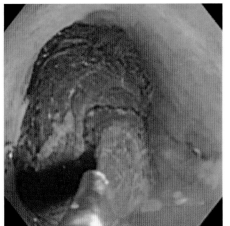
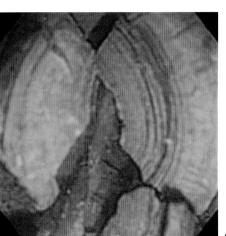

Results of Lithotripsy

▤ Mechanical Lithotripsy (ML)

ML leads to complete bile duct clearance in about 80–90% of patients, but 20–30% require more than one procedure [22–26]. Moreover, ML is less likely to be successful with larger and impacted stones. Nakajima et al. were able to achieve a stone-free rate of 93%, independently of the diameter of the stones, in patients with choledocholithiasis in whom access to the papilla was obtained using only balloon dilation [27]. Cipolletta and colleagues found that the size of the stone was the only important factor involved in the failure of bile duct clearance using ML [24]. They found that bile duct clearance rates were 90% for stones with a diameter less than 10 mm, in comparison with 68% for those over 28 mm in diameter. Subsequently, a prospective study by Garg and colleagues identified only impaction of common duct stones in the bile duct as a factor in the failure of ML [23].

▤ Electrohydraulic Lithotripsy (EHL)

Peroral cholangioscopy–directed EHL has been shown to be highly successful in the treatment of difficult extrahepatic bile duct stones [1,28]. The largest reported study with EHL is that by Binmoeller et al.; EHL was successfully used to fragment stones in 63 of 64 patients, in all of whom previous attempts at ML had failed [29]. Arya and colleagues published a retrospective series of 94 patients in whom stone extraction had failed using standard techniques before peroral cholangioscopy. Overall, the stone clearance rate was 90%, with 90% of the patients requiring one or two EHL sessions and the rest requiring three or more. The complication rate was 17% [28]. In the setting of recurrent pyogenic cholangiohepatitis, intrahepatic bile duct stones pose a special challenge and generally require a more intensive and predominantly percutaneous approach; downstream strictures and acute angulations are more difficult to overcome with a retrograde approach. Although percutaneous choledochoscopy with selective use of EHL can achieve an initial ductal clearance rate of 80–90%, high recurrence rates of 35–50% have been reported due to intrahepatic strictures [30–32].

Our own group reported 114 consecutive patients with hepatolithiasis who were treated with percutaneous choledochoscopy–guided EHL [33]. Despite a mean of 4.8 (1–16) choledochoscopy sessions, ductal clearance was achieved in 90.6%.

Laser Lithotripsy (LL)

Experience with LL is limited to a few centers, and most of the published reports on its use have only included small numbers of patients in nonrandomized studies. Despite these limitations, the reported success rates for clearance of retained bile duct stones using LL in these studies are 64–97% [12,34–38].

Neuhaus et al. reported a 97% success rate after a mean of 1.3 sessions in 38 patients; 18 were treated perorally and 20 via the percutaneous transhepatic route. In this study, both cholangioscopy and fluoroscopy were used to monitor intraductal lithotripsy, without complications [36]. In the largest series to date, Hochberger et al. reported an 80% clearance rate of common duct stones in 50 patients, with an 8% morbidity rate [39].

Maiss et al. reported the first clinical data on LL of CBD stones with a new FREDDY laser system in 22 patients. The results of this study were consistent with our own findings. At the end of treatment, 20 of 22 patients (91%) were free of biliary stones (five patients had additional ML and one patient underwent ESWL). With regard to complications, mild pancreatitis was noted in two patients (9%) [40].

In our own series, including 25 patients treated using transpapillary routes, complete stone removal was achieved in 24 patients (96%). Complete removal of stones required a mean of 1.4 endoscopic sessions (range: one to two). Complete stone removal was achieved in six of the seven patients (85.7%) in whom percutaneous transhepatic approaches were used. The overall success rate for complete stone removal was 93.8% (30 of 32 patients) [41].

Extracorporeal Shock-Wave Lithotripsy (ESWL)

Reported rates of complete clearance of common duct stones following ESWL are in the range of 83–93% [42–45]. The majority of patients require endoscopic extraction of bile stone fragments after ESWL, although approximately 10% of stones may pass spontaneously after treatment [43,46].

Following ESWL, patients subsequently undergo ERC, during which residual stone fragments are extracted using baskets. ESWL was reported to be effective in clearing stones in 80–90% in a series of 310 patients, with only rare complications (cholangitis, hematoma) [43]. In another series including patients with intrahepatic stones, ESWL alone cleared stones in 34% of cases, and in combination with LL the clearance rate increased to 90% [44].

Complications

Basket impaction or rupture of the basket traction wire are potential complications unique to ML. A report from expert centers described complications associated with ML [47], including a total of 46 complications. Complications in the biliary group included trapped/broken basket (n = 15), traction wire fracture (n = 12), broken handle (n = 11), and perforation/duct injury (n = 7).

The majority of complications related to intracorporeal lithotripsy were associated with obtaining pancreaticobiliary access (e. g., ERCP or percutaneous transhepatic access) and included pancreatitis, hemorrhage, perforation, and sepsis [48]. Both EHL and LL

have an overall complication rate of 7–9%, the most common complications being hemobilia, cholangitis, and less commonly ductal perforation [28,49,50]. No complications have been reported with Ho:YAG or FREDDY lasers. However, the published experience is limited and biliary epithelial damage has been noted in vitro with the Ho:YAG device [51,52].

Complications with ESWL for cholelithiasis develop in 30–40% of patients, with the most common complication being biliary colic. About 5% of patients develop biliary obstruction or pancreatitis [53,54]. ESWL for choledocholithiasis is associated with short-term morbidity in approximately 14% of patients, including pain, hemobilia, cholangitis, sepsis, hematomas, pancreatitis, hematuria, ileus, and anesthesia problems.

How to Manage Trapped Baskets

The impaction of Dormia baskets with captured stones or rupture of the basket traction wire during ML are rare complications (0.8–5.9%) during endoscopic treatment for choledocholithiasis [55,56]. Although surgery is the most frequent treatment option, various nonsurgical methods have been used to deal with these problems, including extension of the sphincterotomy, awaiting spontaneous passage of the impacted basket and stone after successful stent placement, use of a second lithotriptor, ESWL [57], LL [58], EHL [59,60], transhepatic lithotripsy [61], and stone dislodgment [57]. With the advent of the Soehendra lithotriptor, stones captured within an impacted basket are either crushed, or the wires of the Dormia basket are broken to release the trapped basket [62]. In a study by Sauter et al. [63], 12 consecutive patients underwent ESWL in an attempt to remove trapped baskets by nonsurgical means. After fragmentation of the bile duct stones, removing all the impacted Dormia baskets was possible, either by traction on the basket wire or by endoscopic extraction [63].

When the entrapped stone resists ML, all four branches of the basket can be stressed, which can result in fracture of the traction wire in up to 5% of cases [63] (**Fig. 39.14**). Fracture of the traction cable is a more severe complication of ML and usually requires additional procedures such as ESWL or surgery. When this occurs with the wire fracture outside the mouth, exchanging the initial 80-cm metal sheath for a shorter one (70, 60, or 50 cm) may allow immediate continuation of lithotripsy in most cases, making this technique time-saving, less expensive, and more successful, and avoiding other unnecessary procedures such as ESWL or surgery. Neuhaus et al. described the use of LL to resolve basket impaction, but this modality is only available in a few centers [64].

Biliary Stent Placement as an Alternative Procedure

Biliary stenting deserves consideration as a quick alternative treatment in elderly and/or frail patients who are unlikely to tolerate prolonged endoscopic attempts at stone extraction. For the treatment of refractory bile duct stones, stent placement has an important role in immediate and subsequent definitive stone treatment. Biliary stent placement may be required on a temporary basis for difficult-to-retrieve common duct stones. Studies have shown that the majority of common duct stones decrease in size following stenting [65].

A potential advantage of pigtail stents over straight stents is that the duodenal portion of the stent comes out at an angle and may keep the biliary orifice open more effectively. If the stent becomes occluded after several months, it still has the potential to keep common duct stones from impacting. The stent probably functions as a wick around which the bile can drain, rather than as a conduit for bile. Some recent evidence has suggested that long-term stent-

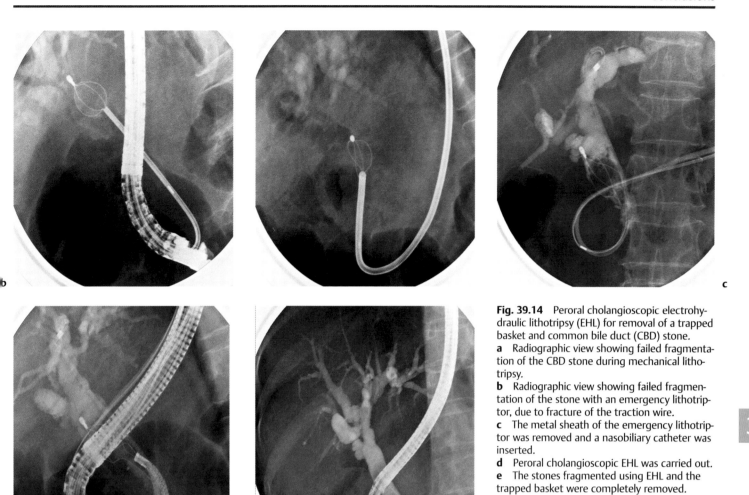

Fig. 39.14 Peroral cholangioscopic electrohydraulic lithotripsy (EHL) for removal of a trapped basket and common bile duct (CBD) stone.
a Radiographic view showing failed fragmentation of the CBD stone during mechanical lithotripsy.
b Radiographic view showing failed fragmentation of the stone with an emergency lithotriptor, due to fracture of the traction wire.
c The metal sheath of the emergency lithotriptor was removed and a nasobiliary catheter was inserted.
d Peroral cholangioscopic EHL was carried out.
e The stones fragmented using EHL and the trapped basket were completely removed.

39

ing may not be necessary and that adding oral ursodeoxycholic acid may dissolve stones. In one report, nine of 10 patients who underwent stenting combined with orally administered ursodeoxycholic acid became stone-free, in comparison with none of 40 patients who received stents alone [66].

Several studies have investigated the role of stent insertion as the sole treatment for common duct stones that could not be removed via ERC. In the study by Bergman and colleagues, 58 of 117 patients had permanent biliary stent insertion as their treatment for common duct stones (i.e., expectant management and stent exchange only if complications occurred). Sixty percent of these patients were alive after a 2-year follow-up period, and 70% of them were symptom-free. However, the overall complication rate was 40% and the mortality rate related to complications of the biliary stent was 16%. Cholangitis and jaundice were considered to be the causes of death in these patients, occurring after a median of 42 months [67]. Jain et al. carried out a prospective study including 20 patients with difficult-to-extract common duct stones. In each case, a pigtail stent (7 Fr) was inserted and ERC was repeated after 6 months. In 20% of the patients, the stones had fragmented and allowed balloon clearance of the duct, and in 35% of patients, the duct had cleared spontaneously [68].

Conclusions

Lithotripsy is a relatively safe and effective treatment for selected difficult bile duct stones. Treatment of difficult biliary stones is generally accomplished using a multimodal approach, with mechanical and/or shock-wave lithotripsy (EHL and LL or ESWL). The presence of large stones, impacted stones, small ducts, ductal strictures, or difficult anatomy—including periampullary diverticula, Billroth II anastomosis, Roux-en-Y anastomosis, and intrahepatic stones—can make the removal of biliary stones very challenging. Most difficult biliary stones can be removed with ML. Stones in which basket extraction fails can be treated with endoscopic intraductal shock-wave lithotripsy. At present, EHL appears to provide the best combination of technical success, low cost, and practicality. Published experience with Ho:YAG laser and FREDDY lithotripsy is limited. EHL and LL usually require direct visualization, which is technically difficult. Recent advances in the development of ultrathin cholangioscopes that fit through the working channel of a standard therapeutic duodenoscope and a pulsed laser with an automatic stone recognition system may allow routine lithotripsy under fluoroscopic guidance in the future.

Peroral and percutaneous cholangioscopic lithotripsy also offer a highly effective and safe alternative to surgery in patients with difficult extrahepatic and intrahepatic ductal stones that are not amenable to routine endoscopic procedures.

References

1. Farrell JJ, Bounds BC, Al-Shalabi S, Jacobson BC, Brugge WR, Schapiro RH, et al. Single-operator duodenoscope assisted cholangioscopy is an effective alternative in the management of choledocholithiasis not removed by conventional methods, including mechanical lithotripsy. Endoscopy 2005;37:542–7.

2. Chen YK, Pleskow DK. SpyGlass single-operator peroral cholangiopancreatoscopy system for diagnosis and therapy of bile duct disorders. A clinical feasibility study. Gastrointest Endosc 2007;65:832–41.

3. Chen YK. Preclinical characterization of the Spyglass peroral cholangio-pancreatoscopy system for direct access, visualization, and biopsy. Gastrointest Endosc 2007;65:303–11.

4. Moon JH, Ko BM, Choi HJ, Hong SJ, Cheon YK, Cho YD, et al. Intraductal balloon-guided direct peroral cholangioscopy with an ultraslim upper endoscope (with videos). Gastrointest Endosc 2009 Apr 24 [Epub ahead of print].

5. Choi HJ, Moon JH, Ko BM, Hong SJ, Koo HC, Cheon YK, et al. Overtube-balloon-assisted direct peroral cholangioscopy by using an ultra-slim upper endoscope (with videos). Gastrointest Endosc 2009;69:935–40.

6. Shim CS, Neuhaus H., Tamada K. Direct cholangioscopy. Endoscopy 2003;35:752–8.

7. Simon T, Fink AS, Zuckerman AM. Experience with percutaneous transhepatic cholangioscopy in the management of biliary tract disease. Surg Endosc 1999;13:1199–202.

8. Bonnel DH, Liguory CE, Cornud FE, Lefebvre JF. Common bile duct and intrahepatic stones: results of transhepatic, electrohydraulic lithotripsy in 50 patients. Radiology 1991;180:345–8.

9. Moon JH, Cho YD, Ryu CB, Kim JO, Cho JY, Kim YS, et al. The role of percutaneous transhepatic papillary balloon dilation in percutaneous choledochoscopic lithotomy. Gastrointest Endosc 2001;54:232–6.

10. DiSario J, Chuttani R, Croffie J, Liu J, Mishkin D, Shah R, et al. Biliary and pancreatic lithotripsy devices. Gastrointest Endosc 2007;65:750–6.

11. Moon JH, Cha SW, Ryu CB, Kim YS, Hong SJ, Cheon YK, et al. Endoscopic treatment of retained bile-duct stones by using a balloon catheter for electrohydraulic lithotripsy without cholangioscopy. Gastrointest Endosc 2004;60:562–6.

12. Lux G, Ell CH, Hochberger J, Müller D, Demling L. The first successful endoscopic retrograde laser lithotripsy of common bile duct stones in man using a pulsed neodymium-YAG laser. Endoscopy 1986;18:144–5.

13. Langhorst J, Neuhaus H. Laser lithotripsy. Dig Endosc 2000;12:8–18.

14. Ell C, Hochberger J, May A, Fleig WE, Bauer R, Mendez L, et al. Laser lithotripsy of difficult bile duct stones by means of a rhodamine-6G laser and an integrated automatic stone–tissue detection system. Gastrointest Endosc 1993;39:755–62.

15. Hochberger J, Wittekind C, Iro H, Mendez L, Ell C. Automatic stone/tissue detection system for dye laser lithotripsy of gallstones—in vivo experiments. Gastroenterology 1992;102:A315.

16. Hochberger J, Tschepe J, Stein R. Frequenzverdoppelter Doppelpuls-Neodym:YAG Laser (FREDDY) für die Lithotripsie von Gallengangssteinen. Ein effektiver und kostengünstiger neuer Festkörperlaser mit piezo-akustischem Stein-Gewebe-Detektionssystem (paSTDS). Lasermedizin 1996;12:51–7.

17. Hochberger J, Tex S, Maiss J, Hahn EG. Management of difficult common bile duct stones. Gastrointest Endosc Clin N Am 2003;13:623–34.

18. Zorcher T, Hochberger J, Schrott KM, Kuhn R, Schafhauser W. In vitro study concerning the efficiency of the frequency-doubled double-pulse neodymium:YAG laser (FREDDY) for lithotripsy of calculi in the urinary tract. Lasers Surg Med 1999;25:38–42.

19. Watanabe Y, Sato M, Tokui K, Nezu K, Shiraishi S, Sato K, et al. Painless lithotripsy by flashlamp-excited dye laser for impacted biliary stones: an experimental and clinical study. Eur J Surg 2000;166:455–8.

20. Tex S, Maiss J, Magdeburg B, Neizamy E, Hahn E, Hochberger J. Preclinical comparative examinations of different laser systems for lithotripsy of common bile duct stones including a new frequency-doubled double-pulse neodymium YAG-laser (FREDDY) [abstract]. Gastrointest Endosc 2002;55:AB170.

21. Choi HJ, Moon JH, Ko BM, et al. Direct peroral cholangioscopic lithotripsy using an ultra-slim upper endoscope. Korean J Gastrointest Endosc 2008;37(Suppl 2):174.

22. Chang WH, Chu CH, Wang TE, Chen MJ, Lin CC. Outcome of simple use of mechanical lithotripsy of difficult common bile duct stones. World J Gastroenterol 2005;11:593–6.

23. Garg PK, Tandon RK, Ahuja V, Makharia GK, Batra Y. Predictors of unsuccessful mechanical lithotripsy and endoscopic clearance of large bile duct stones. Gastrointest Endosc 2004;59:601–5.

24. Cipolletta L, Costamagna G, Bianco MA, Rotondano G, Piscopo R, Mutignani M, et al. Endoscopic mechanical lithotripsy of difficult common bile duct stones. Br J Surg 1997;84:1407–9.

25. Hintze RE, Adler A, Veltzke W. Outcome of mechanical lithotripsy of bile duct stones in an unselected series of 704 patients. Hepatogastroenterology 1996;43:473–6.

26. Schneider MU, Matek W, Bauer R, Domschke W. Mechanical lithotripsy of bile duct stones in 209 patients—effect of technical advances. Endoscopy 1988;20:248–53.

27. Nakajima M, Yasuda K, Cho E, Mukai H, Ashihara T, Hirano S. Endoscopic sphincterotomy and mechanical basket lithotripsy for management of difficult common bile duct stones. J Hepatobiliary Pancreat Surg 1997;4:5–10.

28. Arya N, Nelles SE, Haber GB, Kim YI, Kortan PK. Electrohydraulic lithotripsy in 111 patients: a safe and effective therapy for difficult bile duct stones. Am J Gastroenterol 2004;99:2330–4.

29. Binmoeller KF, Brückner M, Thonke F, Soehendra N. Treatment of difficult bile duct stones using mechanical, electrohydraulic and extracorporeal shock wave lithotripsy. Endoscopy 1993;25:201–6.

30. Hwang MH, Tsai CC, Mo LR, Yang CT, Yeh YH, Yau MP, et al. Percutaneous choledochoscopic biliary tract stone removal: experience in 645 consecutive patients. Eur J Radiol 1993;17:184–90.

31. Huang MH, Chen CH, Yang JC, Yang CC, Yeh YH, Chou DA, et al. Long-term outcome of percutaneous transhepatic cholangioscopic lithotomy for hepatolithiasis. Am J Gastroenterol 2003;98:2655–62.

32. Lee SK, Seo DW, Myung SJ, Park ET, Lim BC, Kim HJ, et al. Percutaneous transhepatic cholangioscopic treatment for hepatolithiasis: an evaluation of long-term results and risk factors for recurrence. Gastrointest Endosc 2001;53:318–21.

33. Bong HK, Cho YD, Shim CS. The efficacy of percutaneous transhepatic choledochoscopic removal of intrahepatic stones. Korean J Gastrointest Endosc 1998;54:778–85.

34. Jakobs R, Maier M, Kohler B, Riemann JF. Peroral laser lithotripsy of difficult intrahepatic and extrahepatic bile duct stones: laser effectiveness using an automatic stone–tissue discrimination system. Am J Gastroenterol 1996;91:468–73.

35. Harris VJ, Sherman S, Trerotola SO, Snidow JJ, Johnson MS, Lehman GA. Complex biliary stones: treatment with a small choledochoscope and laser lithotripsy. Radiology 1996;199:71–7.

36. Neuhaus H, Hoffmann W, Gottlieb K, Classen M. Endoscopic lithotripsy of bile duct stones using a new laser with automatic stone recognition. Gastrointest Endosc 1994;40:708–15.

37. Neuhaus H, Hoffmann W, Zillinger C, Classen M. Laser lithotripsy of difficult bile duct stones under direct visual control. Gut 1993;34:415–21.

38. Ponchon T, Gagnon P, Valette PJ, Henry L, Chavaillon A, Thieulin F. Pulsed dye laser lithotripsy of bile duct stones. Gastroenterology 1991;100:1730–6.

39. Hochberger J, Bayer J, May A, Mühldorfer S, Maiss J, Hahn EG, et al. Laser lithotripsy of difficult bile duct stones: results in 60 patients using a rhodamine 6G dye laser with optical stone tissue detection system. Gut 1998;43:823–9.

40. Maiss J, Tex S, Bayer J, Hahn EG, Hochberger J. First clinical data on laser lithotripsy of common bile duct stones with a new frequency-doubled double-pulse Nd:YAG laser (FREDDY) in 22 patients [abstract]. Endoscopy 2001;33:AB2726.

41. Cho YD, Moon JH, Shim CS. Clinical usefulness and safety of frequency-doubled double-pulsed YAG laser (FREDDY) technology for removing bile duct stones [abstract]. Gastrointest Endosc 2003;57:AB81.

42. Sauerbruch T, Delius M, Paumgartner G, Holl J, Wess O, Weber W, et al. Fragmentation of gallstones by extracorporeal shock waves. N Engl J Med 1986;314:818–22.

43. Sackmann M, Holl J, Sauter GH, Pauletzki J, von Ritter C, Paumgartner G. Extracorporeal shock wave lithotripsy for clearance of bile duct stones resistant to endoscopic extraction. Gastrointest Endosc 2001;53:27–32.

44. Ellis RD, Jenkins AP, Thompson RP, Ede RJ. Clearance of refractory bile duct stones with extracorporeal shockwave lithotripsy. Gut 2000;47:728–31.

45. Meyenberger C, Meierhofer U, Michel-Harder C, Knuchel J, Wirth HP, Bühler H, et al. Long-term follow-up after treatment of common bile duct stones by extracorporeal shock-wave lithotripsy. Endoscopy 1996;28:411–7.

46. Shim CS, Moon JH, Cho YD, Kim YS, Hong SJ, Kim JO, et al. The role of extracorporeal shock wave lithotripsy combined with endoscopic management of impacted cystic duct stones in patients with high surgical risk. Hepatogastroenterology 2005;52:1026–9.

47. Thomas M, Howell DA, Carr-Locke D, Mel Wilcox C, Chak A, Raijman I, et al. Mechanical lithotripsy of pancreatic and biliary stones: complications and available treatment options collected from expert centers. Am J Gastroenterol 2007;102:1896–902.

48. Yoshimoto H, Ikeda S, Tanaka M, Matsumoto S, Kuroda Y. Choledochoscopic electrohydraulic lithotripsy and lithotomy for stones in the common bile duct, intrahepatic ducts, and gallbladder. Ann Surg 1989;210:576–82.

49. Blind PJ, Lundmark M. Management of bile duct stones: lithotripsy by laser, electrohydraulic, and ultrasonic techniques. Eur J Surg 1998;164:403–9.

50. Hochberger J, Tex S, Maiss J, Hahn EG. Management of common bile duct stones. Gastrointest Endosc Clin Am 2003;13:623–34.

51. Teichman JM, Schwesinger WH, Lackner J, Cossman RM. Holmium:YAG laser lithotripsy for gallstones. A preliminary report. Surg Endosc 2001;15:1034–7.

52. Uchiyama K, Onishi H, Tani M, Kinoshita H, Ueno M, Yamaue H. Indication and procedure for treatment of hepatolithiasis. Arch Surg 2002;137:149–53.

53. Sauter G, Kullak-Ublick GA, Schumacher R, Janssen J, Greiner L, Brand B, et al. Safety and efficacy of repeated shockwave lithotripsy of gallstones with and without adjuvant bile acid therapy. Gastroenterology 1997;112:1603–9.

54. Soehendra N, Nam VC, Binmoeller KF, Koch H, Bohnacker S, Schreiber HW. Pulverisation of calcified and non-calcified gallbladder stones: extracorporeal shock wave lithotripsy used alone. Gut 1994;35:417–22.

55. Schneider MU, Matek W, Bauer R, Domschke W. Mechanical lithotripsy of bile duct stones in 209 patients—effect of technical advances. Endoscopy 1988;20:248–53.

56. Neuhaus B, Safrany L. Complications of endoscopic sphincterotomy and their treatment. Endoscopy 1981;13:197–9.

57. Merrett M, Desmond P. Removal of impacted endoscopic basket and stone from the common bile duct by extracorporeal shock waves. Endoscopy 1990;22:92.

58. Martin IG, Curley P, McMahon MJ. Minimally invasive treatment for common bile duct stones. Br J Surg 1993;80:103–6.

59. Josephs LG, Birkett DK. Electrohydraulic lithotripsy for the treatment of large retained common bile duct stones. Am Surg 1990;56:232–4.

60. Arregui ME, Davis CJ, Arkush AM, Nagan RF. Laparoscopic cholecystectomy combined with endoscopic sphincterotomy and stone extraction or laparoscopic choledochoscopy and electrohydraulic lithotripsy for management of cholelithiasis with choledocholithiasis. Surg Endosc 1992;6:10–5.

61. Fujita R, Yamamura M, Fujita Y. Combined endoscopic sphincterotomy and percutaneous transhepatic cholangioscopic lithotripsy. Gastrointest Endosc 1988;34:91–4.

62. Ranjeev P, Goh K. Retrieval of an impacted Dormia basket and stone in situ using a novel method. Gastrointestinal Endosc 2000;51:504–6.

63. Sauter G, Sackmann M, Holl J, Pauletzki J, Sauerbruch T, Paumgartner G. Dormia baskets impacted in the bile duct: release by extracorporeal shock-wave lithotripsy. Endoscopy 1995;27:384–7.

64. Neuhaus H, Hoffman W, Classen M. Endoscopic laser lithotripsy with an automatic stone recognition system for basket impaction in the common bile duct. Endoscopy 1992;24:596–9.

65. Chan AC, Ng EK, Chung SC, Lai CW, Lau JY, Sung JJ, et al. Common bile duct stones become smaller after endoscopic biliary stenting. Endoscopy 1998;30:356–9.

66. Maxton DG, Tweedle DE, Martin DF. Retained common bile duct stones after endoscopic sphincterotomy: temporary and long term treatment with biliary stenting. Gut 1995;36:446–9.

67. Bergman JJ, Rauws EA, Tijssen JG, Tytgat GN, Huibregtse K. Biliary endoprostheses in elderly patients with endoscopically irretrievable common bile duct stones: report on 117 patients. Gastrointest Endosc 1995;42:195–201.

68. Jain SK, Stein R, Bhuva M, Goldberg MJ. Pigtail stents: an alternative in the treatment of difficult bile duct stones. Gastrointest Endosc 2000;52:490–3.

39

40 Percutaneous Endoscopic Gastrostomy and Jejunostomy

Sreeni Jonnalagadda and Steven A. Edmundowicz

Introduction

Many individuals have benefited from this innovative procedure since the first written description of percutaneous endoscopic gastrostomy (PEG) in 1980 by Gauderer and Ponsky at the University Hospitals of Cleveland [1,2]. PEG was rapidly accepted as a favorable alternative to surgical gastrostomy, due to its minimally invasive nature and reduced cost. The widespread dissemination of several standardized techniques for endoscopic gastrostomy placement, commercially available kits, and ease of subsequent gastrostomy tube use after placement have led to the worldwide acceptance of PEG as the procedure of choice in patients requiring intermediate or long-term enteral nutrition. While radiologists and other specialists may perform a fluoroscopically guided percutaneous gastrostomy without using an endoscope, PEG remains the most commonly used method of gastrostomy formation throughout the world.

In the decades after its initial description, two modifications of the original technique were developed. There are currently three general techniques for PEG placement. The "pull" or Ponsky–Gauderer technique [2], the "push" or Sacks–Vine technique [3], and the "introducer" or Russell technique [4] are all effective in creating a gastrostomy, with similar success and complication rates. In certain patients, enteral feeding directly into the jejunum is desired for various reasons. This has led to two techniques of jejunal enteral feeding—jejunostomy through a PEG (JPEG) and direct percutaneous endoscopic jejunostomy (DPEJ) (**Fig. 40.1**).

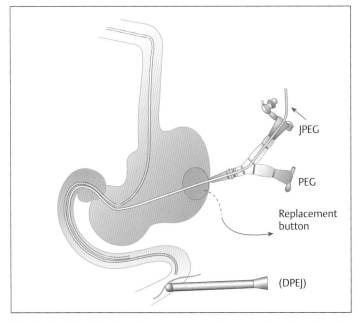

Fig. 40.1 Enteral feeding tubes can be placed in a number of locations for different purposes. DPEJ, direct percutaneous endoscopic jejunostomy; PEG, percutaneous endoscopic gastrostomy; JPEG, jejunal feeding tube through a PEG.

This chapter discusses the indications, contraindications, techniques, and complications of the endoscopic placement of percutaneous feeding tubes.

Indications

Enteral nutrition is the preferred method of feeding in most clinical situations when the gut is functioning and nutrients will be absorbed. Placement of a PEG bypasses the oropharynx and esophagus, and allows nutrients and medications to be instilled directly into the stomach or jejunum. While nasogastric or nasoenteric tubes can be used for short-term situations, PEG should be considered when intermediate (> 3 weeks) or long-term feeding access is desired. The classic indication for PEG is inability to swallow food as a result of oropharyngeal or transfer dysphagia, secondary to a neurological disorder [5]. Other indications for PEG include pharyngeal or esophageal malignancies, facial trauma, and inadequate oral intake in the setting of chronic disease. Rarely, gastric decompression is performed in a terminally ill patient with intra-abdominal malignancies and bowel obstruction, if surgical bypass is not feasible. In this situation, a JPEG, or a PEG combined with a DPEJ, can facilitate gastric decompression while feeding into the jejunum beyond the level of obstruction. Jejunal feeding may also be desired in patients with pancreatic disease, severe gastroparesis, or recurrent large-volume aspiration of gastric contents leading to pneumonia. PEG with gastric feeding does not eliminate the risk for aspiration. Jejunal feeding administered via a jejunal feeding tube passed through a PEG, or a direct percutaneous endoscopic jejunostomy (DPEJ), is better suited for this purpose. In a terminally ill patient, a PEG tube is occasionally required for gastric decompression, while a jejunal feeding tube passed through the PEG into the small bowel can be used simultaneously for feeding. The ethical, legal, and social issues involved when determining whether PEG placement should be undertaken when oral intake is poor secondary to dementia or other irreversible chronic conditions are complex and widely debated [6–8].

Contraindications

Contraindications to PEG can be categorized as absolute and relative. With advances in imaging techniques and increasing experience, there are now few absolute contraindications to PEG (**Table 40.1**).

Relative contraindications include situations in which PEG may be technically possible, but with an increased incidence of morbidity and even mortality. Typical relative contraindications include coagulopathies, which increase the risk of procedure-related bleeding, prior abdominal surgery at the site of PEG placement, which can result in the interposition of the colon between the anterior gastric wall and abdominal wall, and massive obesity, which prevents transillumination. Ongoing systemic infections, fever, abdominal pain, and leukocytosis may mask complications from PEG placement in the immediate postprocedural period, and should be taken into account when determining the optimal timing of PEG place-

Table 40.1 Contraindications to percutaneous endoscopic gastrostomy (PEG) or direct percutaneous endoscopic jejunostomy (DPEJ)

Absolute contraindications
Inability to pass an endoscope into the stomach
Uncorrectable coagulopathy
Peritonitis
Untreatable (loculated) massive ascites
Bowel obstruction (unless for decompression)

Relative contraindications
Massive ascites
Large gastric varices
Extensive abdominal surgery
Subtotal gastrectomy
Morbid obesity
Gastric wall neoplasm

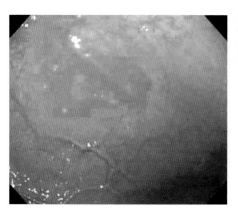

Fig. 40.2 Endoscopic view of the gastric wall in the mid-body of the stomach.

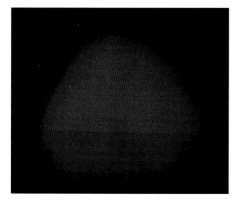

Fig. 40.3 Transillumination from the endoscope through the abdominal wall.

ment, particularly in the acutely ill and hospitalized patient. It should be noted that PEG is rarely absolutely necessary, and rarely an emergency procedure. In most situations, patients can be maintained with nasoenteric feeding, intravenous hydration, or parenteral alimentation if necessary.

PEG has been performed successfully in extreme situations. Cappell and Iocovone treated 28 patients with PEG within 30 days of a myocardial infarction, without a significant increase in morbidity or mortality [9]. PEG has been completed safely in patients with ventriculoperitoneal shunts [10]. Panzer et al. used endoscopic ultrasonography to delineate a path for the needle puncture of the stomach to place a PEG when obesity prevented adequate transillumination or localization for a site [11].

Patient Preparation

To reduce complications related to PEG placement, it is essential to prepare the patient properly. As for any routine upper endoscopy, there should be no oral intake or tube feeding for 6 h before the procedure. The abdominal wall should be inspected for surgical scars that may interfere with the procedure. The coagulation profile should be checked and corrected if necessary. Several studies have confirmed the usefulness of a single dose of broad-spectrum antibiotic (cefazolin 1 g intravenous piggyback, or equivalent) given 30 min before the procedure to reduce the risk of local and systemic infection after PEG placement [12,13].

Procedure

The endoscopist should review the intended procedure with the endoscopy staff and ensure that all of the above prerequisites have been met and that the necessary equipment and materials are available. The procedure will require two operators—an endoscopist to manipulate the endoscope, and an assistant to perform the cutaneous manipulations. The patient is prepared for a standard upper endoscopy, most commonly in a supine position; however, some physicians prefer to start in the left lateral position and rotate the patient after the screening endoscopy. Wrist restraints are commonly used to avoid involuntary contamination of the sterile site by the patient during the procedure. A topical anesthetic, typically a spray (as patients being considered for PEG are often at risk for aspiration) is used to diminish the gag reflex. Intravenous moderate sedation is administered while monitoring key vital signs. The oropharyngeal secretions and any regurgitated material should be promptly suctioned from the oropharynx. The abdominal wall is exposed before or during the procedure, to allow preparation of the skin site. Under direct vision, the gastroscope is passed through the oropharynx, esophagus, and stomach, and into the duodenum. Avoiding oversedation and aspirating all the gastric contents promptly after passage of the endoscope into the stomach decreases the risk of aspiration.

Optimal PEG Site

Regardless of the technique planned for PEG or JPEG, carefully locating the optimal site for the gastrostomy is essential to the success of the procedure. A screening endoscopic examination of the stomach and duodenum is completed to exclude any pathology that would preclude PEG placement. The endoscope is then withdrawn into the fundus of the stomach; air is then instilled until the stomach is fully insufflated. This causes the anterior gastric wall to rest against the abdominal wall after other viscera in the region have been pushed aside. Next, the endoscope tip is directed to face the anterior gastric wall (**Fig. 40.2**). The room lights in the endoscopy suite are dimmed, and an area of maximal transillumination of the light passing through the anterior gastric and abdominal wall is sought (**Fig. 40.3**). Failure to see proper transillumination may indicate the presence of other viscera interposed between the stomach and the abdominal wall. Another reason for poor or absent transillumination may be a subcostal location of the gastric body. The ideal site for the tube placement is further confirmed by digital pressure on the abdominal wall at the site of maximum transillumination (**Fig. 40.4a**) while the gastric indentation is monitored endoscopically. A good site is characterized by a prompt and well-defined indentation corresponding to the external digital pressure (**Fig. 40.4b**). The site is marked with a permanent marker, or other

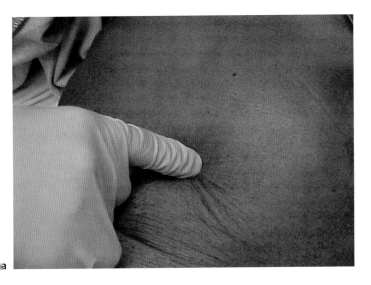

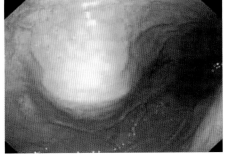

Fig. 40.4
a Digital pressure being applied in the region of transillumination.
b The gastric wall indentation seen with external digital pressure.

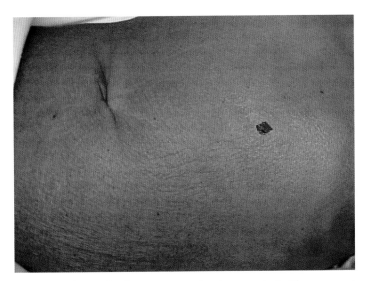

Fig. 40.5 The site for the gastrostomy has been marked with permanent marker.

method (**Fig. 40.5**). It is usually located in the left upper quadrant of the abdomen, 2–4 cm below the left costal margin.

Sometimes the best site is identified closer to the midline at the same level. The area is then prepared with a topical antiseptic, typically containing iodine or Betadine (povidone–iodine). While maintaining a sterile field is not possible given the nature of the procedure, every attempt is made to keep the area clean. The region is covered with a sterile drape. The site is again confirmed by palpation and visualization of the indentation on the anterior wall of the stomach endoscopically. A subcutaneous needle (27 gauge) is used to infiltrate lidocaine into the subcutaneous tissue at the chosen site. Deeper infiltration of local anesthetic and localization of the stomach is then performed using a larger-bore (22 gauge) needle. A key technique for preventing the complication of entering an overlying bowel loop is to advance the longer infiltrating needle slowly while applying negative suction with the syringe (**Fig. 40.6**). The syringe barrel is observed as the needle is advanced toward the stomach. No air should enter the syringe until the needle tip is visualized endoscopically in the stomach. If air bubbles are seen in the syringe before the needle tip is visualized puncturing the gastric wall, then the needle may have entered a bowel lumen that is between the anterior wall of the stomach and the skin. The syringe

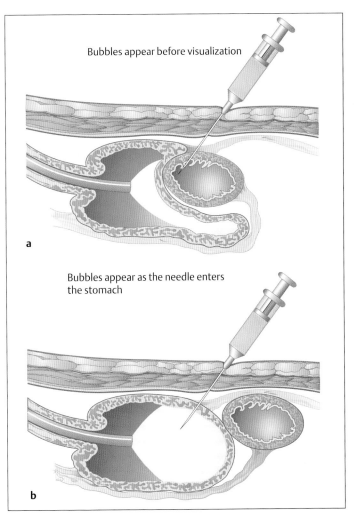

Fig. 40.6 The optimum site for tube placement is selected by transillumination and finger indentation (Fig. 40.4). The skin is prepared with Betadine, and the site for placement is confirmed. The localizing needle (22 gauge, at least 3.8 mm long) and syringe (which is half-filled with lidocaine solution) are advanced through the abdominal wall, with suction being applied once the subcutaneous tissues have been entered. Air bubbles should not appear in the syringe until the needle tip is visualized in the stomach by the endoscopist. If air is seen to enter the syringe before the needle is visualized, then a bowel loop has been entered, and an alternative site for tube placement should be selected
a Bubbles appear before visualization.
b Bubbles appear as the needle enters the stomach.

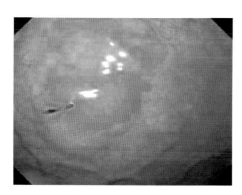

Fig. 40.7 Endoscopic view of the local anesthetic infiltrating needle passing through the abdomen and gastric wall.

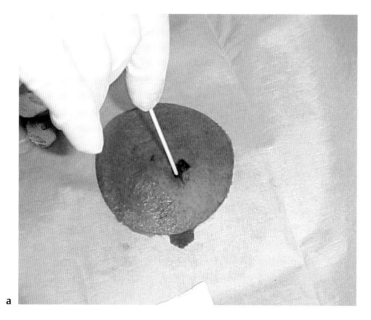

a

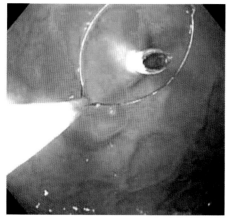

b

Fig. 40.8
a Passage of the cannula and stylet through the incision.
b Endoscopic view of the cannula and stylet being advanced into the stomach. The position of the snare should be noted.

of the selected G-tube is made through the skin and subcutaneous fascia with a scalpel. The cannula and needle assembly are then positioned in the incision and angulated toward the stomach, following the same path the infiltrating needle used. The cannula is then advanced with a quick jab through the incision into the gastric lumen while the site of stomach puncture is observed endoscopically (**Fig. 40.8a**). Slow advancement of the needle may result in the gastric wall moving away as the needle advances. Some endoscopists prefer to pass a snare through the endoscope, opening the loop at the site of intended puncture to facilitate enclosing the snare on the cannula (**Fig. 40.8b**). Once the cannula enters the stomach under direct vision, the procedure will be modified depending on the technique for tube placement that is selected.

▪ Pull-Type (Ponsky–Gauderer) Gastrostomy [2]

This technique is depicted in **Fig. 40.9a**. The snare is positioned to close softly around the cannula. The needle is removed, leaving behind the cannula passing through the abdominal wall into the stomach (**Fig. 40.10**). Insufflation of the stomach is maintained by occluding the external opening of the cannula with finger pressure. A wire (provided in commercially available kits) is passed through the cannula into the stomach (**Fig. 40.11a**). The snare is partially opened and slid down the cannula until the wire is firmly grasped within the snare (**Fig. 40.11b**). With the assistant feeding the wire through the cannula, the scope with snare and grasped wire are gradually withdrawn (**Fig. 40.12**). Once the endoscope has been removed from the patient's mouth, the snare is opened and the wire is secured. The wire is advanced through the skin and withdrawn from the mouth, and it needs to be ensured that the abdominal wall end of the wire is securely held at all times to prevent its passage into the stomach. This results in the wire passing from the assistant's hand, through the abdominal wall into the stomach, and exiting the mouth (**Fig. 40.13**). The tip of the wire exiting the patient's mouth has to be secured to the tip of the PEG tube. In some commercial kits, the tip of the wire is in the form of a loop. The tip of the wire is first passed through the open loop at the tip of the feeding tube (**Fig. 40.14**). Next, the wire loop is opened and the internal bolster of the feeding tube is passed through (**Fig. 40.15**). Thus, the feeding tube and the wire are now enmeshed and cannot be pulled apart. The external surface of the feeding tube is lubricated. The wire is gradually pulled out via the abdominal incision while the feeding tube is guided into the mouth (**Fig. 40.16**). This results in passage of the feeding tube through the esophagus into the stomach. The dilating tip of the feeding tube is pulled through the incision (**Fig. 40.17**). The feeding tube is grasped and pulled through the abdominal wall slowly with firm pressure until resistance is felt (**Fig. 40.18**). While the point of increased resistance is dependent on the thickness of the abdominal wall, this usually occurs when the internal bumper of the tube is less than 4 cm from the skin. The tube is then gently pulled with enough pressure to juxtapose the gastric wall against the abdominal wall using pressure from the internal bolster. An external bolster is placed to prevent migration of the tube into the stomach (**Fig. 40.19a**). After placement of the external bolster, correct positioning will allow the feeding tube to be rotated while gentle torque is applied. Many endoscopists will reintroduce the endoscope at this point to verify and document the correct position of the feeding tube (**Fig. 40.19b**). The feeding tube is then cut from the introducer at the desired distance from the skin, and the feeding adapter or adapters are attached to the tube.

should be withdrawn, and another site should be selected that transilluminates and compresses well. The needle aspiration technique should be repeated until one is certain that the stomach has been entered directly, without entering another bowel loop (**Fig. 40.7**). In obese patients, a 9-cm spinal needle can be used to locate the correct tract to the stomach with the same technique. Once the site for the tube placement has been located, the tract is infiltrated with lidocaine as the needle is withdrawn to the skin. A longitudinal incision that is at least 2 mm longer than the diameter

V

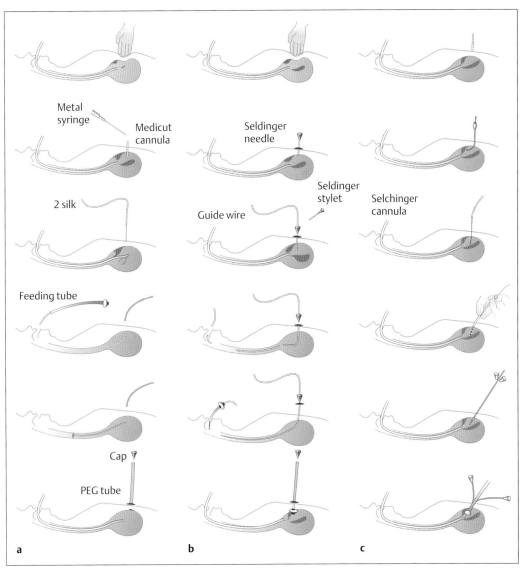

Fig. 40.9
a The pull technique (Ponsky–Gauderer technique).
b The push technique (Sacks–Vine technique).
c The introducer technique (Russell technique).

Metal syringe

Medicut cannula

Seldinger needle

2 silk

Guide wire

Seldinger stylet

Selchinger cannula

Feeding tube

Cap

PEG tube

a

b

c

40

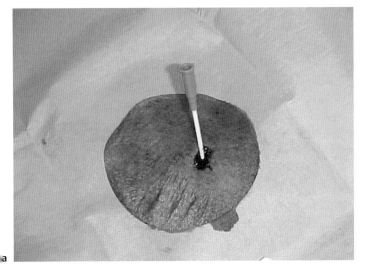

a

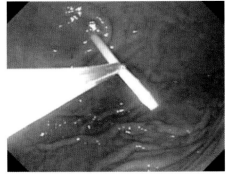

b

Fig. 40.10
a The cannula in place after removal of the stylet.
b Endoscopic view of the cannula being grasped with the snare after removal of the stylet.

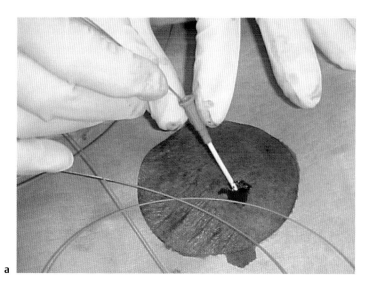

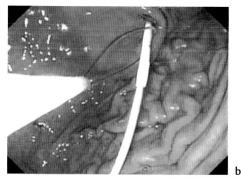

Fig. 40.11
a Passage of the wire through the cannula.
b Endoscopic view of the wire being threaded through the cannula.

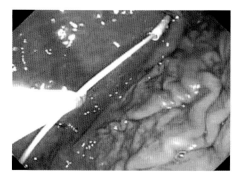

Fig. 40.12 Endoscopic view of the wire being grasped with the snare.

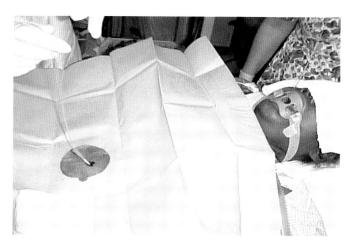

Fig. 40.13 After removal of the endoscope, the wire passes through the incision, stomach, and esophagus, and exits via the mouth.

Push-Type (Sacks–Vine) Gastrostomy [3]

After the snare has been gently closed on the trocar as described with the pull technique above, a push-type guide wire is advanced through the trocar, grasped with the snare, and held in position as the endoscope is withdrawn from the patient (**Fig. 40.9b**). The assistant advances the guide wire through the trocar and skin incision while the endoscope is withdrawn. The guide wire is grasped as it emerges from the patient's oropharynx, and a Kelly clamp is placed on the end of the wire. The wire is further advanced until a length that is longer than the gastrostomy tube and introducer is protruding from the patient's mouth. A second Kelly clamp is then attached to the cutaneous end of the guide wire, to prevent it from migrating into the incision. The guide wire now crosses the gastrostomy site, and will remain in place until the gastrostomy tube is in position. The push-type gastrostomy tube with its attached introducer is then advanced over the guide wire, with the dilating end leading. The feeding tube is lubricated. After the wire has been firmly grasped at both ends to provide tension and prevent migration, the feeding tube is advanced over the wire through the mouth and esophagus, and into the stomach until the dilating tip passes through the abdominal skin incision. The dilating tip is grasped and pulled

through the abdominal wall with firm pressure until only 4–6 cm of tube remains in the stomach. The tube is then gently pulled with enough pressure to juxtapose the gastric wall against the abdominal wall using the internal bolster. An external bolster is placed to prevent migration of the tube into the stomach. After placement of the external bolster, correct positioning will allow the feeding tube to be rotated while gentle torque is applied to the tube. Many endoscopists reintroduce the endoscope into the stomach to verify and document the correct placement of the gastrostomy tube at this point. The feeding tube is then cut from the introducer at the desired distance from the skin, and the feeding adapter is placed into the tube.

Introducer-Type (Russell) Gastrostomy [4]

In certain clinical situations, it is desirable to place a gastrostomy tube directly into the stomach without pulling the internal bumper through the esophagus (**Fig. 40.9c**). This technique can be useful if there is an esophageal stricture, prosthesis, or other abnormality that would allow passage of a pediatric endoscope, but not necessarily a gastrostomy tube bumper. This technique is also used if a

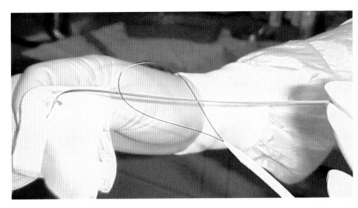

Fig. 40.14 The wire being passed through the loop at the tip of the pull percutaneous endoscopic gastrostomy tube.

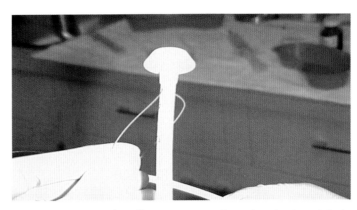

Fig. 40.15 Securing the pull percutaneous endoscopic gastrostomy tube to the wire by passing the bumper through the loop in the wire.

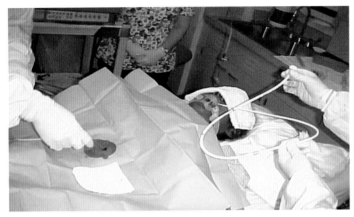

Fig. 40.16 The wire being pulled through the abdominal incision while the percutaneous endoscopic gastrostomy tube is allowed to advance.

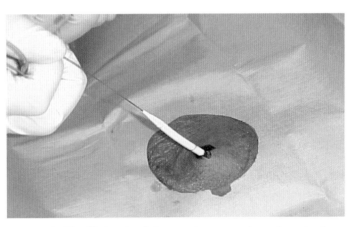

Fig. 40.17 The dilating tip of the percutaneous endoscopic gastrostomy tube is seen externally as the wire is pulled.

40

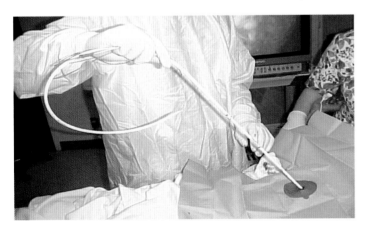

Fig. 40.18 The percutaneous endoscopic gastrostomy tube is pulled into the correct position to approximate the gastric and abdominal walls.

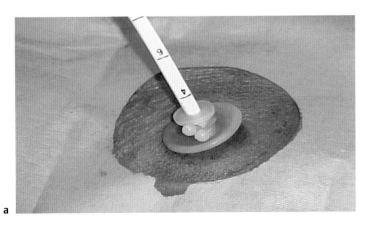

a

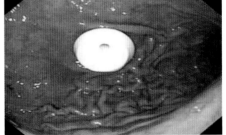

b

Fig. 40.19
a The external bolster and tie after correct placement.
b Endoscopic view of the internal bolster of the percutaneous endoscopic gastrostomy tube after correct placement.

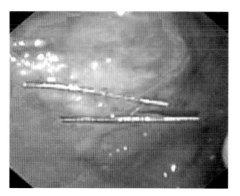

Fig. 40.20 T-fasteners in the stomach.

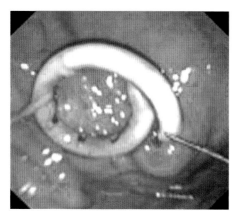

Fig. 40.21 T-fasteners with the introducer percutaneous endoscopic gastrostomy in place (Cope loop tube).

head and neck cancer is present and the endoscopist does not wish to pull the gastrostomy tube through the tumor and abdominal wall, to reduce the risk of tumor seeding of the PEG site [14].

As described above with the other methods, a site is selected, and the needle and cannula assembly is advanced into the stomach under endoscopic guidance. A short guide wire is then advanced into the stomach and coiled in the gastric body. Alternatively, if T-fasteners are going to be used to affix the stomach to the anterior abdominal wall, then they may be placed before tract dilation. While T-fasteners add time and some complexity to the procedure, they ensure that the stomach remains adherent to the abdominal wall even if the gastrostomy tube is removed. This is an important consideration in the introducer technique, as the retention balloon or Cope loop can occasionally fail and result in peritonitis or inadvertent infusion of tube feeding into the peritoneal cavity. If T-fasteners are used, they are passed through the cannula into the stomach lumen, where they are manipulated to form a T that uses a suture and an external pledget to maintain the position of the stomach wall (**Fig. 40.20**). The T-fasteners should be placed in the stomach using the same technique for localization as described above. The fasteners are placed at least 2 cm apart, with the feeding tube site between the two T-fasteners (**Fig. 40.21**).

The exact location for the gastrostomy tube is identified. The skin incision is made, and the needle and cannula are advanced into the stomach under endoscopic guidance. A short guide wire is advanced into the stomach and a dilating catheter with a peel-away sheath is passed over the guide wire. When the sheath is visualized in the stomach, the dilating catheter is removed and the gastrostomy tube is advanced through the sheath into the stomach. The endoscope remains in place, monitoring the process. The gastrostomy tube is fixed in position with either a retention balloon inflated with water

or a Cope loop, depending on the tube design. Finally, the peel-away sheath is removed, the tube position is confirmed by rotation, and the endoscope is withdrawn from the patient. If a retention balloon is used to maintain the gastrostomy tube in the stomach, the balloon channel should be covered with tape or a plastic cap and clearly labeled to avoid inadvertent deflation or rupture due to over-inflation.

Post Procedure

The skin incision is cleaned, and a triple antibiotic cream or Betadine gel is applied. The site is securely bandaged with gauze and tape. An abdominal binder can be placed to limit the patient's access to the gastrostomy tube and prevent premature removal. The timing of starting feeds varies from center to center. While feeds were in the past started 24 h after placement of the feeding tube, there is evidence that it is safe to begin feeds as early as 3 h after placement [14]. Feeding may consist of commercially available canned nutritional supplements. Due to financial considerations, some patients may prefer to blend traditional food to a liquid consistency and instill it via the PEG. Feeding can be given as slow gravity boluses over 30–60 min, or as a continuous drip. More rapid infusion of feeding into the stomach can result in gastroesophageal reflux and aspiration. The feeding tube should be flushed with water after each feed, or at least four times daily if continuous feeds are employed. The incision site should be examined and cleaned daily, and is usually kept covered with a gauze dressing until healing is complete.

Endoscopically Placed Gastrojejunostomy

Occasionally, the need arises for feeds to be delivered directly into the small bowel. This is often performed to decrease the continued aspiration of gastric contents. After placement of a PEG tube as described above, a second catheter (commercially available as a JPEG kit) is threaded through the PEG tube, grasped with a snare or forceps under endoscopic guidance, and advanced into the jejunum. A modification of the procedure involves the initial placement of a wire via the PEG into the small bowel under endoscopic guidance. A jejunal tube is then advanced over the wire into the small bowel. While this is technically feasible, results with JPEG have been disappointing due to tube migration back into the stomach, tube kinking, and obstruction. A plain abdominal radiograph should always be obtained to document proper location of the tube tip before feeding is initiated. Tube migration back into the stomach may occur during use. Techniques such as weighted tips or mucosal clip placement also cannot ensure that the tube will remain in the jejunum.

Direct Percutaneous Endoscopic Jejunostomy

Initially used in patients with partial or total gastrectomy, direct percutaneous endoscopic jejunostomy (DPEJ) is a technique that allows direct endoscopic placement of a feeding tube into the jejunum [15,16]. This eliminates many of the issues that led to failure of the JPEG systems. While technically more difficult than PEG, DPEJ can be accomplished with a success rate of more than 85%, and offers the advantages of direct jejunal feeding with a 20-Fr tube [17]. The technique is essentially the same as the "pull" PEG, except that an enteroscope or pediatric colonoscope is used to intubate the jejunum beyond the ligament of Treitz (**Fig. 40.22**). Fluoroscopy may be useful, especially for orienting the endoscope tip when attempting transillumination. Once the endoscope is in position, transillumination is attempted, and a site for DPEJ is selected.

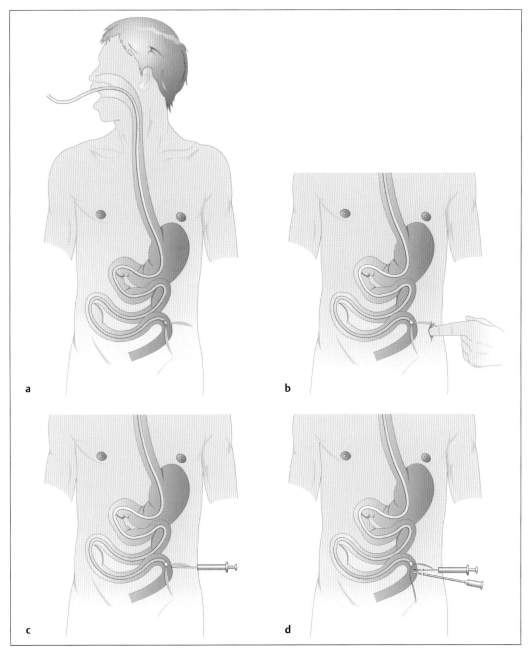

Fig. 40.22e–h ▷

Fig. 40.22 The direct percutaneous endoscopic jejunostomy (DPEJ) placement procedure.
a The enteroscope is advanced until transillumination is achieved.
b A discrete indentation should be reproducible with direct depression at the site of transillumination.
c The sounding/ anesthesia needle is inserted at the site of depression/transillumination, and advanced until it is seen to enter the jejunal lumen under endoscopic visualization.
d The needle/cannula is inserted alongside the sounding needle.

The abdominal wall is prepared, and with careful attention to detail, the infiltrating needle is used to locate the jejunum at the site of endoscopic visualization (**Fig. 40.23**). The infiltrating needle is grasped with a snare to stabilize the small bowel. The cannula is then passed directly into the jejunum alongside the infiltrating needle. The snare is repositioned over the cannula, and a long insertion wire is passed through the cannula and grasped with the snare. The infiltrating needle is then withdrawn. The endoscope is withdrawn as the wire is advanced. The wire is then attached to the 20-Fr pull gastrostomy tube, and with gentle traction on the wire the tube is advanced into the jejunum. The site is dressed, and the external bolster is manipulated into position. Feeding by continuous infusion can be initiated shortly after placement.

Complications

Complications of PEG have been reviewed extensively elsewhere [18,19]. While strict adherence to careful technique may reduce the complications of PEG and percutaneous endoscopic jejunostomy (PEJ), even the most experienced centers have encountered difficulties that are serious, and in some situations life-threatening. Complications of PEG and PEJ are often challenging to manage, as many patients referred for these procedures are poor candidates for operative intervention and respond poorly to aggressive medical care. While there has been no consensus, PEG complications can be classified as major or minor for tracking and reporting purposes. Complications of PEG and PEJ are listed in **Table 40.2**. Common PEG and PEJ complications, along with their etiology, diagnosis, management, and methods of prevention are listed in **Table 40.3**. **Figure 40.24** shows an internal bumper that has eroded through the gastric wall.

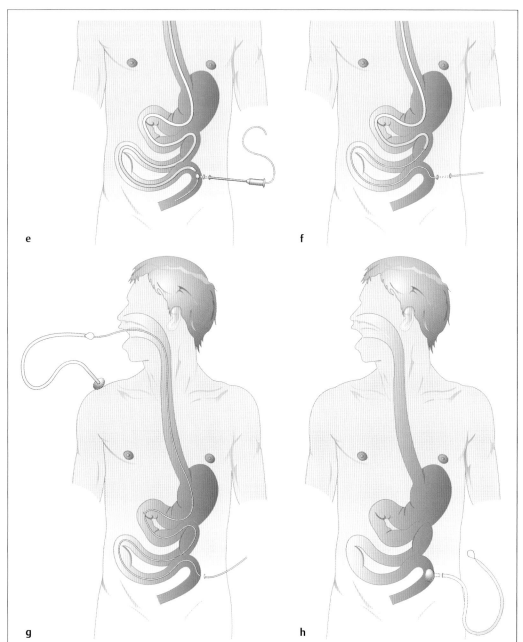

Fig. 40.22e–h
e With the needle removed from within the indwelling cannula, the insertion wire is advanced through the cannula and grasped by the awaiting snare that extends from the tip of the endoscope.
f, g The scope is then removed, and the insertion wire is withdrawn with it so that one end of the insertion wire extends from the mouth and the other end extends from the abdominal wall.
h The attachment loop of the pull-type gastrostomy feeding tube is tethered to the mouth end of the insertion wire, and the assembly is pulled internally until the feeding tube has traversed the jejunal and abdominal walls and is pulled up snugly.

Replacement/Removal of PEG

PEG tract maturity occurs over a variable time (2–6 weeks), and depends on a number of factors, including the patient's nutritional status, steroid use, etc. Before removal or replacement of a gastrostomy tube, one should verify the need for continued enteral nutrition, the type of tube in place, and its ability to be removed without repeat endoscopy.

If removal of the PEG tube is desired, this can usually be accomplished in the office or endoscopy lab without sedation. Many physicians prefer to have the patient prepared for upper endoscopy in case the traction removal is unsuccessful. The patient is placed supine, and the external retaining device on the gastrostomy tube is removed (**Fig. 40.25**). The tube should move easily to and fro through the established tract into the stomach. Lubricant is placed on the external surface of the tube, and it is then advanced into the stomach to lubricate the tract. While firm pressure is being applied on the abdominal wall with one hand to prevent undue tenting, the

tube is grasped with the other hand and pulled out with firm and constant tension. This results in a gradual deformity and collapse of the inner bolster, allowing the tube to be extracted via the tract. When removing a replacement PEG tube, or a PEG tube that has been secured internally by a balloon, the balloon is deflated and the tube is extracted. If the tube is not rapidly replaced by another tube (either a replacement PEG tube or a Foley catheter), the tract will shrink rapidly over the next several hours, and will usually close off in a few days. Replacement PEG tubes have either a balloon that is inflated after passing the tube through the tract, or a mushroom configuration that is straightened for insertion and allowed to reform after passage into the stomach. In either case, after placement, an external bolster is applied to prevent internal migration of the tube. Although it is not usually necessary, a Gastrografin study under fluoroscopy via the newly placed replacement tube will easily confirm correct placement if a question regarding this arises. Alternatively, the old PEG tube can be changed over a standard guide wire by passing it through the PEG tube into the stomach before

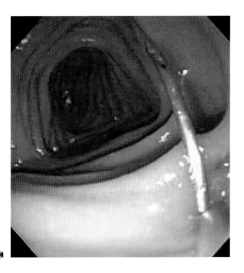
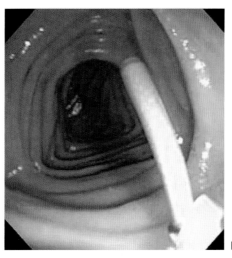

Fig. 40.23
a The infiltrating needle has been grasped with a snare in the small bowel.
b The snare is repositioned on the cannula passed alongside the infiltrating needle into the small bowel. The infiltrating needle has been withdrawn.
c Endoscopic confirmation of successful placement of the percutaneous jejunostomy.

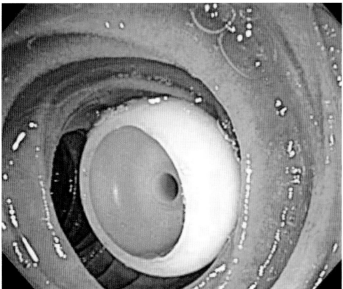

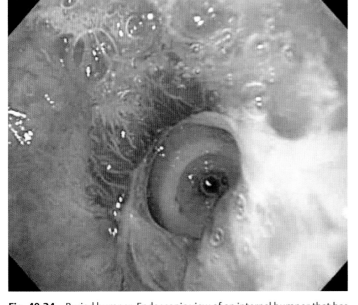

Table 40.2 Complications of percutaneous endoscopic gastrostomy (PEG) and percutaneous endoscopic jejunostomy (PEJ)

Major complications
Aspiration
Peritonitis
Premature removal of the G-tube or J-tube
Tube migration through the gastric or jejunal wall
Perforation
Gastrocolocutaneous fistula
Hemorrhage
Necrotizing fasciitis
Tumor implantation at the PEG stoma

Minor complications
Peristomal wound infections
Tube obstruction or fragmentation
Leakage around feeding tubes
G-tube migration into the duodenum

Fig. 40.24 Buried bumper. Endoscopic view of an internal bumper that has eroded through the gastric wall. The external bolster was loosened and repositioned. The internal bumper was grasped with a forceps and repositioned in the stomach. In the absence of excessive traction, the tract healed around the tube, obviating the need for removal of the percutaneous endoscopic gastrostomy tube.

Table 40.3 Commonly encountered complications of percutaneous endoscopic gastrostomy (PEG) and percutaneous endoscopic jejunostomy (PEJ)

Complication	Etiology	Recognition, symptoms, diagnosis	Management	Considerations for prevention
Aspiration	Oropharyngeal aspiration, reflux of gastric contents	Sx: fever, cough, SOB Dx: new infiltrate on CXR, leukocytosis sputum culture	Antibiotic therapy, treatment of reflux, consider DPEJ or surgical jejunostomy	Attempt to differentiate oropharyngeal aspiration from reflux of gastric contents. *Acute (during procedure)*: Elevate head during endoscopy, frequent oropharyngeal suctioning, avoid excess gastric distention, avoid oversedation *Chronic aspiration*: Elevation of head during feeding, aggressive therapy of reflux disease, frequent monitoring of gastric residuals
Peritonitis	Tract disruption, leakage around tube, premature tube removal, unrecognized perforation of bowel	Sx: abdominal pain, fever, leukocytosis Dx: peritoneal signs on examination, G-tube study with contrast	Antibiotic therapy, surgical consultation, replace PEG if premature removal has occurred	Avoid tract manipulations, abdominal binder to prevent premature tube removal
Premature tube removal	Tube removed before tract maturation	Sx: tube removed and cannot be replaced into stomach easily	Antibiotic therapy, immediate repeat PEG or NG tube placed to suction followed by delayed PEG	Cover tube with binder or dressing, hand restraints for patient if needed, avoid balloon catheters for initial placement or use T-fasteners
Tube migration into the abdominal wall	Excessive tube traction	Sx: difficulty with feeding or leakage around G-tube Dx: G-tube study with contrast or endoscopy	Endoscopic tube replacement or repositioning, surgical consultation if unsuccessful	Avoid excessive traction on inner bumper
Hemorrhage	Ulcers owing to the tube contact with mucosa, peptic ulcer disease	Sx: melena, hematemesis, coffee grounds, or fresh blood in G-tube aspirate Dx: upper endoscopy	Endoscopic therapy of active bleeding, medical therapy of peptic ulcer disease	Avoid excessive traction on inner bumper, medical management of ulcer disease if seen at initial endoscopy
Necrotizing fasciitis	Bacterial translocation during placement	Sx: fever, increased WBC, local wound pain, drainage, discoloration, and/or crepitation Dx: examination, plain radiography, CT scan or ultrasound	Antibiotics and aggressive surgical debridement, hyperbaric oxygen therapy	Prophylactic antibiotics (i.v. cefazolin or equivalent) for all PEGs, adequate abdominal incision length, avoid excessive traction on inner bumper
Peristomal wound infection	Excessive tube traction, tight tube seal	Sx: localized pain, erythema, or fluctuance, fevers	Antibiotic therapy, aggressive wound care	Prophylactic antibiotics (i.v. cefazolin or equivalent) for all PEGs, adequate abdominal incision length, avoid excessive traction on tube
Leakage around the G-tube	Enlarged stoma opening	Sx: localized drainage, skin breakdown at stoma	Gentle increase in bumper tension, short-term tube removal then replacement	Limit tube manipulation

CXR, chest radiography; DPEJ, direct percutaneous endoscopic jejunostomy; Dx, diagnosis; NG, nasogastric; PEG, percutaneous endoscopic gastrostomy; SOB, shortness of breath; Sx, symptoms; WBC, white blood cell (count)

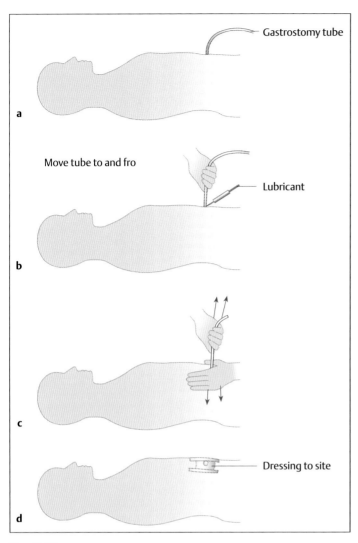

Fig. 40.25

a The patient is supine, and the G-tube is inspected for the type and date of placement.

b The external bolster is removed, and the external surfaces of the tube and tract are lubricated to ease removal.

c One hand is placed on the abdominal wall around the G-tube to apply counterpressure. The other hand grasps the G-tube firmly, and slowly but continuously increases traction until the tube is removed.

d The tube is inspected to ensure that it has been completely removed without fragmentation. A dressing is placed on the removal site if a replacement tube is not to be inserted.

removal. The replacement tube can then be advanced over the guide wire, and its position in the stomach can be confirmed by a Gastrografin tube study if necessary.

Conclusion

Percutaneous endoscopic gastrostomy and jejunostomy have met with widespread acceptance as methods of obtaining long-term feeding access. Barring a few contraindications, placement can be achieved easily in most patients. Ease of placement, simple guidelines for use, and nonendoscopic replacement are the key factors responsible for the extensive use of these techniques today. Careful attention to detail and technique can make this a safe and worthwhile procedure for patients who require intermediate and long-term enteral feeding.

References

1. Safadi BY, Marks JM, Ponsky JL. Percutaneous endoscopic gastrostomy. Gastroenterol Clin N Am 1998;8:551–68.
2. Gauderer MWL, Ponsky JL, Izant RJ Jr. Gastrostomy without laparotomy: a percutaneous endoscopic technique. J Pediatr Surg 1980;15:872–5.
3. Sacks BA, Vine HS, Palestrant AM, Ellison HP, Shropshire D, Lowe R. A nonoperative technique for establishment of a gastrostomy in the dog. Invest Radiol 1983;18:485–7.
4. Russell TR, Brotman M, Forbes N. Percutaneous gastrostomy: a new simplified and cost-effective technique. Am J Surg 1984;148:132–7.
5. Ponsky JL, Gauderer MWL. Percutaneous endoscopic gastrostomy: indications, limitations, techniques and results. World J Surg 1989;13:165–72.
6. Meyers R. Decision making regarding the initiation of tube feeding in the severely demented elderly: a review. J Am Geriatr Soc 1991;39:526–31.
7. Wolfsen HC, Kozarek RA. Percutaneous endoscopic gastrostomy: ethical considerations. Gastrointest Endosc Clin N Am 1992;2:259–71.
8. Ritchie CS, Wilcox CM, Kvale E. Ethical and medicolegal issues related to percutaneous endoscopic gastrostomy placement. Gastrointest Endosc Clin N Am 2007;17:805–15.
9. Cappell MS, Iocovone FM Jr. The safety and efficacy of percutaneous endoscopic gastrostomy after recent myocardial infarction: a study of 28 patients and 40 controls at four university teaching hospitals. Am J Gastroenterol 1996;91:1599–604.
10. Graham SM, Flowers JL, Scott TR, Lin F, Rigamonti D. Safety of percutaneous endoscopic gastrostomy in patients with a ventriculoperitoneal shunt. Neurosurgery 1993;32:932–4.
11. Panzer S, Harris M, Berg W, Ravich W, Kalloo A. Endoscopic ultrasound in the placement of a percutaneous endoscopic gastrostomy tube in the non-transilluminated abdominal wall. Gastrointest Endosc 1995;42:88–90.
12. Jain NK, Larson DE, Schroeder KW, Burton DD, Cannon KP, Thompson RL, et al. Antibiotic prophylaxis for percutaneous endoscopic gastrostomy: a prospective, randomized, double-blind clinical trial. Ann Intern Med 1987;107:824–8.
13. Sharma VK, Howden CW. Meta-analysis of randomized controlled trials of antibiotic prophylaxis before percutaneous endoscopic gastrostomy. Am J Gastroenterol 2000;95:3133–6.
14. Choudhry U, Barde CJ, Markert R, Gopalswamy N. Percutaneous endoscopic gastrostomy: a randomized prospective comparison of early and delayed feeding. Gastrointest Endosc 1996;44:164–7.
15. Shike M, Schroy P, Ritchie MA, Lightdale CJ, Morse R. Percutaneous endoscopic jejunostomy in cancer patients with previous gastric resection. Gastrointest Endosc 1987;33:372–4.
16. Ginsberg GG. Direct percutaneous endoscopic jejunostomy. Tech Gastrointest Endosc 2001;3:42–9.
17. Shike M, Latkany L, Gerdes H, Bloch AS. Direct percutaneous endoscopic jejunostomies for enteral feeding. Gastrointest Endosc 1996;44:536–40.
18. Shapiro GD, Edmundowicz SA. Complications of percutaneous endoscopic gastrostomy. Gastrointest Endosc Clin N Am 1996;6:409–22.
19. Foutch PG. Complications of percutaneous endoscopic gastrostomy and jejunostomy. Recognition, prevention, and treatment. Gastrointest Endosc Clin N Am 1992;2:231–48.

40

41 Therapeutic Endosonography

Jan-Werner Poley and Marco J. Bruno

Introduction

The indications for performing endoscopic ultrasonography (EUS) have changed dramatically with the introduction of curvilinear-array echo endoscopes. From being a solely observational diagnostic tool, EUS has developed into an advanced interventional technique with which it is possible not only to acquire tissue samples by means of fine-needle aspiration (FNA), but also to introduce drugs, for example, using fine-needle injection (FNI). In addition, various accessories such as radiopaque fiducials and guide wires can be advanced through a needle into a target structure or lesion. Using guide wires placed under EUS guidance, advanced types of cyst drainage, as well as biliary and pancreatic drainage procedures, can be carried out. This chapter discusses the indications for and techniques of advanced interventional therapeutic endosonography.

Equipment (see also Chapter 22)

Therapeutic endosonography became possible through the introduction of curvilinear-array echo endoscopes in which the EUS image is parallel to the working channel, allowing instruments to be passed in the same plane with real-time ultrasonographic guidance. **Table 41.1** provides an overview of the curvilinear-array echo endoscopes that are currently available, along with some of their most important features. To facilitate manipulation of FNA needles and other devices, curvilinear-array echo endoscopes, like side-viewing endoscopic retrograde cholangiopancreatography (ERCP) endoscopes, have an elevator. The working channels in curvilinear-array echo endoscopes are as large as 3.8 mm to allow passage of accessories up to 10 Fr. The image resolution and penetration depth of the ultrasound image are inversely related and depend on the frequency. The higher the frequency, the higher the image resolution, but the lower the penetration depth (approximately 2 cm); conversely, the lower the frequency, the lower the image resolution, but the higher the penetration depth (approximately 7 cm). With the exception of a prototype forward-scanning curvilinear-array echo endoscope (Olympus XGIF-UCT160) [1], all devices have endoscopic video imaging oblique to the shaft.

Curvilinear-array echo endoscopes, like radial devices, have a separate channel to allow for water inflation of a disposable balloon mounted at the tip of the instrument. The water-filled balloon improves acoustic coupling for the transmission of ultrasound waves through the gastrointestinal wall. However, as acoustic coupling can also be achieved by gently maneuvering the transducer onto the mucosa, many endosonographers do not use a balloon with curvilinear-array echo endoscopes. A variety of EUS accessories are available, including FNA needles in three different sizes (25, 22, and 19 gauge). For interventional EUS purposes, a 22-gauge needle may suffice in cases in which nonviscous fluids are to be injected. In other cases, and particularly in circumstances in which a guide wire or fiducials are to be introduced, a 19-gauge needle is mandatory. For EUS-guided celiac plexus neurolysis, a special 20-gauge needle device has been developed (Cook Endoscopy, Winston-Salem, North Carolina, USA).

Table 41.1 Electronic curvilinear-array echo endoscopes that are currently commercially available

	Olympus GF-UC140(P)-AL5	Olympus GF-UC160(P)-OL5	Pentax EG-3870UTK
Ultrasound scan angle	180°	150°	120°
Frequency (MHz)	5, 6, 7.5, 10	7.5	5, 7.5, 10
Tip diameter (mm)	14.6 (14.2)	14.6 (14.2)	12.8
Insertion tube (mm)	12.8 (11.8)	12.6 (11.8)	12.8
Channel (mm)	3.7 (2.8)	3.7 (2.8)	3.8
Video: field of view/ direction	100°/55° Forward oblique	100°/55° Forward oblique	120°/50° Forward oblique
Tip deflection: up/down	130°/90°	130°/90°	130°/130°

EUS-Guided Celiac Plexus Neurolysis

A recent meta-analysis by Yan and Myers, including five randomized controlled studies with a total of 302 patients, found that the effectiveness of percutaneous or intraoperative celiac plexus neurolysis (CPN) in pain management was disappointing [2]. There was a statistically significant difference in pain scores in favor of CPN, although with minimal clinical significance. The weighted mean difference in pain scores between conventional treatment (analgesics) and CPN was only 6%. In the light of this disappointing clinical effect, it has been suggested that the limited efficacy of percutaneous CPN may be caused by inadequate targeting of alcohol injection at the site of the celiac plexus. In 1996, Wiersema and Wiersema introduced a new and possibly more effective technique for carrying out CPN with EUS guidance [3]. In this technique, a puncture needle is inserted through the dorsal stomach wall under real-time EUS guidance, immediately adjacent and anterior to the lateral aspect of the aorta at the level of the celiac trunk (**Fig. 41.1**). Once the needle has been positioned, 3–5 mL of bupivacaine (0.25%) is injected for local anesthesia, followed by 10 mL pure alcohol (96%). This is then repeated at the opposite site. Some prefer not to inject bilaterally, and instead inject in the midline anterior to the celiac trunk. There are no data available showing that either of these techniques is superior to the other. The EUS-guided approach is considered to be safer than the traditional percutaneous approach, due to the close approximation to the celiac trunk, avoiding needle puncture alongside the spine or through intra-abdominal organs.

No studies have been published comparing percutaneous CPN with EUS-guided CPN, nor have there been any controlled randomized trials comparing EUS-guided CPN with conventional opioid treatment. EUS-guided CPN has been used in patients with painful chronic pancreatitis and patients with oncologic pain due to inoperable pancreatic carcinoma. For the latter indication, two prospective cohort studies have been published. Gunaratnam and co-workers conducted a study including 58 patients, 78% of whom showed a decline in pain scores after the EUS-guided CPN [4]. This effect lasted for 24 weeks when adjusted for morphine use and adjuvant therapy.

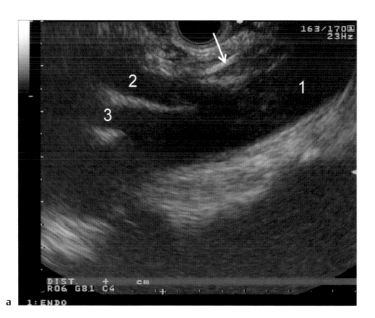

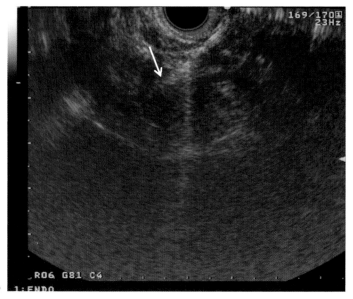

Fig. 41.1 EUS-guided celiac plexus neurolysis.
a 1, abdominal aorta; 2, celiac trunk; 3, superior mesenteric artery. The celiac trunk is visualized by tracing the aorta as the first vessel that branches off the vessel below the diaphragm. The needle (arrow) is advanced just above the celiac trunk.
b The scope is torqued a few degrees laterally, and the needle (arrow) is advanced further alongside the celiac trunk. Once alcohol injection starts, the image becomes blurred. This procedure is repeated on the other side.

Five patients experienced procedure-related transient abdominal pain. No major complications were seen. In the second prospective study, performed by Wiersema and Wiersema, 30 patients (25 with pancreatic carcinoma and five with intra-abdominal metastases) underwent EUS-guided CPN [3]. The pain scores were significantly lower in comparison with baseline scores at 2, 4, 8, and 12 weeks after EUS-CPN. At these follow-up intervals, 82–91% of patients required the same or less pain medication than at baseline, and 79–88% of patients had persistent improvement in their pain score. Complications were minor and consisted of transient diarrhea in four patients. Recently, Levy et al. showed that celiac ganglia can be visualized at EUS [5]. Ganglia were typically seen between the celiac trunk and the left adrenal gland and were hypoechoic, oblong, or normally shaped, often with an irregular edge, and often containing a hyperechoic focus or strands. The size of the ganglia ranged from 2×3 mm to 7×20 mm. The total number of ganglia in patients

ranged between one and four, and more than one ganglion was seen in five out of nine patients. The authors speculated that direct targeting of these ganglia might improve the efficacy of EUS-guided CPN. Whether such an approach would be feasible and lead to an improved outcome in relation to pain control remains to be proved. Recently, Gleeson et al. showed prospectively in a series of 200 patients that celiac ganglia were identified in 81% of cases and were typically located to the left of the celiac artery, anterior to the aorta [6]. Future studies should address the questions of whether EUS-guided CPN is superior to conventional medical treatment and percutaneous CPN and whether direct EUS-guided targeting of celiac ganglia can provide additional treatment benefits.

EUS-Guided FNI in the Treatment of Pancreatic Cancer

On the basis of the safety and feasibility profile of FNA and experiences with EUS-guided CPN, the FNI technique has gradually matured and has expanded the indications for interventional EUS even further. At present, EUS-FNI for intratumoral pancreatic cancer therapy involves antitumoral agents, immunotherapy, and ablative techniques. In recent years, a number of studies have been published describing different agents injected into pancreatic tumors using EUS-FNI, including lymphocyte cultures (Cytoimplant) [7], viral vectors (TNFerade) [8,9], and oncolytic viruses (ONYX-015) [10].

Chang et al. performed a phase 1 trial in which EUS-FNI intratumoral injections of activated allogenic mixed lymphocyte culture (Cytoimplant) were given in eight patients with unresectable pancreatic cancer [7]. Various doses were given using a single injection. There were no procedure-related complications, but grade 3 and 4 toxicities occurred in seven patients, the most frequent one being fever. All toxicities were reversible. On follow-up investigations with computed tomography, a partial response was observed in two patients, a minimal response in one, stable disease in three, and progression of disease in two patients. A randomized trial comparing Cytoimplant with gemcitabine was started, but is currently no longer recruiting patients. The study was stopped prematurely, apparently due to a poorer outcome in the Cytoimplant group, but the results have not been published yet.

TNFerade is a replication-deficient adenovirus vector incorporating the human tumor necrosis factor-α gene, regulated by a radiation-inducible promoter (Egr-1). Animal data from mice provide a rationale for local delivery of human tumor necrosis factor-α in which a host-dependent response to TNFerade was observed both in the primary lesion and in lymph-node metastases [11]. Farrell and co-workers conducted a phase 1/2 multicenter trial in which TNFerade is injected intratumorally using EUS-FNI, computed tomography, or percutaneous ultrasound guidance (PUG) in combination with continuous intravenous infusion of 5-fluorouracil (200 mg/m^2/day, 5 days per week) and radiotherapy (50 Gy) [8]. Preliminary data for 50 patients, 27 of whom had the agent delivered via EUS-FNI and 23 of whom had it delivered using PUG, did not show any significant differences in the treatment response relating to the route of delivery. A partial response was seen in 13% versus 10% of the patients, and stabilization in 73% versus 75%, respectively. Dose-limiting toxicity was seen in three patients after EUS-FNI, with pancreatitis in two and biliary obstruction in one. A multicenter phase 2/3 trial is now being carried out in which patients with unresectable pancreatic adenocarcinoma are randomly assigned to treatment in accordance with standard-of-care therapy alone or TNFerade with standard therapy. Final results are eagerly awaited, following an interim analysis showing a trend toward an improvement in the 1-year and overall survival with TNFerade [9].

ONYX-015 (Onyx Pharmaceuticals, Emeryville, California, USA) is an oncolytic attenuated adenovirus modified selectively to replicate

V

in and kill cells that harbor p53 mutations. Hecht et al. undertook a trial of the feasibility, tolerability, and efficacy of EUS injection of ONYX-015 into unresectable pancreatic carcinomas [10]. Twenty-one patients with locally advanced adenocarcinoma of the pancreas or with metastatic disease but minimal or absent liver metastases underwent eight sessions of ONYX-015 delivered by EUS injection into the primary pancreatic tumor over 8 weeks. The final four treatments were given in combination with gemcitabine. After combination therapy, two patients had partial regression of the treated tumor, two had minor responses, six had stable disease, and 11 had progressive disease or had to withdraw from the study due to treatment toxicity. No clinical pancreatitis occurred despite mild, transient elevations in lipase in a minority of patients. Two patients had sepsis before prophylactic oral antibiotic treatment was instituted. Two patients had duodenal perforations from the rigid endoscope tip; no perforations occurred after the protocol was changed to transgastric injections alone.

There are two related techniques that involve not so much fine-needle injection, but instead consist of fine-needle introduction of an accessory device intended to destroy the tumor mass. One of these techniques is EUS-guided radiofrequency ablation, which was tested several years ago in a porcine model [12]. Although complications were relatively mild and pathology showed a well-demarcated acute coagulation zone of 8–10 mm in all specimens, no subsequent (human) trials have been undertaken to explore the use of this technique further. The same applies to another experimental technique, EUS-guided photodynamic therapy, in which tumor damage is induced by photochemical tissue necrosis after intravenous administration of a photodynamic agent. This was also tested in a porcine model [13]. Three pigs were pretreated with porfimer sodium. Next, a laser fiber with a 1-cm cylindrical light diffuser was passed through a 19-G needle into the liver, kidney, spleen, and pancreas. Energy was delivered to a total of 50 J at 630 nm over 125 s. There were no procedure-related complications. The pathology review showed areas of necrosis measuring approximately 3.5 mm^2, with some hemorrhage and granulation tissue.

Despite initial excitement about the technical feasibility of EUS-guided FNI for treating pancreatic cancer, the technique has not yet become a mainstream indication for EUS. This is mainly due to difficulties in developing effective drugs for intratumoral injections, but progress in this area is eagerly awaited and expected in the coming years.

EUS-Guided Implantation of Radiopaque Markers (Fiducials)

With ongoing developments in radiotherapy, and particularly the value of multiple narrow-beam stereotactic radiosurgery for delivering very high single radiation doses to treat tumors more effectively, the issue of safety in relation to accurate targeting of the radiation beam has become an important issue. For this purpose, these radiotherapy delivery systems use real-time imaging guidance [14]. In some instances, as in brain tumors, for example, anatomical landmarks such as bony structures in the skull can serve as reference points, but for soft-tissue tumors in areas like the chest or abdomen, this is not adequate. In these cases, implantation of radiographic markers, known as "fiducials," has been shown to be a valuable alternative [15]. Traditionally, fiducials were implanted surgically or percutaneously under ultrasonographic or computed tomography (CT) guidance [16]. Since surgery is invasive and some lesions are difficult to access percutaneously, EUS has been proposed as an attractive alternative implant modality [17,18] (**Fig. 41.2**).

Pishvaian et al. performed a prospective study to evaluate the safety and feasibility of placing fiducials in mediastinal and intra-abdominal tumors under EUS guidance in 13 patients scheduled for

high-precision CyberKnife frameless image-guided stereotactic radiosurgery [18]. The fiducials used were cylindrical gold seeds with a length of 3 or 5 mm and a diameter of 0.8 mm, customized to fit into a 19-gauge needle. Under curvilinear-array EUS-guidance, a 19-gauge fine needle was positioned in the target area and the fiducials were placed through the needle lumen. The positioning of the fiducials was verified with EUS and fluoroscopy. To allow accurate fiducial tracking using the CyberKnife system, a minimum of three fiducials were inserted around the tumor area or at the edges of the tumor itself, there was an angle of at least 15° between any two fiducials, and the aim was to achieve a minimum distance between two fiducials of 2 cm. EUS-guided fiducial placement was successful in 11 of 13 patients (84.6%), with tumors in different locations such as the retrocrural area at the dome of the diaphragm, the porta hepatis, gastroesophageal junction, mediastinum, thoracic paraspinal area, and pancreas. A total of three to six fiducials were placed in each patient. No prophylactic antibiotics were administered in the first eight patients. After one patient developed an infectious complication possibly related to the procedure, the following five patients received prophylactic antibiotics at the time of the procedure (ciprofloxacin 400 mg intravenously) followed by a 3-day course of oral ciprofloxacin (500 mg twice a day).

Forward-loading the fiducials and pushing them through the needle can be problematic. Firstly, when the tip of the echo endoscope is angulated, as is commonly the case for pancreatic head tumors, it is often difficult to advance the fiducials through a standard 19-G FNA needle. Secondly, the use of the stylet often introduces air into the tumor, which obscures EUS visualization and may hamper proper delivery of the fiducials. To overcome these problems, Owens and Savides introduced a new technique in which the fiducial is back-loaded into the 19-G needle and held in place with sterile bone wax that allows easy fiducial delivery and avoidance of air introduction [19].

EUS-Guided Drainage of Pancreatic Fluid Collections, Abscesses, and Infected Necroses

The first endoscopic cystogastrostomy and cystoduodenostomy were performed by Sahel et al. and Cremer et al. in 1982 [20,21]. Endoscopic drainage of pseudocysts became an increasingly popular technique, due to its relatively low complication rate in comparison with surgical and percutaneous treatment, with comparable success rates. At an early stage in the development of the technique, it was shown that routine radial EUS undertaken before endoscopic cyst drainage increases the safety of the procedure by determining the optimal access site and avoiding accidental puncture of interposing vessels between the stomach wall and the cyst [22,23]. Equally importantly, carrying out EUS before an attempted cyst drainage can help identify cystic neoplasms in 3–5% of cases [22,24]. Nevertheless, despite the use of radial EUS and marking the optimal site for puncture, endoscopists were still dependent on the bulging of cyst into the lumen of stomach or duodenum.

One of the most important steps in the development of interventional EUS was taken by Grimm et al. in 1992 [25]. They created a fistula between the stomach and cyst with the aid of a linear echo endoscope. Due to the small working channel of only 2.0 mm, the endoscope had to be exchanged for a regular side-viewing endoscope after puncture and guide-wire placement in the pseudocyst under EUS guidance. This procedure was further developed by Giovannini et al., Wiersema et al., and Chak [26–28]. With the introduction of therapeutic linear echo endoscopes with working channels of 3.7 mm (Olympus, Tokyo, Japan) or 3.8 mm (Pentax, Tokyo, Japan), it is now possible to achieve adequate drainage by placing multiple large-bore stents and a nasocystic catheter without changing the endoscope. As a result of these developments, the

41

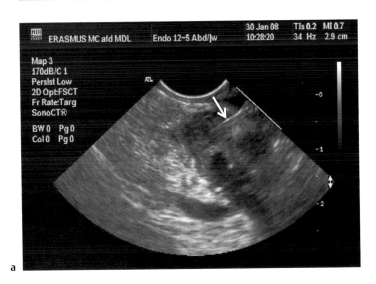
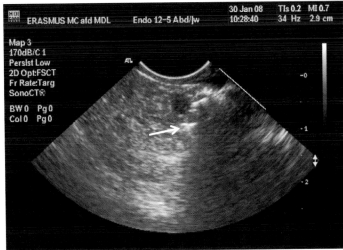
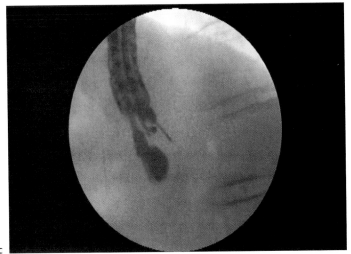
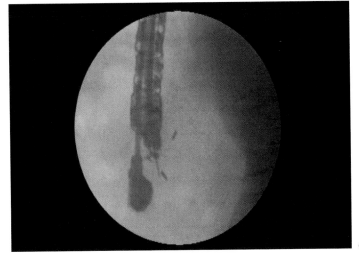

Fig. 41.2 Endoscopic ultrasound (EUS)-guided placement of fiducials to guide CyberKnife radiation in a patient with a small, cytologically confirmed local recurrence of gastric cancer after surgical resection.

a EUS-guided puncture of a malignant mass lesion close to the splenic artery with a 19-G needle (arrow).

b EUS-guided advancement of a fiducial through a 19-G needle with a pusher rod. The fiducial has just disengaged from the needle tip and is visualized as a hyperechoic structure (arrow).

c Radiograph showing a fiducial just being pushed out of the 19-G needle.

d Radiograph showing the tip of the 19-G needle and two fiducials that have already been placed inside the mass lesion.

endoscopist is no longer dependent on a visible bulge to puncture the cyst and is able to choose the safest and shortest puncture route, avoiding blood vessels and other organs under real-time EUS vision.

Several nonrandomized case series have suggested that EUS-guided pseudocyst drainage is safer than traditional "blind" techniques [29,30]. To date, only one randomized trial has been published comparing the two methods [24]. In a series of 30 patients with both bulging and nonbulging cysts, patients randomly assigned to EUS-guided drainage were all treated successfully (100%), whereas this was possible in only five of 15 patients (33%) assigned to conventional drainage. The remaining 10 patients all subsequently underwent successful EUS-guided drainage. There were no differences in the complication rates. Given the study design, potential bias favoring EUS-guided drainage cannot be excluded, but the study does show a 100% success rate, including failed "blind" cases. At present, EUS-guided drainage is the preferred treatment for most pseudocysts in most centers with an interventional endoscopy unit. Only patients in whom endoscopic treatment is not possible due to a location too distant from the stomach or duodenal wall, or those in whom endoscopic treatment fails, are referred for surgical or percutaneous intervention. In our institution, as in other centers, attention has shifted to endoscopic treatment of patients with more complicated diseases—e.g., infected

pseudocysts, pancreatic abscesses, and walled-off pancreatic necrosis [31,32]. Although there have been no randomized trials comparing surgical, percutaneous, and endoscopic treatment, some recent retrospective series have shown that endoscopic treatment of infected necrosis in acute pancreatitis patients may be a viable alternative to surgery [33–35].

Definitions and indications for intervention. There is considerable controversy regarding the nomenclature for peripancreatic fluid collections, despite the attempt to unify terminology with the Atlanta classification system [36]. Most authors agree that peripancreatic fluid collections can be divided into three categories: 1, acute fluid collections; 2, pseudocysts; and 3, walled-off pancreatic necroses (WOPNs) [33]. Acute fluid collections occur early in the course of acute pancreatitis, do not have a defined wall, and usually disappear after several weeks, although they can become very large. Endoscopic interventions are hardly ever necessary. Acute pseudocysts, defined as well-circumscribed, homogeneous lesions with a well-defined wall, require intervention only when symptomatic—i.e., when there is pain, infection, or obstruction of the gastrointestinal tract or bile duct. Size in itself is not an indication for drainage, as spontaneous regression or disappearance is frequently observed. Pseudocysts can also occur in the setting of chronic pancreatitis and

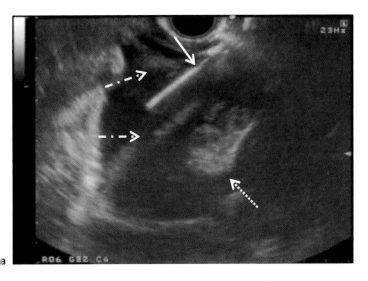
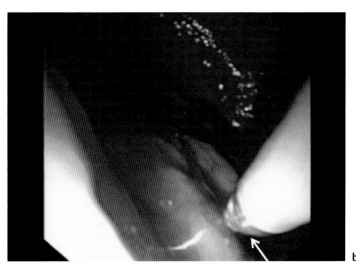
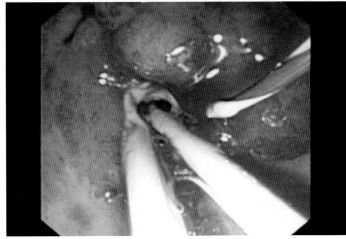
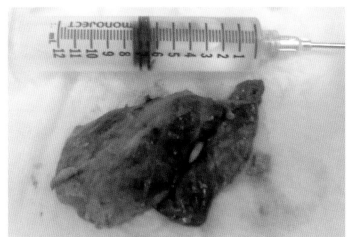

Fig. 41.3 Endoscopic ultrasound (EUS)-guided puncture and drainage of a large pseudocyst using the cystotome.

a The inner 5-Fr catheter (arrow) of the cystotome, with a metal tip, is advanced through the stomach wall into the pseudocyst using electrocautery under EUS guidance. Some electrocautery artifacts are visible (dashed arrows). There is also some blood (dotted arrow) twirling to the bottom of the pseudocyst.

b Using electrocautery at the metal tip (arrow), the 10-Fr outer catheter of the cystotome is advanced over the inner catheter into the pseudocyst.

c The fistulous tract through the stomach and cyst wall created by the 10-Fr electrocautery tip of the outer cystotome catheter is well visualized. Two pigtail stents have already been positioned. The guide wire is advanced into the cyst in order to place a nasocystic catheter for irrigation.

d Forty-eight hours after the initial EUS-guided pseudocyst drainage, the fistula was dilated up to 18 mm and endoscopic debridement was started, removing large chunks of necrotic tissue.

have the same radiographic appearance as acute pseudocysts. Indications for drainage are provided either by symptoms (pain, infection, and obstruction) or size. Most experts advise drainage if the pseudocyst is larger than 6 cm, as this may increase the risk of complications—mainly bleeding and infection [37]. Walled-off pancreatic necrosis (WOPN) is also described as "organized pancreatic necrosis." As long as infection does not occur, treatment is usually conservative. If infection occurs, drainage is mandatory.

Procedure and technique. Antibiotic prophylaxis is generally administered in order to reduce the risk of infectious complications after failed drainage or incomplete drainage of septated or communicating cysts. It is mandatory to have adequate surgical back-up. Drainage can be performed with the patient under moderate sedation, although it may be helpful to carry out the procedure with general anesthesia, especially if multiple cysts need to be drained or the drainage procedure needs to be combined with ERCP. Usually, the procedure is started with the patient in the left lateral position. Depending on local anatomy, it can sometimes be helpful to turn the patient to the prone position. Fluoroscopy is mandatory, even though it is technically feasible to drain a pseudocyst with a single

stent using only EUS guidance. While transgastric or transduodenal drainage of fluid collections has become an established technique, the procedure is quite demanding and usually requires ERCP skills rather than EUS skills. In fact, EUS is required only for the first part of the procedure, to obtain safe access into the fluid collection. There are several different techniques for performing EUS-guided drainage of a pancreatic fluid collection. The choice of technique is largely based on personal preference and experience, but some general considerations are discussed here.

The procedure is started with a therapeutic linear echo endoscope. The optimal site for puncture is chosen on the basis of the distance from the gastric wall and interposing blood vessels. Generally, a distance of 1 cm (or less) is considered safe, although even when the distance between gastric wall and pseudocyst is much larger, up to 2.5 cm, it is often possible to create an endoscopic cystogastrostomy. Access can be achieved either with a specially designed cystotome or with a regular 19-G needle. Potential disadvantages of the cystotome are that EUS visibility of the inner part, which is basically a needle-knife sphincterotome, is sometimes not so clear and that the inner catheter is rather floppy (**Fig. 41.3**). These characteristics sometimes make it more difficult to use. To avoid

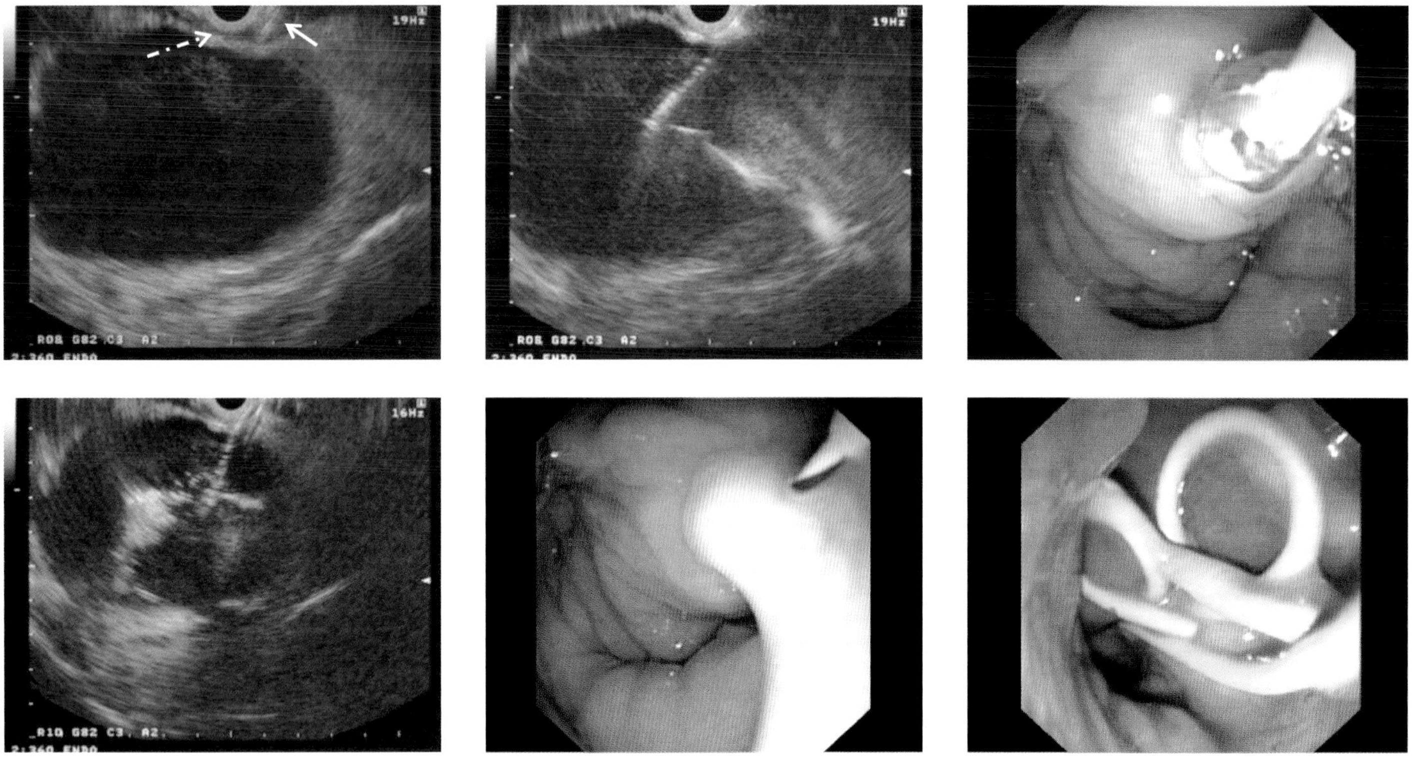

a, b

d, e

Fig. 41.4 Endoscopic ultrasound (EUS)-guided puncture and drainage of a large infected pseudocyst using a 19-G needle.
a A 19-G needle (arrow) is positioned using EUS guidance for transgastric puncture (stomach wall: dashed arrow) of a large pseudocyst.
b The 19-G needle is advanced into the pseudocyst under EUS guidance. The acoustic shadow of the needle is well visible.
c A guide wire has been advanced into the pseudocyst through the 19-G needle. The needle has been removed, and an 8-mm dilation balloon has been introduced over the guide wire into the cyst. Using endoscopy and fluoroscopy, the balloon is adequately positioned to dilate the fistulous tract.

d The guide wire is still safely positioned within the pseudocyst after the balloon has been removed. Some blood can be seen twirling within the cyst cavity after balloon dilation.
e Immediately after the balloon is deflated, pus is seen gushing from the pseudocyst into the stomach.
f Two 7-Fr pigtail stents have already been positioned, and a third stent is being pushed into the pseudocyst.

these problems, a regular 19-G needle can be used to gain access (**Fig. 41.4**). Once the needle is inside the fluid collection, 10 mL of the cyst fluid is aspirated for culture, cytology, and biochemical markers (amylase, carcinoembryonic antigen) and subsequently 10–20 mL of contrast is injected. This sometimes delineates the communication with the pancreatic duct, but more importantly it shows the size and shape of the cyst, making it easier to interpret the position of guide wires later in the procedure. After puncture, a long stiff ERCP guide wire is left in place and dilation of the cystogastrostomy fistula is mandatory. However, if a dilation balloon cannot be passed successfully into the cyst, the outer part of the cystotome can be advanced over the guide wire into the cyst using electrocautery. Use of a regular sphincterotome is associated with an increased risk of bleeding.

It is generally accepted that placing multiple stents reduces the chance of clogging and improves the eventual outcome. Through the outer part of a cystotome or via an 8.5-Fr stent introduction system (One-Action Stent Introduction System, OASIS; Cook Endoscopy, Winston-Salem, North Carolina, USA) a second wire can be placed inside the cyst and two stents can be placed easily [38]. It is advisable to use double-pigtail stents (7 Fr) for drainage, as they are less traumatic to the cyst wall in comparison with straight stents, thereby reducing the chance of bleeding [39]. If there is a clinical suspicion of infection, it is advisable to place a 6-Fr nasocystic catheter and start cyst irrigation with 1 L of water or saline per 24 h, with manual boluses of 100–200 mL every 4 h, depending on the size and appearance of the cyst. If the cyst contains debris and solid or necrotic material, a repeat endoscopic intervention should be considered after 1–2 days, with further dilation of the fistulous tract up to 18 mm and endoscopic debridement using a regular forward-viewing endoscope. Necrosectomy is usually best done with a Dormia basket or Roth net. A grasping forceps can occasionally be useful. Usually, several repeat procedures are necessary until viable tissue in the wall of the cyst is clearly visible. In between these procedures, cyst irrigation is maintained using a nasocystic catheter.

Complications. The main complications of endoscopic drainage of pancreatic fluid collections are infection, bleeding, perforation, stent migration, and stent dysfunction. The frequencies reported in the literature vary markedly, between 11% and 37%, at least partly due to the different patient populations investigated [29,31,39,40]. In general, the risk of complications increases along with increased complexity of the procedure, especially when underlying pancreatic necrosis is present. Infection is probably the most frequent complication after endoscopic drainage. Using prophylactic antibiotics may reduce this risk. The most important risk factor is incomplete drainage, which may be due to stent clogging or migration, noncommunicating cyst compartments, and, most importantly, the presence of pancreatic necrosis. Most cases of infectious complication can be managed endoscopically by transmural necrosectomy [34,41]. Bleeding is less frequently encountered when using EUS-guided drainage. If bleeding occurs from the site of the cystogastrostomy, it can usually be managed endoscopically. Presence of a pseudoaneurysm must be excluded. Overt perforation is rather uncommon, with most series reporting perforation rates below 5%, although in earlier series the figure was somewhat higher [32,39,40,42,43]. Experience is therefore likely to influence the complication rate. Most cases of perforation involve leakage of pancreatic juice into the peritoneum. When the drainage procedure is technically successful and adequate positioning of stents in the cyst cavity is confirmed on CT scan, perforation can usually be managed conservatively. The fistula will mature in 1–3 days and leakage will stop.

Outcome and results. The results are generally best with uncomplicated cysts in chronic pancreatitis. The efficacy of transmural endoscopic drainage in these patients is more than 90%, and the method has therefore become the treatment of choice in centers where this expertise is available, although there have been no prospective controlled series comparing percutaneous, surgical, and endoscopic treatment. A small retrospective case–control study in which surgical cystogastrostomy was compared with EUS-guided endoscopic drainage showed comparable success, repeat intervention, and complication rates [44]. However, due to a shorter mean hospital stay, the endoscopic treatment was more cost-effective. Success rates in infected WOPNs are considerably lower at around 70%, even in centers with considerable experience [31,34].

Drainage of pelvic abscesses. In three published case series including 12, four, and four patients, respectively, it was shown that it is possible to drain pelvic abscesses with the aid of a linear therapeutic echo endoscope [45–47]. In the first study, stent placement was successful in 75% of patients, whereas a 100% technical success rate was achieved in the other two. With the aid of the same techniques as those described above, an overall success rate of approximately 75% was achieved in combination with short-term irrigation of the abscesses. This approach is a promising technique in patients who are sometimes very difficult to manage surgically or radiologically.

Future developments. Some of the difficulties of EUS-guided drainage procedures, especially those relating to the sometimes awkward maneuverability and the oblique direction in which force is exerted, might be overcome by using a prototype forward-viewing linear echo endoscope. Initial clinical experience in a small case series suggests that the endoscope control with this device compares favorably with that of traditional linear echo endoscopes [1]. More trials are awaited to confirm this, and perhaps it will be possible to drain previously inaccessible fluid collections with the aid of this endoscope. With the increasing use of transmural endoscopic necrosectomy, more effective instruments and accessories for evacuating necrotic tissue from the drained cavities are eagerly awaited.

EUS-Guided Drainage of the Biliary System

Most of the biliary system can be visualized with EUS. Only visualization of the right hepatic lobe is limited; the common bile duct, gallbladder, and left hepatic duct are easily identified with a linear echo endoscope. This opened the way for EUS-guided biliary drainage and rendezvous procedures. Although endoscopic treatment of biliary obstruction using ERCP is successful in approximately 90% of patients, cannulation of the major papilla fails in some cases due to local tumor infiltration or (surgically) altered anatomy. Nowadays, almost every patient in whom ERCP fails can be managed using percutaneous transhepatic drainage. However, percutaneous biliary drainage is associated with considerable morbidity due to bleeding, cholangitis, and bile leakage in 10–30% of patients [48]. The search for an endoscopic alternative for percutaneous interventions therefore seems logical, and with the ability of linear EUS to gain access to transmural structures, the development of transgastric and transduodenal EUS-guided biliary drainage was inevitable. Most papers on this subject have focused on the transmural placement of plastic or self-expanding stents, but rendezvous procedures have also been described. This section describes the indications, procedures, complications, and outcomes of EUS-guided hepaticogastrostomy, EUS-guided choledochoduodenostomy, and EUS-guided cholecystostomy.

EUS-Guided Hepaticogastrostomy

Given the excellent visualization of the left lobe of the liver from the stomach, it is not difficult to identify dilated bile ducts. Since the right liver lobe is much more difficult to examine, patients with unilateral dilation of the right biliary system are not candidates for this procedure. In theory, all patients with malignant obstruction after failed ERCP are potential candidates for EUS-guided hepaticogastrostomy. Several case series have shown that the transgastric stenting procedure is technically feasible and promising. However, due to the lack of comparative studies with percutaneous approaches, for example, and the small number of patients included, the technique should still be regarded as an experimental procedure that should only be performed in a clinical research setting [49–55].

Procedure. All patients in published series received antibiotic prophylaxis before the procedure. The biliary system is identified from the stomach at the lesser curvature, and a dilated bile duct is punctured with a 19-G or 22-G needle. A 22-G needle is more flexible and easier to handle, but only allows a soft and floppy 0.018″ guide wire to pass, making subsequent interventions more difficult. After the stylet has been removed from the needle, contrast is injected and a cholangiogram is obtained. The next step is passing a long (480 cm) guide wire through the needle deep into the biliary system, or preferably through the stenosis in the duodenum. If the latter is chosen, a rendezvous procedure could be considered, provided that the papilla can be reached. One of the main concerns in this type of procedure is shearing of the guide wire on the sharp tip of the needle. Modern guidewires are nearly always hybrid wires with a coating and a core. Stripping of the coating can occur, with the risk of loss of part of the guide wire and subsequent failure to exchange accessories over the damaged guide wire. The risk of shearing increases with the stiffness of the wire and increased angulation of the needle. In both circumstances, more force is exerted at the tip of the needle. Obviously, repeated in-and-out movements of the wire during multiple attempts to reach the desired position will also increase the chance of shearing. Some form of dilation is necessary to deploy either a plastic stent or a self-expanding metal stent (SEMS) through the fistula. For this, a sharp-tipped ERCP cannula (4.0 Fr) followed by biliary dilation catheters up to 8.5 Fr can be used, avoiding the use of electrocautery. However, in the studies previously mentioned, small-caliber cystotomes (6 or 8.5 Fr) and needle-knives have also been used successfully. After dilation, deployment of a stent is the final step. Both straight and double-pigtail plastic stents have been used, as well as covered and uncovered SEMS. It is not yet clear which type (or which combination of stents) is the optimal choice in relation to outcome and complications, which mainly involve obstruction with subsequent cholangitis, bile leakage, and migration. Once the fistula has been created and a stent has been in place for several days, it is generally easy to perform a subsequent procedure and exchange or de-obstruct previously placed stents.

Complications. The overall complication risk in the 20 patients described in the literature was 25%, with no mortalities. Complications ranged from cholangitis due to stent migration or obstruction, ileus due to migrated stents, and biloma. Contrary to expectations, bile leakage and subsequent localized peritonitis was not a major clinical problem, although some postprocedural pain was not uncommon.

41

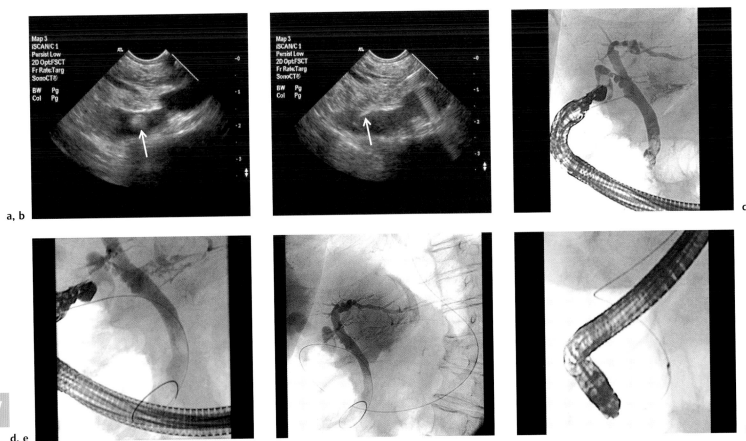

a, b

c

d, e

f

Fig. 41.5 An endoscopic ultrasound (EUS)-guided rendezvous procedure to allow endoscopic retrograde cholangiography (ERC) after a failed attempt to cannulate the papilla of Vater.
a A linear EUS image showing the common bile duct from the duodenal bulb, with a bile stone causing an acoustic shadow (arrow).
b EUS-guided needle puncture (arrow) of the common bile duct.
c Cholangiogram with contrast injection through the EUS puncture needle.

d Advancement of a guide wire through the EUS puncture needle into the common bile duct, across the papilla of Vater into the duodenum.
e The position of the guide wire after removal of the EUS scoop.
f Advancement of a side-viewing ERC scope into the duodenum in front of the papilla. The guide wire has been retrieved through the working channel using a snare. A cannula is advanced over the guide wire into the common bile duct.

Outcome. The outcome and results have generally been good in the published reports, although it should be acknowledged that publication bias may be considerable. The repeat intervention rate was approximately 20%. More data are needed before conclusions can be drawn and definitive recommendations made about the procedure.

EUS-Guided Choledochoduodenostomy

In general, the indications for EUS-guided choledochoduodenostomy are the same as those for hepaticogastrostomy. For this procedure, however, the duodenal bulb has to be preserved and must remain accessible, as it is the point of access—limiting the patients in whom the procedure can be performed. Results for a total of 25 patients have been published in several small case series.

Procedure. As with hepaticogastrostomy, it is common practice to administer preprocedural antibiotic prophylaxis. For transduodenal rendezvous procedures, the therapeutic echo endoscope should be introduced into the duodenum, and after a straight position has been obtained, as in ERCP, the instrument should be slowly withdrawn until the usually dilated bile duct comes into view from the duodenal bulb. The directional view is then toward the ampulla of Vater, making it possible to pass the guide wire after puncture of the common bile duct (**Fig. 41.5**). For EUS-guided choledochoduodenostomy, it is mandatory to introduce the echo endoscope into the duodenal bulb in a long position. From this position, the ultra-

sound view is directed toward the hilum of the liver, allowing transduodenal stent placement. In this position, either a needle-knife or a 19-G needle is introduced into the bile duct, after which a cholangiogram is obtained. Although the hepatic artery and portal vein are close by, avoiding them should not be difficult with the aid of Doppler sonography. A long guide wire is then left in situ, and after this, as in hepaticogastrostomy, dilation of the fistula is performed with a biliary dilation catheter. Next, a plastic stent—most authors have used straight stents—or an SEMS can be placed. Subsequent procedures can be performed with a regular duodenoscope.

Complications. In the 25 patients reported on so far, the complication rate was 19% (five patients). Two cases of biliary leakage led to localized bile peritonitis, and three patients had a pneumoperitoneum after the procedure. Although all cases could be managed conservatively and no procedure-related mortality was observed, this complication rate is rather high, especially when it is considered that the procedures were performed in tertiary referral institutes by expert endoscopists.

Outcome. Procedural success was achieved in 92% of cases (23 of 25). All patients had relief of jaundice and cholestasis. Only one study reported on a long-term follow-up period [56]. In this paper, the average patency period for plastic 8.5-Fr stents was an impressive 211 days. Although this procedure, like EUS-guided hepaticogastrostomy, appears to be a promising and exciting alternative to percutaneous drainage in patients in whom ERCP has failed, it is at

V

present too early for definitive conclusions to be drawn. Further research is awaited, particularly randomized trials comparing EUS-guided choledochoduodenostomy and percutaneous approaches.

▥ EUS-Guided Cholecystostomy

The cornerstone in the management of patients with acute cholecystitis is surgical intervention. In patients deemed unfit for surgery, the most commonly used alternative treatment is percutaneous drainage. As it is usually easy to identify the gallbladder from the gastric antrum and/or the duodenal bulb and it is in close proximity to the enteral wall, the concept of transmural drainage of the gallbladder is a logical extension from other biliary and pancreatic drainage procedures. Internal drainage has potential advantages, as indwelling percutaneous catheters cause considerable patient discomfort.

The EUS-guided cholecystostomy procedure has been described in two case series including a total of 12 patients [57,58]. All patients were deemed unfit for surgery, usually because of severe co-morbidities. The shortest distance to the distended gallbladder was chosen from either the gastric antrum or the duodenal bulb, and the gallbladder was then punctured with a 19-G needle. After contrast injection, a 0.035″ guide wire was placed in the gallbladder. In the Korean series (nine patients), drainage was performed with a 5-Fr nasocholecystic catheter after dilation of the tract to 6 Fr. This catheter was left in situ until elective cholecystectomy in most cases. Surgery was not hampered by the indwelling catheter. In the Belgian series, dilation of the tract was performed with either a 6-Fr or 10-Fr cystotome, with subsequent placement of a nasocholecystic catheter and in one case combined with placement of a double-pigtail stent. In the other two patients, the nasocholecystic catheter was replaced endoscopically with double-pigtail stents several days after the initial drainage. All of the patients did well and had clinical resolution of their cholecystitis within 72 h after the EUS-guided cholecystostomy. There was one case of minor bile leakage and one pneumoperitoneum; both complications were managed conservatively and had no clinical consequences. Although these results are quite promising, prospective randomized trials comparing EUS-guided cholecystostomy with percutaneous drainage obviously need to be performed before any recommendations can be made with regard to the clinical value of EUS-guided cholecystostomy.

EUS-Guided Pancreatic Duct Drainage and Rendezvous

The main principle of endoscopic treatment in patients with chronic pancreatitis is decompression of the duct. It is thought that ductal hypertension due to stones or strictures is one of the key causes of pain in chronic pancreatitis. Endoscopic treatment, if necessary combined with extracorporeal shock-wave lithotripsy (ESWL), using ERCP is quite successful in experienced hands. It can lead to major relief of pain in up to 60–80% of patients if decompression is achieved [59–62]. Although a recent prospectively conducted randomized trial clearly favored surgery over endoscopic treatment [63], endoscopy is still the first-line treatment in many institutions and surgery is only considered when endoscopic treatment fails. Although successful cannulation of the pancreatic duct is achieved in over 90% of cases in expert hands, selective cannulation sometimes fails [64]. Obtaining access can sometimes be impossible, due to altered surgical anatomy, very tight strictures, severe inflammation, or pancreas divisum with orifice stenosis.

After surgical treatment for chronic pancreatitis, recurrent disease and complaints are not infrequent. In some series, drainage is inadequate in up to 20% of patients [65]. Depending on the type of surgical intervention, it may be impossible to continue with endoscopic treatment. Particularly after duodenum-preserving pancreatic head resection using a Beger or Whipple's procedure, it may be impossible to gain access to the pancreatic duct via ERCP. Recurrence after surgery can be caused by recurrent disease or stenosis of the pancreaticojejunostomy. In both cases, this can lead to dilation of the pancreatic duct. As the body and tail of the pancreas are easily identified from the stomach and duodenal bulb even after surgery, puncture and subsequent drainage of the pancreatic duct via linear EUS are possible, or a rendezvous procedure if the papilla can be reached. Four papers (case series, retrospective data, and one prospective study) have been published that evaluate EUS-guided drainage or rendezvous of the pancreatic duct [66–69]. Transluminal drainage was attempted in the papers by Kahaleh et al. [68] and Tessier et al. [69], whereas Mallery and co-workers [66] describe attempted rendezvous procedures. Both techniques were evaluated by Will et al. [67]. A total of 65 patients were described in these papers.

Procedure. All of the patients described received preprocedural prophylactic antibiotic treatment. With the therapeutic linear echo endoscope, the pancreas is examined from the stomach and duodenal bulb (**Fig. 41.6**). The site for puncture needs to be chosen with different parameters being taken into account. The distance to the gastric or duodenal wall is important, but it is also very important to obtain a view of the pancreatic duct longitudinally. This enables the endoscopist to look "into" the pancreatic duct and makes subsequent interventions over a guide wire much easier. Particularly in severe calcifying chronic pancreatitis, the duct may be hard to visualize due to the many acoustic shadows. This is another consideration when determining the puncture site. Finally, every effort should be made to guide the wire toward the pancreatic head and, if at all possible, to pass it into the duodenum or jejunum. This gives the endoscopist more wire to work with and reduces the chance of losing access when exchanging accessories. After successful puncture of the duct, a pancreatogram is obtained after removal of the stylet. As in biliary drainage procedures, it is preferable to use a 19-G needle, since a 0.035″ guidewire facilitates the further procedure due to its inherent stiffness. Particularly during repeated maneuvers when trying to pass a stenosis, the risk of shearing of the guide wire increases, as described in the section on biliary drainage procedures above. The EUS part of the procedure ends when the endoscopist has succeeded in passing the guide wire into the duodenum via the major or minor papilla. It is advisable to place plenty of guide wire in the duodenum, to increase the stability of the position when the duodenoscope is advanced into position.

When transmural drainage is attempted, the next step is dilating the fistula trajectory. Several methods have been described, using either a small-tipped ERCP cannula followed by a biliary dilation catheter and/or a biliary balloon dilation catheter or electrocautery with a cystotome. Our personal preference is to use a small-caliber (6 Fr) cystotome, as it is sometimes very hard, especially when the position of the echo endoscope is not ideal, to advance an accessory into the pancreatic duct, due to the severe fibrosis and scarring that occurs with chronic pancreatitis. When combined cutting/coagulation current is applied to the cystotome, passage into the duct is usually successful. If necessary, intraductal or anastomotic strictures can be dilated with either a biliary balloon dilation catheter or the cystotome. The procedure ends with placement of a 7-Fr straight endoprosthesis. Several weeks later, this can be exchanged for two stents, usually without problems, with the aid of a regular duodenoscope.

Complications. The complication rate with EUS-guided pancreatic duct drainage appears to be quite high; complications may be procedure-related or may develop later. In two series, stent migra-

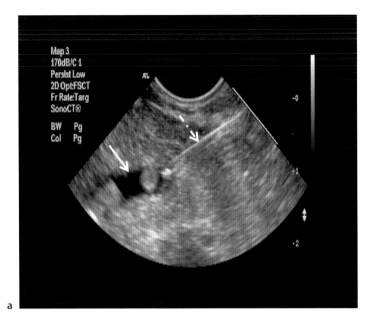

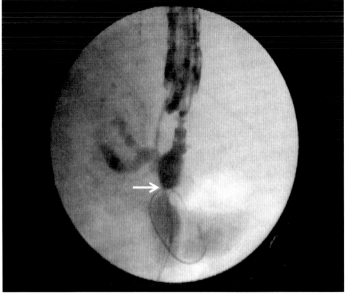

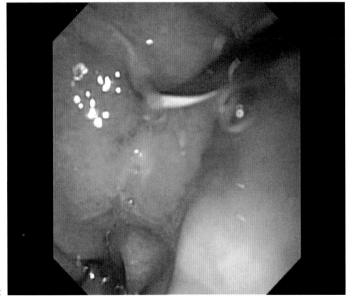

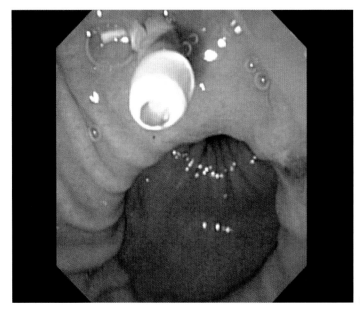

Fig. 41.6 Endoscopic ultrasound (EUS)-guided pancreatic duct gastrostomy in a patient with pain due to a stricture and ductal obstruction after a surgical pancreaticojejunostomy.

a EUS-guided puncture of the dilated pancreatic duct (arrow) with a 19-G needle (dashed arrow).

b Contrast injection through the puncture needle, with filling of the dilated pancreatic duct and the jejunal loop. The anastomotic stricture is nicely visible (arrow). A 6-Fr cystotome is advanced over a guide wire through the stricture into the jejunal loop.

c The puncture hole in the stomach, with a guide wire in position.

d The final situation, with a distal 7-Fr stent tip positioned in the stomach. The stent has been advanced through the stomach wall, pancreatic duct, and stricture, and its proximal tip is located in the jejunal loop.

tion and occlusions occurred in 20–55% of cases [67,69], and stent-induced strictures were also observed during the follow-up in one series [69]. Procedure-related complications varied between 5% and 44%. The most frequent complication was postprocedural pain, but severe pancreatitis, perforations, bleeding, and hematoma have been described. The numbers of patients are too small to judge whether the type of procedure and in particular the dilation modality used influence the complication rate. No procedure-related mortality has been reported.

Outcome. Long-term outcome data are not available. As was to be expected, approximately 65% of the patients experienced pain relief immediately after the procedure, as is seen after successful ERCP for obstructive chronic pancreatitis. The numbers are too small to judge whether a drainage procedure or a rendezvous procedure is more effective in relieving pain. EUS-guided drainage of the pancreatic duct is at present a technically challenging procedure with a relatively high complication rate, both procedure-related and stent-related. Although there is a subset of patients who can definitely benefit from these techniques, there is at present insufficient evidence to recommend the procedure on a routine basis. It should be further explored as part of a research program.

Future Indications for Therapeutic EUS

As shown above, the indications for performing EUS have shifted and are continuing to evolve. As with many other endoscopic interventions, EUS is moving from being a purely diagnostic procedure toward becoming an advanced therapeutic technique. This last section discusses some developments relating to possible future applications of interventional EUS, focusing on vascular interventions and the possible role of EUS in natural orifice transluminal endoscopic surgery (NOTES).

■ EUS and Vascular Interventions

EUS may have a potential role in both detecting and treating various lesions that cause gastrointestinal bleeding. With the detailed images EUS provides, it can potentially be of great value both for identifying the source of bleeding and for directing treatment, specifically through detailed visualization of the local vascular anatomy. This was first shown to be an effective approach in the localization and treatment of Dieulafoy lesions [70]. Another more recent paper described the use of EUS in the management of five patients with refractory bleeding from various sources despite intensive endoscopic and radiological treatment attempts [71]. Real-time EUS visualization was used to inject 99% alcohol into small (1–2 mm) feeding vessels of pseudoaneurysms and Dieulafoy lesions in three patients. In the other two patients, cyanoacrylate was injected into bleeding vessels in patients with a duodenal ulcer and a bleeding gastrointestinal stromal tumor (GIST). Interestingly, it was possible to monitor the efficacy of treatment directly using Doppler ultrasound. During severe gastrointestinal bleeding, it can occasionally be very difficult to visualize the exact source of the bleeding adequately. Since EUS imaging is not hindered by blood, EUS-guided therapy might be a useful adjunct in the endoscopic armamentarium. The development of the forward-viewing linear echo endoscope might overcome problems related to the sometimes awkward handling of the oblique-viewing linear echo endoscope.

EUS has also been used in transmural endovascular interventions. One case report describes the successful insertion of endovascular microcoils through a regular 22-G needle in a patient with ectopic varices refractory to conventional therapy [72]. Several porcine studies have been performed in which angiography of the major abdominal vessels [73], portal vein angiography, and pressure monitoring [74–77], and even cardiac catheterization [78], were performed. Although apparently safe in a porcine model, obvious issues of sterility and bleeding risk need to be assessed before any of these techniques can be used in humans.

■ EUS and NOTES

In addition to safe and effective closure, obtaining reliable and safe access to the (retro)peritoneal cavity is also very important for the further development of NOTES. EUS might be useful here, as it can adequately visualize surrounding structures, organs, and major blood vessels. In a porcine model, it was shown that NOTES incisions, especially in locations other than the anterior gastric wall, are potentially more safe and therefore more versatile when EUS is used [79]. It has been shown in porcine studies that it is possible to perform transmural lymphadenectomy [80], gastropexy [81], and tissue approximation [82] effectively using T-tags, which can be applied through a regular 19-G needle. To date, the most important addition of EUS to NOTES procedures is the identification of the best access point for specific procedures [83].

References

1. Voermans RP, Eisendrath P, Bruno MJ, Le Moine O, Devière J, Fockens P. Initial evaluation of a novel prototype forward-viewing US endoscope in transmural drainage of pancreatic pseudocysts (with videos). Gastrointest Endosc 2007;66:1013–7.
2. Yan BM, Myers RP. Neurolytic celiac plexus block for pain control in unresectable pancreatic cancer. Am J Gastroenterol 2007;102:430–8.
3. Wiersema MJ, Wiersema LM. Endosonography-guided celiac plexus neurolysis. Gastrointest Endosc 1996;44:656–62.
4. Gunaratnam NT, Sarma AV, Norton ID, Wiersema MJ. A prospective study of EUS-guided celiac plexus neurolysis for pancreatic cancer pain. Gastrointest Endosc 2001;54:316–24.
5. Levy M, Rajan E, Keeney G, Fletcher JG, Topazian M. Neural ganglia visualized by endoscopic ultrasound. Am J Gastroenterol 2006;101:1787–91.
6. Gleeson FC, Levy MJ, Papachristou GI, Pelaez-Luna M, Rajan E, Clain JE, et al. Frequency of visualization of presumed celiac ganglia by endoscopic ultrasound. Endoscopy 2007;39:620–4.
7. Chang KJ, Nguyen PT, Thompson JA, Kurosaki TT, Casey LR, Leung EC, et al. Phase I clinical trial of allogeneic mixed lymphocyte culture (cytoimplant) delivered by endoscopic ultrasound-guided fine-needle injection in patients with advanced pancreatic carcinoma. Cancer 2000;88:1325–35.
8. Farrell JJ, Senzer N, Hecht JR, Hanna N, Chung T, Nemunaitis J. Long-term data for endoscopic ultrasound (EUS) and percutaneous (PTA) guided intratumoral TNFerade gene delivery combined with chemoradiation in the treatment of locally advanced pancreatic cancer (LAPC) [abstract]. Gastrointest Endosc 2006;63:AB93.
9. Posner M, Chang KJ, Rosemurgy A, Stephenson J, Khan M, Reid T, et al. Multi-center phase II/III randomized controlled clinical trial using TNFerade combined with chemoradiation in patients with locally advanced pancreatic cancer (LAPC) [abstract]. J Clin Oncol 2007;25(Suppl):4518.
10. Hecht JR, Bedford R, Abbruzzese JL, Lahoti S, Reid TR, Soetikno RM, et al. A phase I/II trial of intratumoral endoscopic ultrasound injection of ONYX-015 with intravenous gemcitabine in unresectable pancreatic carcinoma. Clin Cancer Res 2003;9:555–61.
11. MacGill RS, Davis TA, Macko J, Mauceri HJ, Weichselbaum RR, King CR. Local gene delivery of tumor necrosis factor alpha can impact primary tumor growth and metastases through a host-mediated response. Clin Exp Metastasis 2007;24:521–31.
12. Goldberg SN, Mallery S, Gazelle GS, Brugge WR. EUS-guided radiofrequency ablation in the pancreas: results in a porcine model. Gastrointest Endosc 1999;50:392–401.
13. Chan HH, Nishioka NS, Mino M, Lauwers GY, Puricelli WP, Collier KN, et al. EUS-guided photodynamic therapy of the pancreas: a pilot study. Gastrointest Endosc 2004;59:95–9.
14. Chang BK, Timmerman RD. Stereotactic body radiation therapy: a comprehensive review. Am J Clin Oncol 2007;30:637–44.
15. Shirato H, Harada T, Harabayashi T, Hida K, Endo H, Kitamura K, et al. Feasibility of insertion/implantation of 2.0-mm-diameter gold internal fiducial markers for precise setup and real-time tumor tracking in radiotherapy. Int J Radiat Oncol Biol Phys 2003;56:240–7.
16. Whyte RI, Crownover R, Murphy MJ, Martin DP, Rice TW, DeCamp mm Jr, et al. Stereotactic radiosurgery for lung tumors: preliminary report of a phase I trial. Ann Thorac Surg 2003;75:1097–101.
17. Savides TJ. EUS-guided fine-needle insertion of radiopaque fiducials: X marks the spot. Gastrointest Endosc 2006;64:418–9.
18. Pishvaian AC, Collins B, Gagnon G, Ahlawat S, Haddad NG. EUS-guided fiducial placement for CyberKnife radiotherapy of mediastinal and abdominal malignancies. Gastrointest Endosc 2006;64:412–7.
19. Owens DJ, Savides TJ. EUS placement of metal fiducials by using a back-loaded technique with bone wax seal. Gastrointest Endosc 2009;69:972–3.
20. Sahel J, Bastid C, Pellat B, Schurgers P, Sarles H. Endoscopic cystoduodenostomy of cysts of chronic calcifying pancreatitis: a report of 20 cases. Pancreas 1987;2:447–53.
21. Cremer M, Devière J, Engelholm L. Endoscopic management of cysts and pseudocysts in chronic pancreatitis: long-term follow-up after 7 years of experience. Gastrointest Endosc 1989;35:1–9.
22. Fockens P, Johnson TG, van Dullemen HM, Huibregtse K, Tytgat GN. Endosonographic imaging of pancreatic pseudocysts before endoscopic transmural drainage. Gastrointest Endosc 1997;46:412–6.
23. Norton ID, Clain JE, Wiersema MJ, DiMagno EP, Petersen BT, Gostout CJ. Utility of endoscopic ultrasonography in endoscopic drainage of pancreatic pseudocysts in selected patients. Mayo Clin Proc 2001;76:794–8.

41

24. Varadarajulu S, Christein JD, Tamhane A, Drelichman ER, Wilcox CM. Prospective randomized trial comparing EUS and EGD for transmural drainage of pancreatic pseudocysts (with videos). Gastrointest Endosc 2008;68:1102–11.

25. Grimm H, Binmoeller KF, Soehendra N. Endosonography-guided drainage of a pancreatic pseudocyst. Gastrointest Endosc 1992;38:170–1.

26. Giovannini M, Bernardini D, Seitz JF. Cystogastrotomy entirely performed under endosonography guidance for pancreatic pseudocyst: results in six patients. Gastrointest Endosc 1998;48:200–3.

27. Wiersema MJ, Baron TH, Chari ST. Endosonography-guided pseudocyst drainage with a new large-channel linear scanning echoendoscope. Gastrointest Endosc 2001;53:811–3.

28. Chak A. Endosonographic-guided therapy of pancreatic pseudocysts. Gastrointest Endosc 2000;52:S23–7.

29. Kahaleh M, Shami VM, Conaway MR, Tokar J, Rockoff T, De La Rue SA, et al. Endoscopic ultrasound drainage of pancreatic pseudocyst: a prospective comparison with conventional endoscopic drainage. Endoscopy 2006;38: 355–9.

30. Poley J, Haringsma J, Darwish Murad S, Dees J, van Eijck C, Kuipers E. Endoscopic ultrasound (EUS) guided drainage of pseudocysts: safer and more effective compared to standard endoscopic drainage [abstract]. Gastrointest Endosc 2006;63:AB266.

31. Baron TH, Harewood GC, Morgan DE, Yates MR. Outcome differences after endoscopic drainage of pancreatic necrosis, acute pancreatic pseudocysts, and chronic pancreatic pseudocysts. Gastrointest Endosc 2002; 56:7–17.

32. Hookey LC, Debroux S, Delhaye M, Arvanitakis M, Le Moine O, Devière J. Endoscopic drainage of pancreatic-fluid collections in 116 patients: a comparison of etiologies, drainage techniques, and outcomes. Gastrointest Endosc 2006;63:635–43.

33. Papachristou GI, Takahashi N, Chahal P, Sarr MG, Baron TH. Peroral endoscopic drainage/debridement of walled-off pancreatic necrosis. Ann Surg 2007;245:943–51.

34. Seewald S, Groth S, Omar S, Imazu H, Seitz U, de Weerth A, et al. Aggressive endoscopic therapy for pancreatic necrosis and pancreatic abscess: a new safe and effective treatment algorithm (videos). Gastrointest Endosc 2005;62:92–100.

35. Voermans RP, Veldkamp MC, Rauws EA, Bruno MJ, Fockens P. Endoscopic transluminal debridement of symptomatic organized pancreatic necrosis (with videos). Gastrointest Endosc 2007;66:909–16.

36. Bradley EL 3rd. A clinically based classification system for acute pancreatitis. Summary of the International Symposium on Acute Pancreatitis, Atlanta, Ga, September 11 through 13, 1992. Arch Surg 1993;128:586–90.

37. Bradley EL, Clements JL Jr, Gonzalez AC. The natural history of pancreatic pseudocysts: a unified concept of management. Am J Surg 1979;137: 135–41.

38. Jansen JM, Hanrath A, Rauws EA, Bruno MJ, Fockens P. Intracystic wire exchange facilitating insertion of multiple stents during endoscopic drainage of pancreatic pseudocysts. Gastrointest Endosc 2007;66: 157–61.

39. Cahen D, Rauws E, Fockens P, Weverling G, Huibregtse K, Bruno M. Endoscopic drainage of pancreatic pseudocysts: long-term outcome and procedural factors associated with safe and successful treatment. Endoscopy 2005;37:977–83.

40. Antillon MR, Shah RJ, Stiegmann G, Chen YK. Single-step EUS-guided transmural drainage of simple and complicated pancreatic pseudocysts. Gastrointest Endosc 2006;63:797–803.

41. Baron TH, Thaggard WG, Morgan DE, Stanley RJ. Endoscopic therapy for organized pancreatic necrosis. Gastroenterology 1996;111:755–64.

42. Kruger M, Schneider AS, Manns MP, Meier PN. Endoscopic management of pancreatic pseudocysts or abscesses after an EUS-guided 1-step procedure for initial access. Gastrointest Endosc 2006;63:409–16.

43. Sahel J. Endoscopic drainage of pancreatic cysts. Endoscopy 1991;23: 181–4.

44. Varadarajulu S, Lopes TL, Wilcox CM, Drelichman ER, Kilgore ML, Christein JD. EUS versus surgical cyst-gastrostomy for management of pancreatic pseudocysts. Gastrointest Endosc 2008;68:649–55.

45. Giovannini M, Bories E, Moutardier V, Pesenti C, Guillemin A, Lelong B, et al. Drainage of deep pelvic abscesses using therapeutic echo endoscopy. Endoscopy 2003;35:511–4.

46. Trevino JM, Drelichman ER, Varadarajulu S. Modified technique for EUS-guided drainage of pelvic abscess (with video). Gastrointest Endosc 2008;68:1215–9.

47. Varadarajulu S, Drelichman ER. EUS-guided drainage of pelvic abscess (with video). Gastrointest Endosc 2007;66:372–6.

48. van Delden OM, Lameris JS. Percutaneous drainage and stenting for palliation of malignant bile duct obstruction. Eur Radiol 2008;18:448–56.

49. Artifon EL, Chaves DM, Ishioka S, Souza TF, Matuguma SE, Sakai P. Echo-guided hepatico-gastrostomy: a case report. Clinics 2007;62:799–802.

50. Bories E, Pesenti C, Caillol F, Lopes C, Giovannini M. Transgastric endoscopic ultrasonography-guided biliary drainage: results of a pilot study. Endoscopy 2007;39:287–91.

51. Burmester E, Niehaus J, Leineweber T, Huetteroth T. EUS-cholangio-drainage of the bile duct: report of 4 cases. Gastrointest Endosc 2003;57: 246–51.

52. Fujita N, Noda Y, Kobayashi G, Ito K, Obana T, Horaguchi J, et al. Temporary endosonography-guided biliary drainage for transgastrointestinal deployment of a self-expandable metallic stent. J Gastroenterol 2008;43:637–40.

53. Giovannini M, Dotti M, Bories E, Moutardier V, Pesenti C, Danisi C, et al. Hepaticogastrostomy by echo-endoscopy as a palliative treatment in a patient with metastatic biliary obstruction. Endoscopy 2003;35:1076–8.

54. Puspok A, Lomoschitz F, Dejaco C, Hejna M, Sautner T, Gangl A. Endoscopic ultrasound guided therapy of benign and malignant biliary obstruction: a case series. Am J Gastroenterol 2005;100:1743–7.

55. Will U, Thieme A, Fueldner F, Gerlach R, Wanzar I, Meyer F. Treatment of biliary obstruction in selected patients by endoscopic ultrasonography (EUS)-guided transluminal biliary drainage. Endoscopy 2007;39:292–5.

56. Yamao K, Bhatia V, Mizuno N, Sawaki A, Ishikawa H, Tajika M, et al. EUS-guided choledochoduodenostomy for palliative biliary drainage in patients with malignant biliary obstruction: results of long-term follow-up. Endoscopy 2008;40:340–2.

57. Kwan V, Eisendrath P, Antaki F, Le Moine O, Devière J. EUS-guided cholecystenterostomy: a new technique (with videos). Gastrointest Endosc 2007;66:582–6.

58. Lee SS, Park do H, Hwang CY, Ahn CS, Lee TY, Seo DW, et al. EUS-guided transmural cholecystostomy as rescue management for acute cholecystitis in elderly or high-risk patients: a prospective feasibility study. Gastrointest Endosc 2007;66:1008–12.

59. Delhaye M, Arvanitakis M, Verset G, Cremer M, Devière J. Long-term clinical outcome after endoscopic pancreatic ductal drainage for patients with painful chronic pancreatitis. Clin Gastroenterol Hepatol 2004;2: 1096–106.

60. Dumonceau JM, Costamagna G, Tringali A, Vahedi K, Delhaye M, Hittelet A, et al. Treatment for painful calcified chronic pancreatitis: extracorporeal shock wave lithotripsy versus endoscopic treatment: a randomised controlled trial. Gut 2007;56:545–52.

61. Farnbacher MJ, Muhldorfer S, Wehler M, Fischer B, Hahn EG, Schneider HT. Interventional endoscopic therapy in chronic pancreatitis including temporary stenting: a definitive treatment? Scand J Gastroenterol 2006; 41:111–7.

62. Rösch T, Daniel S, Scholz M, Huibregtse K, Smits M, Schneider T, et al. Endoscopic treatment of chronic pancreatitis: a multicenter study of 1000 patients with long-term follow-up. Endoscopy 2002;34:765–71.

63. Cahen DL, Gouma DJ, Nio Y, Rauws EA, Boermeester MA, Busch OR, et al. Endoscopic versus surgical drainage of the pancreatic duct in chronic pancreatitis. N Engl J Med 2007;356:676–84.

64. Fink AS, Perez de Ayala V, Chapman M, Cotton PB. Radiologic pitfalls in endoscopic retrograde pancreatography. Pancreas 1986;1:180–7.

65. Markowitz JS, Rattner DW, Warshaw AL. Failure of symptomatic relief after pancreaticojejunal decompression for chronic pancreatitis. Strategies for salvage. Arch Surg 1994;129:374–80.

66. Mallery S, Matlock J, Freeman ML. EUS-guided rendezvous drainage of obstructed biliary and pancreatic ducts: Report of 6 cases. Gastrointest Endosc 2004;59:100–7.

67. Will U, Fueldner F, Thieme AK, Goldmann B, Gerlach R, Wanzar I,, et al. Transgastric pancreatography and EUS-guided drainage of the pancreatic duct. J Hepatobiliary Pancreat Surg 2007;14:377–82.

68. Kahaleh M, Hernandez AJ, Tokar J, Adams RB, Shami VM, Yeaton P. EUS-guided pancreaticogastrostomy: analysis of its efficacy to drain inaccessible pancreatic ducts. Gastrointest Endosc 2007;65:224–30.

69. Tessier G, Bories E, Arvanitakis M, Hittelet A, Pesenti C, Le Moine O, et al. EUS-guided pancreatogastrostomy and pancreatobulbostomy for the treatment of pain in patients with pancreatic ductal dilatation inaccessible for transpapillary endoscopic therapy. Gastrointest Endosc 2007;65:233–41.

70. Fockens P, Meenan J, van Dullemen HM, Bolwerk CJ, Tytgat GN. Dieulafoy's disease: endosonographic detection and endosonography-guided treatment. Gastrointest Endosc 1996;44:437–42.

71. Levy MJ, Wong Kee Song LM, Farnell MB, Misra S, Sarr MG, Gostout CJ. Endoscopic ultrasound (EUS)-guided angiotherapy of refractory gastrointestinal bleeding. Am J Gastroenterol 2008;103:352–9.

72. Levy MJ, Wong Kee Song LM, Kendrick ML, Misra S, Gostout CJ. EUS-guided coil embolization for refractory ectopic variceal bleeding (with videos). Gastrointest Endosc 2008;67:572–4.

73. Magno P, Ko CW, Buscaglia JM, Giday SA, Jagannath SB, Clarke JO,, et al. EUS-guided angiography: a novel approach to diagnostic and therapeutic interventions in the vascular system. Gastrointest Endosc 2007;66:587–91.

74. Lai L, Poneros J, Santilli J, Brugge W. EUS-guided portal vein catheterization and pressure measurement in an animal model: a pilot study of feasibility. Gastrointest Endosc 2004;59:280–3.

75. Matthes K, Sahani D, Holalkere NS, Mino-Kenudson M, Brugge WR. Feasibility of endoscopic ultrasound-guided portal vein embolization with Enteryx. Acta Gastroenterol Belg 2005;68:412–5.

76. Giday SA, Clarke JO, Buscaglia JM, Shin EJ, Ko CW, Magno P, et al. EUS-guided portal vein catheterization: a promising novel approach for portal angiography and portal vein pressure measurements. Gastrointest Endosc 2008;67:338–42.

77. Buscaglia JM, Shin EJ, Clarke JO, Giday SA, Ko CW, Thuluvath PJ, et al. Endoscopic retrograde cholangiopancreatography, but not esophagogastroduodenoscopy or colonoscopy, significantly increases portal venous pressure: direct portal pressure measurements through endoscopic ultrasound-guided cannulation. Endoscopy 2008;40:670–4.

78. Fritscher-Ravens A, Ganbari A, Mosse CA, Swain P, Koehler P, Patel K. Transesophageal endoscopic ultrasound-guided access to the heart. Endoscopy 2007;39:385–9.

79. Elmunzer BJ, Schomisch SJ, Trunzo JA, Poulose BK, Delaney CP, McGee MF, et al. EUS in localizing safe alternate access sites for natural orifice transluminal endoscopic surgery: initial experience in a porcine model. Gastrointest Endosc 2009;69:108–14.

80. Fritscher-Ravens A, Mosse CA, Ikeda K, Swain P. Endoscopic transgastric lymphadenectomy by using EUS for selection and guidance. Gastrointest Endosc 2006;63:302–6.

81. Fritscher-Ravens A, Mosse CA, Mukherjee D, Yazaki E, Park PO, Mills T, et al. Transgastric gastropexy and hiatal hernia repair for GERD under EUS control: a porcine model. Gastrointest Endosc 2004;59:89–95.

82. Fritscher-Ravens A, Mosse CA, Mills TN, Mukherjee D, Park PO, Swain P. A through-the-scope device for suturing and tissue approximation under EUS control. Gastrointest Endosc 2002;56:737–42.

83. Fritscher-Ravens A, Ghanbari A, Cuming T, Kahle E, Niemann H, Koehler P, et al. Comparative study of NOTES alone vs. EUS-guided NOTES procedures. Endoscopy 2008;40:925–30.

41

VI

Upper Gastrointestinal Tract Disease

Section editors:
Charles J. Lightdale, Hisao Tajiri, Jaques J.G.J.M. Bergman

42 Esophageal Diseases

Neil Gupta and Prateek Sharma

Anatomy

The esophagus is a muscular tube that connects the pharynx to the stomach. The proximal and distal borders of the esophagus are the upper and lower esophageal sphincter, respectively. The esophagus has a length ranging from 18 to 26 cm and consists of four layers: the mucosa, submucosa, muscularis propria, and adventitia. In contrast to the remainder of the gastrointestinal tract, it has no serosa. The mucosa of the esophagus is made up of squamous epithelium that appears pearly-white during endoscopy. The muscularis propria consists of both skeletal and smooth muscle, with the proximal third of the esophagus containing skeletal muscle, the distal third containing smooth muscle, and the middle third containing a mixture of smooth and skeletal muscle.

There are only a few anatomic landmarks that are visible during esophageal endoscopy. These include compressions from the aortic arch and left atrium, squamocolumnar junction (SCJ), gastroesophageal junction (GEJ), and lower esophageal sphincter (LES). At about 23 cm from the incisors, the aortic arch crosses the esophagus and may cause a visible arterial pulse on the left anterior esophageal wall. About 10 cm distal to the aortic arch, the left atrium may cause visible rhythmic pulsations. The SCJ is the point at which the squamous epithelium of the esophagus abuts the columnar epithelium of the stomach. This is seen during endoscopy as a change from pearly-white mucosa to red, salmon-colored mucosa (**Fig. 42.1**). Adequate distension of the esophagus will produce a straight circumferential line demarcating the borders of the squamous and columnar epithelium. If the lumen is not adequately distended, the SCJ may appear irregular or serrated, and is hence referred to as the Z-line. Normally, the SCJ is located at the distal edge of the LES and at the same level as the diaphragmatic hiatus and the GEJ.

Identification of the exact GEJ is not possible during endoscopy. Instead, luminal anatomy is used as a surrogate landmark to identify the GEJ. Endoscopically, the stomach has longitudinal mucosal folds, while the esophagus does not. Normally, the top of these gastric folds corresponds with the location of the SCJ and the diaphragmatic hiatus. As a result, the top of the gastric folds is an endoscopic landmark that can determine the location of the GEJ. The distal limit of the esophageal palisade vessels has also been used to identify the GEJ, but this is less reliable in comparison with the top of the gastric folds [1,2]. The presence of a hiatal hernia can displace the diaphragmatic hiatus distally, whereas in the setting of Barrett's esophagus the SCJ is displaced proximally.

The distal esophagus also contains two rings, the A and B rings, which provide the proximal and distal borders of the LES. The A ring is a symmetrical band of hypertrophied muscle that constricts the esophageal lumen. It is covered with squamous epithelium and corresponds to the upper end of the LES. The B ring, which is also known as the Schatzki ring, is a thin mucosal membrane composed of only mucosa and submucosa that is seen at the SCJ. It has squamous epithelium on its proximal surface and columnar epithelium on its distal surface. During endoscopy, the proximal margin of the LES can be seen by the presence of four to six smooth mucosal folds that radiate to a central point in the esophageal lumen. This requires a reduction in air inflation during endoscopy. If the esophagus is

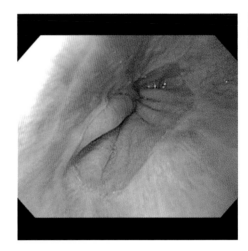

Fig. 42.1 The normal squamocolumnar junction.

distended with air, the mucosal folds will be effaced and the LES will open.

Mucosal Diseases

Reflux Esophagitis

Upper gastrointestinal endoscopy is the diagnostic method of choice when evaluating patients with chronic gastroesophageal reflux disease (GERD) for complications. While an estimated 60–70% of these patients have normal esophageal mucosa on endoscopy, the remainder have visible abnormalities [3–5]. Approximately 5% of patients undergoing upper endoscopy for any indication may have erosive esophagitis [6]. However, higher estimates for the prevalence of erosive esophagitis in the general population have been published, ranging up to 15.5% [3]. The visual appearance of erosive esophagitis can vary between small, subtle erosions involving just the SCJ to severe hemorrhagic ulcerations involving the entire esophageal mucosa (**Fig. 42.2**). In general, erosive esophagitis should begin at the SCJ and progress proximally. If mucosal abnormalities of the proximal or mid-esophagus are seen with a normal-appearing SCJ, then consideration should be given to nonreflux causes of esophagitis.

Unfortunately, the correlation between symptoms of gastroesophageal reflux and the presence of erosive esophagitis is poor. The majority of patients with gastroesophageal reflux symptoms have no visible abnormalities in the esophageal mucosa, and in addition erosive esophagitis can often be found in patients who are asymptomatic [3]. While the clinical characteristics of patients with nonerosive reflux disease and erosive esophagitis are generally the same, patients with erosive esophagitis are more likely to be male and have a hiatal hernia [7]. In addition, obesity increases the risk for having erosive esophagitis on upper endoscopy [8,9]. Recent studies using high-resolution magnification endoscopy and narrow-band imaging (NBI) have challenged the exact prevalence of

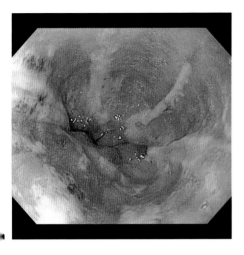 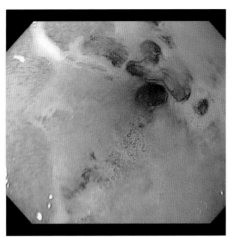

Fig. 42.2
a Mucosal breaks and erosions over multiple folds, consistent with Los Angeles grade C erosive esophagitis.
b Circumferential mucosal breaks and erosions with stricture formation, consistent with Los Angeles grade D erosive esophagitis.

nonerosive reflux disease, as they have found minor visible changes in patients previously characterized as having normal esophageal mucosa [10,11]. As a result, the term "minimal-change esophagitis" has been developed. However, the clinical relevance of this entity has yet to be determined, especially as there are concerns regarding interobserver and intra-observer reliability in identifying these small lesions [12–14].

Multiple endoscopic grading systems have been developed and used for characterizing erosive esophagitis, but none of the available systems is without flaws. The three most widely used scoring systems are the Savary–Miller classification system, the Hetzel–Dent classification system, and the Los Angeles classification system. Of the three systems, the Los Angeles system is the most commonly used in clinical practice and research studies.

- The Savary–Miller system was first published in 1977 [15]. Grades range from 0 to V, with grade 0 representing normal mucosa, grades I–III representing various degrees of esophagitis, and grades IV and V used for complications of esophagitis, including strictures and Barrett's esophagus. This system requires the endoscopist to make determinations of lesion depth and length, which can be difficult. In addition, because complications of esophagitis are grouped into the highest grades irrespective of the presence or absence of mucosal damage, the system is not well suited for documenting healing, as patients with Barrett's esophagus or strictures would remain in the same grade despite mucosal healing.
- The Hetzel–Dent classification was first published in 1988 [16]. Grades range from 0 to IV and are based only on the extent of mucosa that is injured. However, the system fails to recognize the significance of complications of esophagitis.
- In 1991, a more complex system for assessing metaplasia, ulceration, stricture, and esophagitis (MUSE) was developed for research purposes [17]. The system allows for separate assessments of esophagitis and its complications, but is rarely used in clinical practice due to its complexity.
- In response to the lack of a unified system for the assessment of esophagitis that was suitable for clinical practice, the Los Angeles classification was developed in 1996 [18]. Grades range from A to D and are based on the extent, number, and length of lesions seen (**Table 42.1**). Unlike previous systems, the Los Angeles system does not rely on lesion depth, but instead introduced the term "mucosal break" to characterize any mucosal lesion, regardless of depth.

All of the various esophagitis grading systems have been evaluated in multiple trials for both reliability and correlation with clinical outcomes. The Los Angeles, Hetzel–Dent, and MUSE systems have

Table 42.1 Endoscopic grading of erosive esophagitis using the Los Angeles classification

Grade	Description
A	One or more mucosal breaks confined to the mucosal folds, each longer than 5 mm
B	At least one mucosal break more than 5 mm long confined to the mucosal folds but not continuous between the tops of two mucosal folds
C	At least one mucosal break continuous between the tops of two or more mucosal folds but not circumferential (**Fig. 42.2 a**)
D	Circumferential mucosal breaks (**Fig. 42.2 b**)

42

been found to have good interobserver and intra-observer reliability, with the Los Angeles and Hetzel–Dent systems being reliable regardless of the endoscopist's level of experience [19,20]. Preliminary data have revealed that examination with the combination of conventional light and NBI is superior to conventional light alone with regard to interobserver and intra-observer reliability [21]. Both the Hetzel–Dent and Los Angeles systems have been found to correlate with outcomes of acid-suppressant therapy and time needed to heal esophagitis [16].

While most patients with symptoms of GERD can be empirically treated with acid-suppression therapy, endoscopy should be performed if there is a concern for complications of esophagitis, risk factors for Barrett's esophagus, or continued symptoms despite empiric therapy [22]. If visible mucosal abnormalities typical of reflux esophagitis are seen, biopsies are generally not needed unless there is an immunocompromised state, concern for malignancy, or predominance of esophagitis in the proximal or mid-esophagus [22]. Patients with erosive esophagitis should be started on acid-suppression therapy with proton-pump inhibitors (PPI). In the past, repeat endoscopies to evaluate for mucosal healing were not routinely required. However, recent data suggest that in selected patients with erosive esophagitis (especially those with severe grades), a repeat endoscopy may be considered after mucosal healing has been achieved, to exclude the presence of underlying Barrett's esophagus [23,24].

Acid-suppression therapy and antireflux surgery are the mainstays of therapy for patients with GERD. Therapy with a PPI once a day will result in healing of erosive esophagitis in 80–90 % of patients, but complete resolution of GERD symptoms can be achieved in less than 60 % of patients treated with PPI therapy [25]. Once endoscopic healing has occurred, maintenance therapy with a PPI has a relapse rate after 12 months of only 13 %, in comparison with

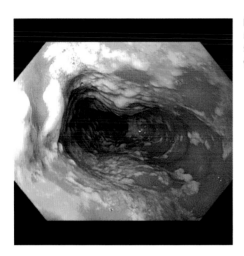

Fig. 42.3 Multiple raised, plaque-like lesions in *Candida* esophagitis.

Table 42.2 Endoscopic grading of **Candida esophagitis**

Grade	Description
I	Raised whitish plaques less than 2 mm in diameter without ulceration
II	Raised whitish plaques greater than 2 mm in diameter without ulceration
III	Confluent linear and nodular plaques with ulceration
IV	Grade III findings with narrowing of the esophageal lumen

VI

relapse rates of 60% and 72% with H_2 antagonists and placebo, respectively [26]. Antireflux surgery in patients with typical GERD symptoms results in symptomatic improvement and esophagitis healing in over 90% of patients [27]. Recent technological advances have allowed the development of different endoscopic therapies, including radiofrequency energy, endoscopic suturing, and injection therapy. However, none of the endoscopic techniques is at present a mainstream therapy for GERD.

▪ Infectious Esophagitis

Esophageal infections are an uncommon finding in immunocompetent individuals. They are more common in immunosuppressed patients, such as those with human immunodeficiency virus infection, hematological malignancy, recent chemotherapy or immunosuppressive therapy, and organ transplantation patients. However, esophageal infections can develop in immunocompetent patients, especially if they have underlying esophageal disease. Patients with esophageal infections generally present with odynophagia and/or dysphagia. Severe cases can result in dehydration and malnutrition. Upper endoscopy is the preferred diagnostic test for esophageal infections, as it allows identification of mucosal lesions and provides an opportunity to obtain samples through tissue biopsy or mucosal brushings.

Candida Esophagitis

Candida is the most common cause of infectious esophagitis. In addition to the immunocompromised states listed earlier, many other conditions can predispose individuals to *Candida* esophagitis, including diabetes mellitus, adrenal insufficiency, alcoholism, advanced age, inhaled glucocorticoid use, and acid-suppression therapy [28,29]. Esophageal diseases that result in luminal stasis have

also been associated with an increased risk for this condition. Not all cases of *Candida* esophagitis are symptomatic, with one series reporting a prevalence of 20% in normal healthy adults, and with up to 40% of immunocompromised patients being asymptomatic [30,31].

The endoscopic appearance of esophageal candidiasis ranges from erythematous, friable mucosa to a white pseudomembrane carpeting the mucosa (**Fig. 42.3**). It can be distributed throughout the esophagus, but the mucosa just proximal to the SCJ is generally less affected. *Candida* plaques cannot be washed away, and when they are brushed there is generally bleeding at the attachment site. Biopsies and brushings should always be obtained to evaluate for coexisting infections, and the severity of *Candida* esophagitis should be graded endoscopically [32] (**Table 42.2**).

Endoscopy is not required in all patients with suspected esophageal candidiasis. The presence of oral candidiasis and esophageal symptoms has a high predictive value for the presence of esophageal candidiasis, and in these patients empiric antifungal therapy is appropriate [31]. If the patient fails to respond, then endoscopy should be performed. On the other hand, the absence of oral thrush does not exclude the presence of *Candida* esophagitis [31]. Patients in whom there is a clinical suspicion for *Candida* esophagitis, but who do not have oral thrush, should therefore undergo endoscopy for diagnosis. All patients diagnosed with symptomatic esophageal candidiasis should receive antifungal therapy.

Herpes Simplex Esophagitis

Herpes simplex (HSV) esophagitis can occur in both immunocompromised and immunocompetent hosts. In immunocompetent patients, the disease is self-limited, but in immunocompromised patients, it can be prolonged and severe. The endoscopic appearance of HSV esophagitis depends on how long the infection has been present. During the early stages, small vesicular lesions with surrounding erythema are seen. The vesicles are fragile, and as the infection progresses they slough and form well-demarcated ulcers with raised edges. If left untreated, the ulcers can coalesce and begin to form inflammatory exudates, which may be misinterpreted as *Candida* esophagitis [33].

Since epithelial cells are needed to make the diagnosis, biopsy samples should be obtained from the ulcer edges and not from the granulation tissue in the center. In immunocompetent patients, the disease is self-limited, and the treatment is therefore mainly supportive. Antiviral therapy is generally not needed, but may hasten recovery if instituted early in the course of the infection [33]. Immunocompromised patients, however, are unlikely to recover spontaneously, and antiviral therapy should therefore be given regardless of symptom duration [33].

Cytomegalovirus Esophagitis

Cytomegalovirus (CMV) esophagitis differs from other types of infectious esophagitis, as it has a more insidious presentation and is generally associated with systemic infection. It can produce different types of esophageal ulceration, varying from large and deep to small and shallow [34]. However, most patients do have multiple lesions. The endoscopist must rely on biopsies for diagnosis, as neither the clinical nor endoscopic presentation is specific enough. The virus typically infects endothelial cells and fibroblasts but spares squamous epithelium, and biopsies must therefore be obtained from the center of the ulcer and not the margins. Up to 8–10 biopsies may be needed to adequately exclude the diagnosis of CMV esophagitis, and cytological brushings generally do not enhance the diagnostic yield [35,36]. All patients with CMV esophagitis should receive antiviral therapy.

Other Infections

In addition to *Candida*, HSV, and CMV, many other pathogens have been found to cause infection in the esophagus (**Fig. 42.4**). These include human immunodeficiency virus, *Mycobacterium tuberculosis*, *Histoplasma capsulatum*, and *Treponema pallidum*. These pathogens can cause a wide variety of esophageal ulcerations. In most cases, tissue biopsies and cytological brushings provide the diagnosis. However, the diagnosis of human immunodeficiency virus (HIV) esophagitis is one of exclusion and requires that other infections (*Candida*, CMV, HSV) are not present.

▦ Pill-Induced Esophagitis

Pharmacotherapy through orally administered tablets and capsules offers a convenient, noninvasive method for medical therapy. However, the high concentration of potent chemicals can result in significant injury to the esophagus. Over 1000 cases of medication-induced esophagitis have been reported in the medical literature, but this is still felt to be an underreported disease process [37]. A multitude of medications have been associated with esophagitis (**Table 42.3**). The exact mechanism of esophagitis for many medications is only speculative, but at least four pathophysiologic processes have been hypothesized. Some agents such as tetracycline, ascorbic acid, and ferrous sulfate produce acidic solutions when dissolved in water, while others such as phenytoin sodium and alendronate produce an alkaline solution. Medications that produce neutral solutions can still cause injury by creating hyperosmolar solutions, or mucosal injury may result from direct drug toxicity.

Patients of all ages are at risk for medication-induced esophagitis [37]. In addition, patients with preexisting anatomic or motility disorders of the esophagus may also have an increased risk; esophageal strictures, esophageal dysmotility, and even extrinsic compression from left atrial enlargement are all documented risk factors. However, most patients have normal esophageal function and anatomy. While this seems counterintuitive, normal individuals have significant pill retention especially if pills are swallowed without water or while the individual is supine [38]. Large pills and those with sticky surfaces are more likely to be retained than those without these features [39]. Finally, several reports have suggested that sustained-release formulations may be more likely to cause esophagitis than standard preparations, but this needs to be investigated further.

Pill esophagitis can present with a variety of symptoms, ranging from the acute onset of severe odynophagia to an almost asymptomatic, chronic esophageal injury. The classic presentation is a sudden onset of odynophagia that is exacerbated by swallowing. With careful questioning, a history of pill ingestion with little to no water or ingestion followed by immediate reclining may be obtained. Patients may even have a sensation of a retained pill in the esophagus. However, others can present with symptoms suggestive of GERD, infectious esophagitis, or progressive esophageal strictures. Hemorrhage can also occur, especially with nonsteroidal anti-inflammatory drugs (NSAIDs), and can be severe if ulcerations penetrate the esophageal wall into the major vessels. The association between medication and esophageal injury can often be missed in these patients, and as a result, medication-induced esophagitis should be considered in patients with esophageal inflammation or stricturing that is difficult to control.

In nonsevere cases, patients with typical symptoms and a history of potentially injurious medication ingestion can forego diagnostic testing and be treated empirically [37]. Those with severe and/or progressive symptoms despite empiric therapy should undergo upper endoscopy [37]. A wide range of endoscopic findings may be seen in pill-induced esophagitis, making the diagnosis based on endoscopic findings alone difficult. Patients can have a few discrete ulcers with normal surrounding mucosa or have circumferential ulcerations involving a large segment of the esophagus (**Fig. 42.5**). Severe cases can present with hemorrhagic ulcerations, stricture formation, and even pseudotumors. Biopsy and brushings of the lesions can help the endoscopist exclude alternative etiologies such as infection and neoplasm. However, no single endoscopic finding is conclusive for pill-induced esophagitis. Finally, no therapy for pill-induced esophagitis has been proven to alter the natural history of the disease. Treatment is directed at avoidance of the offending medication, symptom control, and maintenance of hydration. Topical anesthetics, sucralfate, and antisecretory therapy are often used, despite the absence of clinical data proving their efficacy.

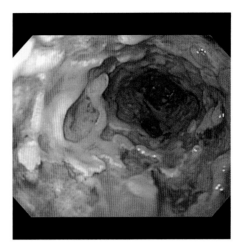

Fig. 42.4 Esophageal ulcerations in human immunodeficiency virus (HIV) infection.

Table 42.3 Medications that cause esophageal injury

Angiotensin-converting enzyme inhibitors
Aspirin
Benzodiazepines
Beta-blockers
Bisphosphonates
Calcium channel blockers
Corticosteroids
Coumarin derivatives
Emepronium bromide
Erythromycin
Ferrous sulfate or succinate
Lincosamides
Methylxanthines
Morphine
Nonsteroidal anti-inflammatory drugs (NSAIDs)
Nucleoside reverse transcriptase inhibitors
Oral contraceptives
Penicillins
Phenytoin
Potassium chloride
Quinidine
Rifampin
Sulfonamide antibiotics
Sulfonylureas
Tetracyclines
Tinidazole
Valproic acid
Vitamins containing minerals

42

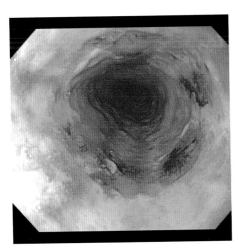

Fig. 42.5 Pill-induced esophagitis due to doxycycline administration.

Pill-induced esophagitis is preventable with proper medication administration. Patients should be instructed to drink at least 120 mL of fluid (4 fluid ounces) with any pill (twice as much for high-risk medications), always take pills when in an upright position, and to remain upright for at least 30 min after pill ingestion [37].

Corrosive Esophagitis

Ingestion of caustic substances can result in severe injury to the esophagus, and while most cases are not life-threatening, such injuries can result in lifelong esophageal disease. The extent of the injury generally depends on the substance and quantity ingested, along with its concentration, physical state, and the duration of exposure. Ingested agents can be separated into two categories—alkaline and acidic. Ingestion of alkaline substances, such as button batteries, lye, bleach, drain cleaners, and other household products are thought to be the most common cases. The primary difference in the pathophysiology of injury between the two substances is that alkaline agents have rapid tissue penetration; these agents have a solvent effect on the lipoprotein lining, causing liquefaction necrosis into the deep layers of the esophagus. In comparison, acidic agents cause a coagulation necrosis that inhibits penetration of the caustic substance. Ingestion of acidic agents is often limited by strong odors and immediate pain on swallowing, whereas alkaline agents are often odorless and tasteless. If the ingested material is solid or granular, the injury is likely to be deeper but focal. Despite pathophysiological differences, some studies have suggested that there is no difference in the rates of esophageal injury between the ingestion of acidic and alkaline substances [40].

Caustic injuries to the esophagus are characterized using the same method as burn injuries to the skin [40,41]. First-degree injuries are superficial and limited to the mucosa of the esophagus. There is generally some edema and erythema of the mucosa that subsequently sloughs off without any scarring or risk for stricture formation. Second-degree injuries are those that penetrate into the submucosa and muscle layers of the esophagus. Erosions, ulcerations, and blisters with and without hemorrhage can be seen in the acute period, with the majority of scar and stricture formation occurring over the next 8 weeks. Second-degree injuries can be further characterized as grade IIA if the ulcerations are patchy or linear and grade IIB if circumferential. Third-degree injuries are full-thickness injuries that carry a high risk for perforation and need for surgical therapy; they can appear as deep ulcerations with black or gray discoloration. Strictures rarely occur in patients with grade I or IIA injuries, but patients with grade IIB and III injuries are at high risk for stricture formation [40–42]. If third-degree injuries are seen

during endoscopy, the endoscope should be immediately withdrawn due to the risk of perforation.

In the acute period, most patients have symptoms including persistent salivation, vomiting, hematemesis, dysphagia, odynophagia, and chest pain. There may be visible injury to the oral cavity and symptoms of upper airway injury, including hoarseness and stridor. Symptoms can progress rapidly, especially in patients with third-degree burns. Patients without symptoms or signs of visible injury on physical examination are unlikely to have significant esophageal injury [43]. Stricture formation does not usually occur until weeks after caustic ingestion and can take up to a year to become clinically apparent.

Initial interventions in the acute setting should be directed toward airway protection, volume resuscitation, and assessment for perforation. Upright chest and abdominal films may reveal evidence of perforation. However, if plain films are normal and perforation is still suspected, imaging with either fluoroscopy or computed tomography (CT), enhanced with orally administered water-soluble contrast, should be obtained to exclude perforation. Due to the poor correlation between symptoms and the degree of injury, upper endoscopy should be performed in all patients with a history of caustic substance ingestion once the patient has been stabilized and perforation has been excluded. The extent of injury may be better assessed if endoscopy is performed within 72 h [40,41]. Regardless of the extent of injury, no therapy—including glucocorticoids, antibiotics, and neutralization of the caustic substance—has been found to reduce the risk for future esophageal disease after ingestion of caustic substances.

Patients with a history of caustic substance ingestion can develop esophageal strictures and are at increased risk for squamous cell carcinoma of the esophagus. Those who develop esophageal strictures should undergo dilation. In comparison with esophageal strictures from other causes, these are more likely to require repetitive and frequent dilations to maintain adequate lumen patency [44,45]. The patients may also be at higher risk for complications including bleeding and perforation [45]. Intralesional steroid injection may improve the efficacy of esophageal dilation [46]. The timing of esophageal dilation is still controversial, as some recommend early dilation despite a potentially increased risk of perforation. Reports of esophageal stent placement for caustic esophageal strictures have been published, but the efficacy and safety of this approach has not been evaluated in a standardized fashion. Patients may require surgery if attempts at endoscopic therapy are unsuccessful. In one series, 13 % of patients requiring surgical therapy for strictures induced by caustic ingestion were found to have esophageal carcinoma after esophagectomy [47]. Despite this risk, there is currently insufficient evidence to recommend upper endoscopy for cancer screening in asymptomatic patients with a history of caustic ingestion.

Radiation Esophagitis

Radiation damage to the esophagus is a major dose-limiting complication, especially for thoracic carcinomas. The amount of radiation exposure required to cause symptomatic esophagitis varies, but the use of organ-specific dose–volume histograms has allowed radiation oncologists to predict esophageal toxicity better [48]. The maximum tolerated dose to the esophagus is 6000 cGy.

Radiation injury can be separated into acute and late complications. Acute radiation esophagitis is characterized by dysphagia and odynophagia. Patients with severe cases may have persistent, substernal chest pain unrelated to swallowing and may require parenteral nutrition. During endoscopy, the esophageal mucosa will appear hyperemic and friable and may contain erosions, ulcers, or exudates. Patients may have associated esophageal infections that require biopsies for diagnosis. The most common late complication of esophageal radiation is stricture formation. It generally takes at least 3 months after the completion of therapy before a stricture forms.

Prevention is the best therapy for radiation injury. Amifostine was found to reduce the risk of radiation-induced esophagitis in an initial small study, but subsequent randomized trials failed to reproduce these results [49,50]. At present, no therapy has been found to be effective in reducing the risk of radiation esophagitis. Treatment for acute radiation esophagitis is generally supportive, with dietary modification, pain control, and radiation dose adjustments. Individuals who develop strictures should undergo dilation; these patients are less likely to respond to dilation and are more likely to require repetitive sessions [51,52]. Intralesional steroid injection at the time of esophageal dilation can increase the symptom-free interval and reduce the need for future dilations [53]. Esophageal stent placement has been performed in refractory cases, but it is associated with high rates of stent migration and response rates of less than 40% [54,55].

Barrett's Esophagus

Epidemiology

Barrett's esophagus is a premalignant condition for esophageal adenocarcinoma, in which the squamous cell mucosa of the distal esophagus undergoes metaplastic transformation. While the transformation is considered to be a response to chronic gastroesophageal reflux, only about 10–15% of GERD patients are found to have Barrett's esophagus [56]. This suggests that unknown factors, both environmental and genetic, probably play a role in who develops Barrett's esophagus and who does not [57,58]. The major concern in patients with Barrett's esophagus is the risk for neoplastic transformation. The majority of esophageal adenocarcinomas are associated with the presence of Barrett's esophagus; estimates for the prevalence of underlying Barrett's esophagus have ranged between 75% and 97% [59]. The length of Barrett's esophagus appears to correlate with the risk for adenocarcinoma, with longer segments of Barrett's esophagus being associated with a higher risk for cancer [60]. In one study, patients with long-segment Barrett's esophagus were estimated to have a 30–125 times increased risk for developing esophageal adenocarcinoma in comparison with those without Barrett's esophagus [61].

Diagnosis

Upper endoscopy is the primary method for visually inspecting the esophagus for mucosal changes and obtaining tissue biopsies. Endoscopically, Barrett's esophagus appears as columnar-lined epithelium with a pink-salmon color (**Fig. 42.6**). As a result, these patients will have displacement of the SCJ proximal to the top of the gastric folds (i.e., the GEJ). When columnar-lined epithelium is seen above the GEJ, biopsies from this epithelium should be obtained to evaluate for metaplastic and dysplastic tissue. In patients with active esophagitis, the SCJ can be blurred by the presence of inflammation masking the presence of columnar-lined epithelium [24]. When visualized, Barrett's esophagus should be endoscopically characterized using a standardized system. The recommended system is the Prague classification system, which includes both the extent of circumferential (C) columnar-lined epithelium and its maximum length (M). The endoscopist should mark the location of the diaphragmatic hiatus, the top of the gastric folds, the top of the columnar-lined epithelium that involves the entire esophageal circumference, and the location of the most proximal edge of the columnar-

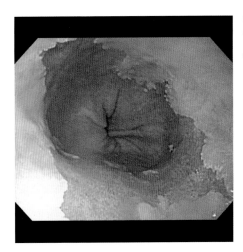

Fig. 42.6 The endoscopic appearance of Barrett's esophagus on white-light imaging.

lined epithelium, excluding any noncontiguous islands. Studies examining this system have reported that it has good interobserver reliability for the location of the GEJ and diaphragmatic hiatus and for characterizing Barrett's esophagus of more than 1 cm in extent [62].

Screening and Surveillance

Screening and surveillance for Barrett's esophagus remains a controversial issue, as its clinical efficacy remains uncertain. On one hand, data suggest that there is a survival benefit in patients who have undergone an upper endoscopy at least 1 year before the diagnosis of esophageal cancer [63,64]. In addition, Barrett's esophagus patients who are enrolled in a surveillance program are more likely to have earlier-stage tumors, a higher resectability rate, and improved mortality [65,66]. On the other hand, other studies have failed to show an overall mortality benefit in patients enrolled in a long-term Barrett's surveillance program [67,68]. Multiple cost-effectiveness studies have been completed examining this issue and have provided mixed results [69–71].

One of the challenges in screening is predicting which patients will have Barrett's esophagus prior to endoscopy. Risk factors include age over 40, presence of heartburn, presence of a hiatal hernia, long duration of GERD symptoms, male gender, obesity, alcohol consumption, and a history of smoking tobacco [72–76]. Despite the identification of these risk factors, some studies have found that up to 45% of Barrett's esophagus patients are asymptomatic [76]. Unfortunately, no risk factors for Barrett's esophagus have been identified in the asymptomatic population, and as a result, screening programs based on currently available risk factors are suboptimal. On the basis of these data, screening for Barrett's esophagus in the general population or even in GERD patients is not recommended. Screening certain high-risk groups may be beneficial, although the exact population has not been determined yet.

Similar to screening, surveillance of Barrett's esophagus also remains controversial. However, surveillance is practiced by the majority of endoscopists in the United States [77,78]. Endoscopists should have a discussion with their patients regarding the risks and benefits of surveillance before enrolling them in such a program. Issues to consider should include the patient's age, estimated survival, the patient's understanding of the potential benefits and limitations of surveillance, and a desire to adhere to surveillance recommendations. Those who choose to enroll in a surveillance program should undergo endoscopy once their symptoms have been controlled on antisecretory therapy. The Barrett's mucosa should be evaluated once any erosive esophagitis is healed, as inflammation can inhibit the visual characterization of Barrett's

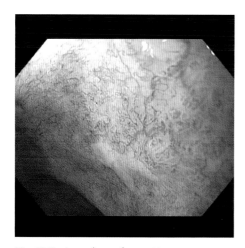

Fig. 42.7 Irregular surface patterns seen on narrow-band imaging in a patient with high-grade dysplasia.

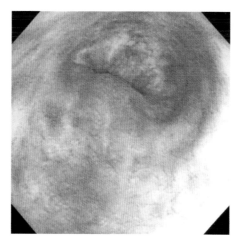

Fig. 42.8 Abnormal purple-appearing areas seen using auto-fluorescence imaging in a patient with dysplastic Barrett's esophagus.

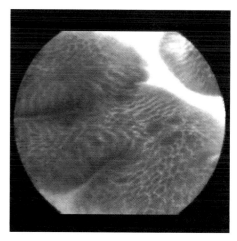

Fig. 42.9 Regular-shaped glands, seen using confocal laser microscopy in a patient with non-dysplastic Barrett's esophagus.

and interfere with the histological assessment for dysplasia [24]. Four-quadrant biopsies should be obtained from every 2 cm of the Barrett's esophagus and additional biopsies should be taken of any visible lesions [79]. In patients with high-grade dysplasia, four-quadrant biopsies should be taken every 1 cm, as taking biopsies using longer intervals (every 2 cm) can be associated with a 50% cancer miss rate [79,80]. The use of large-capacity forceps is advocated, especially in patients with high-grade dysplasia [81]. In addition, biopsies should be taken using the turn-and-suck technique, which brings the biopsy forceps in direct apposition to the mucosa [82]. The specimens from each segment should ideally be submitted to pathology separately to allow for future targeted biopsies if dysplasia is detected. This biopsy protocol only samples a small fraction of the Barrett's mucosa, and as such Barrett's surveillance is subject to a high degree of sampling error.

Novel Imaging Techniques

One of the biggest challenges in surveillance is the inability to detect dysplasia in macroscopically normal-appearing Barrett's esophagus. Several different imaging techniques have been developed to help improve the detection of dysplasia. Some of the more promising technologies that allow targeted biopsies of areas in which there is suspected dysplasia include NBI, autofluorescence imaging (AFI), and confocal laser microscopy. NBI is a technique in which the illuminating light is filtered to two major colors, blue and green, which enhances the visualization of mucosal and blood vessel patterns (**Fig. 42.7**). Multiple studies have found that NBI improves dysplasia prediction in comparison with conventional white-light endoscopy (57% vs. 43%) [83]. In AFI, blue light is used to detect fluorescence from biological tissue. Normal and dysplastic tissue have different fluorescence characteristics, with dysplastic tissue having a dark, violet-purple appearance and nondysplastic tissue appearing light green (**Fig. 42.8**). Several studies have examined the efficacy of AFI and have reported an improved dysplasia and carcinoma detection rate when AFI was combined with conventional four-quadrant biopsy in both short- and long-segment Barrett's esophagus [84]. However, the improvements in dysplasia and carcinoma detection with AFI come with a high false-positive rate. Confocal laser microscopy uses laser imaging to obtain in vivo microscopic analysis of the esophageal mucosa (**Fig. 42.9**). In initial studies, there appears to be good interobserver and intra-observer reliability and a good ability to detect Barrett's associated neoplasia,

with sensitivity and specificity rates reaching up to 92.9% and 98.4%, respectively [85]. However, the high sensitivity has not been reproduced in other studies [86]. While research into various imaging techniques continues, the optimal strategy is likely to involve a combination of different technologies of this type.

Dysplasia

The current recommended intervals for surveillance of patients with Barrett's esophagus depend on the degree of dysplasia. Patients without dysplasia on biopsies should have a repeat endoscopy with biopsy performed within 1 year. If no dysplasia is found, patients should undergo continued surveillance, but the interval can be extended to every 3 years. Despite the absence of dysplasia on two endoscopies, these patients are still at an increased risk for neoplastic transformation. In one cohort, up to 50% of patients who had high-grade dysplasia or esophageal adenocarcinoma were found to have no dysplasia on their first two endoscopies [87]. In all patients who are found to have dysplasia on biopsies, specimens should be reviewed by an expert gastroenterological pathologist, due to the high level of interobserver variability [88]. Patients with low-grade dysplasia should undergo repeat endoscopy in 6 months to exclude the presence of high-grade lesions. However, biopsies obtained in up to 40% of patients with previous low-grade dysplasia will be negative, and approximately 75% of patients will have no progression of dysplasia during the long-term follow-up [89]. Therefore, if no dysplasia is found in these patients at the follow-up examination, then endoscopy should repeated every year until the patient has two consecutive endoscopies with no dysplasia. At this time, the surveillance interval can be increased further.

Patients with high-grade dysplasia are at high risk for developing esophageal adenocarcinoma. The 5-year risk of developing cancer in these patients is estimated to exceed 30%, and it is higher in patients with nodular lesions [90]. Endoscopic mucosal resection (EMR) should be performed in patients with nodular high-grade dysplasia to obtain adequate tissue sampling for a more accurate histological diagnosis. They should also be evaluated for therapeutic interventions, although surveillance with repeat endoscopy every 3 months is reasonable in those who decline treatment or have contraindications to therapy.

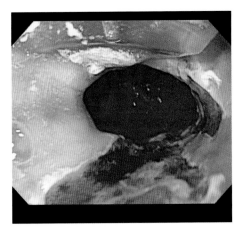

Fig. 42.10 Barrett's esophagus being treated with radiofrequency ablation (focal device).

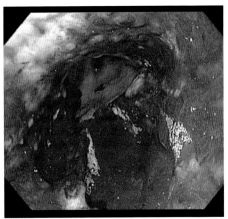

Fig. 42.11 A large esophageal ulcer (covered with blood), caused by nasogastric tube trauma.

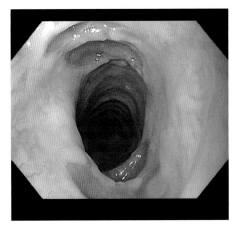

Fig. 42.12 Multiple patches of heterotopic gastric mucosa seen in the proximal esophagus.

Therapy

In patients with Barrett's esophagus, the goal of acid-suppression therapy is to control gastroesophageal reflux symptoms. While studies have shown a decrease in markers of proliferation and development of dysplasia with PPI therapy, a decreased cancer risk has not been found [91,92]. Although there are some case reports of regression of Barrett's esophagus and dysplasia after antireflux surgery, this has not been consistent, and there is no impact on cancer development [93]. Antireflux surgery is effective in controlling gastroesophageal reflux symptoms, but up to 20% of patients may develop recurrent symptoms during the long-term follow-up [94]. Multiple endoscopic therapies have been developed for patients with high-grade dysplasia and early cancer, including mucosal resection, photodynamic therapy, thermal ablation, radiofrequency ablation, and cryotherapy. Endoscopic therapies are generally performed in conjunction with acid suppression. Photodynamic therapy was one of the first treatments found to be effective in patients with high-grade dysplasia. A 5-year follow-up of a clinical trial of 208 patients found a 50% reduction in cancer risk and a similar rate of dysplasia eradication [95]. The use of photodynamic therapy has been limited by the risk of stricture formation, which occurs in approximately 23% of the patients [96]. Radiofrequency ablation is a relatively new technique that has shown promise in initial studies (**Fig. 42.10**). The largest data is from a registry of 142 patients with dysplastic Barrett's esophagus, which showed eradication of high-grade dysplasia and any dysplasia in 90.2% and 80.4% of patients, respectively [97]. However, no trials comparing radiofrequency ablation with photodynamic therapy or long-term follow-up studies are available. In patients with high-grade dysplasia or intramucosal adenocarcinoma, complete eradication of dysplasia and cancer by EMR can be achieved in over 95% of cases [98–100]. Complications including postprocedural bleeding and stricture formation occur in up to 19% and 12% of patients, respectively, but these can be successfully managed endoscopically in most cases [98–100]. There is continuing controversy over whether these patients should be managed with surveillance, endoscopic therapy, or surgical therapy. Treatment decisions should therefore be individualized and based on local expertise, the presence of comorbid conditions, and the patient's preferences.

Nonendoscopic Tube Trauma

The placement of nasogastric tubes is a well-known cause of esophageal injury and can result in direct physical trauma to the esophagus (**Fig. 42.11**). In addition, patients with a nasogastric tube have an increase in esophageal acid exposure, which can lead to erosive esophagitis; furthermore, those who have prolonged tube placement can develop strictures [101]. This injury is not limited to nasogastric tubes, as case reports have also documented esophageal injury with a wide variety of respiratory devices including esophageal–tracheal Combitubes, cuffed tracheal tubes, thoracostomy tubes, and transesophageal echocardiography probes [102–104].

Heterotopic Gastric Mucosa

Heterotopic gastric mucosa is a frequent finding in the cervical esophagus, with an estimated prevalence of 0.1–10% [105]. Such patches of heterotopic mucosa can be found throughout the gastrointestinal tract and have been described in the tongue, small bowel, rectum, and gallbladder [106–110]. Macroscopically, it appears as a red-salmon colored, velvety patch, and when seen in the cervical esophagus, just distal to the upper esophageal sphincter, it is commonly called an "inlet patch" (**Fig. 42.12**). Due to its common location in the cervical esophagus, heterotopic gastric mucosa is probably clinically underestimated [105,111]. The area is not easily visualized during upper endoscopy, as the region is quickly passed during insertion of the endoscope. Only with careful inspection during instrument withdrawal can inlet patches be detected.

While the likely cause of heterotopic gastric mucosa is the entrapment of undifferentiated endodermal cells during development, some have suggested that acid reflux may be a contributing factor [112]. Most patients are asymptomatic, but some may describe pain or dysphagia. In addition, some cases of heterotopic gastric mucosa have led to formation of ulcers, fistulas, high-grade dysplasia, and adenocarcinoma, although no formal surveillance or biopsies are recommended [113]. As symptoms occur rarely, no standardized treatment algorithm has been developed, but most symptomatic patients experience improvement with acid-suppression therapy.

Mallory–Weiss Tears

Mallory–Weiss tears are mucosal lacerations caused by forceful vomiting that are found at the GEJ or gastric cardia. Most patients present with gastrointestinal bleeding; the classic presentation is of violent vomiting or retching followed by hematemesis. An estimated 5–10% of cases of upper gastrointestinal hemorrhage are considered to result from Mallory–Weiss tears [114]. The degree of blood loss can vary, with some patients having significant hemodynamic compromise. Upper endoscopy is recommended for all

42

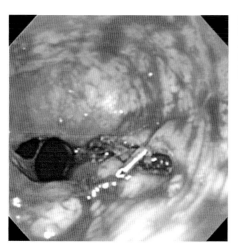

Fig. 42.13 A large Mallory–Weiss tear with active bleeding, treated with endoscopic clip placement.

patients with suspected Mallory–Weiss tears. Most patients will have a single tear, with less than 10% of patients having multiple tears [115]. Bleeding stops spontaneously in up to 90% of patients, and only about 5% have rebleeding [116]. Endoscopy is not only diagnostic, but also allows for therapeutic options if active bleeding is seen (**Fig. 42.13**). In cases in which there is active bleeding or stigmata that represent a high risk for rebleeding, endoscopic therapy with thermal coagulation, epinephrine injection, or hemoclip placement are effective and should be performed.

Rings and Strictures

Schatzki Ring

Schatzki rings are a very common finding during upper endoscopy, with prevalence estimates ranging up to 4% [117]. The etiology of these rings is still not fully understood. While a congenital origin has been hypothesized, other factors such as pill-induced esophagitis and GERD are thought to contribute to their formation [118,119]. Most patients with Schatzki rings are asymptomatic, but when the esophageal lumen diameter is narrowed to less than 13 mm, symptoms can develop. Individuals generally present with intermittent solid food dysphagia or acute food impaction. Barium esophagraphy is the recommended diagnostic test, unless there is a concern regarding acute food impaction. Upper endoscopy is reserved for therapeutic purposes, as it is generally considered to be less sensitive for the detection of Schatzki rings [120]. During upper endo-

scopy, detection is dependent on the degree of lumen compromise, the adequacy of air inflation, and the size of the endoscope used [120]. Small rings can be easily missed if the endoscopist fails to achieve adequate esophageal distension.

Asymptomatic Schatzki rings require no therapy. Patients with dysphagia can be effectively treated with esophageal dilation and dietary modifications. Esophageal dilation performed with the passage of a single, large bougie to mechanically disrupt the ring and has been found to be safe and effective. However, the need for repeat dilation is high, with some studies reporting that over 30% of patients will need repeat dilation within 1 year [121,122]. While the presence of GERD and the ring diameter were speculated to predict dysphagia recurrence, studies have not been conclusive and at present no definitive predictors of recurrence have been established [121,122]. Despite this, clinical trials have found a reduced need for future dilations in patients treated with PPI after undergoing dilation [123,124]. More recent studies comparing electrosurgical incision of the ring with bougie dilation have shown better long-term control of symptoms with electrosurgical incision [124]. However, future studies are needed to confirm these findings.

Peptic Strictures

Peptic strictures are a complication of chronic, uncontrolled gastroesophageal reflux and are estimated to occur in 8% of patients with untreated GERD [125]. Male gender, advanced age, a history of NSAID use, and prolonged duration of symptoms are all risk factors for stricture development [125,126]. Strictures are a result of chronic acid-induced inflammation, which leads to collagen deposition and the creation of irreversible fibrosis. Patients with strictures usually present with new-onset solid food dysphagia and a history of long-standing heartburn. They may have a decrease in the degree of heartburn once dysphagia begins, as the stricture acts as a barrier to further acid reflux. In addition, most patients unknowingly modify their diets, resulting in some weight loss. Dysphagia usually occurs once the esophageal lumen has been reduced to under 13 mm (39 Fr). Upper endoscopy is considered the initial test of choice in patients with a clinical suspicion for a peptic stricture, as it allows both diagnosis and treatment (**Figs. 42.14**). Peptic strictures appear as a smooth, circumferential narrowing, most commonly seen in the lower esophagus; they are generally less than 1 cm long, but may be longer in atypical cases. If a stricture does not have these characteristics, the endoscopist should consider other etiologies or coexisting conditions such as pill esophagitis, malignancy, Zollinger–Ellison syndrome, Schatzki ring, or prolonged na-

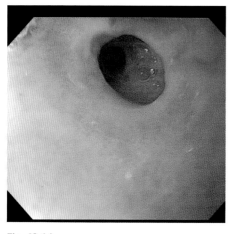
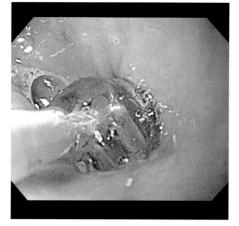
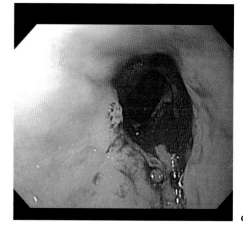

a, b

c

Fig. 42.14
a A peptic stricture in the distal esophagus that developed after healing of erosive esophagitis.
b Dilation of the peptic stricture using a through-the-scope balloon.
c The mucosal tear visualized after balloon dilation.

sogastric intubation. Any stricture with an irregular or nodular appearance should be biopsied to evaluate for malignancy.

Patients with peptic strictures should undergo esophageal dilation to alleviate symptoms, as dilation has a reported effectiveness of over 80 % [127]. Stricture dilation (with or without fluoroscopic guidance) can be performed with Maloney bougies, Savary dilators, or through-the-scope balloons. All of these techniques have been found to be safe and effective, and no technique has been found to be clearly superior in comparison with the others [128,129]. When performing dilation, the "rule of three" has been generally accepted. The initial dilator size should be based on the estimated stricture diameter, and then serial increases are performed until resistance is encountered. However, no more than three consecutive dilators in increments of 1 mm should be used in a single session. In addition, PPI therapy should be initiated, as it reduces the risk for stricture recurrence and the need for repeat dilation from 46 % to 30 % at 1 year [130]. Steroid injection into the peptic stricture before or after dilation may also reduce the need for future dilations, especially in cases of refractory strictures [131]. Initial small lumen size, hiatal hernia > 5 cm, persistent heartburn after dilation, and the number of dilations needed for initial dysphagia relief are all predictors for early stricture recurrence [52].

Eosinophilic Esophagitis

Eosinophilic esophagitis is a distinct clinicopathologic disease characterized by a range of symptoms including dysphagia and food impaction, and the presence of numerous eosinophils on esophageal biopsies. While there are an increasing number of patients being diagnosed with this condition, there are limited clinical trials available to help guide management decisions. Current practice is mostly based on expert opinion and interpretation of the limited data available (predominantly in the pediatric population). The prevalence of eosinophilic esophagitis has been increasing over the past several years. In one cohort study, the prevalence of eosinophilic esophagitis was estimated at up to 6.5 % of patients undergoing upper endoscopy [132]. Known risk factors include male gender, age under 50, a history of asthma, a history of food impactions, and a history of dysphagia [132]. There does not appear to be any predisposition based on ethnic, geographical, socio-economic, or seasonal factors, but the data are limited [133]. Patients with eosinophilic esophagitis can present with various upper gastrointestinal symptoms, including heartburn, chest pain, feeding intolerance in children, dysphagia, odynophagia, and food impactions. Intermittent dysphagia and food impactions are the most common symptoms in adults. Unfortunately, no individual or group of symptoms is specific for eosinophilic esophagitis. As a result, eosinophilic esophagitis should be considered in patients with GERD-like symptoms that are unresponsive to antisecretory therapy, recurrent food impactions, chronic dysphagia, and in children who fail to tolerate oral feeding.

Eosinophilic esophagitis has been associated with a multitude of endoscopic abnormalities, including longitudinal furrowing, friability, edema, longitudinal shearing, raised white specks, whitish exudates, "crepe-paper mucosa," narrow-caliber esophagus, and both transient and fixed rings [133] (**Fig. 42.15**). Unfortunately, almost all of these findings have been associated with other esophageal diseases, making the diagnosis of eosinophilic esophagitis difficult solely on the basis of the endoscopic findings. Furthermore, up to 30 % of patients with eosinophilic esophagitis may have a normal-appearing esophagus on endoscopy [134]. Hence, patients who have clinical and endoscopic features that raise a suspicion for eosinophilic esophagitis should undergo esophageal biopsies during upper endoscopy. The wide range of clinical and endoscopic presentations of eosinophilic esophagitis, along with its many similarities to GERD,

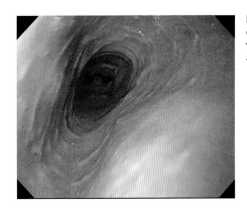

Fig. 42.15 A ringed esophagus in a patient with eosinophilic esophagitis.

can sometimes make distinguishing the two diseases a clinical dilemma. A number of potential mechanisms for the interaction between GERD and eosinophilic esophagitis have been described, but additional research is needed [135]. Both are reported to cause esophageal eosinophilia, making histology an imperfect way to distinguish between the two. As a result, eosinophilic esophagitis is a clinicopathologic diagnosis that requires the presence of esophageal symptoms with severe isolated esophageal eosinophilia. While the sensitivity for detecting eosinophilic esophagitis increases with the number of esophageal biopsies obtained, the optimal number has not yet been determined [136]. At least five to eight biopsies should be taken from the proximal, mid-, and distal esophagus. While no exact histological diagnostic criteria have been developed, a minimum of 15–24 intraepithelial eosinophils per high-powered field is required to classify the esophageal eosinophilia as severe. Biopsies from the stomach and duodenum should be obtained to exclude eosinophilic gastroenteritis and inflammatory bowel disease, as these can both cause esophageal eosinophilia.

While the treatment of eosinophilic esophagitis in the adult population has been understudied, there are a multitude of potential therapies including dietary modification, topical fluticasone, PPIs, and esophageal dilation. A series of 146 children with eosinophilic esophagitis found that 50 % had an identifiable food allergy on skin testing; all of these patients had complete resolution with restrictive diets [137]. Those without an identifiable food allergy may still respond to dietary modification and use of an elemental diet [134,137]. In two series, treatment with topical fluticasone for 4–6 weeks was reported to lead to a response rate of almost 100 % [138,139]. However, over 90 % of these patients develop recurrent symptoms during the long-term follow up [140]. Limited case series have documented the efficacy of PPIs in eosinophilic esophagitis patients, although the response rate is unknown [141]. Esophageal dilation may produce a temporary response rate of almost 85 %, but it may be associated with a high rate of mucosal tears and esophageal perforations [142,143].

Diaphragmatic Hernias

A diaphragmatic hernia occurs when an abdominal organ or structure enters the chest through an opening in the diaphragm. This can occur through the esophageal hiatus, other congenital openings, or post-traumatic defects. The term "hiatal hernia" refers to a diaphragmatic hernia that involves the proximal stomach entering the chest through the esophageal hiatus. In normal individuals, the GEJ, which can be identified by the top of the gastric mucosal folds, is seen at the diaphragmatic pinch. Hiatal hernias are commonly found during endoscopy. While the exact prevalence of hiatal hernias has not been accurately determined, studies have demonstrated that the prevalence is increased in patients with GERD and obesity, and in the elderly [144,145].

42

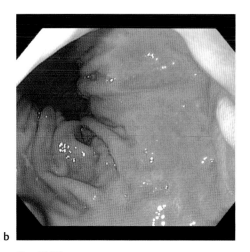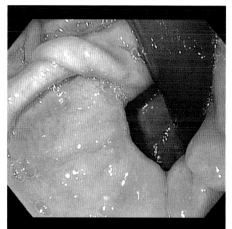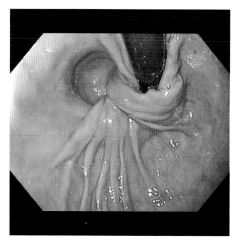

a, b

Fig. 42.16
a Sliding hiatal hernia.
b Sliding hiatal hernia viewed in retroflexion.

Fig. 42.17 A 360° Nissen fundoplication viewed in retroflexion.

The current practice of diagnosing and measuring the size of hiatal hernias during endoscopy relies on the use of distance markings on the endoscope. Unfortunately, there is no standard method of determining the point during respiration when the measurements should be obtained, and there is no certainty that the tip of the endoscope is precisely at the landmark being measured. As a result, endoscopic diagnosis and measurement of hiatal hernias is associated with a degree of inaccuracy. Once the endoscope has been advanced past the hernia pouch and into the stomach, retroflexion should be performed. From this position, further inspection of a hiatal hernia can be conducted. In normal individuals, a ridge of tissue can be seen extending from the GEJ down to a position approximately 3–4 cm along the lesser curvature. This is the angle of His, and in normal individuals it closely approximates the shaft of the endoscope. As a hiatal hernia develops, there is progressive deterioration of the tissue and loosening around the endoscope. While retroflexed in the stomach, the endoscope can be withdrawn to the level of the diaphragmatic hiatus and even into the hernia sac itself, allowing for close inspection.

Sliding Hiatal Hernias

Approximately 95% of all hiatal hernias are type I hernias (**Fig. 42.16**). Type I hiatal hernias, or sliding hiatal hernias as they are commonly called, have been reported in 10–50% of patients undergoing endoscopy [146,147]. These hernias develop when the GEJ enters into the thoracic cavity. Multiple factors are associated with the development and aggravation of GEJ displacement, including age, obesity, weightlifting, pregnancy, and gastroesophageal reflux [145,148]. The majority of patients with type I hiatal hernias are asymptomatic and do not require any treatment. However, these patients may develop symptoms of GERD. In addition, individuals with hiatal hernias can develop iron-deficiency anemia from Cameron ulcers—ulcerations that form within a hernia sac from mechanical trauma, which can cause acute or chronic gastrointestinal bleeding [149].

Paraesophageal Hernias

Paraesophageal hiatal hernias are less common in comparison with sliding hiatal hernias. They represent approximately 5% of all hiatal hernias and are classified as types II, III, and IV. A type II hiatal hernia, or true paraesophageal hernia, occurs when a defect in the phre-

noesophageal membrane of the diaphragm allows herniation of the stomach into the chest while the GEJ remains in its normal position. As the hernia enlarges, the entire stomach may displace into the chest, and gastric volvulus may occur. A type III hiatal hernia is a mixture between a type I and a type II hiatal hernia. As in a type II hiatal hernia, a defect in the phrenoesophageal membrane results in the herniation of the stomach into the chest, but unlike type II hiatal hernias, the GEJ also herniates into the chest, causing some resemblance to a type I hiatal hernia. A type IV hiatal hernia occurs when a defect in the phrenoesophageal membrane is so large that other abdominal organs besides the stomach herniate into the chest. Of the different types of paraesophageal hernias, type III appears to be the most common [150].

Patients with paraesophageal hernias can present with a variety of nonspecific complaints, including postprandial fullness, pain, nausea, vomiting, dysphagia, and respiratory complaints. About one-half of patients with paraesophageal hernias will have GERD [151]. Others may have chronic blood loss, which may be associated with iron-deficiency anemia. While not all patients with paraesophageal hernias will be symptomatic, complications develop in over 20% if left untreated [150]. Surgery is the treatment of choice and is associated with a recurrence rate of about 30% over 10 years with laparoscopic repair [151] (**Fig. 42.17**). Despite the recurrence rate, surgical repair is associated with a significant reduction in symptoms of heartburn, chest pain, regurgitation, and dysphagia [151].

Diverticula

Esophageal diverticula are outpouchings of the esophageal wall that may be congenital or acquired (**Fig. 42.18**). True diverticula are those that involve all layers of the esophagus, while false diverticular (pseudodiverticula) occur when the mucosa and submucosa herniate through the muscular wall. True diverticula are generally assumed to be congenital and false diverticula to be acquired, but this is not always true.

Zenker Diverticula

Zenker diverticulum was first described by Ludlow in 1769. It is an acquired false diverticulum; the pathophysiology behind this is not completely understood, but is hypothesized to be a result of increased intrapharyngeal pressure along with inherent weakness of the esophageal wall between the inferior pharyngeal constrictor muscle and the cricopharyngeus muscle. This space, known as the Killian triangle, is the most common location for the formation of Zenker diverticulum. Zenker diverticula most commonly occur in individuals with advanced age and rarely in those under the age of 40 [152]. While accurate prevalence data are unavailable, primarily due to a large number of asymptomatic cases, this is estimated to be the most common type of esophageal diverticulum, with a prevalence ranging between 0.01 % and 0.11 % [152]. Dysphagia is the most common symptom, although patients can have regurgitation of undigested food, halitosis, hoarseness, chronic cough, and repetitive aspiration. None of these symptoms has high specificity, but the presence of cervical borborygmi is almost pathognomonic of Zenker diverticulum. Symptoms can be present for weeks to years, and if symptoms become severe, weight loss and malnutrition can occur.

If a Zenker diverticulum is suspected clinically, a barium esophagram, especially with lateral views, should be obtained to confirm the diagnosis. Upper endoscopy is generally not required for diagnosis, although diverticula can be found incidentally in patients undergoing endoscopy for other indications. Performing upper endoscopy in patients with large diverticula can be difficult, as the endoscope often enters the pouch during esophageal intubation. The appropriate action at this point is to slowly withdraw the endoscope to the opening of the diverticulum, then apply gentle torque to steer the endoscope tip anteriorly to the esophageal lumen. If this fails, placement of a guide wire into the esophagus under fluoroscopic guidance followed by endoscope insertion over the guide wire may be needed. Treatment is indicated for patients who are symptomatic and is generally in the form of surgical resection. However, as many of these patients are poor surgical candidates, some centers have adopted endoscopic treatment methods. A single series of endoscopic cricopharyngeal myotomy found a success rate of 84 % and a complication rate of less than 5 % [153]. The cricopharyngeal myotomy can be performed using argon plasma coagulation, a needle-knife incision, or monopolar coagulation forceps. The most common serious complications include postprocedural bleeding and microperforation. While the initial results have shown promising success rates, no studies comparing the method with surgical therapy have been conducted.

Other Esophageal Diverticula

Other types of diverticula found within the esophageal body include epiphrenic and traction diverticula. Epiphrenic diverticula are acquired lesions most commonly found in the distal esophagus and are thought to be the consequence of underlying esophageal motility disorders such as achalasia, diffuse esophageal spasm, and hypertensive LES. Traction diverticula are also acquired diverticula, but are more common in the mid-esophagus and are thought to be the result of chronic periesophageal inflammation from diseases including tuberculosis, histoplasmosis, mediastinal fibrosis, and chronic lymphadenopathy. These diverticula are usually asymptomatic, but occasionally they can cause dysphagia, food regurgitation, heartburn, and weight loss. The diagnosis and evaluation of these lesions is best done with a barium esophagram. Those patients who have symptoms that are clearly related to their diverticula should be considered for therapy. Treatment is surgical, but preoperative upper endoscopy and manometry are recommended to evaluate for associated esophageal motility disorders.

Finally, esophageal intramural pseudodiverticula are flask-shaped outpouchings of the esophageal lumen that can appear as diverticula, especially on upper endoscopy. These are acquired diverticula result from dilated ducts of submucosal glands, which can occur throughout the esophagus due to chronic inflammation. GERD, esophageal candidiasis, prior caustic ingestion, esophageal strictures, and esophageal cancer can all be associated with esoph-

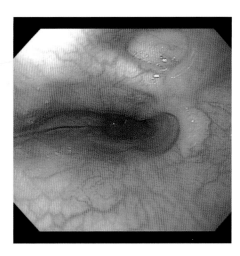

Fig. 42.18 A mid-esophageal diverticulum.

ageal intramural pseudodiverticula. There is no specific treatment for this condition; treatment should be directed at the underlying condition.

Vascular Diseases

Varices

Epidemiology

Esophageal varices are a complication of cirrhosis and a direct result of portal hypertension. Gastroesophageal varices, found in approximately 50 % of individuals with cirrhosis, are the most common and lethal complication of cirrhosis, due to the risk of bleeding from variceal rupture [154]. As the severity of cirrhosis increases, so does the risk of having gastroesophageal varices [154]. While 40 % of patients with Child–Pugh A cirrhosis have varices, they are present in 85 % of patients with Child–Pugh C cirrhosis. Due to the high prevalence of esophageal varices in patients with cirrhosis, current consensus guidelines recommend that all patients with cirrhosis should undergo screening for esophageal varices. Upper gastrointestinal endoscopy is the recommended method for the detection, evaluation, and treatment of esophageal varices. Patients with cirrhosis are at continual risk for the development and progression of esophageal varices. Patients with no varices develop them at the rate of 8 % per year [155]. In these patients, a hepatic venous pressure gradient (HVPG) > 10 mmHg is the strongest predictor of varix development, and the majority of patients have an HVPG of at least 10–12 mmHg [156,157]. Patients with small varices are also at risk for progression to large varices at a rate of 8 % per year. In these patients, the strongest predictors of progression of varices are decompensated cirrhosis (Child–Pugh B/C), alcoholic cirrhosis, and the presence of red wale marks [155]. On the basis of these data, consensus guidelines have been established for the continued screening and surveillance of esophageal varices [158]. In patients with no varices and compensated cirrhosis, upper endoscopy should be performed every 2–3 years. In patients with small varices and compensated cirrhosis, upper endoscopy should be performed every 1–2 years. Patients with decompensated cirrhosis should undergo upper endoscopy every year.

Grading of Varices

Overall, variceal hemorrhage occurs at a rate of 5–15 % per year [159]. Multiple grading systems have been developed for esophageal varices in order to stratify patients according to risk. In an initial

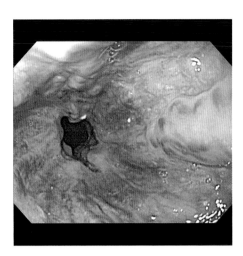

Fig. 42.19 Esophageal varices with multiple red color signs.

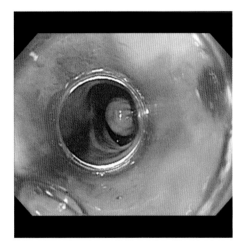

Fig. 42.20 Endoscopic band ligation of esophageal varices.

rate of variceal bleeding. Unfortunately, no single classification system has been found to be superior to any of the others [162].

Despite the presence of multiple classification systems, endoscopic grading remains subjective. Studies conducted to evaluate interobserver reliability in the endoscopic grading of esophageal varices have provided mixed results. Some endoscopic features have been found to have good interobserver reliability, including varix size and presence or absence of red color spots [163]. However, varix length and overall color have poor interobserver reliability [163]. Other studies have found high interobserver variability for all endoscopic features of esophageal varices [164]. Varix size appears not only to be one of the strongest predictors for hemorrhage, but also a characteristic that can be reliably determined endoscopically. Recent consensus guidelines therefore recommend that esophageal varices should be classified by size and should be described as small or large [158]. Esophageal varices should be assessed during withdrawal of the endoscope, with the stomach maximally decompressed, and then the esophagus should be fully insufflated. Varices with an estimated diameter of 5 mm or less are considered small, where those with a diameter greater than 5 mm should be considered large.

Treatment of Varices

The preferred endoscopic treatment for esophageal varices is band ligation therapy. During endoscopic band ligation, a varix is suctioned into an endoscope channel, followed by deployment of a band around the varix, resulting in varix thrombosis (**Fig. 42.20**). The most distal varices should be banded first, and the process should then be repeated in a spiral fashion as the endoscope is withdrawn from the esophagus. Currently available banding devices allow multiple bands to be deployed with a single insertion of the endoscope. Endoscopic band ligation can result in complications including ulcers, strictures, mucosal tears, esophageal perforation, and transient symptoms of chest pain and dysphagia. While proton-pump inhibitor therapy has not been shown to reduce the incidence of ulcer formation or postprocedural bleeding, it does reduce the size of the ulcerations, and prophylactic PPI therapy is still recommended after endoscopic band ligation [165].

Therapy of esophageal varices is indicated in three clinical scenarios: treatment of active variceal hemorrhage, primary prophylaxis of variceal hemorrhage in patients with large varices, and secondary prophylaxis of variceal hemorrhage in all patients. For primary prophylaxis of variceal hemorrhage in patients with large varices, nonselective beta blocker therapy is associated with a reduction in risk of variceal bleeding and mortality [166]. In this patient group, endoscopic band ligation has been found to be as effective as nonselective beta blockade in multiple clinical trials [167]. On the other hand, the evidence supporting the use of endoscopic sclerotherapy for primary prophylaxis has not been as consistent [168,169]. One randomized controlled trial had to be terminated early due to an increased risk of mortality in patients who underwent endoscopic sclerotherapy in comparison with those receiving a placebo [170]. In addition, combination therapy with endoscopic band ligation and nonselective beta blockade has not been found to be superior in reducing the risk for variceal hemorrhage in comparison with endoscopic band ligation alone [171]. As a result, either nonselective beta blockade or endoscopic band ligation should be performed for the primary prophylaxis of variceal hemorrhage in patients with large varices [158].

In patients with acute variceal hemorrhage, upper gastrointestinal endoscopy should be performed as soon as possible so that the diagnosis can be confirmed and endoscopic therapy can be performed. Multiple randomized controlled trials have compared endoscopic band ligation with sclerotherapy for the treatment of acute

study to evaluate the natural history of varices, 75 patients with alcoholic liver disease underwent serial endoscopic assessments for up to 86 months to determine the incidence of variceal bleeding [160]. In this study, varix size and the presence of the characteristic "cherry-red spot," indicating a small varix on top of a large varix, were predictive factors for variceal hemorrhage. The classification system developed by the Japanese Research Society on Portal Hypertension was based on assessing the following varix characteristics: color, red color signs, form, and location. The highest rates of bleeding were associated with the presence of red color signs, including red wale marks, cherry-red spots, hematocystic spots, and diffuse redness [161] (**Fig. 42.19**). Red wale marks represent longitudinal dilated venules on top of a large varix, while a cherry-red spot represents a small red dilated venule on top of a large varix. When multiple dilated venules are seen over a varix, the lesion will appear to have diffuse redness, whereas a hematocystic spot is a single, deep red lesion on a varix that is generally large and over 4 mm in diameter. The predictive value of this classification system was confirmed in a separate study conducted by Beppu et al. including 192 patients with esophageal varices [161]. While multiple endoscopic factors can predict variceal hemorrhage, clinical factors such as severity of liver disease and degree of portal hypertension also play an important role [155]. To address this issue, the North Italian Endoscopic Club (NIEC) for the Study and Treatment of Esophageal Varices created a classification system that includes both endoscopic features and nonendoscopic characteristics of patients [159]. In this system, patients are given a score for varix size, degree of red wale marks, and Child–Pugh classification. The cumulative score is used to create an NIEC score, which corresponds to the

variceal hemorrhage. A meta-analysis of these studies revealed a nonstatistically significant benefit from endoscopic band ligation over sclerotherapy, with a reduced bleeding rate (23% vs. 47%) and mortality rate (10% vs. 32%) [172]. In patients with acute variceal hemorrhage, an HVPG > 20 mmHg is associated with a higher risk of recurrent bleeding, failure to control bleeding, and 1-year mortality [173,174]. Pharmacological therapy to reduce portal hypertension (terlipressin, somatostatin, octreotide, or vasopressin plus nitroglycerin) is effective at controlling variceal bleeding [175]. When endoscopic therapy plus pharmacological therapy is compared to endoscopic therapy alone, there is a reduced risk of continued bleeding (12% vs. 24%) or recurrent bleeding within 5 days (23% vs. 42%) [176]. Current consensus guidelines recommend the combination of endoscopic and pharmacological therapy for patients with acute variceal hemorrhage [158]. Band ligation is the preferred endoscopic treatment modality, but sclerotherapy should be considered if band ligation cannot be technically performed.

Patients who survive an episode of variceal hemorrhage are at high risk for recurrent variceal hemorrhage and death—60% and 33%, respectively, over the subsequent 1–2 years [166,177]. Endoscopic band ligation reduces the risk of recurrent variceal rupture and is more effective and associated with fewer complications than sclerotherapy [172]. The addition of sclerotherapy to band ligation is not superior to endoscopic band ligation alone with regard to the risk of rebleeding or death [178,179]. Endoscopic sclerotherapy is therefore not recommended for secondary prophylaxis of variceal bleeding, either alone or in combination with endoscopic band ligation. However, two randomized controlled trials have demonstrated that endoscopic band ligation plus nonselective beta blocker therapy is superior to endoscopic band ligation alone in preventing recurrent variceal hemorrhage [180,181]. Therefore, patients who survive an episode of variceal hemorrhage should be treated with both endoscopic band ligation and nonselective beta-blockade.

Arteria Lusoria

Vascular anomalies of the mediastinum can cause compression of the esophagus and result in dysphagia. This phenomenon, first described in 1761 by David Bayford, is called dysphagia lusoria [182]. When symptomatic esophageal compression is caused by an aberrant right subclavian artery, it is referred to as arteria lusoria. Arteria lusoria is the most common congenital anomaly of the aortic arch, occurring in approximately 0.4–0.7% of the general population [183]. Instead of arising from the right common carotid artery, the right subclavian artery arises from the left side of the aortic arch and passes posteriorly across the esophagus, causing esophageal compression. While it is commonly stated in the published literature that the artery crosses anterior to the esophagus in approximately 20% of patients with arteria lusoria, this estimate has been challenged by autopsy studies [184]. The majority of patients are asymptomatic, but dysphagia has been reported [183,185]. Endoscopy may reveal a pulsatile extrinsic compression of the esophagus, with normal overlying mucosa [186]. The right radial pulse may also diminish or disappear as the endoscope compresses the right subclavian artery. Confirmation of the diagnosis is generally obtained with CT, magnetic resonance imaging (MRI), angiography, or endoscopic ultrasonography (EUS). Symptoms are generally managed with dietary modifications, but surgical reconstruction may be required in severe or refractory cases.

Mass Lesions of the Esophagus

During upper endoscopy, the endoscopist may encounter several types of mass lesion of the esophagus, both benign and malignant. One of the challenges in assessing these lesions is that they can arise from the different layers of the esophagus; those that arise from the mucosa are easy to visualize and sample with tissue biopsy and brushings, but tumors arising from esophageal layers beneath the mucosa may only appear as a bulge with normal overlying mucosa. In this circumstance, the endoscopist may have difficulty in differentiating between an esophageal mass and extrinsic compression of the esophagus. In addition, tissue biopsies are generally inadequate for submucosal lesions, as they are too deep to sample with standard biopsy forceps. EUS has become an essential tool in the evaluation of these lesions.

Esophageal tumors have a variety of clinical presentations, with dysphagia, weight loss, and gastrointestinal hemorrhage being the most common. The symptoms associated with an esophageal mass depend on its size and location. A mass effect causing a reduction of the esophageal lumen results in progressive dysphagia, weight loss, and even acute food impaction. This can occur with tumors arising from any layer of the esophagus and even mediastinal tumors that cause extrinsic esophageal compression. Gastrointestinal hemorrhage is less common, but occurs when the esophageal mucosa is disrupted by the tumor. Mucosal ulceration generally occurs with tumors arising from the esophageal mucosa, but any tumor can potentially cause mucosal disruption. The degree of gastrointestinal hemorrhage can vary from overt bleeding with hemodynamic compromise to occult bleeding causing mild anemia. Other less common symptoms such as constant substernal pain, regurgitation, and a variety of respiratory complaints can also occur. Barium esophagraphy, CT, upper endoscopy, and EUS can all be used to evaluate esophageal tumors. Each test has its role in diagnosis, staging, and therapy. Barium esophagraphy allows the detection of structural lesions noninvasively. While it provides details regarding the level and degree of lumen compromise, any tumors detected need to be further evaluated using upper endoscopy. Upper endoscopy allows for visual assessment, tissue sampling, and therapy through the use of EMR, ablation therapy, dilation, and stent placement. CT can be helpful if there is a suspicion of a mediastinal mass causing extrinsic compression of the esophagus. In addition, CT is used to evaluate for distant metastases when an esophageal neoplasm has been diagnosed, but it is inadequate for determining local tumor extension. EUS provides a detailed view of the entire esophageal wall and the surrounding structures. With this tool, the endoscopist can assess the origin of the tumor, accurately stage local invasion, and also obtain tissue samples (through guided fine-needle aspiration) to aid in diagnosis.

Benign Tumors

Squamous Papillomas

Squamous papillomas are small, white to pink tumors that are usually detected incidentally during upper endoscopy (**Fig. 42.21**). They are finger-like projections of fibrous connective tissue that arise from the lamina propria and are covered by hyperplastic squamous epithelium. The exact pathogenesis is unknown, but both GERD and human papillomavirus infection may be involved [187]. The diagnosis is made by mucosal biopsy or polypectomy. Once the diagnosis has been made and the lesion removed, no further surveillance is required, as the papillomas have a low risk for malignant transformation [188].

42

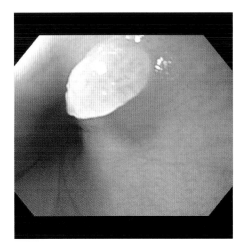

Fig. 42.21 Squamous papilloma of the esophagus.

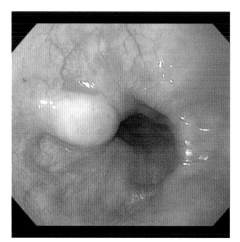

Fig. 42.22 Lipoma of the esophagus.

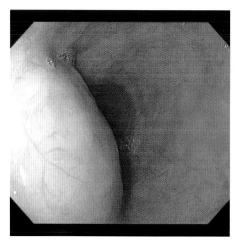

Fig. 42.23 A submucosal lesion in the mid-esophagus. Endoscopic ultrasonography showed that the lesion was a leiomyoma.

Lipomas

Lipomas appear as a pale or yellow lesion with normal overlying mucosa (**Fig. 42.22**). When probed with a blunt instrument, they exhibit easy compressibility, known as the "pillow sign." They are encapsulated tumors of adipose tissue that arise from the submucosa. Tissue biopsies are generally nondiagnostic, as they reveal only normal esophageal mucosa, but if repetitive biopsies are taken over one location, it may be possible to obtain adipose tissue. Tissue diagnosis is usually not required, as the endoscopic appearance is usually convincing and sufficient to make the diagnosis. When viewed with endoscopic ultrasound, esophageal lipomas appear as a homogeneous, hyperechoic lesion with smooth margins arising from the third layer. As the majority of other submucosal tumors are hypoechoic, imaging with endoscopic ultrasound is almost always diagnostic and can be used if there is any doubt with standard upper endoscopy [189]. Lipomas have no malignant potential and are rarely symptomatic; as a result, no therapy or surveillance is required.

Gastrointestinal Stromal Tumors

Gastrointestinal stromal tumors (GISTs) are mesenchymal neoplasms that can affect any part of the gastrointestinal tract. While they are the most common mesenchymal tumor in the gastrointestinal tract, fewer than 5% are found in the esophagus [190]. They have similarities to both smooth-muscle tumors (leiomyomas) and neural-based tumors (schwannomas), making diagnosis by histology alone complicated. The key feature for the diagnosis of GIST is positivity for CD 117 (KIT). Over 95% of GISTs will be KIT-positive, while other mesenchymal tumors (leiomyomas, schwannomas) are KIT-negative [191]. Endoscopically, they appear as a submucosal bulge with normal overlying mucosa (**Fig. 42.23**). Tissue biopsy with standard forceps is inadequate for diagnosis, as it does not obtain tissue from the tumor and almost always reveals normal squamous epithelium. Endoscopic ultrasound is the most accurate method for diagnosing GIST and can be used to obtain tissue. GISTs appear as hypoechoic, homogeneous tumors with sharp margins that most commonly arise from the muscularis propria. They may also be seen arising from the muscularis mucosa, and in these cases can be removed through endoscopic excision.

Symptomatic lesions should be treated with surgical excision or enucleation, although endoscopic excision can be considered when feasible. The management of asymptomatic GISTs is more uncertain.

While these tumors can be benign, the risk of malignant transformation is variable. Tumor size, location, and mitotic rate, along with endoscopic ultrasound features (irregular tumor border, cystic spaces, regional lymphadenopathy) can help predict tumors with an increased malignant potential [192,193].

EMR of esophageal GISTs has been successfully performed using a variety of techniques, but is associated with an increased risk of complications, including bleeding and perforation [194]. Larger case series and long-term follow-up are needed to determine which patients should undergo EMR, along with the efficacy and complication rate of the technique. In approximately 50% of patients with KIT-positive, unresectable or metastatic GIST, imatinib therapy will reduce the total tumor size by at least 50% [195]. However, the impact on overall survival and quality of life, along with the cost-effectiveness of this treatment, has not yet been established.

Granular Cell Tumors

Granular cell tumors are neural-based, submucosal neoplasms that originate from Schwann cells. They appear as pale, nodular lesions with normal overlying mucosa. Tissue biopsies obtained with a bite-on-bite technique can confirm the diagnosis, as the cells will stain strongly positive for S 100 protein [196]. On endoscopic ultrasound, they appear as hypoechoic to isoechoic lesions arising within the submucosa. They have a very low malignant potential, but large tumors and those with increasing size should be considered potentially malignant and should be removed [197].

Hemangiomas

Hemangiomas are a rare finding in the esophagus, but both cavernous and capillary hemangiomas have been reported [198]. They appear as nodular tumors with a blue or red discoloration. Pressure from biopsy forceps can cause the lesion to blanch. They have no malignant potential, but can be a cause of gastrointestinal hemorrhage and rarely dysphagia. Case reports of endoscopic therapy have been published, but patients who are symptomatic should be referred for surgical removal until the safety and efficacy of endoscopic therapy has been established [198].

Inflammatory Fibroid Polyps

Inflammatory fibroid polyp of the esophagus is an uncommon but benign submucosal lesion that is composed of loose connective tissue and vessels without a discrete capsule. They occur as a result of chronic esophageal inflammation, such as from GERD. The diagnosis is generally made with tissue biopsy, and endoscopic resection can be safely performed in patients who are symptomatic.

Fibrovascular Polyps

Fibrovascular polyps generally occur in the upper third of the esophagus, near the upper esophageal sphincter. They are large collections of fibrovascular tissue, adipose cells, and stroma that are covered with normal squamous epithelium. Most patients are asymptomatic, but polyps can cause regurgitation and respiratory symptoms if they reflux into the pharynx. Symptomatic patients should be referred for surgical removal of the polyp [199]. Endoscopic removal has been reported, but this should be done with caution, as these polyps commonly have large feeding vessels [200].

▪ Malignant Tumors

Squamous cell carcinoma and adenocarcinoma of the esophagus account for over 90% of malignant esophageal tumors [201]. While squamous cell carcinoma is the most common esophageal cancer worldwide, the incidence of esophageal adenocarcinoma has increased significantly in the United States and Europe, where it has surpassed squamous cell carcinoma as the predominant esophageal cancer [201]. Several dietary and environmental factors have been linked to squamous cell cancer development, including nitrosamines, hydrocarbon release during coal combustion, certain herbs and teas, tobacco, and alcohol [202]. In the United States, the majority of esophageal squamous cell cancers (over 90%) can be linked to alcohol or tobacco use alone [203]. A number of diseases have also been associated with esophageal squamous cell cancer development, including achalasia, caustic strictures due to lye ingestion, Plummer–Vinson syndrome, tylosis, human papillomavirus infection, Epstein–Barr virus infection, and a family history of squamous cell cancer [204–209]. In contrast, esophageal adenocarcinoma has been linked to GERD, Barrett's esophagus, and obesity, with a negative association with *Helicobacter pylori* infection [59,210].

The majority of patients with esophageal cancer present with symptoms that prompt an evaluation with upper endoscopy. During endoscopy, these tumors can appear as a mass, stricture, or ulcer (**Figs. 42.24, 42.25**). The mucosal origin of these lesions allows the endoscopist to obtain tissue biopsies and cytological brushings, which are effective in establishing a tissue diagnosis. At least six to eight biopsies should be obtained from any lesion that is suspicious for malignancy [211]. Once the diagnosis of esophageal carcinoma has been made, appropriate tumor staging is mandatory in order to provide prognostic information to the patient and formulate a treatment plan (**Table 42.4**). The first step in staging is the evaluation of distant metastases; CT and positron-emission tomography (PET) have accuracy rates of 63% and 84%, respectively [212]. However, both are poor at assessing local invasion by the primary tumor and for detecting metastases to regional lymph nodes. In patients without distant metastases on CT or PET, EUS should be performed to provide accurate T and N staging. The sensitivity and specificity rates for diagnosing T4 lesions are estimated at 92% and 97% respectively, while those for T1 lesions are estimated at 82% and 99%, respectively [213]. When fine-needle aspiration (FNA) is added to EUS, the sensitivity and specificity for N staging are estimated at 85% and 97%, respectively [213].

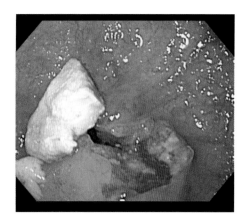

Fig. 42.24 Advanced esophageal squamous cell carcinoma, causing food impaction.

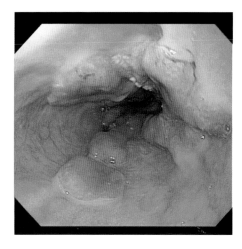

Fig. 42.25 Esophageal adenocarcinoma, diagnosed in a patient with new-onset dysphagia.

42

Table 42.4 TNM staging of esophageal cancer

T	Primary tumor
T0	No evidence of a primary tumor
Tis	Carcinoma in situ
T1	The tumor invades the lamina propria or submucosa, but does not breach the submucosa
T1a	The tumor invades into the mucosa or lamina propria
T1b	The tumor invades into the submucosa
T2	The tumor invades the muscularis propria, but does not breach the muscularis propria
T3	The tumor invades the adventitia, but not the adjacent structures
T4	The tumor invades the adjacent structures
N	**Regional lymph nodes**
Nx	Regional lymph nodes cannot be assessed
N0	No regional lymph-node metastases
N1	Regional lymph-node metastases
M	**Distant metastases**
MX	Distant metastases cannot be assessed
M0	No distant metastases
M1	Distant metastases
Stage	
Stage 0	Tis, N0, M0
Stage I	T1, N0, M0
Stage IIA	T2–T3, N0, M0
Stage IIB	T1–2, N1, M0
Stage III	T3, N1, M0 or T4, any N, M0
Stage IV	Any T, Any N, M1

Patients with disease limited to the mucosa may be candidates for endoscopic therapy, and those with early-stage tumors should undergo surgical resection. The depth of tumor invasion is an important predictor for lymph-node metastasis and can help identify which patients are candidates for endoscopic therapy [214]. EMR in patients with superficial tumors by EUS can provide a more detailed assessment of the depth of tumor invasion and provide a potentially curative resection. Esophagectomy in patients with stage T1 disease is associated with 5-year overall and disease-specific survival rates of 78% and 86%, respectively [215]. There are significant differences in the survival when these lesions are further characterized as T1a and T1b, with a 5-year overall survival of 90% vs. 71% and a 5-year disease-specific survival of 97% vs. 80% [215]. Although there are no randomized controlled studies, retrospective comparisons have found no significant differences in survival rates between EMR with and without other endoscopic ablation procedures and esophagectomy in patients with T1a disease [216,217]. However, prospective comparative studies are needed to further evaluate the long-term efficacy of endoscopic therapy for mucosal tumors. Locally advanced disease does poorly with surgery alone, and these individuals should be assessed for multimodal therapy including chemotherapy and radiotherapy. Therapy with surgery alone or radiotherapy alone is associated with poor survival rates. In these patients, therapy with chemoradiation increases the 5-year overall (26% vs. 0%) [218]. However, phase III trials comparing neoadjuvant chemoradiation plus surgery with surgery alone have shown mixed results [219,220]. As a result, research into the optimal treatment strategy for these patients is ongoing. Patients with local invasion into the vital chest structures or distant metastases should be treated with palliation alone.

Other Malignant Tumors

Other malignant tumors include small cell carcinoma, malignant melanoma, carcinosarcoma, and verrucous carcinoma. The esophagus is the most common extrapulmonary site of small cell cancer, and this accounts for 0.4–2.7% of all esophageal cancers [221]. They metastasize early and have a very poor 1-year survival rate [221]. Primary esophageal melanoma is extremely rare, but the esophagus can be the primary source of metastatic melanoma. Like small cell cancer, it metastasizes early and has a poor survival rate [222]. Carcinosarcoma and verrucous carcinoma are uncommon variants of squamous cell carcinoma. Verrucous carcinomas have a low metastatic potential and a more favorable prognosis, while the prognosis and management in carcinosarcomas are similar to those in squamous cell cancer [223]. Nonepithelial malignancies of the esophagus include lymphoma, leiomyosarcoma, Kaposi's sarcoma, and metastatic disease from a nonesophageal primary cancer. All these rare tumors require EUS-guided FNA in order to confirm the diagnosis.

References

1. Amano Y, Ishimura N, Furuta K, Takahashi Y, Chinuki D, Mishima Y, et al. Which landmark results in a more consistent diagnosis of Barrett's esophagus, the gastric folds or the palisade vessels? Gastrointest Endosc 2006;64:206–11.
2. Ogiya K, Kawano T, Ito E, Nakajima Y, Kawada K, Nishikage T, et al. Lower esophageal palisade vessels and the definition of Barrett's esophagus. Dis Esophagus 2008;21:645–9.
3. Ronkainen J, Aro P, Storskrubb T, Johansson SE, Lind T, Bolling-Sternevald E, et al. High prevalence of gastroesophageal reflux symptoms and esophagitis with or without symptoms in the general adult Swedish population: a Kalixanda study report. Scand J Gastroenterol 2005;40:275–85.
4. Robinson M, Earnest D, Rodriguez-Stanley S, Greenwood-Van Meerveld B, Jaffe P, Silver MT, et al. Heartburn requiring frequent antacid use may indicate significant illness. Arch Intern Med 1998;158:2373–6.
5. Johansson KE, Ask P, Boeryd B, Fransson SG, Tibbling L. Oesophagitis, signs of reflux, and gastric acid secretion in patients with symptoms of gastro-oesophageal reflux disease. Scand J Gastroenterol 1986;21:837–47.
6. Chang CS, Poon SK, Lien HC, Chen GH. The incidence of reflux esophagitis among the Chinese. Am J Gastroenterol 1997;92:668–71.
7. Rosaida MS, Goh KL. Gastro-oesophageal reflux disease, reflux oesophagitis and non-erosive reflux disease in a multiracial Asian population: a prospective, endoscopy based study. Eur J Gastroenterol Hepatol 2004; 16:495–501.
8. Hampel H, Abraham NS, El-Serag HB. Meta-analysis: obesity and the risk for gastroesophageal reflux disease and its complications. Ann Intern Med 2005;143:199–211.
9. Aro P, Ronkainen J, Talley NJ, Storskrubb T, Bolling-Sternevald E, Agreus L. Body mass index and chronic unexplained gastrointestinal symptoms: an adult endoscopic population based study. Gut 2005;54:1377–83.
10. Nakamura T, Shirakawa K, Masuyama H, Sugaya H, Hiraishi H, Terano A. Minimal change oesophagitis: a disease with characteristic differences to erosive oesophagitis. Aliment Pharmacol Ther 2005;21(Suppl 2):19–26.
11. Sharma P, Wani S, Bansal A, Hall S, Puli S, Mathur S, et al. A feasibility trial of narrow band imaging endoscopy in patients with gastroesophageal reflux disease. Gastroenterology 2007;133:454–64; quiz 674.
12. Miwa H, Yokoyama T, Hori K, Sakagami T, Oshima T, Tomita T, et al. Interobserver agreement in endoscopic evaluation of reflux esophagitis using a modified Los Angeles classification incorporating grades N and M: a validation study in a cohort of Japanese endoscopists. Dis Esophagus 2008;21:355–63.
13. Amano Y, Ishimura N, Furuta K, Okita K, Masaharu M, Azumi T, et al. Interobserver agreement on classifying endoscopic diagnoses of nonerosive esophagitis. Endoscopy 2006;38:1032–5.
14. Fock KM, Teo EK, Ang TL, Tan JY, Law NM. The utility of narrow band imaging in improving the endoscopic diagnosis of gastroesophageal reflux disease. Clin Gastroenterol Hepatol 2009;7:54–9.
15. Savary M, Miller G. The esophagus: handbook and atlas of endoscopy. Solothurn, Switzerland: Gussman; 1978.
16. Hetzel DJ, Dent J, Reed WD, Narielvala FM, Mackinnon M, McCarthy JH, et al. Healing and relapse of severe peptic esophagitis after treatment with omeprazole. Gastroenterology 1988;95:903–12.
17. Armstrong D, Blum AL, Savary M. Reflux disease and Barrett's oesophagus. Endoscopy 1992;24:9–17.
18. Armstrong D, Bennett JR, Blum AL, Dent J, De Dombal FT, Galmiche JP, et al. The endoscopic assessment of esophagitis: a progress report on observer agreement. Gastroenterology 1996;111:85–92.
19. Rath HC, Timmer A, Kunkel C, Endlicher E, Grossmann J, Hellerbrand C, et al. Comparison of interobserver agreement for different scoring systems for reflux esophagitis: Impact of level of experience. Gastrointest Endosc 2004;60:44–9.
20. Pandolfino JE, Vakil NB, Kahrilas PJ. Comparison of inter- and intraobserver consistency for grading of esophagitis by expert and trainee endoscopists. Gastrointest Endosc 2002;56:639–43.
21. Lee YC, Lin JT, Chiu HM, Liao WC, Chen CC, Tu CH, et al. Intraobserver and interobserver consistency for grading esophagitis with narrow-band imaging. Gastrointest Endosc 2007;66:230–6.
22. Standards of Practice Committee, Lichtenstein DR, Cash BD, Davila R, Baron TH, Adler DG, et al. Role of endoscopy in the management of GERD. Gastrointest Endosc 2007;66:219–24.
23. Rodriguez S, Mattek N, Lieberman D, Fennerty B, Eisen G. Barrett's esophagus on repeat endoscopy: should we look more than once? Am J Gastroenterol 2008;103:1892–7.
24. Hanna S, Rastogi A, Weston AP, Totta F, Schmitz R, Mathur S, et al. Detection of Barrett's esophagus after endoscopic healing of erosive esophagitis. Am J Gastroenterol 2006;101:1416–20.
25. Zheng RN. Comparative study of omeprazole, lansoprazole, pantoprazole and esomeprazole for symptom relief in patients with reflux esophagitis. World J Gastroenterol 2009;15:990–5.
26. Caro JJ, Salas M, Ward A. Healing and relapse rates in gastroesophageal reflux disease treated with the newer proton-pump inhibitors lansoprazole, rabeprazole, and pantoprazole compared with omeprazole, ranitidine, and placebo: evidence from randomized clinical trials. Clin Ther 2001;23:998–1017.
27. Omura N, Kashiwagi H, Yano F, Tsuboi K, Ishibashi Y, Kawasaki N, et al. Prediction of recurrence after laparoscopic fundoplication for erosive reflux esophagitis based on anatomy-function-pathology (AFP) classification. Surg Endosc 2007;21:427–30.

VI

28. Mimidis K, Papadopoulos V, Margaritis V, Thomopoulos K, Gatopoulou A, Nikolopoulou V, et al. Predisposing factors and clinical symptoms in HIV-negative patients with *Candida* oesophagitis: are they always present? Int J Clin Pract 2005;59:210–3.

29. Underwood JA, Williams JW, Keate RF. Clinical findings and risk factors for *Candida* esophagitis in outpatients. Dis Esophagus 2003;16:66–9.

30. Andersen LI, Frederiksen HJ, Appleyard M. Prevalence of esophageal *Candida* colonization in a Danish population: special reference to esophageal symptoms, benign esophageal disorders, and pulmonary disease. J Infect Dis 1992;165:389–92.

31. Bianchi Porro G, Parente F, Cernuschi M. The diagnosis of esophageal candidiasis in patients with acquired immune deficiency syndrome: is endoscopy always necessary? Am J Gastroenterol 1989;84:143–6.

32. Kodsi BE, Wickremesinghe C, Kozinn PJ, Iswara K, Goldberg PK. *Candida* esophagitis: a prospective study of 27 cases. Gastroenterology 1976; 71:715–9.

33. Ramanathan J, Rammouni M, Baran J Jr, Khatib R. Herpes simplex virus esophagitis in the immunocompetent host: an overview. Am J Gastroenterol 2000;95:2171–6.

34. Wilcox CM, Straub RF, Schwartz DA. Prospective endoscopic characterization of cytomegalovirus esophagitis in AIDS. Gastrointest Endosc 1994; 40:481–4.

35. Wilcox CM, Straub RF, Schwartz DA. Prospective evaluation of biopsy number for the diagnosis of viral esophagitis in patients with HIV infection and esophageal ulcer. Gastrointest Endosc 1996;44:587–93.

36. Wilcox CM, Rodgers W, Lazenby A. Prospective comparison of brush cytology, viral culture, and histology for the diagnosis of ulcerative esophagitis in AIDS. Clin Gastroenterol Hepatol 2004;2:564–7.

37. Kikendall JW. Pill esophagitis. J Clin Gastroenterol 1999;28:298–305.

38. Bonavina L, DeMeester TR, McChesney L, Schwizer W, Albertucci M, Bailey RT. Drug-induced esophageal strictures. Ann Surg 1987;206:173–83.

39. Hey H, Jorgensen F, Sorensen K, Hasselbalch H, Wamberg T. Oesophageal transit of six commonly used tablets and capsules. Br Med J (Clin Res Ed) 1982;285:1717–9.

40. Cheng HT, Cheng CL, Lin CH, Tang JH, Chu YY, Liu NJ, et al. Caustic ingestion in adults: the role of endoscopic classification in predicting outcome. BMC Gastroenterol 2008;8:31.

41. Zargar SA, Kochhar R, Mehta S, Mehta SK. The role of fiberoptic endoscopy in the management of corrosive ingestion and modified endoscopic classification of burns. Gastrointest Endosc 1991;37:165–9.

42. Poley JW, Steyerberg EW, Kuipers EJ, Dees J, Hartmans R, Tilanus HW, et al. Ingestion of acid and alkaline agents: outcome and prognostic value of early upper endoscopy. Gastrointest Endosc 2004;60:372–7.

43. Betalli P, Falchetti D, Giuliani S, Pane A, Dall'Oglio L, de Angelis GL, et al. Caustic ingestion in children: is endoscopy always indicated? The results of an Italian multicenter observational study. Gastrointest Endosc 2008; 68:434–9.

44. Pereira-Lima JC, Ramires RP, Zamin I Jr, Cassal AP, Marroni CA, Mattos AA. Endoscopic dilation of benign esophageal strictures: report on 1043 procedures. Am J Gastroenterol 1999;94:1497–501.

45. Broor SL, Raju GS, Bose PP, Lahoti D, Ramesh GN, Kumar A, et al. Long term results of endoscopic dilatation for corrosive oesophageal strictures. Gut 1993;34:1498–501.

46. Kochhar R, Ray JD, Sriram PV, Kumar S, Singh K. Intralesional steroids augment the effects of endoscopic dilation in corrosive esophageal strictures. Gastrointest Endosc 1999;49:509–13.

47. Kim YT, Sung SW, Kim JH. Is it necessary to resect the diseased esophagus in performing reconstruction for corrosive esophageal stricture? Eur J Cardiothorac Surg 2001;20:1–6.

48. Kahn D, Zhou S, Ahn SJ, Hollis D, Yu X, D'Amico TA, et al. "Anatomically-correct" dosimetric parameters may be better predictors for esophageal toxicity than are traditional CT-based metrics. Int J Radiat Oncol Biol Phys 2005;62:645–51.

49. Movsas B, Scott C, Langer C, Werner-Wasik M, Nicolaou N, Komaki R, et al. Randomized trial of amifostine in locally advanced non-small-cell lung cancer patients receiving chemotherapy and hyperfractionated radiation: radiation therapy oncology group trial 98–01. J Clin Oncol 2005; 23:2145–54.

50. Komaki R, Lee JS, Milas L, Lee HK, Fossella FV, Herbst RS, et al. Effects of amifostine on acute toxicity from concurrent chemotherapy and radiotherapy for inoperable non-small-cell lung cancer: report of a randomized comparative trial. Int J Radiat Oncol Biol Phys 2004;58:1369–77.

51. Ahlawat SK, Al-Kawas FH. Endoscopic management of upper esophageal strictures after treatment of head and neck malignancy. Gastrointest Endosc 2008;68:19–24.

52. Said A, Brust DJ, Gaumnitz EA, Reichelderfer M. Predictors of early recurrence of benign esophageal strictures. Am J Gastroenterol 2003;98: 1252–6.

53. Kochhar R, Makharia GK. Usefulness of intralesional triamcinolone in treatment of benign esophageal strictures. Gastrointest Endosc 2002; 56:829–34.

54. Holm AN, de la Mora Levy JG, Gostout CJ, Topazian MD, Baron TH. Self-expanding plastic stents in treatment of benign esophageal conditions. Gastrointest Endosc 2008;67:20–5.

55. Dua KS, Vleggaar FP, Santharam R, Siersema PD. Removable self-expanding plastic esophageal stent as a continuous, non-permanent dilator in treating refractory benign esophageal strictures: a prospective two-center study. Am J Gastroenterol 2008;103:2988–94.

56. Csendes A, Smok G, Burdiles P, Quesada F, Huertas C, Rojas J, et al. Prevalence of Barrett's esophagus by endoscopy and histologic studies: a prospective evaluation of 306 control subjects and 376 patients with symptoms of gastroesophageal reflux. Dis Esophagus 2000;13:5–11.

57. Munitiz V, Parrilla P, Ortiz A, Martinez-de-Haro LF, Yelamos J, Molina J. High risk of malignancy in familial Barrett's esophagus: presentation of one family. J Clin Gastroenterol 2008;42:806–9.

58. Akiyama T, Inamori M, Iida H, Mawatari H, Endo H, Hosono K, et al. Alcohol consumption is associated with an increased risk of erosive esophagitis and Barrett's epithelium in Japanese men. BMC Gastroenterol 2008;8:58.

59. Theisen J, Stein HJ, Dittler HJ, Feith M, Moebius C, Kauer WK, et al. Preoperative chemotherapy unmasks underlying Barrett's mucosa in patients with adenocarcinoma of the distal esophagus. Surg Endosc 2002;16:671–3.

60. Weston AP, Sharma P, Mathur S, Banerjee S, Jafri AK, Cherian R, et al. Risk stratification of Barrett's esophagus: updated prospective multivariate analysis. Am J Gastroenterol 2004;99:1657–66.

61. Cameron AJ, Ott BJ, Payne WS. The incidence of adenocarcinoma in columnar-lined (Barrett's) esophagus. N Engl J Med 1985;313:857–9.

62. Sharma P, Dent J, Armstrong D, Bergman JJ, Gossner L, Hoshihara Y, et al. The development and validation of an endoscopic grading system for Barrett's esophagus: the Prague C & M criteria. Gastroenterology 2006; 131:1392–9.

63. Cooper GS, Yuan Z, Chak A, Rimm AA. Association of prediagnosis endoscopy with stage and survival in adenocarcinoma of the esophagus and gastric cardia. Cancer 2002;95:32–8.

64. Kearney DJ, Crump C, Maynard C, Boyko EJ. A case–control study of endoscopy and mortality from adenocarcinoma of the esophagus or gastric cardia in persons with GERD. Gastrointest Endosc 2003;57:823–9.

65. Corley DA, Levin TR, Habel LA, Weiss NS, Buffler PA. Surveillance and survival in Barrett's adenocarcinomas: a population-based study. Gastroenterology 2002;122:633–40.

66. Bani-Hani K, Sue-Ling H, Johnston D, Axon AT, Martin IG. Barrett's oesophagus: results from a 13-year surveillance programme. Eur J Gastroenterol Hepatol 2000;12:649–54.

67. Conio M, Blanchi S, Lapertosa G, Ferraris R, Sablich R, Marchi S, et al. Long-term endoscopic surveillance of patients with Barrett's esophagus. Incidence of dysplasia and adenocarcinoma: a prospective study. Am J Gastroenterol 2003;98:1931–9.

68. Dulai GS, Shekelle PG, Jensen DM, Spiegel BM, Chen J, Oh D, et al. Dysplasia and risk of further neoplastic progression in a regional Veterans Administration Barrett's cohort. Am J Gastroenterol 2005;100:775–83.

69. Provenzale D, Schmitt C, Wong JB. Barrett's esophagus: a new look at surveillance based on emerging estimates of cancer risk. Am J Gastroenterol 1999;94:2043–53.

70. Inadomi JM, Sampliner R, Lagergren J, Lieberman D, Fendrick AM, Vakil N. Screening and surveillance for Barrett's esophagus in high-risk groups: a cost-utility analysis. Ann Intern Med 2003;138:176–86.

71. Gerson LB, Groeneveld PW, Triadafilopoulos G. Cost-effectiveness model of endoscopic screening and surveillance in patients with gastroesophageal reflux disease. Clin Gastroenterol Hepatol 2004;2:868–79.

72. Eloubeidi MA, Provenzale D. Clinical and demographic predictors of Barrett's esophagus among patients with gastroesophageal reflux disease: a multivariable analysis in veterans. J Clin Gastroenterol 2001;33: 306–9.

73. Conio M, Filiberti R, Blanchi S, Ferraris R, Marchi S, Ravelli P, et al. Risk factors for Barrett's esophagus: a case–control study. Int J Cancer 2002;97:225–9.

74. El-Serag HB, Kvapil P, Hacken-Bitar J, Kramer JR. Abdominal obesity and the risk of Barrett's esophagus. Am J Gastroenterol 2005;100:2151–6.

75. Edelstein ZR, Bronner MP, Rosen SN, Vaughan TL. Risk Factors for Barrett's esophagus among patients with gastroesophageal reflux disease: a com-

42

munity clinic-based case–control study. Am J Gastroenterol 2009;104: 834–42.

76. Ronkainen J, Aro P, Storskrubb T, Johansson SE, Lind T, Bolling-Sternevald E, et al. Prevalence of Barrett's esophagus in the general population: an endoscopic study. Gastroenterology 2005;129:1825–31.

77. Falk GW, Ours TM, Richter JE. Practice patterns for surveillance of Barrett's esophagus in the united states. Gastrointest Endosc 2000;52:197–203.

78. Gross CP, Canto MI, Hixson J, Powe NR. Management of Barrett's esophagus: a national study of practice patterns and their cost implications. Am J Gastroenterol 1999;94:3440–7.

79. Reid BJ, Weinstein WM, Lewin KJ, Haggitt RC, VanDeventer G, DenBesten L, et al. Endoscopic biopsy can detect high-grade dysplasia or early adenocarcinoma in Barrett's esophagus without grossly recognizable neoplastic lesions. Gastroenterology 1988;94:81–90.

80. Reid BJ, Blount PL, Feng Z, Levine DS. Optimizing endoscopic biopsy detection of early cancers in Barrett's high-grade dysplasia. Am J Gastroenterol 2000;95:3089–96.

81. Schafer TW, Hollis-Perry KM, Mondragon RM, Brann OS. An observer-blinded, prospective, randomized comparison of forceps for endoscopic esophageal biopsy. Gastrointest Endosc 2002;55:192–6.

82. Levine DS, Reid BJ. Endoscopic biopsy technique for acquiring larger mucosal samples. Gastrointest Endosc 1991;37:332–7.

83. Wolfsen HC, Crook JE, Krishna M, Achem SR, Devault KR, Bouras EP, et al. Prospective, controlled tandem endoscopy study of narrow band imaging for dysplasia detection in Barrett's Esophagus. Gastroenterology 2008; 135:24–31.

84. Borovicka J, Fischer J, Neuweiler J, Netzer P, Gschossmann J, Ehmann T, et al. Autofluorescence endoscopy in surveillance of Barrett's esophagus: a multicenter randomized trial on diagnostic efficacy. Endoscopy 2006; 38:867–72.

85. Kiesslich R, Gossner L, Goetz M, Dahlmann A, Vieth M, Stolte M, et al. In vivo histology of Barrett's esophagus and associated neoplasia by confocal laser endomicroscopy. Clin Gastroenterol Hepatol 2006;4:979–87.

86. Pohl H, Rösch T, Vieth M, Koch M, Becker V, Anders M, et al. Miniprobe confocal laser microscopy for the detection of invisible neoplasia in patients with Barrett's oesophagus. Gut 2008;57:1648–53.

87. Sharma P, Falk GW, Weston AP, Reker D, Johnston M, Sampliner RE. Dysplasia and cancer in a large multicenter cohort of patients with Barrett's esophagus. Clin Gastroenterol Hepatol 2006;4:566–72.

88. Kerkhof M, van Dekken H, Steyerberg EW, Meijer GA, Mulder AH, de Bruïne A, et al. Grading of dysplasia in Barrett's oesophagus: substantial interobserver variation between general and gastrointestinal pathologists. Histopathology 2007;50:920–7.

89. Lim CH, Treanor D, Dixon MF, Axon AT. Low-grade dysplasia in Barrett's esophagus has a high risk of progression. Endoscopy 2007;39:581–7.

90. Buttar NS, Wang KK, Sebo TJ, Riehle DM, Krishnadath KK, Lutzke LS, et al. Extent of high-grade dysplasia in Barrett's esophagus correlates with risk of adenocarcinoma. Gastroenterology 2001;120:1630–9.

91. Ouatu-Lascar R, Fitzgerald RC, Triadafilopoulos G. Differentiation and proliferation in Barrett's esophagus and the effects of acid suppression. Gastroenterology 1999;117:327–35.

92. El-Serag HB, Aguirre TV, Davis S, Kuebeler M, Bhattacharyya A, Sampliner RE. Proton pump inhibitors are associated with reduced incidence of dysplasia in Barrett's esophagus. Am J Gastroenterol 2004;99:1877–83.

93. Chang EY, Morris CD, Seltman AK, O'Rourke RW, Chan BK, Hunter JG, et al. The effect of antireflux surgery on esophageal carcinogenesis in patients with Barrett's esophagus: a systematic review. Ann Surg 2007;246:11–21.

94. Hofstetter WL, Peters JH, DeMeester TR, Hagen JA, DeMeester SR, Crookes PF, et al. Long-term outcome of antireflux surgery in patients with Barrett's esophagus. Ann Surg 2001;234:532–9.

95. Overholt BF, Wang KK, Burdick JS, Lightdale CJ, Kimmey M, Nava HR, et al. Five-year efficacy and safety of photodynamic therapy with Photofrin in Barrett's high-grade dysplasia. Gastrointest Endosc 2007;66:460–8.

96. Yachimski P, Puricelli WP, Nishioka NS. Patient predictors of esophageal stricture development after photodynamic therapy. Clin Gastroenterol Hepatol 2008;6:302–8.

97. Ganz RA, Overholt BF, Sharma VK, Fleischer DE, Shaheen NJ, Lightdale CJ, et al. Circumferential ablation of Barrett's esophagus that contains high-grade dysplasia: a U.S. multicenter registry. Gastrointest Endosc 2008;68: 35–40.

98. Larghi A, Lightdale CJ, Ross AS, Fedi P, Hart J, Rotterdam H, et al. Long-term follow-up of complete Barrett's eradication endoscopic mucosal resection (CBE-EMR) for the treatment of high grade dysplasia and intramucosal carcinoma. Endoscopy 2007;39:1086–91.

99. Lopes CV, Hela M, Pesenti C, Bories E, Caillol F, Monges G, et al. Circumferential endoscopic resection of Barrett's esophagus with high-grade dysplasia or early adenocarcinoma. Surg Endosc 2007;21:820–4.

100. Giovannini M, Bories E, Pesenti C, Moutardier V, Monges G, Danisi C, et al. Circumferential endoscopic mucosal resection in Barrett's esophagus with high-grade intraepithelial neoplasia or mucosal cancer. Preliminary results in 21 patients. Endoscopy 2004;36:782–7.

101. Manning BJ, Winter DC, McGreal G, Kirwan WO, Redmond HP. Nasogastric intubation causes gastroesophageal reflux in patients undergoing elective laparotomy. Surgery 2001;130:788–91.

102. Vezina MC, Trepanier CA, Nicole PC, Lessard MR. Complications associated with the esophageal-tracheal Combitube in the pre-hospital setting. Can J Anaesth 2007;54:124–8.

103. Shapira OM, Aldea GS, Kupferschmid J, Shemin RJ. Delayed perforation of the esophagus by a closed thoracostomy tube. Chest 1993;104:1897–8.

104. Arora S, Chakravarthy M, Srinivasan V. Delayed manifestation of a mid-esophageal tear with profuse hemorrhage after transesophageal echocardiogram. Echocardiography 2008;25:328–30.

105. Azar C, Jamali F, Tamim H, Abdul-Baki H, Soweid A. Prevalence of endoscopically identified heterotopic gastric mucosa in the proximal esophagus: endoscopist dependent? J Clin Gastroenterol 2007;41:468–71.

106. Melato M, Ferlito A. Heterotopic gastric mucosa of the tongue and the oesophagus. ORL J Otorhinolaryngol Relat Spec 1975;37:244–54.

107. Mann NS, Mann SK, Rachut E. Heterotopic gastric tissue in the duodenal bulb. J Clin Gastroenterol 2000;30:303–6.

108. Caruso ML, Marzullo F. Jejunal adenocarcinoma in congenital heterotopic gastric mucosa. J Clin Gastroenterol 1988;10:92–4.

109. Xeropotamos N, Skopelitou AS, Batsis C, Kappas AM. Heterotopic gastric mucosa together with intestinal metaplasia and moderate dysplasia in the gall bladder: report of two clinically unusual cases with literature review. Gut 2001;48:719–23.

110. Jordan FT, Mazzeo RJ, Soiderer MH. Heterotopic gastric mucosa of the rectum. A rare cause of rectal bleeding. Arch Surg 1983;118:878–80.

111. Maconi G, Pace F, Vago L, Carsana L, Bargiggia S, Bianchi Porro G. Prevalence and clinical features of heterotopic gastric mucosa in the upper oesophagus (inlet patch). Eur J Gastroenterol Hepatol 2000;12:745–9.

112. von Rahden BH, Stein HJ, Becker K, Liebermann-Meffert D, Siewert JR. Heterotopic gastric mucosa of the esophagus: literature-review and proposal of a clinicopathologic classification. Am J Gastroenterol 2004;99: 543–51.

113. Klaase JM, Lemaire LC, Rauws EA, Offerhaus GJ, van Lanschot JJ. Heterotopic gastric mucosa of the cervical esophagus: a case of high-grade dysplasia treated with argon plasma coagulation and a case of adenocarcinoma. Gastrointest Endosc 2001;53:101–4.

114. Enestvedt BK, Gralnek IM, Mattek N, Lieberman DA, Eisen G. An evaluation of endoscopic indications and findings related to nonvariceal upper-GI hemorrhage in a large multicenter consortium. Gastrointest Endosc 2008;67:422–9.

115. Younes Z, Johnson DA. The spectrum of spontaneous and iatrogenic esophageal injury: perforations, Mallory–Weiss tears, and hematomas. J Clin Gastroenterol 1999;29:306–17.

116. Bharucha AE, Gostout CJ, Balm RK. Clinical and endoscopic risk factors in the Mallory–Weiss syndrome. Am J Gastroenterol 1997;92:805–8.

117. Mitre MC, Katzka DA, Brensinger CM, Lewis JD, Mitre RJ, Ginsberg GG. Schatzki ring and Barrett's esophagus: do they occur together? Dig Dis Sci 2004;49:770–3.

118. Marshall JB, Kretschmar JM, Diaz-Arias AA. Gastroesophageal reflux as a pathogenic factor in the development of symptomatic lower esophageal rings. Arch Intern Med 1990;150:1669–72.

119. Jamieson J, Hinder RA, DeMeester TR, Litchfield D, Barlow A, Bailey RT Jr. Analysis of thirty-two patients with Schatzki's ring. Am J Surg 1989;158: 563–6.

120. Ott DJ, Chen YM, Wu WC, Gelfand DW, Munitz HA. Radiographic and endoscopic sensitivity in detecting lower esophageal mucosal ring. AJR Am J Roentgenol 1986;147:261–5.

121. Sgouros SN, Vassiliadis K, Bergele C, Vlachogiannakos J, Stefanidis G, Mantides A. Single-session, graded esophageal dilation without fluoroscopy in outpatients with lower esophageal (Schatzki's) rings: a prospective, long-term follow-up study. J Gastroenterol Hepatol 2007;22:653–7.

122. Groskreutz JL, Kim CH. Schatzki's ring: long-term results following dilation. Gastrointest Endosc 1990;36:479–81.

123. Sgouros SN, Vlachogiannakos J, Karamanolis G, Vassiliadis K, Stefanidis G, Bergele C, et al. Long-term acid suppressive therapy may prevent the relapse of lower esophageal (Schatzki's) rings: a prospective, randomized, placebo-controlled study. Am J Gastroenterol 2005;100:1929–34.

VI

124. Wills JC, Hilden K, Disario JA, Fang JC. A randomized, prospective trial of electrosurgical incision followed by rabeprazole versus bougie dilation followed by rabeprazole of symptomatic esophageal (Schatzki's) rings. Gastrointest Endosc 2008;67:808–13.

125. El-Serag HB, Sonnenberg A. Associations between different forms of gastro-oesophageal reflux disease. Gut 1997;41:594–9.

126. El-Serag HB, Sonnenberg A. Association of esophagitis and esophageal strictures with diseases treated with nonsteroidal anti-inflammatory drugs. Am J Gastroenterol 1997;92:52–6.

127. Raymondi R, Pereira-Lima JC, Valves A, Morales GF, Marques D, Lopes CV, et al. Endoscopic dilation of benign esophageal strictures without fluoroscopy: experience of 2750 procedures. Hepatogastroenterology 2008;55: 1342–8.

128. Scolapio JS, Pasha TM, Gostout CJ, Mahoney DW, Zinsmeister AR, Ott BJ, et al. A randomized prospective study comparing rigid to balloon dilators for benign esophageal strictures and rings. Gastrointest Endosc 1999;50: 13–7.

129. Saeed ZA, Winchester CB, Ferro PS, Michaletz PA, Schwartz JT, Graham DY. Prospective randomized comparison of polyvinyl bougies and through-the-scope balloons for dilation of peptic strictures of the esophagus. Gastrointest Endosc 1995;41:189–95.

130. Smith PM, Kerr GD, Cockel R, Ross BA, Bate CM, Brown P, et al. A comparison of omeprazole and ranitidine in the prevention of recurrence of benign esophageal stricture. Restore Investigator Group. Gastroenterology 1994;107:1312–8.

131. Ramage JI Jr, Rumalla A, Baron TH, Pochron NL, Zinsmeister AR, Murray JA, et al. A prospective, randomized, double-blind, placebo-controlled trial of endoscopic steroid injection therapy for recalcitrant esophageal peptic strictures. Am J Gastroenterol 2005;100:2419–25.

132. Veerappan GR, Perry JL, Duncan TJ, Baker TP, Maydonovitch C, Lake JM, et al. Prevalence of eosinophilic esophagitis in an adult population undergoing upper endoscopy: a prospective study. Clin Gastroenterol Hepatol 2009;7:420–6.

133. Furuta GT, Liacouras CA, Collins MH, Gupta SK, Justinich C, Putnam PE, et al. Eosinophilic esophagitis in children and adults: a systematic review and consensus recommendations for diagnosis and treatment. Gastroenterology 2007;133:1342–63.

134. Liacouras CA, Spergel JM, Ruchelli E, Verma R, Mascarenhas M, Semeao E, et al. Eosinophilic esophagitis: a 10-year experience in 381 children. Clin Gastroenterol Hepatol 2005;3:1198–206.

135. Spechler SJ, Genta RM, Souza RF. Thoughts on the complex relationship between gastroesophageal reflux disease and eosinophilic esophagitis. Am J Gastroenterol 2007;102:1301–6.

136. Gonsalves N, Policarpio-Nicolas M, Zhang Q, Rao MS, Hirano I. Histopathologic variability and endoscopic correlates in adults with eosinophilic esophagitis. Gastrointest Endosc 2006;64:313–9.

137. Spergel JM, Andrews T, Brown-Whitehorn TF, Beausoleil JL, Liacouras CA. Treatment of eosinophilic esophagitis with specific food elimination diet directed by a combination of skin prick and patch tests. Ann Allergy Asthma Immunol 2005;95:336–43.

138. Arora AS, Perrault J, Smyrk TC. Topical corticosteroid treatment of dysphagia due to eosinophilic esophagitis in adults. Mayo Clin Proc 2003;78: 830–5.

139. Remedios M, Campbell C, Jones DM, Kerlin P. Eosinophilic esophagitis in adults: clinical, endoscopic, histologic findings, and response to treatment with fluticasone propionate. Gastrointest Endosc 2006;63:3–12.

140. Helou EF, Simonson J, Arora AS. 3-yr-follow-up of topical corticosteroid treatment for eosinophilic esophagitis in adults. Am J Gastroenterol 2008;103:2194–9.

141. Ngo P, Furuta GT, Antonioli DA, Fox VL. Eosinophils in the esophagus—peptic or allergic eosinophilic esophagitis? Case series of three patients with esophageal eosinophilia. Am J Gastroenterol 2006;101:1666–70.

142. Croese J, Fairley SK, Masson JW, Chong AK, Whitaker DA, Kanowski PA, et al. Clinical and endoscopic features of eosinophilic esophagitis in adults. Gastrointest Endosc 2003;58:516–22.

143. Cohen MS, Kaufman AB, Palazzo JP, Nevin D, Dimarino AJ Jr, Cohen S. An audit of endoscopic complications in adult eosinophilic esophagitis. Clin Gastroenterol Hepatol 2007;5:1149–53.

144. Furukawa N, Iwakiri R, Koyama T, Okamoto K, Yoshida T, Kashiwagi Y, et al. Proportion of reflux esophagitis in 6010 Japanese adults: prospective evaluation by endoscopy. J Gastroenterol 1999;34:441–4.

145. Wilson LJ, Ma W, Hirschowitz BI. Association of obesity with hiatal hernia and esophagitis. Am J Gastroenterol 1999;94:2840–4.

146. Kim JH, Hwang JK, Kim J, Lee SD, Lee BJ, Kim JS, et al. Endoscopic findings around the gastroesophageal junction: an experience from a tertiary hospital in Korea. Korean J Intern Med 2008;23:127–33.

147. Dickman R, Mattek N, Holub J, Peters D, Fass R. Prevalence of upper gastrointestinal tract findings in patients with noncardiac chest pain versus those with gastroesophageal reflux disease (GERD)-related symptoms: results from a national endoscopic database. Am J Gastroenterol 2007;102:1173–9.

148. Smith AB, Dickerman RD, McGuire CS, East JW, McConathy WJ, Pearson HF. Pressure-overload-induced sliding hiatal hernia in power athletes. J Clin Gastroenterol 1999;28:352–4.

149. Ruhl CE, Everhart JE. Relationship of iron-deficiency anemia with esophagitis and hiatal hernia: hospital findings from a prospective, population-based study. Am J Gastroenterol 2001;96:322–6.

150. Sihvo EI, Salo JA, Rasanen JV, Rantanen TK. Fatal complications of adult paraesophageal hernia: a population-based study. J Thorac Cardiovasc Surg 2009;137:419–24.

151. White BC, Jeansonne LO, Morgenthal CB, Zagorski S, Davis SS, Smith CD, et al. Do recurrences after paraesophageal hernia repair matter? Ten-year follow-up after laparoscopic repair. Surg Endosc 2008;22:1107–11.

152. Ferreira LE, Simmons DT, Baron TH. Zenker's diverticula: pathophysiology, clinical presentation, and flexible endoscopic management. Dis Esophagus 2008;21:1–8.

153. Visosky AM, Parke RB, Donovan DT. Endoscopic management of Zenker's diverticulum: factors predictive of success or failure. Ann Otol Rhinol Laryngol 2008;117:531–7.

154. Zardi EM, Uwechie V, Caccavo D, Pellegrino NM, Cacciapaglia F, Di Matteo F, et al. Portosystemic shunts in a large cohort of patients with liver cirrhosis: detection rate and clinical relevance. J Gastroenterol 2009;44: 76–83.

155. Merli M, Nicolini G, Angeloni S, Rinaldi V, De Santis A, Merkel C, et al. Incidence and natural history of small esophageal varices in cirrhotic patients. J Hepatol 2003;38:266–72.

156. Groszmann RJ, Garcia-Tsao G, Bosch J, Grace ND, Burroughs AK, Planas R, et al. Beta-blockers to prevent gastroesophageal varices in patients with cirrhosis. N Engl J Med 2005;353:2254–61.

157. Garcia-Tsao G, Groszmann RJ, Fisher RL, Conn HO, Atterbury CE, Glickman M. Portal pressure, presence of gastroesophageal varices and variceal bleeding. Hepatology 1985;5:419–24.

158. Garcia-Tsao G, Sanyal AJ, Grace ND, Carey W. Prevention and management of gastroesophageal varices and variceal hemorrhage in cirrhosis. Hepatology 2007;46:922–38.

159. North Italian Endoscopic Club for the Study and Treatment of Esophageal Varices. Prediction of the first variceal hemorrhage in patients with cirrhosis of the liver and esophageal varices. A prospective multicenter study. N Engl J Med 1988;319:983–9.

160. Dagradi AE. The natural history of esophageal varices in patients with alcoholic liver cirrhosis. An endoscopic and clinical study. Am J Gastroenterol 1972;57:520–40.

161. Beppu K, Inokuchi K, Koyanagi N, Nakayama S, Sakata H, Kitano S, et al. Prediction of variceal hemorrhage by esophageal endoscopy. Gastrointest Endosc 1981;27:213–8.

162. Rigo GP, Merighi A, Chahin NJ, Mastronardi M, Codeluppi PL, Ferrari A, et al. A prospective study of the ability of three endoscopic classifications to predict hemorrhage from esophageal varices. Gastrointest Endosc 1992; 38:425–9.

163. Calès P, Zabotto B, Meskens C, Caucanas JP, Vinel JP, Desmorat H, et al. Gastroesophageal endoscopic features in cirrhosis. Observer variability, interassociations, and relationship to hepatic dysfunction. Gastroenterology 1990;98:156–62.

164. Bendtsen F, Skovgaard LT, Sorensen TI, Matzen P. Agreement among multiple observers on endoscopic diagnosis of esophageal varices before bleeding. Hepatology 1990;11:341–7.

165. Shaheen NJ, Stuart E, Schmitz SM, Mitchell KL, Fried MW, Zacks S, et al. Pantoprazole reduces the size of postbanding ulcers after variceal band ligation: a randomized, controlled trial. Hepatology 2005;41:588–94.

166. D'Amico G, Pagliaro L, Bosch J. Pharmacological treatment of portal hypertension: an evidence-based approach. Semin Liver Dis 1999;19:475–505.

167. Gluud LL, Klingenberg S, Nikolova D, Gluud C. Banding ligation versus beta-blockers as primary prophylaxis in esophageal varices: systematic review of randomized trials. Am J Gastroenterol 2007;102:2842–8.

168. D'Amico G, Pagliaro L, Bosch J. The treatment of portal hypertension: a meta-analytic review. Hepatology 1995;22:332–54.

169. Pagliaro L, D'Amico G, Sörensen TI, Lebrec D, Burroughs AK, Morabito A, et al. Prevention of first bleeding in cirrhosis. A meta-analysis of randomized trials of nonsurgical treatment. Ann Intern Med 1992;117:59–70.

170. [No authors listed]. Prophylactic sclerotherapy for esophageal varices in men with alcoholic liver disease. A randomized, single-blind, multicenter

42

clinical trial. The Veterans Affairs Cooperative Variceal Sclerotherapy Group. N Engl J Med 1991;324:1779–84.

171. Sarin SK, Wadhawan M, Agarwal SR, Tyagi P, Sharma BC. Endoscopic variceal ligation plus propranolol versus endoscopic variceal ligation alone in primary prophylaxis of variceal bleeding. Am J Gastroenterol 2005;100:797–804.

172. Laine L, Cook D. Endoscopic ligation compared with sclerotherapy for treatment of esophageal variceal bleeding. A meta-analysis. Ann Intern Med 1995;123:280–7.

173. Moitinho E, Escorsell A, Bandi JC, Salmerón JM, García-Pagán JC, Rodés J, et al. Prognostic value of early measurements of portal pressure in acute variceal bleeding. Gastroenterology 1999;117:626–31.

174. Monescillo A, Martínez-Lagares F, Ruiz-del-Arbol L, Sierra A, Guevara C, Jiménez E, et al. Influence of portal hypertension and its early decompression by TIPS placement on the outcome of variceal bleeding. Hepatology 2004;40:793–801.

175. D'Amico G, Pietrosi G, Tarantino I, Pagliaro L. Emergency sclerotherapy versus vasoactive drugs for variceal bleeding in cirrhosis: a Cochrane meta-analysis. Gastroenterology 2003;124:1277–91.

176. Bañares R, Albillos A, Rincón D, Alonso S, González M, Ruiz-del-Arbol L, et al. Endoscopic treatment versus endoscopic plus pharmacologic treatment for acute variceal bleeding: a meta-analysis. Hepatology 2002;35:609–15.

177. Bosch J, Garcia-Pagan JC. Prevention of variceal rebleeding. Lancet 2003;361:952–4.

178. Singh P, Pooran N, Indaram A, Bank S. Combined ligation and sclerotherapy versus ligation alone for secondary prophylaxis of esophageal variceal bleeding: a meta-analysis. Am J Gastroenterol 2002;97:623–9.

179. Karsan HA, Morton SC, Shekelle PG, Spiegel BM, Suttorp MJ, Edelstein MA, et al. Combination endoscopic band ligation and sclerotherapy compared with endoscopic band ligation alone for the secondary prophylaxis of esophageal variceal hemorrhage: a meta-analysis. Dig Dis Sci 2005;50:399–406.

180. Lo GH, Lai KH, Cheng JS, Chen MH, Huang HC, Hsu PI, et al. Endoscopic variceal ligation plus nadolol and sucralfate compared with ligation alone for the prevention of variceal rebleeding: a prospective, randomized trial. Hepatology 2000;32:461–5.

181. de la Peña J, Brullet E, Sanchez-Hernández E, Rivero M, Vergara M, Martin-Lorente JL, et al. Variceal ligation plus nadolol compared with ligation for prophylaxis of variceal rebleeding: a multicenter trial. Hepatology 2005;41:572–8.

182. Asherson N. David Bayford. His syndrome and sign of dysphagia lusoria. Ann R Coll Surg Engl 1979;61:63–7.

183. De Luca L, Bergman JJ, Tytgat GN, Fockens P. EUS imaging of the arteria lusoria: case series and review. Gastrointest Endosc 2000;52:670–3.

184. Beabout JW, Stewart JR, Kincaid OW. Aberrant right subclavian artery: dispute of commonly accepted concepts. Am J Roentgenol Radium Ther Nucl Med 1964;92:855–64.

185. Balaji MR, Ona FV, Cheeran D, Paul G, Nanda N. Dysphagia lusoria: a case report and review of diagnosis and treatment in adults. Am J Gastroenterol 1982;77:899–901.

186. Janssen M, Baggen MG, Veen HF, Smout AJ, Bekkers JA, Jonkman JG, et al. Dysphagia lusoria: clinical aspects, manometric findings, diagnosis, and therapy. Am J Gastroenterol 2000;95:1411–6.

187. Odze R, Antonioli D, Shocket D, Noble-Topham S, Goldman H, Upton M. Esophageal squamous papillomas. A clinicopathologic study of 38 lesions and analysis for human papillomavirus by the polymerase chain reaction. Am J Surg Pathol 1993;17:803–12.

188. Mosca S, Manes G, Monaco R, Bellomo PF, Bottino V, Balzano A. Squamous papilloma of the esophagus: long-term follow up. J Gastroenterol Hepatol 2001;16:857–61.

189. Gress F, Schmitt C, Savides T, Faigel DO, Catalano M, Wassef W, et al. Interobserver agreement for EUS in the evaluation and diagnosis of submucosal masses. Gastrointest Endosc 2001;53:71–6.

190. Miettinen M, Lasota J. Gastrointestinal stromal tumors—definition, clinical, histological, immunohistochemical, and molecular genetic features and differential diagnosis. Virchows Arch 2001;438:1–12.

191. Rubin BP, Singer S, Tsao C, Duensing A, Lux ML, Ruiz R, et al. KIT activation is a ubiquitous feature of gastrointestinal stromal tumors. Cancer Res 2001;61:8118–21.

192. Palazzo L, Landi B, Cellier C, Cuillerier E, Roseau G, Barbier JP. Endosonographic features predictive of benign and malignant gastrointestinal stromal cell tumours. Gut 2000;46:88–92.

193. Dematteo RP, Gold JS, Saran L, Gönen M, Liau KH, Maki RG, et al. Tumor mitotic rate, size, and location independently predict recurrence after resection of primary gastrointestinal stromal tumor (GIST). Cancer 2008;112:608–15.

194. Ponsaing LG, Hansen MB. Therapeutic procedures for submucosal tumors in the gastrointestinal tract. World J Gastroenterol 2007;13:3316–22.

195. Wilson J, Connock M, Song F, Yao G, Fry-Smith A, Raftery J, et al. Imatinib for the treatment of patients with unresectable and/or metastatic gastrointestinal stromal tumours: systematic review and economic evaluation. Health Technol Assess 2005;9:1–142.

196. Stefansson K, Wollmann RL. S-100 protein in granular cell tumors (granular cell myoblastomas). Cancer 1982;49:1834–8.

197. De Rezende L, Lucendo AJ, Alvarez-Arguelles H. Granular cell tumors of the esophagus: report of five cases and review of diagnostic and therapeutic techniques. Dis Esophagus 2007;20:436–43.

198. Sogabe M, Taniki T, Fukui Y, Yoshida T, Okamoto K, Okita Y, et al. A patient with esophageal hemangioma treated by endoscopic mucosal resection: a case report and review of the literature. J Med Invest 2006;53:177–82.

199. Kanaan S, DeMeester TR. Fibrovascular polyp of the esophagus requiring esophagectomy. Dis Esophagus 2007;20:453–4.

200. Pham AM, Rees CJ, Belafsky PC. Endoscopic removal of a giant fibrovascular polyp of the esophagus. Ann Otol Rhinol Laryngol 2008;117:587–90.

201. Trivers KF, Sabatino SA, Stewart SL. Trends in esophageal cancer incidence by histology, United States, 1998–2003. Int J Cancer 2008;123:1422–8.

202. Wang JM, Xu B, Rao JY, Shen HB, Xue HC, Jiang QW. Diet habits, alcohol drinking, tobacco smoking, green tea drinking, and the risk of esophageal squamous cell carcinoma in the Chinese population. Eur J Gastroenterol Hepatol 2007;19:171–6.

203. Brown LM, Hoover R, Silverman D, Baris D, Hayes R, Swanson GM, et al. Excess incidence of squamous cell esophageal cancer among US Black men: role of social class and other risk factors. Am J Epidemiol 2001;153:114–22.

204. Zendehdel K, Nyrén O, Edberg A, Ye W. Risk of esophageal adenocarcinoma in achalasia patients, a retrospective cohort study in Sweden. Am J Gastroenterol 2007 [Epub ahead of print].

205. Kochhar R, Sethy PK, Kochhar S, Nagi B, Gupta NM. Corrosive induced carcinoma of esophagus: report of three patients and review of literature. J Gastroenterol Hepatol 2006;21:777–80.

206. Larsson LG, Sandstrom A, Westling P. Relationship of Plummer–Vinson disease to cancer of the upper alimentary tract in Sweden. Cancer Res 1975;35:3308–16.

207. Risk JM, Mills HS, Garde J, Dunn JR, Evans KE, Hollstein M, et al. The tylosis esophageal cancer (TOC) locus: more than just a familial cancer gene. Dis Esophagus 1999;12:173–6.

208. Wu MY, Wu XY, Zhuang CX. Detection of HSV and EBV in esophageal carcinomas from a high-incidence area in Shantou China. Dis Esophagus 2005;18:46–50.

209. Chang-Claude J, Becher H, Blettner M, Qiu S, Yang G, Wahrendorf J. Familial aggregation of oesophageal cancer in a high incidence area in China. Int J Epidemiol 1997;26:1159–65.

210. Lofdahl HE, Lu Y, Lagergren J. Sex-specific risk factor profile in oesophageal adenocarcinoma. Br J Cancer 2008;99:1506–10.

211. Graham DY, Schwartz JT, Cain GD, Gyorkey F. Prospective evaluation of biopsy number in the diagnosis of esophageal and gastric carcinoma. Gastroenterology 1982;82:228–31.

212. Luketich JD, Friedman DM, Weigel TL, Meehan MA, Keenan RJ, Townsend DW, et al. Evaluation of distant metastases in esophageal cancer: 100 consecutive positron emission tomography scans. Ann Thorac Surg 1999;68:1133–7.

213. Puli SR, Reddy JB, Bechtold ML, Antillon D, Ibdah JA, Antillon MR. Staging accuracy of esophageal cancer by endoscopic ultrasound: a meta-analysis and systematic review. World J Gastroenterol 2008;14:1479–90.

214. Endo M, Yoshino K, Kawano T, Nagai K, Inoue H. Clinicopathologic analysis of lymph node metastasis in surgically resected superficial cancer of the thoracic esophagus. Dis Esophagus 2000;13:125–9.

215. Altorki NK, Lee PC, Liss Y, Meherally D, Korst RJ, Christos P, et al. Multifocal neoplasia and nodal metastases in T1 esophageal carcinoma: implications for endoscopic treatment. Ann Surg 2008;247:434–9.

216. Schembre DB, Huang JL, Lin OS, Cantone N, Low DE. Treatment of Barrett's esophagus with early neoplasia: a comparison of endoscopic therapy and esophagectomy. Gastrointest Endosc 2008;67:595–601.

217. Pacifico RJ, Wang KK, Wongkeesong LM, Buttar NS, Lutzke LS. Combined endoscopic mucosal resection and photodynamic therapy versus esophagectomy for management of early adenocarcinoma in Barrett's esophagus. Clin Gastroenterol Hepatol 2003;1:252–7.

218. Cooper JS, Guo MD, Herskovic A, Macdonald JS, Martenson JA Jr, Al-Sarraf M, et al. Chemoradiotherapy of locally advanced esophageal cancer: long-

VI

term follow-up of a prospective randomized trial (RTOG 85–01). Radiation Therapy Oncology Group. JAMA 1999;281:1623–7.

219. Urba SG, Orringer MB, Turrisi A, Iannettoni M, Forastiere A, Strawderman M. Randomized trial of preoperative chemoradiation versus surgery alone in patients with locoregional esophageal carcinoma. J Clin Oncol 2001;19:305–13.

220. Tepper J, Krasna MJ, Niedzwiecki D, Hollis D, Reed CE, Goldberg R, et al. Phase III trial of trimodality therapy with cisplatin, fluorouracil, radiotherapy, and surgery compared with surgery alone for esophageal cancer: CALGB 9781. J Clin Oncol 2008;26:1086–92.

221. Lv J, Liang J, Wang J, Wang L, He J, Xiao Z, et al. Primary small cell carcinoma of the esophagus. J Thorac Oncol 2008;3:1460–5.

222. Li B, Lei W, Shao K, Zhang C, Chen Z, Shi S, et al. Characteristics and prognosis of primary malignant melanoma of the esophagus. Melanoma Res 2007;17:239–42.

223. Iascone C, Barreca M. Carcinosarcoma and pseudosarcoma of the esophagus: two names, one disease—comprehensive review of the literature. World J Surg 1999;23:153–7.

42

43 Gastric Diseases

Kristien M.A.J. Tytgat and Guido N.J. Tytgat

Normal Stomach—Anatomical Variants—Mucosal Prolapse and Tearing

Normal Stomach

Normal stomachs have a variety of shapes. Some are long and vertical, others are transverse. At endoscopy, the stomach is gently inflated with air so that the entire mucosal surface can be inspected. Observations are made of the color of the mucosa, the degree of luster, and whether blood vessels can be seen in a not overly distended stomach. The rugae or folds are inspected for caliber, regularity, and pliability, and whether they flatten and disappear as the stomach is inflated. The entire gastric surface is inspected for lesions, including erosions, ulcers, nodules, polyps, tumors, tears, etc.

The stomach has three compartments: the antrum, gastric body (corpus), and fundus. The fundus is the dome-shaped area immedi-ately above the gastric body and abutting the diaphragm. The folds or rugae begin in the upper part of the stomach, and run distally toward the antrum (**Fig. 43.1 a**). Folds or rugae are normally soft and pliable. Usually, they will almost completely flatten with distension of the stomach. Four vertical fairly straight parallel folds run along the lesser curve toward the angle.

The antrum is usually smooth and free of folds. Gastric peristalsis begins in the mid-gastric body, and progresses down to the antrum (**Fig. 43.1 b**). The pylorus is usually open. When the contraction wave reaches it, the pylorus closes. This is probably important for mixing and grinding of food, and to allow only liquid and small particles to pass into the duodenum. Peristaltic contractions nor-mally occur at a frequency of three per minute. It is useful to watch a contraction wave move from the gastric body to the antrum, to determine whether there is a lack of symmetry or whether there is an area that is less pliable. The pylorus opening is normally round or oval (**Fig. 43.1 c**). Occasionally, a fold traverses the opening. Pas-sage of the instrument into the bulb usually occurs after gentle

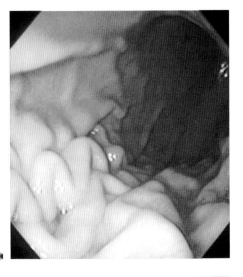
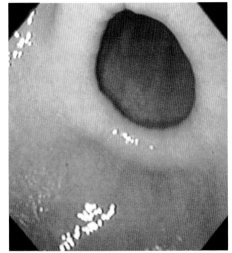
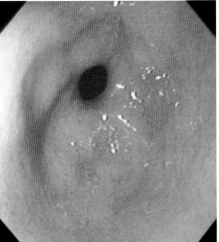
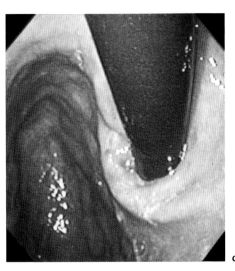

Fig. 43.1
a The normal fold pattern in the gastric body.
b A circular concentric peristaltic wave on its way to the pylorus.
c The normal antrum, with a normal pyloric opening.
d Retroflexed view of the cardia and upper part of the stomach.

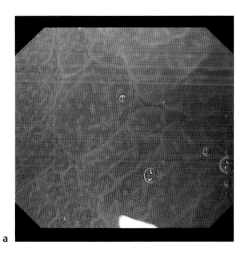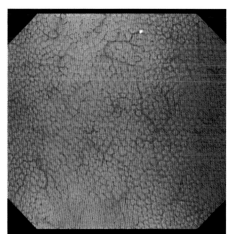

Fig. 43.2
a The sulcular or grooved pit pattern.
b The foveolar or round pit pattern, with a honey-comb-like subepithelial capillary network.

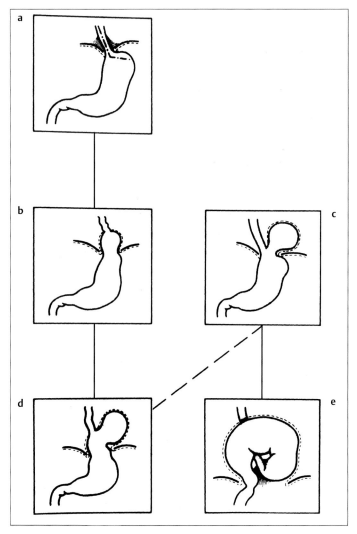

Fig. 43.3 The various forms of hiatal hernia.
a Normal anatomy.
b Axial sliding hiatal hernia.
c Paraesophageal hiatal hernia.
d Combined hiatal hernia.
e Upside-down stomach.

pressure is exerted with the well-centered tip of an end-viewing endoscope into the pyloric channel. This maneuver may occasionally have to be repeated several times, because of displacement of the flexible tip as a consequence of antral motor activity.

When the endoscope is retroflexed, detailed observation of the lesser curvature, cardia, and fundus is possible. The retroflexed endoscope can be pulled up close to the cardia and upper fundus (**Fig. 43.1 d**).

Visualization of the antrum and pylorus is occasionally not immediately apparent after introduction of the endoscope, especially when there is acute angulation of the antrum and gastric body. Problems with orientation also occur when there is cascade formation, in which the upper part of the stomach appears to be separated from the distal part by a tissue bridge. With some maneuvering of the endoscope, it is usually possible to advance the instrument along the lesser curve into the distal stomach and antrum.

There are several organs adjacent to the stomach that can cause extrinsic compression on the gastric lumen. Impression by the spleen is usually seen in the posterior greater curvature area.

Normally, the gastric lining has a uniform salmon color. With careful inspection, one can observe the areae gastricae, and with high magnification the pit pattern. The pit pattern is different in the antrum (with a sulcus or grooved pit pattern) in comparison with the gastric body (with a foveolar or round pit pattern) (**Fig. 43.2**). The areae gastricae are irregular or absent in patients with atrophic gastritis or with intestinal metaplasia, and enlarged in patients with acid hypersecretion. Blood vessels are normally not seen in a healthy stomach.

Hiatal Hernia

The normal cardia fits snugly around the endoscope when viewed in retroflection. When there is a hiatal hernia, this snug apposition is lost, and a pouch or cupola may be seen entering the thorax through the hiatal ring (**Figs. 43.3–43.5**). A commonly used definition of hiatal hernia is based on dislocation of the esophagogastric junction above the pinchcock of the diaphragm during quiet breathing and in the absence of retching or vomiting. Three landmarks are helpful in indentifying the esophagogastric junction: the proximal extent of the gastric folds, the distal extent of the esophageal palisade vessels, and the pinch of the lower esophageal sphincter. A ring-like narrowing, causing dysphagia when the diameter is less than 13 mm, at the level of the squamocolumnar mucosal junction is called a Schatzki ring (**Fig. 43.6**). A hiatal hernia is often combined with evidence of reflux esophagitis or esophageal columnar metaplasia. Mild inflammatory changes may also be seen around the proximal extent of the gastric folds in the hiatal sac. In rare circumstances, there is polypoid thickening of this fold—known as the "sentinel polyp" (**Fig. 43.7**). Riding ulcers (Cameron ulcers) may develop as a consequence of the constant to-and-fro movement of the gastric mucosa across the pinchcock of the diaphragm, causing mechanical

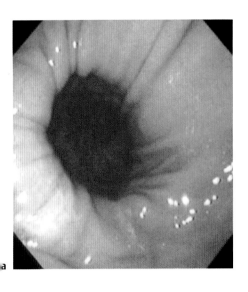

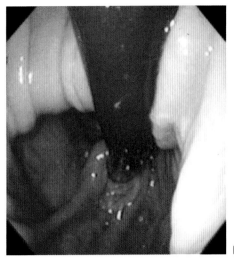

Fig. 43.4 Sliding hiatal hernia, seen from the esophageal side (**a**) and in retroflexion from the stomach (**b**).

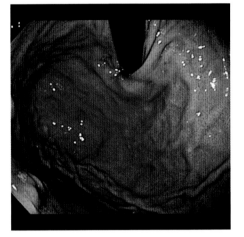

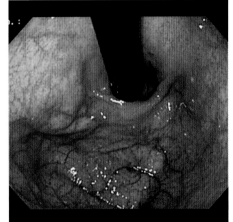

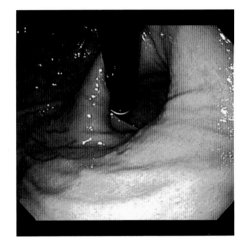

Fig. 43.5 Gradation of severity of hiatal hernia.
a None.

b Mild.

c Severe.

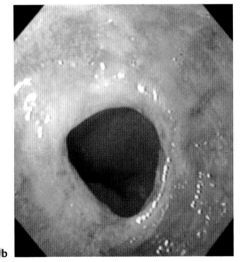

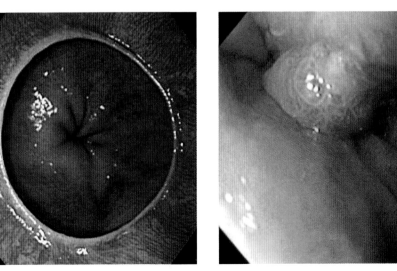

Fig. 43.6
a A Schatzki ring in a patient with hiatal hernia.
b Schatzki ring located at the distal level of the palisade vessel zone.

Fig. 43.7 A sentinel polyp in a hiatal hernia merging with the squamous mucosa.

43

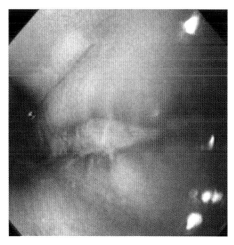
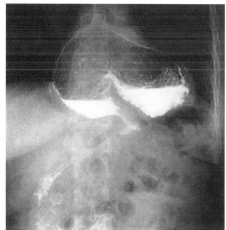
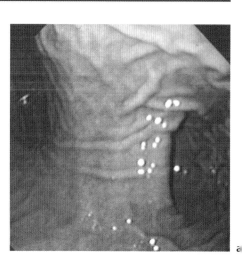

Fig. 43.8 Cameron ulcers in a hiatal hernia, not uncommonly a cause of chronic intermittent bleeding.

Fig. 43.9 Upside-down stomach.
a Radiographic image.
b Endoscopic image.

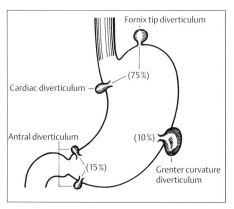
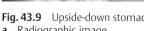

Fig. 43.10 The locations of various types of gastric diverticulum.

damage (**Fig. 43.8**). Such riding ulcers may cause chronic blood loss and anemia [1].

Paraesophageal Hernia

In a paraesophageal hernia, the cardia remains in its normal position across the diaphragm, but a hernial sac develops along the cardia into the left thorax. A proper endoscopic diagnosis can only be made after retroflexion of the endoscope in the stomach. Adjacent to the cardia, which fits snugly around the endoscope, a pouch may be seen extending into the left thorax. Entering the paraesophageal pouch with the endoscope should be avoided, to prevent impaction. This can even happen inadvertently during retching. A paraesophageal hernia may lead to complications (incarceration, strangulation, ulceration, ischemic necrosis, chronic bleeding, etc.).

Mixed Axial and Paraesophageal Herniation

A combination of a sliding and paraesophageal hernia can occur, allowing a variable part of the stomach to enter the mediastinum—known as "thoracic stomach." After the cardia has been passed, a large part of the stomach may be observed toward the left before crossing the diaphragm. Depending on the extent of the hernia, symptoms of postprandial fullness, dysphagia, recurrent singultus, or cardiac symptoms may occur.

Upside-Down Stomach

An upside-down stomach is the consequence of axial rotation and paraesophageal herniation in which the entire stomach is dislocated into the chest, bringing the pylorus next to the cardia (**Fig. 43.9**). The endoscopist should always be aware of this possibility whenever difficulties in orientation are encountered, or if it becomes impossible to identify or reach the pylorus. Usually, the endoscope slides along the greater curvature, creating a loop prohibiting further passage into the pylorus and duodenum. An upside-down stomach should in principle be treated surgically. However, when surgery is not possible, endoscopic correction of the volvulus may be attempted, usually with fixation of the anterior gastric wall with a percutaneous gastrostomy.

Gastric Diverticula

The most common location of a congenital gastric diverticulum is the subcardial lesser curvature area (**Fig. 43.10**). Usually, a gastric diverticulum is covered with normal-looking mucosa. Complications include ulceration due to stagnant food residue or trapping of drugs.

Gastroesophageal Prolapse

Recurrent retching may lead to gastric prolapse, known as "prolapse gastropathy." A plug of edematous and congested gastric folds may be seen prolapsing into the esophagus during retching and vomiting (**Fig. 43.11**). Prolapse trauma causes a circumscribed region 1–3 cm wide at or below the cardia, which is congested and edematous and occasionally frankly hemorrhagic. In addition, erosions and even frank ulceration may be present. Friction and compression of the gastric folds against the esophagogastric junction, or vascular strangulation of the prolapsing knuckle, may cause petechial or ecchymotic hemorrhages [2].

Mallory–Weiss Tears

Mucosal tearing, as seen in Mallory–Weiss syndrome, is also a consequence of excessive retching or vomiting [3] (**Fig. 43.12**). The sudden distension of the upper part of the stomach in the presence

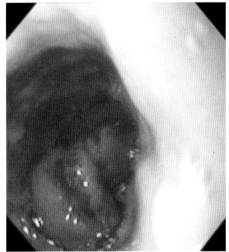
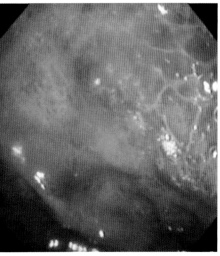
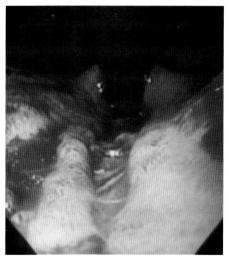

Fig. 43.11 a Congested gastric folds entering the esophagus during the prolapsing phase.
b Congested erythematous gastric mucosa as a consequence of gastroesophageal prolapse.

Fig. 43.12 Mallory–Weiss syndrome, with mucosal tearing and bleeding.

of a tightly closed lower esophageal sphincter during retching presumably predisposes to mucosal tearing. This contrasts with gastric mucosal prolapse, which is more likely to occur when the esophagogastric junction is patulous.

Gastritis

Increasingly, the modified Sydney–Houston system is being used to stage and grade gastric inflammation. This system has endoscopic and histological aspects.

▓ Endoscopic Aspects

It is notoriously difficult to provide a precise and reproducible description of endoscopic inflammatory changes of the stomach. Endoscopic inflammation may be diagnosed when some or all of the following abnormalities are unequivocally present: edema, erythema, exudate, evidence of mucosal breaks, intramural bleeding spots, rugal changes, etc.

Edema or *swelling* is obvious when it is pronounced, but is rather difficult to detect reliably when mild.

Erythema or redness is diagnosed when there is patchy or more diffuse red discoloration, contrasting with the normal pink color of the adjacent mucosa. Presumably, a combination of capillary engorgement and mucus depletion alters the light transmission and reflection from the mucosal surface, producing a redder appearance. Mild erythema represents minimal but obvious change; moderate erythema is in between; and severe or marked erythema is diagnosed when the color change is beefy red in intensity. On close inspection, erythema often appears as innumerable tiny, slightly raised dots of redness, compatible with reddened areae gastricae. Separating these erythematous dots are delicate yellow-white lines, the lineae gastricae.

Exudate may be seen as tiny whitish-grayish punctate spots or gray-yellowish flecks, adherent to lusterless mucosa.

Erosion is a visible break in the mucosal integrity. Erosions are called flat when present within the level of the mucosa, and raised or varioliform when elevated on mounds of inflamed mucosa. Flat erosions vary in size from pinpoint up to 1 cm in diameter. They may be solitary or multiple. Endoscopic detection is easy, particularly when the base is covered with necrotic fibrinous material. By definition, erosions do not breach the muscularis mucosae.

Hyperrugosity or fold enlargement is diagnosed when folds are prominent (5–10 mm), or large (over 10 mm) in diameter. Such enlarged folds do not flatten during insufflation.

Fold atrophy is characterized by flattening, thinning, and ultimate disappearance of the gastric rugae.

Visibility of the vascular pattern develops after the mucosa becomes markedly thin and atrophic, allowing the ramifying vessels to become apparent.

Intramural bleeding spots occur after disruption of the capillary integrity, leading to extravasation of erythrocytes. The latter will be seen as punctate red spots (petechiae) in a congestive mucosa, or as larger red-brownish or darker ecchymotic areas.

Granularity is diagnosed when a fine or coarsely nodular alteration of the normally smooth lining is present.

Compiling the macroscopic features and highlighting the most conspicuous abnormality leads to the following endoscopic classifications in the Sydney system [4,5].

Endoscopic erythematous–exudative gastritis is diagnosed when patchy erythema, fine granularity, loss of shininess, and discrete punctate exudate is visible (**Fig. 43.13 a, b**). This form of gastritis can be mild, moderate, or severe, and may involve the antrum, or both the antrum and gastric body. Occasionally, reddish streaks may be observed in the antrum, running radially toward the pylorus (**Fig. 43.13 c**). These need to be differentiated from antral vascular ectasia. Occasionally, there is conspicuous antral nodularity, especially in chronic *Helicobacter pylori* gastritis, due to massive accumulation of lymphoid aggregates (**Fig. 43.14**).

Endoscopic erosive gastritis is diagnosed when flat or raised (varioliform) erosions are visible as the dominant abnormality—either solitary or multiple, and limited to the antrum or located throughout the antrum and gastric body (**Fig. 43.15**). Mucofibrinoid exudate may cover the erosive defects. Occasionally, there is linear alignment of the erosions along folds that run toward the pylorus.

Endoscopic atrophic gastritis is diagnosed when the vascular ramifications are visible when the stomach is not overdistended (**Figs. 43.16**). Additional pearly-whitish mucosal discoloration is common, as is flattening or absence of the fold pattern in the gastric body. Occasionally, nodularity may be present, accentuated with dye scattering (**Fig. 43.17**). Areas of intestinal metaplasia may be visible as grayish-whitish, slightly raised opalescent patches, which may even have a villous appearance on close inspection (**Fig. 43.18**). Methylene blue chromoscopy may be useful for determining the presence and extent of intestinal metaplasia [6]. After application of a solution of acetylcysteine (Mucomyst) to dissolve gastric mucus,

43

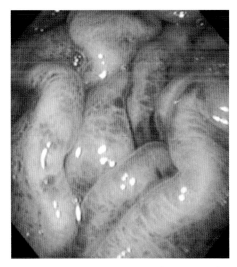
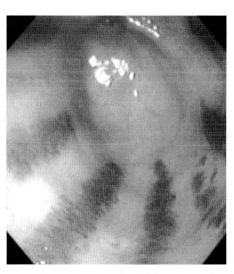

a, b

c

Fig. 43.13
a   Endoscopic erythematous exudative gastritis of the antrum.
b   Endoscopic erythematous exudative gastritis of the gastric body.

c   Endoscopic erythematous exudative gastritis, with reddish streaks radiating toward the pylorus.

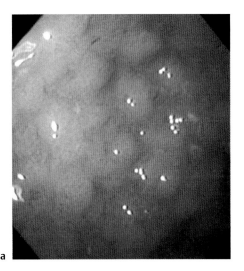
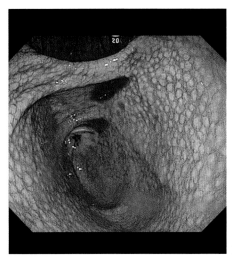

a

b

Fig. 43.14
a   Conspicuous nodular deformity or coarse granularity in the antrum.
b   The nodularity is accentuated with chromoscopy.

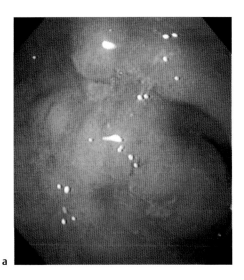
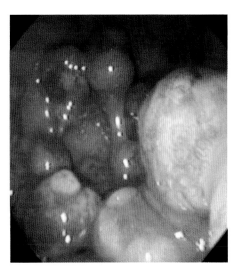

a

b

Fig. 43.15
a   Flat erosive gastritis in the antrum.
b   Raised erosive gastritis.

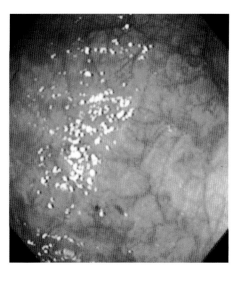

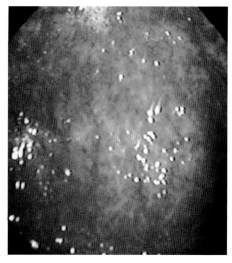

Fig. 43.16
a Atrophic gastritis of the antrum, with visible vascular ramifications.
b Atrophic gastritis of the gastric body, with absent rugae and a visible vascular pattern.

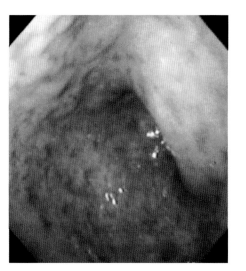

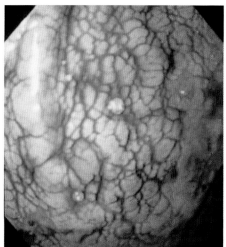

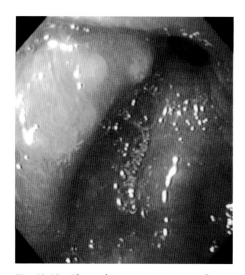

Fig. 43.17
a Advanced atrophic gastritis with nodular deformity.
b Dye staining accentuates the nodular deformity.

Fig. 43.18 The endoscopic appearance of patches of intestinal metaplasia in atrophic gastritis.

0.01 % methylene blue solution is sprayed onto the gastric mucosa. Mucosal staining via absorbed methylene blue may be absent, focally present, or diffusely present. Collections of lipid-filled macrophages, known as xanthelasma, may become visible in severe atrophic gastritis (**Fig. 43.19**).

Endoscopic hemorrhagic gastritis is diagnosed when punctate or ecchymotic, reddish, or brown-blackish discoloration is present in the gastric wall as the dominant abnormality (**Fig. 43.20**). Bleeding may be intramural, or combined intramural and intraluminal, visible as adherent dark-stained material.

Endoscopic hyperplastic gastritis is diagnosed when hyperrugosity is the dominant abnormality (**Fig. 43.21**). Pliancy of the folds should be assessed by means of mucosal tenting, to rule out infiltrative disorders. Occasionally, the folds may reveal caliber changes, superimposed polypoid bulges, or concomitant erosions on top of the folds. Abundant mucus often covers the enlarged folds in Ménétrier's disease. In gastrinoma, there is conspicuous accentuation of the areae gastricae in the gastric body, with copious production of clear, highly acidic gastric juice.

Endoscopic enterogastric reflux gastritis is characterized by severe swelling and erythema, with fiercely red discoloration of the mucosa, stained with refluxed bile. In particular, the area of the stoma is markedly swollen and beefy red in patients with partial gastric resection (**Fig. 43.22**).

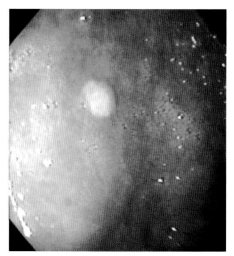

Fig. 43.19 Gastric xanthelasma, with a peculiar yellowish discoloration.

The Research Society for Gastritis in Japan recommends the use of five endoscopic types of gastritis: superficial, erosive, verrucous, atrophic, and special types [7].

43

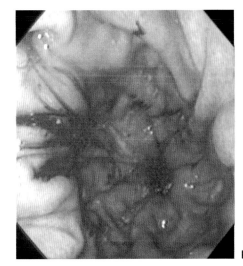

Fig. 43.20
a Hemorrhagic gastritis, with petechial intramural bleeding.
b Hemorrhagic gastritis, with ecchymotic discoloration.

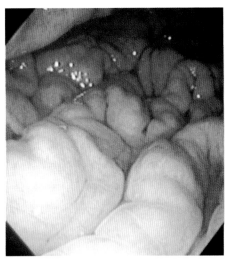
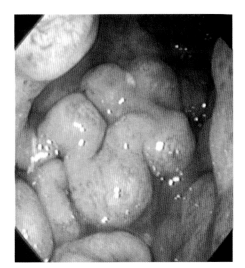
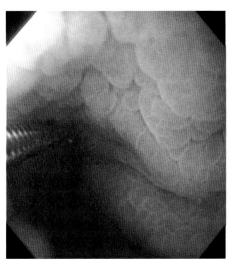

Fig. 43.21
a Hyperplastic gastritis, with conspicuously enlarged folds.

b Hyperplastic gastritis, with fold thickening and superimposed inflammatory changes.
c Accentuation of the areae gastricae in a patient with gastrinoma.

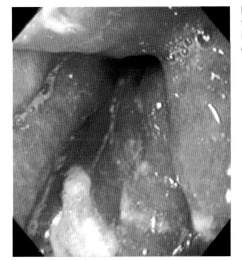

Fig. 43.22 Enterogastric reflux gastritis, with beefy red discoloration of the mucosa.

Histological Aspects [8]

The Sydney system with the Houston modification is increasingly being used to grade gastric inflammation. The Sydney system was designed as a working matrix for both reporting and classification (**Fig. 43.23**). The system incorporates a logical combination of etiology, topography, and morphology. The morphological component includes the basic pattern and topographical distribution of the abnormalities. An essential aspect of the system is recognition of the topographical distribution as antrum-predominant, gastric body–predominant, or pangastritis. Three basic morphologies are distinguished: acute gastritis, chronic gastritis, and special forms. Another important feature is the standard grading scale applicable to a selected number of morphological variables (mild, moderate, and severe). Variables to be graded are: chronic inflammation, polymorphonuclear activity, atrophy, intestinal metaplasia, and density of *H. pylori* organisms. Special forms of gastritis include granulomatous gastritis, vasculitides, eosinophilic, lymphocytic, reactive gastritis, etc.

In the Houston update [9], gastritis is distinguished into two major categories, based on the presence or absence and topographic distribution of atrophy (**Fig. 43.24**). In addition, several special

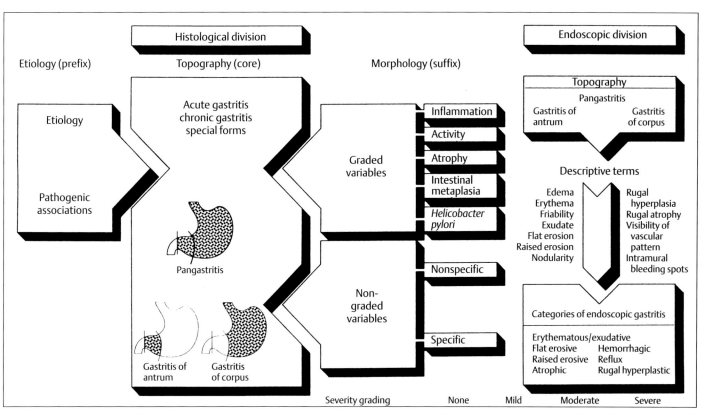

Fig. 43.23 The histologic aspects of the Sydney system.

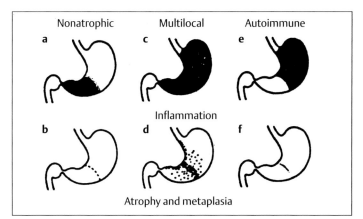

Fig. 43.24 The Houston modification of the Sydney system, showing the distribution of inflammation and atrophy in different types of atrophic and nonatrophic chronic gastritis [10]. In nonatrophic *Helicobacter pylori* gastritis, the inflammation is either predominantly antral or almost uniformly distributed in the antrum and gastric body (**a**), and there is no significant atrophy (**b**). In atrophic *H. pylori* gastritis (**c**), the inflammation is usually less intense and is similar in the antrum and gastric body. Patches of atrophy with intestinal metaplasia arise initially in the area of the angular notch and in the transitional zone and may expand proximally and distally to form confluent patches of atrophic metaplastic mucosa (**d**). In autoimmune gastritis, both inflammation (**e**) and atrophy (**f**) are virtually restricted to the gastric body.

forms are also enumerated (**Table 43.1**) [4,9]. A standardized visual analogue scale is provided to assist in grading relevant features of the chronic inflammatory process (**Fig. 43.25**).

Grading atrophy in the presence of inflammation proves to be exceedingly difficult [10–12]. Atrophy is the final loss of glandular tissue. Atrophy leads to thinning of the mucosa. Loss of glands may be followed by fibrous replacement, or by a collapse of the supporting matrix. Separation of glands by chronic inflammation and fibrosis may make it difficult to recognize antral gland atrophy. Atrophy in the oxyntic mucosa is closely linked to loss of acid secretion and to the development of intestinal metaplasia. However, atrophy can occasionally be found in the absence of intestinal metaplasia, particularly in autoimmune gastritis. Intestinal metaplasia has several subtypes, summarized in **Table 43.2** [13,14]. Type I is complete, types II and III are incomplete.

Where to biopsy. Two biopsies from the antrum and two from the gastric body should be obtained routinely (**Fig. 43.26**) [13]. One specimen each should be obtained from the lesser and greater curvature of the antrum, both within 2–3 cm of the pylorus. One gastric body biopsy should be taken about 4 cm proximal to the angle, and one from the middle portion of the greater curvature approximately 8 cm from the cardia. It is advisable to take one additional biopsy from the angular notch. Degrees of atrophy and intestinal metaplasia are consistently most pronounced in this region.

Nosological Causes of Gastric Inflammation

From a nosological point of view, gastric inflammatory conditions can be subdivided into several categories [15]: infectious gastritides; autoimmune; drug-associated; rugal hyperplastic; granulomatous; enterogastric reflux; physicochemical caustic; stress-associated; primary vascular and ischemic; and a miscellaneous residual group.

Table 43.1 Classification of gastritis (updated Sydney system) [4,9]

Type of gastritis	Etiological factors	Gastritis synonyms
Nonatrophic	Helicobacter pylori	Superficial
		? Other factors
		Diffuse antral gastritis (DAG)
		Chronic antral gastritis (CAG)
		Interstitial follicular
		Hypersecretory
		Type B*
Atrophic	Autoimmunity	Type A*
Autoimmune		Diffuse corporeal
		Pernicious anemia-associated
Multifocal atrophic	H. pylori	Type B,* Type AB*
	Dietary	Environmental
	? Environmental factors	Metaplastic
Special forms	Chemical irritation	Reactive
Chemical †	Bile	Reflux
	NSAIDs	NSAID
	? Other agents	Type C 1
Radiation	Radiation injury	
Lymphocytic	Idiopathic, ? immune mechanisms	Varioliform (endoscopic)
	Gluten	Celiac disease–associated
	Drug (ticlopidine)	
	? H. pylori	
Noninfectious	Crohn's disease	Isolated granulomatous
Granulomatous	Sarcoidosis	
	Wegener granulomatosis and other vasculitides	
	Foreign substances	
	Idiopathic	
Eosinophilic	Food sensitivity	Allergic
	? Other allergies	
Other infectious gastritides	Bacteria (other than H. pylori)	Phlegmonous
	Viruses	
	Fungi	
	Parasites	

*Alphabetic designations of gastritis were abandoned in the original presentation of the Sydney system. That approach is also recommended here. "Type B," used to denote either atrophic or nonatrophic gastritis, is particularly misleading.
† Many favor substitution of the term "gastropathy" for "gastritis" to describe conditions that result from chemical injury.

Table 43.2 The classification of intestinal metaplasia

Type I	Goblet cells with sialomucins. Mature nonsecretory absorptive cells
Type II	Goblet cells with sialomucins. Intermediate cells with neutral and acid sialomucins
	No absorptive cells
Type III	Goblet cells with sialomucins and sulfomucins
	Intermediate cells with sulfomucins
	No absorptive cells
	Disrupted architecture

Infectious Gastritis

H. pylori–associated gastritis. By far the most common form of infectious gastritis is H. pylori colonization. Very little is known about the acute stage of the infection. Presumably, an acute inflammatory reaction with plentiful polymorphs develops both in the antrum and the gastric body. This is then gradually followed by a more chronic phase of the infection. Depending on the adequacy of the immune response and the host's prior acid-secretory potential, the inflammatory reaction becomes largely antrum-predominant, or remains pangastritic. Modified Giemsa, Genta, silver stains, etc., are superior to hematoxylin–eosin staining for detecting the organisms, which live close to the mucosal surface. Organisms can usually be identified due to their characteristic curved or spiral shape. In severe forms of inflammation, the epithelium has a rather immature appearance, with a paucity of mucous granules. Focally, there may be epithelial degeneration, with shedding of inflammatory cells at the luminal surface. Occasionally, lymphoid follicles may develop.

The majority of infected individuals show no obvious endoscopic abnormalities, or only limited abnormalities. With high-resolution and magnification endoscopy, however, subtle changes may be seen (**Fig. 43.27**) [16], the most common of which is erythematous/exudative gastritis. Rather rare in adults, in contrast to children, is nodular deformity, especially of the antrum, or the appearance of endoscopic flat or raised erosive gastritis [17]. Another fairly exceptional finding is the development of rugal hyperplastic hypersecretory gastritis [18].

It is commonly accepted that long-standing H. pylori infection may lead to atrophic changes, with intestinal metaplasia. Development of atrophy is a slow process, which may last up to 20 or more years. Atrophy may occur in about 40–50% of infected individuals. Atrophic changes occur particularly in the antrum, but also in the gastric body, especially in patients receiving acid suppression. The extent to which acid suppression induced by proton-pump inhibitors (PPIs) accelerates the development of atrophy, particularly in the gastric body, remains a controversial issue. The current estimates are that the degree of progression is less than initially suggested [19]. Atrophic changes and metaplasia are at least partially reversible after eradication of the organism [20]. Chronic H. pylori infection is an important precursor of gastric cancer and mucosa-associated lymphoid tissue (MALT) lymphoma [21,22]. Whether screening and surveillance of H. pylori–related atrophic gastritis is advisable remains a moot point [23].

H. heilmannii is a variant of H. pylori and is thought to be transmitted from dogs and cats.

Other infectious forms of gastritis. Several viral and bacterial microorganisms can infect the stomach. The most important relate to cytomegalovirus gastritis, herpetic gastritis, and opportunistic infections in patients with acquired immune deficiency syndrome (AIDS), such as Cryptosporidium infection. Cytomegalovirus gastritis

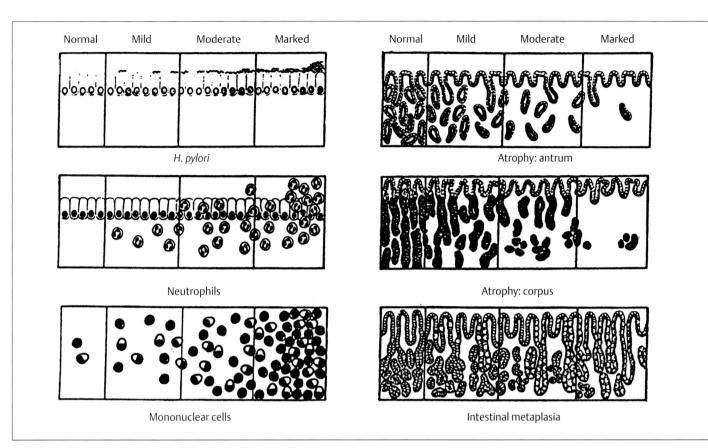

Normal   Mild   Moderate   Marked

H. pylori

Neutrophils

Mononuclear cells

Normal   Mild   Moderate   Marked

Atrophy: antrum

Atrophy: corpus

Intestinal metaplasia

43

Fig. 43.25 The visual analogue scale for grading inflammatory changes in the Houston modification of the Sydney system [10]. The observer should attempt to evaluate one feature at a time. The most prevalent appearance on each slide should be matched with the graded panel that resembles it most closely. It should be borne in mind that these drawings are not intended to represent the histopathological appearance of the gastric mucosa realistically; instead, they provide a schematic representation of the magnitude of each feature, and therefore have certain limitations. For example, the decreasing thickness of the mucosa usually observed with increasing atrophy is not depicted realistically. Particularly with *Helicobacter pylori* and neutrophils, there may be considerable variation of intensity within the same biopsy sample; in such cases, the observer should attempt to average the different areas and score the specimen accordingly.

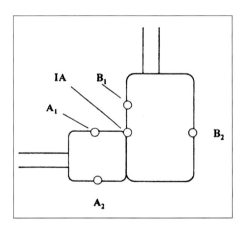

Fig. 43.26 Recommended biopsy sites. One biopsy specimen each should be obtained from the lesser curvature (A1) and the greater curvature (A2) of the antrum, both within 2–3 cm of the pylorus; from the lesser curvature of the gastric body, about 4 cm above the angle (B1); from the greater curvature of the gastric body, about 8 cm from the cardia (B2); and from the angular notch (incisura angularis, IA).

is so rare in immunocompetent adults that its finding suggests an occult malignancy or immune deficiency [24]. Cytomegalovirus infection tends to occur in the gastric body/fundus area, and may cause erythema, hyperrugosity, ulceration, hemorrhage, and even perforation (**Fig. 43.28**). Histology reveals inflammation, particularly of the deeper portions of the mucosa, and cytomegalic cells

with inclusion bodies both in epithelial and endothelial cells, as well as in the base of ulcerations. Herpes simplex gastritis may cause patchy erosions, often in immunocompromised patients [25].

Tuberculosis [26] and syphilis [27], etc., are nowadays rare. A high index of suspicion is mandatory in order not to miss such lesions. The endoscopic presentation is highly variable, but ulcers and fistulas are often present (**Figs. 43.29, 43.30**). Not uncommonly, these infections may mimic malignancy.

Fungal infections such as candidiasis, mucormycosis, histoplasmosis, blastomycosis, and actinomycosis are uncommon. The endoscopic appearance is variable (**Fig. 43.31**).

Parasitic infections are also uncommon. Gastric giardiasis [28] is essentially a histologic diagnosis, in contrast to infestation with the herring worm (anisakiasis) [29]. The common initial symptoms in anisakiasis are severe epigastric pain, nausea, vomiting, chills, and urticaria. Distinct endoscopic findings include impressive focal edema with bleeding spots in the center, often along the greater curvature and the presence of *Anisakis* worms (**Fig. 43.32**). Stomach wall thickening is mainly due to thickening of the submucosal layer as seen endosonographically. Attempts to remove the penetrating worm using a biopsy forceps are always indicated.

Acute phlegmonous or suppurative, occasionally emphysematous gastritis is an uncommon, rapidly progressive and, if untreated, fatal infection, often with Gram-positive and hemolytic streptococci, *Clostridium,* or other pyogenic organisms [30]. Debilitated patients or immunosuppressed individuals are especially at risk. Two types prevail: a diffuse type, in which the whole stomach is involved; and a less common localized type, in which usually the

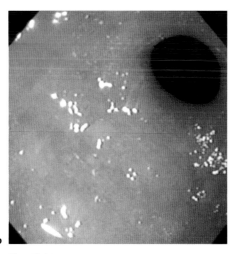 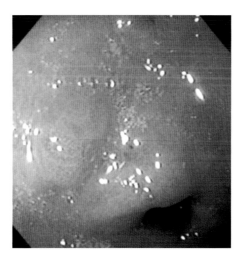 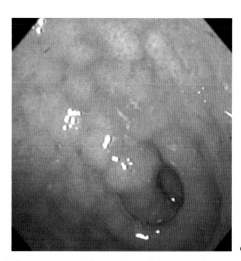

a, b   c

Fig. 43.27
a Discrete antral erythematous exudative gastritis in *Helicobacter pylori* infection.
b More pronounced antral endoscopic erythematous exudative gastritis in *H. pylori* infection.

c Conspicuous nodular deformity in an adult patient with long-standing *H. pylori* infection.

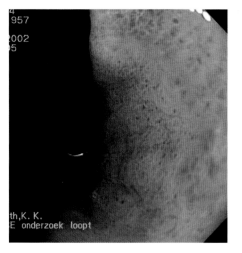 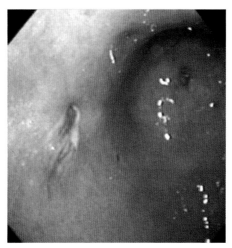 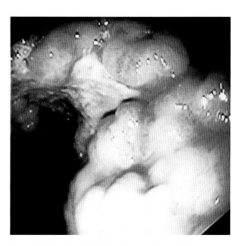

Fig. 43.28 Cytomegalovirus gastritis.

Fig. 43.29 Tuberculous involvement of the stomach, with fistulization.

Fig. 43.30 Syphilitic inflammation of the stomach, with deep ulceration and nodularity in the surrounding mucosa.

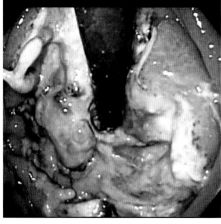 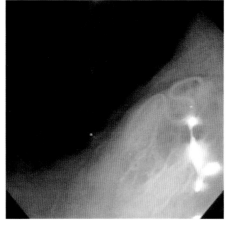

a,

Fig. 43.31 Extensive gastric *Actinomyces* infection, mimicking malignancy. The abundant yellowish exudate should be noted. Sulfur granules are typical at histology.

Fig. 43.32 Anisakiasis of the stomach.
a A worm-like structure on top of swollen erythematous mucosa.
b Endoscopic extraction of the worm with a biopsy forceps.

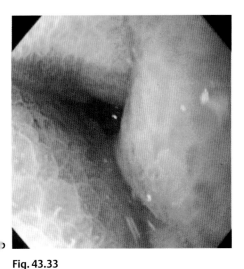
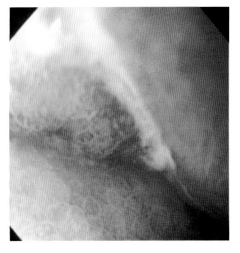
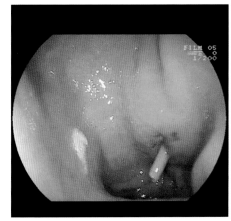

Fig. 43.33
a Phlegmonous gastritis, with massive swelling and near-obliteration of the gastric lumen.
b Phlegmonous gastritis, with pus exuding from the biopsy site.

Fig. 43.34 Localized gastric wall abscess due to a penetrating toothpick. With kind permission of Elsevier. Ruiz-Rebello ML. Gastric wall abscess caused by an ingested toothpick. Gastrointest Endosc 1997;65:518.

Fig. 43.35 a–d Gastric malacoplakia with massive swelling and erythema. The histological findings showed histiocytic infiltration, revealing Michaelis–Gutmann bodies.

43

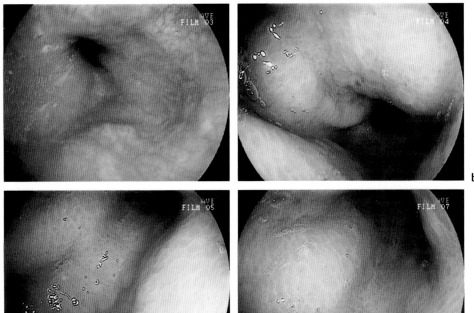

antrum is affected, known as gastric wall abscess [31]. Usually, the gastric lumen is severely narrowed because of impressive mucosal swelling (**Fig. 43.33**). Necrotic areas are focally present within a fiercely erythematous, swollen, and conspicuously friable mucosa. Not uncommonly, purulent material exudes from the mucosal surface at the biopsy site. Extensive ulceration and even perforation may develop during follow-up, if left untreated. The endoscopic abnormalities in the localized form, or gastric wall abscess, are more mitigated. Not uncommonly, a wall abscess is caused by a penetrating foreign body (**Fig. 43.34**). Emphysematous gastritis is an exceedingly rare form of infection of the stomach with gas-forming organisms. The mucosa shows diffuse edema, erythema, friability, and widespread erosions or whitish plaque-like lesions. The milder type (type 1) is characterized by striking swelling of the gastric wall, with a velvet-like mucosal appearance and with markedly decreased distensibility, but without erosions. The hemorrhagic type

(type 2) is diagnosed when, in addition, hemorrhagic spots and erosive defects develop. The severe type (type 3) is characterized by the addition of extensive necrotic mucosal areas, accompanied by bleeding.

Malakoplakia, a chronic mural infection, particularly with *Escherichia coli*, is exceedingly rare. The most conspicuous finding is mural edematous thickening, which is sometimes polypoidal (**Fig. 43.35**) [32].

▦ Autoimmune Gastritis

The link between the immune system and some forms of chronic gastritis was established with the identification of circulating autoantibodies to gastric intrinsic factor (blocking type in 70%, binding type in 30%) and to gastric parietal cells, particularly the H^+,K^+-

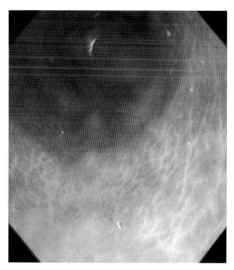
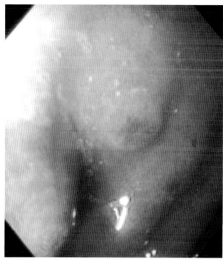
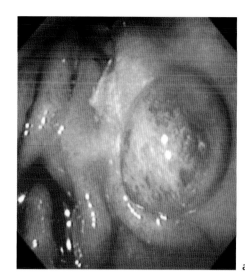

a, b

Fig. 43.36 Autoimmune gastritis with advanced atrophy in the gastric body, contrasting with the normal appearance of the antrum in the upper part of the figure.

Fig. 43.37
a Microcarcinoid in autoimmune gastritis.
b A larger carcinoid or ECLoma in autoimmune gastritis.

ATPase. Such antibodies are present in 80–90% of patients with pernicious anemia. Parietal cell antibody–positive gastritis is also common in relatives of patients with pernicious anemia, in several endocrine disorders, and in vitiligo. Antibodies directed toward the proton pump may also develop in predisposed H. pylori–infected individuals, perhaps through mimicry with epitopes in the H. pylori lipopolysaccharide or Lewis antigens [33]. In general, however, patients with established autoimmune gastritis appear to be less frequently colonized by H. pylori, since advanced atrophic gastritis creates an unfavorable or hostile microenvironment for the organism. Which overall percentage of the autoimmune gastritides has H. pylori infection at its origin remains speculative. As a consequence of severe oxyntic glandular atrophy, anacidity develops, leading to a substantial rise in fasting serum gastrin, often exceeding 500 pmol/ L. Gastrin rises due to the removal of the negative feedback control of gastric acid on the antral G cell. However, in patients with concomitant severe antral atrophic gastritis, serum gastrin levels may remain in the normal range.

Autoimmune gastritis is in principle a histological diagnosis, since clear-cut endoscopic abnormalities are unusual except in advanced disease. When the presentation is classic, there is marked atrophic change in the gastric body mucosa, leaving the antrum essentially intact, especially in idiopathic autoimmune gastritis, but less so in presumed H. pylori–induced autoimmune gastritis (**Fig. 43.36**). The rugae are thin, or may even have disappeared, and the vascular pattern becomes readily visible due to mucosal thinning. Chromoscopy with Congo red staining may show an absence of acid secretion [34]. Histology shows severe atrophic gastric body gastritis, with an absence of parietal cells. Extensive pseudo-pyloric metaplasia and variable amounts of intestinal metaplasia are common. Not uncommonly, tiny, slightly raised nodules with a yellowish hue may be observed in the atrophic gastric body/fundus mucosa. These minute yellowish nodules usually represent enterochromaffin-like (ECL) cell clusters, or even microcarcinoids or ECLomas (**Fig. 43.37**). Rarely, larger carcinoids may be observed. ECL cell hyperplasia is often classified as normal, diffuse hyperplasia, linear hyperplasia, micronodular hyperplasia, adenomatoid hyperplasia, dysplasia, and carcinoid [35]. These lesions are an expression of the trophic drive of hypergastrinemia toward the ECL cell. In contrast to these type I tumors, type II tumors are associated with gastrinoma, whereas sporadic type III carcinoids are gastrin-independent [36].

Autoimmune gastritis is usually clinically silent until vitamin B_{12} deficiency becomes manifest, unless other endocrinopathy alerts the clinician. Only 15–20% of patients with parietal cell antibodies will ultimately progress to pernicious anemia. The onset is usually insidious, and symptoms are often vague, delaying the diagnosis. Subacute combined degeneration of the spinal cord is less common, but the symptoms may antedate the macrocytic anemia. Serum vitamin B_{12} is low. Pernicious anemia responds to parenteral administration of vitamin B_{12}. The risk of gastric cancer is variably increased, up to three or four times, in areas with a high prevalence of gastric malignancy. Cancers are usually located in the gastric body/ fundus area, and are often multicentric and polypoid in appearance. Adenocarcinoma should not be confused with carcinoid tumor.

■ Drug-Induced Gastric Mucosal Damage

Drug-induced gastric mucosal abnormalities are common in everyday practice. Both aspirin and nonsteroidal anti-inflammatory drugs (NSAIDs) are leading causes of mucosal damage [37]. There are two different isoforms of cyclooxygenase: COX-1 and COX-2. Whereas COX-1 is found in most of the body's tissues, COX-2 is only encountered at sites of inflammation, and is normally not abundantly present in the stomach. All currently available nonselective NSAIDs inhibit COX-1 and -2 and hence prostaglandin production. Aspirin inhibits COX-1 irreversibly, whereas other NSAIDs cause a dose-dependent reversible inhibition. The spectrum of endoscopic abnormalities is wide, varying from endoscopic hemorrhagic gastritis to widespread erosions and ultimately extensive deep ulceration (**Figs. 43.38**). The Lanza score is often used to grade the endoscopic abnormalities (**Table 43.3**) [38,39].

Acute aspirin-induced mucosal injury characteristically consists of multiple, small (less than 5 mm), shallow, white-based erosive lesions. The antrum is most commonly involved, although the lesions can occur in any area of the stomach. Intramural hemorrhages occur within 2 h of ingestion, followed by development of erosions after 8 h or more. When necrotic lesions are sharply delineated, punched-out and particularly deep in the center, they are called ulcerations rather than erosions. White-based erosions and focal zones of erythema often occur together. In between the lesions, the mucosa may appear normal. Acute aspirin ingestion causes enhanced back-diffusion of hydrogen ions, contributing to local injury.

VI

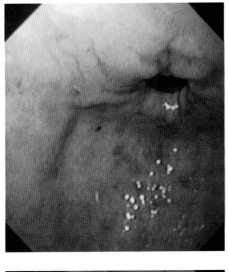
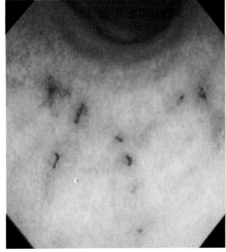
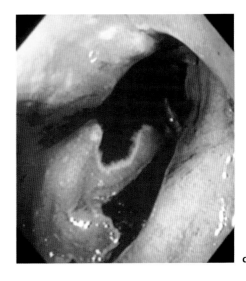

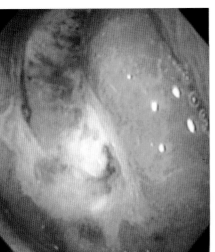
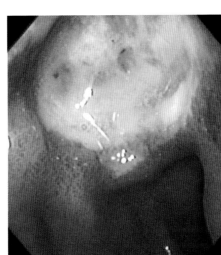

Fig. 43.38
a Drug-induced erosive gastritis.
b Mild drug-induced hemorrhagic gastritis.
c Extensive drug-induced hemorrhagic gastritis.
d Extensive drug-induced ulceration along the greater curvature.
e Extensive drug-induced ulceration in the duodenal bulb.

43

NSAIDs are weak acids that can freely cross cell membranes in the stomach after protonation. They then accumulate intracellularly, being trapped after ionization, and become toxic to cells. In addition to this topical caustic injury, NSAIDs weaken the mucosal defense mechanisms via systemic inhibition of COX-1 and -2. NSAID/acetyl-salicylic acid–induced erosions may be diagnosed histologically when there is homogeneous eosinophilic ischemic necrosis blending into the adjoining lamina propria. By contrast, erosions not induced by drugs but rather by *H. pylori* infection are characterized by heterogeneous necrotic debris, with fibrin and inflammatory cells [40]. While NSAID-induced damage does not require the presence of *H. pylori* for its development, in adults there is evidence that the infection enhances the risk of mucosal injury. Individuals who have a history of peptic ulcer and who require NSAID therapy should also have treatment directed at eradication of the organism and prophylaxis with acid suppressants [41].

Alcohol-induced gastritis. Concentrated alcohol is a well-recognized gastric mucosal irritant that disrupts the mucosal barrier to acid back-diffusion. The endoscopic abnormalities caused by excessive use of concentrated alcohol are variable [42]. The earliest injurious effects of alcohol appear to be directed against the gastric vasculature, resulting in mucosal capillary dilation, stasis, and the extravasation of erythrocytes within the superficial lamina propria.

The most conspicuous finding is vascular congestion, causing diffuse erythema and swelling. Occasionally, there is evidence of focal intramural bleeding [43]. A grading system for alcohol injury is given in **Table 43.4** [44].

Table 43.3 Evaluation scale for gastric injury (Lanza score) [39]

Grade	Description
0	Normal
1	One submucosal hemorrhage or superficial ulceration
2	More than one submucosal hemorrhage or superficial ulceration, but not numerous or widespread
3	Numerous areas with submucosal hemorrhages or superficial ulcerations
4	Widespread involvement of the stomach, with submucosal hemorrhage or superficial ulceration, invasive* ulcer of any size

* "Invasive" ulcer is defined as a lesion that produces an actual crater—i. e., a depression below the normal plane of the mucosal surface.

Table 43.4 Tarnawski endoscopic grading system for alcohol injury [44]

0	Normal mucosa
1	Marked diffuse hyperemia
2	Single hemorrhagic lesion (1 mm or larger)
3	2–5 hemorrhagic lesions
4	6–10 hemorrhagic lesions
5	>10 hemorrhagic lesions, or larger area of confluent hemorrhage

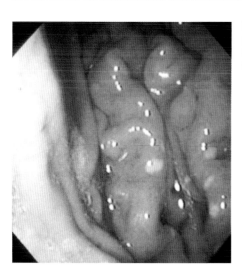

Fig. 43.39 Rugal hyperplastic gastritis, with superimposed flat erosive lesions.

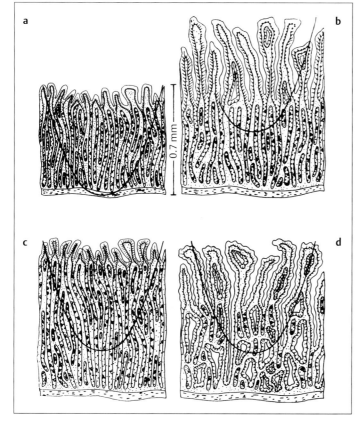

Fig. 43.40 The various forms of hypertrophic–hyperplastic gastritis.
a Normal gastric body mucosa.
b Ménétrier's disease, with superficial hyperplasia.
c Glandular hyperplasia.
d Ménétrier's disease, with reduced glandular parenchyma.

Hypertrophic–Hyperplastic Gastritis

Gastric rugae are considered enlarged when the folds are wider than 10 mm. Truly enlarged or giant folds do not flatten during distension of the stomach with air. Occasionally, such folds reveal caliber changes or superimposed polypoid irregularities. Giant folds may involve the entire stomach, but are usually predominantly present only in the gastric body–fundus area. Fold enlargement may begin and end abruptly, or more gradually. The pliancy should be assessed using the mucosal tenting sign, to rule out infiltrating malignancy. In some patients, there may be additional evidence of flat erosive destruction of the mucosa on top of the folds (**Fig. 43.39**). Histology is essential for proper diagnosis (**Fig. 43.40**). Biopsy with a standard 7-Fr or large-caliber 9-Fr biopsy forceps may be insufficiently deep to demonstrate full-depth foveolar or glandular hyperplasia. Alternatively, a macroparticle biopsy taken with a diathermy snare may yield a specimen that extends into the submucosa. Prior to transection, lifting of the mucosal layer may be carried out with submucosal injection of saline. After snaring, the enlarged fold is lifted up and away from the gastric wall to limit the depth of coagulation damage during transection. The mucosal sample is grasped, either with the snare, a Dormia basket, a retrieval probe, or a net. The most common causes of hyperrugosity are Ménétrier's disease, hypertrophic hypersecretory gastritis, gastrinoma, and infiltrative disorders such as lymphoma, carcinoma, amyloidosis and in particular gastric fundus varices. The latter are usually the expression of a block in the splenic vein, with splenic venous hypertension and formation of segmental collateral circulation.

Ménétrier's disease or hypertrophic hyposecretory gastritis is characterized by impressive fold enlargement, often covered by a thick layer of mucus due to foveolar and glandular elongation with hyperplasia of mucus producing cells. The foveolar part of the mucosa is larger than 0.3 mm. This type of hyperplasia is often accompanied with cystic dilation of the glands, filled with mucus. In addition, there is conspicuous regression of the oxyntic glands. Characteristically, there is overexpression of transforming growth factor-α.

In a variant of Ménétrier's disease, there is superimposed lymphocytic gastritis, with conspicuous infiltration of the epithelial layer with lymphocytes [45].

As there is a certain risk of malignant degeneration, which in some series may occur in about 10 % of patients, endosonographic investigation of the wall layers is recommended in order to rule out infiltrative pathology. However, the endosonographic differential diagnosis between Ménétrier's disease and lymphoma or linitis plastica may be difficult, as all three abnormalities produce a more or less similar echo pattern, with massive thickening of the second layer and preservation of the other layers.

Hypertrophic hypersecretory gastritis (Schindler's disease) has a similar endoscopic appearance (**Fig. 43.41**) to that of Ménétrier's disease, but is histologically characterized by hypertrophy of the oxyntic glandular area [46]. This type of giant fold formation can also occur in *H. pylori* infection [47]. Disappearance of the giant folds can occur after successful eradication of the organisms.

Gastrinoma. In gastrinoma or Zollinger–Ellison syndrome, the glandular hyperplasia is considered to be caused by the trophic action of gastrin. The mucosal thickness may increase up to 2–3 mm. In most patients, fold enlargement is not excessive. The folds are usually covered with copious amounts of clear highly acidic fluid. Occasionally, the folds are slightly irregular or finely nodular. There may be a conspicuous increase in the size of the areae gastricae. Concomitant gastric ulceration is rare, except when there is delayed gastric emptying and stasis. The latter may occur when there is a distal ulceration or scarring in the duodenal bulb or postbulbar duodenum. Not uncommonly, large, deep ulcers may be present both in the bulb or the postbulbar duodenum, up to and even beyond the duodenojejunal angle of Treitz.

Granulomatous Gastritis

Many conditions may lead to granuloma formation in the gastric wall [48]. In Crohn's disease, upper digestive tract involvement is not uncommon, usually in conjunction with involvement elsewhere in the bowel. Endoscopic abnormalities may include focal erythema, mucosal nodularity, aphthoid erosions, and linear cleft-like or ser-

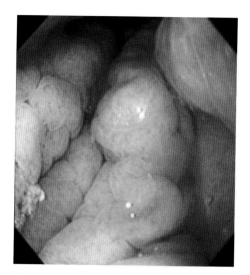

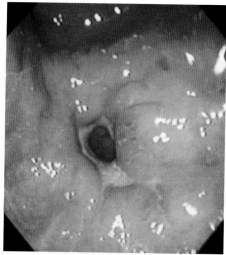

a, b

Fig. 43.41 Rugal hyperplasia in hypertrophic hypersecretory gastritis.

Fig. 43.42
a Crohn's disease of the gastric antrum, with nodular deformity, aphthoid lesions, and ulceration.
b Pronounced abnormalities in Crohn's disease of the stomach, with nodularity and coalescent ulceration.

piginous ulcers. The mucosa intervening between aphthoid erosions or ulcers may be either normal or may appear nodular, creating a cobblestone or bamboo-like appearance (**Fig. 43.42**). The prepyloric antrum is commonly involved, leading to antral deformity. Antral peristalsis may be sluggish, and stricturing may lead to gastric outlet obstruction. Aphthoid erosions and small or large serpiginous ulcers may also occur in the gastric body, or may develop around a gastrojejunostomy. Occasionally, enlarged folds are seen with regularly spaced transverse fissures, particularly along the lesser curve of the proximal stomach. A rather exceptional finding is severe pangastritis with impressive swelling, erythema, and coalescent superficial ulceration. The biopsy yield of granulomas is rather low, although the frequency with which specific features are observed in biopsies (granulomas, giant cells, focal deep inflammation) varies with the number of biopsies taken and the adequacy of the examination [49]. Even when no overt endoscopic abnormalities are visible, random biopsies may reveal focal accumulations, particularly of lymphocytes, more in the antrum than in the gastric body, in a substantial percentage of patients with Crohn's disease elsewhere in the intestinal tract. This is known as focally enhanced gastritis [50].

Another cause of granulomatous inflammation is sarcoidosis affecting the stomach. The antrum is usually involved, with prominent folds, sometimes with superimposed erosions or ulcerations and lack of distensibility. Pronounced antral nodularity may even mimic an infiltrating malignancy.

Granulomatous gastric inflammation is termed idiopathic when no cause can be detected. Idiopathic granulomatous gastritis is a diagnosis made by excluding other causes such as infection, foreign bodies, or systemic granulomatous diseases.

Enterogastric or Biliary Reflux Gastritis

Excessive exposure of the stomach to bile-containing fluid may cause mucosal injury, with pronounced edema, striking erythema, and occasionally erosions and even hemorrhage [51,52]. Enterogastric reflux is most severe after partial gastric resection. A conspicuous finding is the severely swollen, fiercely or beefy red mucosa. Histologically, edema, dilation of superficial capillaries, foveolar hyperplasia, and splaying of muscle fibers in the lamina propria are the dominant abnormalities. This is termed "reactive" gastritis. Acute or chronic inflammation is minimal, or even lacking.

Physical-Chemical and Caustic Gastritis

Caustic injury. Caustic gastric damage is due to the accidental or suicidal intake of injurious agents. Common caustic agents include acetic, sulfuric, and hydrochloric acids. Lye burns are usually due to caustic soda and bleach [53]. Endoscopy provides information on the extent and severity of the injury. Endoscopy is safe in the absence of evidence of perforation or transmural necrosis. Detailed examination of the oropharynx and hypopharynx should always precede endoscopy. The presence of an oropharyngeal burn is a clue to the possibility of esophageal or gastric caustic damage. However, there is no correlation between pharyngeal involvement and the presence or severity of lesions in the stomach. Gastric involvement is usually most severe along the lesser curve and in the region of the antrum, probably because of pyloric spasm and subsequent pooling of secretions (**Fig. 43.43**). Often, but not always, the duodenum is spared, presumably because of pyloric spasm or because of rapid neutralization of the acid by the alkaline content of the duodenum.

Caustic damage to the gastric mucosa may be graded into three stages. In grade I, the only abnormalities consist of focal or linear streaks of erythema. In grade II, a few ulcerations are visible in addition to striking erythema. These ulcers are usually smaller than 5 mm in diameter, and the areas of necrosis are usually superficial and limited to a portion of the stomach. There may be slight hemorrhage. In grade III, there is extensive necrosis of the gastric lining, involving large segments of the stomach. In addition to deep ulceration, there may be evidence of massive hemorrhage. The gastric wall is covered with a thick layer of blackish debris and exudate. The most important late complications are gastric perforation and particularly extensive scarring and retraction, with gastric outlet obstruction.

Radiation-induced gastritis. Radiotherapy delivered to the upper abdomen may cause damage to the gastric wall. Radiation damage is characterized by varying degrees of erythema and friability and prominent gastric folds, with diminished pliability and distensibility (**Fig. 43.44**). On close inspection, the mucosal erythema consists of multiple red dots separated by pale-appearing interconnecting furrows. Ulcerations, both superficial and deep, commonly develop and have a slow tendency to heal. In late stages, there may be evidence of telangiectasia and marked deformity and retraction due to scarring, occasionally leading to gastric outlet obstruction [54].

43

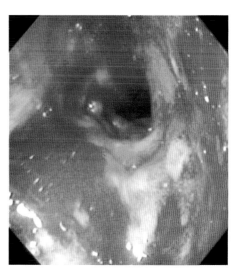

Fig. 43.43 Severe gastric mucosal necrosis, inflammation, and bleeding due to caustic injury.

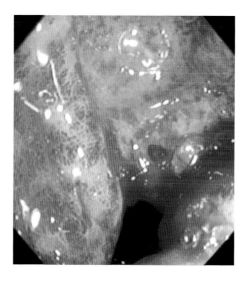

Fig. 43.44 Radiation-induced gastritis, with swelling and erythema and superficial sloughing of the mucosa.

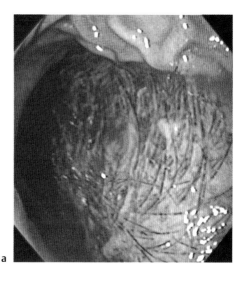

a

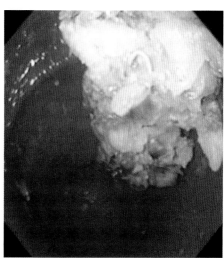

b

Fig. 43.45
a Gastric trichobezoar.
b Phytobezoar in a postoperative stomach.

It is sometimes difficult to differentiate between late radiation damage and recurrent malignancy. Prominent folds with superimposed erosions or ulcers, of a rubbery consistency and with poor mucosal tenting, are common to both radiation damage and recurrent malignancy, particularly lymphoma. Endosonography and multiple biopsies may be helpful in this difficult differential diagnosis.

Mechanical trauma. Mechanical trauma as a cause of mucosal injury and inflammation is rather rare. Nasogastric suction may cause focal mucosal injury, with trauma-induced intramural bleeding and even erosions. Pressure-related trauma may be seen after trichobezoars and phytobezoars (**Fig. 43.45**), intragastric balloons, transpyloric feeding tubes, etc. Ingested foreign bodies, particularly when penetrating the gastric wall, also lead to local inflammation and abscess formation.

Stress-Induced Gastritis

Stress-related gastric mucosal damage is usually associated with severe trauma, hypotension, shock, sepsis, jaundice, renal failure, respiratory failure, major surgical procedures, major burns (Curling's ulcer), or intracranial trauma or surgery (Cushing's ulcer). Acute stress-related mucosal damage is usually preceded by shock, with concomitant decreased gastric mucosal blood flow in the microcirculation [55].

Acute stress-related lesions often begin within minutes or hours after the trauma, critical illness or shock, in the form of shallow erosions in the gastric body/fundus region. During the following 24 h, petechiae develop, and the number of shallow red based erosions increases. By 48 h, the erosions become deeper and black-based, with raised margins. Gradually, such erosions spread to involve the entire stomach. When the necrotizing process extends into the submucosal layer, ulcers of variable size and shape ensue. These deeper lesions are more likely to be associated with significant bleeding, as large-caliber blood vessels are present in the submucosa.

Patients with stress-related pathology are usually in the intensive-care unit and often intubated and receiving assisted ventilation when examined. Some experience is necessary to insert a small-caliber endoscope past an endotracheal tube. Inspection with a laryngoscope may assist the passage of the endoscope through the upper esophageal sphincter when introduction of the endoscope is unsuccessful.

Ischemia and Vasculitis

Ischemia and mucosal injuries such as vasculitis or cholesterol emboli from atheroma cause erosions or ulcers. In exceptional circumstances, with occlusion of all major arterial blood supply to the abdomen, ischemia may develop, involving large segments of the

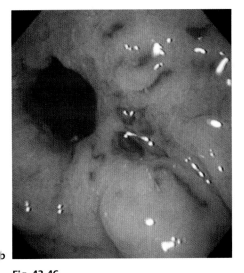
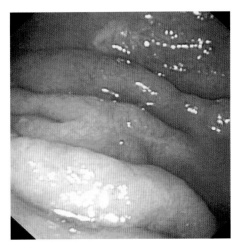
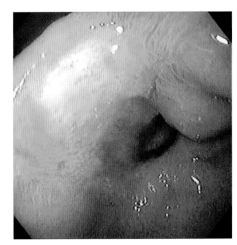

Fig. 43.46
a Bizarre vascular structures due to vasculitis.
b Irregular vascular structures due to vasculitis.
c Superficial ulceration due to vasculitis.

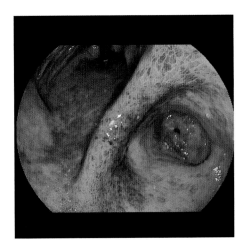
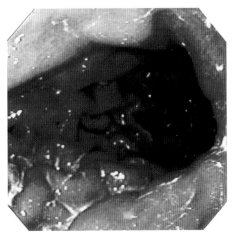
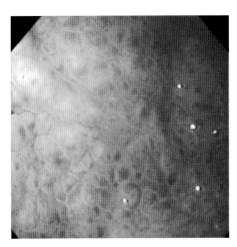

Fig. 43.47 Henoch–Schönlein involvement of the stomach.

Fig. 43.48 Impressive swelling of the gastric wall due to hereditary angioedema (reproduced with permission from [57]).

Fig. 43.49 Idiopathic erythematous gastritis, with normal histological findings on repeated tests.

stomach. There is usually extensive necrosis of the superficial layers, with a sharp transition to uninvolved segments.

Vasculitis involving the stomach is a rare condition. Most often, one sees patchy-shaped erythematous and edematous changes, together with clusters of bizarre vascular structures. There may be superimposed erosive defects and evidence of intramural bleeding (**Fig. 43.46**).

Henoch–Schönlein gastritis is rarely seen, and reveals focal edema and erythema, with raised blebs 3–5 mm in diameter. There are often superimposed punctate bleeding spots and yellow-based erosions (**Fig. 43.47**). Biopsies may show leukocytoclastic vasculitis [56].

Hereditary angioedema involving the stomach causes diffuse edema and erythema, with prominent submucosal bulges [57] (**Fig. 43.48**).

Miscellaneous Idiopathic Conditions

There is a whole spectrum of less common inflammatory conditions for which the etiology and pathogenesis remain obscure and which are therefore termed idiopathic. Occasionally, striking erythematous, flat, or raised erosive gastritis is seen for which no cause can be found (**Fig. 43.49**).

Erosive gastritis. Idiopathic raised erosive (varioliform) gastritis is an uncommon disorder of unknown etiology [58]. The endoscopic appearance is dominated by innumerable nodules, often in the upper part of the stomach and on the crests of irregularly thickened folds, often with a conspicuous umbilicated central necrotic crater. Biopsies of the lesions and surrounding mucosa usually reveal intense chronic active inflammation, with peculiar foveolar hyperplasia. Some patients with idiopathic raised erosive gastritis have histological evidence of lymphocytic infiltration of the epithelium, known as lymphocytic gastritis [59,60]. Celiac disease or prior/current infection with *H. pylori* [61] is possible, but the way in which the gastric abnormalities develop remains enigmatic. Healed erosions may ultimately evolve into hyperplastic polyps, presumably due to

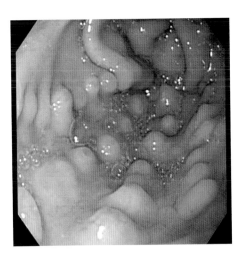

Fig. 43.50 Eosinophilic gastritis, showing antral nodular lesions with apical erythema.

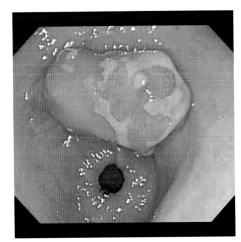

Fig. 43.51 An inflammatory fibrinoid polyp with patchy whitish exudate. Reprinted by kind permission of Elsevier: Tanaka et al. Anemia caused by a gastric inflammatory fibroid polyp. Gastrointest Endosc 2008;67:345.

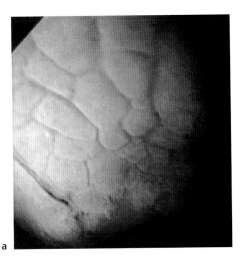

a

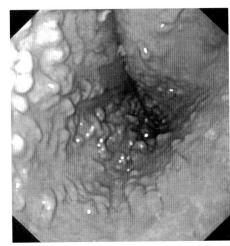

b

Fig. 43.52
a Massive amyloid deposition in the stomach, leading to a coarse areae gastricae pattern.
b Massive amyloidosis, with nodular polypoid deformity in the gastric lining.

foveolar hyperplasia in the borders of the lesion. A red fleck at the top of the lesion is reminiscent of the site of the previous epithelial necrosis, now covered with a thin layer of regenerative epithelium.

Eosinophilic gastroenteritis. Patients with diffuse eosinophilic gastroenteritis affecting the stomach usually present with symptoms of gastric outlet obstruction due to involvement of the prepyloric antrum and pyloric channel. The antral wall loses flexibility and distensibility. The mucosa appears dull and inflamed with swelling, erythema, and friability. When the deeper layers are involved, scattered nodularity and ulceration may supervene (**Fig. 43.50**). The endoscopic appearance is somewhat similar to that seen in Crohn's disease, and may even mimic infiltrating malignancy.

Focal eosinophilic gastritis may present as a polypoid structure, usually located in the antrum. The lesion is occasionally also termed "eosinophilic granuloma" or "inflammatory fibroid polyp." The mucosa covering the polypoid lesion is usually fairly inconspicuous. Occasionally, erosive defects may be present (**Fig. 43.51**). Histologically, areas of dense eosinophilic infiltration are seen, especially in the submucosal layer.

Immunodeficiency may lead to idiopathic chronic gastritis. Approximately 40 % of patients with primary common variable immunodeficiency display chronic gastric inflammation. Panhypogammaglobulinemia and repeated bacterial infections are characteristic features in this disorder. Endoscopic erythematous/exudative gastritis is the dominant presentation. The gastric abnormality is usu-ally seen as pangastritis, with involvement of both antrum and gastric body mucosa. Plasma cells are conspicuously absent from the inflammatory infiltrate. Systemic gastric autoantibodies are not detectable. The pathogenesis of this uncommon form of chronic gastritis has not been established.

Graft-versus-host disease (GVHD) after hematopoietic stem cell transplantation may lead to endoscopic alterations varying from subtle erythema and edema to frank mucosal sloughing, with bleeding. Severe GVHD does not resemble any other disease. GVHD needs to be differentiated from toxic drug reaction and infections in such immunocompromised patients.

Collagenous gastritis, characterized by subepithelial deposition of collagen [62], is mainly a histological diagnosis, with few if any typical macroscopic features. The etiology is unknown.

Amyloidosis. Not strictly inflammatory, but related, is amyloidosis of the stomach. Massive deposition of amyloid causes conspicuous alteration of the areae gastricae pattern and of the gastric contours (**Fig. 43.52**).

Extramedullary hematopoiesis. Another very rare condition is extramedullary hematopoiesis with gastric localization (**Fig. 43.53**).

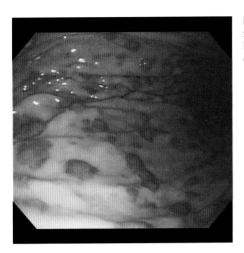

Fig. 43.53 Multiple sessile reddish polypoid lesions due to extramedullary hematopoiesis.

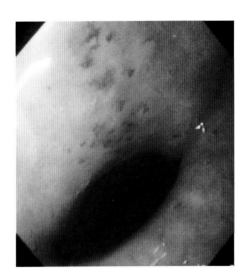

Fig. 43.54 Gastric vascular ectasia or angiodysplasia.

Vascular Disorders

A variety of vascular abnormalities may occur in the stomach. These range from diminutive lesions such as angiodysplasia to large and extensive arteriovenous malformations (**Table 43.5**).

Gastric angiectasia or angiodysplasia may be encountered at any location, but these lesions tend to occur primarily within the gastric body. It is important to distend the stomach adequately in order not to miss lesions that are located between folds. Smaller lesions are usually flat; larger lesions approaching 10 mm may be slightly raised (**Fig. 43.54**). The lesions are clearly composed of abnormally shaped ectatic vascular structures. They are usually sharply circumscribed and may be round, stellate, spider-like, or have discrete dendritic tufts. A distinctive pale halo may surrounds the lesion. Lesions may blanch on pressure from a biopsy forceps. They often cluster along the crests of the longitudinal folds. The mucosa may be unusually mobile, with a tendency to prolapse. A mucosal biopsy can provide reasonable portions of dilated vessels. Endoscopic therapy can be carried out with any ablative thermal modality. The entire vascular lesion should be coagulated. Treatment of larger lesions should begin at the periphery and continue towards the center, where the feeding arteriole is often encountered and bleeding precipitated.

Hereditary hemorrhagic telangiectasia (Osler–Weber–Rendu syndrome), a disorder inherited as an autosomal-dominant trait with an incidence of about five per 100 000, is characterized by vascular anomalies due to mutations in *SMAD4* and in endoglin and activin receptor-like kinase, both binding to transforming growth factor-β (TGF-β), involved in regulation of angiogenesis. The endoscopic appearance mimics that of lesions visible on other mucous membranes (buccal, oral, nasopharyngeal, or lingual mucosa), hand, face, etc. The lesions are bright cherry red, flat or slightly elevated, varying in diameter from pinpoint up to 10 mm. Histologically, irregular ectatic tortuous blood cavities are seen, lined with a single row of endothelial cells and supported by a fine layer of fibrous connective tissue. Arteries show intima proliferation and may have thrombi. Venules are thickened and have prominent muscle cells. Endoscopic ablation may reduce the transfusion requirements [63].

Dieulafoy lesion. A Dieulafoy lesion is an exposed caliber-persistent artery—an artery that fails to undergo the usual ramifications and the tapering into the minute size of the mucosal capillary microvasculature. A caliber-persistent Dieulafoy artery ranges from 1 to 3 mm and is situated subepithelially. The exposed artery is usually associated with a tiny mucosal defect, 2–5 mm in size. There is no

Table 43.5 Vascular malformations in the stomach

Commonly recognized
Angiodysplasia
Phlebectasia
Watermelon stomach (gastric antral vascular ectasia, GAVE)
Radiation telangiectasia
Portal hypertensive intestinal vasculopathy
Osler–Weber–Rendu syndrome
Hemangioma
Congenital arteriovenous malformation
Blue rubber bleb nevus syndrome
Less commonly recognized
Von Willebrand disease
Ehlers–Danlos syndrome
Pseudoxanthoma elasticum
Marfan syndrome
Klippel–Trenaunay syndrome

43

evidence of inflammation, sclerosis, or aneurysmal dilation. The stomach is the site of predilection, with the vast majority of lesions developing within 6–8 cm from the cardia [64]. This may perhaps be due to the fact that the arterial blood supply in this area arises directly from the left gastric artery. A Dieulafoy lesion is responsible for 2 % of upper gastrointestinal hemorrhages. A Dieulafoy lesion is notoriously difficult to identify, and repeat endoscopy is commonly needed. Timing the endoscopy as close as possible to a rebleeding event improves the chances of detection. Endoscopic therapy should be the first line of therapy and is aimed at eliminating the exposed vessel; it can be repeated in case of rebleeding. This can be accomplished by coagulation, rubber band ligation, or the injection of necrotizing agents such as polidocanol or alcohol. The latter technique is associated with a recognized risk of perforation, especially when used in the gastric fundus. Band ligation is rapidly becoming a favored option in the stomach [65,66] (**Fig. 43.55**).

Gastric antral vascular ectasia (GAVE), or watermelon stomach—occasionally confused with severe or hemorrhagic antral gastritis—is characterized by prominent antral stripes of ectatic vascular structures radiating out from the pylorus (**Fig. 43.56**). Histopathologically, GAVE corresponds to dilated mucosal capillaries with focal thrombosis, dilated tortuous submucosal vessels, and fibromuscular hyperplasia in the lamina propria. On close inspection, the spoke-

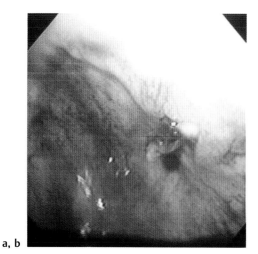
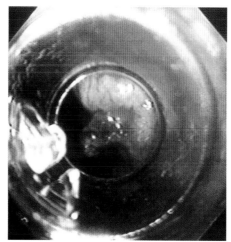
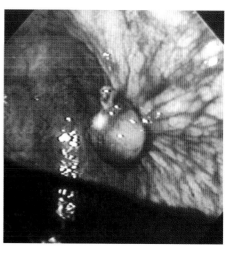

a, b

Fig. 43.55 Band ligation of a Dieulafoy lesion in the stomach.
a A tiny exulceration, with a small protuberant coagulum.
b The lesion is approached with a cap-fitted endoscope.

c The strangulated lesion with the rubber band (not visible) below the vascular abnormality.

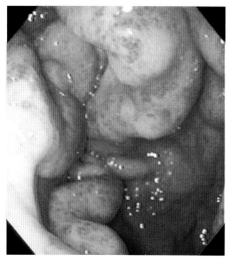
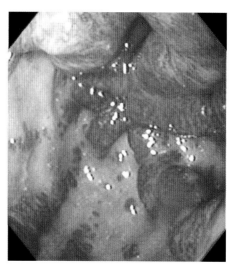

a, b

Fig. 43.56
a Mild gastric antral vascular ectasia.

b Lush gastric antral mucosa, with vascular ectasia.
c Ectatic vascular stripes radiating towards the pylorus.

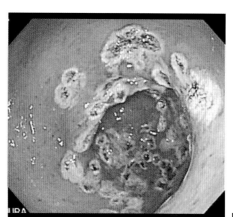

a

b

Fig. 43.57 Gastric antral vascular ectasia (GAVE).
a Before argon plasma coagulation.
b After argon plasma coagulation.

like red stripes can be flat and/or associated with raised convoluted folds, mimicking a watermelon. Less commonly, the antrum contains innumerable and diffusely scattered ectatic vascular lesions instead of stripes. GAVE can also have a honeycomb-like appearance, with coalescence of many vascular lesions. The proximal stomach may be involved in up to 30% of patients. Often, this is in association with a hiatal hernia. The remainder of the gastric mucosa may have an overall atrophic appearance [67].

Argon plasma coagulation, bipolar electrocoagulation, heater probe coagulation, and injection sclerotherapy have all been used successfully to eradicate the lesions and to control bleeding (**Figs. 43.57, 43.58**). The antrum should be treated first in patients with

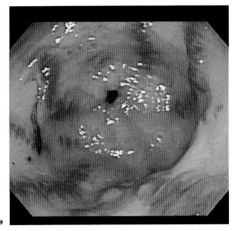 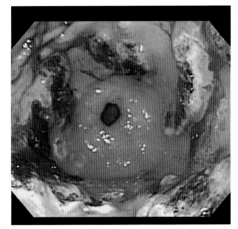 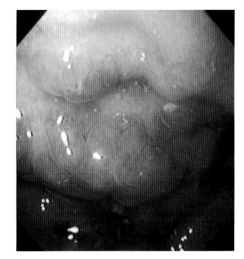

Fig. 43.58 Gastric antral vascular ectasia (GAVE).
a Before argon plasma coagulation.
b After argon plasma coagulation.

Fig. 43.59 Portal hypertensive gastropathy.

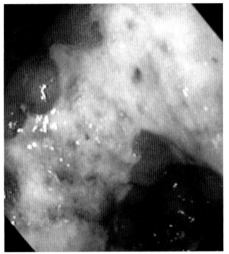 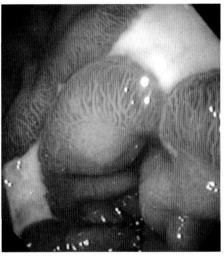 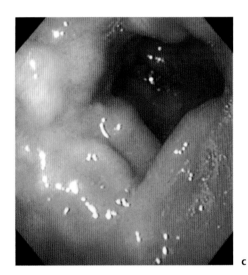

Fig. 43.60 A large gastric ulcer of unknown etiology.
a The initial appearance of the extensive ulceration.

b Partial healing.
c End-stage healing.

extensive disease. If the patient continues to lose blood and the antral abnormalities have for the most part cleared up, then the more proximal vascular lesions should be treated [68].

GAVE should be distinguished from portal hypertensive gastropathy in patients with chronic liver disease. The latter may have a similar appearance in the antrum. Such lesions however do not respond to endoscopic therapy.

Portal hypertensive gastropathy. Portal hypertensive gastropathy has a complex pathophysiology, in part related to sustained portal hypertension. Portal hypertensive gastropathy may occur in the presence or absence of gastric fundus varices. The latter are seen as discrete, moderate or massive tortuous vascular bulges, with a grayish-bluish hue, projecting from the fundic wall. Portal hypertensive endoscopic findings vary from mild, with a mosaic pattern of 2–5 mm erythematous patches separated by a fine white lattice (**Fig. 43.59**); to severe, typified by the presence of cherry-red spots or even intramural confluent hemorrhages [69,70]. The innumerable discrete, punctate, friable mucosal red spots correspond to the ectatic vessels. Endoscopic therapy is usually ineffective in controlling the bleeding. Benefit has been reported from beta-blockade and liver transplantation.

Gastric Ulcer

Gastric ulcer is by definition a defect or tissue loss that extends through the muscularis mucosae into the submucosal layer. Deep ulcers may extend even into the muscularis propria and beyond. Many conditions can cause gastric ulceration, such as *H. pylori* and other infections, drug-induced injury, mucosal resection, ischemia, injection of necrotizing agents, caustic injury, radiation injury, and idiopathic ulceration. Endoscopy is the imaging method of choice, not only for visual detection but also for accurate histopathological confirmation of the benign nature of the lesion. An upper intestinal radiographic series is currently considered inappropriate due to the poor sensitivity of barium radiography, especially for detecting small gastric ulcers.

Gastric ulcers are usually single. Multiple ulcers and/or ulcers located along the greater curvature are most often seen as a consequence of ulcerogenic drugs such as aspirin or nonsteroidal anti-inflammatory drugs (NSAIDs). Most gastric ulcers are 3 cm or less in diameter. Occasionally, a giant ulcer is encountered, with a diameter greater than 3 cm (**Fig. 43.60**).

Most benign gastric ulcers are found in the distal part of the stomach or close to the gastric angle, the angular notch [71]. Benign

43

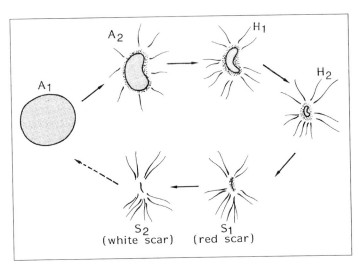

Fig. 43.61 The various phases of healing of a gastric ulcer (adapted from Sakita and Fukutomi [73]). A1, A2: active stages; H1, H2: healing stages; S 1, S 2, scar stages (red scar, white scar).

gastric ulcers can be divided into three major subtypes, depending on their location:

- Type 1 ulcers are located at the level of the angular notch, or above. This is usually in the area of the transitional zone between the antrum and gastric body, which may rise along the lesser curve as a function of age [72].
- Type 2 ulcers are in the same location, but occur in association with evidence of actual or prior duodenal ulcer disease.
- Type 3 ulcers are in the prepyloric region, usually within 2.5 cm of the pylorus. Nowadays this subdivision is rarely used.

The most prominent feature of an ulcer is its base. Granulation tissue covering the crater has a whitish or grayish-white appearance. The crater may be shallow or deep. During the early phase of development, the base of an ulcer is typically round or oval and regular, with a smooth, punched-out appearance. If the ulcer is exceptionally large, as in drug-induced injury, the base may appear irregular. Occasionally, the base may be covered with an adherent clot or may be stained with dark spots reminiscent of prior bleeding, or a vessel stump often covered with fibrin may be visible.

Benign gastric ulcers have smooth, usually slightly raised margins. In the early phases of development, the margin is regular and the mucosa has an inconspicuous appearance. Scarring from previous ulceration may give the margin a distorted appearance. Usually, the gastric folds can be followed right up to the ulcer base.

The healing process passes through various phases, illustrated schematically in **Fig. 43.61** [73]. During the initial phases of healing, an erythematous rim develops surrounding the ulcer base. The whitish coating of the base of the ulcer becomes smaller and thinner, and the regenerating epithelium is seen to extend into the ulcer base. The ulcer base shrinks in a concentric fashion, but healing may occasionally occur linearly, or the ulcer defect may be divided by a mucosal bridge (**Fig. 43.60 b**). As healing continues, the ulcer base loses its punched-out appearance and becomes irregular and less well defined. The erythematous margins become slightly nodular. Gradually regenerating epithelium almost completely covers the ulcer floor, and the whitish base shrinks further and ultimately becomes linear and disappears altogether.

Regenerating epithelium is initially red due to the presence of many capillaries, and this is therefore termed the "red scar stage." Months later, the reddish appearance fades out and the mature epithelium becomes indistinguishable from the surrounding mucosa, and this is therefore known as the "white scar stage." Converging folds at the point where the ulcer was previously located remain as the only evidence of a prior but now healed ulcer. If the fibrotic process is intense, scarring may produce conspicuous retraction, surrounded by diverticular outpouching.

H. pylori–associated gastric ulcer. Genuine *H. pylori*–associated gastric ulcers are nowadays rare. Such ulcers develop in the antrum–gastric body transitional zone in the area of the angular notch. As a function of age, this transitional zone may gradually move upward toward the cardia, and so does the position of the gastric ulcers along the lesser curve. Usually, the background mucosa reveals pangastritis, often with a substantial degree of atrophy. Numerous factors may contribute to focalizing the ulcer in the area of the angle (intensity of inflammation, enhanced acid production, restricted blood supply particularly during postprandial distension of the stomach, etc).

Drug-induced gastric ulceration. A whole spectrum of drugs can damage the gastric mucosa and ultimately lead to ulceration [74]. Currently, the most common cause of drug-induced injury is aspirin-related and NSAID-related, but bisphosphonates and dendronates should also be considered. Multiple ulcers are often the consequence of such ulcerogenic drugs. Although drug-induced ulcers may occur throughout the stomach, most often the distal stomach is involved (**Fig. 43.62**). Not only the lesser curvature area, but also the other quadrants of the circumference may be injured. In contrast to *H. pylori*–associated ulcer, the surrounding mucosa in drug-induced ulceration often looks unremarkable, both endoscopically and even histologically. Many giant ulcers are drug-induced. Occasionally,

Fig. 43.62 Gastric ulcer.
a The gastric ulcer stage, with sharp demarcation.
b The healing stage, with retraction of the surrounding wall.

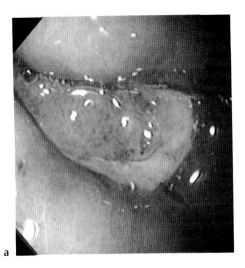

a

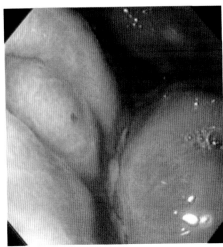

b

drug-induced ulcers show a tendency to coalesce, creating irregular serpiginous defects. Rarely, very extensive areas of the distal stomach are denuded.

A feared complication is ulcer bleeding, particularly after NSAID ulceration. Endoscopic hemostasis is usually possible with injection, clipping, coagulation, etc. If all endoscopic attempts fail, selective vascular embolization may be tried. A rare complication is migration of the endovascular coils into the stomach (**Fig. 43.63**).

Differential diagnosis. The distinction between benign and malignant gastric ulcers is of major clinical importance. Several criteria, summarized in **Fig. 43.64**, can help the endoscopist establish a suspicion that a gastric ulcer is malignant. Although the base tends to be irregular in malignant gastric ulcers, there is so much variation that this criterion is of limited usefulness. In early gastric cancer, the tumor may be confined to the ulcer margin, leaving the base smooth and regular, whereas large benign ulcers may have an irregular or even nodular base. The appearance of the ulcer margin may be more helpful. Normally, smooth mucosa of a uniform color without nodularity or irregularity meets the ulcer base in a benign ulcer. Any pattern other than this normal appearance should suggest possible malignancy. The findings most suggestive of malignancy are distinct nodularity in the ulcer margin, irregular mucosal discoloration, and lack of a clear, regular areae gastricae and lineae gastricae pattern. In addition, the mucosa may be patchily and irregularly eroded. In a benign ulcer, the folds characteristically terminate at the base, or if the ulcer is very large, merge with the margin. In malignancy, folds may end at a distance from the base, or end with a clubbed or piled-up appearance. A plateau-like ulcer margin that obliterates the surrounding folds also suggests malignancy.

However, despite all of the helpful discriminating features listed above, it is often impossible from an endoscopic point of view to differentiate confidently between benign and malignant ulceration. Because of this limitation, the standard advice is to take multiple biopsies from all quadrants of the margin and from the base in order to rule out malignancy, both adenocarcinoma and lymphoma. The accuracy of multiple biopsies is high. As malignant ulcers may also heal after acid-suppressant therapy, it is usually advised to take biopsies from the ulcer scar after healing as well. It is occasionally only at this stage that tiny foci of malignancy may be detected.

Gastric Polyps

Gastric polyps are detected in up to 3% of upper intestinal endoscopies—often incidentally, as such lesions rarely cause symptoms. Polyps are well circumscribed, sharply delineated tissue masses that project above the level of the surrounding mucosa. The insertion base can be sessile, pedunculated, or in between. In roughly one-third of cases, polyps may be multiple and clustered together, or spread out over a larger surface area of the stomach. When more than 50 polyps are present, the condition is known as gastric polyposis.

Most of the polyps are small, with a diameter of less than 10 mm. In approximately 30%, the polyps are larger, with a diameter up to 3–5 cm. Usually, polyps are equally frequent in the antrum and gastric body, but only 10% are present in the cardia [75–78].

Polyps may be neoplastic or nonneoplastic. Neoplastic polyps include adenoma, polypoid carcinoma, and some unusual lesions such as neuroendocrine tumors. About 80–90% of gastric polyps are nonneoplastic. They can be divided into epithelial and nonepithelial lesions. The epithelial lesions include hyperplastic polyps—the most commonly seen polyp in the stomach—and polyps seen in the various polyposis syndromes, including juvenile polyposis, familial polyposis coli, Peutz–Jeghers syndrome [79], Cronkhite–Canada syndrome, etc. Endoscopically, such polyps may appear similar,

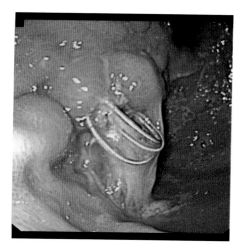

Fig. 43.63 Migration of endovascular coils into the stomach, adjacent to a large varix.

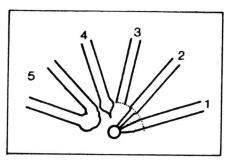

Fig. 43.64 Ulcer features suggesting malignancy: 1, rigidity; 2, narrowing; 3, sharp break; 4, thickening of the proximal end in the area of the break; 5, convergence.

43

except that Peutz–Jeghers polyps are usually larger than the others. Another common epithelial polyp in the stomach is the fundic gland or cystic gland polyp, seen in patients with familial polyposis coli, or during or after proton-pump inhibitor therapy. These fundic gland polyps consist of cystically dilated foveolae and glandular structures [80–83].

▪ Epithelial Lesions

Neoplastic epithelial polyps. *Adenomatous polyps.* Adenomas are uncommon, responsible for 5–10% of polypoid lesions in the stomach. Up to 40% of gastric adenomas may contain a focus of cancer, particularly in larger villous-type lesions. Not only may the polyps become malignant over time, but the adjacent mucosa surrounding them also has a higher risk of cancer development. It would appear prudent after polyp removal to examine the remaining gastric mucosa carefully as well and to biopsy any surface abnormalities. Gastric adenomas are usually larger than hyperplastic polyps. Their average size is 3–4 cm. Adenomatous polyps are often slightly reddish in color. The surface may be smooth and glistening, or multilobulated and superficially eroded (**Figs. 43.65, 43.66**). The latter appearance may be indicative of an increased risk of malignant degeneration. Adenomatous polyps are usually sessile, but may have a pedicle. Exceptionally, adenomas may be flat or even depressed. They occur most often in the antrum, and less frequently in the gastric body. The histological configuration of adenomas may be tubular, villous, or mixed tubulovillous.

Villous polyps are often large, sessile, antrum-predominant, and superficially eroded. Dysplasia and carcinomatous changes occur more frequently in villous adenomas.

Adenomas may also occur in patients with familial adenomatous polyposis (FAP), although the majority of the gastric polyps in FAP are fundic gland polyps. Virtually all gastric cancers in FAP originate from preexisting antral adenomas.

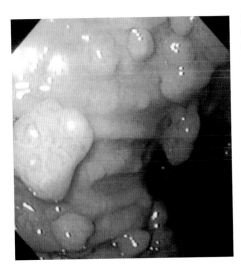

Fig. 43.65 Adenomatous polyps in the stomach.

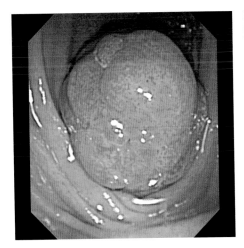

Fig. 43.66 Antral villous adenoma, prolapsing through the pylorus.

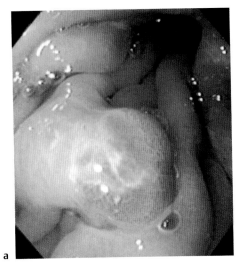

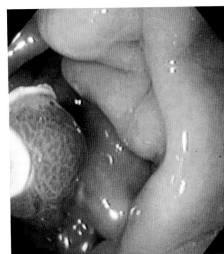

Fig. 43.67 Gastric adenoma.
a Before polypectomy.
b After polypectomy.

a

b

Adenomatous polyps need to be differentiated from type I or type II early gastric cancer, as well as from polypoid advanced carcinoma. Adenomatous lesions also need to be differentiated from polypoid ectopic pancreas, etc. There is a consensus that all adenomatous polyps have to be removed, due to their malignant potential (**Figs. 43.67, 43.68**).

Nonneoplastic epithelial polyps. *Hyperplastic polyps.* Hyperplastic polyps are by far the most common polypoid lesions in the stomach, together with fundic gland polyps. They can occur throughout the stomach. Their size is usually less than 1.5 cm (**Fig. 43.69**). Hyperplastic polyps may be single or multiple, and may be sessile or pedunculated. Occasionally, a long stalk may be seen. The mucosa covering the polyp may appear normal, but in larger polyps the mucosa is often red and friable, and there may be evidence of small erosions or ulcerations at the top as a consequence of twisting. If there are more than 10 polyps, the chance of associated atrophic gastritis may be as high as 30%. The 10–20% of hyperplastic polyps that are larger than 2 cm may be confused with adenomatous or carcinomatous lesions. Not uncommonly, hyperplastic polyps may be present in the antrum and may cause bizarre polypoid configurations. Because of local trauma, there is often a whitish cap of granulation tissue on the top of these polyps. The mucosa in which hyperplastic polyps develop may appear inflamed and atrophic.

The healing stage of raised erosive gastritis or varioliform gastritis may lead to polypoid deformity, resembling hyperplastic pol-

yps histologically because of the foveolar hyperplasia. Anecdotal reports indicate that eradication of *H. pylori* may lead to polyp regression. Hyperplastic polyps need to be differentiated from other nonneoplastic polypoid lesions such as juvenile polyps (**Fig. 43.70**), Peutz–Jeghers polyps, gastric heterotopia (**Fig. 43.71**), etc.

Fundic gland polyps. Fundic gland polyps are small, hemispherical lesions, mainly in the middle and proximal part of the stomach. They routinely appear to be of the same color as normal gastric mucosa, but they are sometimes paler. Fundic gland polyps may be single, but are usually multiple in closely spaced clusters, or may present as a carpet of polyps in the gastric body/fundus area. The polyps are made up of cystically enlarged glands and foveolar areas. They occur particularly in patients with FAP (**Fig. 43.72**), but also in those with Peutz–Jeghers syndrome. They may also develop during long-term therapy with proton-pump inhibitors [83]. Proton-pump inhibitor–related gastric polyps are generally small (< 1 cm), sessile, multiple, and whitish-pink, with a mottled, partly translucent surface. Because of their small size, such polyps are often hidden between rugae and only become visible when the stomach is fully distended. Polyps are sometimes seen in clusters (**Fig. 43.73**). Not uncommonly, there is associated parietal cell hyperplasia and pseudohypertrophy or parietal cell protrusion [81]. Such polyps have no neoplastic potential, although mutations have recently been described—*APC* gene in FAP and *CDH1* (E-cadherin) in PPI-associated lesions [81]. Microscopic foci of adenomatous transformation can occasionally be seen [84,85]. This is reminiscent of the neoplastic

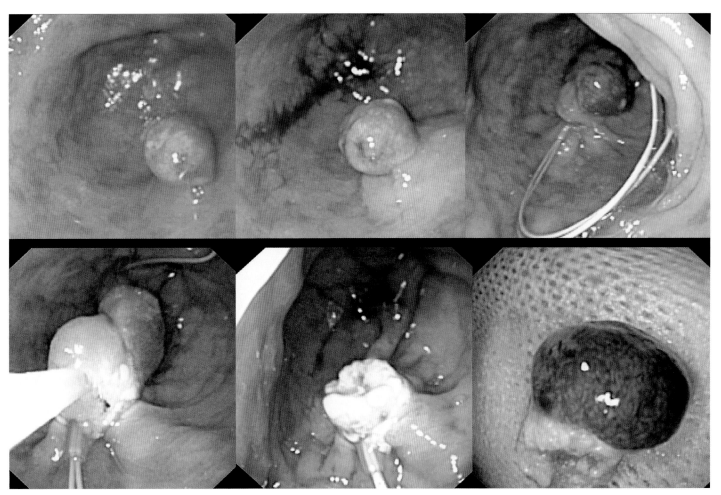

Fig. 43.68 Removal of a tubulovillous adenoma using an endoloop.

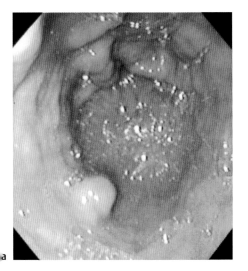

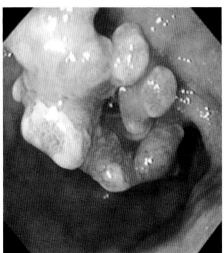

Fig. 43.69
a A small antral hyperplastic polyp.
b A large antral hyperplastic polyp, with granulation tissue on the surface.

43

VI

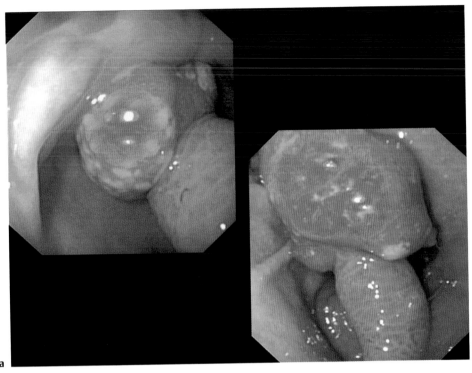

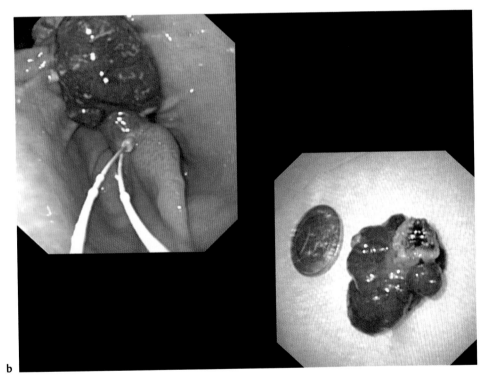

Fig. 43.70 A pedunculated gastric juvenile polyp.
a Before placement of an Endoloop.
b After Endoloop placement, before transection.

Fig. 43.71 A polypoid lesion due to gastric gland heterotopia. By kind permission of Elsevier. Oshima T. Gastric gland heterotopia in muscularis mucosa treated by endoscopic polypectomy.Gastrointest Endosc 2004;60: 664–7.

change that has occasionally been seen in hyperplastic polyps [86,87].

Neuroendocrine, enteroendocrine, or carcinoid tumors. Carcinoids make up 1–2% of all gastric polyps. Type I is associated with autoimmune atrophic gastritis, type II with multiple endocrine neoplasia type I, and type III is sporadic. The cells stain strongly for chromogranin A. Such polypoid lesions are usually small and sessile (**Fig. 43.74**), made up of enterochromaffin-like (ECL) cells. Carcinoids develop in patients with autoimmune gastritis and extensive mucosal atrophy with antral G cell hyperplasia and hypergastrinemia. They vary from tiny yellowish and slightly raised dots to well developed polypoid structures. The mucosa is usually intact when

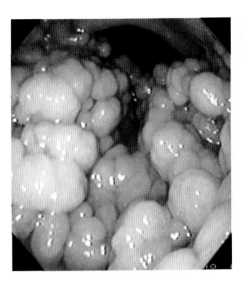

Fig. 43.72 Fundic gland polyps in a patient with familial adenomatous polyposis coli.

the lesion is small, but in larger lesions, ulceration at the top may develop.

Any gastric epithelial polypoid lesion should be removed or biopsied (**Fig. 43.75**). All polyps less than 2 cm in size should in principle be removed endoscopically. When multiple polyps are encountered, the largest polyps should be biopsied or excised, and representative biopsies should be taken from some other polyps, which may or may not need removal. Additional biopsies of the surrounding mucosa are advisable in a search for *H. pylori* infection, atrophy, and intestinal metaplasia. Polyps larger than 2 cm should only be excised endoscopically whenever this is feasible and considered safe. If standard endoscopic polypectomy is not possible and biopsies reveal adenomatous tissue, endoscopic submucosal excision or (minimally invasive) surgical excision needs be considered. Otherwise, careful follow-up may be appropriate when repetitive biopsies only reveal hyperplastic tissue.

Carrying out surveillance endoscopy 1 year after the removal of adenomatous polyps is reasonable in order to assess recurrence at the excision site and identify any new or previously missed lesions

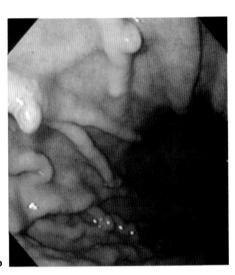
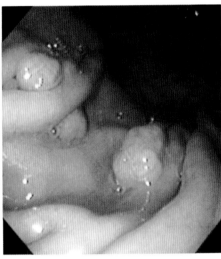
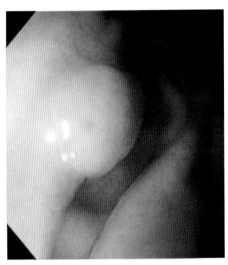

Fig. 43.73
a   Small fundic gland polyps induced by proton-pump inhibitors (PPIs).

b   Somewhat larger fundic gland polyps induced by PPIs.
c   Large fundic gland polyps induced by PPIs.

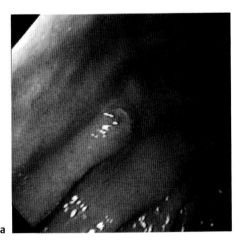
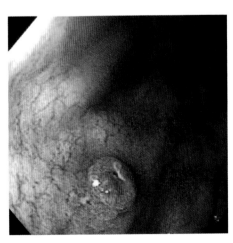

Fig. 43.74 a, b Carcinoid tumor, before (**a**) and after (**b**) chromoscopy. The central depression should be noted.

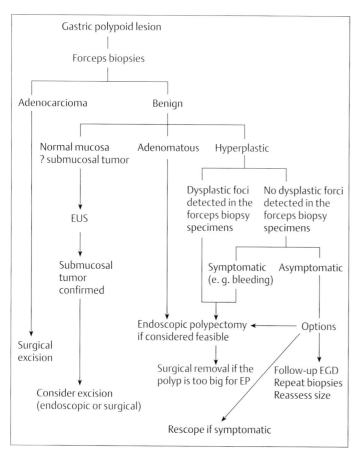

Fig. 43.75 Algorithm for the management of the main types of gastric polypoid lesion. EP, endoscopic polypectomy; EGD, esophagogastroduodenoscopy; EUS, endoscopic ultrasonography.

and/or supervening malignancy in the adjacent mucosa. Further surveillance may be carried out at intervals of 3–5 years.

Subepithelial Mesenchymal Polypoid Lesions

There is a range of subepithelial polypoid lesions in the stomach, including gastrointestinal stromal tumors (GISTs), ectopic pancreatic tissue, leiomyomas, adenomyomas, hamartomatous polyps, lipomas, and other stromal tumors [75]. Usually, such lesions are small

and occasionally difficult to distinguish from hyperplastic or adenomatous polyps. In principle, the bulges are covered with normal-looking mucosa (**Fig. 43.76**). Occasionally, a central depression may be seen in the lesion. The cause of the central depression is usually necrosis as a result of the tumor outgrowing its blood supply. There are often bridging folds on either side of the polypoid mass. The subepithelial or submucosal mass is usually sharply delineated from the surrounding gastric wall. Gastric submucosal tumors that ulcerate may cause acute bleeding. Bleeding may arise from a very deep location within the lesion, inaccessible to endoscopic therapy. Treatment is in general surgical for bleeding lesions, when endoscopic hemostasis is impossible.

Gastrointestinal stromal tumors (GISTs) expressing c-*kit* (CD 117) arise predominantly in the stomach, perhaps originating from the interstitial cells of Cajal. Gastric GISTs may vary in size and shape. Occasionally, the overlying mucosa is eroded or frankly ulcerated. Malignant potential is based on mitotic count as well as size. Small lesions may be endoscopically removed through enucleation [88]. Larger lesions may require minimally invasive surgical removal. Metastatic disease may respond to imatinib mesylate [89,90] (**Fig. 43.77**).

Leiomyomas. Leiomyomas are usually small, less than 1–2 cm in diameter, and they are preferentially located in the proximal stomach (**Fig. 43.78**). Rarely, the tumors are large and extend outside the gastric contours. The covering mucosa is easily tented using a biopsy forceps. In larger lesions, there may be a central depression or a central necrotic area, presumably secondary to infarction. Bridging folds are often observed. Endosonography is the standard imaging modality for further characterizing such lesions.

Endoscopic biopsy is in principle not indicated. Small lesions are often only followed up, but larger lesions may require endoscopic or surgical resection. The differential diagnosis includes GIST tumors, schwannomas, leiomyoblastoma, and rarely leiomyosarcoma.

Miscellaneous polyps. Several other polypoid lesions may develop in the stomach, such as vascular tumors, lipomas, fibromas, neurofibromas, adenomyomas, hamartomatous lesions, and ectopic pancreas. Lipomas are typically yellow, and they are often associated with lipomas elsewhere in the gastrointestinal tract. They may be pedunculated or sessile. Occasionally, lipomas may be large and may invaginate through the pyloric channel. Ectopic pancreatic tissue is usually located in the distal stomach and almost always reveals a ductular opening in the center (**Fig. 43.79**).

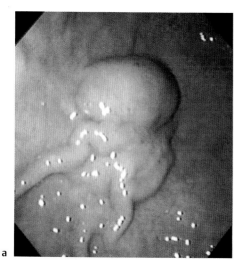

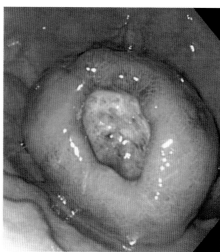

Fig. 43.76 a A subepithelial polyp, covered with normal-appearing mucosa.
b A gastrointestinal stromal tumor (GIST) with central ulceration.

a

b

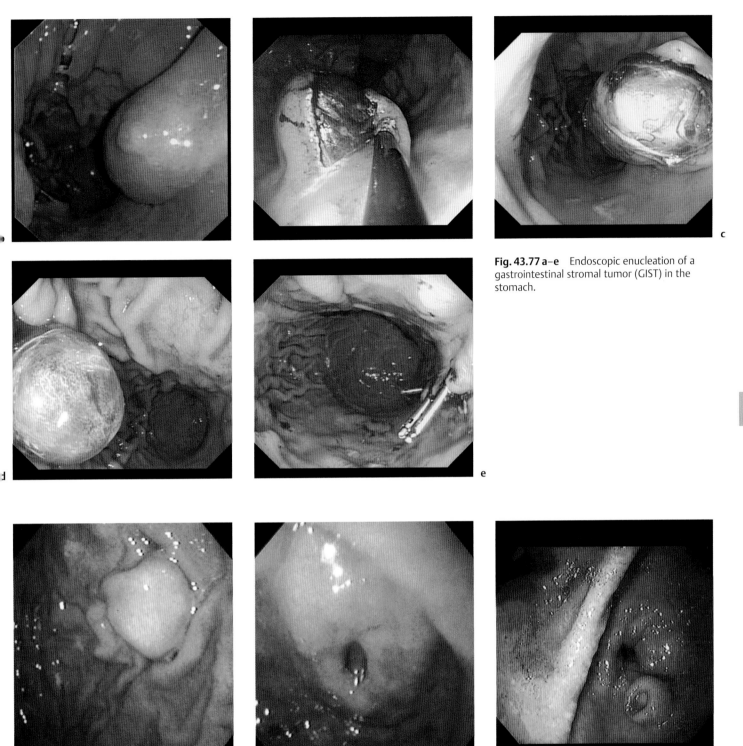

Fig. 43.77 a–e Endoscopic enucleation of a gastrointestinal stromal tumor (GIST) in the stomach.

Fig. 43.78 A leiomyoma in the proximal stomach, covered with normal mucosa.

Fig. 43.79
a Ectopic pancreas in the distal stomach, with a central depression leading to a ductular structure.
b Ectopic pancreas with a central depression, close to the pyloric opening.

Malignant Epithelial Tumors, Gastric Cancer

On a global scale, gastric cancer is the second leading cause of cancer-related deaths. It is now generally accepted that chronic *H. pylori* infection is of predominant importance in up to 80 % of gastric cancer cases [21,22]. The sequence of events encompasses chronic active inflammation, development of atrophic gastritis, intestinal metaplasia, dysplasia, and ultimately invasive malignancy. Biliary reflux, a high-salt diet and several other factors may contribute to the development of cancer, whereas nutrition rich in antioxidants is presumed to slow down such development.

For practical purposes, a distinction should be made between early gastric cancer, which has an excellent prognosis, and advanced gastric cancer, which has a dismal prognosis.

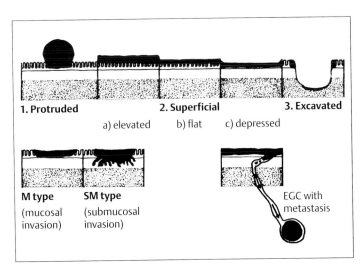

Fig. 43.80 The classification of early gastric cancers according to the Japanese Society for Gastrointestinal Endoscopy. EGC, early gastric cancer.

Early Gastric Cancer

Early gastric cancer, as originally described by the Japanese Society for Gastroenterological Endoscopy, is defined as malignancy limited to the mucosa and submucosa, with or without evidence of lymph-node metastasis [91,92]. Ultimate proof of the degree of invasion can only be provided through careful histological examination. The overall 5-year survival for early gastric cancer is excellent and well over 90 % [93–95].

According to the Japanese and Paris classifications [96], early gastric cancer can be distinguished macroscopically into three basic types, summarized in **Fig. 43.80**. Type 1 is a protruding type; type 2 is a superficial type, with three subcategories—2 a elevated, 2 b flat, and 2 c flat-depressed; and type 3 is the excavated type. Often, several types are combined; the dominant form is given first and the additional forms are given second—for example, 2 c + 2 a. Early gastric cancers with a diameter of less than 1 cm are often designated as "minute cancer" (**Fig. 43.81**).

The protruding type 1 needs to be differentiated from benign polypoid lesions. Size by itself does not allow a distinction between benign and malignant.

Type 2 a may mimic a flat sessile villous polyp. Macroscopically most conspicuous is the discoloration and/or granular surface area of the polypoid lesion. Type 2 b in particular may be difficult to

detect. Only changes in color or minute nodular deformities can raise a suspicion of malignancy. In particular, patchy areas of irregular but well-demarcated redness, irregular and uneven discoloration, and spotty bleeding should raise suspicion for a type 2 b lesion. An increased number of capillaries is responsible for the redness [97]. Chromoscopy with indigo carmine or methylene blue is usually helpful in detecting such lesions. Since type 2 b lesions are rarely symptomatic, they are usually found incidentally. The distinction between type 3 early gastric cancer and a benign gastric ulcer may be extraordinarily difficult (**Fig. 43.64**). Not uncommonly, the pathologist finds a minute area of malignancy in what otherwise looks like a benign gastric ulcer. This is a consequence of the so-called "malignant cycle" of gastric ulceration (**Fig. 43.82**) [98]. Adequate histological diagnosis in such cases is only possible if extensive biopsy sampling is carried out in all four quadrants, both of the ulcer base and of the edges and the scarred area after healing [99]. Up to 5 % of macroscopically benign-looking gastric ulcers turn out to be early gastric cancers. When the ulcer crater heals, a type 3 lesion may develop into a type 2 c, the latter being again amenable to extensive biopsy. After healing, the malignant tissue remains vulnerable and easily damaged by acid peptic attack, allowing the malignant cycle to be repeated.

The overall detection and staging accuracy of endoscopy in early gastric cancer is approximately 70 % [100]. Not uncommonly, early gastric cancers may be overlooked. Moreover, about one in five endoscopically identified "mucosal" cancers may have limited submucosal invasion. Fortunately, the rate of progression of early gastric cancer is often rather slow, allowing detection of the lesion at a later but still early stage.

Biopsy technique. It is generally advised that at least 6–10 biopsies should be taken from any gastric ulceration, not only from the base but also from the four quadrants of the edges. The yield of malignancy from the margins is obviously higher than from the necrotic crater, but the latter needs to be biopsied to detect the occasional patient with signet-ring cell cancer. It is also advisable to take biopsies from the ulcer scar after healing, as it is occasionally only at this time that remaining foci of malignancy become detectable.

Endoscopic mucosal resection. Endoscopic mucosal or submucosal resection (EMR) of early gastric cancer is preferable to endoscopic thermal ablation, as the resected specimen can be retrieved for full histological examination. Complete en-bloc resection of the lesion is preferable to piecemeal removal (**Fig. 43.83**).

Several modalities are currently available for mucosal resection [100–107]. Mucosal resection with a cap-fitted endoscope is often

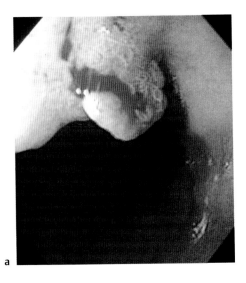

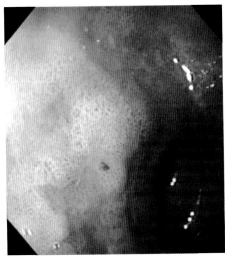

Fig. 43.81
a Early gastric cancer, type 1.
b Early gastric cancer, types 2 a and 2 b.

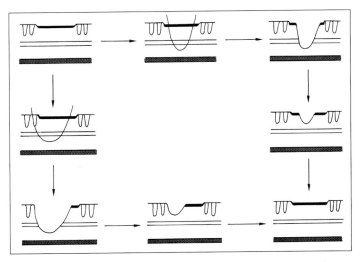

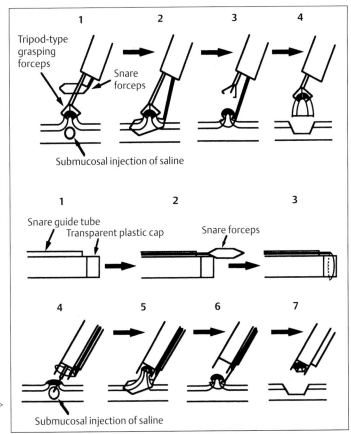

Fig. 43.82 The malignant cycle of gastric ulceration, according to Sakita et al. [98].

Fig. 43.83 Endoscopic mucosal resection using a two-channel endoscope ▷ or a cap-fitted endoscope.

preferred (**Fig. 43.84**). A transparent plastic cap is attached to the tip of a single-channel endoscope. The lesion is aspirated into the cap and resected with a snare that is passed through a guide tube fitted onto the endoscope. After injection of saline or other substances into the submucosa, the raised mucosa with the demarcated suspicious area is suctioned into the cap and the snare is closed. A variant method uses a variceal ligating device to suction the raised mucosa, followed by the application of a ligating band to create a pseudo-polyp for snare resection.

Soehendra et al. [104] introduced a simple mucosectomy technique that does not require any accessory devices except for a monofilament stainless-steel snare with a diameter of 0.4 mm and

a large-channel endoscope. The latter provides adequate suction alongside the inserted snare. The open snare loop is pressed onto the target mucosa and a pseudopolyp is created while suction is applied. The monofilament snare creates adequate counterpressure during suction of the target mucosa. Alternatively, a double-channel endoscope may be used to further lift the target area with a biopsy forceps inserted inside the open snare (**Fig. 43.85**) [102].

The usual indications for EMR are mainly intestinal-type intramucosal cancers less than 20 mm in size (type 1 protruding lesions, types 2 a and 2 b), and mucosal cancer without ulceration less than 10 mm in size. Endoscopic mucosal resection is in general contraindicated when the lesion is larger than 2 cm in diameter, except

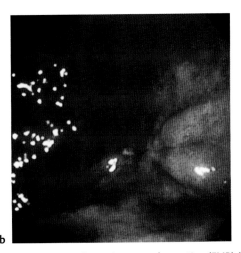

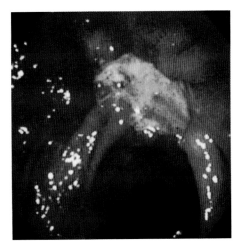

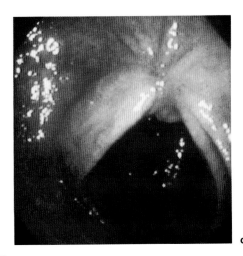

b

c

Fig. 43.84 Endoscopic mucosal resection (EMR) (reproduced with permission from Noda et al. [102].
a Early gastric cancer before resection.

b The defect after EMR.
c The healing phase, with retraction, after EMR.

VI

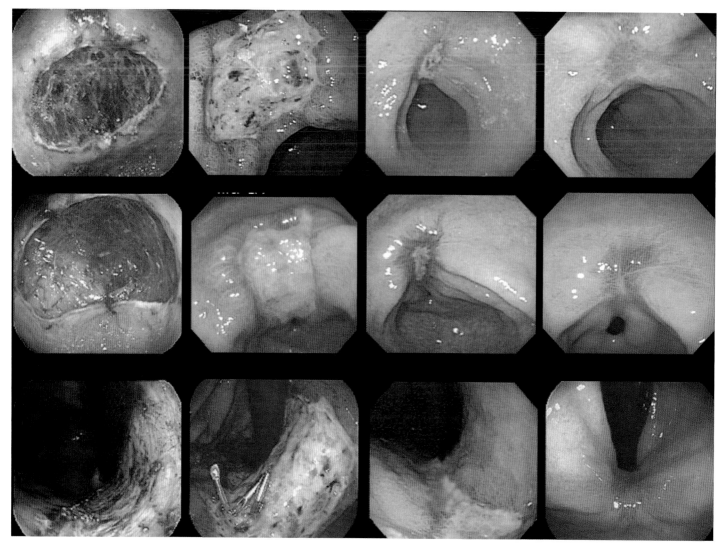

Fig. 43.85 Healing phases after endoscopic mucosectomy of early gastric cancers.

when endoscopic submucosal dissection (ESD) is being considered or when the lesion is depressed (type 2 c) or excavated (type 3) [105]. Particularly in Japan, submucosal dissection of early gastric cancers is increasingly being performed (**Fig. 43.86**) [108–111].

On average, 75% of early gastric cancers can be completely resected. Complete resection of lesions in the proximal and middle third of the stomach is somewhat more difficult. Lesions along the posterior wall of the proximal stomach and in the region of the cardia are generally approached in retroflexion. The most important complications are bleeding and perforation, usually occurring in a few percent of cases. Bleeding is usually treated with hemoclipping [105]. If resection is incomplete, additional endoscopic treatment is indicated, such as repeat EMR or tissue-ablative therapy with argon plasma coagulation, laser photocoagulation, bipolar electrocautery, heater probe, etc., or surgical resection.

■ Advanced Gastric Cancer

Advanced gastric cancer is usually diagnosed in patients over 50 years of age. Japan, Chile, Finland, parts of the former USSR, China, and Colombia have especially high incidence rates of gastric carcinoma.

Conditions associated with an increased incidence of gastric cancer include previous gastric surgery [112], adenomatous gastric polyps [113], autoimmune gastritis with pernicious anemia, and end-stage atrophic gastritis with intestinal metaplasia and miscellaneous conditions such as Ménétrier's disease. The signs and symptoms and differential diagnosis are summarized in **Tables 43.6** and **43.7**.

Previously, advanced gastric cancers were divided into four categories according to Borrmann's classification [114] (**Fig. 43.87**). Type 1 corresponds to a large polypoid cauliflower-like mass projecting into the gastric lumen, without substantial necrosis or ulceration (**Fig. 43.88**). Type 2 corresponds to an ulcerated mass or fungating lesion with sharp margins. Cancerous tissue is present in the periphery and in the center of the ulceration (**Fig. 43.89**). Type 3 is a diffusely infiltrating type, with superimposed ulcerations (**Fig. 43.90**). Type 3 lesions often have indistinct margins. Type 4 corresponds to a diffuse infiltrating linitis plastica–type malignancy (**Fig. 43.91**).

The staging and grading are currently based on the TNM system (**Table 43.8**) [115]. **Figure 43.92** illustrates the lymph-node stations currently resected. Occasionally, an R classification is used to denote residual disease after surgery. R0 is no residual disease, and R1 and R2 are microscopic and macroscopic residual disease, respectively. The staging is summarized in **Fig. 43.93**.

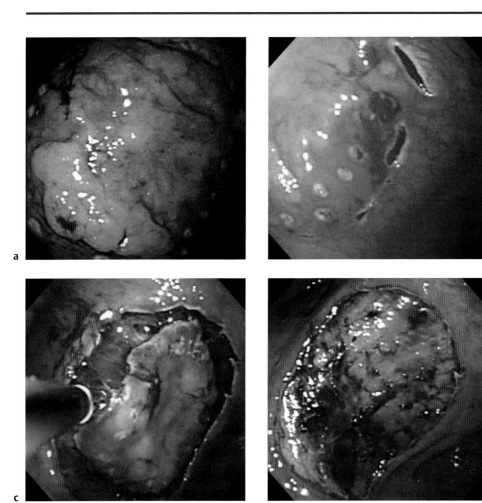

Fig. 43.86 Early gastric cancer treated with submucosal dissection.
a Submucosal injection to lift the lesion.
b Start of the incision into the mucosa.
c Submucosal connective tissue beneath the lesion.
d The lesion has been completely removed from the muscle layer.

43

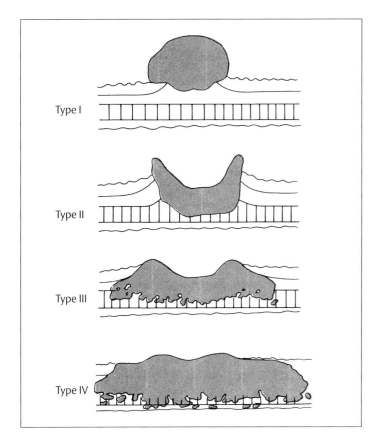

Fig. 43.87 The classification of gastric cancer into four categories, according to Borrmann [114].7

Table 43.6 Signs and symptoms of gastric cancer (nonspecific and late in onset)

Early gastric cancer
Asymptomatic or silent
Epigastric discomfort or dyspepsia
Anorexia, nausea, or vomiting
Early satiety
Weight loss
Gastrointestinal blood loss
Disseminated gastric cancer
Dysphagia (involvement of the esophagogastric junction)
Gastric outlet obstruction (involvement of pylorus or duodenum)
Abdominal mass or hepatomegaly
Node involvement • Supraclavicular (Virchow node) • Left anterior axillary (Irish node)
Peritoneal involvement • Umbilical (Sister Mary Joseph's node) • Ascites • Rectal shelf (Blumer shelf) • Enlarged ovary (Krukenberg tumor)

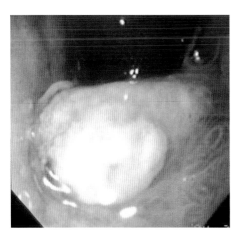

Fig. 43.88 Borrmann type I gastric adenocarcinoma.

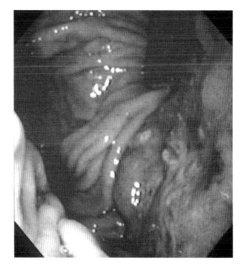

Fig. 43.89 Borrmann type II, with superimposed ulceration.

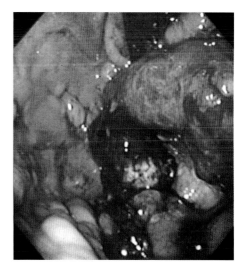

Fig. 43.90 Borrmann type III, with superimposed ulceration.

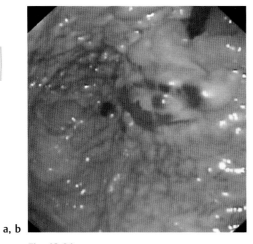

a, b

Fig. 43.91
a Peculiar appearance of limited linitis plastica.
b Typical appearance of diffuse linitis plastica.

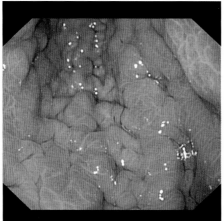

c

c Borrmann type IV, with diffusely infiltrating carcinoma, linitis plastica type.

Table 43.7 Differential diagnosis of gastric cancer

Dyspepsia
Peptic ulcer disease
Nonulcer dyspepsia
Gastric tumors
Metastases to the stomach

Gastric mass or ulcer
Peptic ulcer disease
Gastric adenocarcinoma
Gastric polyp
Gastric lymphoma
Gastric leiomyoma or leiomyosarcoma
Gastric carcinoid
Metastases to the stomach
Ménétrier's disease
Pancreatic remnant
Miscellaneous tumors

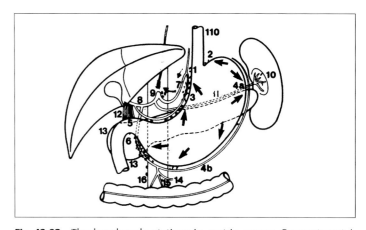

Fig. 43.92 The lymph-node stations in gastric cancer. Compartment I, (perigastric): 1, right paracardiac; 2, left paracardiac; 3, lesser curvature; 4, greater curvature—(a) upper, (b) lower; 5, suprapyloric; 6, infrapyloric. Compartment II (adjacent extraperigastric): 7, left gastric artery; 8, common hepatic artery; 9, celiac artery; 10, splenic hilum; 11, splenic artery; 12, hepatoduodenal; 13, retropancreatic. Compartment III (distant extraperigastric): 14, mesenteric; 15, transverse mesocolic; 16, para-aortic.

Table 43.8 TNM classification of gastric carcinoma [115]

Primary tumor (T)

TX	Primary tumor cannot be assessed
T0	No evidence of primary tumor
Tis	Carcinoma in situ: intraepithelial tumor without invasion of the lamina propria
T1	Tumor invades lamina propria or submucosa
T2	Tumor invades muscularis propria or subserosa*
T2 a	Tumor invades muscularis propria
T2 b	Tumor penetrates subserosa
T3	Tumor penetrates serosa (visceral peritoneum) without invasion of adjacent structures †, ‡
T4	Tumor invades adjacent structures †, ‡

Regional lymph nodes (N)

NX	Regional lymph node(s) cannot be assessed
N0	No regional lymph node metastasis §
N1	Metastases in 1–6 regional lymph nodes
N2	Metastases in 7–15 regional lymph nodes
N3	Metastases in more than 15 regional lymph nodes

Distant metastasis (M)

MX	Distant metastasis cannot be assessed
M0	No distant metastasis
M1	Distant metastasis

Stage grouping

0	Tis	N0	M0
IA	T1	N0	M0
IB	T1	N1	M0
	T2 a/b	N0	M0
II	T1	N2	M0
	T2 a/b	N1	M0
	T3	N0	M0
IIIA	T2 a/b	N2	M0
	T3	N1	M0
	T4	N0	M0
IIIB	T3	N2	M0
IV	T4	N1–3	M0
	T1–3	N3	M0
	Any T	Any N	M1

*A tumor may penetrate the muscularis propria with extension into the gastrocolic or gastro-hepatic ligaments, or into the greater or lesser omentum, without perforation of the visceral peritoneum covering these structures. In this case, the tumor is classified T2. If there is perforation of the visceral peritoneum covering the gastric ligaments or the omentum, the tumor should be classified T3.

†The adjacent structures of the stomach include the spleen, transverse colon, liver, diaphragm, pancreas, abdominal wall, adrenal gland, kidney, small intestine, and retroperitoneum.

‡Intramural extension to the duodenum or esophagus is classified by the depth of greatest invasion in any of these sites, including the stomach.

§A designation of pN0 should be used if all examined lymph nodes are negative, regardless of the total number removed and examined.

		M0				M1	
		N0	N1	N2	N3		
M0	T1	IA	IB	II	IV	IV	
	T2	IB	II	IIIA	IV	IV	
	T3	II	IIIA	IIIB	IV	IV	
	T4	IIIA	IIIB	IV	IV	IV	
M1		IV	IV	IV	IV	IV	

Stage	5-year survival (%)
IA	95
IB	90
II	45
IIIA	15
IIIB	5
IV	1

Fig. 43.93 Staging of gastric malignancy.

Table 43.9 The Ann Arbor classification system for extranodal lymphomas, as modified by Musshoff (adapted from [118])

EI	Lymphoma restricted to gastrointestinal tract on one side of the diaphragm; no nodal involvement
EI 1	Infiltration limited to the mucosa and submucosa
EI 2	Lymphoma extending beyond the submucosa
EII	Lymphoma additionally infiltrating lymph nodes on the same side of the diaphragm
EII 1	Infiltration of regional lymph nodes (involvement of contiguous nodes)
EII 2	Infiltration of lymph nodes beyond regional (but sub-diaphragmatic)
EIII	Lymphoma infiltrating gastrointestinal tract and/or lymph nodes on both sides of the diaphragm
EIV	Localized infiltration of associated lymph nodes, together with diffuse or disseminated involvement of extragastro-intestinal organs

Malignant Nonepithelial Tumors

Gastric lymphoma. Some 0.5–8.0% of gastric malignancies are caused by lymphoma. Primary gastric lymphoma includes extranodal non-Hodgkin's lymphoma and less commonly Hodgkin's lymphoma. The most common is primary gastric mucosa-associated lymphoid tissue (MALT)-type lymphoma, which is almost always related to *H. pylori* infection. Partial and often complete remission of low-grade *H. pylori* MALT lymphoma, limited to the wall of the stomach, is possible after curing of the *H. pylori* infection through removal of the antigenic drive, particularly in the absence of chromosomal translocations such as t(1;14) and t(11;18) [116,117].

Full staging of the lymphoma usually requires extensive investigation. Among the many staging systems, the Ann Arbor classification system is often used (**Table 43.9**) [118].

Characteristically, gastric lymphoma occurs as an infiltrating lesion, often associated with ulceration. In some patients, there is peculiar polypoid nodularity in the invaded area. Single or multiple ulcers may be seen in association with areas of infiltration and nodularity. Occasionally, the lymphomatous growth may resemble

43

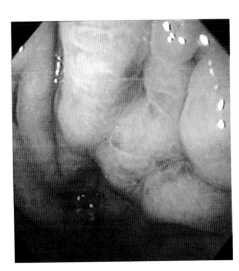

Fig. 43.94 Gastric mucosa-associated lymphoid tissue (MALT) lymphoma with conspicuous fold enlargement.

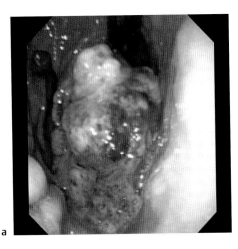

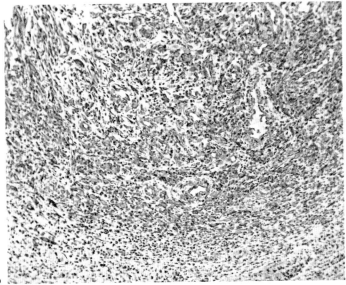

Fig. 43.95
a Extensive sarcoma of the cardia.
b Positive vimentin staining.

an infiltrating adenocarcinoma, as seen in linitis plastica. Also common are infiltrated folds with diffuse ulceration (**Fig. 43.94**) and irregular nodularity. Lymphomas may also appear as single or multiple masses. There are essentially three main patterns: ulceration (48%), polypoid mass (30%), and diffuse infiltration (16%) [119,120]. In approximately 75% of cases, the endoscopic abnormalities are

sufficiently bizarre to suggest malignancy. In about one-quarter, the initial impression is that of benign disease.

Firm histological diagnosis is mandatory. The yield of multiple biopsies is often disappointing. However, with extensive biopsies mapping the entire stomach, it is usually possible to reach a correct diagnosis in 70–80% of cases. Areas with the highest yield of positivity are ulcers, nodules, or frankly abnormal-appearing mucosa. Endoscopically guided sheathed brush cytology may also be helpful. Rarely, needle cytology is necessary under endosonographic guidance.

Proper staging of the lymphomatous involvement of the stomach with endosonography is currently the standard diagnostic methodology. Endosonography is essential to select those patients with MALT lymphoma in whom antimicrobial therapy is suitable.

Endoscopy is also indicated to monitor the effect of therapy, whether with *H. pylori* eradication, chemotherapy, radiotherapy, or combinations of these.

Gastric sarcoma. Sarcomas account for roughly 2% of gastric malignancies. Such mesenchymal tumors usually present as large masses, over 4 cm in diameter. Not uncommonly, the mass extends outside the contours of the stomach. In at least 20% of the patients, there is a central depression in the surface of the mass lesion caused by central necrosis, leading to overt gastrointestinal bleeding (**Fig. 43.95**). Smaller lesions may appear similar to any stromal tumor such as GIST or leiomyoma.

Histologically, the most common sarcoma is leiomyosarcoma (**Fig. 43.96**), followed by fibrosarcoma. Histological examination by biopsy or cytology can be problematic. Characteristic findings are spindle cells, with evidence of increased mitotic activity.

Kaposi's sarcoma. Kaposi's sarcoma is usually a generalized disease also involving the skin and other parts of the gastrointestinal tract. The lesion is usually seen in patients with human immunodeficiency virus (HIV) infection and AIDS. It is due to infection with herpes-type virus (HHV-8), mainly involving the endothelial cells.

Endoscopically, there are three dominant types of appearance: single or multiple maculopapular lesions; polypoid lesions; and ulcerating lesions (**Fig. 43.97**). Occasionally, Kaposi's lesions may appear in a diffuse form rather than in isolated maculopapular abnormalities. Characteristically, the lesions are intensely red, corresponding to the underlying histopathology. Findings at biopsy are mesenchymal-type tissue with vascular spaces or slits, and numerous endothelial cells amongst the spindle cells. All such lesions need to be differentiated from other rare malignancies such as plasmacytoma (**Fig. 43.98**) or extragonadal embryonic germline tumors (**Fig. 43.99**).

Metastatic gastric disease. Not uncommonly, cancer of the lung and breast or melanoma metastasize to the stomach. Tumors of the pancreas, testis, thyroid, or female genital tract metastasize to the stomach more rarely. The discovery of a gastric lesion is sometimes the first manifestation of metastatic spread [121].

Metastases usually present as multiple submucosal lesions 1–2 cm in size. Less commonly, they project into the lumen or may present with central ulceration and overt blood loss. Characteristic pigmentation may be noted in cases of melanoma, although the lesions are not uncommonly amelanotic. Metastatic breast cancer may appear as a diffuse infiltration, with superimposed tiny polypoid or sessile nodules.

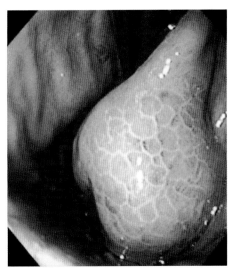

Fig. 43.96 A large gastric leiomyosarcoma in the fundus.

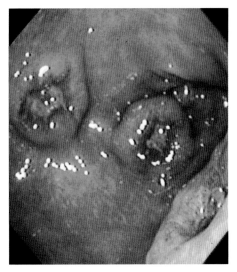

Fig. 43.97 Gastric Kaposi's sarcomatous lesions.

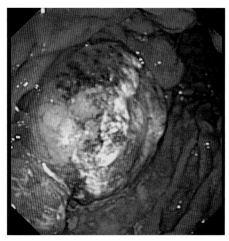

Fig. 43.98 Plasmacytoma of the stomach.

Fig. 43.99 An extragonadal germ cell tumor.

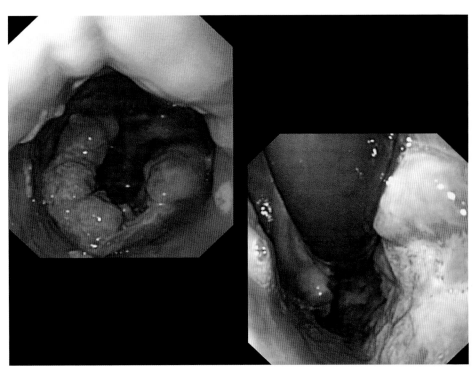

43

Postoperative Stomach

Gastric resection for benign disease is now almost never used. Billroth I and Billroth II operations and highly selective, selective, or truncal vagotomy are now only rarely performed. Despite the rarity of the procedures, the endoscopist should be aware of anatomic variations that may result from surgical intervention. A wide range of postoperative changes are possible. Some of these changes occur early after surgery, while others develop later on.

Postoperative edema. Early after surgery, there is impressive swelling and erythema at the level of the surgical anastomosis, regardless of the type of surgery that has been carried out. Edema may be so pronounced that it seems to obliterate the lumen.

Suture granuloma. Suture material is often visible in the area of the anastomosis. Usually, residual suture material is surrounded by inflamed, partially eroded mucosa. It is doubtful whether suture material should be removed endoscopically using a biopsy forceps or scissors. Suture material often disappears spontaneously, but it may take a long time.

Pyloroplasty. A pyloroplasty can be carried out in several ways. The defect created by a Heineke–Mikulicz procedure resembles an open pyloric ring, through which another ring-like structure may be seen. Detection of recurrent ulcer in this type of pyloroplasty may be difficult.

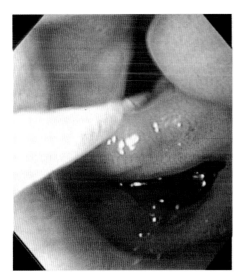

Fig. 43.100 A split or double pylorus, with a catheter lifting the barrier between the two openings.

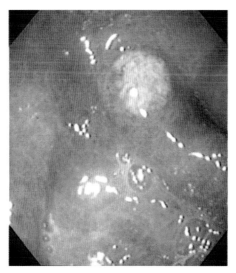

Fig. 43.101 Swollen erythematous mucosa caused by biliary reflux gastritis. A xanthelasma is also present.

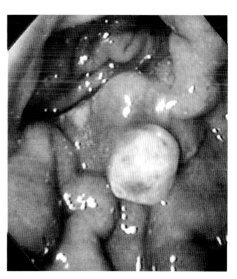

Fig. 43.102 A granulation polyp at the level of the stoma.

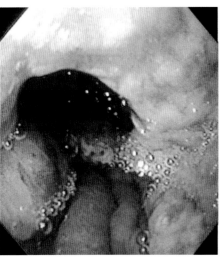

Fig. 43.103 Whitish areas around the stoma, suggesting intestinal metaplasia.

Split pylorus or double pylorus. When a deep ulcer—often an NSAID-induced ulcer—creates a fistulous tract between the antrum and duodenal bulb, a double or split pylorus is created that mimics the defect seen after a surgical gastroduodenostomy. The scope can be advanced through both openings lining a mucosal bridge, to enter the duodenal bulb (**Fig. 43.100**).

Billroth I and II partial gastrectomy. Rugal folds terminate circumferentially and abruptly around the stoma in Billroth I gastrectomy. In Billroth II gastrectomy, the stoma is usually located 15–20 cm below the esophagogastric junction. The transition between the redder gastric mucosa and the more yellowish-gray small-bowel mucosa is easily identified. The opening of the efferent loop is usually somewhat larger, and connects more directly with the gastric anastomosis than does the opening of the afferent loop. Not uncommonly, the blindly closed inverted end of the afferent loop resembles a polyp. Biopsies should be obtained from the very end of the afferent loop when the presence of retained antral mucosa is suspected clinically.

The mucosa in the gastric remnant is usually fiercely erythematous due to biliary reflux (**Fig. 43.101**). Biopsies reveal reactive or chemical gastritis. Not uncommonly, polypoid excrescences may be seen around the anastomosis, together with granulation polyps

(**Fig. 43.102**) and areas of discoloration suggestive of intestinal metaplasia (**Fig. 43.103**).

Stomal ulceration or ulcus jejuni pepticum is a feared complication of gastric surgery (**Fig. 43.104**). Stomal ulcers are usually located within 2 cm on either side of the stoma. A jejunal ulcer is similar in appearance to a bulbar ulcer, with a whitish-grayish crater and erythematous inflamed edges. Occasionally, such ulcers are large and multiple. Bleeding is a serious complication. Exceptionally, such ulcers may perforate into the colon, creating a gastrojejunal-colonic fistula.

Stomal or retrograde jejunogastric intussusception is a rare and serious complication. Endoscopically, an erythematous mass made up of jejunal folds is seen projecting through the stoma into the lumen of the gastric remnant. Patches of severe erythema may be seen in the small bowel after resolution of the intussusception.

Bezoar formation. Dysmotility of the gastric remnant predisposes to bezoar formation. Usually, the bezoar is made up of vegetable food remnants and is known as a phytobezoar (**Fig. 43.105**). Occasionally, the bezoar may partly obstruct the gastric outlet. Various methods are usually used in an attempt to break up such bezoars. Combinations of flushing and suction, and removal of fragments with baskets or polypectomy snares, should be attempted. An overtube around the endoscope can be used to facilitate repetitive insertion of the endoscope [122].

Postgastrectomy neoplasms. Patients with partial gastrectomy, particularly Billroth II gastrectomy, have a slightly increased risk of malignant degeneration some 10–20 years after surgery. Progressively worsening dysplasia is usually evident before the development of overt cancer. Early malignancy is usually not associated with symptoms and is often an incidental finding. Common appearances are small polypoid masses, areas of discoloration, or minor erosive defects. In particular, the area within 2 cm of the stoma is predisposed to this type of malignant degeneration [123,124]. Gastric remnant cancers are usually far advanced at the time of diagnosis when detected in the symptomatic stage. Some of these cancers are of the linitis plastica type and not only involve the remnant but also spread into the esophagus.

Bariatric surgery. Various bariatric surgical procedures are currently performed [125]. Adjustable silicone gastric banding is commonly used (**Fig. 43.106**). For morbid obesity, gastric bypass is often

VI

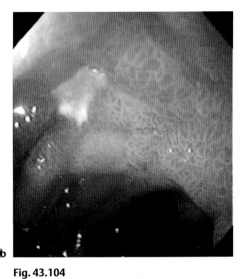

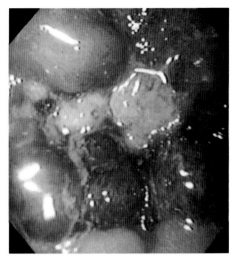

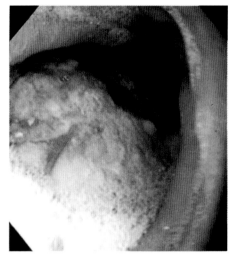

Fig. 43.104
a A small ulcer in the small intestine, in a patient with Billroth I resection.
b Ulcus jejuni pepticum after Billroth II resection.

Fig. 43.105 A phytobezoar in a patient with gastric resection.

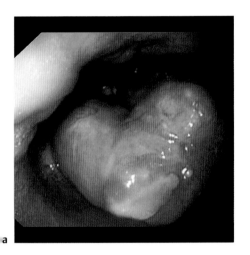

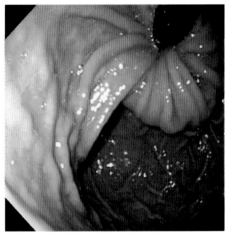

Fig. 43.106
a The endoscopic appearance after gastric banding.
b Retrograde view of the ring-like compression of the endoscope. (Reproduced courtesy of J. Weber).

43

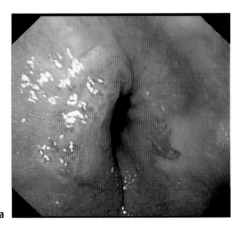

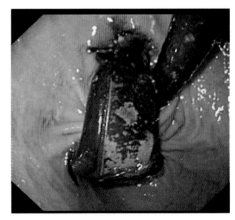

Fig. 43.107
a Ineffective closure after gastric banding.
b A migrated and perforated gastric band. (Reproduced courtesy of J. Weber).

used. Endoscopy is indicated to analyze the causes of failure and to identify and correct complications [126]. Common complications are inefficient gastric banding (**Fig. 43.107 a**), stricturing causing food bolus obstruction and requiring dilation, anastomotic ulcers after bypass surgery, and migration and perforation of gastric bands (**Fig. 43.107 b**).

The authors gratefully acknowledge the superb cooperation of the following colleagues in providing unique picture material:

Drs. Kamada & Tanaka, Japan (**Fig. 43.14b**), Lee & Kim, South Korea (**Fig. 43.31**), Ruiz-Rebello (**Fig. 31.34**), Han, Korea (**Fig. 43.35**), Ueo, Japan (**Fig. 43.47**), Tanioka & Machida, Japan (**Fig. 43.50**),Hamada & Tanaka, Japan (**Fig. 43.51**), Janczewska, Sweden (**Fig. 43.52b**), Suk & Tiong, Taiwan (**Fig. 43.53**), Nakamura, Japan (**Fig. 43.57a,b**), Kupkova, Czech Republic (**Fig. 43.63**), Oshima, Japan (**Fig. 43.71**), Jun, Korea (**Fig. 43.76b**), Kakushima & Yahagi, Japan (**Fig. 43.85**),Yamamoto, Japan (**Fig. 43.86**), Negreanu, Romania (**Fig. 43.91a**), Weber, Luxemburg (**Fig. 43.106–107**).

References

1. Cameron AJ, Higgins JA. Linear gastric erosion. Gastroenterology 1986;91:338–42.
2. Shepherd HA, Harvey J, Jackson A, Colins-Jones DG. Recurrent retching with gastric mucosal prolapse: a proposed prolapse gastropathy syndrome. Dig Dis Sci 1984;29:121–8.
3. Mallory GK, Weiss S. Hemorrhages from lacerations of the cardiac orifice of the stomach due to vomiting. Am J Med Sci 1929;178:506–15.
4. Tytgat GNJ. The Sydney system: endoscopic division, endoscopic appearance in gastritis/duodenitis. J Gastroenterol Hepatol 1991;6:223–34.
5. Tytgat GNJ. Endoscopic gastritis and duodenitis. Endoscopy 1992;24:34–40.
6. Fennerty MB, Sampliner RE, McGee DL, Hixson LJ, Garewal HS. Intestinal metaplasia of the stomach: identification by a selective mucosal staining technique. Gastrointest Endosc 1992;38:696–8.
7. Kaminishi M, Yamaguchi H, Nomura S, Oohara T, Sakai S, Fukutomi H, et al. Endoscopic classification of chronic gastritis based on a pilot study by the Research Society for Gastritis. Dig Endosc 2002;14:138–51.
8. Price AB. The Sydney system: histological division. J Gastroenterol Hepatol 1991;6:209–22.
9. Dixon MF, Genta RH, Yardley JH, Correa P. Classification of gastritis. The updated Sydney System – International Workshop on Histopathology of gastritis. Houston 1994. Am J Surg Pathol 1996;20:1161–81.
10. Genta RM. Gastric atrophy and atrophic gastritis: nebulous concepts in search of a definition. Aliment Pharmacol Ther 1998;12(Suppl 1):17–23.
11. Rugge M, Genta RM. Staging and grading of chronic gastritis. Human Pathol 2005;36:228–33.
12. Rugge M, Meggio A, Pennelli G, Piscioli F, Giacomelli L, De Pretis G, et al. Gastritis staging in clinical practice: the OLGA staging system. Gut 2007;56:631–6.
13. Craanen ME, Blok P, Dekker W, Ferwerda J, Tytgat GNJ. Prevalence of subtypes of intestinal metaplasia in gastric antral mucosa. Dig Dis Sci 1991;36:1529–36.
14. Carpenter HA, Talley NJ. Gastroscopy is incomplete without biopsy: clinical relevance of distinguishing gastropathy from gastritis. Gastroenterology 1995;108:917–24.
15. Haber MM. Gastric biopsies: Increasing the yield. Clin Gastroenterol Hepatol 2007;5:160–5.
16. Anagnostopoulos GK, Yao K, Kaye P, Fogden E, Fortun P, Shonde A, et al. High-resolution magnification endoscopy can reliably identify normal gastric mucosa, Helicobacter pylori–associated gastritis, and gastric atrophy. Endoscopy 2007;39:202–7.
17. Stolte M, Eidt S. Chronic erosions of the antral mucosa: a sequela of Helicobacter pylori–induced gastritis. Z Gastroenterol 1992;30:846–50.
18. Nishibayashi H, Kanayama S, Kiyohara T, Yamamoto K, Miyazaki Y, Yasunaga Y, et al. Helicobacter pylori–induced enlarged-fold gastritis is associated with increased mutagenicity of gastric juice, increased oxidative DNA damage, and increased risk of gastric carcinoma. J Gastroenterol Hepatol 2003;18:1384–91.
19. Rindi G, Fiocca R, Morocutti A, Jacobs A, Miller N, Thjodleifsson B, et al. Effect of 5 years of treatment with rabeprazole on the gastric mucosa. Eur J Gastroenterol Hepatol 2005;17:559–66.
20. Mera R, Fontham ETH, Bravo LE, Piazuelo MB, Camargo MC, Correa P. Long term follow up of patients treated for Helicobacter pylori infection. Gut 2005;54:1536–40.
21. Wang C, Yuan Y, Hunt RH. The association between Helicobacter pylori infection and early gastric cancer: a meta-Analysis. Am J Gastroenterol 2007;102:1789–98.
22. Correa P, Houghton J. Carcinogenesis of Helicobacter pylori. Gastroenterology 2007;133:659–72.
23. Nardone G, Rocco A, Compare D, De Colibus P, Autiero G, Pica L, et al. Is screening for and surveillance of atrophic gastritis advisable? Dig Dis 2007;25:214–7.
24. Goodgame RW. Gastrointestinal cytomegalovirus disease. Ann Intern Med 1993;119:924–35.
25. Howiler W, Goldberg HI. Gastroesophageal involvement in herpes simplex. Gastroenterology 1976;70:775–8.
26. Subei I, Attar B, Schmitt G, Levendoglu H. Primary gastric tuberculosis: a case report and literature review. Am J Gastroenterol 1987;82:769–72.
27. Long BW, Johnston JH, Wetzel W, Flowers RH, Haick A. Gastric syphilis: endoscopic and histological features mimicking lymphoma. Am J Gastroenterol 1995;90:1504–7.
28. Oberhuber G, Stolte M, Bethke B, Ritter M, Eidt H. Gastric giardiasis: analysis of biopsy specimens from 191 patients infected with Giardia lamblia. Eur J Gastroenterol Hepatol 1993;5:357–60.
29. Kakizoe S, Kakizoe H, Kakizoe K, Kakizoe Y, Maruta M, Kakizoe T, et al. Endoscopic findings and clinical manifestation of gastric anisakiasis. Am J Gastroenterol 1995;90:761–3.
30. Schultz MJ, Van der Hulst RWM, Tytgat GNJ. Acute phlegmonous gastritis. Gastrointest Endosc 1996;44:80–3.
31. Will U, Masri R, Bosseckert H, Knopke A, Schönlebe J, Justus J. Gastric wall abscess, a rare endosonographic differential diagnosis of intramural tumors: successful endoscopic treatment. Endoscopy 1998;30:432–5.
32. Kim JB, Han DS, Lee HL, Park JY, Jeon YC, Sohn JH, et al. Malacoplakia of the stomach: case report and review. Gastrointest Endosc 2003;58:441–5.
33. Faller G, Winter M, Steininger H, Konturek P, Konturek SJ, Kirchner T. Antigastric autoantibodies and gastric secretory function in Helicobacter pylori–infected patients with duodenal ulcer and non-ulcer dyspepsia. Scand J Gastroenterol 1998;33:276–82.
34. Tòth E, Sjölund K, Fork FT, Lindström C. Chronic atrophic fundic gastritis diagnosed by a modified Congo red test. Endoscopy 1995;27:654–8.
35. Solcia E, Bordi C, Creutzfeldt W, Dayal Y, Dayan AD, Falkmer S, et al. Histopathological classification of nonantral gastric endocrine growths in man. Digestion 1988;41:185–200.
36. Burkitt MD, Pritchard DM. Review article: pathogenesis and management of gastric carcinoid tumours. Aliment Pharmacol Ther 2006;24:1305–20.
37. American Gastroenterological Association, Wilcox CM, Allison J, Benzuly K, Borum M, Cryer B, et al. Consensus development conference on the use of nonsteroidal anti-inflammatory agents, including cyclooxygenase-2 enzyme inhibitors and aspirin. Clin Gastroenterol Hepatol 2006;4:1082–9.
38. Lanza FL, Aspinall RL, Swabb EA, Davis RE, Rack MF, Rubin A. Double-blind, placebo-controlled endoscopic comparison of the mucosal protective effects of misoprostol versus cimetidine on tolmetin-induced mucosal injury to the stomach and duodenum. Gastroenterology 1988;95:289–94.
39. Lanza FL, Nelson RS, Rack MF. A controlled endoscopic study comparing the toxic effects of sulindac, naproxen, aspirin, and placebo on the gastric mucosa of health volunteers. J Clin Pharmacol 1984;24:89–95.
40. Stolte M, Panayiotou S, Schmitz J. Can NSAID/ASA-induced erosions of the gastric mucosa be identified at histology? Pathol Res Pract 1999;195:137–42.
41. Hooper L, Brown TJ, Elliott R, Payne K, Roberts C, Symmons D. The effectiveness of five strategies for the prevention of gastrointestinal toxicity induced by non-steroidal anti-inflammatory drugs: systemic review. BMJ 2004;329:948.
42. Laine L, Weinstein WM. Histology of alcoholic hemorrhagic gastritis: a prospective evaluation. Gastroenterology 1988;94:1254–62.
43. Knoll MR, Kölbel CB, Teyssen S, Singer MV. Action of pure ethanol and some alcoholic beverages on the gastric mucosa in healthy humans: a descriptive endoscopic study. Endoscopy 1998;30:293–301.
44. Tarnawski A, Hollander D, Stachura J, Klimczyk B, Mach T, Bogdal J. Alcohol injury to the normal human gastric mucosa: endoscopic, histologic and functional assessment. Clin Invest Med 1987;10:259–63.
45. Haot J, Bogomoletz W, Jouret A, Mainguet P. Ménétrier's disease with lymphocytic gastritis: an unusual association with possible pathogenic implications. Hum Pathol 1991;22:379–86.
46. Overholt BF, Jeffries GH. Hypertrophic, hypersecretory protein-losing enteropathy. Gastroenterology 1970;58:80–7.
47. Bayerdörffer E, Ritter MM, Hatz R, Brooks W, Stolte M. Ménétrier's disease and Helicobacter pylori. N Engl J Med 1993;329:60.
48. Ectors NL, Dixon MF, Geboes KJ, Rutgeerts PJ, Desmet VJ, van Trappen GR. Granulomatous gastritis: a morphological and diagnostic approach. Histopathology 1993;23:55–61.
49. Wright CL, Riddell RH. Histology of the stomach and duodenum in Crohn's disease. Am J Surg Pathol 1998;22:383–90.
50. Oberhuber G, Püspök A, Oesterreicher C, Novacek G, Zauner C, Burghuber M, et al. Focally enhanced gastritis: a frequent type of gastritis in patients with Crohn's disease. Gastroenterology 1997;112:698–706.
51. Sobala GM, King RF, Axon AT, Dixon MF. Reflux gastritis in the intact stomach. J Clin Pathol 1990;43:303–6.
52. Girelli CM, Cuvello P, Limido E, Rocca F. Duodenogastric reflux: an update. Am J Gastroenterol 1996;91:648–53.
53. Byrne WJ. Foreign bodies, bezoars, and caustic ingestion. Gastrointest Clin N Am 1994;4:99–120.
54. McDonald GB, Rees GM. Approach to gastrointestinal problems in the immunocompromised patient. In: Yamada T, editor. Textbook of gastroenterology. 2nd ed. Philadelphia: Lippincott; 1995. p. 988–1022.

VI

55. Vorder Bruegge WF, Peura DA. Stress-related mucosal damage: review of drug therapy. J Clin Gastroenterol 1990;12(Suppl 2):S 35–40.

56. Kato S, Shibuya H, Naganuma H, Nakagawa H. Gastrointestinal endoscopy in Henoch–Schönlein purpura. Eur J Pediatr 1992;11:482–4.

57. Hara T, Shiotani A, Matsunaka H, Yamanishi T, Oka H, Ishiguchi T, et al. Hereditary angioedema with gastrointestinal involvement: endoscopic appearance. Endoscopy 1999;31:322–4.

58. Gallagher CG, Lennon JR, Crowe JP. Chronic erosive gastritis: a clinical study. Am J Gastroenterol 1987;82:302–6.

59. Haot J, Jouret A, Willette M, Gossuin A, Mainguet P. Lymphocytic gastritis—prospective study of its relationship with varioliform gastritis. Gut 1990;31:282–5.

60. Jones EA, Fléjou JF, Potet F, Muzeau F, Molas G, Rotenberg A, et al. Lymphocytic gastritis: a clinicopathological study of 32 patients. Eur J Gastroenterol Hepatol 1990;2:367–72.

61. Dixon MF, Wyatt JI, Burke DA, Rathbone BJ. Lymphocytic gastritis: relationship to *Campylobacter pylori* infection. J Pathol 1988;154:125–32.

62. Colletti RB, Trainer TD. Collagenous gastritis. Gastroenterology 1989;97:1552–5.

63. Longacre AV, Gross CP, Gallitelli M, Henderson KJ, White RI Jr, Proctor DD. Diagnosis and management of gastrointestinal bleeding in patients with hereditary hemorrhagic telangiectasia. Am J Gastroenterol 2003;98:59–65.

64. Stark ME, Gostout CJ, Balm RK. Clinical features and endoscopic management of Dieulafoy's disease. Gastrointest Endosc 1992;38:545–50.

65. McGrath K, Mergener K, Branch S. Endoscopic band ligation of Dieulafoy's lesion: report of two cases and review of the literature. Am J Gastroenterol 1999;94:1087–90.

66. Romãozinho JM, Pontes JM, Lérias C, Ferreira M, Freitas D. Dieulafoy's lesion: Management and long-term outcome. Endoscopy 2004;36:416–20.

67. Gostout CJ, Viggiano TR, Ahlquist DA, Wang KK, Larson MV, Balm R. The clinical and endoscopic spectrum of the watermelon stomach. J Clin Gastroenterol 1992;15:256–63.

68. Lecleire S, Ben-Soussan E, Antonietti M, Goria O, Riachi G, Lerebours E, et al. Bleeding gastric vascular ectasia treated by argon plasma coagulation: a comparison between patients with and without cirrhosis. Gastrointest Endosc 2008;67:219–25.

69. Viggiano TR, Gostout CJ. Portal hypertensive intestinal vasculopathy: a review of the clinical, endoscopic, and histopathologic features. Am J Gastroenterol 1992;87:944–54.

70. de Franchis R. Evolving consensus in portal hypertension. Report of the Baveno IV consensus workshop on methodology of diagnosis and therapy in portal hypertension. J Hepatol 2005;43:167–76.

71. Veldhuyzen van Zanten SJO, Dixon MF, Lee A. The gastric transitional zones: neglected links between gastroduodenal pathology and *Helicobacter* ecology. Gastroenterology 1999;116:1217–29.

72. Kawai K, Ida K, Akasaka Y, Nakujima M, Misaki F, Miyaoka T. Location of gastric ulcer and the fundopyloric border [in Japanese]. Gastroenterol Endosc 1973;15:142–5.

73. Sakita T, Fukutomi H. Endoscopy of gastric ulcer. In: Yoshitoshi Y, editor. Peptic ulcer. Tokyo: Nankodo; 1971. p. 198–208.

74. Aabakken L. Clinical symptoms, endoscopic findings and histologic features of gastroduodenal non-steroidal anti-inflammatory drugs lesions. Ital J Gastroenterol Hepatol 1999;31(Suppl 1):S 19–22.

75. Stolte M, Sticht T, Eidt S, Ebert D, Finkenzeller G. Frequency, location, and age and sex distribution of various types of gastric polyp. Endoscopy 1994;26:659–65.

76. Oberhuber G, Stolte M. Gastric polyps: an update of their pathology and biological significance. Virchow Arch 2000;437:581–90.

77. Stolte M. Clinical consequences of the endoscopic diagnosis of gastric polyps. Endoscopy 1995;27:32–7.

78. Schmitz JM, Stolte M. Gastric polyps as precancerous lesions. Gastrointest Endosc Clin N Am 1997;7:1–18.

79. Giardello FM, Trimbath JD. Peutz–Jeghers syndrome and management recommendations. Clin Gastroenterol Hepatol 2006;4:408–15.

80. Choudhry U, Boyce HW, Coppola D. Proton pump inhibitor–associated gastric polyps: a retrospective analysis of their frequency and endoscopic, histologic, and ultrastructural characteristics. Am J Clin Pathol 1998;110:615–21.

81. Driman DK, Wright C, Tougas G, Riddell RH. Omeprazole produces parietal cell hypertrophy and hyperplasia in humans. Dig Dis Sci 1996;41:2039–47.

82. Abraham SC, Park SJ, Mugartegui L, Hamilton SR, Wu TT. Sporadic fundic gland polyps with epithelial dysplasia: evidence for preferential targeting for mutations in the adenomatous polyposis coli gene. Am J Pathol 2002;161:1735–42.

83. Jalving M, Koornstra JJ, Wesseling J, Boezen HM, DE Jong S, Kleibeuker JH. Increased risk of fundic gland polyps during long-term proton pump inhibitor therapy. Aliment Pharmacol Ther 2006;24:1341–8.

84. Bertoni G, Sassatelli R, Nigrisoli E, Pennazio M, Tansini P, Arrigoni A, et al. Dysplastic changes in gastric fundic gland polyps of patients with familial adenomatous polyposis. Ital J Gastroenterol Hepatol 1999;31:192–7.

85. Wu TT, Kornacki S, Rashid A, Yardley JH, Hamilton SR. Dysplasia and dysregulation of proliferation in foveolar and surface epithelia of fundic gland polyps from patients with familial adenomatous polyposis. Am J Surg Pathol 1998;22:293–8.

86. Hizawa K, Fuchigami T, Iida M, Aoyagi K, Iwashita A, Daimaru Y, et al. Possible neoplastic transformation within gastric hyperplastic polyp: application of endoscopic polypectomy. Surg Endosc 1995;9:714–8.

87. Zea-Iriarte WL, Sekine I, Itsuno M, Makiyama K, Naito S, Nakayama T, et al. Carcinoma in gastric hyperplastic polyps. A phenotypic study. Dig Dis Sci 1996;41:377–86.

88. Park YS, Park SW, Kim TI, Song SY, Choi EH, Chung JB, et al. Endoscopic enucleation of upper-GI submucosal tumors by using an insulated-tip electrosurgical knife. Gastrointest Endosc 2004;59:409–15.

89. Miettinen M, Lasota J. Gastrointestinal stromal tumors—definition, clinical, histological, immunohistochemical, and molecular genetic features and differential diagnosis. Virchows Arch 2001;438:1–12.

90. Hwang JH, Rulyak SD, Kimmey MB. American Gastroenterological Association Institute technical review on the management of gastric subepithelial masses. Gastroenterology 2006;130:217–28.

91. Japanese Gastric Cancer Association. Japanese classification of gastric carcinoma – 2nd English edition. Gastric Cancer 1998;1:10–24.

92. Japanese Gastric Cancer Association. Japanese classification of gastric carcinoma [in Japanese]. 13th ed. Tokyo: Kanehara; 1998.

93. Everett SM, Axon ATR. Early gastric cancer in Europe. Gut 1997;41:142–50.

94. Everett SM, Axon ATR. Early gastric cancer: disease or pseudo-disease? Lancet 1998;351:1350–2.

95. Lambert R. Mass screening programs in Japan: what can we learn in the West? Endoscopy 1998;30:721–3.

96. [No authors listed.] The Paris endoscopic classification of superficial neoplastic lesions: esophagus, stomach, and colon: November 30 to December 1, 2002. Gastrointest Endosc 2003;58(6 Suppl):S 3–43.

97. Honmyo U, Misumi A, Murakami A, Mizumoto S, Yoshinaka I, Maeda M, et al. Mechanisms producing color change in flat early gastric cancers. Endoscopy 1997;29:366–71.

98. Sakita T, Oguro Y, Takasu S, Fukutomi H, Miwa T. Observations on the healing of ulcerations in early gastric cancer. The life cycle of the malignant ulcer. Gastroenterology 1971;60:835–9.

99. Dekker W, Tytgat GN. Diagnostic accuracy of fiberendoscopy in the detection of upper intestinal malignancy: a follow-up analysis. Gastroenterology 1977;73:710–4.

100. Yanai H, Noguchi T, Mizumachi S, Tokiyama H, Nakamura H, Tada M, et al. A blind comparison of the effectiveness of endoscopic ultrasonography and endoscopy in staging early gastric cancer. Gut 1999;44:361–5.

101. Chonan A, Mochizuki F, Ando M, Atsumi M, Mishima T, Fujita N, et al. Endoscopic mucosal resection (EMR) of early gastric cancer: usefulness of aspiration EMR using a cap-fitted scope. Dig Endosc 1998;10:31–6.

102. Noda M, Kodama T, Atsumi M, Nakajima M, Sawai N, Kashima K, et al. Possibilities and limitations of endoscopic resection for early gastric cancer. Endoscopy 1997;29:361–5.

103. Inoue H, Tani M, Nagai K, Kawano T, Takeshita K, Endo M, et al. Treatment of esophageal and gastric tumors. Endoscopy 1999;31:47–55.

104. Soehendra N, Binmoeller KF, Bohnacker S, Seitz U, Brand B, Thonke F, et al. Endoscopic snare mucosectomy in the esophagus without any additional equipment: a simple technique for resection of flat early cancer. Endoscopy 1997;29:380–3.

105. Kojima T, Parra-Blanco A, Takahashi H, Fujita R. Outcome of endoscopic mucosal resection for early gastric cancer: review of the Japanese literature. Gastrointest Endosc 1998;48:550–3.

106. Tani M, Takeshita K, Kawano T. Characteristics and role of endoscopic mucosal resection using cap-fitted panendoscope for early gastric cancer. Dig Endosc 2005;17:17–20.

107. Soetikno R, Kaltenbach T, Yeh R, Gotoda T. Endoscopic mucosal resection for early cancers of the upper gastrointestinal tract. J Clin Oncol 2005;23:4490–8.

108. Oda I, Gotoda T, Hamanaka H, Eguchi T, Saito Y, Matsuda T, et al. Endoscopic submucosal dissection for early gastric cancer: technical feasibility,

43

operation time and complications from a large consecutive series. Dig Endosc 2005;17:54–8.

109. Yokoi C, Gotoda T, Hamanak H, Oda I. Endoscopic submucosal dissection allows durative resection of locally recurrent early gastric cancer after prior endoscopic mucosal resection. Gastrointest Endosc 2006;64:212–8.

110. Watanabe K, Ogata S, Kawazoe S, Watanabe K, Koyama T, Kajiwara T, et al. Clinical outcomes of EMR for gastric tumors: historical pilot evaluation between endoscopic submucosal dissection and conventional resection. Gastrointest Endosc 2006;63:776–82.

111. Takeuchi Y, Uedo N, Iishi H, Yamamoto S, Yamamoto S, Yamada T, et al. Endscopic submucosal dissection with insulated-tip knife for large mucosal early gastric cancer: a feasibility study (with videos). Gastrointest Endosc 2007;66:186–93.

112. Offerhaus GJ, Tersmette AC, Huibregtse K, van de Stadt J, Tersmette KW, Stijnen T, et al. Mortality caused by stomach cancer after remote partial gastrectomy for benign conditions: 40 years of follow up of an Amsterdam cohort of 2633 postgastrectomy patients. Gut 1988;29:1588–90.

113. Antonioli DA. Precursors of gastric carcinoma: a critical review with a brief description of early (curable) gastric cancer. Hum Pathol 1994;25:994–1005.

114. Borrmann R. Das Wachstum und die Verbreitungswege des Magencarcinoms vom anatomischen und klinischen Standpunkt. Jena: Fischer, 1911 (Supplementband zu Mitteilungen aus den Grenzgebieten der Medizin und Chirurgie).

115. Greene FL, Page DL, Fleming ID, Fritz A, Balch CM, Haller DG, et al. AJCC cancer staging manual. American Joint Committee on Cancer. 6th ed. New York: Springer, 2002.

116. Bayerdörffer E, Neubauer A, Rudolph B, Thiede C, Lehn N, Eidt S, et al. Regression of primary gastric lymphoma of mucosa-associated lymphoid tissue type after cure of *Helicobacter pylori* infection. Lancet 1995;345:1591–4.

117. Sackmann M, Morgner A, Rudolph B, Neubauer A, Thiede C, Schulz H, et al. Regression of gastric MALT lymphoma after eradication of *Helicobacter pylori* is predicted by endosonographic staging. Gastroenterology 1997;113:1087–90.

118. Bayerdörffer E, Miehlke S, Neubauer A, Stolte M. Gastric MALT-lymphoma and *Helicobacter pylori* infection. Aliment Pharmacol Ther 1997;11 (Suppl 1):89–94.

119. Taal BG, den Hartog Jager FCA, Tytgat GNJ. The endoscopic spectrum of primary non-Hodgkin's lymphoma of the stomach. Endoscopy 1987;19:190–2.

120. Taal BG, Boot H, van Heerde P, de Jong D, Hart AAM, Burgers JMV. Primary non-Hodgkin's lymphoma of the stomach: endoscopic pattern and prognosis in low versus high grade malignancy in relation to the MALT concept. Gut 1996;34:556–61.

121. Taal BG, den Hartog Jager FCA, Steinmetz R, Peterse H. The spectrum of gastrointestinal metastases of breast carcinoma, 1: stomach. Gastrointest Endosc 1992;38:130–5.

122. Delpre G, Glanz I, Neeman A, Avidor I, Kadish U. New therapeutic approach in postoperative phytobezoars. J Clin Gastroenterol 1984;6:231–7.

123. Offerhaus GJA, Stadt J, Huibregtse K, Tytgat GNJ. Endoscopic screening for malignancy in the gastric remnant: the clinical significance of dysplasia in gastric mucosa. J Clin Pathol 1984;37:748–54.

124. Pickford IR, Craven JL, Hail R, Thomas G, Stone WD. Endoscopic examination of the gastric remnant 31–39 years after subtotal gastrectomy for peptic ulcer. Gut 1984;25:393–7.

125. Elders KA, Wolfe BM. Bariatric surgery: a review of procedures and outcomes. Gastroenterology 2007;132:2253–71.

126. Weber J, Azagra-Goergen M, Strock P, Azagra J. Endoscopy after bariatric surgery. Acta Endosc 2007;37:27–37.

VI

44 Duodenal and Small-Intestinal Diseases

Blair S. Lewis

Diseases of the small intestine have been divided into several categories here, to make it easier for readers to absorb and organize the information. The categories are listed in **Table 44.1**. Another way of looking at the pathologies involved is in relation to bleeding—a common presentation (**Table 44.2**).

Small-Bowel Tumors

Small-bowel tumors account for only 5% of all gastrointestinal tract tumors [1]. Approximately 60% of these tumors are benign. In 1995, 4600 new cases of small-intestinal cancer were reported, along with 1120 deaths [2]. Certain illnesses increase the risk of developing small-bowel malignancy. Celiac disease increases the risk of both adenocarcinoma and lymphoma. Crohn's disease increases the risk of developing adenocarcinoma, as does familial polyposis and Peutz– Jeghers syndrome. Human immunodeficiency virus (HIV) infection increases the risk of small-bowel lymphoma and Kaposi's sarcoma.

Tumors of the small bowel, both benign and malignant, classically present with symptoms of pain, bleeding, and weight loss. On examination, patients often have signs of obstruction or a palpable mass. Before the advent of enteroscopy, computed-tomographic enterography, and capsule endoscopy, presentation and diagnosis were usually late. The tumors are typically missed with most standard radiographic tests, and the prognosis consequently used to be dismal. In 1980, Herbsman et al. reported that survival for more than 6 months after a diagnosis of adenocarcinoma of the small bowel was rare [3]. In 2006, 5420 new cases were reported, along with 1070 deaths [4]. It has been shown that early diagnosis improves survival. In a study including 71 patients treated for obscure gastrointestinal bleeding, Szold et al. reported 19 patients with tumors detected early using enteroscopy [5]. In this series, 13 patients were long-term survivors and six died of metastatic disease. In a retrospective review of 144 patients with primary cancer of the small intestine, the overall 5-year survival was 57% and the median survival was 52 months [6]. Not surprisingly, survival was best with early-stage tumors and those that could be completely resected.

Failure to diagnose tumors at an early stage is the result of two major factors. The first reason is that physicians fail to consider tumors as a source of a patient's symptoms. Tumors typically present with vague early symptoms, and there is an absence of physical findings. Anemia is present in 88% of patients. Since bleeding is often the sole symptom when a tumor initially presents, the diagnosis is overlooked. Gross bleeding is the presenting symptom in 25–53% of patients with small-bowel tumors. Tumors are the second most common cause of small-intestinal hemorrhage after vascular lesions [1,7] and account for 5–10% of all cases of small-intestinal hemorrhage [8,9]. The patients are generally younger than those with angiectasias of the small bowel, with an average age of 51 compared to 69 [10]. In 1987, Thompson et al. reported on 37 patients with obscure gastrointestinal bleeding [11]. Fifteen of the patients were younger than 50 years of age, and a small-bowel tumor was identified as the culprit lesion in all but one. This finding led the authors to advocate early surgery in young patients with obscure bleeding. Berner et al. reported another series also suggest-

Table 44.1 Diseases of the Small Intestine

Tumors
Stromal tumors
Adenomas and adenocarcinoma
Inflammatory polyps
Lipomas
Carcinoid
Lymphoma
Kaposi's sarcoma
Metastatic disease
Ulcerative/erosive diseases
Crohn's disease
Zollinger–Ellison syndrome
Infections
Medication effects
Vasculitis
Radiation injury
Ischemia
Graft-versus-host disease
Congenital lesions
Diverticula
Meckel's diverticula
Duplication cysts
Vascular lesions
Angiectasia
Venous ectasias
Telangiectasias
Hemangiomas
Arteriovenous malformations
Malabsorption
Celiac disease
Whipple's disease
Amyloid

ing that small-bowel tumors must be searched for in younger patients [12]. The average age of patients with a tumor was 51. Although angiectasias were present in all age groups, they were more common in elderly patients. In addition, young patients with small-bowel tumors tend to require fewer transfusions, presumably because they tolerate the anemia. It can therefore be suggested that tumors should be searched for in younger patients with obscure bleeding, even if the effect on the patient's quality of life seems mild. Lewis et al. reported gross bleeding as the presentation in 62% of 13 patients with small-bowel tumors, while 38% presented with occult blood in the stool [10]. According to Lewis et al., the type of bleeding—whether frank blood loss or occult blood in the stool—is not an effective means of differentiating between bleeding secondary to angiectasia and a small-bowel tumor [10]. Patients often go on to

Table 44.2 Obscure gastrointestinal bleeding: causes of small-bowel bleeding

Brisk bleeding	Occult bleeding
Angiectasia	Angiectasia
Leiomyoma/leiomyosarcoma	Adenocarcinoma
Jejunal diverticula	Lymphoma
Crohn's disease	Carcinoid
Aortoenteric fistula	Crohn's disease
Meckel's diverticulum	Zollinger–Ellison syndrome
Duplication cyst	Vasculitis
Hemangioma	Medications (e.g., nonsteroidal anti-inflammatory drugs, potassium, 6-mercaptopurine)
	Infectious causes
	Ulcerative jejunoileitis

develop symptoms as the disease progresses. The most frequent symptoms are abdominal pain, weight loss, nausea, vomiting, bleeding, jaundice and anorexia [13]. Patients present with pain 16% of the time and with intussusception 12% of the time. While benign lesions are more likely to cause pain with small-bowel obstruction and intussusception, malignant lesions tend to cause pain syndromes that are less specific for small-bowel pathology. Unfortunately, by the time they are diagnosed, most small-bowel malignancies have advanced beyond the early stage of neoplasm.

The second reason that tumors of the small bowel are not diagnosed early is that until recently the diagnostic modalities for investigating small-intestinal pathology were suboptimal. Due to the inaccessibility of the small bowel to conventional diagnostic modalities, the diagnosis and localization of small-bowel tumors was a clinical challenge. Small-bowel series were long regarded as being the mainstay in the evaluation of the small intestine. However, the data show a relatively low yield of positive findings for patients with occult bleeding or iron deficiency. It is estimated that only approximately 5% of small-bowel follow-through examinations detect an intestinal bleeding site. Rabe et al. reported a yield of 5.6% in a series of 215 small-bowel series performed for obscure bleeding [14]. Fried et al. made no diagnoses in 28 examinations [15]. Gordon et al. made diagnoses in three of 46 patients (6.5%) with iron-deficiency anemia who underwent small-bowel follow-through examinations [16]. These included one patient with a jejunal ulcer and two with an abnormal terminal ileum. Rockey and Cello evaluated 29 patients with iron-deficiency anemia and negative esophagogastroduodenoscopy and colonoscopy using enteroclysis in 26 and small-bowel series in three. No lesions were identified [17]. Noninvasive barium studies have a particularly low yield for diagnosing the source of obscure gastrointestinal bleeding. Although better than small-bowel series, enteroclysis is reported to have a yield of only 10–20% [18]. Bleeding scans and angiography, although superior to barium studies, require active bleeding at the time of testing. While computed tomography (CT) may be useful in diagnosing extraluminal and metastatic spread of small-bowel malignancies, its role in detecting small intraluminal and mucosal lesions is limited, with a diagnostic yield as low as 20% [19].

The two most effective imaging modalities are capsule endoscopy and CT enterography. Capsule endoscopy is a relatively new tool for investigating the small bowel [20]. It is already recognized as the state-of-the-art method for examining the small bowel, and it is clear that capsule endoscopy allows early diagnosis of tumors when all other modalities have failed. The first study describing the diagnosis of small-bowel tumors using capsule endoscopy, including 130 patients, reported a 3.8% rate of primary tumors [21]. In describing the five cases of small-bowel tumor detected, the authors concluded that the accuracy of capsule endoscopy in diagnosing the tumors appeared to be superior to that of other methods. Several case reports have also attested to the ability of capsule endoscopy to diagnose tumors [22–25]. Cobrin et al. reported that the prevalence of small-bowel tumors may be higher than was predicted in the pre–capsule endoscopy era [26]. Their data suggest that 9% of obscure gastrointestinal bleeding is due to small-bowel tumors. The calculated number of capsule studies needed to diagnose a small-bowel tumor in a patient with obscure gastrointestinal bleeding was 12. A pooled analysis of 24 studies included a total of 530 patients, 310 of whom had obscure gastrointestinal bleeding [27]. The patients had undergone an average of 7.4 diagnostic tests before being diagnosed. Eighty-six of the 1349 pathologies identified at capsule endoscopy (6.4%) were intestinal neoplasms. Another pooled analysis, including only patients with tumors diagnosed by capsule endoscopy, was reported by Schwartz and Barkin [28]. Eighty-nine tumors were identified, including 87 small-bowel tumors, one cecal cancer, and one gastric tumor. The patients underwent an average of 4.6 negative examinations before the diagnosis was made using capsule endoscopy. The other evaluations conducted included 40 small-bowel series, 24 CT scans, 26 push enteroscopies, 16 enteroclyses, and six angiographies. Malignant tumors represented 61% of the lesions identified. Capsule endoscopy has also been used to evaluate patients with polyposis syndromes, including familial polyposis and Peutz–Jeghers syndrome [29–31]. Again, capsule endoscopy appears to be superior to small-bowel series and magnetic resonance enterography for detecting these lesions.

Multidetector CT scanning provides high-resolution cross-sectional imaging of the abdomen and the small bowel. It allows identification of small-bowel tumors and can demonstrate signs of small-bowel obstruction, as well as the mural and extramural extent of small-bowel malignancies. This aids planning for surgical resection. In addition, liver metastases or peritoneal seeding can be detected with CT [32].

Obscure bleeding, a common indication for capsule endoscopy, is also a common sign of a small-bowel tumor. In the report by Martin et al. of 25 small-bowel tumors, 88% presented with anemia as the primary symptom, while weight loss was seen in only 28%, abdominal pain in 16%, and intussusception in 12% [8]. Tumors are the second most common cause of small-bowel bleeding, ranked behind small intestinal vascular lesions. It is estimated that small-bowel tumors account for 5–10% of all cases of small intestinal hemorrhage and approximately 0.3% of all cases of gastrointestinal bleeding. As shown by the data presented by Martin et al., bleeding and resultant anemia are the presenting symptoms in the majority of patients with small-bowel tumors [8]. Frank bleeding is most common, with either melena or maroon blood per rectum. Lewis et al. reported this presentation in 62% of 13 patients with small-bowel tumors, while 38% presented with occult blood in the stool [10]. According to Lewis et al., the type of bleeding—whether frank blood loss or occult blood in the stool—is not an effective means of differentiating between bleeding secondary to angiectasia and a small-bowel tumor [10].

There are several different types of tumor of the small intestine (**Table 44.3**) [1]. These pathologies are located in different areas of the small intestine. Some distal locations may make diagnosis difficult. In addition, many small-bowel tumors are submucosal, making diagnosis on the basis of the gross appearance difficult. Furthermore, endoscopic biopsy via the enteroscope frequently will not yield diagnostic tissue samples from submucosal lesions. The endoscopist may only be able to state that a tumor is present. Submucosal tumors include leiomyomas, carcinoids, lipomas, and metastatic disease. Typically, the endoscopist identifies a tumor as submucosal by the presence of normal overlying mucosa and the presence of a vascular pattern across the tumor (**Fig. 44.1**). Visualization of bridging folds across the tumor may also be useful in diagnosing a submucosal mass. Correct identification of abnormalities on capsule endoscopy is not an easy task. Unlike standard endoscopy, the capsule reader has to diagnose disease states on the basis of a few images alone. The lesion identified cannot be palpated with a biopsy forceps, biopsies cannot be obtained, and a variety of views are often not available. In addition, the images obtained at capsule endoscopy differ from those in traditional endoscopy, as there is no air distension of the bowel wall and the capsule is at times located within millimeters of the mucosa. The procedure thus provides a kind of "physiologic endoscopy" in which the bowel is not altered by the examination process [33].

Correct diagnosis of a submucosal lesion can be particularly difficult, as a bulge may mimic such lesions. Bulges are indentations into the small-bowel wall created by another loop of bowel overlying the loop being inspected. There are visual cues that make it possible to distinguish between a bulge and a true mass. Most importantly, the stream of video images needs to be reviewed, rather than simply relying on a single image. Bulges from adjacent loops of bowel will show peristaltic movement. Peristalsis through the area confirms that the lesion in question is not solid and is therefore not truly a mass. In addition, inspecting the overlying mucosa can provide clues for differentiating a mass from a bulge. Bulges will have a normal villous pattern over the surface, while most submucosal masses will have stretched the mucosa, making it look thin and translucent (**Figs. 44.1, 44.2**). A mass lesion can also change the color of the mucosa, since when it is stretched the underlying whiteness or grayness of the mass may be apparent [34]. The presence of "bridging folds"—valvulae conniventes that stop at the edge of the mass edge and re-form on the other side—suggests a submucosal process. Simple bulges would not make intestinal folds disappear.

At the International Conference on Capsule Endoscopy (Miami and Paris, 2006), a consensus group proposed using a series of endoscopic features in an attempt to improve the diagnosis of tumors at capsule endoscopy. These are listed in **Table 44.4** [35]. They were divided into major and minor features and classified into high, intermediate, and low probabilities. Algorithms were developed depending on the probability of a tumor being present on the basis of these features. All patients should have cross-sectional imaging with CT, CT enterography, or magnetic resonance imaging (MRI) to assess for extraluminal involvement or metastatic disease. A patient with high or intermediate probability of a tumor should undergo either double-balloon enteroscopy or laparoscopy. With a low-probability lesion and if no abnormality is seen on CT, the further management depends on the clinician's assessment of the significance of the lesion.

Stromal Tumors

Stromal cell tumors were previously called leiomyomas and leiomyosarcomas. The term was changed due to the variation in the content of these tumors, which include more than smooth-muscle fibers. These tumors can be located throughout the small bowel and are the most common tumors that bleed. Bleeding, which may be brisk, occurs in these submucosal smooth-muscle tumors when there is central tumor necrosis and subsequent ulceration of the overlying mucosa (**Fig. 44.2**). Gradual, chronic blood loss is more commonly associated with other small-bowel tumors, including carcinoid, adenocarcinomas, and lymphomas. Leiomyomas can vary in size and the endoscopic appearance does not predict the extent of the extramucosal component. The diagnosis of a gastro-intestinal stromal tumor (GIST) is made pathologically along with staining for expression of *KIT*, a gene that codes for tyrosine kinase [36]. The prognosis is determined on the basis of the National Institutes of Health (NIH) consensus classification system, which

Table 44.3 Small-bowel tumors: prevalence by site [1]

Site, type	%
Duodenum (n = 310)	
Carcinoma	72
Carcinoid	15
Sarcoma	8
Lymphoma	5
Jejunum (n = 447)	
Carcinoma	54
Sarcoma	23
Lymphoma	16
Carcinoid	7
Ileum (n = 808)	
Carcinoid	44
Carcinoma	22
Lymphoma	21
Sarcoma	13

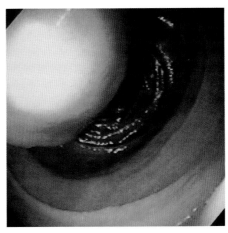

Fig. 44.1 Biopsies of this jejunal mass revealed normal mucosa. A stromal cell tumor was discovered at surgery.

44

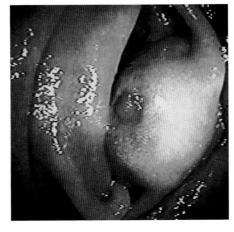

Fig. 44.2 Central ulceration of a stromal cell tumor is commonly seen.

uses tumor size and mitotic count. This, along with the presence of tumor rupture, can help predict tumor recurrence [37].

Adenoma and Adenocarcinoma

Adenomatous polyps and adenocarcinomas are most frequently found in the proximal bowel, with 90% of lesions located in the duodenum and the first 20 cm of the jejunum. Tubular, tubulovil-

Table 44.4 Classification of mass lesions seen on capsule endoscopy (based on Mergener et al. [35]).

Probability of tumor	Major					Minor		
	Bleeding	Mucosal disruption	Irregular surface	Polypoid appearance	Color	Delayed passage (≥ 30 min)	White villi	Invagination
High	++	++	++	++	++	++	++	++
Intermediate	+ / –	+	+	+	+			
Low	–	–	–	+ / –	–	–	–	–

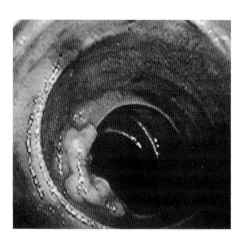

Fig. 44.3   A solitary tubular adenoma of the proximal jejunum.

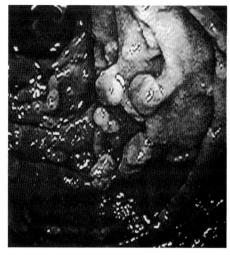

Fig. 44.4   Multiple duodenal polyps in a patient with Gardner's syndrome.

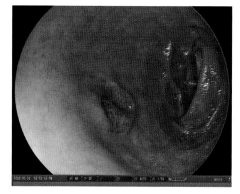

Fig. 44.5   Duodenal cancer in the anterior wall of the duodenal bulb (white/light image).

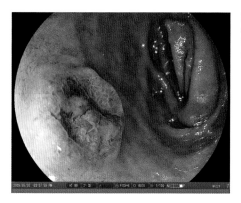

Fig. 44.6   Duodenal cancer at low magnification, with surface structures enhanced by FICE.

lous, and villous adenomas are seen (**Fig. 44.3**). These lesions are generally identified within reach of push enteroscopy. Endoscopic biopsy is recommended, and polypectomy is readily accomplished even with flat lesions. One helpful guideline for therapy in the small bowel is to consider it similar to therapies delivered in the cecum. Both organs are thin-walled and perforate more easily than other areas of the gastrointestinal tract. Adenomas of the small bowel are associated with familial polyposis and Gardner's syndrome. Polyps may be multiple (**Fig. 44.4**) or superficially spreading. Up to 90% of patients with these diseases will have adenomas of the duodenum (**Fig. 44.5**, **Fig. 44.6**) [38]. Periampullary adenomas and adenocarcinomas are most typical in Gardner's syndrome. Most authors suggest surveillance of these patients with a combination of push enteroscopy and duodenoscopy using a side-viewing endoscope [39]. Small-intestinal adenocarcinoma is also more common in patients with small-intestinal Crohn's disease, as well as in patients with celiac disease.

Adenocarcinoma of the small bowel is often circumferential and quite exophytic. It has an apple-core appearance, similar to cancers in the colon. If a cancer is seen in the duodenum, the differential diagnosis should also include invasive pancreatic cancer (**Fig. 44.8**). Due to the liquid nature of food in the small bowel, cancers are typically quite advanced before the development of obstructive symptoms. This late diagnosis contributes to the relatively poor outcomes in these patients, with 5-year survival rates of less than 25%.

Nonneoplastic Polyps

Hyperplastic and hamartomatous polyps can occur in the small bowel. These tend to be pedunculated—in marked contrast to adenomatous polyps in the small bowel, which tend to be sessile. These polyps can occur de novo, or can be associated with a polyposis syndrome such as Peutz–Jeghers (**Fig. 44.9**). Endoscopic polypectomy of these pedunculated lesions is readily accomplished.

Lipomas

Lipomas of the small bowel are also seen. Typically, these polyps are yellow in color and are quite soft and pliable on manipulation with the biopsy forceps (**Fig. 44.10**). When the tip of the forceps is pushed into the body of a lipomatous polyp, the lipoma is easily "indented—the so-called "pillow sign." Lipomas are usually asymptomatic unless they grow to a large size. Lipomas are the most common cause of intussusception among adults, and they may also ulcerate and cause bleeding (**Fig. 44.11**). Endoscopic polypectomy is not performed in these patients, due to the high risk of perforation or snare entrapment within the fatty tissue.

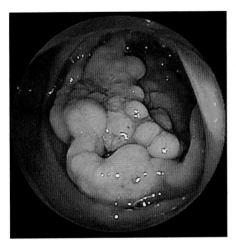

Fig. 44.7 Follicular lymphoma in the jejunum. Multiple whitish nodules aggregated in the proximal jejunum.

▥ Carcinoid

Next to the appendix, the small intestine is the most common location for carcinoid tumors, and they tend to be located distally in the small bowel, with the ileum being the most common location. Size of the lesions is an important predictor of metastatic spread; lesions less than 1 cm in size are uncommonly associated with metastatic disease. Carcinoid tumors appear as small submucosal nodules, which are often umbilicated. As these tumors grow in size, ulceration may occur, with the potential for bleeding.

▥ Lymphoma

Primary lymphoma of the small bowel is generally a discrete tumor in the United States and developed countries, and tends to involve the distal jejunum or ileum (**Fig. 44.7**). Primary lymphoma of the

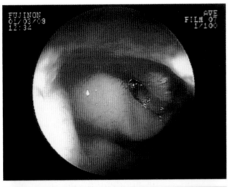
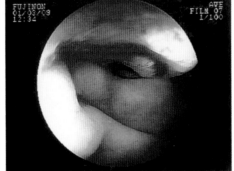
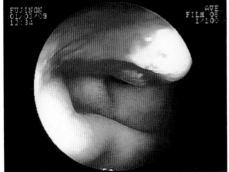
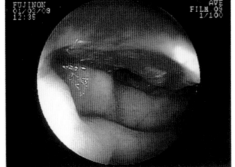

Fig. 44.8 Pancreatic cancer infiltrating and stricturing the duodenal lumen. Bleeding. Diagnosis by biopsy from the lesion.

44

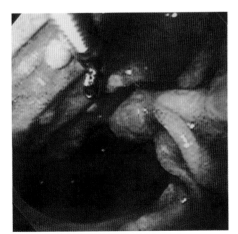
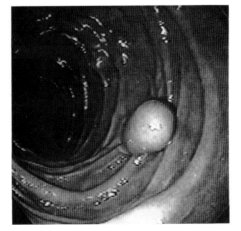
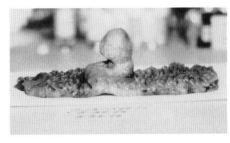

Fig. 44.9 Jejunal polyps in a patient with Peutz–Jeghers syndrome.

Fig. 44.10 A lipoma of the jejunum.

Fig. 44.11 Surgical specimen of a large lipoma that ulcerated and led to internal bleeding.

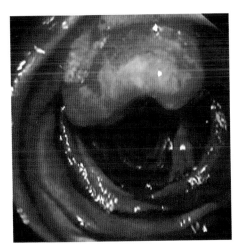

Fig. 44.12 A renal cell carcinoma metastatic to the jejunum.

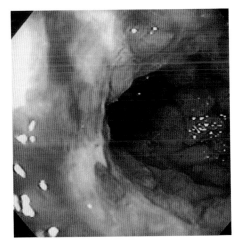

Fig. 44.13 An area of jejunal Crohn's disease is clearly identified, with ulceration and cobblestoning.

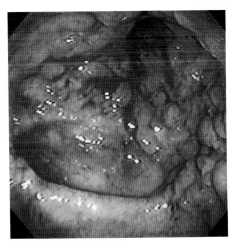

Fig. 44.14 An area of cobblestoning in the distal jejunum. Stricture can be seen in the distance.

small bowel is uncommon and may be associated with celiac disease or HIV infection. Celiac disease is associated with T cell lymphomas, while HIV-associated lymphomas are generally B cell lymphomas, which almost always present in extranodal sites and involve the gastrointestinal tract in approximately 25% or more of cases. Most primary small-bowel lymphomas not associated with celiac disease are B cell lymphomas and have been termed mucosa-associated lymphoid tissue (MALT) lymphomas.

In developing countries, a diffuse primary small-intestinal lymphoma known as immunoproliferative small-intestinal disease (IPSID) occurs. This disease is also known by other terms such as Mediterranean lymphoma or α-chain disease. It is characterized by an intense infiltration of the lamina propria with lymphocytes and plasma cells, and extensive follicular lymphoid hyperplasia. Over a number of years, frank lymphoma can develop. Infection is thought to play an important role in the development of IPSID, and the disease is reversible if treated with antibiotics (tetracycline) in its early stages.

Lymphomas can have several different appearances. A classification of these appearances has been developed and includes a nodular pattern, an infiltrative pattern, and an ulcerating pattern [40]. Halphen et al., in a review of 120 patients with primary small-bowel lymphoma, found that the infiltrative pattern, in which the mucosa is firm and motionless, is most indicative of lymphoma [41]. The other patterns may be mimicked by celiac disease and radiation enteritis, among others. While only limited, discrete regions of the small intestine are generally involved in primary small-intestinal lymphoma, the involved area is extensive in IPSID.

Kaposi's Sarcoma

Kaposi's sarcoma also may involve any part of the small intestine. These lesions are generally asymptomatic. As they enlarge, ulceration may occur, leading to gastrointestinal bleeding. Large lesions also have the potential to cause obstruction or intussusception.

Metastatic Disease

Metastatic disease can also migrate to the small bowel. Melanoma, breast cancer, and lung cancer are the most common lesions metastasizing to the small intestine [42]. Metastases may present clinically with bleeding (from ulceration), intussusception, or rarely obstruction. Metastatic melanoma can often be suspected on the

basis of its pigmented nature. Pigmentation is not necessary, however, and amelanotic melanoma may be seen. Often, the typical bull's-eye appearance seen in the stomach is not observed in the small bowel. Other tumors that migrate to the small bowel include colon cancer, renal cell cancer, osteogenic sarcoma, Merkel's cell carcinoma of the skin, and germ cell cancers (**Fig. 44.12**). As mentioned above, pancreatic cancer can directly invade the duodenum and present with bleeding or obstruction.

Ulcerative and Erosive Diseases of the Small Bowel

Crohn's Disease

Ulcerative and erosive diseases in the small intestine are another group of entities that cause small-bowel bleeding. In this category, Crohn's disease is the most common. Gross bleeding is unusual in Crohn's disease, occurring in 4–10% of patients with ileitis [43–45]. Transmural inflammation, the pathologic hallmark of the disease, can lead to erosion of large submucosal vessels, causing massive bleeding. These episodes are usually self-limited and do not recur [26]. Bleeding is not usually the sole symptom in these patients, since most also have the more common symptoms of Crohn's disease such as diarrhea and abdominal pain [26]. The diagnosis is virtually always made on small-bowel radiography series. The typical findings on barium studies can also be observed endoscopically. Ulceration, stricture formation, and fistulization can be identified (**Fig. 44.13**). Cobblestoning, a pattern of raised nodules, can also be readily identified endoscopically (**Fig. 44.14**). Linear ulcers may be seen outlining the nodules, but are not required for an endoscopic diagnosis of cobblestoning.

Zollinger–Ellison Syndrome

Zollinger–Ellison syndrome (gastrinoma) can also cause small-bowel ulcerations. Postbulbar ulcerations occur in gastrinomas, with ulcers described not only in the second portion of the duodenum, but also in the third and fourth portions and in the jejunum. It has been reported that postbulbar ulcerations in the duodenum occur in 14%, and jejunal ulcers occur in 11%. of patients with Zollinger–Ellison syndrome [46].

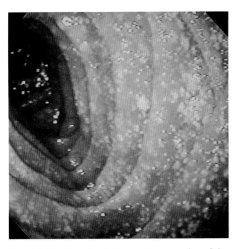

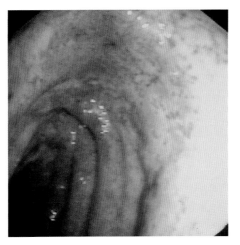

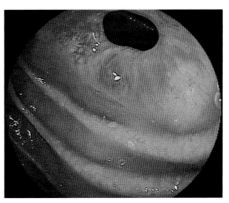

Fig. 44.15 *Mycobacterium avium* complex of the jejunum.

Fig. 44.16 *Strongyloides* infection of the duodenum, leading to mucosal edema and malabsorption.

Fig. 44.17 Jejunal stricture due to NSAIDs use in a 47-year-old woman with rheumatoid arthritis. The stricture with a 5 mm opening can be seen at the duodenojejunal junction.

The duodenum is the most common extrapancreatic site of gastrinomas. These may be identified with endoscopy or endoscopic ultrasound, or both, although intraoperative endoscopic transillumination appears to be the most sensitive technique for diagnosing duodenal gastrinomas.

Infections

Small-bowel infections with mycobacteria, syphilis, typhoid, and histoplasmosis can cause ulcerations and bleeding. Tuberculosis typically involves the distal ileum, although isolated involvement of the duodenum and jejunum have been described [47]. Other abnormalities in the small bowel apart from ulceration include obstruction secondary to enlarged lymph nodes, and fistulization.

Mycobacterium avium complex (MAC) infection occurs in the small intestine in patients with HIV disease. MAC typically presents with weight loss, fever, diarrhea, and abdominal pain. The duodenum is most commonly involved, in up to 88% of cases [48]. Endoscopically, MAC and *M. tuberculosis* infection can be suspected by the presence of tiny, punctate white nodules or exudate (**Fig. 44.15**). Both illnesses can cause ulcers, bleeding, diarrhea, and malabsorption. The histology results with small-intestinal endoscopic biopsies may be confused with the findings in Whipple's disease. Foamy macrophages can be seen in both MAC and Whipple's disease [49].

Strongyloides infections can cause upper gastrointestinal symptoms as well as malabsorption due to the marked edema of the bowel (**Fig. 44.16**). *Strongyloides* hyperinfection is a multiorgan system disease that occurs in patients with decreased cell-mediated immunity (e.g., transplants, steroid therapy, and hematologic malignancies). This can also lead to bowel involvement and may cause severe gastrointestinal symptoms.

Medication Effects

Medications such as potassium, nonsteroidal anti-inflammatory drugs (NSAIDs) and 6-mercaptopurine can also cause small-bowel ulcerations and bleeding. The mechanism of injury by potassium appears to be secondary to its effect on the mesenteric circulation. In high doses, potassium decreases mesenteric blood flow, and stenosing ulcers of the small intestine have been found to have the pathologic features of ischemic injury [50].

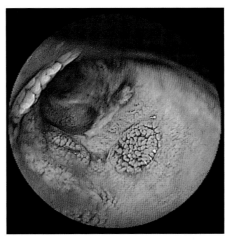

Fig. 44.18 Jejunal stricture after endoscopic balloon dilation up to 1500 mm using double-balloon enteroscopy (same patient as **Fig. 44.17**).

44

NSAIDs can cause ulcerations and erosions throughout the small bowel and may account for unexplained blood loss in patients without lesions identified in the upper gastrointestinal tract. Sonde enteroscopy was used to evaluate chronic occult bleeding in 15 patients receiving NSAIDs who had nondiagnostic upper endoscopies and colonoscopies; it was found that 47% of the patients had ulcerations or erosions in the jejunum or ileum [51]. A subsequent study showed that misoprostol therapy was associated with an improvement in the anemia in this group of patients with proven NSAID enteropathy [52]. In addition, long-term NSAID use has been associated with the development of multiple small-bowel strictures [53] (**Figs. 44.17, 44.18**). These strictures are thin diaphragms associated with inflammation and submucosal fibrosis.

Vasculitis

Vasculitis can affect the bowel in several different ways [54]. A patient's presentation depends on the size of the vessels involved. While large artery vasculitis such as giant cell arteritis, which may involve the aorta as well as medium-sized vessels, can lead to arterial occlusion and subsequent bowel gangrene and perforation, venulitis and obstruction of venous return leads to mucosal edema and malabsorption. Vasculitis of medium and small arteries (e.g., polyarteritis nodosa, Churg–Strauss disease) may cause gastrointes-

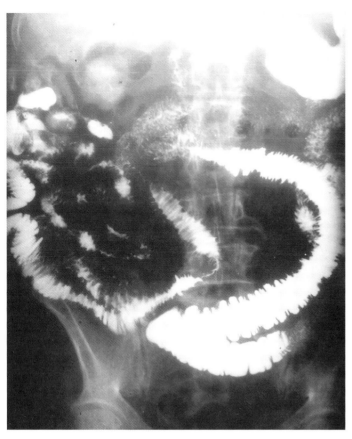

Fig. 44.19 A small-bowel series revealing stricturing and bowel wall separation, suggesting vasculitis in a patient with lupus erythematosus.

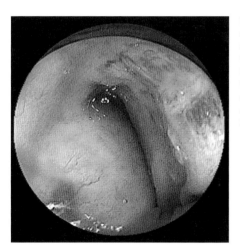

Fig. 44.20 Radiation enteritis and proctitis in a 50-year-old woman with hematochezia, 9 months after radiation therapy for cervical cancer. Radiation proctitis: A shallow ulcer with surrounding redness.

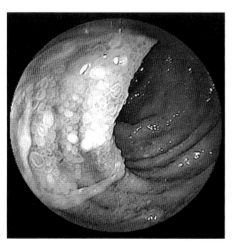

Fig. 44.21 Radiation enteritis seen in the same patient as **Fig. 44.20**. Inflamed mucosa of the ileum with shallow villi and bleeding.

tinal bleeding secondary to ischemia and subsequent ulceration (**Fig. 44.19**). Medium-sized arteries may also develop aneurysms, which can rupture and bleed massively, as seen in polyarteritis nodosa. Other necrotizing vasculitides of the bowel are seen in rheumatoid arthritis (though usually affecting the colon), systemic lupus erythematosus, Behçet disease, Wegener granulomatosis, and cryoglobulinemia. Vasculitis of small arteries, the vasa recta, or the intramural arterioles presents with pain, fever, and occult bleeding. Hypersensitivity vasculitis—a vasculitis usually affecting the small vessels in response to a specific antigen—is seen in Henoch–Schönlein purpura.

Radiation Injury

Radiation injury to the bowel can cause mucosal injury, ulceration, vascular injury with endothelial inflammation, and dilation of vessels (telangiectasias) (**Figs. 44.20, 44.21**). Diarrhea is a common manifestation, and bleeding may occur. Late injury usually occurs approximately 6–24 months after radiation treatment, as a consequence of vascular injury and progressive ischemia [55]. Injury rarely occurs with total doses of less than 30–40 Gy; greater amounts of radiation increase the risk of radiation injury, as do low-flow states of mesenteric circulation (such as congestive heart failure or vasoconstrictive drug therapy), previous abdominal surgery (which immobilizes bowel loops), and chemotherapy. Endoscopic findings include edema, friability, and hemorrhage; erosion or ulceration; and stricture of the small bowel. Fistulas and even perforation can also occur with progressive vascular occlusion.

Mesenteric Ischemia

Mesenteric ischemia may occur as a result of arterial embolus (e.g., atrial fibrillation) or arterial thrombosis (e.g., preexisting atherosclerotic lesions), or mesenteric venous thrombosis—either occlusive (e.g., hypercoagulable states) or nonocclusive, such as splanchnic vasoconstriction due to congestive failure, shock, or vasoconstrictive medications (e.g., digoxin). Endoscopic examination of the small intestine is virtually never employed in the evaluation of patients with suspected mesenteric ischemia. However, endoscopic findings would include the spectrum of changes due to ischemia—edematous, friable, and hemorrhagic mucosa, and erosions or ulcers (**Figs. 44.22, 44.24**). With increasing severity of ischemia, the bowel may appear cyanotic or bluish and may eventually develop a blue-black appearance. Relatively discrete segments of intestinal involvement are consistent with ischemic injury.

Graft-versus-Host Disease (GVHD)

With the increasing use of bone marrow transplantation, gastroenterologists are seeing more cases of GVHD. This illness occurs secondary to undetectable histocompatibility differences between donor and host, with infiltration of a variety of tissues by donor lymphocytes. Clinically, patients typically develop skin rash, diarrhea, and jaundice. On biopsy, an increased number of CD8 T cells are found in the intestinal mucosa. The intestinal mucosa can ulcerate or completely desquamate, leading to severe diarrhea, malabsorption, and bleeding (**Fig. 44.25**). GVHD occurs in up to 50% of bone marrow transplant patients and can contribute to mortality [56]. Treatment is directed at suppressing the immune response.

VI

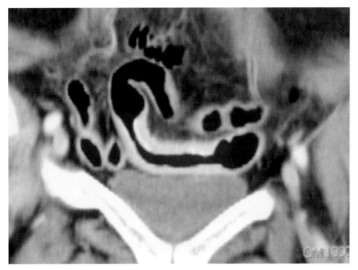

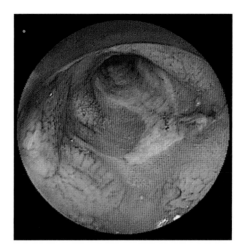

Fig. 44.22 Ischemic enteritis in a 73-year-old woman with atrial fibrillation. Clinical picture: Abdominal pain, nausea, and vomiting. CT detected a thickened ileal wall.

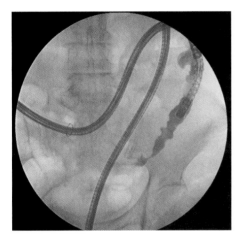

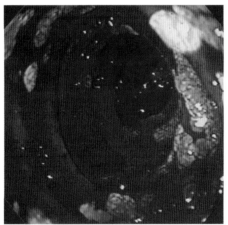

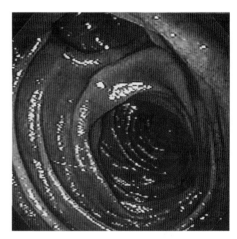

Fig. 44.24 Retrograde balloon enteroscopy with selective contrast radiography: Irregular narrowed segment of the ileum (same patient as **Fig. 44.22**).

Fig. 44.25 Severe graft-versus-host disease has led to desquamation of the jejunal mucosa.

Fig. 44.26 A jejunal diverticulum.

Congenital Lesions

▥ Diverticula and Duplication Cysts

Congenital duodenal diverticula are commonly identified on routine endoscopy. They are almost always asymptomatic and usually occur in the second portion of the duodenum, within 2 cm of the ampulla of Vater. Acquired duodenal diverticula may occur in the duodenal bulb in connection with peptic ulcer disease.

Jejunal diverticula can cause small-bowel bleeding and bacterial overgrowth. These are acquired pseudodiverticula that develop on the mesenteric border of the intestine at the site of perforating blood vessels. Jejunal diverticula, found in 1–2% of individuals in autopsy studies, are usually asymptomatic (**Fig. 44.26**). Jejunal diverticula most often present with symptoms of bacterial overgrowth such as diarrhea and abdominal bloating. It is estimated that less than 5% of those with jejunal diverticula actually bleed from them. When discovered on a small-bowel series, small-bowel diverticula should be considered incidental findings, since angio-graphic or radionuclide scanning evidence of active bleeding is necessary to conclude that the diverticula are the site of blood loss. When bleeding does occur from jejunal diverticula, it is often massive and can be associated with a mortality as high as 20%.

▥ Meckel's Diverticulum

Meckel's diverticulum is a remnant of the vitelline duct and is usually located within 100 cm of the ileocecal valve (**Fig. 44.27**). This anomaly occurs in 2% of the population and is more common in men than women. It is the cause of bleeding in two-thirds of men under the age of 30 presenting with small-bowel bleeding [57]. Bleeding is almost always brisk, resulting from ulceration in the diverticulum or the adjoining ileum secondary to acid production from ectopic gastric mucosa lining the diverticulum. Preoperative diagnosis is uncommon, although radionuclide scanning using ^{99m}Tc pertechnetate allows identification of the gastric mucosa (**Fig. 44.28**). Endoscopic diagnosis is rarely made. Ulceration in the

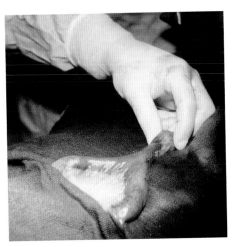

Fig. 44.27 A Meckel's diverticulum discovered at surgery.

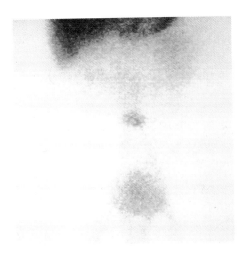

Fig. 44.28 A positive Meckel's scan.

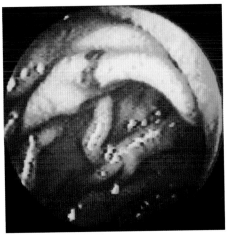

Fig. 44.29 Angiectasia in the jejunum.

Table 44.5 Classification of vascular anomalies [59]

I	Angiectasia (vascular ectasia)
	a Sporadic
	b Associated with renal failure
	c Associated with von Willebrand disease
	d Congestive gastropathy
	e Watermelon stomach
II	Venous ectasia
III	Telangiectasia
IV	Hemangiomas
V	Arteriovenous malformation
VI	Caliber-persistent artery (Dieulafoy lesion)

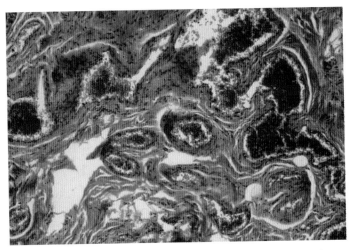

Fig. 44.30 A pathologic specimen, showing an angiectasia with its characteristic dilated capillaries.

adjacent ileal mucosa can lead to suspicion of a Meckel's diverticulum. Intussusception of the diverticulum can also be seen endoscopically.

Duplication Cysts

An intestinal duplication cyst can also be lined with ectopic gastric mucosa, leading to ulceration and bleeding. Unlike a Meckel's diverticulum, these congenital cysts may be located anywhere in the bowel.

Vascular Anomalies

Vascular anomalies are the most common cause of intestinal bleeding, accounting for 70–80% of cases [58]. Vascular lesions of the bowel are not all the same. Although most vascular lesions appear endoscopically similar and can be a cause of bleeding, they consist of various pathologic identities (**Table 44.5**) [38]. Lewis et al. reported on the yield of standard pathologic examinations when vascular lesions in the small intestine are identified endoscopically and then resected [59]. All lesions appeared similarly endoscopically (**Fig. 44.29**). The yield of routine pathologic examination was 57%. Pathologic examination of 14 patients' lesions revealed eight identifiable vascular lesions, including five angiectasias, one capillary hemangioma, one venous hemangioma, and one arteriovenous malformation (AVM). True angiectasias accounted for only 63% of identifiable lesions.

- *Angiectasias* are dilated vessels, including capillaries, and contain no dysplastic tissue [60] (**Fig. 44.30**). These lesions can be found throughout the bowel and appear to recur and develop with aging. They are thought to be the most common vascular lesion, and the term "angiectasia" is therefore typically applied to all small vascular lesions. The term used for these lesions has changed over the years, and the older term "angiodysplasia" has now been replaced by angiectasia, as pathologic examination of the lesions fails to show dysplasia, and "ectasia" is more descriptive.
- *Venous ectasias*, also called phlebectasias, differ from angiectasias and varices pathologically and clinically. These lesions consist of dilated submucosal veins, usually with thin overlying mucosa. These venous varicosities have a normal endothelial lining and are nonneoplastic. They are not associated with liver disease. Endoscopically, they appear as multiple bluish-red nodules and occur predominantly in the rectum and esophagus. Small-bowel lesions have been described [61]. Clinically they are an uncommon cause of bleeding and are usually asymptomatic.

- *Telangiectasias* differ from angiectasias in their diffuse nature, their known tendency to recur, and in having associated skin or mucous membrane lesions. Pathologically, these hereditary lesions have dilated blood vessels throughout the bowel wall, not just mucosally or submucosally as seen in angiectasias. Thinning of the arterial muscular layer is also considered specific for these lesions. Hereditary hemorrhagic telangiectasia (HHT) syndrome (Rendu–Osler–Weber syndrome) is the most common cause of intestinal telangiectasias. This illness is inherited as an autosomal-dominant condition. Initially, patients present with mucocutaneous lesions in the second and third decades of life, and epistaxis is the most common presenting symptom. Gastrointestinal bleeding, which occurs in approximately 15% of patients, develops later in life [62]. Lesions tend to occur in the stomach and proximal small intestine (**Fig. 44.31**). Turner syndrome has also been associated with telangiectasias. The occurrence of bleeding in these patients is quite low, reported in four of 56 patients by Haddad and Wilkins [63] and none of 48 patients by Engel and Forbes [64]. Telangiectasias also occur in the syndrome of calcinosis, Raynaud phenomenon, sclerodactyly, and telangiectasia (CRST). Although lesions usually occur on the hands, face, and mouth, gastric and small-bowel telangiectasias may form and be a cause of bleeding [65].
- *Hemangiomas* are neoplastic tumors made up of proliferating blood vessels and are rarely malignant (**Fig. 44.32**). The lesions may be single or multiple, but once they are treated, recurrence of bleeding is rare. Pathologically, these lesions are divided into capillary, cavernous, and mixed forms. Hemangiomas are also associated with skin lesions such as the cavernous hemangiomas of the skin in blue rubber bleb nevus syndrome, or the cutaneous hemangiomas and soft-tissue hypertrophy of Klippel–Trenaunay–Weber syndrome [66].
- *Arteriovenous malformation* (AVM) is a term formerly used to describe angiectasias. True AVMs are congenital lesions characterized by thick-walled arteries and veins without intervening capillaries, forming a true arteriovenous fistula [67] (**Fig. 44.33**). Muscular hypertrophy and eccentric intimal thickening are also seen. These lesions tend to occur in younger patients and may be located anywhere in the gastrointestinal tract, although they are most commonly found in the stomach and small intestine. Like hemangiomas, the lesions tend to be single and do not recur.

Angiectasias are classically described as occurring in the right colon. Colonic angiectasias were initially described angiographically by Baum et al. [68] and Boley et al. [69]. The colonic ectasias described by Boley et al. were small and located predominantly in the cecum and ascending colon. Patients were over the age of 60, and there was no sex predilection. All lesions in this series were diagnosed by angiography, and 12 were further studied using stereomicroscopy after injection of the vasculature of the resected colon with a silicone–rubber compound. The angiographic and injection studies correlated well, showing the evolution from early to late lesions. Early lesions showed dilated tortuous submucosal veins on injection and late-emptying veins on angiography. The so-called capillary tuft on angiography was shown by injection studies to consist of clusters of dilated arterioles. Late lesions consisted of arteriovenous fistulas and were evidenced on angiography by the presence of an early-filling vein. On the basis of these findings, Boley et al. suggested that angiectasias develop as a consequence of the normal, intermittent distension of the cecum and right colon, causing recurrent obstruction to venous outflow where veins perforate the muscularis propria. The cecal location of the lesions was explained by the relatively large diameter of the cecum, producing relatively high wall pressures in accordance with Laplace's law. With venous outflow obstruction, increased pressure would be transmitted to the capillary bed, dilating it. Over time, pressure would be transmitted to the

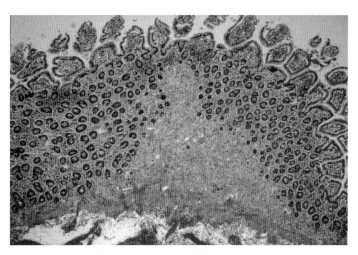

Fig. 44.31 A bleeding vascular lesion of the jejunum.

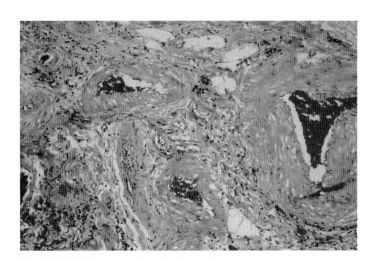

Fig. 44.32 High-power view of a hemangioma.

44

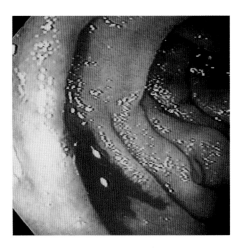

Fig. 44.33 Multiple telangiectasias in a patient with hereditary hemorrhagic telangiectasia.

precapillary sphincters, which in turn could become incompetent, creating an arteriovenous fistula. Boley et al. therefore believed that angiectasias were a common degenerative disease of aging. This theory was supported when they examined 15 patients over the age of 60 without bleeding or obstruction who had undergone right hemicolectomies for cancer. Eight of the 15 had submucosal ectasias and four had mucosal lesions. Other studies suggest that angiectasia are an incidental finding at colonoscopy in 2% of nonbleeding individuals over the age of 60 [70,71].

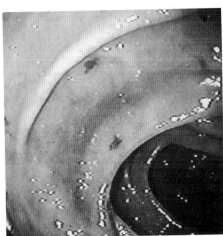

Fig. 44.34 A true arteriovenous malformation contains thick-walled vessels.

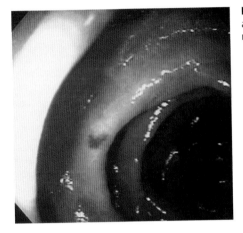

Fig. 44.35 A jejunal angiectasia with an anemic halo.

VI

Although these postulates have been accepted, they remain only conjectural. Clinically, it has not been shown that pressures generated in the cecum and right colon are enough to cause obstruction to venous outflow. More recent research has revealed less mucosal vascular collagen type IV in colons with angiectasias than in normal colons [72]. This deficiency of collagen may place the colon at risk for the development of the vascular lesions. In other avenues of research, it has been shown that there are fibroblast and endothelial growth factors in the colons of patients with angiectasias, in marked contrast to the findings in normal colons [73]. These new data suggest that colonic vascular ectasias are not formed by the degeneration of blood vessels, but rather by angiogenesis.

Research into the pathogenesis of HHT also points to angiogenesis as the cause. HHT is a systemic hereditary illness associated with bleeding telangiectasias of every organ. The condition has been linked with the presence of mutations on chromosome 9. It is postulated that the mutation alters endoglin, a transforming growth factor-β (TGF-β) binding protein [74]. Endoglin is an integral membrane glycoprotein in endothelial cells of capillaries, arterioles, and venules. Endoglin binds transforming growth factor, and this in turn leads to tissue growth, differentiation, motility, and remodeling. It is thought that the initiating event that leads to telangiectasia formation in patients with altered endoglin is tissue injury leading to abnormal tissue repair. Research has shown that patients with HHT are a very heterogeneous group [75]. At present, two HHT diseases are recognized—HHT1 and HHT2. HHT1 is the disease created by mutations on chromosome 9. At least 20 different mutations have been identified in 20 different families. Most simply, mutations in the q3 region are not associated with pulmonary vascular lesions, while mutations in the q34 region are associated

with pulmonary disease. HHT2 is the disease created by mutations on chromosome 12 in the q13 region. This area codes for the activin receptor-like kinase gene. At least 14 different mutations have been described for this disease.

There have been no injection studies of small-bowel angiectasias to help explain their pathophysiology. Since the time of early reports, vascular ectasias have been identified in the stomach and small intestine, though far less commonly than in the colon. Quintero was the first to describe angiectasia in the stomach and duodenum with an appearance similar to that of colonic lesions [76]. Meyer et al. [77] reviewed 218 angiectasias found at postmortem examinations; 2.3% were located in the duodenum, 10.5% in the jejunum, and 8.5% in the ileum. Small-bowel angiectasias are usually diagnosed endoscopically during either enteroscopy or intraoperative endoscopy. Angiography rarely diagnoses small-intestinal vascular lesions. This is secondary to the multiple arterial arcades that feed the small bowel, limiting the identification of a late-emptying or early-filling vein, or even a vascular tuft. Some form of pathophysiology other than the theory behind colonic vascular ectasias may be explain the occurrence of angiectasias in the small bowel. Another difficulty in understanding angiectasias of the small intestine is that the various pathologies discussed above present with similar clinical scenarios and similar endoscopic findings.

Vascular lesions of the small bowel can present with either brisk or occult bleeding (**Fig. 44.34**). Patients may have only positive fecal occult blood testing or melena. Red or maroon blood per rectum is uncommon. Lewis et al. reported that melena was the presenting sign in 64% of 102 patients with bleeding small-bowel angiectasias, while 36% had occult blood in the stool [10]. The reason why angiectasias bleed also remains unclear. Some postulate that bleeding results from high pressure bursting the thin-walled capillary, or is due to food abrading the mucosa. It has been noted pathologically that bleeding lesions are associated with thinning of the overlying mucosa and ulceration in some cases. The fistula may cause localized ischemia of the mucosa, leading to thinning and ulceration of the mucosa, the final pathway to bleeding [69]. This theory also correlates with the endoscopic finding of "anemic halos" associated with angiectasias (**Fig. 44.35**). A ring of pale mucosa is seen endoscopically around some angiectasias, similar to the anemic halos dermatologists describe with telangiectasias of the skin. These pale rings are thought to be secondary to the shunting of blood [78]. Their presence endoscopically confirms the vascular nature of the lesion seen.

Angiectasias have been associated with several other clinical disorders, including aortic stenosis and chronic renal failure. Aortic stenosis has long been implicated as a cause of bleeding from the right colon and, by inference, the formation of angiectasias [79]. While the cardiac lesion may not be etiologically involved in the formation of angiectasias, it may be causative in their bleeding due to the change in pulse pressure [69]. Although some studies report a cessation of bleeding after aortic valve replacement, the long-term follow-up has not substantiated that claim [80,81]. Imperiale and Ransohoff [82] reviewed the literature and found only four controlled studies addressing the association of idiopathic gastrointestinal bleeding and aortic stenosis [83–86]. None addressed the presence of angiectasias directly. They also found major methodological deficiencies in these studies, including nonblinded data collection, noncomparable diagnostic work-up between groups, nonblinded ascertainment of exposure, and noncomparable demographic susceptibility. Mehta et al. [87] performed echocardiography in 29 patients with colonic angiectasia. Although 76% of the patients had a systolic murmur, it was thought that the murmurs were related to flow, and none of the patients had evidence of true aortic stenosis. Thus, there is little evidence that aortic stenosis is an independent risk factor for the development of, or bleeding from, angiectasias.

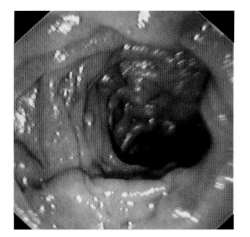

Fig. 44.36 Jejunal varices.

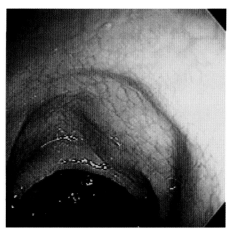

Fig. 44.37 The duodenum in a patient with celiac disease, showing a loss of valvulae conniventes and a mosaic pattern in the mucosa.

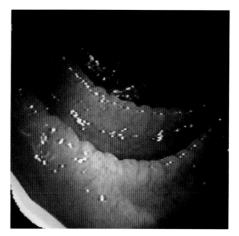

Fig. 44.38 Notching of duodenal folds in a patient with celiac disease.

The natural history of angiectasias is also still not known. It is estimated that less than 10% of patients with colonic angiectasia will eventually bleed. Foutch et al. followed eight patients with incidentally found colonic angiectasia for a mean of 3 years, and none developed bleeding [88]. Richter et al. reported on 15 patients with incidental ectasias diagnosed at colonoscopy, who were followed for a mean of 23 months, and none developed bleeding [89]. Once lesions have bled, the likelihood that they will rebleed is also not fully known. Although physicians are eager to treat these lesions, it may be that up to 50% will not rebleed. Hutcheon et al. reported on six patients who were treated with only blood transfusions after having a transfusion-dependent bleed from colonic vascular lesions [90]. There was a 91% decrease in transfusions during the follow-up period. Richter et al. reported 36 patients treated conservatively after having documented bleeding from colonic angiectasia. Twenty-six percent had re-bled at 1 year, and 46% had re-bled at 3 years. In a cohort study of medical therapy for bleeding angiectasia, Lewis et al. [91] reported spontaneous cessation of bleeding in 44% of patients with small-bowel angiectasia during a mean follow-up period of 13.1 months. In all of these studies, the propensity for rebleeding was not dependent on the type of bleeding the patient experienced.

There are several other vascular lesions that may cause bleeding in the small bowel. Small-bowel varices rarely may be a cause of major bleeding (**Fig. 44.36**) [92]. In patients without a history of abdominal surgery, these lesions are usually located in the duodenum and proximal jejunum [93]. They are much less likely to rupture and cause bleeding than esophageal varices, as they are located more deeply in the gut wall. Patients who have undergone abdominal surgery more commonly develop varices in adhesions or at the site of an enterostomy. For example, varices can occur in the ileum in cirrhotic patients following ileostomy or ileocolic resection. It is postulated that shunts form in the adhesions between the mesentery and the abdominal wall. It is estimated that only 1–3% of patients with cirrhosis and portal hypertension develop small-bowel varices. Although they uncommonly occur secondary to intrahepatic disease, small-bowel varices occur more often with extrahepatic causes of portal hypertension such as malignancy, mesenteric vein thrombosis, and pancreatitis [94]. Familial varices of the colon and small bowel have also been reported [95,96]. In this situation, it is postulated that congenital vascular abnormalities combined with portal hypertension produce the varices.

Malabsorption

Celiac Disease

Endoscopic small-bowel biopsies have long been used to diagnose celiac disease. Pathologic confirmation of villous atrophy is the hallmark of diagnosis. There are characteristic endoscopic findings in this illness that are quite specific. The typical changes of celiac disease include loss of valvulae conniventes, scalloping of folds, a mosaic pattern in the mucosa, and visualization of a vascular pattern in the proximal small bowel (**Figs. 44.37, 44.38**). In a study of 100 patients with celiac disease, Maurino et al. found that these findings were sensitive and specific, with a positive predictive value of 84% [97]. The reduction or loss of folds was the most reliable sign of sprue. These endoscopic changes have been confirmed in children as well [98], in whom the endoscopic findings correlated with the severity of the histologic findings, but not with the level of malabsorption. Thus, the endoscopic appearance of celiac disease may be used not only for diagnosis, but also to grossly gauge the histologic severity. These endoscopic findings are less important when dealing with a patient with known malabsorption, or when endoscopic biopsy is planned. Knowledge of these changes is important in patients with subclinical cases of sprue in whom endoscopy is carried out without planned biopsy. Subclinical sprue is increasingly recognized, and endoscopic evaluation of first-degree relatives of celiac disease patients is recommended by some authors [99].

These changes also come into play when evaluating patients with iron-deficiency anemia. In some cases of sprue, anemia may be the only sign [100]. Often, gastrointestinal bleeding is suspected in these patients and endoscopy is performed. It is important to consider celiac disease when no potential bleeding sites are identified; endoscopic changes of celiac disease should be specifically sought, and small-intestinal biopsies should be considered. Repeat endoscopic evaluation is often necessary in cases of refractory sprue, and enteroscopy has been used to diagnose or exclude small-bowel lymphomas and ulcerative jejunitis [101].

Whipple's Disease

Whipple's disease is a chronic small-intestinal infection with a variety of extraintestinal manifestations [102]. The infection has recently been identified as a new genus of *Actinomyces*, a Gram-

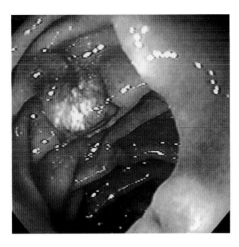

Fig. 44.39 Amyloid deposits in the jejunum.

positive bacillus. This infection typically presents in middle-aged men. Typical symptoms include weight loss, diarrhea, arthralgias, and abdominal pain; fever, neurologic abnormalities (e.g., dementia, ophthalmoplegia, myoclonus), and cardiovascular involvement (e.g., pericarditis, endocarditis) may also occur. Endoscopically, most patients have normal-appearing mucosa. Infection can produce small (1–2 mm) yellow-white plaques, or a yellow granular coating of the mucosa; folds may be thickened. The endoscopic changes may be suggestive of Whipple's disease, but can also be noted in cases of MAC, lymphangiectasia, histoplasmosis, and Waldenström macroglobulinemia. Biopsies are usually diagnostic, showing positive macrophages on periodic acid–Schiff (PAS) staining; however, infrequently these PAS-positive macrophages may be seen with MAC, histoplasmosis, or macroglobulinemia. Villi are intact, and lipid accumulation is seen.

Amyloid

Amyloid is deposited in the small bowel more frequently than in the stomach and colon. Endoscopic findings of amyloid include a granular appearance, polypoid protrusions, erosions, ulcerations, and mucosal friability [103,104] (**Fig. 44.39**). The first two of these findings do not change over time. They can be found in up to 84% of cases with biopsy-proven amyloid. Discrete mass lesions due to amyloid are seen and they have been termed "amyloidomas." Biopsies reveal amyloid deposits in the vascular walls, lamina propria, mucosa, muscularis mucosa, and submucosa.

References

1. Conn M. Tumors of the small intestine. In: DiMarino A, Benjamin S, editors. Gastrointestinal disease. Oxford: Blackwell Science; 1997. p. 551–66.
2. Wingo G, Tong T, Bolden S. Cancer statistics 1995. Cancer 1995;45:8–30.
3. Herbsman H, Wetstein L, Rosen Y, Orces H, Alfonso AE, Iyer SK, et al. Tumors of the small intestine. Curr Probl Surg 1980;17:121–82.
4. American Cancer Society. Cancer facts and figures. Atlanta, GA: American Cancer Society, 2005.
5. Szold A, Katz LB, Lewis BS. Surgical approach to occult gastrointestinal bleeding. Am J Surg 1992;163:90–3.
6. North JH, Pack MS. Malignant tumors of the small intestine: a review of 144 cases. Am Surg 2000;66:46–51.
7. Rossini F, Risio M, Pennazio M. Small bowel tumors and polyposis syndromes. Gastrointest Endosc Clin North Am 1999;9:93–114.
8. Martin L, Max M, Richardson J, Peterson G. Small bowel tumors: continuing challenge. South Med J 1980;73:981–5.
9. Ashley S, Wells S. Tumors of the small intestine. Semin Oncol 1988;15:116–28.
10. Lewis B, Kornbluth A, Waye J. Small bowel tumors: the yield of enteroscopy. Gut 1991;32:763–5.
11. Thompson JN, Salem RR, Hemingway AP, Rees HC, Hodgson HJ, Wood CB, et al. Specialist investigation of obscure gastrointestinal bleeding. Gut 1987;28:47–51.
12. Berner JS, Mauer K, Lewis BS. Push and sonde enteroscopy for the diagnosis of obscure gastrointestinal bleeding Am J Gastroenterol 1994;89:2139–42.
13. Torres M, Matta E, Chinea B, Dueno MI, Martinez-Souss J, Ojeda A, et al. Malignant tumors of the small intestine. J Clin Gastroenterol 2003;37:372–80.
14. Rabe FE, Becker GJ, Besozzi MJ, Miller RE. Efficacy study of the small-bowel examination. Radiology 1981;140:47–50.
15. Fried A, Poulos A, Hatfield D. The effectiveness of the incidental small-bowel series. Radiology 1981;140:45–6.
16. Gordon SR, Smith RE, Power GC. The role of endoscopy in the evaluation of iron deficiency anemia in patients over the age of 50. Am J Gastroenterol 1994;89:1963–7.
17. Rockey DC, Cello, JP. Evaluation of the gastrointestinal tract in patients with iron-deficiency anemia. N Engl J Med 1993;329:1691–5.
18. Lewis B, Goldfarb N. Review article: the advent of capsule endoscopy—a not-so-futuristic approach to obscure gastrointestinal bleeding. Aliment Pharmacol Ther 2003;17:1085–96.
19. Hara AK, Leighton JA, Sharma VK, Fleisher DE. Small bowel: preliminary comparison of capsule endoscopy with barium study and CT. Radiology 2004;230:260–5.
20. O'Loughlin C, Barkin JS. Wireless capsule endoscopy: summary. Gastrointest Endosc Clin North Am 2004;14:229–37.
21. de Mascarenhas-Saraiva MNG, da Silva Araujo Lopes LM. Small-bowel tumors diagnosed by capsule endoscopy: report of five cases. Endoscopy 2003;35:865–8.
22. Kimchi NA, Broide E, Zehavi S, Halevy A, Scapa E. Capsule endoscopy diagnosis of celiac disease and ileal tumors in a patient with melena of obscure origin. Isr Med Assoc J 2005;7:412–3.
23. Kruger S, Noack F, Blochle C, Feller AC. Primary malignant melanoma of the small bowel: a case report and review of the literature. Tumori 2005;91:73–6.
24. Coates SW Jr, DeMarco DC. Metastatic carcinoid tumor discovered by capsule endoscopy and not detected by esophagogastroduodenoscopy. Dig Dis Sci.2004;49:639–41.
25. Forner A, Mata A, Puig M, Varela M, Rodriguez F, Llach J, et al. Ileal carcinoid tumor as a cause of massive lower-GI bleeding: the role of capsule endoscopy. Gastrointest Endosc 2004;60:483–5.
26. Cobrin G, Pittman R, Lewis B. Increased diagnostic yield of small bowel tumors with capsule endoscopy. Cancer 2006;107:22–7.
27. Eisen G, Lewis BS, Friedman S. A pooled analysis to evaluate results of capsule endoscopy trials. Endoscopy 2005;37:960–5.
28. Schwartz G, Barkin J. Small bowel tumors. Gastrointest Endosc Clin N Am 2006;16:267–75.
29. Soares J, Lopes L, Vilas Boas G, Pinho C. Wireless capsule endoscopy for evaluation of phenotypic expression of small-bowel polyps in patients with Peutz–Jeghers syndrome and in symptomatic first-degree relatives. Endoscopy 2004;36:1060–6.
30. Caspari R, von Falkenhausen M, Krautmacher C, Schild H, Heller J, Sauerbruch T. Comparison of capsule endoscopy and magnetic resonance imaging for the detection of polyps of the small intestine in patients with familial adenomatous polyposis or with Peutz–Jeghers syndrome. Endoscopy 2004;36:1054–9.
31. De Palma GD, Rega M, Ciamarra P, Di Girolamo E, Patrone F, Mastantuono L, et al. Small-bowel polyps in Peutz–Jeghers syndrome: diagnosis by wireless capsule endoscopy. Endoscopy 2004;36:1039.
32. Sailer J, Zacherl J, Schima W. MDCT of small bowel tumours. Cancer Imaging 2007;7:224–33.
33. Lewis B. Evaluation of capsule endoscopic images. In: Keuchel M, Hagenmuller F, Fleischer D, editors. Atlas of video capsule endoscopy. Berlin: Springer; 2006. p. 14–23.
34. Lewis B, Keuchel M, Caselitz J. Malignant tumors of the small intestine. In: Keuchel M, Hagenmuller F, Fleischer D, editors. Atlas of video capsule endoscopy. Berlin: Springer; 2006. p. 172–90.
35. Mergener K, Ponchon T, Gralnek I, Pennazio M, Gay G, Selby W, et al. Literature review and recommendations for clinical application of small-bowel capsule endoscopy, based on a panel discussion by international experts. Endoscopy 2007;39:895–909.
36. Kitamura Y. Gastrointestinal stromal tumors: past, present and future. J Gastroenterol 2008;43:499–508.

37. Joensuu H. Risk stratification of patients with gastrointestinal stromal tumor. Hum Pathol 2008;39:1411–9.

38. Lewis B. Vascular anomalies. Adv Gastrointest Dis 1992;3:105–12.

39. Iida M, Matsui T, Itoh H, Mibu R, Fujishima M. The value of push-type jejunal endoscopy in familial adenomatosis coli/Gardner's syndrome. Am J Gastroenterol 1990;85:1346–8.

40. Barakat M. Endoscopic features of primary small bowel lymphoma: a proposed endoscopic classification. Gut 1982;23:36–41.

41. Halphen M, Najjar T, Jaafoura H, Cammoun M, Tufrali G. Diagnostic value of upper intestinal fiber endoscopy in primary small intestinal lymphoma. A prospective study by the Tunisian-French Intestinal Lymphoma Group. Cancer 1986;58:2140–5.

42. Kadakia S, Parker A, Canalses L. Metastatic tumors to the upper gastrointestinal tract: endoscopic experience. Am J Gastroenterol 1992;87:1418–23.

43. Farmer R, Hawk W, Turnbull R. Clinical patterns in Crohn's disease: a statistical study of 615 cases. Gastroenterology 1975;68:627–35.

44. Gryboski J, Spiro H. Prognosis in children with Crohn's disease. Gastroenterology 1978;74:807–17.

45. Sparberg M, Kirsner J. Recurrent hemorrhage in regional enteritis: report of 3 cases. Am J Dig Dis 1966;8:652–7.

46. Ellison E, Wilson S. The Zollinger–Ellison syndrome: reappraisal and evaluation of 260 registered cases. Ann Surg 1964;160:512–5.

47. Nair KV, Pai CG, Rajagopal KP, Bhat VN, Thomas M. Unusual presentations of duodenal tuberculosis. Am J Gastroenterol 1991;86:756–60.

48. Gray J, Rabeneck L. Atypical mycobacterial infection of the gastrointestinal tract in AIDS patients. Am J Gastroenterol 1989;84:1521–4.

49. Maliha GM, Hepps KS, Maia DM, Gentry KR, Fraire AE, Goodgame RW. Whipple's disease can mimic chronic AIDS enteropathy. Am J Gastroenterol 1991;86:79–81.

50. Boley SJ, Allen AC, Schultz L, Schwartz S. Potassium-induced lesions of the small bowel. I. Clinical aspects. JAMA 1965;193:997–1000.

51. Morris A, Madhok R, Sturrock RD, Capell HA, MacKenzie J. Enteroscopic diagnosis of small bowel ulceration in patients receiving non-steroidal anti-inflammatory drugs. Lancet 1991;337:520.

52. Morris AJ, Murray L, Sturrock RD, Madhok R, Capell HA, Mackenzie JF. The effect of misoprostol on the anaemia of NSAID enteropathy. Aliment Pharmacol Ther 1994;8:343–6.

53. Matsuhashi N, Yamada A, Hiraishi M, Konishi T, Minota S, Saito T, et al. Multiple strictures of the small intestine after long-term nonsteroidal anti-inflammatory drug therapy. Am J Gastroenterol 1992;87:1183–6.

54. Harris M, Lewis B. Systemic diseases affecting the mesenteric circulation. Surg Clin N Am 1992;72:245–9.

55. Sher M, Bauer J. Radiation-induced enteropathy. Am J Gastroenterol 1990;85:121–8.

56. Mahendra P, Bedlow AJ, Ager S, Ancliff PJ, Wraight EP, Marcus RE. Technetium (99mTc)-labelled white cell scanning, ^{51}Cr-EDTA and ^{14}C-mannitol-labelled intestinal permeability studies: non-invasive methods of diagnosing acute intestinal graft-versus-host disease. Bone Marrow Transplant 1994;13:835–7.

57. Brown C, Olshaker J. Meckel's diverticulum. Am J Emerg Med 1988;6:157–64.

58. Lewis B. Vascular diseases of the small intestine. In: DiMarino A, Benjamin S, editors. Gastrointestinal disease. Oxford: Blackwell Science; 1997. p. 541–50.

59. Lewis B, Mauer K, Harpaz N, Katz L, Morris P. The correlation of endoscopically identified vascular lesions to their pathologic diagnosis. Gastrointest Endosc 1993;39:344.

60. Harford W. Gastrointestinal angiodysplasia: clinical features. Endoscopy 1988;20:144–8.

61. Peoples J, Kartha R, Sharif S. Multiple phlebectasia of the small intestine. Am Surg 1981;47:373–6.

62. Shigematsu A, Iida M, Hatanaka M, Kohrogi N, Matsui T, Fujishima M, et al. Endoscopic diagnosis of lymphangioma of the small intestine. Am J Gastroenterol 1988;83:1289–93.

63. Haddad H, Wilkins L. Congenital anomalies associated with gonadal aplasia; review of 53 cases. Pediatrics 1959;23:885–902.

64. Engel E, Forbes A. Cytogenetic and clinical findings in 48 patients with congenitally defective or absent ovaries. Medicine 1965;44:135–64.

65. Rosekrans PC, de Rooy DJ, Bosman FT, Eulderink F, Cats A. Gastrointestinal telangiectasia as a cause of severe blood loss in systemic sclerosis. Endoscopy 1980;12:200–4.

66. Golitz LE. Heritable cutaneous disorders which affect the gastrointestinal tract. Med Clin North Am 1980;64:829–46.

67. Ottinger L, Vickery A. A 30 year history of recurrent gastrointestinal bleeding. N Engl J Med 1981;305:211–8.

68. Baum S, Athanasoulis CA, Waltman AC, Galdabini J, Schapiro RH, Warshaw AL, et al. Angiodysplasia of the right colon: a cause of gastrointestinal bleeding. AJR Am J Roentgenol 1977;129:789–94.

69. Boley SJ, Sammartano R, Adams A, DiBiase A, Kleinhaus S, Sprayregen S. On the nature and etiology of vascular ectasias of the colon. Degenerative lesions of aging. Gastroenterology 1977;72:650–60.

70. Hochter W, Weingart W, Kuhner E, Frimberg R, Ottenjann R. Angiodysplasia in the colon and rectum—endoscopic morphology, localization, and frequency. Endoscopy 1985;17:182–5.

71. Heer M, Sulser H, Hany A. Angiodysplasia of the colon: an expression of occlusive vascular disease. Hepatogastroenterology 1987;34:127–31.

72. Roskell D, Biddolph S, Warren B. Apparent deficiency of mucosal vascular collagen type IV associated with angiodysplasia of the colon. J Clin Pathol 1998;51:18–20.

73. Junquera F, Saperas E, de Torres I, Vidal MT, Malagelada JR. Increased expression of angiogenic factors in human colonic angiodysplasia. Am J Gastroenterol 1999;94:1070–6.

74. McAllister KA, Grogg KM, Johnson DW, Gallione CJ, Baldwin MA, Jackson CE, et al. Endoglin, a TGF-beta binding protein of endothelial cells, is the gene for hereditary haemorrhagic telangiectasia type 1. Nat Genet 1994;8:345–51.

75. Marchuk D, Guttmacher A, Penner J, Ganguly P. Report on the workshop on hereditary hemorrhagic telangiectasia, July 10–11, 1997. Am J Med Genet 1998;76:269–73.

76. Quintero E. Upper gastrointestinal bleeding caused by gastroduodenal vascular malformations. Dig Dis Sci 1986;31:897–905.

77. Meyer C, Troncale F, Galloway S, Sheahan D. Arteriovenous malformations of the bowel: an analysis of 22 cases and a review of the literature. Medicine 1981;60:36–48.

78. Brandt L. Anemic halos around telangiectasias. Gastroenterology 1987;92:1282.

79. Weaver G, Alpern H, Davis J, Ramsey W, Reichelderfer M. Gastrointestinal angiodysplasia associated with aortic valve disease: part of a spectrum of angiodysplasia of the gut. Gastroenterology 1979;77:1–11.

80. Scheffer S, Leatherman L. Resolution of Heyde's syndrome of aortic stenosis and gastrointestinal bleeding after aortic valve replacement. Ann Thorac Surg 1986;42:477–80.

81. Cappell M, Lebwohl O. Cessation of recurrent bleeding from gastrointestinal angiodysplasias after aortic valve replacement. Ann Intern Med 1986;105:54–7.

82. Imperiale T, Ransohoff D. Aortic stenosis, idiopathic gastrointestinal bleeding and angiodysplasia: is there an association? Gastroenterology 1988;95:1670–6.

83. Williams R. Aortic stenosis and unexplained gastrointestinal bleeding. Arch Intern Med 1961;108:859–64.

84. Schoenfeld Y, Eldar M, Bedazovsky B, Levy M, Pinkhas J. Aortic stenosis associated with gastrointestinal bleeding. A survey of 612 patients. Am Heart J 1980;100:179–82.

85. McNamara J, Austen W. Gastrointestinal bleeding occurring in patients with acquired valvular heart disease. Arch Surg 1968;97:538–40.

86. Cody MC, O'Donovan TP, Hughes RW Jr. Idiopathic gastrointestinal bleeding and aortic stenosis. Am J Dig Dis 1974;19:393–8.

87. Mehta P, Heinsimer J, Bryg R, Jaszewski R, Wynne J. Reassessment of the association between gastrointestinal arteriovenous malformations and aortic stenosis. Am J Med 1989;86:275–7.

88. Foutch P, Rex D, Lieberman D. Prevalence and natural history of colonic angiodysplasia among healthy asymptomatic people. Am J Gastroenterol 1995;90:564–7.

89. Richter J, Christensen M, Colditz G. Angiodysplasia: natural history and efficacy of therapeutic interventions. Dig Dis Sci 1989;34:1542–6.

90. Hutcheon D, Kabelin J, Bulkley G, Smith G. Effect of therapy on bleeding rates in gastrointestinal angiodysplasia. Am Surg 1987;53:6–9.

91. Lewis B, Salomon P, Rivera-MacMurray S, Kornbluth A, Wenger J, Waye J. Does hormonal therapy have any benefit for bleeding angiodysplasia? J Clin Gastroenterol 1992;15:99–103.

92. Philippakis M, Karkanias G, Sakorafas GH, Pontikis I, Gavalas M. Massive gastrointestinal bleeding secondary to intestinal varices. Eur J Surg 1992;158:379–81.

93. Lewis B, Waye J. Duodenal varices. IM Intern Med Spec 1989;10:19.

94. Lein B, McCombs P. Bleeding varices of the small bowel as a complication of pancreatitis. World J Surg 1992;16:1147–9.

95. Atin V, Sabas J, Cotano J, Madariago M, Galan D. Familial varices of the colon and small bowel. Int J Colorectal Dis 1993;8:4–8.

96. Morini S, Caruso F, DeAngelis P. Familial varices of the small and large bowel. Endoscopy 1993;25:188–90.

44

97. Mauriño E, Capizzano H, Niveloni S, Kogan Z, Valero J, Boerr L, et al. Value of endoscopic markers in celiac disease. Dig Dis Sci 1993;38:2028-33.

98. Corazza GR, Caletti GC, Lazzari R, Collina A, Brocchi E, Di Sario A, et al. Scalloped duodenal folds in childhood celiac disease. Gastrointest Endosc 1993;39:543-5.

99. Corazza GR, Frisoni M, Treggiari EA, Valentini RA, Filipponi C, Volta U, et al. Subclinical celiac sprue. Increasing occurrence and clues to its diagnosis. J Clin Gastroenterol 1993;16:16-21.

100. Gostout C. Enteroscopy for unexplained iron-deficiency anemia: identifying the patient with sprue. Gastrointest Endosc 1993;39:76-79.

101. Green J, Barkin J, Gregg P, Kohen K. Ulcerative jejunitis in refractory celiac disease: enteroscopic visualization. Gastrointest Endosc 1993;39:584-5.

102. Gaist D, Ladefoged K. Whipple's disease. Scand J Gastroenterol 1994;29: 97-101.

103. Tada S, Iida M, Iwashita A, Matsui T, Fuchigami T, Yamamoto T, et al. Endoscopic and biopsy findings of the upper digestive tract in patients with amyloidosis. Gastrointest Endosc 1990;36:10-4.

104. Tada S, Iida M, Yao T, Kawakubo K, Yao T, Okada M, Fujishima M. Endoscopic features in amyloidosis of the small intestine: clinical and morphologic differences between chemical types of amyloid protein. Gastrointest Endosc 1994;40:45-50.

VI

45 Diseases of the Ampulla

Nalini M. Guda and Joseph E. Geenen

Introduction

The ampulla of Vater was first described in 1720 by the German anatomist Abraham Vater (1684–1751). Endoscopically, the ampulla/papilla is seen as a smooth, spherical, nipple-like structure of varying size and shape. It is usually located on the posteromedial wall of the second portion of the duodenum. However, it may be seen anywhere between the pylorus and the ligament of Treitz. It typically has a horizontal duodenal fold as a hood, which can serve as a landmark. Mucin-producing glands are present throughout the biliary tree, but these are prominent near the ampulla, where they interdigitate with the smooth muscle fibers of the sphincter [1,2]. The bile duct and the main pancreatic duct join together at the ampulla to drain either by separate orifices or through a common channel (in 60–70% of cases). A separate bile duct opening may be seen, with bilious fluid flowing from the apex separately from a clear flow from the pancreatic duct. If separate, the distinct orifices can sometimes be discernible, but this distinction is not always feasible (**Fig. 45.1**). Diseases of the biliary tree or head of the pancreas, or processes involving the duodenum, can affect the ampulla. There are certain diseases that are specific to the ampulla that may also affect biliary and pancreatic drainage.

Anatomic Variations

In patients who have previously undergone an endoscopic sphincterotomy, the bile duct opening is at the apex of the ampulla, appearing as an elongated and patent opening. In patients with biliary pancreatitis, the bile duct orifice appears erythematous and traumatic, suggesting the passage of a stone. Sometimes the opening of the bile duct is obstructed by a stone. A "fishmouth" appearance with mucous secretions from the pancreatic duct is suggestive of intraductal papillary mucinous neoplasms (**Fig. 45.2**). Certain parasitic diseases of the liver and gastrointestinal tract may sometimes be identified by an examination of the ampulla, as in hydatid cysts or *Ascaris* worms protruding through the ampulla.

Duodenal diverticula are not uncommon. Periampullary diverticula are more common in elderly patients and may lead to difficulty in cannulating the biliary and pancreatic ducts (**Fig. 45.3**). The relation of the ampulla to the diverticulum may vary; the ampulla may be found within the rim of the diverticulum or at its base (intradiverticular papilla). In one study, the papilla was not visualized in up to 8% of patients with periampullary diverticula undergoing ERCP, although this is quite uncommon in the present authors' experience [3]. The papilla may also occasionally be seen in between two diverticula. Periampullary diverticulum may result in bile stasis and an increased risk for choledocholithiasis. Although it has been suggested that periampullary diverticula may result in an increased risk of complications during ERCP and sphincterotomy, recent studies have shown that there is no increase in postprocedural complications [3,4]. Rarely, a small diverticulum can be seen arising out of the ampulla of Vater as a small sack-like protrusion from the distal end of the common bile duct; this may be visible on opacification of the common bile duct at ERCP [1]. Periampullary diverticula with inspissated food may sometimes give the appearance of a possible tumor or soft-tissue density on conventional cross-sectional imaging [5]. At endoscopy, the presence of a soft, compressible periampullary mass-like structure should raise the possibility of a duodenal duplication cyst. The findings can be distinguished using imaging techniques including computed tomography (CT) and endoscopic ultrasonography (EUS).

A choledochocele forms as a result of the prolapse or herniation of the intramural segment of the distal common bile duct and can be seen as a protruding ampulla with an eccentric biliary orifice. Choledochoceles can be identified by magnetic resonance cholangio-

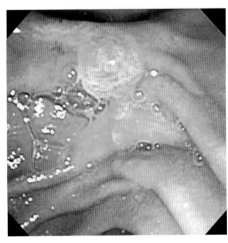

Fig. 45.1 A normal papilla seen with a duodenoscope at endoscopic retrograde cholangiopancreatography.

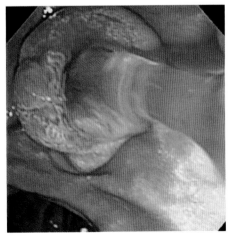

Fig. 45.2 Mucous drainage from a pancreatic duct with a characteristic "fishmouth" appearance, suggestive of intraductal papillary mucinous neoplasia.

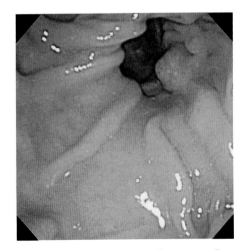

Fig. 45.3 Endoscopic image of a periampullary diverticulum. The altered angle of the papilla should be noted.

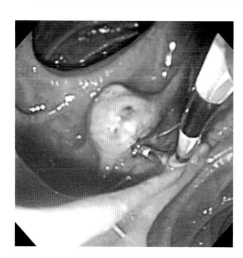

Fig. 45.4 Endoscopic image of a choledocho-cele.

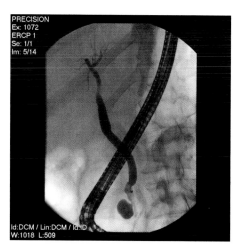

Fig. 45.5 Fluoroscopic image of a choledocho-cele.

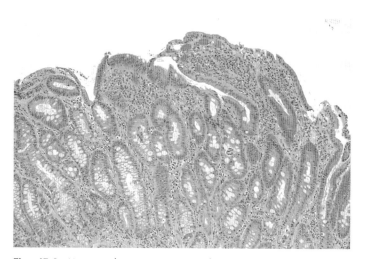

Fig. 45.6 Hematoxylin–eosin staining of a papilla with inflammatory changes.

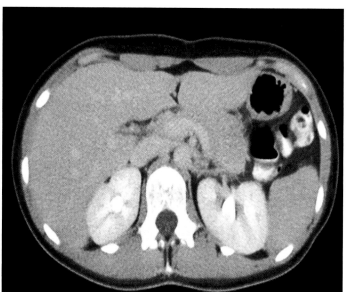

Fig. 45.7 Computed tomogram showing a bulky, "sausage-shaped" pancreas (courtesy of Martin L. Freeman, MD).

pancreatography (MRCP) and sometimes with EUS. Direct cholangiography is often needed in order to identify this condition (**Figs. 45.4, 45.5**), which rarely causes symptoms and is often overlooked [1]. It may be the cause of unexplained pancreatitis in some patients.

Papillitis

Inflammatory conditions in the biliary or pancreatic duct, as well as in the duodenum, may affect the papilla and cause papillary inflammation. Passage of a stone or iatrogenic causes can result in a benign inflammatory process involving the papilla (**Fig. 45.6**). This can at times be seen with reactive changes, as in a post-sphincterotomy state. Although infectious etiologies are less common in immunocompetent patients, unusual infectious etiologies should be a concern in those who are immunocompromised.

Cytomegalovirus can cause inflammatory changes in the papilla, leading to abnormal liver function tests and jaundice. Particular attention should be given to obtaining biopsies in relevant clinical settings, such as in patients with human immunodeficiency virus (HIV) and post-transplant patients receiving immunosuppressive therapy. Biliary or pancreatic duct aspirates for microbiological examination can be useful as well [6–9]. Papillitis can also be seen secondary to infections from *Cryptosporidium* or infiltration from Kaposi's sarcoma. Treatment in these situations generally involves sphincterotomy and usually results in biliary drainage in patients with cholestasis.

Autoimmune pancreatitis, especially involving the head of the pancreas, can cause subtle inflammatory changes in the ampulla, which may or may not be visually evident. This may be difficult to distinguish from infiltration of tumors involving the pancreatic head. If autoimmune pancreatitis is suspected, it may be useful to take biopsies of the ampulla and stain the specimen with immunoglobulin G4 (IgG4). Preliminary data suggest that IgG4 stains are positive in autoimmune pancreatitis and can help distinguish papillary involvement with tumors, particularly in patients with negative serology [10] (**Figs. 45.7–45.9**).

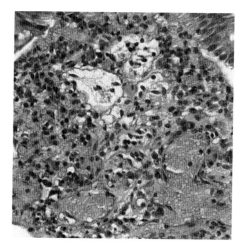

Fig. 45.8 Hematoxylin–eosin staining of the papilla in a patient with suspected autoimmune pancreatitis (courtesy of Martin L. Freeman, MD).

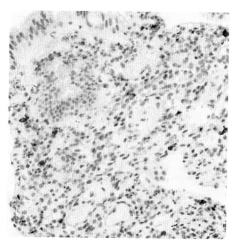

Fig. 45.9 Immunoglobulin G4 (IgG4) stain of the papilla in a patient with suspected autoimmune pancreatitis (courtesy of Martin L. Freeman, MD).

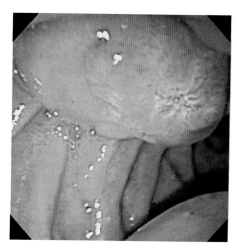

Fig. 45.10 Endoscopic appearance of an ampullary adenoma.

Tumors of the Ampulla of Vater

Adenomatous lesions of the small intestine are not uncommon and account for about 25% of small-bowel tumors. The ampulla of Vater is a very common site. The lesions are often detected incidentally in patients undergoing endoscopy/radiologic imaging for other reasons, and may also be a source of occult blood loss. Symptoms of biliary or pancreatic duct obstruction, including jaundice and pancreatitis, are not uncommon. Rarely, intussusception secondary to ampullary adenomas has also been reported [11]. Patients with familial adenomatous polyposis are particularly susceptible to ampullary adenomas and are at risk of adenocarcinoma developing; they should therefore receive routine endoscopic surveillance. Endoscopic resection of adenomas in these individuals is often effective and should be undertaken before more invasive surgical procedures are considered [12]. Other less common lesions include stromal tumors and neuroendocrine tumors. Ectopic pancreas may mimic an ampullary tumor [13].

The majority of ampullary lesions are adenomatous (**Figs. 45.10, 45.11**). However, as with colonic polyps, they may progress to adenocarcinoma through the adenoma–carcinoma sequence (**Figs. 45.12–45.14**). Appropriate evaluation is warranted before excision, as accurate diagnosis and staging are crucial before definitive therapy can be offered. Endoscopic excision of ampullary adenomas is now done routinely and has reduced the need for more invasive surgery. However, it should be assessed whether there is any involvement of the biliary and/or pancreatic ducts by neoplastic tissue before endoscopic excision is carried out. In selected cases, particularly patients who have a poor surgical risk, endoscopic excision and ablation of the involved ducts can be considered. Endoscopic ultrasound is routinely performed in addition to conventional cross-sectional imaging. Routine cross-sectional imaging methods, including transabdominal ultrasonography and CT scanning, have poor sensitivity and specificity in evaluating ampullary tumors, in comparison with standard endoscopic ultrasound [14]. Intraductal ultrasound using a miniprobe through the ERCP scope appears to have better sensitivity and specificity in comparison with conventional ultrasonography, although it may overestimate the T staging [15,16]. Most referring institutions now have facilities for endoscopic ultrasound, and EUS examinations have become standard practice in the diagnosis and staging of ampullary tumors. Through-the-scope miniprobes are not commonly used, as they

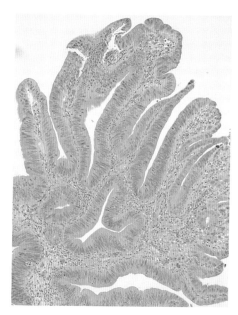

Fig. 45.11 Histopathology of an ampullary adenoma.

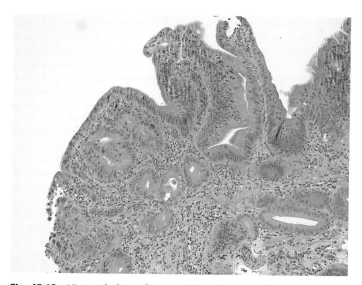

Fig. 45.12 Histopathology of an ampullary adenoma with high-grade dysplasia.

45

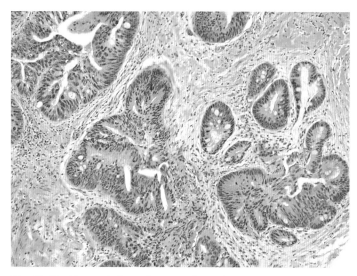

Fig. 45.13 Histopathology of an ampullary adenocarcinoma.

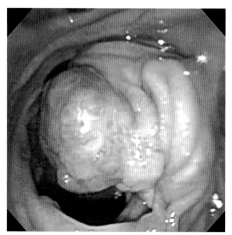

Fig. 45.14 Endoscopic appearance of an ampullary adenocarcinoma.

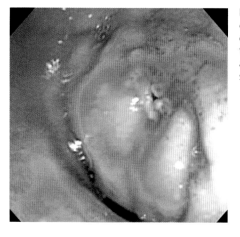

Fig. 45.15 Cholecystoduodenal fistula. An opening in the bulb of the duodenum is seen in a patient with Mirizzi syndrome.

out invasion of the biliary/pancreatic duct by the tumor. The presence of high-grade dysplasia or carcinoma in situ is not an absolute contraindication to ampullectomy, and the procedure may be appropriate in patients who are poor candidates for surgery. Placing a pancreatic duct stent after ampullectomy has been shown to reduce the risk of postprocedural pancreatitis [17,18]. Procedural techniques and indications are described elsewhere. In patients with adenocarcinoma or intraductal extension who are good candidates for surgery, resection generally consists of a Whipple's procedure. There has been some debate on whether a pylorus-sparing or conventional Whipple's procedure should be carried out; a recent systematic review found no differences between the two procedures with regard to mortality, morbidity, or survival rates [19].

Periampullary Fistula

In rare instances, an opening in the duodenum separate from the papilla may be seen, representing a fistulous communication from which bile is sometimes draining. The fistulous tract may involve a communication between the bile duct and the duodenal wall (choledochoduodenal fistula) or between the gallbladder and duodenum (cholecystoduodenal fistula) (**Fig. 45.15**). It often forms as a result of spontaneous passage of a common bile duct stone or gallbladder stone through an abnormal course, creating a false tract. Fistulous tracts are not infrequently seen in patients with ampullary tumors, particularly ampullary carcinoma. Fistulas resulting from blunt abdominal trauma, iatrogenic fistulas secondary to trauma from instruments or migration of endobiliary prostheses, and fistulas due to the erosion of duodenal ulcers into the bile duct have also been described. Therapy usually involves surgical repair of the common duct and closure of the fistula and may involve sphincterotomy or stenting of the common duct. In patients without choledocholithiasis, routine sphincterotomy and extension fistulotomy have not been shown to be of significant benefit [20].

In patients with papillary carcinoma, treatment to create a periampullary fistula between the distal common bile duct and the duodenum—choledochoduodenal fistulotomy—results in biliary drainage. In these patients, a suprapapillary bulge is visible endoscopically, and a fistulotomy can be created with a needle-knife [21]. Techniques using EUS-guided drainage or the use of magnets to create a fistulotomy are being developed, and preliminary studies in animals have been promising. No studies in humans have been reported yet.

Sphincter of Oddi Dysfunction

The sphincter of Oddi is a smooth muscle at the distal end of the bile duct, first described about 120 years ago by the Italian physician Ruggiero Oddi (1864–1913). It is a complex structure that has a choledochal sphincter and a pancreatic sphincter, as well as interconnecting fibers. Physiological studies have shown that the sphincter has a role in the controlling the flow of bile and pancreatic duct outflow and also prevents reflux of duodenal contents. The sphincter of Oddi is a dynamic structure with a basal pressure that is higher than the intraductal pressure, although measured bile duct pressures do not correlate with the sphincter pressure. Superimposed on the basal pressure, there are rhythmically appearing phasic contractions that occur at the rate of five to eight per minute. Although there are dynamic abnormalities relating to the intensity, frequency, and propagation of these waves, basal pressure is generally measured clinically, with good interobserver reliability and reproducibility. The basal pressure is thought to be stable over time, and it correlates with clinical responses [22–25]. The sphincter pressure can be measured using manometry. Various manometry catheters

are fragile and conventional EUS is capable of identifying ductal involvement quite accurately.

Ampullary tumors can be resected surgically or endoscopically. Surgical resection methods include pancreatoduodenectomy and transduodenal ampullectomy. With growing expertise, resection is increasingly being carried out endoscopically, with less morbidity. Endoscopic ultrasound should be carried out for staging and to rule

are available, including a triple-lumen perfusion catheter; an aspiration catheter, in which one of the perfusion leads is dispensed with in order to allow aspiration of perfused saline in an effort to reduce post-ERCP pancreatitis; a solid-state manometry catheter; and a newly developed sleeve catheter [26].

Standard values have been established on the basis of pressure measurements in normal individuals and symptomatic "normal" patients. The normal basal pressures are in the range of 5–20 mmHg. A sustained basal pressure >40 mmHg is currently considered to be abnormal for both the biliary and pancreatic sphincter. On the basis of the nature of the pain, laboratory findings, and radiological abnormalities, patients with sphincter of Oddi dysfunction (SOD) are classified into three types (**Table 45.1**). The nature of the pain may help determine whether the patient has biliary sphincter SOD or pancreatic sphincter SOD. Biliary pain is typically described as being located in the epigastric area or right upper quadrant, as lasting from several minutes to less than a few hours, and as resembling the pain experienced in biliary colic. Pancreatic pain, on the other hand, is described as radiating to the back, as in pancreatitis, and is usually associated with elevated amylase and/or lipase values.

On the basis of the available data, it appears reasonable to offer sphincterotomy to patients with type 1 SOD. The need for manometry in these patients has been questioned, as there appears to be stenosis of the sphincter in this group, and normal manometry does not preclude sphincter stenosis [23]. There is good evidence from randomized controlled trials that there is a persisting symptomatic response to sphincter division in patients with type 2 SOD [22–25]. Some data have suggested that empirical sphincterotomy without manometry should be carried out in patients with type 2 SOD. There is at present insufficient evidence for recommendations to be made; in the view of the present authors, manometry should be carried out in patients in whom there is a suspicion of type 2 SOD, and treatment with sphincter division should be offered only to those in whom elevated sphincter pressures are found [23]. Type 3 SOD is a matter of controversy, as there are no objectively abnormal findings and the responses to sphincter division are variable [23,27]. Given the risk of post-ERCP pancreatitis, which is high in these individuals, patients should be selected very carefully and sphincter division treatment should only be offered to those with manometrically documented abnormalities. The available evidence is weak [23]. A randomized, sham-controlled multicenter study is currently being conducted, the results of which should provide better guidance. In general, ERCP should be avoided as an initial investigation, and alternative imaging methods including magnetic resonance pancreatography and EUS should be used to rule out other etiologies for the pain before manometry and ERCP are performed in these individuals.

The National Institutes of Health conference statement and clinical practice in advanced centers broadly support the performance of pancreatic sphincterotomy in patients with pancreatic sphincter hypertension and appropriate symptoms, whether at initial ERCP or at a follow-up ERCP if there is no response to initial biliary sphincterotomy. Prospective studies are currently being conducted to assess the responses to various strategies [28].

Diseases of the Minor Papilla

The minor papilla is seen proximal and medial to the ampulla of Vater. The dorsal pancreatic duct drains through this orifice and is usually quite inconspicuous, except in patients with pancreas divisum, in whom it may be prominent due to the pancreatic drainage, or in certain situations involving obstruction of the ventral pancreatic duct, as in calcareous pancreatitis or tumor. Diseases affecting the major papilla may also affect the minor papilla, although these

Table 45.1 The Hogan–Geenen (Milwaukee) classification for sphincter of Oddi dysfunction (SOD)

Patient group	Criteria
Biliary type 1	Biliary-type pain
	Serum AST or ALP > 2 × normal on two or more occasions
	Delayed contrast drainage at ERCP > 45 min
	CBD dilated > 12 mm
Biliary type 2	Biliary-type pain
	One or two of the other three criteria
Biliary type 3	Biliary-type pain alone, in the absence of any objective criteria

ALP, alkaline phosphatase; AST, aspartate aminotransferase; CBD, common bile duct; ERCP, endoscopic retrograde cholangiopancreatography.

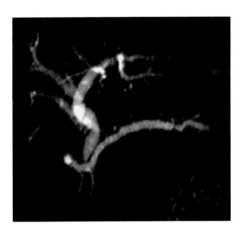

Fig. 45.16 Secretin-enhanced magnetic resonance cholangiopancreatography, showing a Santorinicele (courtesy of Martin L. Freeman, MD).

are uncommon. Adenoma and adenocarcinoma involving the minor papilla have been reported [29,30]. Endoscopic snare excision of minor papilla adenoma appears to be feasible and safe [31]. Secretin-enhanced MRCP may be useful for identifying the ductal anatomy. A Santorinicele of the minor papilla, similar to choledochocele, has been described (**Fig. 45.16**).

References

1. Venu RP, Geenen JE. Diagnosis and treatment of diseases of the papilla. Clin Gastroenterol 1986;15:439–56.
2. Crawford JM. The liver and the biliary tract. In: Cotran RS, Kumar V, Collins T, editors. Robbins pathologic basis of disease. 6th ed. Philadelphia: Saunders; 1999. p. 892–901.
3. Panteris V, Vezakis A, Filippou G, Filippou D, Karamanolis D, Rizos S. Influence of juxtapapillary diverticula on the success or difficulty of cannulation and complication rate. Gastrointest Endosc 2008;68:903–10.
4. Tham TC, Kelly M. Association of periampullary duodenal diverticula with bile duct stones and with technical success of endoscopic retrograde cholangiopancreatography. Endoscopy 2004;36:1050–3.
5. Clemente G, Sarno G, Giordano M, De Rose AM, Nuzzo G. Intramural duodenal diverticulum mimicking a periampullary neoplasm. Am J Surg 2008;196:e31–2.
6. Kim YS, Cho YD, Lee JS, Jin SY, Shim CS. Cytomegalovirus infection in an HIV patient with duodenal papillitis. Endoscopy 2007;39(Suppl 1):E23.
7. Papachristou GI, Smyrk TC, Baron TH. Cytomegalovirus infection in a liver transplant patient identified by endoscopically severe duodenal papillitis. Clin Gastroenterol Hepatol 2006;4(4):xxxii.
8. Keaveny AP, Karasik MS. Hepatobiliary and pancreatic infections in AIDS: part II. AIDS Patient Care STDS 1998;12:451–6.
9. Schneiderman DJ, Cello JP, Laing FC. Papillary stenosis and sclerosing cholangitis in the acquired immunodeficiency syndrome. Ann Intern Med 1987;106:546–9.

45

10. Kamisawa T, Tu Y, Egawa N, Tsuruta K, Okamoto A. A new diagnostic endoscopic tool for autoimmune pancreatitis. Gastrointest Endosc 2008;68:358–61.

11. Ijichi H, Kawabe T, Isayama H, Yamagata M, Imai Y, Tada M, et al. "Duodenal intussusception" due to adenoma of the papilla of Vater. Hepatogastroenterology 2003;50:1399–402.

12. Ouaïssi M, Panis Y, Sielezneff I, Alves A, Pirrò N, Robitail S, et al. Long-term outcome after ampullectomy for ampullary lesions associated with familial adenomatous polyposis. Dis Colon Rectum 2005;48:2192–6.

13. Hsu SD, Chan DC, Hsieh HF, Chen TW, Yu JC, Chou SJ. Ectopic pancreas presenting as ampulla of Vater tumor. Am J Surg 2008;195:498–500.

14. Chen CH, Tseng LJ, Yang CC, Yeh YH. Preoperative evaluation of periampullary tumors by endoscopic sonography, transabdominal sonography, and computed tomography. J Clin Ultrasound 2001;29:313–21.

15. Menzel J, Hoepffner N, Sulkowski U, Reimer P, Heinecke A, Poremba C, et al. Polypoid tumors of the major duodenal papilla: preoperative staging with intraductal US, EUS, and CT—a prospective, histopathologically controlled study. Gastrointest Endosc 1999;49:349–57.

16. Ito K, Fujita N, Noda Y, Kobayashi G, Horaguchi J, Takasawa O, et al. Preoperative evaluation of ampullary neoplasm with EUS and transpapillary intraductal US: a prospective and histopathologically controlled study. Gastrointest Endosc 2007;66:740–7.

17. Catalano MF, Linder JD, Chak A, Sivak MV Jr, Raijman I, Geenen JE, et al. Endoscopic management of adenoma of the major duodenal papilla. Gastrointest Endosc 2004;59:225–32.

18. Harewood GC, Pochron NL, Gostout CJ. Prospective, randomized, controlled trial of prophylactic pancreatic stent placement for endoscopic snare excision of the duodenal ampulla. Gastrointest Endosc 2005;62:367–70.

19. Diener MK, Knaebel HP, Heukaufer C, Antes G, Buchler MW, Seiler CM. A systematic review and meta-analysis of pylorus-preserving versus classical pancreaticoduodenectomy for surgical treatment of periampullary and pancreatic carcinoma. Ann Surg 2007;245:187–200.

20. Ohtsuka T, Tanaka M, Inoue K, Nabae T, Takahata S, Yokohata K, et al. Is peripapillary choledochoduodenal fistula an indication for endoscopic sphincterotomy? Gastrointest Endosc 2001;53:313–7.

21. Park JJ, Kim SS, Kim YK, Jung MK, Park HC, Kim JH, et al. Biliary drainage by endoscopic choledochoduodenal fistulotomy in patients with papillary carcinoma. Gastrointest Endosc 2002;55:730–5.

22. Geenen JE, Hogan WJ, Dodds WJ, Toouli J, Venu RP. The efficacy of endoscopic sphincterotomy after cholecystectomy in patients with sphincter-of-Oddi dysfunction. N Engl J Med 1989;320:82–7.

23. Petersen BT. Sphincter of Oddi dysfunction, part 2: Evidence-based review of the presentations, with "objective" pancreatic findings (types I and II) and of presumptive type III. Gastrointest Endosc 2004;59:670–87.

24. Smithline A, Hawes R, Lehman G. Sphincter of Oddi manometry: interobserver variability. Gastrointest Endosc 1993;39:486–91.

25. Toouli J, Roberts-Thomson IC, Kellow J, Dowsett J, Saccone GT, Evans P, et al. Manometry based randomised trial of endoscopic sphincterotomy for sphincter of Oddi dysfunction. Gut 2000;46:98–102.

26. Kawamoto M, Geenen J, Omari T, Schloithe AC, Saccone GT, Toouli J. Sleeve sphincter of Oddi (SO) manometry: a new method for characterizing the motility of the sphincter of Oddi. J Hepatobiliary Pancreat Surg 2008;15:391–6.

27. Petersen BT. An evidence-based review of sphincter of Oddi dysfunction: part I, presentations with "objective" biliary findings (types I and II). Gastrointest Endosc 2004;59:525–34.

28. Cohen S, Bacon BR, Berlin JA, Fleischer D, Hecht GA, Loehrer PJ Sr, et al. National Institutes of Health State-of-the-Science Conference Statement: ERCP for diagnosis and therapy, January 14–16, 2002. Gastrointest Endosc 2002;56:803–9.

29. Wakatsuki T, Irisawa A, Takagi T, Koyama Y, Hoshi S, Takenoshita S, et al. Primary adenocarcinoma of the minor duodenal papilla. Yonsei Med J 2008;49:333–6.

30. Nakamura Y, Tajiri T, Uchida E, Aimoto T, Taniai N, Katsuno A, et al. Adenoma of the minor papilla associated with pancreas divisum. Hepatogastroenterology 2007;54:1841–3.

31. Trevino JM, Wilcox CM, Varadarajulu S. Endoscopic resection of minor papilla adenomas (with video). Gastrointest Endosc 2008;68:383–6.

VI

46 Upper Gastrointestinal Bleeding Disorders

Shiv K. Sarin, Vikram Bhatia, Justin C.Y. Wu, and Joseph J.Y. Sung

Variceal Bleeding in Cirrhosis

Shiv K. Sarin and Vikram Bhatia

▪ Anatomy of Esophageal and Gastric Varices

The venous drainage that is involved in the formation of gastro-esophageal varices can be divided into four zones. From below upward, these are [1]:

- The *gastric zone*, which extends for 2–3 cm below the gastro-esophageal junction, where the veins join and drain into the short gastric and left gastric veins.
- The *palisade zone*, which extends for 2–3 cm in the lower esophagus.
- The *perforating zone*, where the network of submucosal veins connects via perforating veins to the periesophageal veins, which then drain into the azygous system. These perforating veins have valves that normally direct blood flow toward the periesophageal veins. In portal hypertension, the valves of the perforating veins are incompetent and allow retrograde flow toward the intramural veins [2].
- The *truncal zone*, which is approximately 10 cm long and has four longitudinal venous columns. Over 80% of variceal bleeding arises within the distal 2–5 cm of the esophagus, and interventional strategies therefore need to be focused in this zone.

The afferent veins of gastric varices are the left gastric vein, posterior gastric vein, short gastric veins, and gastroepiploic vein. Most gastric varices are formed by the left gastric or posterior gastric veins [3]. The left gastric vein enters the stomach wall at the cardia, approximately 2–3 cm from the gastroesophageal junction, and then diverges into multiple branches running throughout the cardia. Gastric varices of the left gastric vein are therefore frequently located at the cardia and sometimes extend cephalad to coalesce with the paraesophageal collaterals. Varices of the posterior gastric vein and short gastric veins are usually located in the fundus of the stomach and drain into a major gastrosystemic shunt. Varices of the gastroepiploic vein are rare and often occur after treatment of other gastric varices. Gastric varices can be supplied by a single afferent vein or multiple afferent veins [4].

▪ Classification Systems

Esophageal Varices

Dagradi suggested one of the first classifications of esophageal varices, by dividing them into grades 1–5 based on their diameter. This system was devised using the rigid esophagoscope [5]. With a fiberoptic endoscope, the size of the varices is assessed during withdrawal of the instrument. As much air as possible should be aspirated from the stomach, while the distal esophagus must be insufflated with air while the variceal size is being assessed. As a point of reference, any varix larger in diameter than an open punch-biopsy forceps is likely to be over 5 mm in diameter. Palmer and Brick

classified varices on the basis of their length and diameter. Varices were classified by their diameter as mild (diameter > 3 mm), moderate (diameter 3–6 mm), and severe (diameter > 6 mm) [6]. According to Conn, the size of the varices can be graded as follows (**Fig. 46.1**): 1+, small varices only detectable on performing a Valsalva maneuver; 2+, small varices (approximately 1–3 mm in diameter) that are visible without a Valsalva maneuver; 3+, varices of moderate size (3–6 mm in diameter); and 4+, large varices (over 6 mm) [7]. The Japanese Research Society for Portal Hypertension proposed a classification system based on five features, including the basic color of the varices (white or blue), red color signs (red wale markings, cherry-red spots, hematocystic spots, and diffuse redness), shape (small straight, tortuous, coil-like), location or longitudinal extent, and additional findings such as erosions [8]. The red wale markings refer to longitudinal dilated venules resembling whip marks on the variceal surface. Cherry-red spots (also called "varices upon varices" by Dagradi) refer to small, flat, red dots about 2 mm in diameter on the surface of the varices. Hematocystic spots refer to round, dark red, raised spots about 4 mm or larger in diameter. The North Italian Endoscopic Club (NIEC) classification divides varices into small, medium, and large, based on variceal sizes of > 30%, 30–60%, and > 60% of their maximum potential size, namely half of the esophageal lumen. The size of the largest varix is used to define the grade [9]. However, all of these systems have a potential for interobserver and intraobserver variability. At a recent consensus conference held by the Asia–Pacific Association for the Study of the Liver (APASL), the grading of variceal size was therefore simplified to either small or large, with large varices being those over 5 mm in diameter [10]. In this grading, large varices are further qualified as "high-risk" varices if red color signs are present over them.

Gastric Varices

Gastroesophageal varices (GEVs) are classified on the basis of their location and relationship to esophageal varices, as in the classification presented by Sarin and Kumar [11]. Large esophageal varices extending for 3–5 cm onto the lesser curvature are called GEV1, and those extending toward the greater curvature are termed GEV2. Isolated gastric varices (IGVs) are located either in the fundus (IGV1) or in other sites in the stomach or first part of duodenum (IGV2) [11]. GEV2 and IGV1 include fundic varices (**Figs. 46.2, 46.3**).

▪ Local and Systemic Hemodynamics

Factors influencing variceal wall tension can be described using Laplace's law as: $T = Pr/w$, where T is variceal wall tension, P is the transmural pressure gradient between the variceal lumen and esophageal lumen, r is the variceal radius, and w is the variceal wall thickness. When the variceal wall thins and the varix increases in diameter and pressure, the variceal wall tension increases and the varix may rupture. These physiologic principles explain why larger varices (r) in sites with limited soft-tissue support (w) such as the

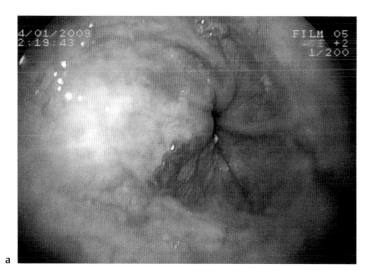

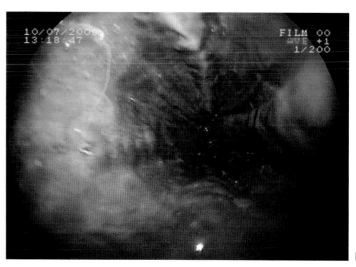

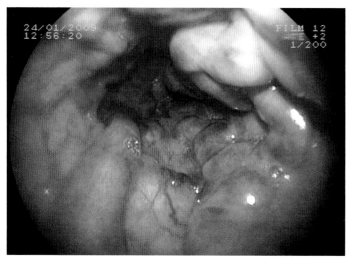

Fig. 46.1 The grading of esophageal varices according to Conn [7].
a Grade 1 esophageal varices, only detectable on performing a Valsalva maneuver.
b Grade 2 esophageal varices, 1–3 mm in diameter.
c Grade 3 esophageal varices. The varices are moderately large, approximately 3–6 mm in diameter.

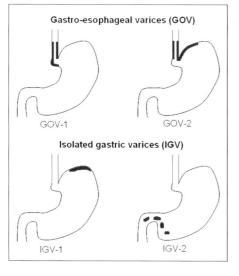

Fig. 46.2 Gastric varices according to the Sarin classification.

gastroesophageal junction, and with elevated portal pressure (P), tend to be at greatest risk for rupture.

Portal hypertension is defined by an increase in the pressure gradient between the portal vein and the inferior vena cava to more than 5 mmHg, measured as the hepatic venous pressure gradient (HVPG). HVPG, a marker of sinusoidal pressure, is determined by subtracting the free hepatic venous pressure (FHVP) from the

wedged hepatic venous pressure (WHVP), measured using a balloon catheter.

Assessment of HVPG is useful for predicting the outcome in both compensated and decompensated stages of cirrhosis. HVPG values between 5 and 9 mmHg correspond to preclinical portal hypertension. Clinically significant portal hypertension (CSPH) is diagnosed when clinical manifestations of the disease appear or when the portal pressure gradient (measured as its equivalent HVPG in cirrhosis) exceeds a threshold value of 10 mmHg. In a compensated cirrhotic patient, an HVPG value of 10 mmHg or more is the most important predictor of the development of varices [12]. In decompensated cirrhotic patients with variceal bleeding, an HVPG value of 20 mmHg or more within 48 h of admission is associated with increased rates of rebleeding and mortality [13–15]. In patients with medium or large esophageal varices, reduction of HVPG by > 10–20% reduces the incidence of first variceal bleeding, and if HVPG is reduced to > 12 mmHg, the risk of esophageal variceal bleeding is virtually eliminated [16]. HVPG measurement is highly recommended in the management of patients with variceal bleeding, as it provides important prognostic information and also helps in making treatment decisions.

Predictors of First Variceal Bleed

The severity of liver disease, variceal size, and the presence or absence of red color signs on endoscopy have been used by the North Italian Endoscopic Club (NIEC) to provide an index for predicting the first variceal bleeding. A patient with Child's C cirrhosis and large varices with red signs has a more than 76% risk of hemorrhage within 1 year. In contrast, a patient with Child's A cirrhosis and small varices without red signs has a less than 10% likelihood of bleeding [9]. However, as only one-third of patients who present with variceal hemorrhage have these risk factors, more accurate predictive factors need to be defined. According to the recently published APASL consensus statement, factors associated with the risk of bleeding from varices include size and wall thickness, presence of endoscopic stigmata such as red signs, the severity of the liver disease, and portal pressure [10].

Natural History

Esophageal Varices

When cirrhosis is first diagnosed, varices are present in about 30–40% of compensated patients and in 60% of decompensated patients. In cirrhotic patients without varices, the incidence of new varices ranges from 5% to 10% annually. In patients with small varices, the rate of progression to large varices is 5–30% per year. The rate of first variceal bleeding among patients with medium to large varices is 15% per year without treatment [17]. Overall, about one-third of patients with varices experience a variceal hemorrhage [18]. The lifelong risk of variceal bleeding is close to 50%. In portal vein obstruction, the bleeding rate is even higher than in cirrhosis, with a lifetime bleeding risk of 80%. Approximately half of all bleeds in this condition occur before the age of 5 years.

Only 40–50% of active variceal bleeds cease spontaneously [19]. The incidence of very early rebleeding (within first 2–5 days of the index bleed) ranges from 30% to 40%. Early rebleeding after 5 days and within 42 days occurs in a further 30–40% of patients. After 6 weeks, the risk of further bleeding becomes virtually equal to that before bleeding [20]. Graham and Smith reported in 1981 that following an initial variceal bleed, approximately one-third of patients died during the initial hospitalization, a further third had a second bleed within 6 weeks, and only one-third survived 1 year or more [20]. Current treatment modalities have reduced the 6-week rebleeding rate to 20% [19]. The mortality from variceal bleeding has also decreased during the last two decades to the current mortality rate of 15–20% [11].

The immediate mortality from uncontrolled variceal bleeding is in the range of 4–8%, but any death occurring within 6 weeks of hospital admission for variceal bleeding should be considered as a bleeding-related death [11]. At present, most of the mortality among patients with variceal bleeding is caused by liver failure, infections, and hepatorenal syndrome. Preventing the deterioration of liver and renal function should therefore be an integral part of the care provided for these patients.

The presence of varices and variceal bleeding has important prognostic value and has been used to define four stages of cirrhosis, based on the 1-year mortality data in a large cohort of untreated patients. The first two stages occur in compensated cirrhosis and are defined by the absence (stage 1) or presence (stage 2) of varices. The other two stages occur in decompensated cirrhosis and are defined by the presence of ascites (with or without varices, stage 3), and by variceal hemorrhage (with or without ascites, stage 4). The 1-year mortality rates in these four stages are 1%, 3%, 20%, and 57%, respectively [21].

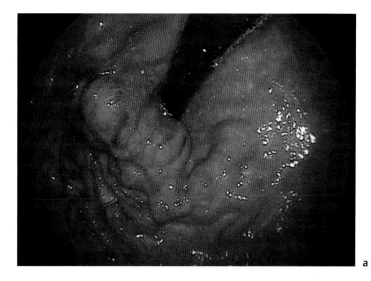

a

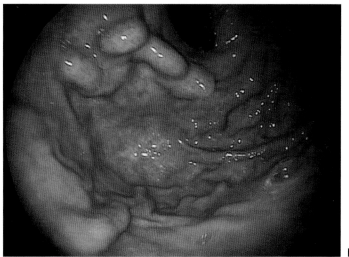

b

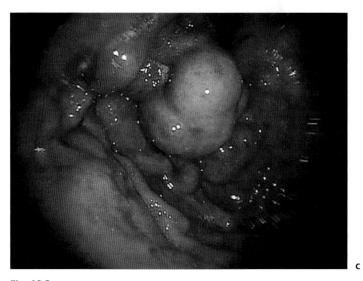

c

Fig. 46.3
a A type 2 gastroesophageal varix (GEV2), extending toward the greater curvature.
b An elongated isolated gastric varix located in the fundus (IGV1).
c A large, globular isolated gastric varix (IGV1).

46

Table 46.1 Assessing the severity of gastrointestinal bleeding

Patient's hemodynamic status (vital signs)	Blood loss (% of intravascular volume)*	Severity of bleeding
Resting hypotension	20–25	Massive
Orthostatic hypotension †	10–20	Moderate
Normal	< 10	Minor

* Blood volume (mL): 70 ×weight (in kg).
† Orthostatic hypotension is defined as a systolic blood pressure decrease of > 20 mmHg or an increase in pulse rate by > 20 beats/min from recumbency to standing.

Table 46.2 Target parameters for resuscitation in a patient with acute variceal bleeding

Parameter	Optimal target
Heart rate	< 100/min
Blood pressure	90–100 mmHg systolic
Hematocrit	21–24% (hemoglobin level: 7–8 g/dL)
Central venous pressure	0–5 mmHg

Table 46.3 Checklist before endoscopy

Patient
Vital signs
Two intravenous lines
Volume resuscitation measures on supplemental oxygen
Endoscopy room
Check endoscope (air–water channel, suction, knobs etc.)
Suction device
Patient resuscitation cart
Patient monitor
Accessories
Availability of alternative therapy
Interventional radiologist
Gastrointestinal surgeon
Sengstaken–Blakemore tube

Gastric Varices

Gastric varices occur in approximately 20% of patients with portal hypertension. Some 5–10% of patients with gastric varices may not have esophageal varices. Gastric variceal bleeding has been reported to account for 3–30% of all acute variceal bleeding episodes. The risk of bleeding from gastric varices depends on their location. Although GEV1 varices constitute more than 70% of gastric varices, only 11% of GEV1s ever bleed. After obliteration of esophageal varices, GEV1s disappeared in 59% of the patients. In contrast, even though IGV1s constitute less than 8% of all gastric varices, 78% of IGV1s bleed. IGV2s are rare (4.7% of all gastric varices) and are located in the antrum (53%), duodenum (32%), at both sites (11%), or in the gastric body (4%) [22]. IGV2s are predominantly (84.9%) secondary in origin, developing a mean of 8.2 months after esophageal variceal obliteration in patients with cirrhosis. Bleeding due to IGV2 varices was seen only in 5.7% of patients during a mean follow-up period of 36.3 ± 12.1 months [23]. Overall, gastric varices bleed less frequently but more severely than esophageal varices.

Treatment of Acute Esophageal Variceal Hemorrhage

The first step in the management of a patient with gastrointestinal bleeding is to assess the severity of bleeding and the patient's hemodynamic status (**Table 46.1**). Immediate and ongoing assessment of vital signs helps guide resuscitation efforts, provides important prognostic information, and assists with triage of patients to assign them to the appropriate intervention.

Resuscitation (ABC: airway, breathing, and circulation) should precede endoscopy in patients presenting with shock or hemodynamic instability. The systolic blood pressure should be above 70 mmHg before endoscopy. Two large-bore intravenous catheters should be placed immediately. The airway should be protected with endotracheal intubation if the patient has altered mental status. The target hemodynamic parameters are listed in **Table 46.2**, and a preendoscopy checklist is given in **Table 46.3**. There have been no reports specifically comparing crystalloids versus colloids in bleeding cirrhotic patients. The preferred blood product is leukocyte-depleted red cells (packed red blood cells, PRBC). Transfusion of whole blood carries a higher risk of febrile nonhemolytic reactions, infections, and immune depression. The hematocrit value, when determined soon after the onset of bleeding, may not accurately reflect the degree of blood loss. The hematocrit value will fall as extravascular fluid enters the vascular space to restore volume, a process that is not complete for 24–72 h. Overhydration can falsely depress the hematocrit. Hence, although serial hematocrit estimations are helpful, they should be integrated with the hemodynamic assessment. It is recommended that the hematocrit should be measured at least every 6 h for the first 2 days, and then every 12 h from days 3 to 5. The usual transfusion rate should be approximately one unit of PRBC per hour. Transfusion to replace the total estimated blood loss could lead to a rebound rise in portal pressure and precipitate rebleeding, as shown in experimental cirrhotic animals [24,25]. In a randomized study, 25 cirrhotic patients who were transfused aggressively with at least two units of PRBC had significantly higher rates of rebleeding in comparison with 25 similar cirrhotic patients who were transfused conservatively only for shock or hemoglobin level > 8 g/dL [26]. It is therefore advisable to use caution and transfuse blood slowly to maintain the hemoglobin around 7–8 g/dL. The use of vasopressin and somatostatin analogues may blunt an increase in portal pressure induced by volume expansion [27]. Avoiding prolonged hypotension is also equally important to prevent hepatic ischemia, infection, renal failure, and deterioration of liver function. Vital signs and urine output should be monitored closely, and in selected situations (e.g., patients with underlying cardiopulmonary disease), central venous monitoring is helpful.

The role of fresh frozen plasma (FFP) and platelet transfusions in the management of acute variceal bleeding is unclear. Generally, one unit of FFP is transfused for every four units of PRBC transfused, to replace lost coagulation factors. Mild thrombocytopenia (50 000–90 000 platelets/µL) does not usually aggravate bleeding. Recombinant activated factor VII (rVIIa, Novoseven1), which corrects prothrombin time in cirrhotic patients, has been evaluated in two randomized trials with conflicting results and is not recommended [27,28].

Nasogastric tube placement and saline lavage are generally not recommended unless endoscopic facilities are not available. It is recommended that endoscopy should be carried out as soon as possible and with therapeutic intent in patients with variceal bleeding.

Variceal bleeding can precipitate hepatic encephalopathy. However, there are no data supporting the use of prophylactic lactulose or lactitol to prevent it [29].

VI

Up to 20% of cirrhotic patients hospitalized for gastrointestinal bleeding already have a bacterial infection on admission, and another 50% develop infections during hospitalization. Short-term antibiotic prophylaxis in patients with variceal hemorrhage reduces bacterial infection [30], variceal rebleeding [31], and the risk of death [32]. Antibiotic prophylaxis significantly improves survival after acute variceal bleeding, with a mean improvement rate of 9.1% [32]. Administration of a short course of antibiotic prophylaxis (for 5–7 days) with intravenous ceftriaxone (2–4 g/day) is recommended [32].

Pharmacologic treatment of esophageal variceal hemorrhage. In suspected variceal bleeding, vasoactive drugs should be started as soon as possible, preferably within 30 min of presentation and before endoscopy [31]. Early administration of a vasoactive drug facilitates endoscopy, improves control of bleeding, and reduces the 5-day rebleeding rate. No randomized trials have compared the different pharmacologic agents. The optimal duration of vasoactive drug use is also not well established. An appropriate length of therapy would be between 2 and 5 days, to cover the duration of the highest risk of early rebleeding [33]. The only vasoactive drug shown to improve survival is terlipressin [34]. Terlipressin is associated with a significant reduction in all-cause mortality in comparison with placebo (with a 34% relative risk reduction) [35]. The combination of pharmacologic treatment with endoscopic band ligation (EBL) is the current standard of care for acute variceal hemorrhage.

Endoscopic treatment of esophageal variceal hemorrhage. Endoscopic therapy is carried out as soon as the patient is hemodynamically stable, within 6–12 h after admission [31]. Two randomized trials specifically compared EBL and sclerotherapy in acute variceal bleeding [36,37]. In one of the trials, all patients also received pharmacological therapy with somatostatin [38]. EBL was found to be more effective than sclerotherapy for the initial control of bleeding, and was associated with fewer adverse events and improved mortality. Additionally, there may be a sustained increase in portal pressure after sclerotherapy, but not EBL [39]. EBL is therefore the recommended therapy for acute esophageal bleeding, although sclerotherapy can be used in the acute setting if ligation is technically difficult [31]. Triantos et al. compared sclerotherapy and EBL for acute variceal bleeding in a recent meta-analysis including 12 trials, with 1309 patients. They found only a small increase in efficacy of 2.5% (95% CI, 0.4% to 4.6%) for EBL, but no survival difference between the two modalities [38].

Endoscopic Sclerotherapy

The injection of sclerosing solutions into esophageal varices is a method that has been used for many years [40–42]. There are two basic techniques in sclerotherapy—intravariceal injection and paravariceal injection of sclerosants.

Intravariceal injection. The objective of intravariceal injections is to initiate thrombosis and necrotizing inflammation within varices [43]. Usually, the needle catheter is advanced from 1 to 2 cm beyond the endoscope, so that any retching or sudden movement will be absorbed by the flexibility of the injector (**Fig. 46.4**). At a single site, 0.5–3.0 mL of the sclerosant is injected. Injections are usually begun at the gastroesophageal junction, working in a circumferential pattern and proceeding in a cephalad direction. Only varices in the distal third of the esophagus need to be injected [44].

Paravariceal injection. The purpose of paravariceal injections is to generate fibrosis of the esophageal mucosa overlying the varices, thus preventing them from rupturing [45]. Formation of a bleb or

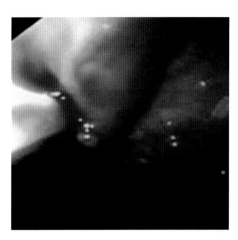

Fig. 46.4 Injection sclerotherapy. The needle is positioned inside the varix; the adjacent white fibrin clot indicates the site of recent active bleeding.

submucosal swelling is indicative of a paravariceal injection. This technique, introduced by Paquet, involves the submucosal injection of a small volume (0.5 mL) of sclerosant next to variceal columns beginning at the gastroesophageal junction [46]. Volumes of 30 to 40 mL are usually injected at each session.

Intravariceal and paravariceal sclerotherapy techniques were compared in a randomized trial including 54 patients by Sarin et al. Sclerotherapy was performed every 3 weeks. Intravariceal sclerotherapy was more effective for control of active bleeding, required fewer treatment sessions, and led to faster variceal eradication, compared to paravariceal sclerotherapy. The complication rate was the same for both groups. However, the variceal recurrence rate was lower in the paravariceal group [47]. Currently, most endoscopists prefer the intravariceal technique.

Needles and sclerosants. Needles are available in 23- and 25-G diameters and with lengths of 4 or 5 mm, and with a short bevel to prevent deep sclerosant injection. The available sclerosants are: absolute alcohol, sodium tetradecyl sulfate, sodium morrhuate, polidocanol, and ethanolamine oleate. More potent agents such as alcohol or sodium morrhuate should be used in smaller quantities. The injection of any sclerosant is optimal when an area of about 1 cm around the injection site becomes blanched. None of the sclerosants has any clear advantage over the others.

Sclerotherapy-induced esophageal wall changes. The earliest changes in the esophageal wall within the first 24 h after sclerosant injection are thrombosis in varices, submucosal edema, and minor areas of tissue necrosis. During the first week, mucosal ulceration and a marked acute polymorphonuclear leukocyte inflammatory response occur [48]. Most ulcers are limited to the submucosa or inner layer of the muscularis propria, while a few extend more deeply into the muscularis propria, particularly if the needle was positioned more deeply and the volume of the agent was more than optimal. This ulceration may persist for up to 3 weeks. This is followed by intense macrophage and fibroblast infiltration. The fibrosis is usually limited to the submucosa and the inner muscularis propria, but may occur as diffuse transmural fibrosis. Marked thickening of the esophageal wall is seen in some patients after variceal sclerotherapy [46].

Sclerotherapy schedule. The interval between treatment sessions varies between 1 and 4 weeks. Sarin et al. found that weekly sclerotherapy sessions with alcohol resulted in earlier eradication of varices in comparison with 3-weekly injections (7.1 vs. 14.9 weeks) and less recurrent bleeding. Mucosal ulceration was observed in 68% in the weekly treatment group, in comparison with 12% in the group treated every 3 weeks. However, there was no difference

46

VI

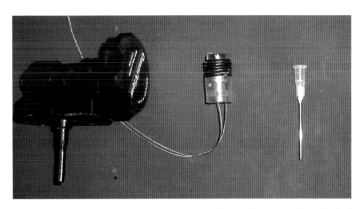

Fig. 46.5 The ligator handle, transparent cylindrical cap with six loaded bands and attached tripwire, and an adaptor for irrigating the accessory channel during endoscopy.

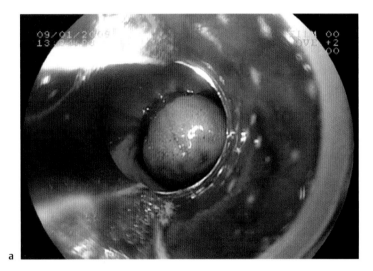

a

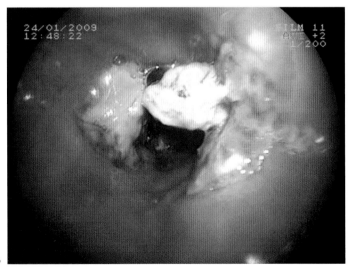

b

Fig. 46.6
a An esophageal varix that has just been banded. The band encircling the varix is seen at its base.
b The same varix after 1 week. The band is being sloughed off. A shallow ulcer has replaced the varix, which will heal by reepithelialization.

between the groups with regard to stricture formation, chest pain, or fever. The authors concluded that weekly sclerotherapy sessions with injection of a small volume at each site was the most effective schedule [44]. Usually, approximately six sclerotherapy sessions at intervals of 2 weeks are necessary to obliterate the varices.

Complications. Approximately 10% of patients undergoing sclerotherapy develop a major complication. Transient fever lasting for 24–48 h due to chemical phlebitis occurs in 25–40% of patients after sclerotherapy. If the fever persists for more than 2 days, a search for a septic or local esophageal complication is mandatory.

In 5–20% of patients, bleeding recurs before obliteration of the varices, and in another 5–20% of patients, there is recurrent bleeding after eradication of varices due to gastric varices or portal gastropathy. After obliteration, varices tend to recur over time in about 50% of individuals [49,50].

Superficial ulcers resulting from tissue necrosis are present in 90% of patients on the day after endoscopic sclerotherapy and in 70% at 1 week [51].

Endoscopic Band Ligation (EBL)

An endoscopic variceal banding device was initially introduced in 1986 by Gregory Stiegmann [52]. Band deployment at the base of a varix leads to vascular occlusion and subsequent thrombosis, necrosis, and sloughing of the varix. In experimental studies, variceal banding leads to ischemic necrosis limited to the mucosa and submucosa, with intact muscularis propria. Later, the entire submucosa at the treated sites is replaced by dense mature scar tissue, with an intact underlying muscular wall [53]. The ulcers induced by variceal banding are shallower than sclerotherapy-induced ulcers and heal faster.

Banding devices. Commercially available endoscopic banding devices include single-band and multiple-band devices. The former require the use of an overtube for repeated intubation. The components of all endoscopic band ligating devices are: a short transparent cylindrical cap that carries 1, 4, 5, 6, 7, or 10 stretched bands, a tripwire that runs from the cap through the accessory channel to the control handle, a ligator handle with a retracting spool that is fixed to the biopsy port for attachment and firing of the trip wire, and an irrigation adapter or catheter that allows irrigation of the accessory channel (**Fig. 46.5**) [54]. The transparent cap with the loaded bands attaches via friction fitting of its base to the leading end of the endoscope. The visibility with the newer transparent caps has improved by nearly 30%. The bands are made of rubber, latex free rubber, or neoprene.

Variceal banding technique. The endoscopist identifies a target varix and advances the endoscope under direct vision until the banding cylinder is in full 360° contact with the targeted varix. Once full contact is made, endoscopic suction is activated to draw the varix into the banding chamber. When the target varix has filled the chamber, as evidenced by a complete "red-out" of the visual field, the tripwire is pulled to deploy the band at the base of the varix. Suction continues in order to hold the banded varix in the chamber for a few additional seconds to allow the band to seat firmly at the base of the varix and prevent it from slipping (**Fig. 46.6a**). Bands are initially deployed distally, followed by progressive proximal placement over a length of 6–8 cm within the palisade and perforating zones. Varices in the mid-esophagus or proximal esophagus do not need to be banded. EBL can be repeated at 1-week to 4-week intervals until the varices are obliterated. The combination of EBL and sclerotherapy appears to offer no advantage over EBL alone.

Number of bands. Up to six bands can be deployed in each session. There is no advantage to deploying a higher number of bands in each session.

Complications. Common complications associated with EBL include chest pain, bleeding, dysphagia, and rarely stricture formation and perforation. Shallow ulcers at the site of banding are frequent (**Fig. 46.6b**). In a randomized and double-blinded study, it was found that patients receiving pantoprazole after elective EBL had significantly smaller post-banding ulcers on follow-up endoscopy than those receiving placebo. However, the total ulcer numbers and patient symptoms did not differ between the groups [55]. Bacteremia and infectious complications are also less frequent with EBL. EBL is difficult to perform in children who weigh less than around 8–10 kg or are under 1 year of age.

Rescue Therapies for Esophageal Variceal Bleeding

According to the Baveno IV consensus workshop, any one of the following criteria defines failure to control bleeding:
- Fresh hematemesis over 2 h after the start of specific drug treatment or therapeutic endoscopy. For patients with a nasogastric tube in place, aspiration of more than 100 mL of fresh blood represents failure.
- A drop in hemoglobin of > 3 g/dL (or a hematocrit decrease of > 9%) without transfusion.
- Adjusted blood transfusion requirement index (ABRI) > 0.75 at any time point. The ABRI is defined by: units of blood transfused / [(final hematocrit – initial hematocrit) + 0.01].

With the current recommended treatment combining vasoactive drugs, emergency EBL, and prophylactic antibiotics, 5-day therapeutic failure occurs in only 10–15% of cases. A second attempt at endoscopy and more intensive pharmacologic treatment (doubling the dose of somatostatin, or shifting to terlipressin) are justified in case of rebleeding. Failures of first-line treatment are best managed by transjugular intrahepatic portosystemic shunt (TIPS) with covered stents. Emergency shunt surgery may be an option in Child's class A patients.

Transjugular intrahepatic portosystemic shunt (TIPS) and surgical shunts. TIPS or surgical shunts (distal splenorenal shunt or 8-mm H-graft) are effective for patients with Child's class A and B cirrhosis in whom endoscopic and pharmacologic treatment have failed. A small study suggested that early TIPS placement within 24 h of hemorrhage is associated with a significant improvement in survival in patients with HVPG > 20 mmHg [56]. Early TIPS in high-risk patients may have a role and needs to be investigated. In those who are not candidates for surgery, TIPS is the only option. However, a patient with a Child–Pugh score over 13 will rarely survive in the long term after TIPS without transplantation.

Balloon tamponade. Balloon tamponade using triple lumen Sengstaken–Blakemore tube or a four-lumen Minnesota tube stops acute variceal bleeding as efficiently as sclerotherapy. The Zimmon tube allows endoscopy through the inflated rim of the balloon, which abuts the gastroesophageal junction and compresses the bleeding varices. With the widespread use of therapeutic endoscopy, the use of balloon tamponade is now very limited and the procedure is restricted to rescue therapy in patients with rebleeding or uncontrolled bleeding.

Treatment of Acute Gastric Variceal Hemorrhage

While GEV1s disappear with obliteration of esophageal varices in nearly 60% of patients, GEV2s and IGV1s require specific therapy [24]. The risk of bleeding from IGV1 was shown to correlate with variceal size (> 10 mm), Child's class, and the presence of red color

Table 46.4 Tips and tricks for gastric variceal obturation with cyanoacrylate glue

1 Preendoscopy checklist
• Cyanoacrylate glue loaded (diluted with lipiodol or undiluted) into 2-mL syringes
• Multiple syringes of distilled water loaded into 2-mL syringes
• Needle catheters of 21 G or 23 G (at least two)
• Acetone to remove accidental glue sticking to the endoscope
• Scissors to cut the injection catheter at the hub, if needed
• Goggles for endoscopist, assistants, and patient, for eye protection
• Insertion tube of the endoscope lubricated with Lipiodol, silicone oil, or Vaseline oil to prevent glue sticking
• Sengstaken–Blakemore or Linton–Nachlas tube readily available in case of uncontrolled bleeding during injection
2 Trim the injection catheter at its distal tip and advance the needle to just within the catheter tip before introduction into the endoscope *
3 The needle catheter is advanced to just beyond scope tip before retroflexion *
4 Continuous air insufflation is carried out during injection†
5 No suction during and for 20 s after the injection†
6 Slow injection of the glue‡
7 The flush volume is limited to the dead space volume of the injection catheter ‡
8 The injection volume is limited to up to 2 mL per injection ‡
9 Prompt removal of the needle from the varix after injection§

To allow easy advancement of the needle out of the injection catheter in a retroflexed endoscope position.
† To keep any spilled glue away from the endoscope.
‡ To reduce the risk of glue embolization.
§ To prevent needle impaction in the injected varix.

signs on varices [25]. Vasoactive drugs may be used initially as in acute esophageal variceal bleeding, although they have not been tested specifically in this setting. Sclerotherapy, gastric variceal obturation (GVO) with glue, thrombin, elastic band ligation, and ligation with large detachable snares have been reported in gastric variceal bleeding. Endoscopic injection of cyanoacrylate glue for gastric variceal bleeding was first reported in 1986 by Soehendra et al. and is the preferred method for treating gastric varices (**Table 46.4**) [57]. Recently, a pilot study using undiluted 2-octyl cyanoacrylate glue to obturate gastric varices has been reported [58].

Cyanoacrylate Glue

In its liquid form, cyanoacrylate consists of monomers of cyanoacrylate molecules. It rapidly undergoes exothermic polymerization in the presence of water (specifically hydroxide ions). The double bonds in the monomer become single bonds, causing them to link together in long chains, changing the liquid to a hard, brittle acrylic plastic.

Preinjection preparation. There are many different variations of the injection techniques. N-butyl-2-cyanoacrylate is injected either in undiluted form or mixed with Lipiodol to prevent premature polymerization. Undiluted glue minimizes the embolization risk, but premature solidification in the needle and needle impaction in the varix are potential problems. The glue can also be mixed with Lipiodol at a ratio of 0.5 to 0.8 mL [59]. At this dilution, polymerization of the glue is delayed by about 5–20 s [60]. Overdilution of the glue prolongs the polymerization process and thus increases the risk of embolization.

Injection catheters 23-G in size for Lipiodol-mixed glue and 21-G for undiluted glue are ideal. Before injection of undiluted glue, some endoscopists flush the needle with Lipiodol followed by air to allow Lipiodol coating of the catheter lumen so that glue polymerization

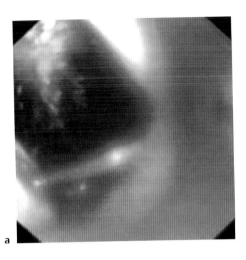

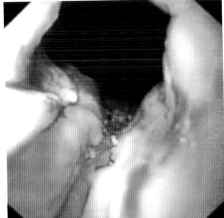

Fig. 46.7
a A GEV2 ("junctional") varix with spurting bleeding.
b Cyanoacrylate glue is being injected in an antegrade position to achieve hemostasis.

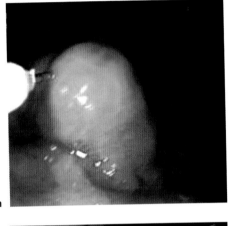

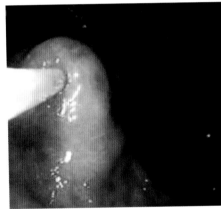

Fig. 46.8 Gastric variceal obturation with cyanoacrylate glue.
a The gastric varix is approached with a needle catheter.
b The varix is punctured, and glue is injected.
c The needle is retracted into the sheath, with continued flushing of the catheter. Note the small amount of glue spillage.
d The needle is withdrawn away from the injected varix. Some extravasated glue is visible on the varix.

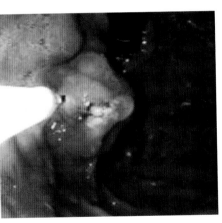

within the needle can be prevented. When Lipiodol is mixed with the glue, this step is probably not necessary. Lipiodol, silicone oil, or vaseline oil can also be used to lubricate the insertion tube of the endoscope and the injection catheter to prevent sticking of the glue to the endoscope. The needle sometimes does not exit the catheter with the scope in the retroflexed position. This can be avoided by trimming the sheath by a few millimeters, advancing the needle to just within the catheter tip before introduction, preloading the catheter before scope retroflexion, and gently jiggling the catheter after pushing it out of the scope.

Cyanoacrylate glue injection—technique. Injection can be carried out using an "end-on" endoscopic view for GEV1s and some patients with GEV2s (**Fig. 46.7**). For injection of most GEV2s or IGV1s, however, a retroflexed endoscopic approach is recommended. After the gastric varices have been punctured, the glue (or mixture) is in-

jected, followed by distilled water to deliver the entire glue from the catheter into the varix. The volume of distilled water should be equal to slightly more than the dead space of the needle catheter. The entire injection process must be slow and controlled to prevent glue embolization. Although cyanoacrylate has a viscosity similar to that of water, the addition of Lipiodol increases the viscosity considerably. A 2-mL syringe should be used for the injection to allow rapid injection of the glue. The needle is retracted, followed by continued flushing with distilled water to keep it patent. During the injection process, the endoscopist should continuously insufflate air and avoid suction to keep any excess glue from getting sucked into the endoscope. The needle should be withdrawn immediately after the glue injection to prevent it from impacting in the tissue adhesive (**Fig. 46.8**).

To minimize the risk of embolism, no more than 2.0 mL of the *N*-butyl-2-cyanoacrylate–Lipiodol mixture is injected into the varix each time. The injections can be repeated several times, but the volume of each injection is limited to 2.0 mL. The glue injection must be strictly intravariceal to prevent tissue ulceration.

Postinjection evaluation. Obturation of the gastric varices is assessed by blunt palpation of the varices with the injection catheter. If the varix remains soft, the injection is repeated. An attempt is made to obliterate all varices in the same session. A repeat endoscopy is carried out after 3–4 days. This is because 3–4 days after injection, mucosal necrosis develops around the site of injection and rebleeding may occur from any remaining patent gastric varices. Ultimately, the glue is extruded as a cast from the gastric varices after several months, and the injection site reepithelializes with scar formation (**Fig. 46.9**) [60].

Complications of glue injection. Although rare, the complications of GVO include pulmonary, cerebral, and coronary embolization, and clinicians should have a high index of suspicion for embolism in the setting of tachycardia, chest pain, cough, dyspnea, or hypoxia after a patient undergoes endoscopic injection therapy with cyanoacrylate glue. Other complications include portal vein, splenic vein, and left renal vein thrombosis, splenic infarction, bacteremia, and the needle becoming stuck in the varix [60]. Care needs to be taken to protect the eyes of all personnel as well as the patient, with goggles being used during the injection process.

With GVO, the rate of control of active bleeding has been reported to range from 93% to 100% of patients, and the rate of recurrent bleeding is generally very low. Huang et al. reported a 94% hemostasis rate in 90 patients with active or recent variceal bleeding from fundal varices. Tumorous gastric varices had a higher rebleeding rate than the tortuous and nodular-type ones (34.4% versus 17.2%) [61]. The largest series of GVO using cyanoacrylate glue was reported recently by Seewald et al. from two centers in Germany and Egypt, including 131 patients. The mean number of sessions for GVO was one (range one to three). The mean total volume of glue mixture used was 4.0 mL (range 1–13 mL). There were no procedure-related complications or bleeding-related deaths. At 1, 3, and 5 years, 94.5%, 89.3%, and 82.9% of the patients, respectively, were free of bleeding [62].

A single randomized controlled trial has compared GVO and sclerotherapy with alcohol [63], and two randomized controlled trials have compared GVO and EBL in bleeding gastric varices [64,65]. All three trials show that GVO was more effective in controlling acute hemorrhage and was associated with lower rebleeding and complication rates. EBL of gastric varices can be performed in both retroflexed and nonretroflexed scope positions. Most authors have applied up to four bands in one session. Esophageal varices have also been banded in the same session. Although effective in controlling active gastric variceal bleeding, endoscopic sclerotherapy or banding of a gastric varix does not achieve complete thrombosis of gastric varices, and may induce massive rebleeding. Gastric varices are usually two or three times larger than esophageal varices and are directly connected to dilated left gastric or posterior gastric veins [66]. The volume of blood flow through gastric varices is greater than that through the esophageal varices. If blood flow in the gastric varices cannot be stopped completely, bleeding may recur from the site of the resultant post-EBL ulcer. It may therefore be dangerous to treat gastric varices using EBL.

Endoscopic ligation [67] and detachable snares [68] have also been used by some groups to control acute gastric variceal bleeding. However, limited efficacy data are available.

Kojima et al. suggested the combined use of 5% ethanolamine as a sclerosant with vasopressin infusion, which improved the retention of the ethanolamine in the gastric varices. After the needle was removed, the puncture site was additionally sprayed with thrombin glue to prevent puncture-site bleeding [69]. In another recent study,

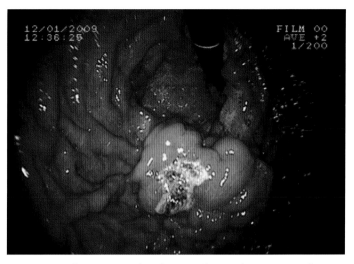

Fig. 46.9 A glue cast extruding from an obturated gastric varix that was injected several months previously.

paravariceal injections of hypertonic glucose solutions were used to obliterate residual small gastric varices and prevent recurrence after initial GVO with cyanoacrylate glue [70].

Thrombin Glue

Fibrin sealants are derived from blood plasma and contain fibrinogen and thrombin. Fibrin clots formed from fibrin sealants are similar to normal blood clots. Bovine thrombin was originally used, but owing to the risk of prion transmission, human thrombin has since been adopted.

Assembly and injection. Thrombin injections need time for preparation and assembly of the injection system. The Beriplast-P Combi-Set (Aventis Behring Ltd., Marburg, Germany) is available in packages of 0.5, 1.0, and 3.0 mL. Each set contains two parts: one containing 500 IU of thrombin as a lyophilized powder (in a red vial) with its reconstituent, and the other containing 90 mg of fibrinogen as a lyophilized powder (in a blue vial) with its reconstituent. Thrombin injection sets should be stored in the refrigerator at 2–8 °C and need a period of time to reach room temperature (4 min for the 1-mL size and 30 min for the 3-mL pack) before they can be used. After reconstitution, the thrombin and fibrinogen are loaded into their respective color-coded syringes. The syringes are loaded into a syringe holder and connected with a Y-piece, which is then connected to the injector. Both thrombin and fibrinogen are injected together after accurate needle placement into the varix. Beriplast-P forms a fibrin clot at the needle tip immediately after injection through a double-lumen needle.

Efficacy. Three uncontrolled case series with human thrombin have been reported. Dutta et al. used Beriplast in 15 patients with acute gastric variceal bleeding. Bleeding was controlled in 11 patients in a single session and in three patients with two sessions. None of the patients had any injection-induced complications [71]. Heneghan et al. reported that with a median dose of 6 mL, Beriplast injection achieved immediate hemostasis in seven of 10 patients (70%) with acute gastric variceal bleeding, with a single injection. After a median follow-up period of 8 months, there had been no episodes of recurrent bleeding from the gastric varices [72]. Yang et al. reported Beriplast injection in 12 patients who presented with acute gastric variceal bleeding. Hemostasis in the acute setting was successful in nine patients. The patients received one to four sessions, with a mean total dose of 1833 U (range: 800–4000 U) [73].

46

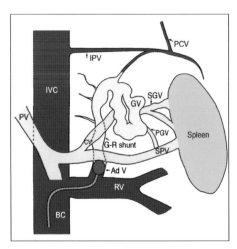

Fig. 46.10 Balloon-occluded retrograde transvenous obliteration (BRTO). BC, balloon catheter; CV, coronary or left gastric vein; G–R shunt, gastrorenal shunt; GV, gastric varices; IPV, inferior phrenic vein; IVC, inferior vena cava; PCV, posterior cardiophrenic vein; PGV, posterior gastric vein; PV, portal vein; RV, left renal vein; SGV, short gastric veins; SPV, splenic vein.

Safety. No adverse reactions have been reported in any of the series. In particular, no thrombosis distant from the injection site has been reported.

Rescue Therapies for Gastric Variceal Bleeding

Balloon tamponade. The gastric balloon with the Sengstaken-Blakemore tube has an inflated volume of 200–250 mL and may not be effective for tamponading gastric varices. The Linton–Nachlas balloon, which has a volume of 600 mL, has been shown to be more effective for achieving hemostasis in gastric variceal bleeding.

Transjugular intrahepatic portosystemic shunt (TIPS). TIPS has been recommended for acute bleeding from gastric varices when GVO is unavailable or has failed. TIPS is very effective in the treatment of bleeding gastric varices, with a success rate of more than 90% for initial hemostasis and a low rebleeding rate [74,75].

Balloon-occluded retrograde transvenous obliteration (BRTO). BRTO is performed by inserting a balloon catheter into the outflow shunt of the gastric varices (gastrorenal or gastrocaval shunt) via the femoral or internal jugular vein (**Fig. 46.10**). Any additional large collateral draining veins are occluded with coils or small amounts of sclerosants first. The balloon is inflated in the outflow shunt, and a test dose of contrast is injected to determine the optimal volume of sclerosant that will be required. Five percent ethanolamine oleate is slowly injected to fill the shunt and the varix. Long-term eradication of gastric varices that have been treated has been reported by most centers, without recurrences [76].

Since BRTO also obliterates the large portosystemic shunt, additional benefits such as decreased blood ammonia levels and improved encephalopathy are sometimes observed. On the other hand, due to the elevation of the portal pressure, transient ascites, increase of ascites, pleural effusion, and the appearance or enlargement of esophageal varices may be seen [70]. Many researchers believe that BRTO should be used only after initial hemostasis of bleeding gastric varices either with GVO or tamponade by a gastric balloon.

Transportal obliteration. Percutaneous transhepatic obliteration and transileocolic vein obliteration can be used.

Partial splenic artery embolization. The femoral arterial route is used for superselective catheterization of the splenic artery. The catheter tip is placed distally in either the splenic hilum or in an intrasplenic artery. Embolization is achieved by injecting gelatin sponge cubes suspended in saline.

Prophylaxis

Prevention of Development of Varices: Pre-Primary Prophylaxis

A large multicenter placebo-controlled trial showed that nonselective beta-blockers such as timolol are not effective in preventing the development of varices in patients with portal hypertension (HVPG > 6 mmHg) [14]. There is no indication at present to treat patients to prevent the formation of varices.

Prevention of Growth of Varices: Early Primary Prophylaxis

Variceal size progresses at a rate of 5–12% per year, and the rate is higher in patients with severe liver disease. In a randomized trial, the growth of small esophageal varices was shown to be slower in patients treated with nadolol [77]. Non-selective beta-blocker prophylaxis to prevent variceal enlargement or bleeding may be started in patients with compensated cirrhosis with small varices [12]. There is no role for EBL in preventing enlargement or bleeding in patients with small varices. Since high-risk small esophageal varices (with red signs or Child–Turcotte–Pugh class C status) can bleed at a similar rate to large varices, these patients should receive non-selective beta-blockers [78].

Prevention of First Variceal Hemorrhage: Primary Prophylaxis

Non-selective beta-blockers cause a decrease in portal pressure and collateral blood flow via the blockade of both the β_1-adrenoreceptors, causing a reduction in cardiac output, and the β_2-adrenoreceptors in the splanchnic vasculature, causing splanchnic vasoconstriction. The starting dose of propranolol is 20 mg twice a day, which is incrementally increased to achieve a target heart rate reduction to 55 beats per minute. The starting dose of nadolol is 40 mg once daily, and the dose can be increased to 160 mg once daily.

In patients with large esophageal varices, both non-selective beta-blockers and EBL are effective. Non-selective beta-blockers reduce the risk of bleeding from 25% to 15%, with a relative risk reduction of 40%. The number needed to treat (NNT) with non-selective beta-blockers to prevent variceal hemorrhage in one patient is 10 [79]. Non-selective beta-blockers may have additional benefits of preventing bleeding from portal hypertensive gastropathy and gastric varices, and may also reduce the incidence of spontaneous bacterial peritonitis [80]. However, an adequate hemodynamic response to non-selective beta-blocker is seen in only 20–30% of patients. Another 10–20% patients cannot tolerate these drugs. EBL reduces the risk of bleeding from 23% to 14%, with an NNT of 11. A large number of trials and several meta-analyses have confirmed the benefits of EBL and its superiority over non-selective beta-blockers in preventing first variceal bleeds [81]. EBL is associated with a significantly lower incidence of first variceal hemorrhage in comparison with non-selective beta-blocker therapy; however, there is no mortality benefit.

A combination of non-selective beta-blockers and EBL or non-selective beta-blockers and nitrates does not confer any added advantage for primary prevention of esophageal variceal hemorrhage over non-selective beta-blockers alone or EBL alone [81,82].

There is a lack of data regarding the risk of bleeding from gastric varices after an episode of bleeding from esophageal varices—whether eradication of esophageal varices increases the risk of subsequent bleeding from gastric varices, and whether nonbleeding gastric varices that accompany bleeding esophageal varices should be prophylactically treated. No firm recommendations can therefore be given regarding prophylactic treatment of gastric varices, and treatment protocols vary from center to center. At present, decision-making on whether to treat gastric varices prophylactically should take into account their size, the presence of red color signs, Child grade, and the patient's access to cyanoacrylate treatment in the event of sudden hemorrhage [33].

There are now some data suggesting that BRTO could be offered to patients with large gastric varices in order to prevent the first variceal bleed. Akahoshi et al. reported that among 48 patients with risky gastric varices who received prophylactic BRTO treatment, the 8-year cumulative bleeding rate was 0% [82].

Prevention of Recurrent Variceal Hemorrhage: Secondary Prophylaxis

Our group observed faster variceal eradication, but a higher recurrence rate, with EBL in comparison with sclerotherapy for secondary prophylaxis [83]. A higher rate of variceal recurrence with EBL probably results from the fact that ligation does not occlude the perforators. The incidence of portal hypertensive gastropathy was higher after sclerotherapy than after EBL (20.5% versus 2.3%).

For secondary prophylaxis of variceal hemorrhage, the options include EBL alone, non-selective beta-blockers alone, a combination of EBL and non-selective beta-blockers, and a combination of nitrates with non-selective beta-blockers.

In comparison with sclerotherapy, EBL reduces the relative risk of rebleeding by 37% and the absolute risk by 13%, with an NNT of eight [84]. Non-selective beta-blockers reduce the relative risk of bleeding by 33%, with an NNT of 4.8 [79]. A combination of nitrates with non-selective beta-blockers was found by Sarin et al. to have similar efficacy to that EBL alone [85]. Two randomized controlled trials have demonstrated that a combination of non-selective beta-blockers plus EBL is superior to EBL alone in preventing recurrent variceal bleeding [50,86]. A recent meta-analysis including 23 trials with a total of 1860 patients concluded that a combination of endoscopic and drug therapy reduces variceal rebleeding in cirrhosis more than either therapy alone. The additive effects were independent of the endoscopic procedure (sclerotherapy or EBL) [87]. Non-selective beta-blockers can protect against rebleeding before complete variceal obliteration and may also prevent variceal recurrence. However, in a recent large trial, a combination of both non-selective beta-blockers and nitrates with EBL was not found to be superior to EBL alone in preventing variceal rebleeding [88].

There is no agreement on the optimal interval between banding sessions. The "interbanding interval" has varied from 1 week [89] to 1 month [90] among the reported series. Generally, a 2–3-week interval between EBL sessions is chosen in practice.

Many researchers have evaluated a combination of EBL with sclerotherapy during the same session (synchronous combination) for obliteration of esophageal varices. Laine et al. [91] and Saeed et al. [92] found that ligation alone was as effective, with fewer complications. On the other hand, to reduce the high rate of variceal recurrence after EBL, the concept of complementing EBL with sclerotherapy in metachronous fashion has found support [93].

After variceal eradication, follow-up endoscopy should be performed after 1–3 months, then 3 months later, and then at 6–12-monthly intervals, depending on variceal recurrence [81]. For patients on non-selective beta-blockers alone for secondary prophylaxis, a baseline and repeat HVPG needs to be done to assess the response to therapy. Follow-up endoscopies may be indirectly helpful if a distinct reduction in variceal size is observed.

TIPS provides a salvage therapy for those who experience recurrent bleeding despite secondary prophylaxis with EBL and non-selective beta-blocker. A large multicenter trial of TIPS versus distal splenorenal shunt showed similar rates of rebleeding, encephalopathy, and mortality in patients with Child's class A and B cirrhosis in whom pharmacologic and endoscopic treatment had failed. A higher rate of shunt dysfunction was found in the TIPS group [94].

In summary, our understanding of the pathophysiology of portal hypertension and variceal bleeding has significantly improved during the last 10 years. This has translated into more aggressive use of vasoactive agents and endoscopic procedures to treat variceal bleeding. Control of both esophageal and gastric variceal bleeding is now very effective with current treatments, and the frequency of rebleeding has been modestly reduced. However, post-EBL ulcers and the limited response to current non-selective beta-blocker drugs in the prevention of development, growth, or first bleeding from varices are still major challenges. The overall mortality from variceal bleeding has shown a decline, and it is hoped that with the wider availability and application of hemodynamic criteria such as HVPG, the treatment of variceal bleeding will substantially improve in the future.

Nonvariceal Upper Gastrointestinal Bleeding

Justin C.Y. Wu and Joseph J.Y. Sung

46

Introduction

Upper gastrointestinal bleeding refers to bleeding in the gastrointestinal tract anywhere from the proximal esophagus to the duodenum above the Ampulla of Vater. It is one of the most common gastrointestinal emergencies throughout the world and is associated with significant morbidity and mortality. Peptic ulcer is the most important cause of nonvariceal upper gastrointestinal bleeding (**Figs. 46.11–46.14**). Other less common causes included Mallory–Weiss syndrome, gastroduodenal erosions, esophagitis and esophageal ulcers, Dieulafoy lesions, and gastroesophageal tumors.

Preendoscopy Management

The initial evaluation involves an assessment of hemodynamic stability, resuscitation, management of complications secondary to bleeding, and exclusion of contraindications of endoscopy such as

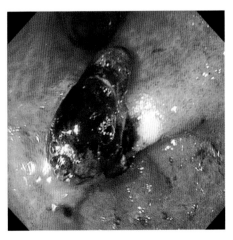

Fig. 46.11 An angular ulcer with clots.

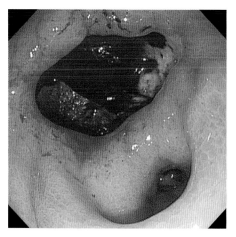
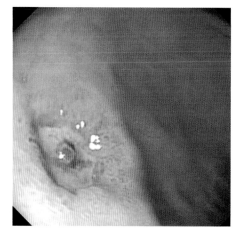
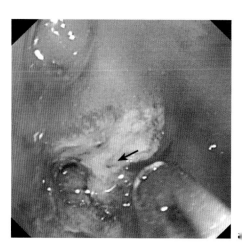

Fig. 46.12 An antral ulcer.

Fig. 46.13
a A gastric ulcer with a visible vessel.
b The same ulcer after heater-probe treatment.

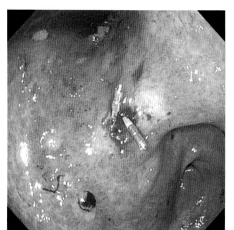

Fig. 46.14 Hemoclips on an ulcer.

Table 46.5 Stigmata of recent hemorrhage for peptic ulcer [101]

Type	Endoscopic appearance
Ia	Spurting
Ib	Active oozing
IIa	Visible vessel (no active bleeding)
IIb	Adherent clot (no visible vessel)
IIc	Pigmented spot
III	Clean base

Table 46.6 Outcome of bleeding peptic ulcers relative to the endoscopic appearance [103]

	Prevalence % (range)	Rebleeding % (range)	Surgery % (range)	Mortality % (range)
Clean base	42 (19–52)	5 (0–10)	0.5 (0–3)	2 (0–3)
Flat pigmented spot	20 (0–42)	10 (0–13)	6 (0–10)	3 (0–10)
Adherent clot	17 (0–49)	22 (14–36)	10 (5–12)	7 (0–10)
Protuberant vessel	17 (4–35)	43 (0–81)	34 (0–56)	11 (0–21)
Active bleeding	18 (4–26)	55 (17–100)	35 (20–69)	11 (0–23)

perforation [95]. Endoscopy remains the most important tool for diagnosis and intervention and should be performed within 24 h after admission. There are many scoring systems for risk stratification of patients in order to predict various clinical outcomes, such as the need for early endoscopic hemostasis, rebleeding after endoscopy, the safety of early discharge, and mortality [96]. The Rockall score is the most widely used risk score and includes clinical variables such as age, presence of shock, and comorbidity, as well as endoscopic variables such as diagnosis and stigmata of recent hemorrhage (SRH) [97]. The Rockall score has been shown to be accurate in predicting mortality, but it is less well validated for predicting rebleeding. The Blatchford score uses preendoscopic clinical and laboratory variables only to predict the need for clinical intervention [98]. It has been shown to be more sensitive than the Rockall score for identifying patients in need of endoscopic intervention. In addition, nasogastric tube lavage that yields blood or material resembling coffee-grounds predicts the presence of high-risk lesions. On the basis of these assessments, patients who are at low risk for rebleeding can be safely discharged early after endoscopy. It has been shown that a single dose of intravenous erythromycin 1–2 h before endoscopy in patients with recent hematemesis promotes gastric emptying of blood, improves visibility, and shortens the endoscopy time, thereby reducing the need for a repeat procedure [99].

Peptic Ulcer

Peptic ulcer disease is the most common cause of nonvariceal upper gastrointestinal bleeding. *Helicobacter pylori* infection and nonsteroidal anti-inflammatory drugs (NSAIDs) are the two most common causes of peptic ulcer. Stress-related ulcer is also a common cause of upper gastrointestinal bleeding in hospitalized patients with severe medical conditions. Peptic ulcer may rarely be caused by Zollinger–Ellison syndrome. Peptic ulcer bleeding stops spontaneously in 80% of cases, and most patients do not rebleed during hospitalization. A subset of patients with recurrent or massive hematemesis, age over 60, comorbid illness, bleeding that develops after hospital admission for another medical condition, and those with coagulopathy are at higher risk of rebleeding and have a higher mortality rate [100].

The endoscopic appearance of ulcers is strongly predictive of the risk of recurrent bleeding, requirement for surgery, and mortality. Large ulcers (> 2 cm) are more likely to rebleed. The Forrest classification further stratifies patients and predicts the risk of rebleeding on the basis of various stigmata of recent hemorrhage (SRH) (**Tables 46.5, 46.6**) [101–103]. While there is excellent agreement regarding spurting and oozing bleeding, interobserver agreement on the endoscopic assessment of nonbleeding visible vessels, adherent clot, and flat pigmented spots is very poor even among experienced endoscopists [104].

Endoscopic hemostasis is the first-line therapy for ulcers with stigmata of hemorrhage. Injection, thermocoagulation, and hemoclips can successfully stop bleeding in 85–90% of cases. Current evidence suggests that there are no significant differences in the rates of initial hemostasis, rebleeding, surgical intervention, or mortality between these modalities [105,106]. High-dose intravenous infusion of proton-pump inhibitors (PPIs) has revolutionized the management of peptic ulcer bleeding. Preemptive administration of intravenous PPIs before endoscopy accelerates the resolution of stigmata of hemorrhage and reduces the need for endoscopic therapy [107]. It has also been shown to be a cost-effective strategy [108]. After endoscopic treatment of bleeding peptic ulcers, intravenous PPIs substantially reduce the risk of recurrent bleeding [109]. A scheduled second-look endoscopy and repeat treatment may further reduce the risk of rebleeding in patients with Forrest I and IIa ulcers [110].

Despite the effectiveness of endoscopic hemostasis and intravenous PPIs, ulcer rebleeding occurs in about 10–15% of cases. A second attempt at endoscopic treatment is still successful in three-quarters of patients with rebleeding. However, large ulcers (> 2 cm) and the presence of hypotension when rebleeding occurs are predictive of the failure of endoscopic treatment, and early surgery is preferable [111]. Angiographic intervention with transcatheter arterial infusion of vasoconstrictive agents (e.g., vasopressin) or embolization of particulate matter has been shown to be as effective as surgery for treatment of rebleeding with failure of endoscopic hemostasis [112]. This approach has a long-term clinical success rate of about 60–80% and may be associated with lower rate of major complications.

Proton-pump inhibitors are the treatment of choice for healing of bleeding peptic ulcers. Eradication of *H. pylori* prevents the recurrence of both duodenal and gastric ulcer bleeding, and long-term acid-suppressive therapy is not required after successful eradication of the bacterium [113]. For patients with aspirin-induced ulcer bleeding, *H. pylori* eradication alone effectively prevents recurrent ulcer bleeding without the need for proton-pump inhibitors [114]. For patients who do not have *H. pylori* infection, aspirin in combination with a proton-pump inhibitor is superior to clopidogrel in preventing recurrent ulcer bleeding [115]. In contrast to aspirin-related peptic ulcer bleeding, prophylactic cotherapy with proton-pump inhibitors or misoprostol is necessary for NSAID-related ulcer bleeding [114]. Cyclooxygenase-2 (COX-2) inhibitors have a better gastrointestinal toxicity profile in comparison with nonselective NSAIDs [116]. Combination treatment with a COX-2 inhibitor and a proton-pump inhibitor provides the most effective prevention for patients who are at very high risk for recurrent NSAID ulcer bleeding [117]. However, long-term use of COX-2 inhibitors is limited by the associated increase in cardiovascular risk [118].

Gastric and Duodenal Erosion and Hemorrhage

The histological definition of an erosion is a break in the mucosa that does not penetrate the muscularis mucosae into the submucosa. However, endoscopy is unable to predict the depth of erosion reliably. This is reflected in an interobserver agreement rate of only 55% with regard to the types of lesion present in patients receiving NSAIDs [119]. In practice, most endoscopists define an erosion as an area of adherent hemorrhage or a defect in the mucosa with a necrotic base that is less that 3 mm in depth. At endoscopy, the lesions are generally multiple, with white bases, and they are commonly encircled by erythematous mucosa. In general, larger lesions

(> 5 mm) are more likely to involve the muscularis mucosae, while small lesions (≤ 3 mm) are more likely to be superficial erosions. Subepithelial or intramural hemorrhage refers to an appearance of discrete petechiae or bright red streaks and patches that are not associated with any visible break in the mucosa.

Important causes of gastroduodenal erosion and hemorrhage include alcohol, corrosive agents, nasogastric tube injury, severe medical conditions such as burns, medications such as NSAIDs, aspirin, bisphosphonate, potassium chloride, iron, chemotherapeutic agents, and cocaine. Aspirin and NSAIDs are the most important causes of acute bleeding from hemorrhagic and erosive gastritis. In recent years, bariatric procedures have become a common cause of gastric erosions. Vertical-banded gastroplasty and laparoscopic adjustable gastric banding have been reported to cause erosion of the bands into the gastric wall, and this is further complicated with bleeding [120].

Gastritis and erosions account for 15–20% of cases of upper gastrointestinal hemorrhage, but the bleeding is rarely serious or life-threatening, as subepithelial hemorrhage and erosion are confined to the gastric mucosa, in which the vessels are usually small. Exposure to noxious agents should be avoided. H_2-receptor antagonists and proton-pump inhibitors are effective in healing gastroduodenal erosions.

Mallory–Weiss Syndrome

Mallory–Weiss syndrome refers to longitudinal mucosal tears in the distal esophagus at the gastroesophageal junction, with bleeding originating from submucosal veins or arteries underlying the lacerations. It is usually associated with forceful retching and vomiting. Other rare causes include epileptic convulsions, blunt abdominal injury, and gastroscopy. Heavy alcohol intake and presence of hiatus hernia may predispose to Mallory–Weiss tears. The condition accounts for approximately 5% of cases of acute upper gastrointestinal bleeding.

Mallory–Weiss syndrome usually presents with hematemesis preceded by a history of bloodless vomiting or retching. The bleeding stops spontaneously in 90% of patients, and in most cases the mucosal tear heals spontaneously within 24–48 h. However, massive bleeding is not uncommon, especially in patients with portal hypertension and coagulopathy. Endoscopic therapy is required when there are risk factors such as a bleeding diathesis, evidence of active bleeding such as hematemesis and hemodynamic instability, or presence of stigmata of recurrent bleeding such as visible vessels or adherent clots. Endoscopic injection of epinephrine or saline has been the treatment of choice for Mallory–Weiss tears. Endoscopic clipping has been shown to have a comparable success rate for initial hemostasis and even a lower rebleeding rate in comparison with injection [121,122]. It may be the preferred treatment when there is deeper extension of Mallory–Weiss tears, with esophageal perforation. Other less commonly used modalities include electrocoagulation and ligation. However, thermal coagulation is contraindicated in patients with portal hypertension, as it may provoke variceal bleeding. It is also important to apply less tamponade force and total energy in order to avoid transmural burning and esophageal perforation. Angiographic arterial embolization and surgical oversewing of the bleeding vessel are occasionally used to control severe bleeding.

Esophagitis and Esophageal Ulcers

Gastroesophageal reflux disease (GERD) accounts for the majority of cases of esophagitis (**Fig. 46.15**) and ulcers. Other causes include nasogastric tube injury, corrosives, irradiation, infection (e.g., with

46

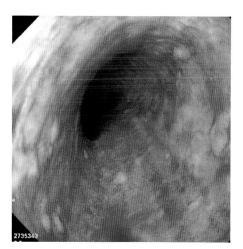

Fig. 46.15 Circumferential esophagitis.

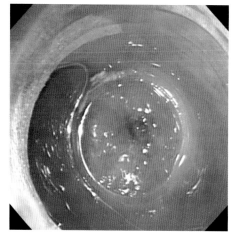
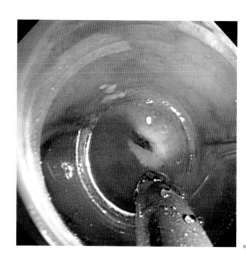

Fig. 46.16
a An antral Dieulafoy lesion.
b The same lesion after heater-probe treatment.

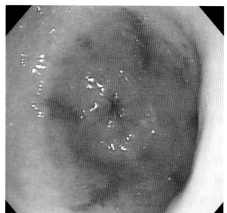

Fig. 46.17 Gastric antral vascular ectasia (GAVE).

Candida species, herpesvirus, cytomegalovirus), and drug-induced injury (tetracycline, bisphosphonate, iron tablets). Injection sclerotherapy and variceal ligation almost always produce esophageal ulcers and occasionally bleeding. Idiopathic esophageal ulcer can be complicated by severe bleeding in patients with human immunodeficiency virus infection of any status. Esophagitis itself seldom causes severe upper gastrointestinal bleeding. On the other hand, severe bleeding may result from large esophageal ulcers due to cytomegalovirus infection and radiation injuries. Endoscopic injection therapy is the mainstay of treatment for bleeding.

Dieulafoy Lesion

A Dieulafoy lesion is a dilated aberrant submucosal vessel eroding into the mucosal surface in the absence of an ulcer. Dieulafoy lesions are typically located in the proximal stomach, along the lesser curvature or gastric fundus, but they may also occur in other parts of the gastrointestinal tract such as the esophagus, duodenum, and colon. The etiology of Dieulafoy lesions is probably ischemic, and bleeding is more commonly seen in patients with cardiovascular comorbidities or NSAID use. Dieulafoy lesions account for less than 1% of all cases of upper gastrointestinal bleeding. The condition is often self-limiting, but life-threatening arterial bleeding occurs in approximately 10% of cases.

Endoscopic diagnosis of Dieulafoy lesions may be difficult, as there is no ulcer base indicating the source of bleeding and the lesion may be obscured by profuse bleeding. The condition presents with active bleeding from relatively normal-looking mucosa, or with a raised nipple or visible vessel without an associated ulcer in the absence of active bleeding. Endoscopic ultrasonography (EUS) may be useful in confirming the diagnosis by detecting the aberrant vessel [123].

Epinephrine injection followed by thermal coagulation is the treatment of choice for acute hemostasis [124] (**Fig. 46.16**). However, rebleeding may occur in up to 40% of cases, and tattooing with Indian ink is therefore helpful for locating the site if rebleeding occurs. Hemoclips, band ligation, and argon plasma coagulation have all been described for control of bleeding from Dieulafoy lesions [125–127]. Surgical wedge resection of the involved gut segment is reserved for bleeding that is refractory to endoscopic treatment.

Gastric Antral Vascular Ectasia

Gastric antral vascular ectasia (GAVE), also known as watermelon stomach, is a variant of gastric vascular ectasia. These lesions represent ectatic mucosal vessels and resemble those in portal hypertensive gastropathy. Most cases of GAVE are idiopathic, but it has been associated with cirrhosis and systemic sclerosis [128]. There are two distinct endoscopic forms of GAVE [129,130]. The classic form is characterized by multiple linear flat, reddish stripes radiating from the pylorus into the antrum (**Fig. 46.17**). Punctate-type vascular ectasia tends to have diffuse antral angiomas and is strongly associated with cirrhosis. GAVE primarily affects patients over the age of 70. It accounts for less than 1% of all cases of upper gastrointestinal bleeding. Patients usually present with iron-deficiency anemia and a positive fecal occult blood test. The diagnosis can be confirmed using endoscopic biopsy, which shows vascular ectasia in the antral mucosa, fibrohyalinosis, and spindle cell proliferation [131]. Bleeding from GAVE can also be localized by red cell scan.

Bleeding from GAVE can be managed conservatively by transfusion. The vascular ectasia can also be obliterated by various endoscopic treatment methods such as heater probe, argon plasma coagulation, or band ligation [132]. Despite its association with cirrhosis and portal hypertension, TIPS and portosystemic shunts often fail to control bleeding from GAVE. Antrectomy is the surgical treatment of choice for patients in whom endoscopic treatment fails.

Upper Gastrointestinal Tumors

Acute bleeding is often a complication of advanced gastric neoplasia, when the tumor causes mucosal ulceration or erodes into a blood vessel. Gastric carcinoma is the cause of the majority of cases of bleeding gastric tumor. Gastric lymphoma and gastrointestinal stromal tumor (GIST) account for the remaining cases [133,134]. Endoscopic methods for controlling bleeding include injection therapy, thermal coagulation, and laser therapy, but these measures are only temporary and recurrent bleeding is common [135]. The prognosis is poor for advanced gastric carcinoma, but low-grade lymphomas of the large cell type and GISTs have a better prognosis. Palliative resection of gastric carcinoma is the treatment of choice for recurrent bleeding. Surgery or radiotherapy is indicated for advanced local lymphoma. Segmental surgical resection is generally indicated for GISTs > 2 cm in size, as they have an increased malignant potential and risk of complications. Tyrosine kinase inhibitors such as imatinib or sunitinib reduce the recurrence rate and progression in patients with GIST [136].

Other Rare Causes of Nonvariceal Upper Gastrointestinal Bleeding

Hemobilia, or bleeding from the hepatobiliary tract, should be considered in a patient with liver parenchymal or biliary tract pathology, injury, or following procedures such as liver biopsy, percutaneous transhepatic cholangiography, and angioembolization. Other features of hemobilia include biliary colic and obstructive jaundice [137]. Hemosuccus pancreaticus refers to bleeding from the pancreatic duct. It occurs when a pancreatic lesion such as a pseudocyst or tumor erodes into a vessel, creating a communication between the pancreatic duct and a blood vessel [138]. It is also rarely caused by diseases of retroperitoneal structures such as splenic artery aneurysms. Transcatheter angiography and intervention are the treatment of choice for bleeding into the biliary tree or pancreatic duct. Aortoenteric fistulas may be caused by atherosclerotic aortic aneurysms, infected prosthetic abdominal aortic vascular grafts, penetrating peptic ulcer, tumor invasion, radiotherapy, and foreign-body perforation. The distal duodenum is the most common site for aortoenteric fistulas, which should be considered with a high index of suspicion in patients with a history of aortic aneurysm or prosthetic vascular grafting who present with massive upper gastrointestinal bleeding and exsanguination [139].

References

1. Vianna A, Hayes PC, Moscoso G, Driver M, Portmann B, Westaby D, et al. Normal venous circulation of the gastroesophageal junction. A route to understanding varices. Gastroenterology 1987;93:876–89.
2. McCormack TT, Smith PM, Rose JD, Johnson AG. Perforating veins and blood flow in oesophageal varices. Lancet 1983;2:1442–46.
3. Kimura K, Ohto M, Matsutani S, Furuse J, Hoshino K, Okuda K. Relative frequencies of portosystemic pathways and renal shunt formation through the "posterior" gastric vein: portographic study in 460 patients. Hepatology 1990;12:725–8.
4. Kiyosue H, Mori H, Matsumoto S, Yamada Y, Hori Y, Okino Y. Transcatheter obliteration of gastric varices. Part 1. Anatomic classification. Radiographics 2003;23:911–20.
5. Dagradi AE. The natural history of esophageal varices in patients with alcoholic liver cirrhosis. An endoscopic and clinical study. Am J Gastroenterol 1972;57:520–40.
6. Palmer ED, Brick IB. Correlation between the severity of esophageal varices in portal cirrhosis and their propensity toward hemorrhage. Gastroenterology 1956;30:85–90.
7. Conn HO. Ammonia tolerance in the diagnosis of oesophageal varices. A comparison of the endoscopic, radiologic and biochemical techniques. J Lab Clin Med 1967;70:442–51.
8. Beppu K, Inokuchi K, Koyanagi N, Nakayama S, Sakata H, Kitano S, et al. Prediction of variceal hemorrhage by esophageal endoscopy. Gastrointest Endosc 1981;27:213–8.
9. North Italian Endoscopic Club for the Study and Treatment of Esophageal Varices. Prediction of the first variceal hemorrhage in patients with cirrhosis of the liver and esophageal varices. N Engl J Med 1988;319:983–9.
10. Sarin SK, Kumar A, Angus PW, Baijal SS, Chawla YK, Dhiman RK, et al. APASL Working Party on Portal Hypertension. Prophylaxis of gastroesophageal variceal bleeding: consensus recommendations of the Asian Pacific Association for the Study of the Liver. Hepatol Int 2008;2:429–39.
11. Sarin SK, Kumar A. Gastric varices: profile, classification, and management. Am J Gastroenterol 1989;84:1244–9.
12. Groszmann RJ, Garcia-Tsao G, Bosch J, Grace ND, Burroughs AK, Planas R, et al. Beta-blockers to prevent gastroesophageal varices in patients with cirrhosis. N Engl J Med 2005;353:2254–61.
13. Moitinho E, Escorsell A, Bandi JC, Salmerón JM, García-Pagán JC, Rodés J, et al. Prognostic value of early measurements of portal pressure in acute variceal bleeding. Gastroenterology 1999;117:626–31.
14. Avgerinos A, Armonis A, Stefanidis G, Mathou N, Vlachogiannakos J, Kougioumtzian A, et al. Sustained rise of portal pressure after sclerotherapy, but not band ligation, in acute variceal bleeding in cirrhosis. Hepatology 2004;39:1623–30.
15. Villanueva C, Ortiz J, Miñana J, Soriano G, Sàbat M, Boadas J, et al. Somatostatin treatment and risk stratification by continuous portal pressure monitoring during acute variceal bleeding. Gastroenterology 2001;121:110–17.
16. Bosch J, García-Pagán JC. Prevention of variceal rebleeding. Lancet 2003;361:952–4.
17. Bosch J, Abraldes JG, Berzigotti A, Garcia-Pagan JC. Portal hypertension and gastrointestinal bleeding. Semin Liver Dis 2008;28:3–25.
18. Luketic VA, Sanyal AJ. Esophageal varices. I. Clinical presentation, medical therapy, and endoscopic therapy. Gastroenterol Clin North Am 2000;29:337–85.
19. Sanyal AJ, Bosch J, Blei A, Arroyo V. Portal hypertension and its complications. Gastroenterology 2008;134:1715–28.
20. Graham DY, Smith JL. The course of patients after variceal hemorrhage. Gastroenterology 1981;80:800–9.
21. Garcia-Tsao G, D'Amico G, Abraldes JG, Schepis F, Merli M, Kim WR, et al. predictive models in portal hypertension. In: de Franchis R, editor. Portal hypertension IV. Proceedings of the Fourth Baveno International Consensus Workshop on Methodology of Diagnosis and Treatment. Oxford: Blackwell Science; 2006. p. 47–100.
22. Sarin SK, Lahoti D, Saxena SP, Murthy NS, Makwana UK. Prevalence, classification and natural history of gastric varices: a long-term follow-up study in 568 portal hypertension patients. Hepatology 1992;16:1343–9.
23. Sarin SK, Jain AK, Lamba GS, Gupta R, Chowdhary A. Isolated gastric varices: prevalence, clinical relevance and natural history. Dig Surg 2003;20:42–7.
24. Kravetz D, Bosch J, Arderiu M, Pilar Pizcueta M, Rodés J. Hemodynamic effects of blood volume restitution following a hemorrhage in rats with portal hypertension due to cirrhosis of the liver: influence of the extent of portal-systemic shunting. Hepatology 1989;9:808–14.
25. Morales J, Moitinho E, Abraldes JG, Fernández M, Bosch J. Effects of the V1a vasopressin agonist F-180 on portal hypertension-related bleeding in portal hypertensive rats. Hepatology 2003;38:1378–83.
26. Blair SD, Janvrin SB, McCollum CN, Greenhalgh RM. Effect of early blood transfusion on gastrointestinal haemorrhage. Br J Surg 1986;73:783–5.
27. Bosch J, Thabut D, Bendtsen F, D'Amico G, Albillos A, González Abraldes J, et al. Recombinant factor VIIa for upper gastrointestinal bleeding in patients with cirrhosis: a randomized, double-blind trial. Gastroenterology 2004;127:1123–30.
28. Bosch J, Thabut D, Albillos A, Carbonell N, Spicak J, Massard J, et al. International Study Group on rFVIIa in UGI Hemorrhage. Recombinant factor VIIa for variceal bleeding in patients with advanced cirrhosis: a randomized, controlled trial. Hepatology 2008;47:1604–14.
29. de Franchis R. Evolving consensus in portal hypertension. Report of the Baveno IV consensus workshop on methodology of diagnosis and therapy in portal hypertension. J Hepatol 2005;43:167–76.
30. Bernard B, Grangé JD, Khac EN, Amiot X, Opolon P, Poynard T. Antibiotic prophylaxis for the prevention of bacterial infections in cirrhotic patients with gastrointestinal bleeding: a meta-analysis. Hepatology 1999;29:1655–61.

46

31. Hou MC, Lin HC, Liu TT, Kuo BI, Lee FY, Chang FY, et al. Antibiotic prophylaxis after endoscopic therapy prevents rebleeding in acute variceal hemorrhage: a randomized trial. Hepatology 2004;39:746–53.

32. Asian Pacific Association for the Study of the Liver. APASL consensus on acute variceal bleeding 2009: consensus recommendations of the Asian Pacific Association for the Study of the Liver. Hepatol Int [in press].

33. Garcia-Tsao G, Bosch J, Groszmann RJ. Portal hypertension and variceal bleeding—unresolved issues. Summary of an American Association for the study of liver diseases and European Association for the study of the liver single-topic conference. Hepatology 2008;47:1764–72.

34. Levacher S, Letoumelin P, Pateron D, Blaise M, Lapandry C, Pourriat JL. Early administration of terlipressin plus glyceryl trinitrate to control active upper gastrointestinal bleeding in cirrhotic patients. Lancet 1995;346:865–8.

35. Ioannou G, Doust J, Rockey DC. Terlipressin for acute esophageal variceal hemorrhage. Cochrane Database Syst Rev 2003;(1):CD002147.

36. Lo GH, Lai KH, Cheng JS, Lin CK, Huang JS, Hsu PI, et al. Emergency banding ligation versus sclerotherapy for the control of active bleeding from esophageal varices. Hepatology 1997;25:1101–4.

37. Villanueva C, Piqueras M, Aracil C, Gómez C, López-Balaguer JM, Gonzalez B, et al. A randomized controlled trial comparing ligation and sclerotherapy as emergency endoscopic treatment added to somatostatin in acute variceal bleeding. J Hepatol 2006;45:560–7.

38. Triantos CK, Goulis J, Patch D, Papatheodoridis GV, Leandro G, Samonakis D, et al. An evaluation of emergency sclerotherapy of varices in randomized trials: looking the needle in the eye. Endoscopy 2006;38:797–807.

39. Avgerinos A, Armonis A, Stefanidis G, Mathou N, Vlachogiannakos J, Kougioumtzian A, et al. Sustained rise of portal pressure after sclerotherapy, but not band ligation, in acute variceal bleeding in cirrhosis. Hepatology 2004;39:1623–30.

40. Crafoord C, Frenckner P. Nonsurgical treatment of varicose veins in the esophagus. Acta Otolaryngol 1939;27:422–9.

41. Moersch HJ. Further studies on the treatment of esophageal varices by injection of a sclerosing solution. Ann Otol Rhinol Laryngol 1941;50:1233–46.

42. Williams KG, Dawson JL. Fibreoptic injection of oesophageal varices. Br Med J 1979;2:766–7.

43. Kage M, Korula J, Harada A, Mucientes F, Kanel G, Peters RL. Effects of sodium tetradecyl sulfate endoscopic variceal sclerotherapy on the esophagus. A prospective clinical and histopathologic study. J Clin Gastroenterol 1987;9:635–43.

44. Sarin SK, Sachdev G, Nanda R, Batra SK, Anand BS. Comparison of the two time schedules for endoscopic sclerotherapy: a prospective randomised controlled study. Gut 1986;27:710–13.

45. Paquet KJ, Oberhammer E. Sclerotherapy of bleeding oesophageal varices by means of endoscopy. Endoscopy 1978;10:7–12.

46. Paquet KJ. Endoscopic paravariceal injection sclerotherapy of the esophagus—indications, technique, complications: results of a period of 14 years. Gastrointest Endosc 1983;29:310–5.

47. Sarin SK, Nanda R, Sachdev G, Chari S, Anand BS, Broor SL. Intravariceal versus paravariceal sclerotherapy: a prospective, controlled, randomised trial. Gut 1987;28:657–62.

48. Helpap B, Bollweg L. Morphological changes in the terminal oesophagus with varices, following sclerosis of the wall. Endoscopy 1981;13:229–33.

49. Waked I, Korula J. Analysis of long-term endoscopic surveillance during follow-up after variceal sclerotherapy from a 13-year experience. Am J Med 1997;102:192–9.

50. Lo GH, Lai KH, Cheng JS, Chen MH, Huang HC, Hsu PI, et al. Endoscopic variceal ligation plus nadolol and sucralfate compared with ligation alone for the prevention of variceal rebleeding: a prospective, randomized trial. Hepatology 2000;32:461–5.

51. Sarin SK. Endoscopic sclerotherapy for esophagogastric varices: a critical reappraisal. Aust N Z J Med 1989;19:162–71.

52. Van Stiegmann G, Cambre T, Sun JH. A new endoscopic elastic band ligating device. Gastrointest Endosc 1986;32:230–3.

53. Stiegmann GV, Sun JH, Hammond WS. Results of experimental endoscopic esophageal varix ligation. Am Surg 1988;54:105–8.

54. Liu J, Petersen BT, Tierney WM, Chuttani R, Disario JA, Coffie JM, et al. Endoscopic banding devices. Gastrointest Endosc 2008;68:217–21.

55. Shaheen NJ, Stuart E, Schmitz SM, Mitchell KL, Fried MW, Zacks S, et al. Pantoprazole reduces the size of postbanding ulcers after variceal band ligation: a randomized, controlled trial. Hepatology 2005;41:588–94.

56. Monescillo A, Martínez-Lagares F, Ruiz-del-Arbol L, Sierra A, Guevara C, Jiménez E, et al. Influence of portal hypertension and its early decompression by TIPS placement on the outcome of variceal bleeding. Hepatology 2004;40:793–801.

57. Soehendra N, Nam VC, Grimm H, Kempeneers I. Endoscopic obliteration of large esophagogastric varices with bucrylate. Endoscopy 1986;18:25–6.

58. Rengstorff DS, Binmoeller KF. A pilot study of 2-octyl cyanoacrylate injection for treatment of gastric fundal varices in humans. Gastrointest Endosc 2004;59:553–8.

59. Seewald S, Sriram PV, Naga M, Fennerty MB, Boyer J, Oberti F, et al. Cyanoacrylate glue in gastric variceal bleeding. Endoscopy 2002;34:926–32.

60. Soehendra N, Grimm H, Maydeo A, Nam VC, Eckmann B, Brückner M. Endoscopic sclerotherapy—personal experience. Hepatogastroenterology 1991;38:220–3.

61. Huang YH, Yeh HZ, Chen GH, Chang CS, Wu CY, Poon SK, et al. Endoscopic treatment of bleeding gastric varices by N-butyl-2-cyanoacrylate (Histoacryl) injection: long-term efficacy and safety. Gastrointest Endosc 2000;52:160–7.

62. Seewald S, Ang TL, Imazu H, Naga M, Omar S, Groth S, et al. A standardized injection technique and regimen ensures success and safety of N-butyl-2-cyanoacrylate injection for the treatment of gastric fundal varices. Gastrointest Endosc 2008;68:447–54.

63. Sarin SK, Jain AK, Jain M, Gupta R. A randomized controlled trial of cyanoacrylate versus alcohol injection in patients with isolated fundic varices. Am J Gastroenterol 2002;97:1010–5.

64. Lo GH, Lai KH, Cheng JS, Chen MH, Chiang HT. A prospective, randomized trial of butyl cyanoacrylate injection versus band ligation in the management of bleeding gastric varices. Hepatology 2001;33:1060–4.

65. Tan PC, Hou MC, Lin HC, Liu TT, Lee FY, Chang FY, et al. A randomized trial of endoscopic treatment of acute gastric variceal hemorrhage: N-butyl-2-cyanoacrylate injection versus band ligation. Hepatology 2006;43:690–7.

66. Hashizume M, Kitano S, Sugimachi K, Sueishi K. Three-dimensional view of the vascular structure of the lower esophagus in clinical portal hypertension. Hepatology 1988;8:1482–7.

67. Shiha G, El-Sayed SS. Gastric variceal ligation: a new technique. Gastrointest Endosc 1999;49:437–41.

68. Yoshida T, Harada T, Shigemitsu T, Takeo Y, Miyazaki S, Okita K. Endoscopic management of gastric varices using a detachable snare and simultaneous endoscopic sclerotherapy and O-ring ligation. J Gastroenterol Hepatol 1999;14:730–5.

69. Kojima K, Imazu H, Matsumura M, Honda Y, Umemoto N, Moriyasu H, et al. Sclerotherapy for gastric fundal variceal bleeding: is complete obliteration possible without cyanoacrylate? J Gastroenterol Hepatol 2005;20:1701–6.

70. Kuo MJ, Yeh HZ, Chen GH, Poon SK, Yang SS, Lien HC, et al. Improvement of tissue-adhesive obliteration of bleeding gastric varices using adjuvant hypertonic glucose injection: a prospective randomized trial. Endoscopy 2007;39:487–91.

71. Datta D, Vlavianos P, Alisa A, Westaby D. Use of fibrin glue (Beriplast) in the management of bleeding gastric varices. Endoscopy 2003;35:675–8.

72. Heneghan MA, Byrne A, Harrison PM. An open pilot study of the effects of a human fibrin glue for endoscopic treatment of patients with acute bleeding from gastric varices. Gastrointest Endosc 2002;56:422–6.

73. Yang WL, Tripathi D, Therapondos G, Todd A, Hayes PC. Endoscopic use of human thrombin in bleeding gastric varices. Am J Gastroenterol 2002;97:1381–5.

74. Chau TN, Patch D, Chan YW, Nagral A, Dick R, Burroughs AK. "Salvage" transjugular intrahepatic portosystemic shunts: gastric fundal compared with esophageal variceal bleeding. Gastroenterology 1998;114:981–7.

75. Barange K, Péron JM, Imani K, Otal P, Payen JL, Rousseau H, et al. Transjugular intrahepatic portosystemic shunt in the treatment of refractory bleeding from ruptured gastric varices. Hepatology 1999;30:1139–43.

76. Yoshida H, Mamada Y, Taniai N, Tajiri T. New methods for the management of gastric varices. World J Gastroenterol 2006;12:5926–31.

77. Merkel C, Marin R, Angeli P, Zanella P, Felder M, Bernardinello E, et al. A placebo-controlled clinical trial of nadolol in the prophylaxis of growth of small esophageal varices in cirrhosis. Gastroenterology 2004;127:476–84.

78. Garcia-Tsao G, Sanyal AJ, Grace ND, Carey WD. Prevention and management of gastroesophageal varices and variceal hemorrhage in cirrhosis. Am J Gastroenterol 2007;102:2086–102.

79. D'Amico G, Pagliaro L, Bosch J. Pharmacological treatment of portal hypertension: an evidence-based approach. Semin Liver Dis 1999;19:475–505.

80. Turnes J, Garcia-Pagan JC, Abraldes JG, Hernandez-Guerra M, Dell'Era A, Bosch J. Pharmacological reduction of portal pressure and long-term risk of first variceal bleeding in patients with cirrhosis. Am J Gastroenterol 2006;101:506–12.

VI

81. Khuroo MS, Khuroo NS, Farahat KL, Khuroo YS, Sofi AA, Dahab ST. Meta-analysis: endoscopic variceal ligation for primary prophylaxis of oesophageal variceal bleeding. Aliment Pharmacol Ther 2005;21:347–61.

82. Akahoshi T, Hashizume M, Tomikawa M, Kawanaka H, Yamaguchi S, Konishi K, et al. Long-term results of balloon-occluded retrograde transvenous obliteration for gastric variceal bleeding and risky gastric varices: a 10-year experience. J Gastroenterol Hepatol 2008;23:1702–9.

83. Sarin SK, Govil A, Jain AK, Guptan RC, Issar SK, Jain M, et al. Prospective randomized trial of endoscopic sclerotherapy versus variceal band ligation for esophageal varices: influence on gastropathy, gastric varices and variceal recurrence. J Hepatol 1997;26:826–32.

84. Laine L, Cook D. Endoscopic ligation compared with sclerotherapy for treatment of esophageal variceal bleeding. A meta-analysis. Ann Intern Med 1995;123:280–7.

85. Sarin SK, Wadhawan M, Gupta R, Shahi H. Evaluation of endoscopic variceal ligation (EVL) versus propranolol plus isosorbide mononitrate/nadolol (ISMN) in the prevention of variceal rebleeding: comparison of cirrhotic and noncirrhotic patients. Dig Dis Sci 2005;50:1538–47.

86. de la Peña J, Brullet E, Sanchez-Hernández E, Rivero M, Vergara M, Martin-Lorente JL, et al. Variceal ligation plus nadolol compared with ligation for prophylaxis of variceal rebleeding: a multicenter trial. Hepatology 2005;41:572–8.

87. Gonzalez R, Zamora J, Gomez-Camarero J, Molinero LM, Bañares R, Albillos A. Meta-analysis: combination endoscopic and drug therapy to prevent variceal rebleeding in cirrhosis. Ann Intern Med 2008; 149:109–22.

88. Kumar A, Jha SK, Sharma P, Dubey S, Tyagi P, Sharma BC, et al. Endoscopic variceal ligation plus propranolol and isosorbide mononitrate versus endoscopic variceal ligation alone for secondary prophylaxis of variceal bleeding: A randomized controlled trial. Gastroenterology 2009 [in press].

89. Schepke M, Kleber G, Nürnberg D, Willert J, Koch L, Veltzke-Schlieker W, et al. Ligation versus propranolol for the primary prophylaxis of variceal bleeding in cirrhosis. Hepatology 2004;40:65–72.

90. Jutabha R, Jensen DM, Martin P, Savides T, Han SH, Gornbein J. Randomized study comparing banding and propranolol to prevent initial variceal hemorrhage in cirrhotics with high-risk esophageal varices. Gastroenterology 2005;128:870–81.

91. Laine L, Stein C, Sharma V. Randomized comparison of ligation versus ligation plus sclerotherapy in patients with bleeding esophageal varices. Gastroenterology 1996;110:529–33.

92. Saeed ZA, Stiegmann GV, Ramirez FC, Reveille RM, Goff JS, Hepps KS, et al. Endoscopic variceal ligation is superior to combined ligation and sclerotherapy for esophageal varices: a multicenter prospective randomized trial. Hepatology 1997;25:71–4.

93. Lo GH, Lai KH, Cheng JS, Lin CK, Huang JS, Hsu PI, et al. The additive effect of sclerotherapy to patients receiving repeated endoscopic variceal ligation: a prospective, randomized trial. Hepatology 1998;28:391–5.

94. Henderson JM, Boyer TD, Kutner MH, Galloway JR, Rikkers LF, Jeffers LJ, et al. Distal splenorenal shunt versus transjugular intrahepatic portal systematic shunt for variceal bleeding: a randomized trial. Gastroenterology 2006;130:1643–51.

95. Barkun A, Bardou M, Marshall JK. Consensus recommendations for managing patients with nonvariceal upper gastrointestinal bleeding. Ann Intern Med 2003;139:843–57.

96. Das A, Wong RC. Prediction of outcome of acute GI hemorrhage: a review of risk scores and predictive models. Gastrointest Endosc 2004;60:85–93.

97. Rockall TA, Logan RF, Devlin HB, Northfield TC. Selection of patients for early discharge or outpatient care after acute upper gastrointestinal haemorrhage. National Audit of Acute Upper Gastrointestinal Haemorrhage. Lancet 1996;347:1138–40.

98. Blatchford O, Murray WR, Blatchford M. A risk score to predict need for treatment for upper-gastrointestinal haemorrhage. Lancet 2000;356:1318–21.

99. Frossard JL, Spahr L, Queneau PE, Giostra E, Burckhardt B, Ory G, et al. Erythromycin intravenous bolus infusion in acute upper gastrointestinal bleeding: a randomized, controlled, double-blind trial. Gastroenterology 2002;123:17–23.

100. Fleischer D. Etiology and prevalence of severe persistent upper gastrointestinal bleeding. Gastroenterology 1983;84:538–43.

101. Forrest JA, Finlayson ND, Shearman DJ. Endoscopy in gastrointestinal bleeding. Lancet 1974;2:394–7.

102. Katschinski B, Logan R, Davies J, Faulkner G, Pearson J, Langman M. Prognostic factors in upper gastrointestinal bleeding. Dig Dis Sci 1994; 39:706–12.

103. Laine L, Peterson WL. Bleeding peptic ulcer. N Engl J Med 1994;331:717–27.

104. Lau JY, Sung JJ, Chan AC, Lai GW, Lau JT, Ng EK, et al. Stigmata of hemorrhage in bleeding peptic ulcers: an interobserver agreement study among international experts. Gastrointest Endosc 1997;46:33–6.

105. Sung JJ, Tsoi KK, Lai LH, Wu JC, Lau JY. Endoscopic clipping versus injection and thermo-coagulation in the treatment of non-variceal upper gastrointestinal bleeding: a meta-analysis. Gut 2007;56:1364–73.

106. Yuan Y, Wang C, Hunt RH. Endoscopic clipping for acute nonvariceal upper-GI bleeding: a meta-analysis and critical appraisal of randomized controlled trials. Gastrointest Endosc 2008;68:339–51.

107. Lau JY, Leung WK, Wu JC, Chan FK, Wong VW, Chiu PW, et al. Omeprazole before endoscopy in patients with gastrointestinal bleeding. N Engl J Med 2007;356:1631–40.

108. Tsoi KK, Lau JY, Sung JJ. Cost-effectiveness analysis of high-dose omeprazole infusion before endoscopy for patients with upper-GI bleeding. Gastrointest Endosc 2008;67:1056–63.

109. Lau JY, Sung JJ, Lee KK, Yung MY, Wong SK, Wu JC, et al. Effect of intravenous omeprazole on recurrent bleeding after endoscopic treatment of bleeding peptic ulcers. N Engl J Med 2000;343:310–6.

110. Chiu PW, Lam CY, Lee SW, Kwong KH, Lam SH, Lee DT, et al. Effect of scheduled second therapeutic endoscopy on peptic ulcer rebleeding: a prospective randomised trial. Gut 2003;52:1403–7.

111. Lau JY, Sung JJ, Lam YH, Chan AC, Ng EK, Lee DW, et al. Endoscopic retreatment compared with surgery in patients with recurrent bleeding after initial endoscopic control of bleeding ulcers. N Engl J Med 1999;340:751–6.

112. Millward SF. ACR Appropriateness criteria on treatment of acute non-variceal gastrointestinal tract bleeding. J Am Coll Radiol 2008;5:550–4.

113. Sung JJ, Chung SC, Ling TK, Yung MY, Leung VK, Ng EK, et al. Antibacterial treatment of gastric ulcers associated with *Helicobacter pylori*. N Engl J Med 1995;332:139–42.

114. Chan FK, Chung SC, Suen BY, Lee YT, Leung WK, Leung VK, et al. Preventing recurrent upper gastrointestinal bleeding in patients with *Helicobacter pylori* infection who are taking low-dose aspirin or naproxen. N Engl J Med 2001;344:967–73.

115. Chan FK, Ching JY, Hung LC, Wong VW, Leung VK, Kung NN, et al. Clopidogrel versus aspirin and esomeprazole to prevent recurrent ulcer bleeding. N Engl J Med 2005;352:238–46.

116. Bombardier C, Laine L, Reicin A, Shapiro D, Burgos-Vargas R, Davis B, et al. Comparison of upper gastrointestinal toxicity of rofecoxib and naproxen in patients with rheumatoid arthritis. VIGOR Study Group. N Engl J Med 2000;343:1520–8.

117. Chan FK, Wong VW, Suen BY, Wu JC, Ching JY, Hung LC, et al. Combination of a cyclo-oxygenase-2 inhibitor and a proton-pump inhibitor for prevention of recurrent ulcer bleeding in patients at very high risk: a double-blind, randomised trial. Lancet 2007;369:1621–6.

118. Bresalier RS, Sandler RS, Quan H, Bolognese JA, Oxenius B, Horgan K, et al. Cardiovascular events associated with rofecoxib in a colorectal adenoma chemoprevention trial. N Engl J Med 2005;352:1092–102.

119. Hudson N, Everitt S, Hawkey CJ. Interobserver variation in assessment of gastroduodenal lesions associated with non-steroidal anti-inflammatory drugs. Gut 1994;35:1030–2.

120. Rao AD, Ramalingam G. Exsanguinating hemorrhage following gastric erosion after laparoscopic adjustable gastric banding. Obes Surg 2006; 16:1675–8.

121. Yamaguchi Y, Yamato T, Katsumi N, Morozumi K, Abe T, Ishida H, et al. Endoscopic hemoclipping for upper GI bleeding due to Mallory–Weiss syndrome. Gastrointest Endosc 2001;53:427–30.

122. Huang SP, Wang HP, Lee YC, Lin CC, Yang CS, Wu MS, et al. Endoscopic hemoclip placement and epinephrine injection for Mallory–Weiss syndrome with active bleeding. Gastrointest Endosc 2002;55:842–6.

123. Squillace SJ, Johnson DA, Sanowski RA. The endosonographic appearance of a Dieulafoy's lesion. Am J Gastroenterol 1994;89:276–7.

124. Sone Y, Kumada T, Toyoda H, Hisanaga Y, Kiriyama S, Tanikawa M. Endoscopic management and follow up of Dieulafoy lesion in the upper gastrointestinal tract. Endoscopy 2005;37:449–53.

125. Matsui S, Kamisako T, Kudo M, Inoue R. Endoscopic band ligation for control of nonvariceal upper GI hemorrhage: comparison with bipolar electrocoagulation. Gastrointest Endosc 2002;55:214–8.

126. Yamaguchi Y, Yamato T, Katsumi N, Imao Y, Aoki K, Morita Y, et al. Short-term and long-term benefits of endoscopic hemoclip application for Dieulafoy's lesion in the upper GI tract. Gastrointest Endosc 2003;57:653–6.

127. Iacopini F, Petruzziello L, Marchese M, Larghi A, Spada C, Familiari P, et al. Hemostasis of Dieulafoy's lesions by argon plasma coagulation (with video). Gastrointest Endosc 2007;66:20–6.

46

128. Watson M, Hally RJ, McCue PA, Varga J, Jimenez SA. Gastric antral vascular ectasia (watermelon stomach) in patients with systemic sclerosis. Arthritis Rheum 1996;39:341–6.

129. Ito M, Uchida Y, Kamano S, Kawabata H, Nishioka M. Clinical comparisons between two subsets of gastric antral vascular ectasia. Gastrointest Endosc 2001;53:764–70.

130. Dulai GS, Jensen DM, Kovacs TO, Gralnek IM, Jutabha R. Endoscopic treatment outcomes in watermelon stomach patients with and without portal hypertension. Endoscopy 2004;36:68–72.

131. Payen JL, Cales P, Voigt JJ, Barbe S, Pilette C, Dubuisson L, et al. Severe portal hypertensive gastropathy and antral vascular ectasia are distinct entities in patients with cirrhosis. Gastroenterology 1995;108:138–46.

132. Wells CD, Harrison ME, Gurudu SR, Crowell MD, Byrne TJ, Depetris G, et al. Treatment of gastric antral vascular ectasia (watermelon stomach) with endoscopic band ligation. Gastrointest Endosc 2008;68:231–6.

133. Koch P, del Valle F, Berdel WE, Willich NA, Reers B, Hiddemann W, et al. Primary gastrointestinal non-Hodgkin's lymphoma: I. Anatomic and histologic distribution, clinical features, and survival data of 371 patients registered in the German Multicenter Study GIT NHL 01/92. J Clin Oncol 2001;19:3861–73.

134. Miettinen M, Sobin LH, Lasota J. Gastrointestinal stromal tumors of the stomach: a clinicopathologic, immunohistochemical, and molecular genetic study of 1765 cases with long-term follow-up. Am J Surg Pathol 2005;29:52–68.

135. Savides TJ, Jensen DM, Cohen J, Randall GM, Kovacs TO, Pelayo E, et al. Severe upper gastrointestinal tumor bleeding: endoscopic findings, treatment, and outcome. Endoscopy 1996;28:244–8.

136. Demetri GD, von MM, Blanke CD, Van den Abbeele AD, Eisenberg B, Roberts PJ, et al. Efficacy and safety of imatinib mesylate in advanced gastrointestinal stromal tumors. N Engl J Med 2002;347:472–80.

137. Bloechle C, Izbicki JR, Rashed MY, el-Sefi T, Hosch SB, Knoefel WT, et al. Hemobilia: presentation, diagnosis, and management. Am J Gastroenterol 1994;89:1537–40.

138. Risti B, Marincek B, Jost R, Decurtins M, Ammann R. Hemosuccus pancreaticus as a source of obscure upper gastrointestinal bleeding: three cases and literature review. Am J Gastroenterol 1995;90:1878–80.

139. Saers SJ, Scheltinga MR. Primary aortoenteric fistula. Br J Surg 2005;92:143–52.

VI

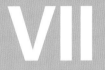

VII

Lower Gastrointestinal Tract Diseases

Section editors:
Charles J. Lightdale, Guido N.J. Tytgat, Alexander Meining

47 Colorectal Disorders

Witold Bartnik, Jacek Pachlewski, and Jaroslaw Regula

Colorectal Polyps

Gastrointestinal tract polyps are typically limited protrusions that form on the mucosal lining. The majority of colorectal polyps are sporadic and solitary. However, some are hereditary—particularly multiple polyps—and give rise to polyposis syndromes. The clinical description of polyps and their treatment includes several elements, including the shape (pedunculated, sessile, or flat), size (in centimeters), location (the region of the colon or the distance from the anus on withdrawal of a colonoscope), the technique of polyp removal, and its endoscopic completeness. For a more detailed shape description, the Paris–Japanese classification, including depressed lesions, can be used (**Table 47.1**) [1].

Three main groups of polyps can be distinguished histopathologically: neoplastic, nonneoplastic, and submucosal (**Table 47.2**). Single, nonneoplastic polyps do not have malignant potential. Hyperplastic polyps occur most frequently. Diminutive hyperplastic polyps (< 5 mm) located in the rectum have no clinical significance; however, it is important to distinguish them from adenomas by histopathology. In contrast, large hyperplastic polyps may have malignant potential. A hyperplastic polyposis syndrome is suspected when hyperplastic polyps are numerous (n > 20), large (> 1 cm), and localized in the right colon.

Among intestinal polyps, adenomas are the most important from the clinical point of view [2]. Adenomas represent 70 % of all polyps removed during colonoscopy. Four types of adenoma can be distinguished histopathologically: tubular, tubulovillous, villous, and "serrated" (**Table 47.2**). A common feature among adenomas is epithelial cell dysplasia, which involves cytological and architectural changes that unequivocally indicate a neoplastic abnormality. Dysplasia is divided into low-grade and high-grade types. Cells with high-grade dysplasia may penetrate through the muscularis mucosa into the submucosal layer, resulting in invasive carcinoma.

Colorectal adenomas can be diagnosed at any age, but there is a clear increase in the incidence among adults over 30, and the incidence increases to about one-third in those over the age of 50. Colorectal adenomas are significant, as they are regarded as precancerous lesions in the large bowel. The majority of adenomas are less than 1 cm in diameter, with low malignant potential. The potential is significantly increased in advanced adenomas that are 1 cm or larger in diameter, contain a villous element (at least 20 %), or show high-grade dysplasia. It is estimated that development into a medium-sized adenoma takes roughly 5 years, while development to invasive cancer takes about 10 years. In an asymptomatic population of adults over 50 years old, the incidence of advanced adenoma is about 5–10 %, while that of invasive cancer is about 1 %. Advanced adenoma plus cancer is known as advanced neoplasia.

The most frequent symptom of polyps is rectal bleeding. Less frequently reported symptoms include mild anemia, tenesmus, or the presence of mucus in the stool. The majority of polyps are completely asymptomatic, especially when small (< 1 cm in diameter). Polyps can be diagnosed with endoscopy or radiography. The barium enema has limited diagnostic value, particularly when performed without using the double-contrast method. Even in referral centers, the sensitivity is not more than 60–70 % for lesions 1 cm or

Table 47.1 The Paris–Japanese classification of the morphology of polypoid lesions [1]

Polyp type	Description
Protruding	
Ip	Pedunculated
Isp	Semipedunculated
Is	Sessile
Superficial	
IIa	Flat, elevation
IIa + IIc	Flat, elevation + depression
IIb	Flat; no elevation or depression
Depressed	
IIc	Mucosal depression
IIc + IIa	Depression + elevated edges

Table 47.2 Classification of colorectal polyps

Mucosal polyps		Submucosal polyps
Neoplastic	**Nonneoplastic**	
Adenomas:	Hyperplastic	Lymphoid collection
Tubular	Inflammatory	Pneumatosis cystoides intestinalis
Tubulovillous	Hamartomas:	Colitis cystica profunda
Villous	Juvenile	Lipoma
"Serrated"	Peutz–Jeghers	Neuroendocrine (carcinoid)
		Hemangioma
		Leiomyoma

larger. Better results can be obtained with computed-tomographic colonography; spiral computed tomography (CT) allows detection of 90 % of polyps 1 cm or larger, but it is not widely used for polyp diagnosis. Endoscopy is most commonly used to diagnose adenomatous polyps and makes it possible to carry out treatment with endoscopic polypectomy simultaneously. Approximately two-thirds of adenomas lie within reach of flexible sigmoidoscopy, which is also used for screening purposes, especially in the United Kingdom. Small polyps (< 7 mm) that are detected during flexible sigmoidoscopy screening are biopsied to examine the histology. According to current opinion, when only hyperplastic polyps without adenomas are detected, the diagnostic process is completed; the risk of advanced proximal adenoma is estimated to be only 1–3 %. However, when an adenoma is detected in the rectum or sigmoid colon, independent of its diameter, the risk of advanced proximal adenoma increases to 5–7 %, and a total colonoscopy is indicated. The sensitivity of total colonoscopy is over 90 % for detecting polyps ≥ 7 mm. Characterization of the polyp type (neoplastic, nonneoplastic, type of adenoma, etc.) is based on the histopathologist's assessment and currently cannot be predicted macroscopically with sufficient probability, even with modern visualization techniques.

Detection of a colorectal polyp as a result of diagnostic work-up or incidental discovery nearly always requires its removal. Pedun-

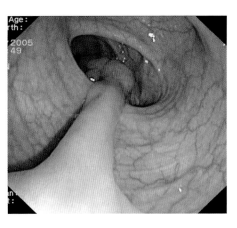

Fig. 47.1 The long stalk of a pedunculated adenoma.

culated and semipedunculated polyps larger than 7 mm should be removed with a diathermic snare. Smaller polyps can be removed with biopsy forceps or cold snaring, which is performed without activating the diathermic current. Other techniques are also available, including piecemeal polypectomy, endoscopic mucosal resection (EMR), or endoscopic submucosal dissection (ESD). Only a minority of polyps (very large polyps with visible signs of malignancy) may require a laparotomy. Typical shapes and sizes of colonic polyps, including pedunculated, semipedunculated, and flat polyps, as well as the value of image enhancement using the narrow-band imaging technique (NBI), are illustrated in **Figs. 47.1–47.5**.

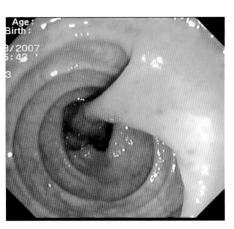
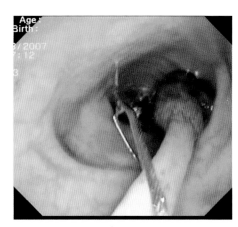
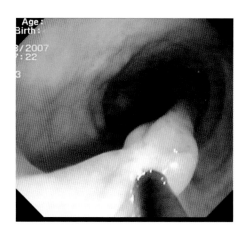

c

Fig. 47.2 A pedunculated adenoma undergoing endoscopic polypectomy.
a The long stalk of the adenoma.
b Placing the snare.
c Closing the snare while applying diathermy current.

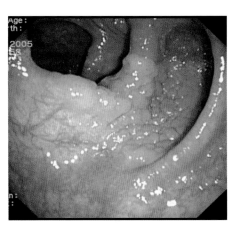
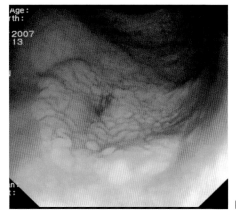

b

Fig. 47.3 Various flat adenomas.
a A flat adenoma in the ascending colon, close to the ileocecal valve.
b A flat rectal adenoma.
c A flat adenoma with an elevated portion.
d A flat adenoma—underwater view.

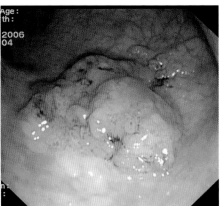
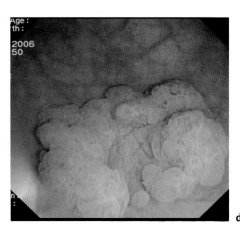

d

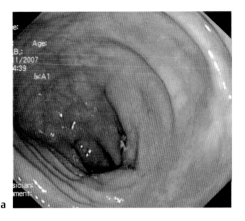
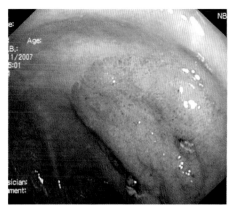

Fig. 47.4 Narrow-band imaging (NBI) improves the visibility of flat lesions.
a A flat adenoma near a splenic flexure.
b The same polyp, with improved visibility using narrow-band imaging.

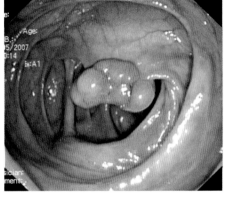
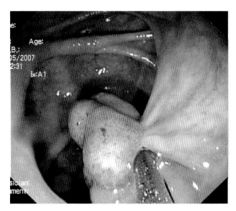
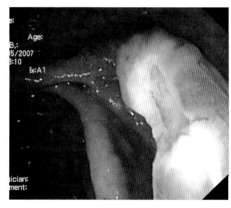

Fig. 47.5 A semipedunculated polyp.
a A hanging semipedunculated adenoma opposite the ileocecal valve.

b A polypectomy snare closed at the base of the polyp.
c The postpolypectomy base.

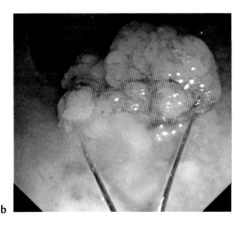
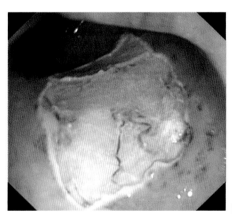

Fig. 47.6 Complete polypectomy without saline injection.
a Snare placement around the polyp with desufflation of the lumen.
b The clean postpolypectomy base after removal of the polyp in two pieces.

The polypectomy technique for large lesions using a piecemeal approach without saline injection is shown in **Figs. 47.6–47.8**. In this approach, firm placement of the snare against the lesion, with air suction allowing complete capture of the area intended to be removed by the snare, is crucial.

Difficult cases of polypectomy of large adenomas are usually time-consuming, require additional maneuvers including saline injection, and may be extremely difficult in cases in which polyp removal has been attempted previously. Such cases are illustrated in **Figs. 47.9–47.13**.

Patients who have adenomas removed using special techniques (mentioned above), especially with the piecemeal method, require follow-up colonoscopies within 2–6 months after the polypectomy to ensure complete removal. A clean postpolypectomy scar, adenoma recurrence, and tattooing to mark the polypectomy site are shown in **Figs. 47.14–47.16**.

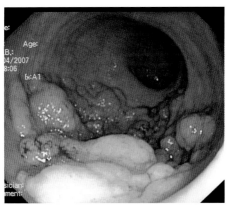
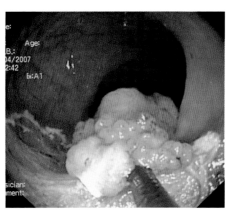
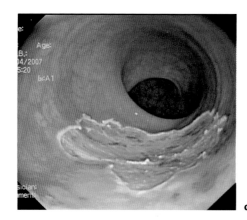

Fig. 47.7 A large rectal adenoma removed using the piecemeal technique.
a The carpet-like rectal adenoma before removal.
b Piecemeal polypectomy.
c The clean postpolypectomy base.

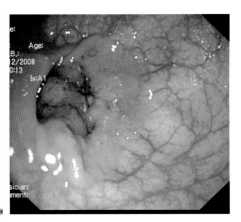
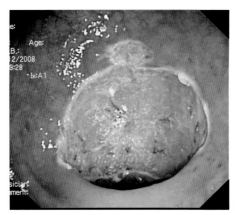

Fig. 47.8 Complete removal of a large polyp.
a The large adenoma in the rectosigmoid before removal.
b The polyp base after removal.

47

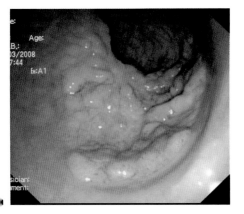
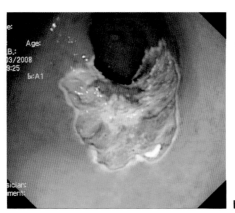

Fig. 47.9 Unsuccessful polypectomy attempts may hamper endoscopic removal.
a A flat adenoma after a previous unsuccessful removal attempt; scarring is visible in the left upper corner.
b An incomplete polypectomy due to scarring caused by previous unsuccessful attempts.

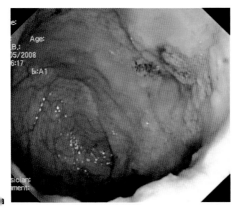
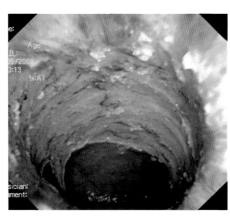

Fig. 47.10 A large rectal flat adenoma requiring the long procedure for removal with a snare.
a The nearly circumferential carpet-like rectal adenoma before removal.
b The endoscopic appearance 2 h after polypectomy.

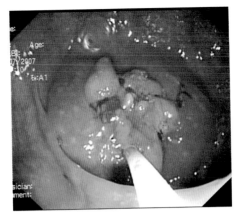

Fig. 47.11 Saline injection as a preparatory maneuver for safe polypectomy.
a A sessile adenoma in the right colon.
b The saline injection is successful (without a nonlifting sign).

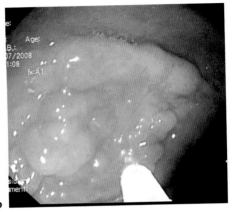
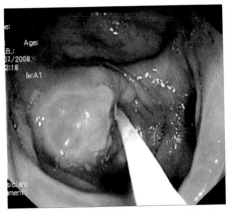
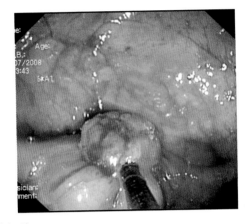

a, b

Fig. 47.12 Saline injection provides safety, especially in the thin-walled parts of the colon.
a A flat adenoma at the bottom of the cecum.
b A successful saline injection.
c Placement of the snare around the saline cushion.

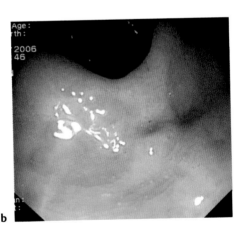
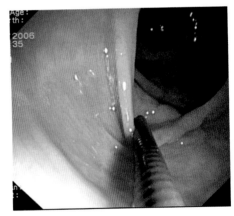
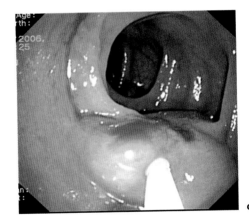

a, b

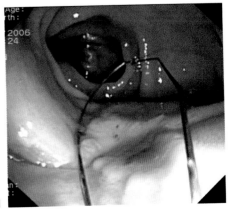
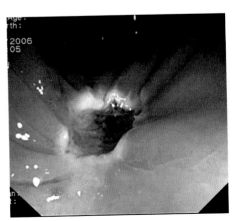

Fig. 47.13 A saline injection sometimes makes it difficult to place the snare properly around the polyp.
a A flat adenoma on both sides of the fold.
b Visualization of the proximal part of the polyp.
c A saline injection.
d Extreme difficulty in placing the snare around the polyp, due to the snare slipping off the saline cushion.
e Successful removal despite difficulties.

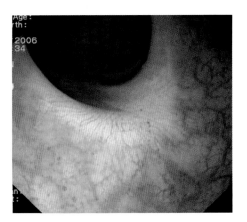

Fig. 47.14 A clean postpolypectomy scar.

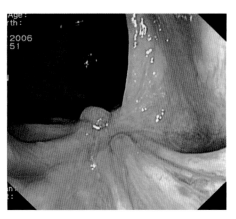

Fig. 47.15 Adenoma recurrence after polypectomy.

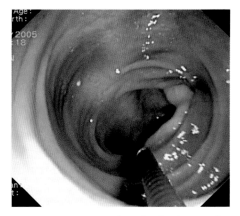

Fig. 47.16 Tattooing the colon for future reference.

Rules that need to be observed during polypectomy include the following:

- All detected polyps should be removed; however, the patient's age and any comorbid conditions should also be taken into account in order to avoid overtreatment.
- Not all polyps have to be removed endoscopically. A small percentage of polyps are better managed surgically; endoscopists should not insist on removing all polyps.
- Endoscopists should be aware of their own abilities and limitations. They should be trained in the use of endoscopic equipment, especially electrosurgical diathermy.
- All polyps should be retrieved for histology, optimally in separate containers.
- Histologists should be provided with high-quality biopsies that are as intact as possible.
- The completeness of removal should be assessed both endoscopically and histologically.
- A polyp should be removed in one piece whenever possible.
- The six-o'clock position rule should be remembered (positioning the polyp within the endoscopic view for removal).
- When cold-snare polypectomy is performed, there is no need to lift the lesion. In fact, lifting should be avoided.
- When hot-snare polypectomy is performed, coagulation or blended current should be used.
- The bowel should always be desufflated before polypectomy.
- Closure of the snare for polypectomy is optimally performed by the endoscopist (rather than by an accompanying nurse).

Different centers may have slightly modified rules, depending on the endoscopist's level of experience the availability of equipment, and other factors.

Following removal, all polyps should be carefully examined histologically. Endoscopic therapy can be regarded as definitive when the histological findings show a benign adenoma. It can also be regarded as definitive when the histology shows invasive carcinoma in an adenoma that is limited to the submucosal layer, provided that: 1, the adenoma was removed completely; 2, the cancer is not undifferentiated; 3, the resection margins are free of cancer (the minimum free margin should be at least 2 mm); and 4, no lymphatic or blood vessels are infiltrated. If any of these criteria is not met, additional surgery is indicated, with segmental resection and lymphadenectomy.

The most common complications of endoscopic polypectomy include perforation (0.1–0.2 %), a local serosal burn syndrome, and bleeding (< 1 %). Perforation requires immediate surgery. Bleeding

Table 47.3 Recommendations for surveillance timing (time of the next control colonoscopy) after polypectomy, provided that a high-quality colonoscopy has been performed and a "clean colon" has been obtained [3]

Low-risk group*	
Hyperplastic, rectal, small polyps	No surveillance
1 or 2 adenomas, less than 1 cm in diameter, tubular histology, low-grade dysplasia	5–10 years
Increased-risk group*	
> 1 cm in diameter or HGD or villous component	3 years
3–10 adenomas all sizes	3 years
> 10 adenomas	< 3 years
Piecemeal or incomplete polypectomy	2–6 months until completeness ensured

* "Low" and "increased" risks refer to the probability of the occurrence of new colorectal adenoma(s) or cancer after polypectomy. HGD, high-grade dysplasia.

may require endoscopy; sometimes bleeding is delayed for as long as 2 weeks. Other complications do not require specific treatment.

Colorectal adenomas recur within 3–5 years after a polypectomy in 30–40 % of the patients. In recent years, recommendations concerning postpolypectomy surveillance have changed toward less intensive surveillance. Recent recommendations developed by the United States Multi-Society Task Force on Colorectal Cancer and the American Cancer Society are presented in **Table 47.3** [3]. These recommendations are valid only when a high-quality colonoscopy is performed, a "clean colon" without polyps is obtained, and the colonoscopy reaches the cecum.

Nonpolypoid flat lesions are currently regarded as an important colorectal abnormality [4]. Recent studies performed in the USA have shown that this type of lesion—flat or depressed—occurs in 9.3 % of patients examined by colonoscopy and may represent 15 % of all neoplastic lesions in the large bowel [5]. Flat lesions are difficult to assess precisely, and several definitions exist. The endoscopic definition describes them as lesions whose height is less than half of their diameter. The histological definition describes them as lesions that are no thicker than twice the thickness of the adjacent normal mucosa, measured from the muscularis mucosa to the top of the lesion. The "laterally spreading tumor" is a special type of flat lesion that is large and flat like a carpet. Nonpolypoid lesions display high-grade dysplasia and contain foci of invasive cancer more fre-

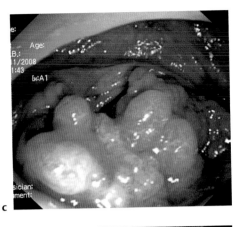

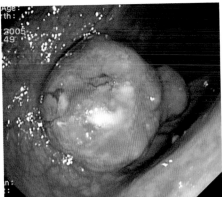

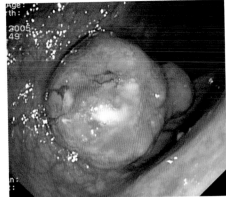

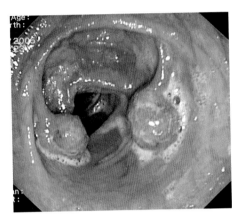

Fig. 47.17 Hamartomatous polyps.
a A juvenile polyp in the cecum.
b A medium-sized Peutz–Jeghers polyp.
c A single small Peutz–Jeghers polyp.
d Twin polyps in Peutz–Jeghers syndrome.

quently than polypoid lesions. In addition, nonpolypoid lesions are smaller and more difficult to detect than polypoid lesions during colonoscopy. CT colonography is generally not able to detect flat colorectal lesions that do not protrude into the lumen. Detection may be facilitated by new technologies, including chromoendoscopy, NBI, and autofluorescence imaging. Novel therapies, including inject-and-cut EMR, can be extremely useful in removing flat lesions over 1 cm in diameter [6]. Lesions that visually suggest cancer or show nonlifting signs after a submucosal injection of saline should only be biopsied on visualization. Cancerous lesions should optimally be removed surgically.

The category of nonneoplastic polyps includes hamartomatous and inflammatory polyps (**Fig. 47.17**). Juvenile polyps are the most frequent type of hamartomatous polyp and the most frequent cause of intestinal bleeding in children. Juvenile polyps are typically solitary lesions located in the rectum or sigmoid colon. They have a tendency to autoamputate or prolapse rectally. Histologically, they appear as dilated and mucus-filled glands that are embedded in the enlarged and edematous lamina propria of the large bowel mucosa. Juvenile polyps can also arise from a heritable juvenile polyposis syndrome. This is described in more detail below.

Peutz–Jeghers polyps may be present in any part of the intestinal tract, but are most frequently located in the small bowel. The main histological abnormality is an "arborous" growth of muscle bundles originating from the muscularis mucosa. These polyps become symptomatic in young adults, causing bleeding, anemia, or intussusception. Peutz–Jeghers syndrome is inherited as an autosomal-dominant disease and involves hamartomatous polyps in the intestine and mucocutaneous pigmentation around the mouth (see below).

Hyperplastic polyps are usually small, whitish, 2–3 mm in diameter, and are composed of elongated and dilated mucosal glands. They are most frequently located in the rectum and can be numer-

ous. When large and numerous hyperplastic polyps (diameter > 1 cm) appear proximal to the sigmoid colon, they may lead to the development of serrated adenomas and may even lead to cancer.

Inflammatory polyps (pseudopolyps) are typically diagnosed in the context of large-bowel inflammatory changes with a different etiology and can be regarded as "witnesses" of past inflammation. Most frequently, they are diagnosed in patients with ulcerative colitis (see Chapter 48).

Single nonneoplastic polyps have no malignant potential. The optimal therapy is endoscopic removal, as for adenomas. After the removal of juvenile polyps, recurrences are extremely rare, and patients (usually children) do not require a follow-up colonoscopy.

Hereditary Colorectal Syndromes

There are two main groups of neoplastic colorectal diseases in which hereditary factors play an important role: syndromes with adenomas and syndromes with hamartomatous polyps (**Table 47.4**).

Familial adenomatous polyposis (FAP) is responsible for about 0.5 % of cases of colorectal cancer. The condition arises from an inherited autosomal-dominant mutation in the adenomatous polyposis coli (*APC*) gene. The disease is characterized by hundreds to thousands of digestive-tract adenomas and a number of extracolonic manifestations. Adenomas begin to appear at about age 15. Cancer develops, not infrequently multifocal, up to the age of 40. About 90 % of patients also develop adenomas in the duodenum, particularly in the periampullary region, which significantly increases the risk of duodenal adenocarcinoma (5 % lifetime risk) [7]. About 50 % of patients also have detectable fundic gland polyps in the stomach, but with no malignant potential per se. The syndrome is characterized by extraintestinal soft-tissue tumors, bone tumors, and congenital hypertrophy of the retinal pigment epithelium. Ab-

VII

dominal or skin desmoid tumors are a serious complication, responsible for a substantial part of the mortality rate (15% of cases). Other complications can include central nervous systems tumors (Turcot syndrome), thyroid tumors, and hepatic tumors. The clinical manifestation depends on the mutation site in the *APC* gene. Polyposis patients and members of their families should be referred for genetic counseling, followed by testing to identify the type and site of the mutation. In classic FAP, mutations in the *APC* gene are found in 80% of the cases. When no *APC* mutation is detected, the patient should be tested for a *MUTYH* mutation [8]. All patients with confirmed FAP syndrome should have annual sigmoidoscopies, starting at age 12, and a prophylactic proctocolectomy before age 20. Those without a known associated mutation do not require endoscopic surveillance. In some patients, the rectum may be preserved; these patients require frequent endoscopic check-up examinations of the rectum (every 3–6 months), due to a 10% risk of rectal cancer. Upper gastrointestinal endoscopies should be performed every 1–3 years. Growth of rectal adenomas can be partially controlled with sulindac or celecoxib [8].

Attenuated FAP syndrome is characterized by a smaller number of adenomas (n < 100) and a lower malignant potential in comparison with classic FAP. The mean age at which FAP-related cancer is detected is about 56. Attenuated FAP is caused by a mutation close to the proximal end of the *APC* gene. Polyposis associated with the *MUTYH* gene mutation is phenotypically similar to attenuated FAP, but it is inherited in an autosomal-recessive fashion.

Hereditary nonpolyposis colorectal cancer (HNPCC), also known as Lynch syndrome (after the name of its discoverer), is responsible for roughly 3% of all colorectal cancers. Lynch I and II syndromes differ in that Lynch I syndrome includes only colorectal cancer, while Lynch II syndrome also features other neoplasms in the endometrium, ovary, stomach, small bowel, skin, and urinary tract. The primary cause of Lynch syndrome is a mutation in one of six mismatch repair genes, including *hMSH2, hMSH6, hMLH1, hMLH3, hPMS 1*, and *hPMS 2*. Approximately 90% of patients with Lynch syndrome have autosomal-dominant mutations in the *hMSH2* or *hMLH1* genes. The most important indicator of this syndrome is the family history. The Amsterdam criteria have been established to identify families at risk (**Table 47.5**).

HNPCC patients have an 80% lifetime risk of sustaining colorectal cancer and a 30% lifetime risk of sustaining endometrial cancer. Unlike FAP, Lynch syndrome exhibits adenomas that are not numerous, are located mainly in the right colon, and often contain a villous component or high-grade dysplasia. Gene mutations are associated with a characteristic DNA abnormality known as microsatellite instability (MSI). MSI is present in more than 90% of patients with HNPCC and can be detected in tumor tissue by polymerase chain reaction (PCR) amplification of a panel of DNA markers. This test should be performed in patients with families that meet any of the revised Bethesda criteria (**Table 47.6**) [9].

In patients who meet the revised Bethesda criteria, tumor tissue should also be tested using immunochemistry staining to identify the protein products of mismatch repair genes. Normal staining and no indication of MSI would indicate that mutations are highly unlikely in the mismatch repair genes, and no further genetic testing is required. However, patients who have negative immunochemistry staining and/or a high level of MSI should be tested further. Confirmation of a mutation in one of the mismatch repair genes in a patient with colorectal cancer is an indication for colonoscopic surveillance in family members. Colonoscopies should be performed every 1–2 years after the age of 25 and in any family members who are within 5 years younger than the youngest patient who has colorectal cancer. In addition, gastric cancer should be investigated, with an upper gastrointestinal endoscopy performed every 2–3 years. Women also require frequent assessments of the endometrium and ovaries, starting at the age of 25–35, with gyne-

Table 47.4 Hereditary polyposis syndromes

Syndrome	Mutated gene(s)	Colorectal cancer risk
Syndromes with adenomas		
Familial adenomatous polyposis (FAP)	*APC*	100%
Attenuated FAP	*APC*	100%
MUTYH gene–associated polyposis (MAP)	*MUTYH*	?
Hereditary nonpolyposis colorectal cancer (HNPCC)	MMR genes	80%
Syndromes with hamartomatous polyps		
Peutz–Jeghers syndrome	*STK11* (*LKB1*)	40%
Juvenile polyposis syndrome	*SMAD 4, BRPR1A*	20–60%
Cowden syndrome	*PTEN*	10%

MMR, mismatch repair genes.

Table 47.5 The Amsterdam I and II criteria for the diagnosis of hereditary nonpolyposis colorectal cancer (all criteria must be met)

Amsterdam I criteria
1. Three or more relatives with histologically verified colorectal cancer, one of whom is a first-degree relative of the other two; familial adenomatous polyposis should be excluded
2. Colorectal cancer involving at least two successive generations
3. One or more colorectal cancer cases diagnosed before the age of 50

Amsterdam II criteria
1. Three or more relatives with histologically verified HNPCC-associated cancer (colorectal, endometrial, small bowel, ureter, or renal pelvis), one of whom is a first-degree relative of the other two; familial adenomatous polyposis should be excluded
2. HNPCC-associated cancer involving at least two successive generations
3. One or more cancer cases diagnosed before the age of 50

HNPCC, hereditary nonpolyposis colorectal cancer.

Table 47.6 Revised Bethesda guidelines for microsatellite instability (MSI) testing of colorectal tumors (only one criterion must be met) [9]

Tumors from individuals should be tested for MSI in the following situations
- Colorectal cancer diagnosed in a patient under 50 years of age
- Presence of synchronous or metachronous colorectal, or other HNPCC-associated tumors, regardless of age*
- Colorectal cancer with MSI-H† histology‡ diagnosed in a patient under 60 years of age
- Colorectal cancer diagnosed in one or more first-degree relatives with an HNPCC-related tumor, with one of the cancers being diagnosed under the age of 50
- Colorectal cancer diagnosed in two or more first-degree or second-degree relatives with HNPCC-related tumors, regardless of age

* Colorectal, endometrial, stomach, small bowel, ovarian, pancreas, ureter and renal pelvis, biliary tract, and brain (usually glioblastoma) cancers, sebaceous gland neoplasms (carcinomas, adenomas), and keratoacanthomas.
† MSI-H, microsatellite instability–high; tumors with changes in two or more of the five National Cancer Institute–recommended panels of microsatellite markers.
‡ Presence of tumor-infiltrating lymphocytes, Crohn-like lymphocytic reaction, mucinous/signet-ring differentiation, or medullary growth pattern.
HNPCC, hereditary nonpolyposis colorectal cancer.

47

cological ultrasonography, endometrial biopsy, and CA-125 monitoring. Treatment for Lynch syndrome is the same as that for sporadic colorectal cancer. In patients with colonic cancer, a colectomy with an ileorectal anastomosis is usually advocated. When the rectum is preserved, annual endoscopic check-ups are required.

Hamartomatous polyposis syndromes are responsible for only 0.1% of all colorectal cancers. Peutz–Jeghers syndrome is an autosomal-dominantly inherited mutation of the serine/threonine kinase 11 gene (*STK11*, also known as *LKB1*). The main features are hamartomatous polyps in the gastrointestinal tract and pigmentation of the skin around the mouth, on the lips, and on the buccal mucosa. Polyps occur in the stomach and intestines, but most frequently in the small bowel (95%). As they grow to about 3 cm in diameter, symptoms and complications may appear, including bleeding, intussusception, and ileus. In patients over age 30, cancers can occur in the stomach, pancreas, small bowel, and large bowel. The cumulative risk for these cancers is 40% by the age of 60. The risk of tumors occurring outside the gastrointestinal tract is also relatively high—for example, in the breast (50% risk), endometrium, ovaries, and lungs. Management consists of screening and removal of polyps larger than 1 cm [10]. Small-bowel screening begins at the age of 10, or when symptoms occur, and is repeated annually. Screenings include small-bowel radiography, capsule endoscopy, and balloon-assisted enteroscopy. The large bowel is examined every 2 years, starting at the age of 25. Polyps that cannot be removed by endoscopic methods for various reasons (e.g., size or location) are removed by surgery. During surgery, intraoperative endoscopy may be useful. Balloon-assisted enteroscopy also allows safe polyp removal.

Juvenile polyposis syndrome results from autosomal-dominant mutations in the *SMAD4, BMPR1A,* or *ENG* (rarely) genes. The syndrome is characterized by the presence of hamartomatous polyps in the gastrointestinal tract, mainly in the large bowel (98%), and less frequently in the stomach, duodenum, or small bowel. The syndrome significantly increases the risk of colorectal cancer (up to 60%), and to a lesser extent cancer of the stomach, duodenum, and pancreas. Juvenile polyps may occur as early as infancy to age 10, but the mean age of diagnosis is around 20 years old. The disease results in the formation of tens to hundreds of polyps. The majority of polyps are pedunculated, but smaller polyps, typically in the stomach, are sessile. The presenting symptoms are usually bleeding and anemia. Later, abdominal pain, diarrhea, and intussusception may occur. Surveillance colonoscopy usually begins after diagnosis, but no later than age 15. Colonoscopy with polypectomy should be repeated every 1–2 years and, after removal of all visible polyps, every 3 years. Gastroscopy is indicated every 1–2 years starting at age 25. The small bowel is examined radiologically and/or by enteroscopy or capsule endoscopy. In patients with moderate numbers of polyps in the gastrointestinal tract, endoscopic therapy is usually sufficient. Patients with multiple polyps, anemia, significant hypoproteinemia, high-grade dysplasia, or cancer require a colectomy with an ileorectal anastomosis or a proctocolectomy.

Colorectal Cancer

Colorectal cancer is the fourth most frequent cause of cancer mortality worldwide. The incidence and mortality are decreasing in developed countries, but increasing in most other countries [11]. Colorectal cancer rarely occurs in people under the age of 40. The risk increases after 40 and peaks in the eighth decade of life. Approximately 85% of colorectal cancers are adenocarcinomas, and the majority develop from adenomas.

Development of colorectal cancer is caused by many factors, but the most significant are genetic and environmental. Established precancerous lesions include sporadic adenomas, polyposis syn-

dromes, and inflammatory bowel disease. The majority of sporadic cancers (>90%) arise from adenomas as a result of acquired and accumulated mutations in suppressor genes (*APC, SMAD4, DCC, TP53*) and oncogenes (K-*ras*). The alternative pathway, modeled after hereditary nonpolyposis colorectal cancer (HNPCC), involves inactivation of mismatch repair genes that provide genetic stability in normal conditions. Mutations or silencing of these genes causes uncontrolled growth. Microsatellite instability occurs in nearly all cases of HNPCC and in 15% of sporadic cancers. The most common epigenetic mechanism that leads to functional silencing of genes is DNA hypermethylation in the promoter regions of genes such as *hMLH1* and *APC*. A silent *hMLH1* gene is also characteristic of malignant transformation in serrated, hyperplastic polyps. It is the third most common pathway that leads to cancer in the large bowel.

Differences in the epidemiology of colorectal cancer may be explained by differences in exposure to environmental factors. The most important environmental factor is diet. Colorectal cancer is associated with a diet rich in animal fat and red meat and poor in calcium, selenium, folic acid, and fiber. This type of diet has an unfavorable influence on the bacterial flora of the large bowel, induces synthesis of carcinogenic substances, and prolongs the time of passage of intestinal contents.

Many symptoms of colorectal cancer depend on the location and stage of the disease. However, irrespective of location and stage, the most frequent symptoms are occult bleeding and abdominal pain. The former led to the introduction of fecal occult blood testing for colorectal cancer screening. Abdominal pain, although frequent, is not a specific characteristic. The most frequent symptoms of rectal and left-sided cancer are overt bleeding and a recent change in bowel habits. Cecal and ascending colon cancers frequently present with anemia. Hemorrhage and perforation occur rarely. Mechanical ileus is a presenting symptom in about 6% of patients.

The most useful diagnostic test is colonoscopy because it permits visualization of the tumor, biopsy sampling for histology, and inspection of the entire large bowel to locate synchronous tumors (**Fig. 47.18**). An abdominal ultrasound or a CT scan is useful for detecting metastases to the liver and lymph nodes. Endosonography and magnetic resonance imaging are employed for staging rectal cancers. Positron-emission tomography (PET) is a good method for detecting recurrences of colorectal cancer, but has limited value for primary staging. The differential diagnosis includes diverticular disease, hemorrhoids, colitis, neuroendocrine tumors, and lymphomas.

The mainstay of therapy is bowel resection and regional lymph nodes. Resection is performed by traditional surgery or, in selected cases, with a laparoscopic approach; the two methods have similar long-term results. The prognosis depends on many different factors, but the main one is the pathological stage at the time of surgery. **Table 47.7** presents the Dukes, Astler–Coller, and TNM classifications, with corresponding 5-year survival rates.

Adjuvant chemotherapy consisting of intravenous fluorouracil (5-FU) and folinic acid is advocated for patients with stage III colon cancer. Oral therapy with 5-FU precursors (capecitabine and tegafur–uracil) provides similar efficacy and reduced toxicity in comparison with intravenous 5-FU. The addition of oxaliplatin to standard doses of 5-FU and folinic acid improves the results of therapy. For patients with stage II colon cancer, adjuvant chemotherapy is not routinely recommended.

In contrast to colon cancer, rectal cancer can also be treated with radiotherapy. The efficacy of chemotherapy and radiotherapy has been confirmed for rectal cancers in stages II and III. Currently, the preferred method of radiotherapy is intense, high-dose irradiation (2500 cGy over 5 days) preoperatively. In patients who receive preoperative irradiation, adding 5-FU and folinic acid appears to have no effect on survival, although it significantly decreases the rate of local recurrences [12].

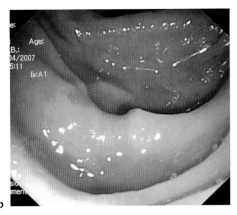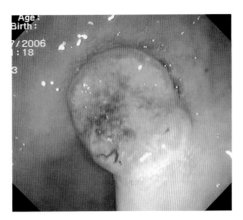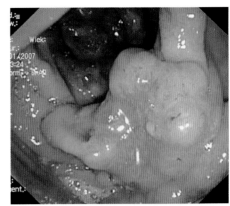

Fig. 47.18 Examples of early cancers in the large bowel.
a A type IIa + IIc cancer in the ascending colon.

b A small asymptomatic cancer.
c A small cancer in the ascending colon.

Advanced, nonresectable colorectal cancers are treated with intravenous 5-FU and folinic acid or oral capecitabine. Other regimens known as FOLFIRI and FOLFOX consist of irinotecan or oxaliplatin added to 5-FU and folinic acid. The newest drugs used for metastatic tumors are monoclonal antibodies against epidermal growth factor receptors (EGFR; cetuximab and panitumumab) and a humanized antibody against vascular endothelial growth factor (VEGF; bevacizumab).

Colorectal strictures can be recanalized palliatively using self-expanding metal stents, laser photocoagulation, or argon plasma coagulation. Hepatic metastases can be resected or destroyed with a percutaneous alcohol injection into the tumor, or with cytostatic drugs administered selectively into appropriate branches of the hepatic artery.

After radical surgery, patients are followed up every 3–6 months for the first 2 years, and less frequently for the next 3 years. Follow-up schedules differ between centers. The prognosis can be improved with yearly CT (or ultrasound) examinations and frequent assessments of the serum carcinoembryonic antigen (CEA) concentration. A colonoscopy is recommended in the perioperative period (to search for synchronic lesions) and then at 1, 3, and 5 years after surgery (to search for metachronous lesions). As mentioned earlier, the prognosis depends on the stage of the disease at the time of surgery (**Table 47.7**). As many as 80 % of tumors are staged B, C, or D; thus, the mean 5-year survival rate is approximately 45 %.

Since the 1980s, it has been well documented that the prognosis in colorectal cancer can be improved by screening the asymptomatic population. The main aim of screening is to reduce the incidence and mortality of colorectal cancer. This can be achieved with early detection and removal of colorectal adenomas. Research into screening strategies has intensified over the last 30 years. Studies have usually included healthy, asymptomatic people over 45 years old. The three dominant screening strategies were fecal occult blood testing, fiber sigmoidoscopy, and total colonoscopy. Each has advantages and disadvantages. The preferred strategy in the United States and some other countries is primary colonoscopy, as it provides the highest sensitivity and specificity for cancer; this is also the only method that allows immediate removal of all polyps detected [13,14]. The value of this approach depends on the quality of the examination, which is measured by the adenoma detection rate, cecal intubation rate, and colonoscope withdrawal time from cecum to rectum (more than 6 min) [15,16]. Other potential screening methods are CT colonography (virtual colonoscopy) and stool testing for mutated genes (APC, K-ras, TP53). All these methods are listed in the latest recommendations prepared by the American Cancer Society, the U.S. Multi-Society Task Force on Colorectal Cancer, and

Table 47.7 Staging of colorectal cancer and corresponding 5-year survival rates

Stage	Dukes[*]/ Astler–Coller classifications	TNM stages[†]	Description	5-year survival rate
0	–	Tis, N0, M0	Cancer limited to the mucosa	100 %
I	A /A and B1	T1–2, N0, M0	Tumor not through the muscularis propria	80–95 %
II	B /B2	T3–4, N0, M0	Through the bowel wall	65–75 %
III	C/C 1 and C 2	T1–4, N1–2, M0	Positive lymph nodes	25–65 %
IV	D	T1–4, N0–2, M1	Distant metastases	0–7 %

[*] According to the Turnbull modification.
[†] N0, negative lymph nodes; N1, one to three positive lymph nodes; N2, four or more positive lymph nodes.

Table 47.8 Screening strategies for early detection of colorectal cancer and adenomatous polyps in asymptomatic adults aged 50 years and older [17]

Tests that detect adenomatous polyps and cancer
Flexible sigmoidoscopy every 5 years
Colonoscopy every 10 years
Double contrast barium enema every 5 years
CT colonography every 5 years

Tests that primarily detect cancer
Guaiac FOBT annually
Immunological FOBT annually
Fecal DNA testing, interval uncertain

CT, computed tomography; FOBT, fecal occult blood test.

the American College of Radiology (**Table 47.8**) [17]. The recommendations group screening tests into those that primarily detect cancer and those that detect cancer and adenomatous polyps, thus providing cancer prevention through polypectomy. In practice, screening should be offered to asymptomatic individuals with an average risk of cancer, aged 50–75 years old; the choice of screening method will depend on local availability, costs, and preferences.

47

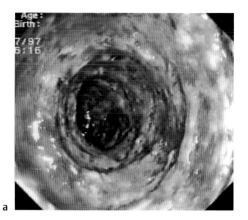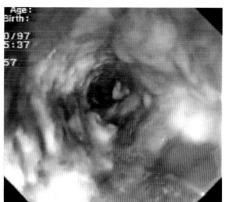

Fig. 47.19 Ischemic colitis.
a An early image, with hemorrhagic mucosa.
b Two weeks later, the image shows necrosis.

Numerous epidemiological studies have shown that regular acetylsalicylic acid consumption was associated with a 40–50 % reduction in the incidence and mortality of colorectal cancer. In addition, sulindac, a nonsteroidal anti-inflammatory drug, reduced the number and size of adenomas in patients with familial adenomatous polyposis. The mechanism underlying the chemopreventive activity of nonsteroidal anti-inflammatory drugs is not completely understood, but one mechanism is related to cyclooxygenase-2 (COX-2) inhibition. For practical reasons, selective COX-2 inhibitors cannot be widely used as chemopreventive agents, due to their cardiovascular complications. Currently, only 300 mg/day acetylsalicylic acid can be regarded as a chemopreventive agent [18]. However, it is not recommended in practice due to the apprehension that its permissive effect on gastrointestinal bleeding might negate any clinical benefits [19].

Ischemic Colitis

Ischemic colitis develops when insufficient blood flows into the bowel wall. It has various degrees of severity and courses, some with poor prognoses. The disease is usually associated with atherosclerosis. The most frequent triggering factors are shock, recent myocardial infarction, and cardiac insufficiency. Other factors include thromboembolism, coagulopathies with excessive coagulation, and use of contraceptives. Intestinal blood flow may also be interrupted as a consequence of abdominal aortic aneurysm surgery or abdominoperineal rectal resection. The most frequently affected segments of the large bowel are the splenic flexure and descending and sigmoid colons. In some patients, the disease is caused by stenosis due to malignancy or diverticulitis. In these situations, ischemic changes occur proximal to the stenosis.

In the majority of cases, ischemic colitis begins subacutely with bleeding and ends after a few weeks, even without any specific therapy. Some patients develop scar stenoses after healing from ischemic colitis. In about 10 % of the cases, the disease starts with acute abdominal pain and hemorrhage. The pain is usually located in the left abdomen. Other symptoms include fever and leukocytosis. The development of intestinal damage is rapid. Necrosis of the bowel wall and perforation with peritonitis may develop within a short period of time. The "thumbprinting" seen on a barium enema may be a sign of early ischemic colitis within a diseased segment of the colon. However, in the early phase of ischemic colitis, a barium enema is usually contraindicated, as is colonoscopy. Nevertheless, one of these two examinations should be performed after clinical stabilization of the patient has been achieved. The endoscopic findings vary depending on the severity of the ischemia and the timing of the examination. Usually, endoscopy should be performed within 48 h of presentation. Typically, segmental colitis with a sharp demarcation between involved and normal colon is seen. Early endoscopic changes include edema and blebs in the mucosa and submucosal hemorrhage. As the hemorrhage is resorbed, friability, necrosis, and ulceration can occur (**Fig. 47.19**). Histologically, vascular congestion with acute or chronic inflammation is commonly seen. Changes more typical of ischemia include mucosal infarction, ghost cells, and hemosiderin-laden macrophages. It is generally difficult to diagnose ischemic colitis in the early stages of the disease. The differential diagnosis includes diverticulitis and colonic cancer with perforation. An abdominal CT is typically performed to rule out other diagnoses. Ischemia and small-bowel infarctions are usually present and are expressed clinically as central abdominal pain without intestinal bleeding.

Initial general supportive measures include intravenous fluids and antibiotics. The subsequent disease course may be uncomplicated without further therapy; however, the most severe cases require surgical resection of the diseased segment. Segmental resection is also the method of choice in patients who develop post-ischemic stenoses.

Pseudomembranous Colitis

Pseudomembranous colitis is an acute diarrheal disease of the small and/or large bowel, characterized by the presence of yellowish pseudomembranes that are evenly distributed on the mucosal surface in the diseased segments of the large bowel. Microscopically, these pseudomembranes are composed of fibrin, mucus, shed epithelial cells, and granulocytes. The epithelium is typically infiltrated with cells characteristic of acute or chronic inflammation.

Pseudomembranous colitis was first described at the end of the 19th century. In the era before antibiotics, the disease was attributed to ischemia of the bowel due to hypotension as a result of abdominal surgery. In the 1950s and 1960s, the same disease was attributed to *Staphylococcus aureus* infection. By 1978, it was known that the disease was caused by the use of wide-spectrum antibiotics and the action of the *Clostridium difficile* toxin. The antibiotics that pose the greatest risk are ampicillin, amoxicillin, clindamycin, lincomycin, and cephalosporins, because they select C. difficile from among the normal bacterial strains of the large bowel. Given a competitive advantage, these bacteria rapidly multiply and produce large amounts of A and B toxins, which cause damage to the large-bowel mucosa. Apart from antibiotics, there are many other conditions that predispose to pseudomembranous colitis, including vertebral column fracture, ileus, colon cancer, leukemia, other neoplasms, severe burn, shock, uremia, severe infections, ischemic colitis, and Hirschsprung disease. In addition, oncological chemotherapy is a very important risk factor. Recently, the incidence and severity of pseudomembranous colitis appear to be increasing, which is attrib-

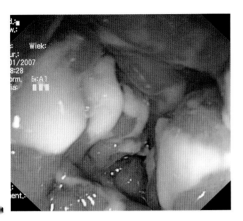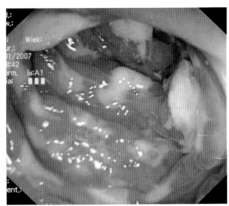

Fig. 47.20 Pseudomembranous colitis.
a Pseudomembranes covering folds of the large bowel.
b Another view in the same patient.

utable to a more virulent strain of C. difficile (BI/NAP1) that produces more toxins [20].

The main symptom of pseudomembranous colitis is diarrhea. It starts during antibiotic therapy or within 1 month after the completion of therapy. The severity of diarrhea can vary from a few liquid stools per day to 30 watery defecations per day. Blood is rarely present in the stool. Other symptoms include abdominal pain, fever, and increased white blood cell counts. Patients with more severe cases may develop dehydration, electrolyte disturbance, hypoalbuminemia, a drop in blood pressure, toxic megacolon, or bowel perforation. In the majority of cases, the course of pseudomembranous colitis is mild and self-limiting; it typically resolves within 5–10 days after elimination of the causative factor.

The diagnosis of pseudomembranous colitis is confirmed by endoscopy and stool examination. Flexible sigmoidoscopy is performed in patients with more severe symptoms when an accurate diagnosis is desired in order to initiate therapy. In patients with mild symptoms, there may be no abnormalities or only patchy or diffuse, nonspecific inflammation of the colonic mucosa. In patients with severe illness, true pseudomembranous colitis is seen. This has a characteristic appearance, with yellow adherent plaques from 2 mm to 2 cm in diameter scattered over the colonic mucosa, interspersed with hyperemic mucosa (**Fig. 47.20**). In 10 % of cases, a colonoscopy may be required due to abnormalities present exclusively in the right colon. During endoscopy, biopsies should be taken. The stool should be cultured to assess for C. difficile and examined for the presence of A and B toxins. The latter procedure is simpler, and the results correlate with clinical severity. The differential diagnosis includes infectious diseases (based on microbiological assessment) and ulcerative colitis.

Mild cases of pseudomembranous colitis may be sufficiently treated by terminating the use of the antibiotics thought to be causing the disease. Antiperistaltic drugs are contraindicated. Patients with severe cases require hospitalization. Typically, intravenous fluids are necessary. If a link to *Clostridium difficile* is confirmed, oral metronidazole (500 mg t.i. d.) or vancomycin (125 mg q.i.d.) is prescribed for 1–2 weeks. In severe cases, the doses may be increased. Other drugs are rarely necessary—e. g., teicoplanin; however, in the most severe cases, systemic steroids are prescribed. Toxic megacolon or perforation requires surgery. Treatment for recurrences requires the same antibiotics, metronidazole or vancomycin. Recently, probiotics *(e. g.,Saccharomyces boulardii)* have been prescribed to prevent recurrences and to maintain and restore the natural intestinal flora [21].

Bacterial Colitis

Bacterial colitis may be caused by a number of pathogens. **Table 47.9** lists the most common of these.

Invasive *Shigella* species are classical pathogens of the large bowel. They enter the epithelial cells and cause damage to the rectum and colon, resulting in tenesmus and bloody diarrhea. *Escherichia coli* (O157:H7), *Campylobacter jejuni*, and *Entamoeba histolytica* belong to the same group of invasive pathogens. Other bacteria typically damage the distal part of the small bowel, but they can also cause inflammation of the colorectum. *Salmonella* and *Yersinia enterocolitica* may also cause fever and symptoms of arthritis. Colorectal inflammation in homosexual individuals may be caused by amebas, gonococci, and chlamydias (*Chlamydia trachomatis*).

In an infection that involves the rectum, rigid or flexible proctosigmoidoscopy can reveal inflammation, hemorrhage, and ulcerations. The endoscopic picture may be indistinguishable from ulcerative colitis. A special type of intestinal infection is known as traveler's diarrhea. It is mainly caused by *E. coli* species that produce enterotoxin (40–75 % of cases). Food and water in developing countries or regions with poor hygiene can cause this type of infection. Symptoms become obvious 1–3 days after the infection. They include watery diarrhea, abdominal pain, nausea, and shivering. The symptoms generally disappear within several days without therapy. Some authors advocate using a novel nonabsorbed antibiotic, rifaximin [22].

47

Table 47.9 Main causes and symptoms of intestinal infections

Pathogen	Incubation time	Main symptoms	Sensitivity to antibiotics
Escherichia coli O157:H7	3–9 days	From asymptomatic to bloody diarrhea, vomiting	Therapy is controversial
Shigella spp.	1–3 days	Tenesmus, watery and later bloody diarrhea	Ciprofloxacin, cotrimoxazole
Salmonella spp.	6–48 h	Watery or bloody diarrhea, general symptoms	Ciprofloxacin, cephalosporin III
Campylobacter jejuni	1–8 days	Headache, muscle pain, fever, bloody diarrhea	Ciprofloxacin, erythromycin
Yersinia enterocolitica	Various	Abdominal pain, fever, diarrhea, arthritis	Ciprofloxacin, tetracycline
Entamoeba histolytica	Various	From asymptomatic to bloody diarrhea	Metronidazole

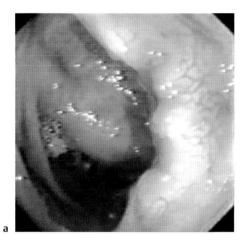
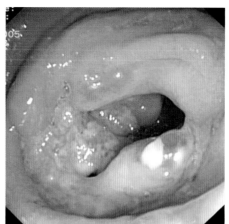

Fig. 47.21 Colonic tuberculosis.
a A transverse ulceration.
b Ileocecal valve involvement.

Most infections of the large bowel are characterized by a mild course. In the developed world, the clinical significance arises from the need to make a differential diagnosis from inflammatory bowel disease, especially ulcerative colitis. Differentiation is most important at the beginning of the disease, when diarrhea is a presenting symptom and the endoscopic picture is not specific. During this period, a conclusive diagnosis is made with microbiological and histological assessments of biopsies taken during proctosigmoidoscopy. Microbiological assessment is based on stool culture, identification of pathogens, and/or serological tests. Recently, it has become possible to use molecular-biological techniques to diagnose intestinal infections. These valuable methods provide rapid diagnosis and improved sensitivity, and are easier in comparison with bacterial culturing.

The microscopic picture of infectious colitis, irrespective of the causative pathogen, includes granulocyte infiltration of the lamina propria. Lymphocytes are rare or absent. There is no distortion of crypt architecture and there is a normal population of goblet cells that produce mucus. These features allow differentiation from inflammatory bowel disease; however, microbiology can only confirm the etiology in 40–60% of acute infection cases, and histological examination is therefore important. Other features include the duration of symptoms and response to antibiotics. When a rectal inflammation does not respond to antibiotics and lasts longer than 1 month, the most likely diagnosis is inflammatory bowel disease.

Approximately 90% of patients with acute infectious diarrhea do not require therapy. The disease is self-limiting and generally disappears within 5–15 days. Antibiotic treatment (**Table 47.8**) is only necessary in more severe and prolonged cases—especially in infections caused by amebas, *Shigella*, *Salmonella typhi* and S. paratyphi, and *E. coli* pathogens in children. Symptomatic antidiarrheal therapy is not contraindicated, but requires care. For example, these drugs are strictly contraindicated for infections with *Salmonella* and *Shigella*.

Tuberculosis

Tuberculosis may involve the entire gastrointestinal tract, but the most common site of abdominal involvement is the ileocecal area. Tuberculosis affected over 400 000 people in Europe in 2002; 1% had intestinal involvement; of those, only 3–4% had colonic involvement. The incidence of colonic tuberculosis in the Western world correlates with increased migration from developing countries and with the regional prevalence of human immunodeficiency virus (HIV) infection.

Mycobacterium tuberculosis (acid-fast bacilli) is the predominant pathogen in intestinal tuberculosis. Another responsible bacterium is M. avium. Abdominal tuberculosis is usually secondary to active pulmonary or miliary tuberculosis. It can be caused by swallowing infected sputum in the active pulmonary form, or by ingesting contaminated milk. The symptoms (and frequency) include fever (40–70%), weight loss (40–90%), abdominal pain (80–95%), and abdominal distention with diarrhea (11–20%). Other less frequent symptoms are anorexia, change in bowel habits, fatigue, and malaise. Ileocecal tuberculosis usually presents with abdominal pain, nausea, vomiting, and symptoms of malabsorption. Rectal tuberculosis presents with hematochezia and constipation in approximately one-third of the patients.

The main diagnostic tool is endoscopy. This reveals lesions mainly in the right colon, including ulcerative lesions, hypertrophic lesions, or both (**Fig. 47.21**). Hypertrophic lesions may mimic a mass lesion. Tuberculosis-related ulcers are usually oriented transversely, with sharp margins and surrounding erythema. Typically, a patulous type of deformation is observed in the ileocecal valve, with heaped-up mucosal folds. Other lesions include fistulas, pseudopolyps, fibrous bands, and strictures. More than half of the patients have multifocal lesions.

Typical histological observations include caseating tuberculous granulomas, which are usually large, confluent, and multiple. However, in many cases, granulomas may not be detectable in biopsy specimens. PCR is highly specific for identifying a pathogen, but it is not very sensitive. A colonic biopsy cultured for *Mycobacterium tuberculosis* is therefore still the gold standard for diagnosis.

For an initial evaluation, plain radiography, barium enema, ultrasonography, and computed tomography are useful. The differential diagnosis includes Crohn's disease, sarcoidosis, periappendiceal abscess, or other infections. Though not specific for tuberculosis, noncaseous granulomas with Langhans giant cells can occur in a colonic biopsy in tuberculosis; caseation is likely to occur only in lymph nodes. On the other hand, observations of aphthoid erosions, linear ulcers, and cobblestoning mucosa are strongly suggestive of Crohn's disease [23].

Typical antituberculosis treatment (isoniazid, pyrazinamide, ethambutol, or rifampicin) for a sufficiently long period is the mainstay of therapy. Additionally, in selected complicated cases, surgery may be necessary.

Viral Colitis

Viral colonic infections—cytomegalovirus (CMV) and herpes simplex virus (HSV)—are most often observed in immunocompromised patients, including patients who have undergone transplantation and those with acquired immunodeficiency syndrome (AIDS), immunosuppressive treatment, or inflammatory bowel disease [24]. Viral infections are rare in immunocompetent individuals.

Cytomegalovirus is the most clinically important of the colonic viral infections. The primary infection presents as a typically self-limiting mononucleosis-like syndrome. Organ involvement usually occurs through reactivation of a latent CMV infection. CMV has an affinity for dysplastic colonic tissue (adenomas and adenocarcinomas). The incidence of CMV infections in patients with inflammatory bowel disease (IBD) is reported to be 0.53–3.4%. The general clinical signs and symptoms of symptomatic CMV infection include fever, leukopenia, and organ involvement. Mortality rates for patients with CMV enterocolitis have been reported to be as high as 71%. Patients with IBD and active CMV infections have a 67% colectomy rate and a 33% mortality rate.

Colonic involvement may cause fever, abdominal pain, diarrhea, gastrointestinal bleeding, and weight loss. Patients with IBD may experience massive hemorrhage, colovesical fistula, toxic megacolon, perforation, and peritonitis. Ischemic colitis due to CMV has been reported in a recipient of an organ transplant. In immunocompetent individuals, the clinical course is usually mild and self-limiting.

Endoscopy can detect CMV colitis, particularly in the right colon, in up to 30% of cases. Typical findings are patchy erythema, exudates, microerosions, mucosal erosions, and deep oval, round ulcers (**Fig. 47.22**). The central regions of ulcers should be biopsied. Histological diagnosis is the gold standard. Microscopically, the classical finding is known as the "owl's eye"—a large eosinophilic intranuclear inclusion body, surrounded by a clear halo. In serological examinations, CMV-specific immunoglobulin M (IgM) antibodies have almost 100% sensitivity and specificity. A PCR test (on organ tissue, whole blood, and stool) is useful for detecting CMV DNA in blood, with a sensitivity of 65–100% and a specificity of 40–92%.

The therapy of choice for CMV colitis is ganciclovir (5 mg/kg i. v. every 12 h). Usually 2 weeks of treatment is recommended. Antiviral treatment is not always necessary in an immunocompetent patient.

Herpes infection predominantly affects homosexuals and presents with severe anorectal pain, tenesmus, and mucus discharge that may be accompanied by difficulty in urinating and inguinal lymphadenopathy. It involves the perianal skin and anal canal, but may extend to the rectum. The endoscopic appearance includes patchy or diffuse erythema and edema with erosions or ulcerations and discrete vesicular or pustular lesions. Oral administration of acyclovir may accelerate resolution of the symptoms.

Diverticular Disease

Diverticula in the large bowel may be inherited or acquired. Inherited diverticula are rare, mainly single lesions located in the right colon; they have little practical significance. In contrast, acquired diverticula occur frequently. They are small hernias of the mucosa that penetrate through the muscularis propria of the colon. Diverticula are among the most frequent human diseases occurring in the fifth decade of life or later. One-third of the population over the age of 60 may have colonic diverticula. Diverticula belong to the group of "diseases of civilization," as they are present mainly in Western societies and are almost unknown in developing countries. The main factor responsible for this distribution is believed to be the content of fiber in food. According to one hypothesis, insufficient

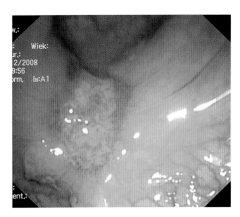

Fig. 47.22 An oval ulcer surrounded by normal mucosa in cytomegalovirus colitis.

dietary fiber causes excessive colonic contractions, hypertrophy of the circular layer of the muscularis propria, and an increase in intracolonic pressure. This pressure causes "expulsion" of the mucosa to the outer abdominal cavity through the points of least resistance—i. e., the points where small vessels penetrate the muscle layer.

Diverticula are typically 5–10 mm in diameter and never occur in the rectum. Their wall is composed of mucosal and serosal layers, and they are therefore also called pseudodiverticula. Diverticula are typically accompanied by hypertrophy of the muscularis layer, thickening of circular muscle layer, and shortening of the teniae. These abnormalities occur mostly in the sigmoid colon (more than 90%) and less frequently in the more proximal parts of the colon.

Large-bowel diverticula are generally asymptomatic and are typically detected incidentally during a barium enema study or colonoscopy. The asymptomatic form of the disease is called diverticulosis. Only about 20–30% of the patients have symptoms that can be attributed to diverticula. The most frequent are left lower abdominal quadrant pain and a change in stool habits, often accompanied by abdominal distension, constipation, or alternating constipation and diarrhea. Symptoms of subocclusion may also occur. All of these symptomatic forms are known as symptomatic diverticular disease. Infrequently, acute diverticulitis develops; this typically starts in a single diverticulum, but may quickly spread along the colon wall, causing a pericolonic abscess. In this situation, microperforation may occur, with symptoms of local peritonitis. Typical signs of diverticulitis include fever, leukocytosis, palpable tumor, and peritonitis in the left lower quadrant. Complications may occur, including occlusion, fistula, intra-abdominal abscess, free perforation, and hemorrhage.

Diverticula are diagnosed on barium enema or endoscopic examinations (**Figs. 47.23–47.25**). In acute cases, and when a complication is suspected, computed tomography is the most useful diagnostic tool. The most frequent findings are bowel wall thickening, inflammatory cell infiltration in the pericolonic fatty tissue, or the presence of an abscess. Abscesses can also be identified by abdominal ultrasound. Bleeding can be confirmed by angiography or isotope scanning. The differential diagnosis of diverticular disease and its complications includes functional diseases of the gastrointestinal tract, colorectal cancer, Crohn's disease, ischemic colitis, acute bacterial colitis, and some gynecological disorders (e. g., ovarian cancer) or urological disorders (e. g., urinary bladder infection).

Therapy for uncomplicated diverticular disease is administered on an outpatient basis and includes dietary fiber, starting with one or two large tablespoons daily. Pharmacotherapy includes antispasmodic drugs (drotaverine) or anticholinergic drugs (oxyphenonium bromide). A nonabsorbed antibiotic, rifaximin, can also be used even in the absence of an overt inflammation [25]. Italian authors

47

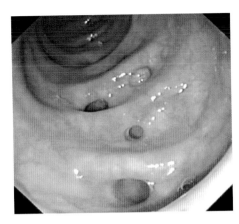

Fig. 47.23 Large-bowel diverticula.

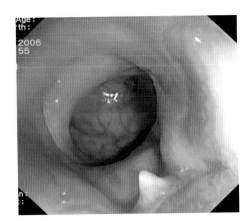

Fig. 47.24 Diverticulitis, with pus evacuation from the inflamed diverticulum.

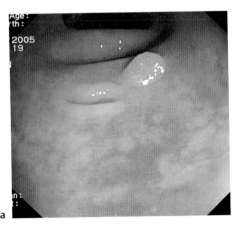

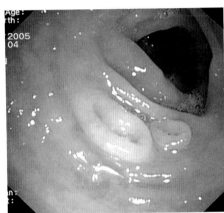

Fig. 47.25 Some small diverticula may look like small polyps at some stages; an attempt to remove them may potentially cause perforation.
a Two diverticula, one inverted, resembling a small polyp.
b It is clear that both lesions are diverticula.

a

b

VII

have described favorable results with the use of mesalazine [26]. Diverticulitis requires a strict diet and oral antibiotics in less severe cases, or parenteral antibiotics in severe cases. The recommended antibiotics include ciprofloxacin and/or metronidazole, but also third-generation cephalosporins or aminoglycosides in combination with metronidazole. The duration of antibiotic therapy should be 7–10 days. Free perforation, intra-abdominal abscess, and ileus require surgery. In septic complications, the most frequent type of surgery is the Hartmann procedure, with reconstruction of bowel continuity in a second stage. Some patients require surgery for recurrent diverticulitis or subocclusion; in these cases, the typical operation is a single-stage segmental sigmoid resection.

Diverticular hemorrhage stops spontaneously in 80% of patients. In life-threatening situations, endoscopic or radiological methods are necessary to arrest the hemorrhage. These include thermal, injection, and mechanical clipping methods, or interventional angiography with a vasopressin injection. The efficacy of these methods is around 90%. A few patients with persistent or recurrent bleeding may require surgical treatment.

Microscopic Colitis

Microscopic colitis occurs in two forms: collagenous and lymphocytic. Each form has distinct microscopic features, but in both, the large bowel is endoscopically and radiologically normal. The number of newly diagnosed cases of microscopic colitis was six per 100 000 in Sweden in the late 1990s. Women aged 60 or over have the highest prevalence of collagenous colitis. Lymphocytic colitis occurs at a similar age, but with no sex bias. Similar data have been recently reported from a large population-based study conducted in Canada [27].

The pathogenesis and causes of microscopic colitis are unknown. No allergic or bacterial factors have been identified to date. Some studies suggest that nonsteroidal anti-inflammatory drugs may play a role in the pathogenesis of collagenous colitis.

The primary microscopic feature of collagenous colitis is a thickening of the collagen layer at the base of the epithelium. This thickening ranges from 15 to 60 μm (normal thickness is up to 10 μm) and is readily visible in histological sections stained with hematoxylin and eosin. Despite this, diagnosis is sometimes hampered by a patchy distribution (more frequently in the colon than the rectum). The primary microscopic feature of lymphocytic colitis is an increased number of intraepithelial lymphocytes, which are CD8$^+$ T cells (the normal density is 20 lymphocytes per 100 epithelial cells). In both diseases, the lamina propria shows mild to moderate infiltrations of lymphocytes and plasmocytes.

Watery diarrhea is the typical symptom of both collagenous and lymphocytic colitis. Diarrhea is typically accompanied by crampy abdominal pain and excessive intestinal gas. Despite the large-volume defecations, general dehydration is rare. Weight loss (mean 5 kg) occurs in the majority of patients. Both types of microscopic colitis are often accompanied by arthritis, various gastrointestinal diseases (celiac disease, Crohn's disease, ulcerative colitis), rheumatoid arthritis, lupus erythematosus, scleroderma, Sjögren syndrome, psoriasis, hepatitis, or diabetes mellitus.

In microscopic colitis, typically no abnormalities are observed in routine laboratory tests or barium studies of the small and large

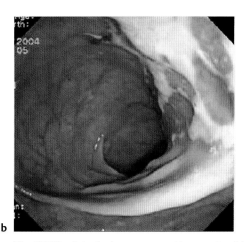
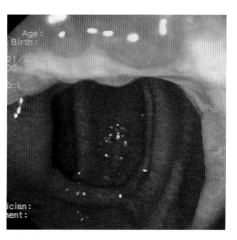
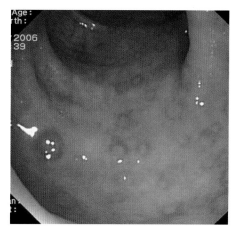

Fig. 47.26 Colonic damage caused by nonsteroidal anti-inflammatory drugs.
a Flat, superficial ulcerations.
b Linear ulcerations along the colonic folds, which may lead to diaphragm-like stenoses (right colon, concomitant melanosis).

Fig. 47.27 Aphthoid-like lesions surrounded by a red "halo" caused by sodium phosphate bowel preparation.

bowel. The colonoscopic findings also appear to be normal, although in some cases mild edema, hyperemia, and petechiae are described. Recently, it was suggested that the "tear sign" (excessive superficial mucosal damage during standard biopsies) can be suggestive of microscopic colitis. In patients with a clinical suspicion of microscopic colitis, biopsies should be taken from the right colon and from the descending or sigmoid colon. The differential diagnosis primarily includes irritable bowel syndrome. Other diseases that have to be taken into account include lactose intolerance, celiac disease, laxative abuse, amyloidosis, neuroendocrine tumors, or abnormalities in bile acid circulation.

Until recently, the only treatment option for microscopic colitis was administration of 5-aminosalicylic acid compounds (sulfasalazine, mesalazine). However, recent studies have indicated the efficacy of budesonide at 9 mg/day for 6–8 weeks [28]. In severe cases, classical corticosteroids can induce improvement in at least 80 % of the patients. Antibiotics (metronidazole, erythromycin) or bismuth compounds are only partially effective. In some patients, an antidiarrheal effect can be obtained with cholestyramine. Loperamide can also inhibit diarrhea when taken in large doses (4 mg per dose). In extreme cases that are refractory to pharmacotherapy, it may be necessary to perform surgical ileostomy. Treatment of lymphocytic colitis is less well established. Sulfasalazine or prednisone may lead to improvement in the majority of cases. Surgery is not indicated for this form of microscopic colitis.

Drug-Induced and Chemical-Induced Colopathy

Nonsteroidal anti-inflammatory drugs (NSAIDs) are the most common cause of drug-induced colopathy in clinical practice. Approximately 10 % of newly diagnosed colitis may be related to these drugs. The most frequently used oral preparations of NSAIDs that may induce colonic injury include enteric-coated aspirin, ibuprofen, diclofenac, naproxen and ketoprofen. NSAID-induced colitis affects older people, without gender preponderance. Although the most common presenting symptom is diarrhea, other symptoms such as rectal bleeding, fever, weight loss, or iron-deficiency anemia can occur. Endoscopically, mucosal erythema, granularity, erosions, or flat ulcerations are seen in the colon (**Fig. 47.26**). Diaphragm-like strictures, occasionally leading to colonic obstruction, may be present in the right colon. Rectal preparations of NSAIDs may cause proctitis, rectal ulcers, and anorectal stenosis. Histological features are typically nonspecific, with ulceration and other inflammatory

changes seen in the colonic mucosa. The treatment of choice is withdrawal of NSAIDs. It should be stressed that the use of NSAIDs may worsen the existing inflammatory bowel disease and is associated with an increased risk of diverticulitis and diverticular perforation.

Sodium phosphate. The use of sodium phosphate solutions for bowel cleansing for colonoscopy causes mucosal injury in 3 % of cases. Lesions are usually found in the left colon and rectum. Endoscopically, the mucosa may appear edematous and erythematous or may look normal, with tiny aphthoid-like lesions ranging from petechial markings to superficial ulcerations (**Fig. 47.27**). Histological examination demonstrates focal neutrophilic cryptitis and the presence of apoptotic bodies within the crypts. Diagnosis is made on the basis of the endoscopic and histological appearance of the mucosa in a patient who has used sodium phosphate solutions for bowel preparation. The sodium phosphate–induced colonic lesions should be distinguished from early aphthoid ulcers in Crohn's disease.

Melanosis Coli

Melanosis is a deposition of brown pigment in the mucosa of the colon. It develops in patients with recurrent constipation who have a long history of using anthracene-containing laxatives. The name for the condition is deceptive, as it mistakenly suggests that the pigment involved might be melanin. However, the pigment arises from lipofuscin, a lipid residue formed by the degradation of colonic epithelial cells. The colonic epithelial cells are damaged by anthraquinones and then stored in macrophages in the lamina propria of the colon. The pigmentation is most intense in the cecum and ascending colon. This is probably due to the higher laxative concentration in the lumen of the proximal colon, or the different mucosal absorption rates of cathartic agents within that part of the colon. The pigmentation in the colonic mucosa may be patchy, with a "starry sky" appearance in regions such as the rectum, which has a high concentration of lymphoid cells that do not accumulate pigment (**Fig. 47.28**). Neoplastic lesions, including adenomas and carcinomas, are easily detected endoscopically because they do not take up the pigment. However, submucosal lesions (e. g., leiomyomas) are concealed by the pigmented mucosa. Melanosis typically resolves spontaneously, following discontinuation of anthracene-containing laxatives.

47

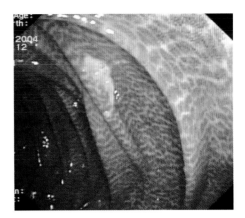

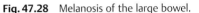

Fig. 47.28 Melanosis of the large bowel.

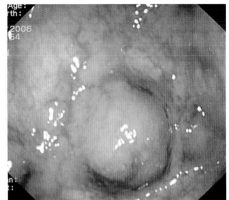

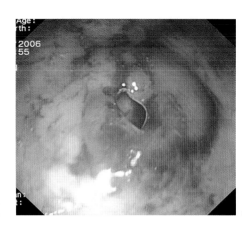

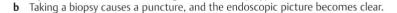

Fig. 47.29 Pneumatosis cystoides intestinalis.
a A pneumatosis lesion resembling a submucosal polyp.
b Taking a biopsy causes a puncture, and the endoscopic picture becomes clear.

Pneumatosis Cystoides Intestinalis

Pneumatosis cystoides intestinalis is the presence of gas in the bowel wall. Typically, this condition shows multiple submucosal or subserosal pneumocysts. The disease was first described by the French pathologist Du Vernoi in the 18th century, in an autopsy specimen. In fact, the term represents a physical or radiographic finding that is the result of an underlying pathological process. Conditions thought to be related include various connective tissue diseases (dermatomyositis, systemic lupus erythematosus, scleroderma), chronic obstructive pulmonary disease, ischemic bowel disease, necrotizing enterocolitis, AIDS, drug therapy (steroids, methotrexate, alpha-glucosidase inhibitors), trichloroethylene exposure, and raised intra-abdominal pressure due to ileus surgery.

The overall incidence of pneumatosis cystoides intestinalis in the general population is estimated to be 0.03%, according to autopsy studies. It occurs more commonly in men than women, and the peak incidence occurs in individuals aged 30–50. The sigmoid colon is the most common site of occurrence.

Patients may be asymptomatic or may present with symptoms of nausea, vomiting, diarrhea, bloody stools, abdominal pain and distention, constipation, weight loss, and tenesmus. Diagnosis is based on plain radiography, abdominal ultrasonography, and preferably a CT scan. The CT scan will reveal a linear or bubbly pattern of gas in the bowel wall. The diagnosis of pneumatosis cystoides intestinalis is established by finding intramural gas parallel to the bowel wall. Pneumatosis cystoides intestinalis typically exhibits a circular collection of gas in the bowel and mesentery. A positive abdominal radiograph is obtained in two-thirds of patients with pneumatosis cystoides intestinalis. The presence of massive intraperitoneal and/or retroperitoneal air can mimic perforated diffuse peritonitis. Occasionally, pneumatosis is first diagnosed on endoscopy, due to the observation of polyp-like lesions that are soft to the touch and can be "punctured" with biopsy forceps (**Fig. 47.29**).

The therapy for pneumatosis cystoides intestinalis is complex. Inspiration of oxygen (70–75% at a flow rate of 8 L/min) from a face mask should be administered to maintain the partial pressure of arterial oxygen above 300 mmHg for at least 48 h after the complete radiological disappearance of all cysts. Unfortunately, discontinuation of therapy leads to recurrence. Other forms of therapy include broad-spectrum antibiotics and elemental diets. Urgent surgery is required for ischemic bowel (mesenteric ischemia), perforation, peritonitis, or abdominal sepsis [29,30].

Solitary Rectal Ulcer Syndrome

Solitary rectal ulcer syndrome is a rare disorder characterized by inflammation of the rectum associated with functional disturbances. The pathophysiology of solitary rectal ulcer syndrome is complex and not fully understood. However, the main factors that contribute to its development appear to be anorectal redundancy, with a lack of mesorectosacral fixation, and rectal hypersensitivity, leading to uncoordinated defecation with excessive straining and occult rectorectal intussusception. The classic symptoms of solitary rectal ulcer syndrome are rectal bleeding (usually mild), mucus discharge, rectal pain, and tenesmus. Patients also usually report constipation, dyschezia (mainly excessive straining or a feeling of incomplete evacuation), and the need for rectal digitation in some cases.

The endoscopic appearance of solitary rectal ulcer syndrome is heterogeneous and includes ulcerated, polypoid, and flat lesions. The term for the disease is misleading, as the lesions may not be solitary or ulcerated. A typical ulcer associated with this syndrome is shallow, with a white slough base, surrounded by a rim of erythematous mucosa, and is situated 4–12 cm from the anal verge on the anterior wall of the rectum. However, ulcers sometimes occur on the lateral or posterior rectal wall and may even be circumferential. There may be multiple lesions. The lesions may also appear as a sessile protruding mass, several broad-based polypoid lesions, or as an erythematous flat area (**Fig. 47.30**).

Generally, the differential diagnosis includes inflammatory bowel disease (e.g., Crohn's disease), infection, or even cancer. Diagnosis is confirmed on the basis of the histopathological examination, which mainly shows fibromuscular obliteration of the lamina propria, upward proliferation and hypertrophy of the muscularis mucosa, and glandular crypt abnormalities, including hyperplasia, branching, elongation, and distortion.

Treatment of solitary rectal ulcer syndrome is difficult. Initial medical therapies should include dietary fiber and bulk laxatives. In view of the behavioral nature of the disease, therapy may include advice on defecation habits or biofeedback defecation re-training to improve symptoms and anorectal function, facilitating healing of the lesions. However, for some refractory patients and for patients with persistent or massive bleeding or obstructive symptoms, surgery could be an option. Abdominal rectopexy is often performed when rectal prolapse is present. Surgical excision provides immediate improvements, but the recurrence rate is high.

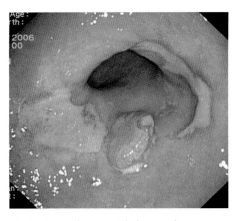
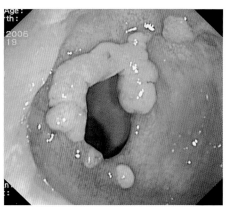
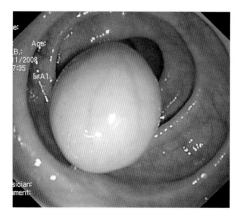

Fig. 47.30 Solitary rectal ulcer syndrome.
a A patient with two ulcers and one polypoid lesion.
b Irregular polypoid elevations.

Fig. 47.31 A large lipoma in the right colon.

Colitis Cystica Profunda

Colitis cystica profunda (CCP) is a rare nonneoplastic lesion characterized by the presence of a mucus-filled cyst, typically situated in the middle or lower rectum or in the sigmoid colon. However, there is also a diffuse form that involves the entire colon, which is frequently associated with inflammatory bowel disease and irradiation. The localized form may be related to solitary rectal ulcer and rectal prolapse syndrome, but its etiology remains unclear. The clinical symptoms of CCP include rectorrhagia, mucorrhea, and abdominal pain.

Endoscopic examination may reveal a polypoid mass, plaques, or nodules, which are suggestive, but not specific for CCP. The differential diagnosis mainly includes mucinous adenocarcinoma of the colon. Transrectal ultrasound is helpful in establishing the diagnosis. The primary sign is multiple cysts in the rectal submucosa that do not infiltrate the muscular layer. An intense signal in the T2 sequences of magnetic resonance images may indicate mucoprotein content in the cysts. The diagnosis of CCP is confirmed by the histological examination of deep biopsy specimens extending into the submucosa, which shows intramural cysts filled with mucus.

Treatment can include endoscopic or surgical resection, but good results have been achieved with a change in bowel habits to avoid straining and introducing a high-fiber diet combined with bulk laxatives.

Stercoral Ulcers

Stercoral ulcers of the colon are caused by pressure from prolonged fecal impaction and are most commonly located in the rectum. Risk factors include immobility and advanced age. Stercoral ulcers are rare, but can lead to colonic perforation or bleeding. The treatment consists of removing fecal stones by manual disimpaction or by softening with mineral-oil enemas. As there is a risk of colonic perforation, all maneuvers should be cautious, and patients should be carefully evaluated after each procedure.

Lipomas

Colonic lipomas are benign, nonepithelial tumors consisting of spherical deposits of adipose tissue in the submucosa. About 10% are subserosal. The incidence of colonic lipoma ranges from 0.035%

to 4.4% in autopsies. They occur up to two times more often in women in the fifth or sixth decade of life than in the general population. The typical site of occurrence is the right colon, particularly the cecum. Colonic lipomas are generally single lesions, but multiple lesions have been reported in 6–26% of cases. Colonic lipomas are usually asymptomatic and are detected incidentally during colonoscopy or imaging examinations. Large lipomas can result in abdominal pain, gastrointestinal bleeding, alterations in bowel movements, bowel obstruction, or intussusception. On colonoscopy, the typical lipoma is a spheroidal, smooth, slightly yellowish polyp of variable size; it can also appear pedunculated (**Fig. 47.31**).

There are three endoscopic signs of lipoma: the cushion sign (pressure on the polyps with closed biopsy forceps produces a pillow-like impression in the polyp); the tenting effect (grasping the overlying mucosa with biopsy forceps creates a tent-like shape); and the naked fat sign (following biopsy, the yellowish fat extrudes from the lesion). In addition, collected specimens usually float in the formalin fixation solution. All of these features are highly reliable for lipoma, but in doubtful cases, a CT can confirm the diagnosis with the appearance of a uniform surface and the absorption density of fat tissue. Lipomas can be removed endoscopically, but an increased risk of perforation is associated with polypectomy of large lesions (> 2 cm or, according to some authors, > 4 cm in diameter) or broad-based, intramural polyps. Surgery is therefore recommended for these types of lesion and for symptomatic tumors.

Large-Bowel Carcinoids

Carcinoids (neuroendocrine tumors) of the large bowel arise in the rectum, colon, and appendix and represent 12.6%, 7.8%, and 4.7% of all carcinoids, respectively. In the rectum, most lesions are small, mobile, submucosal nodules and elevations, covered with normal-appearing mucosa located on the anterior or lateral wall (**Fig. 47.32**). Most rectal carcinoids are asymptomatic and are discovered incidentally during endoscopy. About 80% of rectal carcinoids are small solitary tumors less than 1 cm in diameter. They are rarely malignant, and endoscopic excision is safe and curative. However, an appropriate removal technique must be chosen for complete removal.

The preferred treatment for carcinoids 1–2 cm in diameter for which there is no evidence of lymph-node metastasis is wide local excision. Radical surgery is recommended for lesions larger than

47

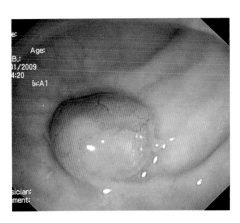

Fig. 47.32 Carcinoid of the rectum: a small, round, sessile elevation covered with normal-appearing mucosa.

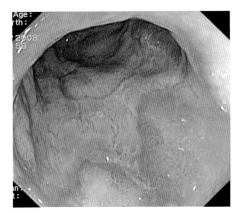

Fig. 47.33 Colonic manifestation of graft-versus-host disease.

2 cm and those associated with spread to the lymph nodes or muscular invasion. Rectal carcinoids have a favorable prognosis. In contrast, colonic carcinoids are associated with the poorest prognosis among all gastrointestinal carcinoid tumors. The symptoms typically include abdominal pain, changes in bowel habit, and bleeding; when found, the tumors are typically large, with metastases already present in 50% of cases. The treatment for colonic carcinoids, especially tumors > 2 cm, is wide bowel resection with lymphadenectomy.

Colonic Endometriosis

Endometriosis affects approximately 15% of menstruating women and can involve the intestines, most commonly the rectosigmoid colon. Endometrial involvement of the colon is often asymptomatic. Symptoms of pelvic endometriosis such as dysmenorrhea, dyspareunia, and infertility are more prominent. Endometrial serosal implants may cause abdominal pain, bloating, low back pain, diarrhea, and rectal bleeding. Intestinal symptoms are not related to the menstrual cycle. Macroscopically, endometrial implants are nodules ranging from 2 mm to 2 cm in diameter, surrounded by mural cysts and fibrosis. Microscopically, characteristic structures of the endometrium are seen. The colonic mucosa is rarely involved, but can demonstrate minor inflammatory changes in areas adjacent to the endometrial nodules. The nodules themselves are located deep in the colonic wall and may not be present in biopsy specimens.

The endoscopic appearance of the colon may be normal in the presence of noninvasive serosal implants. In case of rectal bleeding, the mucosa may be invaded by endometrial tissue or, in case of intestinal obstruction, stricture or extrinsic compression of the lumen may be present.

The diagnosis of colonic endometriosis is confirmed by laparoscopy or laparotomy, and treatment is based on either laparoscopic

ablation of the serosal implants or, in the presence of obstruction, partial resection of the colon.

Metastases to the Large Bowel

Metastases to the colonic or rectal wall are rare. Melanoma, breast cancer, and lung cancer are among the most frequent primary tumors associated with distant metastases to the large bowel. The metastases may occur several years after diagnosis of the primary tumor. Although there is no specific endoscopic appearance, a nodule up to 2 cm in diameter with central depression or ulceration in an individual with a history of malignancy may be suggestive of metastasis. Other notable endoscopic presentations are diffuse thickening of the colonic wall (mimicking linitis plastica) for breast cancer metastases and pigmented brownish nodules for melanoma metastases. Therapy is aimed at palliation, to avoid obstruction.

Other Diseases

Behçet disease is a rare, multisystem vasculitis of unknown origin. It manifests with recurrent oral and genital aphthae, ulceration of the gastrointestinal tract, ocular lesions, neurologic disease, and arthritis. Intestinal lesions are most commonly located in the ileocecal region. Rectal and anal involvement is infrequent. The predominant type of endoscopic presentation is a punched-out ulcer characterized by deep excavation and discrete margins. The range of endoscopic appearances also includes aphthous and geographic ulcers. The endoscopic and histologic appearance may mimic Crohn's disease, and differential diagnosis therefore relies on other clinical signs and symptoms. Although immunosuppressive treatment may be effective, the high recurrence rate and depth of ulcer penetration may result in perforation and bleeding that require surgery [31].

Graft-versus-host disease (GVHD) is a common, life-threatening complication of allogeneic bone-marrow transplantation that often involves the gastrointestinal tract. The clinical presentation of gastrointestinal GVHD is anorexia, vomiting, watery diarrhea, and gastrointestinal bleeding. Endoscopic appearances vary widely, ranging from normal findings or erythema and edema to ulceration, exudate, and bleeding (**Fig. 47.33**). Although the endoscopic findings may be predictive of GVHD, biopsies are needed for a final diagnosis. Whether the biopsies should be taken from the rectum or upper gastrointestinal tract remains a matter of controversy. The mainstay for histological diagnosis of GVHD is the presence of epithelial cell apoptosis [32].

References

1. Endoscopic Classification Review Group. Update on the Paris classification of superficial neoplastic lesions in the digestive tract. Endoscopy 2005;37:570–8.
2. Levine JS, Ahnen DJ. Adenomatous polyps of the colon. N Engl J Med 2006;355:2551–7.
3. Winawer SJ, Zauber AG, Fletcher RH, Stillman JS, O'Brien MJ, Levin B, et al. Guidelines for colonoscopy surveillance after polypectomy: a consensus update by the US Multi-Society Task Force on Colorectal Cancer and the American Cancer Society. CA Cancer J Clin 2006;56:143–59.
4. Kudo S, Lambert R, Allen JI, Fujii H, Fujii T, Kashida H, et al. Nonpolypoid neoplastic lesions of the colorectal mucosa. Gastrointest Endosc 2008;68(Suppl 4):S 3–47.
5. Soetikno RM, Kaltenbach T, Rouse RV, Park W, Maheshwari A, Sato T, et al. Prevalence of nonpolypoid (flat and depressed) colorectal neoplasms in asymptomatic and symptomatic adults. JAMA 2008;299:1027–35.

VII

6. Kaltenbach T, Friedland S, Maheshwari A, Ouyang D, Rouse RV, Wren S, et al. Short- and long-term outcomes of standardized EMR of nonpolypoid (flat and depressed) colorectal lesions ≥ 1 cm (with video). Gastrointest Endosc 2007;65:857–65.

7. Bülow S, Björk J, Christensen IJ, Fausa O, Järvinen H, Moesgaard F, et al. Duodenal adenomatosis in familial adenomatous polyposis. Gut 2004;53:381–6.

8. Maple JT, Boardman LA. Genetics of colonic polyposis. Clin Gastroenterol Hepatol 2006;4:831–5.

9. Umar A, Boland CR, Terdiman JP, Syngal S, de la Chapelle A, Rüschoff J, et al. Revised Bethesda guidelines for hereditary nonpolyposis colorectal cancer (Lynch syndrome) and microsatellite instability. J Natl Cancer Inst 2004;96:261–8.

10. Giardiello FM, Trimbath JD. Peutz–Jeghers syndrome and management recommendations. Clin Gastroenterol Hepatol 2006;4:408–15.

11. Jemal A, Siegel R, Ward E, Hao Y, Xu J, Murray T, et al. Cancer statistics, 2008. CA Cancer J Clin 2008;58:71–96.

12. Bosset JF, Collette L, Calais G, Mineur L, Maingon P, Radosevic-Jelic L, et al. Chemotherapy with preoperative radiotherapy in rectal cancer. N Engl J Med 2006;355:1114–23.

13. Lieberman DA, Weiss DG, Bond JH, Ahnen DJ, Garewal H, Chejfec G. Use of colonoscopy to screen asymptomatic adults for colorectal cancer. N Engl J Med 2000;343:162–168. [Erratum in N Engl J Med 2000;343:1204.]

14. Regula J, Rupinski M, Kraszewska E, Polkowski M, Pachlewski J, Orlowska J, et al. Colonoscopy in colorectal-cancer screening for detection of advanced neoplasia. N Engl J Med 2006;355:1863–72.

15. Rex DK, Petrini JL, Baron TH, Chak A, Cohen J, Deal SE, et al. Quality indicators for colonoscopy. Am J Gastroenterol 2006;101:873–85.

16. Lieberman D, Nadel M, Smith RA, Atkin W, Duggirala SB, Fletcher R, et al. Standardized colonoscopy reporting and data system: report of the Quality Assurance Task Group of the National Colorectal Cancer Roundtable. Gastrointest Endosc 2007;65:757–66.

17. Levin B, Lieberman DA, McFarland B, Andrews KS, Brooks D, Bond J, et al. Screening and surveillance for the early detection of colorectal cancer and adenomatous polyps, 2008: a joint guideline from the American Cancer Society, the US Multi-Society Task Force on Colorectal Cancer, and the American College of Radiology. Gastroenterology 2008;134:1570–95.

18. Chan AT, Giovannucci EL, Meyerhardt JA, Schernhammer ES, Wu K, Fuchs CS. Aspirin dose and duration of use and risk of colorectal cancer in men. Gastroenterology 2008;134:21–8.

19. Dubé C, Rostom A, Lewin G, Tsertsvadze A, Barrowman N, Code C, et al. The use of aspirin for primary prevention of colorectal cancer: a systematic review prepared for the U.S. Preventive Services Task Force. Ann Intern Med 2007;146:365–75.

20. McDonald LC, Killgore GE, Thompson A, Owens RC Jr, Kazakova SV, Sambol SP, et al. An epidemic, toxin gene-variant strain of *Clostridium difficile*. N Engl J Med 2005;353:2433–41.

21. McFarland LV. Meta-analysis of probiotics for the prevention of antibiotic associated diarrhea and the treatment of *Clostridium difficile* disease. Am J Gastroenterol 2006;101:812–22.

22. Adachi JA, DuPont HL. Rifaximin: a novel nonabsorbed rifamycin for gastrointestinal disorders. Clin Infect Dis 2006;42:541–7.

23. Sibartie V, Kirwan WO, O'Mahony S, Stack W, Shanahan F. Intestinal tuberculosis mimicking Crohn's disease: lessons relearned in new era. Eur J Gastroenterol Hepatol 2007;19:347–9.

24. Kandiel A, Lashner B. Cytomegalovirus colitis complicating inflammatory bowel disease. Am J Gastroenterol 2006;101:2857–65.

25. Colecchia A, Vestino A, Pasqui F, Mazzella G, Roda E, Pistoia F, et al. Efficacy of long term cyclic administration of the poorly absorbed antibiotic rifaximin in symptomatic, uncomplicated colonic diverticular disease. World J Gastroenterol 2007;13:264–9.

26. Di Mario F, Comparato G, Fanigliulo L, Aragona G, Cavallaro LG, Cavestro GM, et al. Use of mesalazine in diverticular disease. J Clin Gastroenterol 2006;40(Suppl 3):S 155–9.

27. Williams JJ, Kaplan GG, Makhija S, Urbanski SJ, Dupre M, Panaccione R, et al. Microscopic colitis—defining incidence rates and risk factors: a population-based study. Clin Gastroenterol Hepatol 2008;6:35–40.

28. Nyhlin N, Bohr J, Eriksson S, Tysk C. Systematic review: microscopic colitis. Aliment Pharmacol Ther 2006;23:1525–34.

29. Morris MS, Gee AC, Cho SD, Limbaugh K, Underwood S, Ham B, et al. Management and outcome of pneumatosis intestinalis. Am J Surg 2008;195:679–83.

30. Ho LM, Paulson EK, Thompson WM. Pneumatosis intestinalis in the adults: benign to life-threatening causes. AJR Am J Roentgenol 2007;188:1604–13.

31. Schneider A, Merikhi A, Frank BB. Autoimmune disorders: gastrointestinal manifestations and endoscopic findings. Gastrointest Endoscopy Clin N Am 2006;16:133–51.

32. Cruz-Correa M, Poonawala A, Abraham SC, Wu TT, Zahurak M, Vogelsang G, et al. Endoscopic findings predict the histologic diagnosis in gastrointestinal graft-versus-host disease. Endoscopy 2002;34:808–13.

47

48 Endoscopy of Inflammatory Bowel Disease

Wojciech Blonski, David Kotlyar, and Gary R. Lichtenstein

Introduction

Inflammatory bowel disease (IBD) is a term that encompasses two distinct disorders—ulcerative colitis (UC) and Crohn's disease (CD). Either disease can often be diagnosed with endoscopy by an experienced gastroenterologist in the setting of a suggestive clinical presentation. It is a "first step" in the investigation of persistent or repeated diarrhea. Endoscopy also allows for the sampling and biopsy of areas in the digestive tract in patients with both diseases [1].

Endoscopy in patients with IBD is critically important not only in the initial diagnosis, but also in the assessment of the severity and extent of disease on presentation [1]. In addition, it is vital for monitoring the progression of IBD as well as the response to therapeutic modalities. New forms of endoscopy, including capsule endoscopy, are helpful as an addition to traditional approaches such as lower endoscopy (colonoscopy, flexible sigmoidoscopy) and upper endoscopy (esophagogastroduodenoscopy).

Preparation for Colonoscopy

The effectiveness of colon cleansing before colonoscopy is very important from a diagnostic point of view. There are two major classes of bowel preparation: polyethylene glycol–electrolyte solution (PEG-ELS) and sodium phosphate products. PEG-ELS is an isotonic agent that promotes bowel cleansing through the ingestion of nonabsorbable fluid and requires the administration of large volumes of the solution. Sodium phosphate preparations are hyperosmotic agents that promote bowel cleansing by osmotically drawing fluid into the bowel with a small volume of the preparation.

A meta-analysis of 16 clinical trials, including 1855 patients who received PEG-ELS and 1629 patients who received sodium phosphate solution, observed that patients who received sodium phosphate solutions were significantly ($P = 0.0004$) more likely to have acceptable (good or excellent) bowel cleansing (odds ratio 0.75; 95 % confidence interval, 0.65 to 0.88) [2]. Data pooled from 15 trials showed that patients receiving sodium phosphate (n = 1529) were significantly more likely to complete the preparation than those who received PEG-ELS (n = 1764; 94 % vs. 71 %, $P < 0.00001$) [2]. Data pooled from 12 trials demonstrated that the total number of adverse events did not differ between PEG-ELS and sodium phosphate solutions (OR 0.98; 95 % CI, 0.82 to 1.17; $P = 0.81$) [2]. However, on individual analysis, PEG-ELS was found to be associated with more severe abdominal pain than sodium phosphate (OR 1.67; 95 % CI, 1.36 to 2.04; $P < 0.00001$) [2]. Conversely, sodium phosphate was significantly more likely to cause dizziness than PEG-ELS (OR 0.55; 95 % CI, 0.36 to 0.86; $P = 0.008$) [2]. Studies included in the meta-analysis compared high-volume PEG-ELS with 90 mL of sodium phosphate formulation (n = 12), reduced-volume PEG-ELS with 90 mL of sodium phosphate formulation (n = 2), high-volume PEG-ELS with 80 mL of sodium phosphate formulation (n = 1), and high-volume PEG-ELS with sodium phosphate tablets [2].

The timing of administration of the cleansing agent has been found to be a major factor determining the quality of bowel cleansing [3]. A short interval between intake of the cleansing agent and the colonoscopy resulted in better bowel preparation [3]. Recently, there have been reports of nephrocalcinosis with the use of oral sodium phosphate preparations. This has lessened the enthusiasm for the use of these agents [4–6].

Newer-generation cleansing agents for bowel preparation are better tolerated by patients and have similar efficacy in comparison with the original PEG-ELS formulations. The original PEG-ELS has a salty taste due to sodium sulfate [7,8], which is a major objection to it by patients. Although a study comparing the original PEG-ELS with a sulfate-free PEG-ELS solution showed similar cleansing efficacy with both agents, a sulfate-free PEG-ELS formulation was preferred by three times as many patients as the original PEG-ELS (76 % vs. 24 %; $P \leq 0.001$) [8]. It was also shown that 75 % of patients prefer flavored formulations over unflavored ones during preparation for colonoscopy [9]. Further studies demonstrated that reduced-volume PEG-ELS formulations had a cleansing efficacy comparable with that of high-volume PEG-ELS. A regimen consisting of either low-volume PEG-ELS administered with bisacodyl or high-volume sulfate-free PEG-ELS provided good or excellent colon cleansing in 87–96 % and 92–95 % of patients, respectively [10,11]. However, the low-volume regimen was associated with a significant ($P \leq 0.01$) reduction in preparation-related side effects [10].

Administration of more advanced reduced-volume PEG-ELS with ascorbic acid without the addition of bisacodyl had cleansing effects comparable with the high-volume PEG-ELS formulation (89 % vs. 95 %). However, the low-volume regimen was associated with significantly ($P < 0.025$) better overall acceptability than the high-volume PEG-ELS preparation [12].

Newer-generation sodium phosphate formulations in the form of tablets were found to be as effective as, and more tolerable than, PEG-ELS preparations or traditional sodium phosphate products. Studies have observed that sodium phosphate tablets without microcrystalline cellulose had similar cleansing efficacy and a better acceptability profile than sodium phosphate tablets with microcrystalline cellulose [13,14], and both better cleansing efficacy and tolerability than low-volume PEG-ELS administered with bisacodyl tablets [15].

It should be emphasized that none of the cleaning agents mentioned above has been studied in patients with IBD. Notably, it has been suggested that sodium phosphate preparation may be involved in the development of acute colitis. All cleansing agents should be administered with caution in patients with existing electrolyte disturbances and those with an increased risk for electrolyte disturbances [16].

Endoscopic Evaluation of Disease Activity

Ulcerative Colitis

Several endoscopic indices have been developed for endoscopic assessment of UC activity (**Table 48.1**) [17–26]. However, endoscopy does not appear to be necessary to evaluate the UC activity, as endoscopic parameters do not provide any information additional to that obtained with noninvasive indices [27].

Table 48.1 Endoscopic indexes for ulcerative colitis activity

First author, year [ref.]	Description
Truelove 1955 [17]	Sigmoidoscopic appearance: ● Normal or near-normal (only slight hyperemia or only slight granularity) ● Improved ● Unchanged or worse
Baron 1964 [18]	Baron score ● Normal (0): matt mucosa, ramifying vascular pattern clearly visible throughout, no spontaneous bleeding, no bleeding to light touch ● Abnormal (1): between normal (0) and moderately hemorrhagic (2) ● Moderately hemorrhagic (2): bleeding to light touch, but no spontaneous bleeding seen ahead of instrument on initial inspection ● Severely hemorrhagic: spontaneous bleeding seen ahead of instrument at initial inspection with bleeding to light touch
Feagan 2005 [19]	Modified Baron score: ● Normal mucosa (0) ● Granular mucosa with an abnormal vascular pattern (1) ● Friable mucosa (2) ● Microulceration with spontaneous bleeding (3) ● Gross ulceration (4)
Powel-Tuck 1978 [20]	Sigmoidoscopic appearance: ● Nonhemorrhagic (0): no spontaneous bleeding or bleeding to light touch ● Hemorrhagic (1): no spontaneous bleeding, but bleeding to light touch ● Hemorrhagic (2): spontaneous bleeding ahead of instrument at initial inspection, with bleeding to light touch
Schroeder 1987 [21]	Mayo score (sigmoidoscopic evaluation): ● Normal or inactive disease (0) ● Mild disease (1): erythema, decreased vascular pattern, mild friability ● Moderate disease (2): marked erythema, absent vascular pattern, friability, erosions ● Severe disease (3): spontaneous bleeding, ulceration
Sutherland 1987 [22]	Sutherland Sigmoidoscopic Mucosal Appearance: ● Normal (0) ● Mild friability (1) ● Moderate friability (2) ● Exudation, spontaneous hemorrhage (3)
Rachmilewitz 1989 [23]	Rachmilewitz Index: ● A: granulation scattering reflected light: yes (0), no (2) ● B: vascular pattern: normal (0), faded/disturbed (1), completely absent (2) ● C: vulnerability of mucosa: none (0); slightly increased (contact bleeding) (2); greatly increased (spontaneous bleeding) (4) ● D: mucosal damage (mucus, fibrin, exudates, erosions, ulcer): none (0), slight (2), pronounced (4).
Hanauer 1993 [24]	Sigmoidoscopic Index (0, normal; 1, mild; 2, moderate; 3, severe). ● A: erythema (0–3) ● B: friability (0–3) ● C: granularity/ulceration (0–3) ● D: mucopus (0–3) ● E: lack of mucosal vascular pattern (0–3) The total score is the sum of subscores A through E
Lemann1995 [25], Hanauer 1998 [26]	Sigmoidoscopic Inflammation Grade ● Normal mucosa (0) ● Edema and/or loss of visible mucosal vascularity, granularity (1) ● Friability (visible, contact bleeding on examination), petechiae (2) ● Spontaneous hemorrhage, visible ulcers (3)

A recent prospective case-crossover study also suggested that colonoscopy may be associated with exacerbation of quiescent UC. A multivariate analysis showed that relapse of UC immediately after colonoscopy and a need to increase 5-aminosalicylic acid medication occurred in one in eight and one in 10 patients, respectively [28]. Further studies are needed to further clarify the relationship between preparation for colonoscopy as well as colonoscopy and relapses in UC.

▓ Crohn's Disease

Two endoscopic indices have been developed to evaluate colonic CD activity endoscopically. The first, known as the Crohn's Disease Endoscopic Index of Severity (CDEIS), was proposed by a multicenter group of experts in France (Groupe d'Etudes Thérapeutiques des Affections Inflammatoires du Tube Digestif (GETAID) [29]. The colon was divided into the following five segments: rectum, sigmoid and left colon, transverse colon, right colon, and ileum. Among various mucosal lesions, deep and superficial mucosal ulcerations were given 12 and 6 points in every bowel segment affected, respectively. If no mucosal ulceration was found within a given segment, a score of 0 points was assigned. The scores for deep and superficial ulcerations were multiplied by the number of bowel segments with an identified lesion, divided by the number of endoscopically explored segments. In addition, the presence or absence of bowel stenosis either with or without ulceration at any site during colonoscopy was given 3 or 0 points, respectively. The average area of colon affected by disease and the average area of ulcerated colon were also incorporated into the equation. All of these variables summed together provide the total CDEIS score [29]. Although CDEIS was found to be reproducible, it showed weak correlation with clinical CD activity of as measured by the Crohn's Disease Activity Index (CDAI) ($r = 0.32$) [30]. In addition, the complicated method required to calculate the CDEIS does not encourage its use in the clinical setting. On the other hand, a randomized placebo-controlled clinical trial of infliximab in patients with active CD showed a high correlation between changes in the endoscopic (CDEIS) and clinical (CDAI) indices [31]. It should also be noted that observation of a subgroup of patients who completed the ACCENT I trial has shown that patients who achieved mucosal healing also had longer periods of remission [32]. Patients with CD and endoscopic remission were also found to be hospitalized less often than those without mucosal healing [33].

In 2004, an Italian group developed a second endoscopic index for Crohn's disease, known as the Simple Endoscopic Score for Crohn's Disease (SES-CD) [34]. SES-CD is simple and easy to use in comparison with the CDEIS (**Table 48.2**). This is particularly significant, as endoscopic remission has become important in assessing the efficacy of treatment for Crohn's disease in clinical trials. As in the CDEIS, the colon is divided into five segments in the SES-CD. On the basis of endoscopic parameters (size of ulcers, degree of ulcerated surface, degree of affected surface, and presence of narrowing in the colon) a numerical score of 0–3 is given to each segment of the colon. The sum of all the numeric scores for each endoscopic parameter in each of the five segments of the colon constitutes the SES-CD score. SES-CD was found to be reproducible and correlated strongly with the CDEIS. On the other hand, a weak correlation

Table 48.2 The Simple Endoscopic Score for Crohn's Disease (SES-CD) [34]

Variable	0	1	2	3
Size of ulcers	None	Aphthous ulcers (0.1–0.5 cm)	Large ulcers (0.5–2 cm)	Very large ulcers (>2 cm)
Ulcerated surface	None	<10%	10–30%	>30%
Affected surface	Unaffected segment	<50%	50–75%	>75%
Strictures	None	Single, can be passed	Multiple, can be passed	Cannot be passed

With kind permission from Elsevier: Daperno M, D'Haens G, Van Assche G, Baert F, Bulois P, Maunoury V, et al. Development and validation of a new, simplified endoscopic activity score for Crohn's disease: the SES-CD. Gastrointest Endosc 2004;60:505–12.

($r = 0.32$) was observed between SES-CD and CDAI; this might be explained either by the fact that the appearance of colonic mucosa may not reflect many systemic manifestations of the symptomatic inflammatory process, by the time difference between the clinical and endoscopic course of the disease, or by disease involvement of more proximal segments of the bowel that are not normally visible at colonoscopy [34].

Rutgeerts et al. developed an endoscopic score system to assess ileal lesions in CD [35]. The lesions were graded on a 0–4 scale: no lesions (0); less than five aphthous lesions (1); more than five aphthous lesions and normal mucosa between them or skip areas of larger lesions, or lesions limited to the ileocolonic anastomosis, diffuse aphthous ileitis with diffusely inflamed mucosa (3); and diffuse inflammation with larger ulcers, nodules and/or narrowing (4) [35].

The efficacy of various medications used in the treatment of IBD in relation to mucosal healing has been evaluated in several controlled clinical studies (**Table 48.3**) [31,36–38] and uncontrolled studies (**Table 48.4**) [39–42].

48

Table 48.3 Controlled studies evaluating the efficacy of various medications for mucosal healing in patients with inflammatory bowel disease

First author, year [ref.]	IBD type	Drug 1 (no. of patients)	Patients with complete mucosal healing*	Drug 2 (no. of patients)	Patients with complete mucosal healing*
Rutgeerts 2004 [36]	CD	Infliximab in multiple doses (45)	29%	Infliximab, single dose followed by placebo (29)	3% (P=0.006)
Mantzaris 2008 [37]	CD	Azathioprine (38)	83%	Budesonide (37)	24% (P<0.0001)
Rutgeerts 2005 [38] ACT 1	UC	Infliximab 5 mg/kg (121) Infliximab 10 mg/kg (122)	Week 8: 62% 59%	Placebo (121)	Week 8: 33.9% (P<0.001)
		Infliximab 5 mg/kg (121) Infliximab 10 mg/kg (122)	Week 30: 50.4% 49.2%	Placebo (121)	Week 30: 24.8% (P<0.001)
		Infliximab 5 mg/kg (121) Infliximab 10 mg/kg (122)	Week 54: 45.5% 46.7%	Placebo (121)	Week 54: 16.5% (P<0.001)
ACT 2	UC	Infliximab 5 mg/kg (121) Infliximab 10 mg/kg (120)	Week 8: 60.3% 61.7%	Placebo (123)	Week 8: 30.9% (P<0.001)
		Infliximab 5 mg/kg (121) Infliximab 10 mg/kg (120)	Week 30: 46.3% 56.7%	Placebo (123)	Week 30: 30.1% (P=0.009) (P<0.001)
D'Haens 1999 [31]	CD	Infliximab (22)	CDEIS baseline: 13.0 CDEIS baseline at week 4: 5.3 (P<0.001)	Placebo (8)	CDEIS baseline: 8.4 CDEIS baseline at week 4: 7.5

* Unless otherwise stated.
ACT, Active Ulcerative Colitis Trials (1 and 2); CD, Crohn's disease; CDEIS, Crohn's Disease Endoscopic Index of Severity; IBD, inflammatory bowel disease; UC, ulcerative colitis.

Table 48.4 Uncontrolled studies evaluating the efficacy of various medications for mucosal healing in patients with inflammatory bowel disease

First author, year [ref.]	IBD type	Patients (n)	Drug studied	Patients with mucosal healing (%)
D'Haens 1999 [39]	CD	20	Azathioprine	Colon: • Complete healing 70% • Near-complete healing 10% • Partial healing 15% • no healing 5% Ileum: • Complete healing 54% • Near-complete healing 15% • Partial healing 8% • No healing 15%
Modigliani 1990 [40]	CD	142	Prednisone	Colon: endoscopic remission 27%
Kozarek 1989 [41]	CD	14	Methotrexate	Colon: endoscopic healing 36%
	UC	7	Methotrexate	Colon: endoscopic healing 0%
D'Haens 1997 [42]	CD	15	Azathioprine	Ileum: • Complete healing 40% • Near-complete healing 33.3% • Partial healing 20% • No healing 6.7%

CD, Crohn's disease; IBD, inflammatory bowel disease; UC, ulcerative colitis.

Endoscopic Characteristics of IBD

Colonoscopy

Colonoscopy is regarded as the gold standard in diagnosing UC and colonic CD. It also allows macroscopic and microscopic assessment of endoscopic disease activity and surveillance for colon cancer. It is imperative to examine the entire colon with biopsies taken from regularly spaced regions in the colon, including normal-appearing mucosa. A Cochrane review showed that colonoscopy and surveillance biopsies can also help indirectly to reduce the mortality risk, probably due to early detection of colorectal cancer (CRC) [43,44]. The current Crohn's guidelines require surveillance colonoscopy with random biopsies in patients 8–10 years after the development of CD with involvement of one-third or more of the colon. However, patients with UC and proctitis with less than 15 cm of disease can follow the screening guidelines for the general populace [45].

In general, biopsies should be carried out as four-quadrant biopsies with jumbo forceps every 10 cm [44]. Biopsies of the proximal mucosa may be helpful in assessing for the presence of proximal disease. In these patients, local treatments such as topical mesalamine or enemas may be beneficial, and corticosteroids with fewer systemic effects, such as budesonide, may be useful [46].

Complications

Colonic rupture or perforation is a catastrophic complication that must be assiduously avoided. Patients who are at greatest risk for perforation include males, older patients, and those having colonoscopy performed by an inexperienced operator [47]. The reported incidence is in the range of 0.1–0.85% [47–49]. Other risk factors include colonic obstruction, severe ulcerations or transmural inflammation, abscess, and megacolon [47].

Normal Colonic Mucosa

Normal mucosa has a distinct and clean vascular pattern, with a salmon-pink color, and the presence of a light reflex. The mucosa is smooth, without any irregular polyps or nodules. Normal colonic mucosa can be observed in patients with quiescent UC (**Fig. 48.1**).

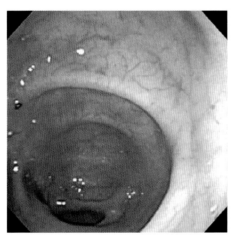

Fig. 48.1 Ulcerative colitis in endoscopic remission, with no evidence of active disease. The vasculature is clear and distinct. A light reflex is present. The biopsies did not show any crypt distortion.

Ulcerative Colitis

Disease begins in the rectum, with proximal retrograde progression that has a continuous and circumferential pattern, without obvious skip lesions [50]. There is usually a sharp border between normal and diseased mucosa [1]. Rectal sparing often occurs in patients with UC and primary sclerosing cholangitis, or in patients treated with topical medications [50]. It should be emphasized that up to 44% of patients with long-standing and medically treated UC may have endoscopic patchiness in the colonic mucosa, which is described either as rectal sparing, patches of distinct normal mucosa within inflamed mucosa, or as more marked inflammation in the proximal than distal colon [51,52]. Initial lesions include loss of vasculature and hyperemia of the colonic mucosa [50]. There is edema of the colonic mucosa with progression of the inflammatory process, leading to granularity of the mucosa, which is described as resembling "wet sandpaper." The colonic mucosa is friable, with bleeding on contact with an endoscope. Discrete ulcers surrounded by inflamed mucosa occur in moderate disease and progress to become large, continuous ulcers with increasing severity of the disease. **Figures 48.2–48.12** illustrate colonic mucosa with quiescent and active UC. Pseudopolyps (**Figs. 48.13–48.17**) may also develop in severe disease [50].

VII

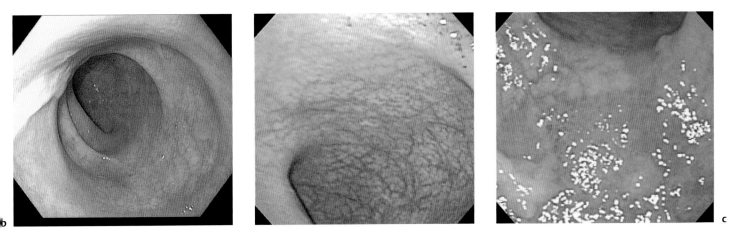

Fig. 48.2 a–c Granular colonic mucosa, with preservation of the vasculature and a light reflex in a patient with ulcerative colitis (mild endoscopic activity, Sutherland score 1).

Fig. 48.3 a–d Granular colonic mucosa with indistinct vasculature in a patient with ulcerative colitis (moderate endoscopic activity, Sutherland score 2).

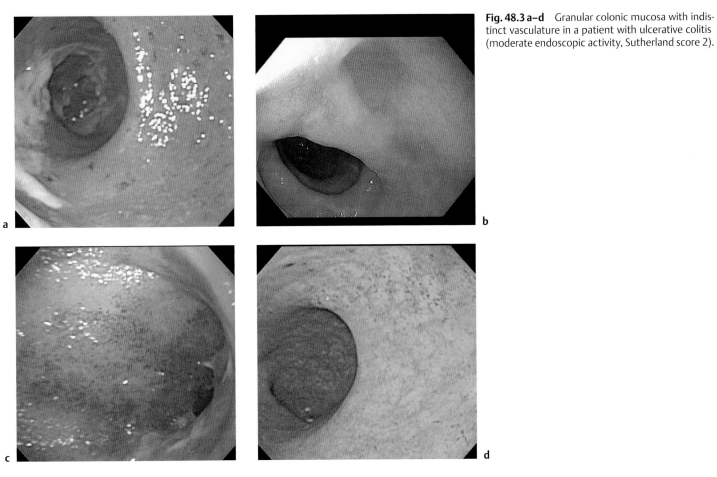

Fig. 48.4 Granular colonic mucosa with hypervascularity in a patient with ulcerative colitis (mild endoscopic activity, Sutherland score 1).

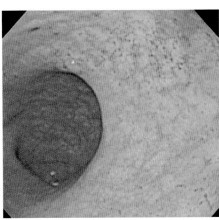

Fig. 48.5 Granular, friable colonic mucosa with hypervascularity in a patient with ulcerative colitis (moderate endoscopic activity, Sutherland score 2).

48

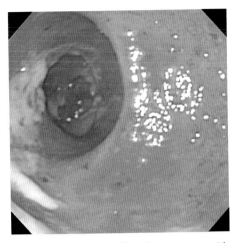

Fig. 48.6 Granular, friable colonic mucosa with indistinct vasculature and mucopus, as well as several areas of spontaneous hemorrhage, in a patient with ulcerative colitis (moderate endoscopic activity, Sutherland score 2). The image shows no evidence of ulceration.

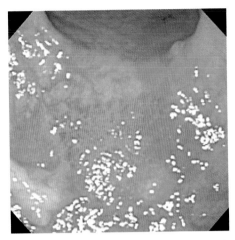

Fig. 48.7 Granular, friable colonic mucosa with mucopus and no evidence of spontaneous hemorrhage or obvious ulceration in a patient with ulcerative colitis (moderate endoscopic activity, Sutherland score 2).

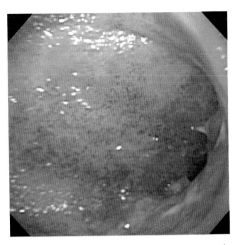

Fig. 48.8 Granular, friable colonic mucosa with indistinct vasculature. There is no obvious ulceration or mucopus (moderate endoscopic activity, Sutherland score 2).

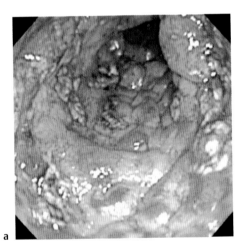

a

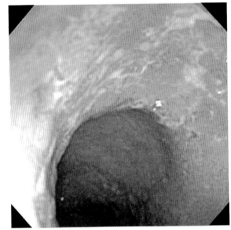

b

Fig. 48.9 a–d Granular, friable colonic mucosa with erosions and a linear ulceration in a patient with ulcerative colitis. There is no evidence of spontaneous hemorrhage (severe endoscopic activity, Sutherland score 3).

c

d

Crohn's Disease

In CD, the colonic mucosa is characterized by areas involved by the disease separated by normal colonic mucosa [50]. Colonic CD is most severe in the cecum and right colon, with rectal sparing. Inflammatory changes are very likely to be localized on the antimesenteric side of the colon. Early lesions in mild CD include small "punched-out" aphthous ulcers. These ulcers adhere as the disease progresses and form stellate ulcers. Ulcers in severe disease may be large and linear, resembling "bear's claw" ulcers or deep serpiginous ulcers. Large areas of linear cobblestone mucosa are visible in severe chronic disease [50]. **Figures 48.18–48.24** illustrate colonic CD.

Pathologically, the colonic mucosa in CD is found to have a monocytic or lymphoid infiltrate that encompasses the entire in-

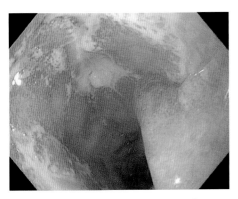

Fig. 48.10 Granular, friable mucosa with exudates overlying it and ulceration in a patient with known ulcerative colitis (severe endoscopic activity, Sutherland score 3).

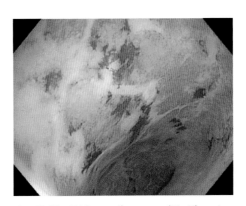

Fig. 48.11 Evidence of severe colitis. There is ulceration and spontaneous bleeding, with granular, friable mucosa (severe endoscopic colitis, Sutherland score 3).

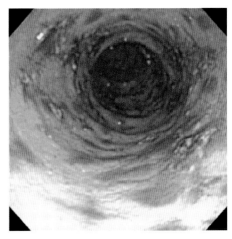

Fig. 48.12 Severe ulcerative colitis with near-circumferential ulceration in the colon, with spontaneous hemorrhage (severe endoscopic activity, Sutherland score 3).

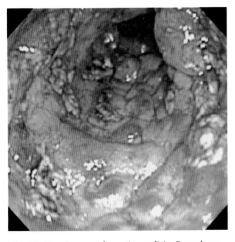

Fig. 48.13 Severe ulcerative colitis. Pseudopolyps, spontaneous hemorrhage, ulceration, and markedly friable mucosa are seen in the rectum (severe endoscopic activity, Sutherland score 3).

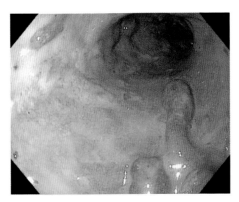

Fig. 48.14 Active ulceration in granular, friable colonic mucosa with pseudopolyps in a patient with ulcerative colitis (severe endoscopic activity, Sutherland score 3).

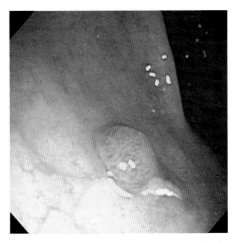

Fig. 48.15 A pseudopolyp in a region in which inflammatory bowel disease was previously found. The colonic mucosa has an appearance consistent with inactive ulcerative colitis.

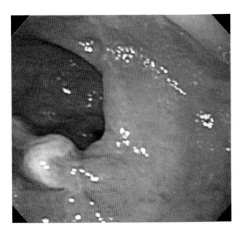

Fig. 48.16 A pseudopolyp in a patient with long-standing ulcerative colitis in remission. A biopsy showed acute inflammatory changes, with granulation tissue.

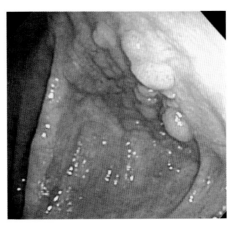

Fig. 48.17 Multiple pseudopolyps in the cecum in a patient with ulcerative colitis. There is no evidence of active disease.

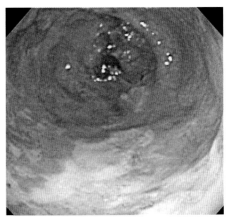

Fig. 48.18 Severe ulceration in the rectosigmoid region in a patient with known Crohn's disease. There is evidence of large ulcerations, with no visible vasculature and granular, friable colonic mucosa.

48

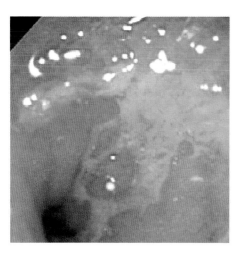

Fig. 48.19 A large, irregular ulceration in the region of the mid-transverse colon, associated with luminal narrowing more proximally due to scarring and ulceration in a patient with Crohn's disease.

testinal wall [53]. In addition, noncaseating granulomas are often associated with CD, although more often early in the progression of the disease [54]. Granulomas can be found in CD anywhere from the mouth to the anus, and so upper endoscopy with biopsy can be very helpful in the diagnosis of CD. Transmural inflammation predisposes patients with Crohn's disease to the development of fistulas. A population-based study in Olmsted County in Minnesota observed that fistulas developed in 35% of patients with Crohn's disease [55] over the course of the disease. Fifty-four percent of the fistulas were perianal, 24% were enteroenteric, 9% were rectovaginal, and 13% were others [55]. An example of a fistula between the sigmoid colon and the urinary bladder is shown in **Fig. 48.25**. Colonoscopic findings in UC and CD are listed in **Table 48.5**.

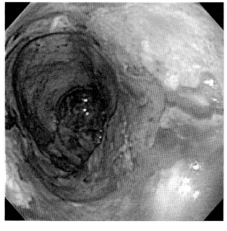
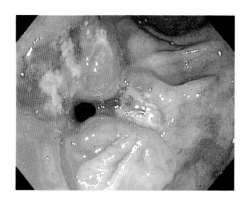
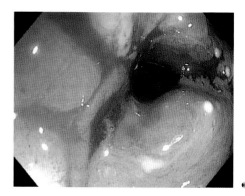

a, b

Fig. 48.20 a–c Severe Crohn's disease with stricture formation in a patient with long-standing colonic Crohn's disease. Many ulcerations and spontaneous hemorrhage are visible.

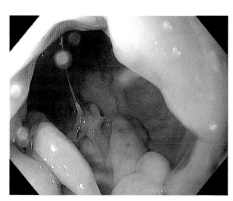
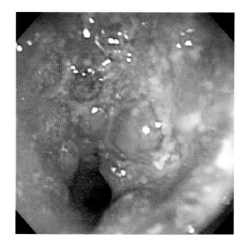
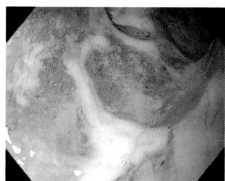

Fig. 48.21 Large filiform polyps in the area proximal to a colonic stricture in a patient with Crohn's disease. The polyps showed no evidence of any active inflammation. They represent an area of previous inflammation.

Fig. 48.22 Severe Crohn's disease, with cobblestone-like colonic mucosa.

Fig. 48.23 Severe ulceration in the sigmoid colon with granular, friable mucosa and absent vasculature. These findings are typical of severe Crohn's colitis.

VII

Table 48.5 Colonoscopic features of ulcerative colitis and Crohn's disease

	Ulcerative colitis	Crohn's disease
Nature of mucosal lesions		
Erythema	+++	++
Blurred vascular pattern	+++	+
Granularity, friability	+++	+
Cobblestoning	–	++
Pseudopolyps	+++	++
Aphthoid ulcers	–	+++
Superficial ulcers	+	+++
Serpiginous deep ulcers	–	+++
Strictures	++	+++
Mucosal bridges	++	++
Distribution of lesions		
Rectal involvement	++++	++
Continuous and symmetrical involvement	++++	+
Patchiness	– *	+++
Skip areas	–	+++
Ileal ulcerations	–	+++

Key: –, almost never; +, rare; ++, possible; +++, frequent; ++++, almost constant.
* With the exception of periappendicular inflammation, and occasionally patients receiving rectal treatment.

Upper Endoscopy

Ulcerative Colitis

Upper endoscopy is not routinely performed in patients with UC.

Crohn's Disease

Upper endoscopy is frequently performed in patients with known or suspected CD. Symptomatic CD of the upper gastrointestinal tract has been reported in fewer than 5 % of CD patients [56,57]. The presenting symptoms include heartburn, dysphagia, vomiting, and epigastric pain. The most commonly affected sites are the gastric antrum and duodenum [50]. The endoscopic findings include the presence of erythema, erosions, ulcers, or complications such as strictures or fistulas [58]. Ulcers may also be present in the oral cavity, with sporadic involvement of the esophagus and pharynx [50]. A report from the Mayo Clinic identified 0.2 % of patients with esophageal CD out of 9900 patients with CD who had been evaluated at the center over a 22-year period [58]. An example of a CD ulcer in the esophagus is shown in **Fig. 48.26**. Biopsies from the stomach and duodenum revealed epithelioid cell granulomas in 83 % and 33 % of evaluated patients, respectively [59]. It is imperative to take multiple biopsies in patients with suspected CD or

48

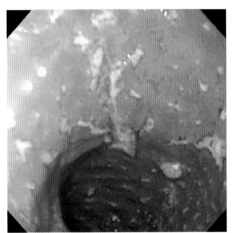

Fig. 48.24 Multiple aphthous ulcers near the terminal ileum in a patient with a transverse colon anastomosis. Aphthous ulceration indicates a recurrence of active Crohn's disease in this segment of bowel.

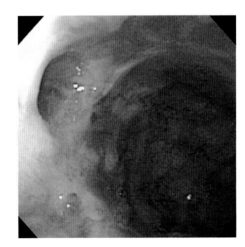

Fig. 48.25 A fistula orifice in a patient with Crohn's disease in the sigmoid.

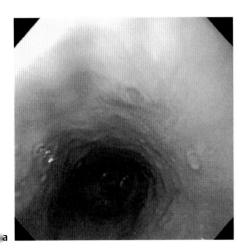

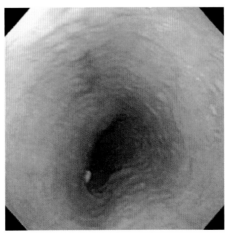

Fig. 48.26 a, b Aphthous ulceration in Crohn's disease in the distal part of the esophagus.

a

b

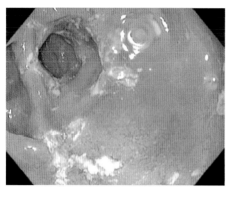

a

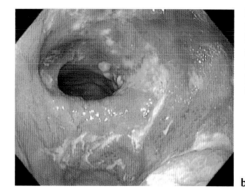

b

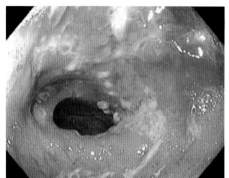

c

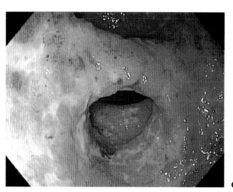

d

Fig. 48.27 a–d   An ileal pouch–anal anastomosis (IPAA). The pouch has a J-pouch configuration. The images were obtained during flexible sigmoidoscopic evaluation using an esophagogastroduodenoscope. There is evidence of ulceration in the pouch itself, with indistinct vasculature and evidence of pseudopolyps.

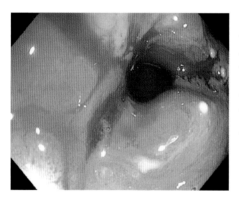

Fig. 48.28   An ileoanal J pouch. There is evidence of severe pouchitis, with large ulcerations throughout the pouch. The ulcerations are not deep and are serpiginous. The rectum is inflamed—a finding consistent with cuffitis.

Pouchitis is diagnosed by endoscopy (flexible pouchoscopy) with biopsy. The mucosa is friable and erythematous (**Fig. 48.28**). One study found that clinical symptoms did not significantly correlate with the endoscopic and histological findings [66]. The appearance of aphthous ulcers heralds the possibility of CD, which must be excluded. It is therefore necessary for the endoscopic examination to include the ileum and to take biopsies. Flexible pouchoscopy is a very effective and safe technical method of evaluating pouch dysfunction, with a high diagnostic yield, and does not require sedation [67].

The rectum may also be involved. On occasion, the rectal cuff after IPAA with stapling may develop inflammation, known as "cuffitis." Topical mesalamine appears to have improved the condition in one study, with improvements in the clinical symptoms, histology, and endoscopic appearance [68]. In addition, dysplasia may occur in the rectal mucosa, and patients with IPAA therefore need regular sigmoidoscopy and biopsy of the rectum to monitor for possible dysplasia. Strictures can also present a problem, but endoscopic balloon dilation of pouch strictures has been shown to be safe and effective treatment [69].

indeterminate colitis during upper endoscopy, even in cases of normal-appearing mucosa, as histologic findings of focal cryptitis or granulomas may make the diagnosis of CD more likely [60–62]. Upper endoscopy also allows therapeutic interventions in the upper gastrointestinal tract, such as treatment for bleeding or pneumatic dilation of strictures.

Surgery for IBD

▥ Pouchitis

After surgery for refractory IBD or dysplasia or carcinoma—often involving a restorative proctocolectomy with ileal pouch–anal anastomosis (IPAA) (**Fig. 48.27**)—the pouch that is left behind often develops chronic inflammation, a condition known as "pouchitis" [63]. Up to 60% of patients with an IPAA may develop pouchitis. Clinically, this is accompanied by frequent stools, liquid stools, urgency, abdominal pain, and/or incontinence [63]. Women may be more frequently affected than men (74% of women vs. 47% of men in one study) [64]. Smoking may reduce the severity of pouchitis, but this is not recommended [65].

▥ Postoperative Recurrence of Crohn's Disease

Endoscopic recurrence of CD following colectomy or ileocolectomy occurs in 73–93% of patients within 1 year after surgery and in 85–100% of patients within 3 years after surgery [35,70]. Clinical recurrence of CD affects 20% and 34% of patients at 1 and 3 years after surgery, respectively [35]. The presence of diffuse recurrent ileal lesions 1 year after surgery (Rutgeerts score 3–4) was found to be predictive of early recurrence of symptoms and development of complications in subsequent years [35]. It is therefore not unreasonable to carry out an assessment of the neoterminal ileum within 1 year after surgery in order to identify patients with an increased risk of recurrence [71].

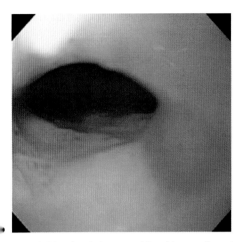
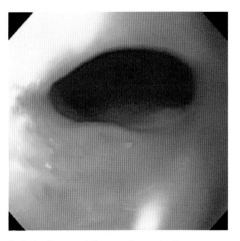

Fig. 48.29 a, b   Strictures with evidence of previous Crohn's disease at the anastomosis site.

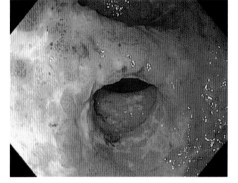

Fig. 48.30   A stricture 15 mm in diameter in the ascending colon, with active ulceration.

Complications of Crohn's Disease

Strictures

It is thought that the strictures seen in IBD often result from the healing response after a flare. Strictures can occur in UC, but they are seen most often in CD secondary to transmural inflammation (**Fig. 48.29**). In CD, strictures may occur throughout the gastrointestinal tract, although they are most frequent in the colon [72] (**Fig. 48.30**). It is thought that an excessive smooth muscle cell and fibroblast response to injury results in the formation of transmural fibrosis, leading to strictures [73]. Nearly 10% of patients with CD develop strictures [74,75]. Strictures may also develop into dysplastic and ultimately malignant lesions. While strictures in UC are less common, those that appear are more frequently malignant, with up to 25% being cancerous in UC, while approximately 10% are malignant in CD [76,77]. When a lesion cannot be biopsied in UC, some authors have suggested that surgical resection should be considered [77]. It is necessary to differentiate between benign and malignant strictures; biopsies should always be obtained from strictures in order to rule out malignancy.

Various methods are available for treating strictures, including balloon dilation. A disadvantage of the balloon method is that there is a risk of perforation, with rates of up to 11% reported [1,78]. Patients who are least at risk for perforation include those without active inflammation at the site of the stricture [1].

Most authors recommend a target diameter of 15–20 mm with either multiple dilation sessions or a single session [1,78–80]. Strictures that are short (< 8 cm) and localized are often most suitable for endoscopic therapy. The success rate of dilation was 86% in one meta-analysis including 13 studies examining its efficacy. With a mean follow-up period of 33 months, the long-term success rate was approximately 58%. A systematic review of 34 studies including 347 patients with CD who underwent endoscopic dilation showed technical success in 86% of cases and responses (surgery-free) in 58% of the patients during a mean follow-up period of 33 months [73]. A single dilation session was beneficial in 59% of responders, whereas benefit was seen in 22% after two dilations and in 19% after more than two sessions. In addition, the study found that a stricture length of less than 4 cm was significantly associated with a surgery-free outcome; on the other hand, local steroid injection was of no benefit. The overall complication rate was low (2%), with bowel perforation being the most common procedural complication]. However, two studies reported complication rates of more than 10% [73].

Acute Lower Gastrointestinal Bleeding

Acute bleeding from the lower part of the gastrointestinal tract occurs rarely (0.9–6.0%) in the course of CD [81–83]. A group in Belgium described the largest cohort of 34 CD patients who experienced such acute bleeding [84]. Acute lower gastrointestinal bleeding occurred more frequently in patients with colonic involvement than in those with small-bowel involvement (85% vs. 15%; $P < 0.0001$). Among patients with acute bleeding, 65% had a quiescent CD, whereas 35% had active disease. Notably, acute bleeding was the first manifestation of CD disease in 23.5% of the patients. Patients underwent colonoscopy (n = 30) or angiography (n = 4). The bleeding site was identified in 22 patients (65%). Colonoscopy detected the bleeding site in 60% of the patients. In the remaining patients, the bleeding site was detected by angiography (n = 3) or at surgery (n = 1). In 95% of cases, the bleeding was caused by an ulcer, with the ulcers mainly being located in the left colon. Medical treatment was initiated in 22 patients (70%); endoscopic treatment was carried out in seven patients (20.5%) and consisted of either laser coagulation, bipolar coagulation, or polypectomy of pseudopolyps in the sigmoid. Endoscopic treatment was successful in five patients. Seven patients were referred for surgery. The rate of recurrent bleeding was 35% during a mean follow-up period of 3 years, with three patients being referred for surgery. The authors suggested a conservative approach to acute bleeding in CD as first-line therapy, due to its therapeutic potential and the lack of mortality [84].

Differential Diagnosis

IBD has to be differentiated from other causes of colitis (**Table 48.6**), including infectious conditions (bacterial, viral, parasitic, fungal) and noninfectious conditions (ischemic colitis, diverticulitis, solitary ulcer of the rectum, drug-induced colitis, and others).

The common clinical symptoms of IBD and infectious colitis are abdominal pain and bloody diarrhea (acute self-limited colitis) [85]. Among patients with suspected IBD presenting with bloody diarrhea, 38% were found to have infectious colitis [86]. In 45 patients hospitalized over a 4-year period due to acute colitis, identified pathogens included *Yersinia enterocolitica* (46%), *Campylobacter jejuni* (20%), *Salmonella* species (13%), less virulent strains of *Shigella* (9%), *Entamoeba histolytica* (7%), and cytomegalovirus (4%) [87]. Colitis due to *Salmonella* and *E. histolytica* was characterized by diffuse colonic lesions, thus resembling UC, whereas the other

48

Table 48.6 Differential diagnosis of inflammatory bowel disease from other causes of colitis

Infectious colitis

Bacterial
  Actinomyces israelii
  Balantidium coli
  Campylobacter jejuni
  Chlamydia trachomatis
  Escherichia coli O157:H7
  Klebsiella oxytoca
  Mycobacterium tuberculosis
  Neisseria gonorrhoeae
  Salmonella spp.
  Shigella dysenteriae
  Treponema pallidum
  Yersinia enterocolitica

Viral
  Cytomegalovirus
  Herpes simplex virus

Fungal
  Aspergillus fumigatus
  Blastomyces spp.
  Candida albicans
  Cryptococcus
  Histoplasma capsulatum

Parasitic
  Entamoeba histolytica
  Schistosoma mansonii
  Strongyloides stercoralis

Noninfectious colitis

Chemical colitis due to glutaraldehyde

Diverticulitis

Ischemic colitis

Solitary ulcer of the rectum

Drug-induced
  Chemotherapy
  Gold salts
  Isotretinoin
  Methotrexate, NSAIDs
  Oral sodium phosphate
  Radiotherapy

Other

Acute intestinal graft-versus-host disease

Behçet's disease

Cap polyposis

Colon cancer

Diversion colitis

Kaposi's sarcoma

Microscopic colitis

Portal hypertension

Post-traumatic

NSAID, nonsteroidal anti-inflammatory drug.

pathogens lead to focal colitis, which had to be differentiated from CD [87]. However, *Salmonella* colitis mimicking CD, with colonic ulcerations, mucosal edema, friability, and a loss of normal vascularity has also been described [88]. In order to differentiate between inflammatory and infectious etiologies of colitis, stool cultures (typical *Salmonella, Shigella, Yersinia, Campylobacter, Escherichia coli,* and *Clostridium difficile*) and the duration of the diarrhea are usually taken into consideration [85]. Usually, IBD can be diagnosed if stool cultures are negative and clinical symptoms last longer than 2 weeks. However, it has been reported that stool tests in acute diarrhea have sensitivities of 40–80 % [85]. Pathogens such as *Campylobacter* or *Clostridium* may also cause exacerbation of symptoms in patients with UC [85,87]. Some studies have also reported cases of infectious diarrhea that have lasted more than 30 days [89].

Mantzaris et al. suggested that the endoscopic appearance of the colon may help differentiate between IBD and acute infectious colitis in patients presenting with acute bloody diarrhea [90]. Among 114 patients studied, 60 % had infectious colitis (52 % of whom had positive stool cultures), 37 % had UC, and 3 % had CD. Significant differences in the endoscopic appearance of the colon in UC and infectious colitis included the presence of patchy erythema (0 % vs. 100 %), diffuse erythema (100 % vs. 25 %), granularity (100 % vs. 8 %), friability (100 % vs. 12 %), hemorrhagic spots (0 % vs. 100 %), evident bleeding (100 % vs. 57 %), microaphthoid ulcers (0 % vs. 100 %), aphthoid ulcers (0 % vs. 17 %), irregular ulcers (0 % vs. 8 %), large regular ulcers (38 % vs. 0 %), deep ulcers (15 % vs. 0 %), denuded areas (5 % vs. 0 %), mucosal bridging (10 % vs. 0 %), and pseudopolyps (15 % vs. 0 %). On the other hand, mucosal edema, spontaneous bleeding, erosions, small superficial ulcers, and luminal exudate were found in the same proportions of patients with UC and infectious colitis. Patients with UC always had severe inflammation of the rectum and sigmoid colon, with symmetric and continuous distribution of endoscopic lesions in the involved colonic area and nonadherent exudate. On the other hand, patients with infectious colitis had a characteristic pattern of lesions with rectal sparing, the most severe and continuous lesions in the distal colon and less severe and patchy lesions in the proximal colon, small islands of disease-free mucosa within severely inflamed colonic mucosa, and adherent exudate [90].

The value of histopathologic examination of biopsied colonic samples in differentiating between infectious colitis and IBD has been evaluated in several studies. Surawicz et al. identified several histologic characteristics of rectal biopsy samples that make it possible to differentiate between IBD and infectious colitis [91]. Features with a positive predictive value (PPV) of 87–100 % in IBD include distortion of crypt architecture and atrophy, mixed lamina propria cellularity, villous surfaces, granulomas, and basal lymphoid aggregates or giant cells. In contrast, normal crypt architecture, superficial giant cells and crypt abscesses have a PPV of 67–84 % for infectious colitis [91]. Nostrant et al. recommended that biopsy specimens should be obtained within the first 4 days from the start of symptoms in order to be diagnostic [92]. Histologic features found only in cases of chronic ulcerative colitis included the presence of plasmocytosis within the lamina propria and mucosal distortion [92]. It is thus worth emphasizing that histologic examination is very accurate in differentiating between IBD and infectious colitis. The endoscopic appearance of infectious colitis is illustrated in **Figs. 48.31–48.36**.

Noninfectious causes of colitis should also be taken into account when considering a diagnosis of IBD. It is necessary to obtain a detailed medical history from the patient in order to have a broad picture and identify potential etiologic factors that may have contributed to the development of colonic inflammation. Endoscopic examples of noninfectious colitis are shown in **Figs. 48.37–48.42**.

VII

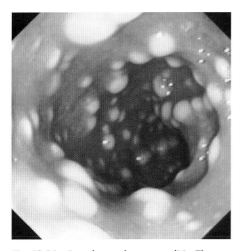

Fig. 48.31 Pseudomembranous colitis. There are multiple yellow coalescent and tenacious plaques throughout the colon. In some areas around the yellow plaques, edema is present, manifested by loss of the normal vascular pattern. This appearance is characteristic of *Clostridium difficile* colitis.

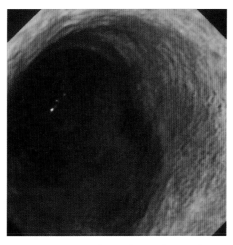

Fig. 48.32 Postantibiotic hemorrhagic colitis related to *Klebsiella oxytoca*. The colonic mucosa is characterized by friability, erosions, and mainly diffuse, intense hemorrhage. This appearance is usually associated with *Klebsiella oxytoca* infection.

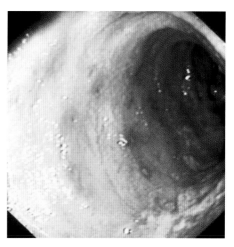

Fig. 48.33 Aphthoid ulceration at the ileum. This appearance was associated with *Yersinia enterocolitica* infection.

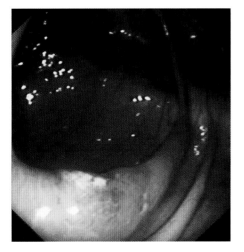

Fig. 48.34 Erythema and exudate located at the ileocecal valve. This appearance is relatively characteristic of amebiasis infection, but it can also be suggestive of Crohn's disease.

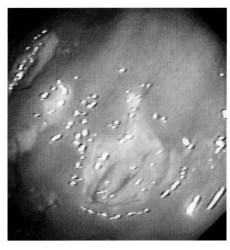

Fig. 48.35 Cytomegalovirus colitis. Well-circumscribed ulceration in the descending colon. The surrounding mucosa is mildly erythematous and edematous.

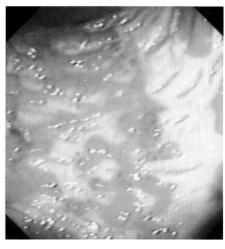

Fig. 48.36 Cytomegalovirus colitis. Severe colitis with deep confluent ulcerations reaching the striation of the muscle layer. These findings may also be seen with other inflammatory diseases, such as severe Crohn's disease or ulcerative colitis.

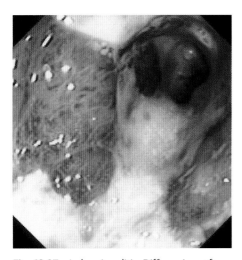

Fig. 48.37 Ischemic colitis. Diffuse circumferential disease with ulcerations, resembling *Clostridium difficile* colitis. Segmental circumferential disease is typical of ischemia.

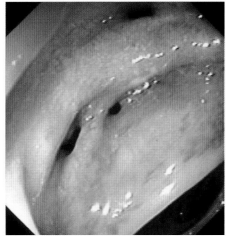

Fig. 48.38 Sigmoiditis associated with diverticular disease. Edema, subepithelial hemorrhage, and mucopus are seen surrounding diverticula.

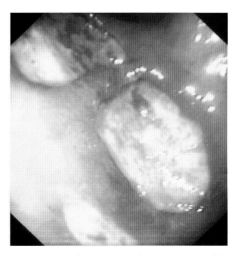

Fig. 48.39 Colonic lesions due to nonsteroidal anti-inflammatory drugs. Multiple well-circumscribed ulcerations are seen throughout the colon. The ulcers have a punched-out appearance, with normal-appearing intervening mucosa.

48

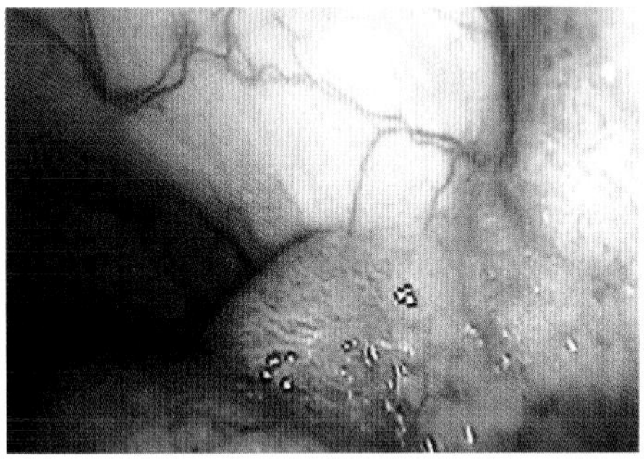

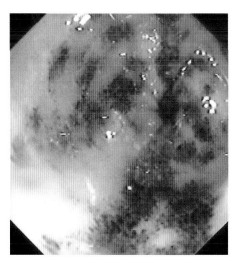

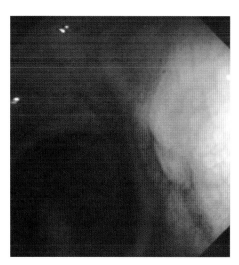

Fig. 48.40 Solitary ulceration of the distal rectum. A large, well-circumscribed ulceration with a clean base is associated with edema of the proximal margin. This elderly patient had no evidence of infection, ischemia, or anorectal trauma.

Fig. 48.41 Glutaraldehyde colitis. These patchy, multiple erythematous lesions, with submucosal hemorrhage, have to be distinguished from inflammatory bowel disease.

Fig. 48.42 A large, well-circumscribed, deep ulcer is seen in the distal rectum.

Cancer and IBD

Risk of Colorectal Cancer

Patients with IBD have a greater risk of colorectal cancer (CRC) than the general population. A population-based study including 5529 patients with IBD observed a similarly increased incidence rate of CRC for patients with both Crohn's disease (2.64) and ulcerative colitis (2.75) in comparison with non-IBD controls [93]. The incidence of rectal carcinoma was significantly increased only in patients with UC (1.9), whereas the rate of small-intestinal carcinoma was significantly increased only in patients with Crohn's disease (17.4) in comparison with non-IBD controls [93]. These data suggesting an increased risk of CRC in patients with IBD were further supported by other studies. A study by Gillen et al. showed a similar 18–19-fold increase in the risk of CRC in patients with extensive colonic Crohn's disease or extensive ulcerative colitis, respectively, in comparison with the general population [94]. There were similar absolute cumulative risks for CRC in patients with extensive ulcerative colitis (8 % after 22 years of disease) and extensive colonic Crohn's disease (7 % after 20 years' duration). The risk of CRC was increased 109-fold or 57-fold, respectively, in patients with ulcerative colitis or colonic Crohn's disease when their IBD began before they were 25 years old [94]. A meta-analysis of 116 studies reported an overall prevalence of 3.7 % for CRC in patients with UC and a prevalence of 5.4 % for CRC among patients with UC pancolitis [95]. The cumulative probability of CRC increased with disease duration, irrespective of the disease extent (2 % at 10 years, 8 % at 20 years, and 18 % at 30 years) [95]. The risk of CRC in patients with IBD has been found to be associated with early onset of the disease [93,96,97], disease duration [95] and extent [96], severity of colonic inflammation [98], a family history of CRC [99,100], a history of postinflammatory pseudopolyps [101], backwash ileitis [102], and primary sclerosing cholangitis [103] (with a predilection for right-colon cancer [104]) . Factors that appear to reduce the risk of CRC in patients with UC include surveillance colonoscopy, smoking, use of corticosteroids, aspirin, nonsteroidal anti-inflammatory drugs (NSAIDs), and 5-ASA [101].

Dysplasia

Dysplasia in the colon has been defined as unequivocal neoplastic alteration of the colonic epithelium [105] and is regarded as a precursor lesion in the pathway leading to the development of invasive colon carcinoma in patients with IBD [106]. Dysplastic epithelium may itself be a marker for malignancy in nearby underlying tissue [105]. Dysplasia in the colon is found in approximately 20 % of patients with ulcerative colitis undergoing surveillance colonoscopy with biopsies [107]. According to a consensus statement dating from 1983, colonic biopsy specimens are classified on microscopic examination into one of the following categories: negative for dysplasia, indefinite for dysplasia, low-grade dysplasia (LGD), high-grade dysplasia (HGD), or invasive cancer [105]. From the endoscopic point of view, dysplasia may be either invisible (flat dysplasia) or visible (raised dysplasia, dysplasia-associated lesion or mass, DALM) [108,109]. Flat dysplasia occurs most often in macroscopically normal mucosa and represents 95 % of the dysplasia found [107]. Occasionally, flat dysplasia may be macroscopically visible as thickened mucosa with mild discoloration and a velvety appearance, with evidence of nodularity [107]. Raised dysplastic lesions, which account for 5 % of the dysplasia found, belong to a heterogeneous group of lesions and can be further divided into adenoma-like DALMs and non–adenoma-like DALMs on the basis of their endoscopic appearance [110]. Adenoma-like DALMs have been defined as grossly discrete, well-defined, sessile or pedunculated polyps, similar to sporadic adenomas found in non-IBD patients. Non–adenoma-like DALMs are irregular plaques or mass-like lesions [110] (**Fig. 48.43**).

Endoscopic Surveillance

One screening surveillance strategy is presented in **Fig. 48.44** [111]. A diagnosis of dysplasia should be confirmed by an experienced second gastrointestinal pathologist [45]. If flat dysplasia is found on biopsy, immediate colectomy is recommended. Studies have shown that the presence of flat LGD or HGD is associated with a high rate of synchronous and metachronous adenocarcinoma [112–115]. If adenoma-like DALMs are found on colonoscopy inside the area of colitis, the patient should undergo complete polypectomy and

VII

four biopsies should be taken adjacent to the raised lesion [45]. If the biopsy results are negative for adenocarcinoma and there is no flat dysplasia adjacent to the lesion or anywhere in the colon, then the patient requires regular endoscopic surveillance, with the first follow-up examination within 6 months [45]. Adenoma-like DALMs found outside the area of colitis should be treated with polypectomy. On the other hand, non–adenoma-like DALMs are strong indicators for colectomy.

The approach to DALMs (**Fig. 48.45**) in patients with IBD is based on the results of several studies [116]. A prospective study by Rubin et al. found that in 48 IBD patients with chronic colitis and no flat dysplasia who were followed up for a mean of 4 years, endoscopic polypectomy of adenoma-like DALMs was as effective as in non-colitic colons [117]. Although follow-up colonoscopies revealed additional polyps in 48% of the patients, no colon cancer or flat dysplasia was found at surgery or in biopsy specimens [117]. These data were further supported by a prospective study by Odze et al., which followed up a cohort of 34 patients with ulcerative colitis and adenoma-like DALMs who had undergone polypectomy, with surveillance continuing for a mean of 82 months, and compared them with a group of 49 non-IBD patients treated similarly for sporadic adenomas [118]. During the follow-up, at least one further adenoma-like DALM was found in 20 of the 34 ulcerative colitis patients (58.8%). Flat dysplasia and adenocarcinoma were found in one patient each. A subgroup analysis of patients with ulcerative colitis found no significant differences in the prevalence of polyp development between 24 patients with adenoma-like DALMs located in the area of colitis and 10 patients with adenoma-like DALMs located outside the area of active inflammation in the colon (62.5% vs. 50%). The prevalence of new sporadic adenomas in non-IBD patients was similar to that observed in the ulcerative colitis group (49%; $P > 0.05$) [118]. A recent retrospective study from our own center followed up a nine patients with adenoma-like DALMs and HGD without synchronous flat dysplasia who had undergone endoscopic polypectomy and found that none of these patients developed either cancer or flat dysplasia in surveillance biopsies or resection specimens [119].

The presence of non–adenoma-like DALMs in patients with IBD mandates colectomy, as these lesions are indeed associated with

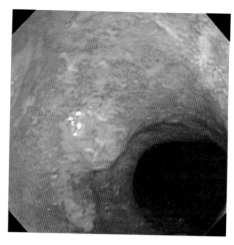

Fig. 48.43 A dysplasia-associated lymphoid mass (DALM) in a patient with ulcerative colitis. There is active colitis in the presence of a neoplastic polypoid lesion in the rectum. Biopsy demonstrated intramucosal carcinoma.

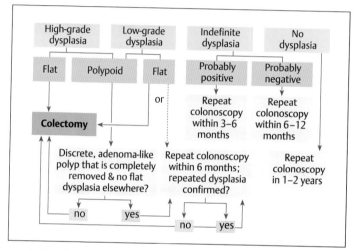

Fig. 48.44 Suggested surveillance strategy. The duration of short-term surveillance has not been established [111]. With kind permission from Elsevier: Itzkowitz SH, Harpaz N. Diagnosis and management of dysplasia in patients with inflammatory bowel diseases. Gastroenterology 2004;126:1634–48.

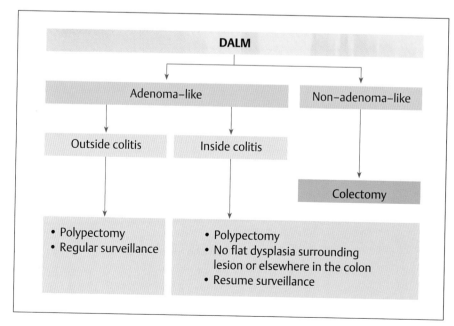

Fig. 48.45 A proposed management scheme for dysplasia-associated lymphoid masses (DALM) in patients with inflammatory bowel disease [116]. With kind permission from Elsevier: Farraye FA, Waye JD, Moscandrew M, Heeren TC, Odze RD. Variability in the diagnosis and management of adenoma-like and non-adenoma-like dysplasia-associated lesions or masses in inflammatory bowel disease: an Internet-based study. Gastrointest Endosc 2007;66:519–29.

Table 48.7 Suggested surveillance colonoscopy procedures for diagnosis and management of dysplasia in patients with inflammatory bowel diseases [111]

- Obtain four biopsy specimens of flat mucosa every 10 cm (consider sampling every 5 cm in the rectosigmoid)
- Place each quadruplicate set in a separate specimen jar (as opposed to pooling biopsy specimens from several colonic segments)
- Sample suspicious lesions or polyps
- Make sure to biopsy flat mucosa around the base of any suspicious polyp and submit the specimen in a separate container
- Consider suppressing symptoms of active inflammation with medical therapy before surveillance colonoscopy
- In Crohn's colitis, strictures may require a thinner-caliber colonoscope
- Consider brush cytology or barium enema to evaluate impassable strictures

With kind permission from Elsevier: Itzkowitz SH, Harpaz N. Diagnosis and management of dysplasia in patients with inflammatory bowel diseases. Gastroenterology 2004;126:1634–48.

colon cancer. A study dating from the early 1980s by Blackstone et al., who followed 112 patients with chronic ulcerative colitis over a 4-year period, found non–adenoma-like DALMs in 12 patients; invasive carcinoma was detected in seven of these 12 patients (58.3%) [108]. The authors described DALMs as a "single polypoid mass," "a plaque-like lesion," or "multiple sessile polyps," which is consistent with the definition of non–adenoma-like DALMs [108]. A study by Bernstein et al. analyzing 10 prospective studies of endoscopic surveillance in patients with ulcerative colitis found that, of 40 patients with ulcerative colitis with DALMs detected during colonoscopy, 17 (43%) already had cancer at immediate colectomy [114]. However, DALMs were defined by the authors as "the equivalent of small sessile tumors," which is consistent with the current definition of non–adenoma-like DALMs [114].

The current guidelines of American Society for Gastrointestinal Endoscopy recommend that surveillance colonoscopy should be carried out in patients with extensive or left-sided ulcerative colitis of at least 8–10 years' duration, in patients with IBD and a family history of CRC or primary sclerosing cholangitis, and in those with extensive Crohn's colitis, every 1–2 years starting after 8–10 years of disease [71]. Suggested methods for surveillance colonoscopy are presented in **Table 48.7** [111]. It has been suggested that a finding of normal-appearing colonic mucosa at colonoscopy in patients with IBD reduces the risk of colon cancer developing to that seen in the general population; reducing the endoscopic surveillance interval to 5 years might therefore be considered in such cases [120]. It has been recommended that four-quadrant jumbo biopsies of the colon should be obtained every 10 cm between the rectum and the cecum, for a total of 40–50 random biopsies per colonoscopy, in patients with ulcerative colitis. One study observed that at least 56 jumbo biopsies during colonoscopy are required in order to provide 95% confidence of identifying dysplasia; 64 jumbo biopsies are required in order to detect cancer with 95% confidence; and 18 jumbo biopsies are required in order to detect either cancer or dysplasia with 95% confidence [121].

Endoscopic Features Associated with Dysplasia

Kudo et al. developed a pit pattern classification in which lesions with pit patterns of type 1 or 2 were non-tumors and those with types 3–5 were neoplastic tumors [122]. Recently, Matsumoto et al. presented a classification of dysplastic lesions of the colon into five categories on the basis of their endoscopic appearance: protruding lesions, slightly elevated lesions, flat lesions, depressed lesions, and mixed-type lesions [123]. Protruding lesions are the ones most commonly seen. The presence of DALM, surface irregularity, or uneven redness within protruding lesions strongly suggests dys-

plastic changes. Slightly elevated lesions displaying irregular granular surfaces and uneven redness warrant biopsy. Areas of reddish mucosa with a defined boundary are indicative of flat dysplasia. Depressed lesions are not frequently seen and are usually associated with the presence of slightly elevated lesions. These lesions can be identified by chromoendoscopy, rather than conventional colonoscopy. Finally, the majority of mixed lesions have the appearance of protruding lesions accompanying slightly elevated lesions [123].

Endoscopic Detection of Colonic Neoplasia

Although it was earlier suggested that dysplastic lesions are macroscopically visible only occasionally [107], three recent studies have reported that most dysplastic lesions are visible at colonoscopy in IBD patients [124–126]. The macroscopically visible dysplastic lesions accounted for 58.5–87.9% of all detected dysplastic sites [124–126]. The study by Rutter et al. found that only 5.9% of endoscopically visible dysplastic lesions were flat [124], whereas a study from our own institution observed that 23.5% of all visible dysplastic lesions were flat [126].

The question of random biopsies in patients with IBD continues to be a matter of controversy. Chromoendoscopy (endoscopic dye spraying) allows more accurate identification of areas that should be biopsied in the colon, thus reducing the necessity for random biopsies. Three classes of dye are used in chromoendoscopy: contrast dyes, absorptive dyes, and reactive dyes [127]. Contrast dyes (indigo carmine) coat the colonic mucosa, do not react with it, and are nonabsorbable. Once sprayed, the colonic mucosa has a typical appearance of "tiny pits and whorls of parallel 'innominate' grooves" resembling fingerprints. Absorptive dyes (methylene blue) are absorbed more rapidly by normal mucosa, as opposed to inflamed or dysplastic colonic mucosa. Reactive dyes cause color changes by reacting either with the colonic epithelium or with mucosal secretions [127].

Chromoendoscopy appears to be superior to standard colonoscopy for surveillance, although it takes longer to perform. According to the SURFACE guidelines, chromoendoscopy should be performed in patients with a confirmed diagnosis of UC with a history of at least 8 years and clinically quiescent disease (strict selection); with excellent bowel cleansing (*u*nmasking the mucosal surface); with peristaltic waves reduced by administering spasmolytic medication (*r*educe peristaltic waves); with pancolonic staining (*f*ull-length staining of the colon); with additional use of 0.4% indigo carmine or 0.1% methylene blue (*a*ugmented detection with dyes); with a complete analysis of mucosal lesions in accordance with the pit pattern guidelines (*c*rypt architecture analysis); and with biopsies obtained from all mucosal lesions (*e*ndoscopic targeted biopsies) [128]. Rutter et al. indicated that none of 2904 untargeted colonic biopsies detected dysplasia in 100 patients with ulcerative colitis, whereas a targeted biopsy protocol in conjunction with pancolonic chromoendoscopy using indigo carmine dye spraying detected dysplastic changes in 7% of the patients (*P* = 0.02) [129]. Use of a targeted biopsy protocol with dye spraying showed a trend toward a statistically larger number of patients having dysplasia detected in comparison with a targeted biopsy protocol alone (7% vs. 2%; *P* = 0.06). The authors concluded that careful examination of the colonic mucosa enhanced by chromoendoscopy may be superior to untargeted colonic biopsies for detecting dysplastic changes [129]. These data were supported recently by Marion et al., who found that biopsies targeted with methylene blue dye spraying identified significantly more patients with dysplastic changes (16.7%) than untargeted biopsies (2.9%; *P* = 0.001) and more than targeted biopsies without dye spraying (8.8%; *P* = 0.057) [130]. In a randomized and controlled study, Kiesslich et al. demonstrated that chromoendoscopy using methylene blue staining allows more ac-

VII

Table 48.8 Prospective studies comparing panchromoendoscopy with white-light endoscopy for surveillance of patients with long-standing ulcerative colitis [135]

First author, year [ref].]	Patients (n)	Method	Increase in diagnostic yield
Kiesslich 2003 [131]	165	Methylene blue staining	3-fold (per lesion)
Hurlstone 2004 [134]	162	Indigo carmine staining	4-fold (per lesion)
Rutter 2004 [129]	100	Indigo carmine staining	4.5-fold (per lesion)
Hurlstone 2005 [132]	700	Indigo carmine	3-fold (per lesion)
Kiesslich 2007 [133]	161	Methylene blue staining and endomicroscopy	4.75-fold (per lesion)
Marion 2007 [130]	102	Methylene blue staining	1.5-fold (per patient)

With kind permission from Elsevier: Kiesslich R, Galle PR, Neurath MF. Endoscopic surveillance in ulcerative colitis: smart biopsies do it better. Gastroenterology 2007;133:742–5.

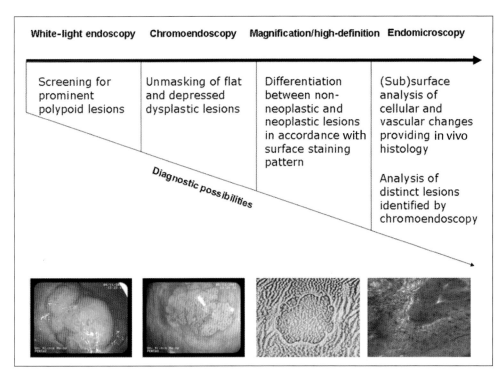

Fig. 48.46 Diagnostic options for surveillance in patients with ulcerative colitis [135]. With kind permission from Elsevier: Kiesslich R, Galle PR, Neurath MF. Endoscopic surveillance in ulcerative colitis: smart biopsies do it better. Gastroenterology 2007;133:742–5.

48

curate diagnosis of the extent and severity of the inflammatory activity in ulcerative colitis in comparison with conventional colonoscopy [131]. Chromoendoscopy allowed more targeted biopsies to be obtained and made it possible to detect a statistically significantly larger number of intraepithelial neoplasias than conventional colonoscopy (32 vs. 10; $P=0.003$) [131]. Chromoendoscopy with magnifying endoscopes was shown to be capable of identifying significantly more intraepithelial neoplastic colonic lesions in patients with ulcerative colitis than conventional colonoscopy (69 vs. 24; $P<0.0001$) [132]. The diagnostic yields for detecting intraepithelial neoplasia with chromoendoscopy combined with magnifying colonoscopy were 0.16% and 8% for untargeted and targeted biopsies, respectively. The corresponding diagnostic yields for identifying intraepithelial neoplasia with untargeted and targeted biopsies with conventional colonoscopy were 0.14% and 1.6%, respectively [132]. Kiesslich et al. recently reported that combined chromoendoscopy and endomicroscopy increased the diagnostic yield for detecting intraepithelial neoplasia in the colon in patients with ulcerative colitis 4.75-fold in comparison with conventional colonoscopy with random biopsies ($P=0.005$), with a simultaneous 50% reduction in the number of biopsies required ($P=0.008$) [133]. **Table 48.8** presents the results of six prospective studies [129–134] comparing the diagnostic yield of panchromoendoscopy with white-light endoscopy [135]. While chromoendoscopy helps unmask flat lesions in the colon, targeted endomicroscopy makes it possible to detect neoplastic changes, identifying which colonic lesions should

be biopsied [133]. On the basis of these findings, the authors modified one of the SURFACE criteria (endomicroscopy and endoscopically targeted biopsies) and recommended that endomicroscopy should be performed on all stained lesions, followed by targeted biopsies of all mucosal changes [135]. Diagnostic options for surveillance in patients with UC are shown in **Fig. 48.46**.

Another new modality, narrow-band imaging (NBI), for detecting colonic neoplasia has also been proposed [136]. The NBI system makes it possible to visualize neoplastic lesions in the colon on the basis of improved contrast imaging of the capillary pattern in the superficial layer [137]. Published studies show that NBI does not improve detection of neoplasia in the colon or differentiation between neoplastic and nonneoplastic colonic polyps, and its diagnostic yield is comparable with that of chromoendoscopy [138]. Pooled data from six studies showed that the NBI system and chromoendoscopy had comparable sensitivity (92% vs. 91%), specificity (86% vs. 89%), and overall accuracy (89% vs. 91%) rates in differentiating between neoplastic and nonneoplastic colonic lesions [138]. Another technique, autofluorescence imaging (AFI), was shown to be significantly superior to white-light colonoscopy in detecting colonic dysplasia in 50 patients with long-standing UC [139]. The reported adenoma miss rates for AFI and standard colonoscopy were 0% and 50%, respectively ($P=0.036$) [139]. Future randomized studies including larger numbers of patients are needed in order to further evaluate the diagnostic yield of NBI and other modalities in detecting colonic neoplasia.

Capsule Endoscopy

Video capsule endoscopy (VCE) is a new modality that allows minimally invasive evaluation of the small bowel. VCE is generally contraindicated in patients with known or suspected gastrointestinal obstruction, strictures, or fistulas, and in pregnant women [140]. However, it has been suggested that small-bowel obstruction and stricture are not contraindications to VCE [141]. Conversely, retention of the video capsule might help identify small-bowel lesions requiring surgery in patients with suspected small-bowel obstruction. VCE examinations in 19 patients with suspected small-bowel obstruction did not lead to the development of acute small-bowel obstruction [141]. VCE is relatively contraindicated in patients with dysphagia, Zenker diverticulum, colonic diverticulosis, extensive Crohn's enteritis, and prior pelvic or abdominal surgery [140]. It has been reported that VCE examinations can be safely performed in patients with pacemakers [140,142]. The rate of VCE retention is significantly higher in patients with previously diagnosed CD (13%; 95% CI, 5.6% to 28%) than in those tested due for suspected CD (1.6%; 95% CI, 0.2% to 10%) [143]. However, patients in whom suspected CD has been confirmed by VCE appear to have a similar rate (12.5%) of capsule retention to those with known CD [143]. Performance of VCE in CD patients in whom small-bowel strictures had been excluded on the basis of previous small-bowel imaging led to an overall capsule retention rate of 5.1% (seven of 136 patients in whom small-bowel strictures had been ruled out with small-bowel radiography), due to the presence of strictures that had not been identified with radiography [143–146]. Patients with retained capsules should undergo surgery, which allows capsule removal and excision of the small-bowel stricture, thus improving the patient's preexisting condition [143,147]. There are no published data regarding conservative treatment for capsule retention using anti-inflammatory medication (steroids, infliximab), prokinetics, or cathartics to promote passage of the capsule through the stricture [147].

A recent meta-analysis compared the yield of VCE with other diagnostic modalities in patients with suspected or established nonstricturing small-bowel Crohn's disease [148]. The yield of VCE was significantly superior to small-bowel barium radiography (78% vs. 32%; $P<0.001$), colonoscopy with ileoscopy (86% vs. 60%; $P=0.002$), computed-tomographic (CT) enterography (68% vs. 38%; $P<0.001$), and push enteroscopy (incremental yield of 69%; $P<0.001$) for diagnosing recurrence of small-bowel Crohn's disease in patients with a previously established diagnosis of Crohn's disease. It was demonstrated that VCE had a number needed to test (NNT) of three in order to yield one additional diagnosis of Crohn's disease in comparison with small-bowel barium radiography, and an NNT of seven in comparison with colonoscopy with ileoscopy [148]. A recently published small study from Spain reported that VCE had a diagnostic yield of 85.7% in patients with previously established small-bowel CD and that the capsule-endoscopic findings resulted in a change in CD therapy in 64% of the patients [149].

The use of VCE as a first-line modality for initial diagnosis of CD is limited. Data from a meta-analysis demonstrated that the yield of VCE was not significantly superior to small-bowel barium radiography (43% vs. 13%; $P=0.09$), colonoscopy with ileoscopy (33% vs. 26%; $P=0.48$), CT enterography (70% vs. 21%; $P=0.07$), or push enteroscopy (incremental yield of 8%; $P=0.51$) for diagnosing small-bowel Crohn's disease in patients with suspected Crohn's disease [148]. In addition, its lower specificity and the necessity for small-bowel radiography beforehand in order to exclude any small-bowel obstruction mean that VCE is not capable of being used as a first-line diagnostic method in CD [150]. Although the sensitivity of VCE for diagnosing CD (83%) is not significantly different from that of CT enterography (83%), ileocolonoscopy (74%), and small-bowel follow-through (65%), its specificity (53%) is signifi-

cantly lower than that of other tests ($P<0.05$) [150]. It should be emphasized that there are no uniform criteria for diagnosing CD with VCE [71]. Small-bowel ulcerations mimicking CD may be caused by infection, ischemia, radiation injury, and drugs such as NSAIDs [71,151]. In addition, capsule endoscopy may also identify small-bowel mucosal lesions in up to 14% of healthy individuals [151]. Future studies including large numbers of patients are needed in order to further evaluate the diagnostic yield of VCE as a first-line diagnostic tool in suspected CD.

In patients with a diagnosis of ulcerative colitis or indeterminate colitis, 16% of patients were found to have features consistent with small-bowel Crohn's disease on VCE [152]. Patients with prior colectomy were more likely to have abnormal findings on VCE than those with an intact colon (33% vs. 12%; $P=0.04$). It was therefore suggested that VCE should be considered in patients with ulcerative colitis and atypical clinical symptoms, particularly after colectomy [152].

Recently, Gal et al. developed and validated a new capsule endoscopy Crohn's disease activity index (CECDAI) [153]. The CECDAI evaluates the following parameters measured in the proximal (1) and distal (2) segments of the small bowel:
- A. Inflammation, rated on a scale of 0 (none) to 5 (large ulcer, >2 cm)
- B. Extent of disease, rated on a scale of 0 (none) to 3 (diffuse)
- C. Presence of strictures, rated from 0 (none) to 3 (obstruction)*

The segmental score is calculated using the formula $(A \times B + C)$ for the proximal and distal segments of the small bowel, and the sum of the segmental scores constitutes the total CECDAI score: $(A1 \times B1 + C1) + (A2 \times B2 + C2)$. In a group of 20 patients with Crohn's disease included in the study, the score ranged from 0 to 26 points. The index was found to be easy to calculate, reproducible, and with low intraobserver variability ($\kappa = 0.867$) [153]. VCE findings in patients with suspected Crohn's disease are illustrated in **Figs. 48.47–48.51.**

* With kind permission from Springer Science+Business Media: Dig Dis Sci. Assessment and validation of the new capsule endoscopy Crohn's disease activity index (CECDAI). Vol. 53, 2008, pages 1933–7, Gal E, Geller A, Fraser G, Levi Z, Niv Y.

Enteroscopy

Push Enteroscopy

This technique has limited usefulness in patients with IBD [71]. It allows endoscopic examination of the small intestine up to 160 cm beyond the ligament of Treitz [154–156]. It is currently recommended as an adjuvant technique to VCE for treatment of lesions located in the proximal small bowel identified by VCE [157].

Double-Balloon Enteroscopy

The small bowel is approximately 430 cm long. Conventional push enteroscopy allows examination of only the proximal 160 cm of the small bowel beyond the ligament of Treitz [154,156]. In double-balloon enteroscopy (DBE), developed by Yamamoto et al., balloons are attached to the tip of a flexible overtube and to the tip of the endoscope [158]. DBE makes it possible to examine the entire small-bowel mucosa, with the tip of the enteroscope being inserted beyond the ileocecal valve [158]. The endoscopes can be inserted either orally or anally [159]. The balloon on the overtube is deflated, and the overtube is advanced over the endoscope after it has been inserted to the maximum possible depth]. At this point, the balloon on the endoscope is inflated to prevent the endoscope from sliding.

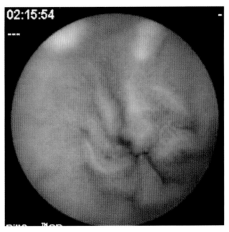
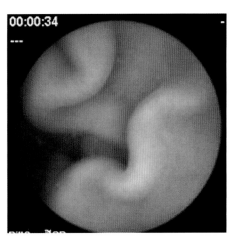
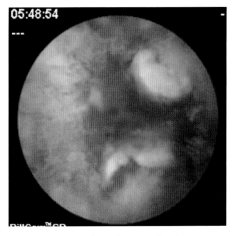

a, b

Fig. 48.47 a, b Capsule endoscopy images showing normal small-bowel mucosa.

Fig. 48.48 Capsule endoscopy showing a terminal ileal area of ulceration with luminal narrowing, consistent with Crohn's disease of the small intestine.

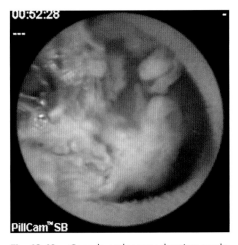
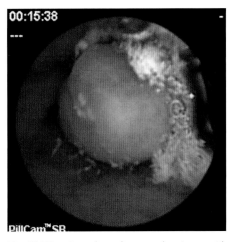
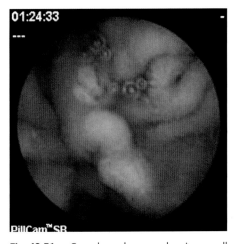

Fig. 48.49 Capsule endoscopy showing a polypoid exophytic mass lesion with mucoid material in a patient with Crohn's disease. The lesion was identified as an adenocarcinoma in an area of severe ulceration and inflammation in the ileum.

Fig. 48.50 Capsule endoscopy showing a mid-jejunal benign lipoma in a patient with long-standing ulcerative colitis.

Fig. 48.51 Capsule endoscopy showing small aphthous ulcers in the distal ileum in a patient with Crohn's disease.

48

Alternating inflation and deflation of the two balloons makes it possible to advance the endoscope through the small intestine. The maneuvers cause shortening of the small intestine, allowing for deep advancement of the instrument. Movement of the endoscope is controlled at the point at which the balloon on the overtube grips the small bowel [159]. DBE is currently indicated in patients with mid-gastrointestinal bleeding, small-bowel strictures, and small-bowel tumors, as well as for removing foreign bodies from the small intestine and for endoscopic examination and therapy following VCE findings [160].

DBE has been shown to be an effective and safe method for treating small-bowel strictures. The first series of small-bowel stricture dilations with DBE showed that it was possible to improve small-intestinal strictures using the enteroscope up to 180 cm from the pylorus and 270 cm from the colon in 10 patients [161]. Dilation was not attempted in nine patients, due to either severe inflammation (n = 6) or for anatomic reasons (n = 3). Of the 10 patients who underwent DBE dilation, technical success, defined as balloon inflation and advancement of the endoscope through the dilated part of the bowel, was achieved in 80 % and 60 % of cases, respectively, and the patients experienced symptomatic improve-

ment, with avoidance of surgery, after a follow-up period of 10 months [161].

Perioperative Endoscopy

In this procedure, performed during surgery, the endoscope is advanced in a retrograde fashion from the enterotomy up to the ligament of Treitz. A recent study in Japan found that 42 % of intestinal Crohn's strictures detected on intraoperative enteroscopy had not been identified during preoperative examinations [162]. It has also been reported that perioperative endoscopy allows accurate evaluation of the luminal status of the small bowel at the site of the stricture, ileocecal valve, or previous operation, so that it is helpful in decision-making during surgery in patients with Crohn's disease [162]. However, an earlier study by Esaki et al. claimed that although more small-bowel lesions can be detected during perioperative endoscopy, the findings are not predictive of postoperative recurrence of CD [163].

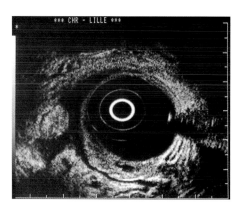

Fig. 48.52 Ultrasonography showing a rectal fistula in a patient with Crohn's disease.

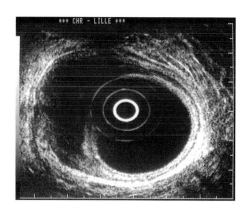

Fig. 48.53 Ultrasonography showing an anal abscess in a patient with Crohn's disease.

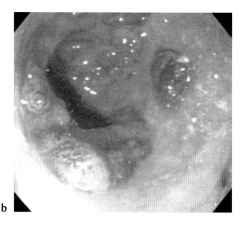

a, b

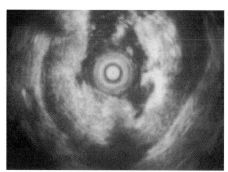

Fig. 48.54 A 56-year-old man with left-sided ulcerative colitis who underwent surgery [178]. With kind permission from Elsevier: Yoshizawa S, Kobayashi K, Katsumata T, Saigenji K, Okayasu I. Clinical usefulness of EUS for active ulcerative colitis. Gastrointest Endosc 2007;65:253–60.
a The conventional colonoscopic view shows deep ulcers in the descending colon. Only island-shaped regions of mucosa are left.
b Endoscopic ultrasonography shows a markedly thickened bowel wall, with a poorly demarcated structure from the first to fourth layers, suggesting that the intestinal inflammation extends to the muscularis propria.

Endoscopic Retrograde Cholangiopancreatography

Primary sclerosing cholangitis (PSC), a type of chronic inflammation and fibrosis of the bile ducts [164,165], affects approximately 5 % of patients with IBD [166]. Ninety percent of patients with PSC have accompanying IBD [166]. Endoscopic retrograde cholangiopancreatography (ERCP) is the gold standard for diagnosing PSC. The typical cholangiogram shows a diffuse distribution of annular and multifocal strictures of the intrahepatic and extrahepatic bile ducts, displaying a "beaded" appearance [167,168]. ERCP allows endoscopic therapy for benign biliary strictures, either by balloon dilation or stent placement [169]. The technique also makes it possible to take biopsies and perform brush cytology of the bile ducts in order to differentiate between benign and malignant lesions [170–172].

Endoscopic Ultrasonography (EUS)

Transrectal EUS is a useful diagnostic tool for evaluating perianal fistulas in patients with CD [173–175]. Fistulas are visible as hyperechoic tracks or beads within a larger hypoechoic tract consistent with surrounding inflammation [176]. Transrectal EUS has an accuracy of 91 % in detecting perianal fistulas in patients with CD [173]. The EUS findings allow effective medical and surgical management of perianal fistulas. A retrospective analysis of 21 patients who developed perianal fistulas in the course of CD reported high short-term (86 %) and long-term (76 %) fistula response rates. The authors also suggested that the EUS findings may make it possible to discontinue infliximab treatment without recurrent fistula development in up to 64 % of patients [174]. A randomized, prospective, and controlled trial reported improved long-term outcomes (at week

54) in patients in whom the medical and surgical therapy was guided by the EUS findings in comparison with those without such guidance, with complete cessation of fistula drainage in 80 % and 20 %, respectively. The poor outcome in the control group was probably due to fistulas or abscesses that had been missed during surgical evaluation, or premature seton removal before the fistula became inactive [175]. **Figures 48.52** and **48.53** illustrate EUS imaging in patients with CD.

EUS has also been evaluated in patients with UC (**Fig. 48.54**). In a pilot study, Higaki et al. reported that the mean thickness of the first three layers of the rectal wall on EUS was significantly larger in patients with active disease (1.97 mm for Baron score 1, 2.46 mm for Baron score 2, and 2.74 mm for Baron score 3) than in normal control individuals (1.24 mm) ($P < 0.05$) [177]. There was a significant difference in the mean thickness of the rectal wall between patients with mild and severe endoscopic activity of UC ($P < 0.05$). A larger mean initial thickness of the three layers of the rectal wall on EUS was predictive of relapse of UC (2.73 mm vs. 1.79 mm; $P = 0.0001$) [177]. EUS evaluation of 13 colectomy specimens showed a strong correlation between the EUS findings and the histologic examination of the specimens [178]. The results of EUS performed in vivo showed that significantly more patients who underwent surgery had inflammation confined to the muscularis propria than those who were treated medically (62 % vs. 19 %; $P = 0.002$) [178]. Future studies are needed in order to further validate these promising findings.

Conclusions

Endoscopy is critical in both the diagnosis and management of IBD. Lower gastrointestinal endoscopy with biopsy is a vital tool for differentiating between CD and UC. With the advent of balloon dilation to treat strictures, endoscopy can also be used to provide

VII

treatment. Colonoscopy also serves as an outstanding screening tool for monitoring dysplasia and preventing cancer. The colonoscopic findings can allow accurate management, diagnosis, and monitoring of IBD.

Acknowledgment

Table 48.5 and **Figs. 48.31–48.42, 48.52**, and **48.53** are reproduced from the chapter on inflammatory bowel disease in the previous edition of the present volume, by Yoram Bouhnik, Marc Lémann, Vincent Maunoury, Alain Bitoun, and Jean-Frédéric Columbel.

References

1. Simpson P, Papadakis KA. Endoscopic evaluation of patients with inflammatory bowel disease. Inflamm Bowel Dis 2008;14:1287–97.
2. Tan JJ, Tjandra JJ. Which is the optimal bowel preparation for colonoscopy—a meta-analysis. Colorectal Dis 2006;8:247–58.
3. Church JM. Effectiveness of polyethylene glycol antegrade gut lavage bowel preparation for colonoscopy—timing is the key! Dis Colon Rectum 1998;41:1223–5.
4. Gonlusen G, Akgun H, Ertan A, Olivero J, Truong LD. Renal failure and nephrocalcinosis associated with oral sodium phosphate bowel cleansing: clinical patterns and renal biopsy findings. Arch Pathol Lab Med 2006;130:101–6.
5. Heher EC, Thier SO, Rennke H, Humphreys BD. Adverse renal and metabolic effects associated with oral sodium phosphate bowel preparation. Clin J Am Soc Nephrol 2008;3:1494–503.
6. Ori Y, Herman M, Tobar A, Chernin G, Gafter U, Chagnac A, et al. Acute phosphate nephropathy—an emerging threat. Am J Med Sci 2008;336:309–14.
7. Davis GR, Santa Ana CA, Morawski SG, Fordtran JS. Development of a lavage solution associated with minimal water and electrolyte absorption or secretion. Gastroenterology 1980;78:991–5.
8. DiPalma JA, Marshall JB. Comparison of a new sulfate-free polyethylene glycol electrolyte lavage solution versus a standard solution for colonoscopy cleansing. Gastrointest Endosc 1990;36:285–9.
9. Diab FH, Marshall JB. The palatability of five colonic lavage solutions. Aliment Pharmacol Ther 1996;10:815–9.
10. DiPalma JA, Wolff BG, Meagher A, Cleveland M. Comparison of reduced volume versus four liters sulfate-free electrolyte lavage solutions for colonoscopy colon cleansing. Am J Gastroenterol 2003;98:2187–91.
11. Ker TS. Comparison of reduced volume versus four-liter electrolyte lavage solutions for colon cleansing. Am Surg 2006;72:909–11.
12. Ell C, Fischbach W, Bronisch HJ, Dertinger S, Layer P, Runzi M, et al. Randomized trial of low-volume PEG solution versus standard PEG + electrolytes for bowel cleansing before colonoscopy. Am J Gastroenterol 2008;103:883–93.
13. Rex DK, Schwartz H, Goldstein M, Popp J, Katz S, Barish C, et al. Safety and colon-cleansing efficacy of a new residue-free formulation of sodium phosphate tablets. Am J Gastroenterol 2006;101:2594–604.
14. Wruble L, Demicco M, Medoff J, Safdi A, Bernstein J, Dalke D, et al. Residue-free sodium phosphate tablets (OsmoPrep) versus Visicol for colon cleansing: a randomized, investigator-blinded trial. Gastrointest Endosc 2007;65:660–70.
15. Johanson JF, Popp JW Jr, Cohen LB, Lottes SR, Forbes WP, Walker K, et al. A randomized, multicenter study comparing the safety and efficacy of sodium phosphate tablets with 2 L polyethylene glycol solution plus bisacodyl tablets for colon cleansing. Am J Gastroenterol 2007;102:2238–46.
16. Lichtenstein G. Bowel preparations for colonoscopy: a review. Am J Health Syst Pharm 2009;66:27–37.
17. Truelove SC, Witts LJ. Cortisone in ulcerative colitis: final report on a therapeutic trial. Br Med J 1955;ii:1041–8.
18. Baron JH, Connell AM, Lennard-Jones JE. Variation between observers in describing mucosal appearances in proctocolitis. Br Med J 1964;i:89–92.
19. Feagan BG, Greenberg GR, Wild G, Fedorak RN, Pare P, McDonald JW, et al. Treatment of ulcerative colitis with a humanized antibody to the alpha4-beta7 integrin. N Engl J Med 2005;352:2499–507.
20. Powell-Tuck J, Bown RL, Lennard-Jones JE. A comparison of oral prednisolone given as single or multiple daily doses for active proctocolitis. Scand J Gastroenterol 1978;13:833–7.
21. Schroeder KW, Tremaine WJ, Ilstrup DM. Coated oral 5-aminosalicylic acid therapy for mildly to moderately active ulcerative colitis. A randomized study. N Engl J Med 1987;317:1625–9.
22. Sutherland LR, Martin F, Greer S, Robinson M, Greenberger N, Saibil F, et al. 5-Aminosalicylic acid enema in the treatment of distal ulcerative colitis, proctosigmoiditis, and proctitis. Gastroenterology 1987;92:1894–8.
23. Rachmilewitz D. Coated mesalazine (5-aminosalicylic acid) versus sulphasalazine in the treatment of active ulcerative colitis: a randomised trial. BMJ 1989;298:82–6.
24. Hanauer S, Schwartz J, Robinson M, Roufail W, Arora S, Cello J, et al. Mesalamine capsules for treatment of active ulcerative colitis: results of a controlled trial. Pentasa Study Group. Am J Gastroenterol 1993;88:1188–97.
25. Lemann M, Galian A, Rutgeerts P, Van Heuverzwijn R, Cortot A, Viteau JM, et al. Comparison of budesonide and 5-aminosalicylic acid enemas in active distal ulcerative colitis. Aliment Pharmacol Ther 1995;9:557–62.
26. Hanauer SB, Robinson M, Pruitt R, Lazenby AJ, Persson T, Nilsson LG, et al. Budesonide enema for the treatment of active, distal ulcerative colitis and proctitis: a dose-ranging study. U.S. Budesonide enema study group. Gastroenterology 1998;115:525–32.
27. Higgins PD, Schwartz M, Mapili J, Zimmermann EM. Is endoscopy necessary for the measurement of disease activity in ulcerative colitis? Am J Gastroenterol 2005;100:355–61.
28. Menees S, Higgins P, Korsnes S, Elta G. Does colonoscopy cause increased ulcerative colitis symptoms? Inflamm Bowel Dis 2007;13:12–8.
29. Mary JY, Modigliani R. Development and validation of an endoscopic index of the severity for Crohn's disease: a prospective multicentre study. Groupe d'Etudes Thérapeutiques des Affections Inflammatoires du Tube Digestif (GETAID). Gut 1989;30:983–9.
30. Cellier C, Sahmoud T, Froguel E, Adenis A, Belaiche J, Bretagne JF, et al. Correlations between clinical activity, endoscopic severity, and biological parameters in colonic or ileocolonic Crohn's disease. A prospective multicentre study of 121 cases. The Groupe d'Etudes Thérapeutiques des Affections Inflammatoires Digestives. Gut 1994;35:231–5.
31. D'Haens G, Van Deventer S, Van Hogezand R, Chalmers D, Kothe C, Baert F, et al. Endoscopic and histological healing with infliximab anti-tumor necrosis factor antibodies in Crohn's disease: A European multicenter trial. Gastroenterology 1999;116:1029–34.
32. D'Haens G, Noman M, Baert F, Hiele M, Van Assche G, Daperno M, et al. Endoscopic healing after infliximab treatment for Crohn's disease provides longer time to relapse [abstract]. Gastroenterology 2002;122:A100.
33. Rutgeerts P, Malchow H, Vatn M, Yan S, Bala M, Van Deventer S. Mucosal healing in Crohn's disease patients is associated with reduction in hospitalizations and surgeries [abstract]. Gastroenterology 2002;123:A43.
34. Daperno M, D'Haens G, Van Assche G, Baert F, Bulois P, Maunoury V, et al. Development and validation of a new, simplified endoscopic activity score for Crohn's disease: the SES-CD. Gastrointest Endosc 2004;60:505–12.
35. Rutgeerts P, Geboes K, Vantrappen G, Beyls J, Kerremans R, Hiele M. Predictability of the postoperative course of Crohn's disease. Gastroenterology 1990;99:956–63.
36. Rutgeerts P, Feagan BG, Lichtenstein GR, Mayer LF, Schreiber S, Colombel JF, et al. Comparison of scheduled and episodic treatment strategies of infliximab in Crohn's disease. Gastroenterology 2004;126:402–13.
37. Mantzaris GJ, Christidou A, Sfakianakis M, Roussos A, Koilakou S, Petraki K, et al. Azathioprine is superior to budesonide in achieving and maintaining mucosal healing and histologic remission in steroid-dependent Crohn's disease. Inflamm Bowel Dis 2008;15:375–82.
38. Rutgeerts P, Sandborn WJ, Feagan BG, Reinisch W, Olson A, Johanns J, et al. Infliximab for induction and maintenance therapy for ulcerative colitis. N Engl J Med 2005;353:2462–76.
39. D'Haens G, Geboes K, Rutgeerts P. Endoscopic and histologic healing of Crohn's (ileo-)colitis with azathioprine. Gastrointest Endosc 1999;50:667–71.
40. Modigliani R, Mary JY, Simon JF, Cortot A, Soule JC, Gendre JP, et al. Clinical, biological, and endoscopic picture of attacks of Crohn's disease. Evolution on prednisolone. Groupe d'Etudes Thérapeutiques des Affections Inflammatoires Digestives. Gastroenterology 1990;98:811–8.
41. Kozarek RA, Patterson DJ, Gelfand MD, Botoman VA, Ball TJ, Wilske KR. Methotrexate induces clinical and histologic remission in patients with refractory inflammatory bowel disease. Ann Intern Med 1989;110:353–6.
42. D'Haens G, Geboes K, Ponette E, Penninckx F, Rutgeerts P. Healing of severe recurrent ileitis with azathioprine therapy in patients with Crohn's disease. Gastroenterology 1997;112:1475–81.

48

43. Mpofu C, Watson AJ, Rhodes JM. Strategies for detecting colon cancer and/or dysplasia in patients with inflammatory bowel disease. Cochrane Database Syst Rev 2004;(2):CD 000 279.

44. Ahmadi A, Polyak S, Draganov PV. Colorectal cancer surveillance in inflammatory bowel disease: the search continues. World J Gastroenterol 2009;15:61–6.

45. Itzkowitz SH, Present DH. Consensus conference: colorectal cancer screening and surveillance in inflammatory bowel disease. Inflamm Bowel Dis 2005;11:314–21.

46. Klotz U, Schwab M. Topical delivery of therapeutic agents in the treatment of inflammatory bowel disease. Adv Drug Deliv Rev 2005;57:267–79.

47. Rabeneck L, Paszat LF, Hilsden RJ, Saskin R, Leddin D, Grunfeld E, et al. Bleeding and perforation after outpatient colonoscopy and their risk factors in usual clinical practice. Gastroenterology 2008;135:1899–1906.

48. Anderson ML, Pasha TM, Leighton JA. Endoscopic perforation of the colon: lessons from a 10-year study. Am J Gastroenterol 2000;95:3418–22.

49. Lohsiriwat V, Sujarittanakarn S, Akaraviputh T, Lertakyamanee N, Lohsiriwat D, Kachinthorn U. Colonoscopic perforation: a report from World Gastroenterology Organization endoscopy training center in Thailand. World J Gastroenterol 2008;14:6722–5.

50. Lee SD, Cohen RD. Endoscopy in inflammatory bowel disease. Gastroenterol Clin North Am 2002;31:119–32.

51. Bernstein CN, Shanahan F, Anton PA, Weinstein WM. Patchiness of mucosal inflammation in treated ulcerative colitis: a prospective study. Gastrointest Endosc 1995;42:232–7.

52. Kim B, Barnett JL, Kleer CG, Appelman HD. Endoscopic and histological patchiness in treated ulcerative colitis. Am J Gastroenterol 1999;94:3258–62.

53. Rehberger A, Puspok A, Stallmeister T, Jurecka W, Wolf K. Crohn's disease masquerading as aphthous ulcers. Eur J Dermatol 1998;8:274–6.

54. Potzi R, Walgram M, Lochs H, Holzner H, Gangl A. Diagnostic significance of endoscopic biopsy in Crohn's disease. Endoscopy 1989;21:60–2.

55. Schwartz DA, Loftus EV Jr, Tremaine WJ, Panaccione R, Harmsen WS, Zinsmeister AR, et al. The natural history of fistulizing Crohn's disease in Olmsted County, Minnesota. Gastroenterology 2002;122:875–80.

56. Haggitt RC, Meissner WA. Crohn's disease of the upper gastrointestinal tract. Am J Clin Pathol 1973;59:613–22.

57. Lossing A, Langer B, Jeejeebhoy KN. Gastroduodenal Crohn's disease: diagnosis and selection of treatment. Can J Surg 1983;26:358–60.

58. Decker GA, Loftus EV Jr, Pasha TM, Tremaine WJ, Sandborn WJ. Crohn's disease of the esophagus: clinical features and outcomes. Inflamm Bowel Dis 2001;7:113–9.

59. Tanaka M, Kimura K, Sakai H, Yoshida Y, Saito K. Long-term follow-up for minute gastroduodenal lesions in Crohn's disease. Gastrointest Endosc 1986;32:206–9.

60. Meining A, Bayerdorffer E, Bastlein E, Raudis N, Thiede C, Cyrus B, et al. Focal inflammatory infiltrations in gastric biopsy specimens are suggestive of Crohn's disease. Crohn's Disease Study Group, Germany. Scand J Gastroenterol 1997;32:813–8.

61. Parente F, Cucino C, Bollani S, Imbesi V, Maconi G, Bonetto S, et al. Focal gastric inflammatory infiltrates in inflammatory bowel diseases: prevalence, immunohistochemical characteristics, and diagnostic role. Am J Gastroenterol 2000;95:705–11.

62. Danelius M, Ost A, Lapidus AB. Inflammatory bowel disease-related lesions in the duodenal and gastric mucosa. Scand J Gastroenterol 2008;44:441–5.

63. Pardi DS, Shen B. Endoscopy in the management of patients after ileal pouch surgery for ulcerative colitis. Endoscopy 2008;40:529–33.

64. Simchuk EJ, Thirlby RC. Risk factors and true incidence of pouchitis in patients after ileal pouch–anal anastomoses. World J Surg 2000;24:851–6.

65. Merrett MN, Mortensen N, Kettlewell M, Jewell DO. Smoking may prevent pouchitis in patients with restorative proctocolectomy for ulcerative colitis. Gut 1996;38:362–4.

66. Shen B, Achkar JP, Lashner BA, Ormsby AH, Remzi FH, Bevins CL, et al. Endoscopic and histologic evaluation together with symptom assessment are required to diagnose pouchitis. Gastroenterology 2001;121:261–7.

67. McLaughlin SD, Clark SK, Thomas-Gibson S, Tekkis PP, Ciclitira PJ, Nicholls RJ. Guide to endoscopy of the ileo-anal pouch following restorative proctocolectomy with ileal pouch–anal anastomosis; indications, technique, and management of common findings. Inflamm Bowel Dis 2009 Jan 29 [Epub ahead of print].

68. Shen B, Lashner BA, Bennett AE, Remzi FH, Brzezinski A, Achkar JP, et al. Treatment of rectal cuff inflammation (cuffitis) in patients with ulcerative colitis following restorative proctocolectomy and ileal pouch–anal anastomosis. Am J Gastroenterol 2004;99:1527–31.

69. Shen B, Fazio VW, Remzi FH, Delaney CP, Achkar JP, Bennett A, et al. Endoscopic balloon dilation of ileal pouch strictures. Am J Gastroenterol 2004;99:2340–7.

70. Olaison G, Smedh K, Sjodahl R. Natural course of Crohn's disease after ileocolic resection: endoscopically visualised ileal ulcers preceding symptoms. Gut 1992;33:331–5.

71. Leighton JA, Shen B, Baron TH, Adler DG, Davila R, Egan JV, et al. ASGE guideline: endoscopy in the diagnosis and treatment of inflammatory bowel disease. Gastrointest Endosc 2006;63:558–65.

72. Legnani PE, Kornbluth A. Therapeutic options in the management of strictures in Crohn's disease. Gastrointest Endosc Clin N Am 2002;12:589–603.

73. Hassan C, Zullo A, De Francesco V, Ierardi E, Giustini M, Pitidis A, et al. Systematic review: endoscopic dilatation in Crohn's disease. Aliment Pharmacol Ther 2007;26:1457–64.

74. Waye JD. Endoscopy in inflammatory bowel disease. Clin Gastroenterol 1980;9:279–96.

75. Danzi JT, Farmer RG, Sullivan BH Jr, Rankin GB. Endoscopic features of gastroduodenal Crohn's disease. Gastroenterology 1976;70:9–13.

76. Yamazaki Y, Ribeiro MB, Sachar DB, Aufses AH Jr, Greenstein AJ. Malignant colorectal strictures in Crohn's disease. Am J Gastroenterol 1991;86:882–5.

77. Gumaste V, Sachar DB, Greenstein AJ. Benign and malignant colorectal strictures in ulcerative colitis. Gut 1992;33:938–41.

78. Erkelens GW, van Deventer SJ. Endoscopic treatment of strictures in Crohn's disease. Best Pract Res Clin Gastroenterol 2004;18:201–7.

79. Couckuyt H, Gevers AM, Coremans G, Hiele M, Rutgeerts P. Efficacy and safety of hydrostatic balloon dilatation of ileocolonic Crohn's strictures: a prospective long-term analysis. Gut 1995;36:577–80.

80. Sabate JM, Villarejo J, Bouhnik Y, Allez M, Gornet JM, Vahedi K, et al. Hydrostatic balloon dilatation of Crohn's strictures. Aliment Pharmacol Ther 2003;18:409–13.

81. Cirocco WC, Reilly JC, Rusin LC. Life-threatening hemorrhage and exsanguination from Crohn's disease. Report of four cases. Dis Colon Rectum 1995;38:85–95.

82. Driver CP, Anderson DN, Keenan RA. Massive intestinal bleeding in association with Crohn's disease. J R Coll Surg Edinb 1996;41:152–4.

83. Robert JR, Sachar DB, Greenstein AJ. Severe gastrointestinal hemorrhage in Crohn's disease. Ann Surg 1991;213:207–11.

84. Belaiche J, Louis E, D'Haens G, Cabooter M, Naegels S, De Vos M, et al. Acute lower gastrointestinal bleeding in Crohn's disease: characteristics of a unique series of 34 patients. Belgian IBD Research Group. Am J Gastroenterol 1999;94:2177–81.

85. Bousvaros A, Antonioli DA, Colletti RB, Dubinsky MC, Glickman JN, Gold BD, et al. Differentiating ulcerative colitis from Crohn disease in children and young adults: report of a working group of the North American Society for Pediatric Gastroenterology, Hepatology, and Nutrition and the Crohn's and Colitis Foundation of America. J Pediatr Gastroenterol Nutr 2007;44:653–74.

86. Tedesco FJ, Hardin RD, Harper RN, Edwards BH. Infectious colitis endoscopically simulating inflammatory bowel disease: a prospective evaluation. Gastrointest Endosc 1983;29:195–7.

87. Rutgeerts P, Geboes K, Ponette E, Coremans G, Vantrappen G. Acute infective colitis caused by endemic pathogens in western Europe: endoscopic features. Endoscopy 1982;14:212–9.

88. Vender RJ, Marignani P. *Salmonella* colitis presenting as a segmental colitis resembling Crohn's disease. Dig Dis Sci 1983;28:848–51.

89. Drake AA, Gilchrist MJ, Washington JA 2nd, Huizenga KA, Van Scoy RE. Diarrhea due to *Campylobacter fetus* subspecies *jejuni*. A clinical review of 63 cases. Mayo Clin Proc 1981;56:414–23.

90. Mantzaris GJ, Hatzis A, Archavlis E, Petraki K, Lazou A, Ladas S, et al. The role of colonoscopy in the differential diagnosis of acute, severe hemorrhagic colitis. Endoscopy 1995;27:645–53.

91. Surawicz CM, Belic L. Rectal biopsy helps to distinguish acute self-limited colitis from idiopathic inflammatory bowel disease. Gastroenterology 1984;86:104–13.

92. Nostrant TT, Kumar NB, Appelman HD. Histopathology differentiates acute self-limited colitis from ulcerative colitis. Gastroenterology 1987;92:318–28.

93. Bernstein CN, Blanchard JF, Kliewer E, Wajda A. Cancer risk in patients with inflammatory bowel disease: a population-based study. Cancer 2001;91:854–62.

94. Gillen CD, Walmsley RS, Prior P, Andrews HA, Allan RN. Ulcerative colitis and Crohn's disease: a comparison of the colorectal cancer risk in extensive colitis. Gut 1994;35:1590–2.

95. Eaden JA, Abrams KR, Mayberry JF. The risk of colorectal cancer in ulcerative colitis: a meta-analysis. Gut 2001;48:526–35.

96. Ekbom A, Helmick C, Zack M, Adami HO. Ulcerative colitis and colorectal cancer. A population-based study. N Engl J Med 1990;323:1228–33.

97. Karlen P, Lofberg R, Brostrom O, Leijonmarck CE, Hellers G, Persson PG. Increased risk of cancer in ulcerative colitis: a population-based cohort study. Am J Gastroenterol 1999;94:1047–52.

98. Rutter M, Saunders B, Wilkinson K, Rumbles S, Schofield G, Kamm M, et al. Severity of inflammation is a risk factor for colorectal neoplasia in ulcerative colitis. Gastroenterology 2004;126:451–9.

99. Nuako KW, Ahlquist DA, Mahoney DW, Schaid DJ, Siems DM, Lindor NM. Familial predisposition for colorectal cancer in chronic ulcerative colitis: a case–control study. Gastroenterology 1998;115:1079–83.

100. Askling J, Dickman PW, Karlen P, Brostrom O, Lapidus A, Lofberg R, et al. Family history as a risk factor for colorectal cancer in inflammatory bowel disease. Gastroenterology 2001;120:1356–62.

101. Velayos FS, Loftus EV Jr, Jess T, Harmsen WS, Bida J, Zinsmeister AR, et al. Predictive and protective factors associated with colorectal cancer in ulcerative colitis: a case–control study. Gastroenterology 2006;130:1941–9.

102. Heuschen UA, Hinz U, Allemeyer EH, Stern J, Lucas M, Autschbach F, et al. Backwash ileitis is strongly associated with colorectal carcinoma in ulcerative colitis. Gastroenterology 2001;120:841–7.

103. Soetikno RM, Lin OS, Heidenreich PA, Young HS, Blackstone MO. Increased risk of colorectal neoplasia in patients with primary sclerosing cholangitis and ulcerative colitis: a meta-analysis. Gastrointest Endosc 2002;56:48–54.

104. Claessen MM, Lutgens MW, van Buuren HR, Oldenburg B, Stokkers PC, van der Woude CJ, et al. More right-sided IBD-associated colorectal cancer in patients with primary sclerosing cholangitis. Inflamm Bowel Dis 2009 Feb 19 [Epub ahead of print].

105. Riddell RH, Goldman H, Ransohoff DF, Appelman HD, Fenoglio CM, Haggitt RC, et al. Dysplasia in inflammatory bowel disease: standardized classification with provisional clinical applications. Hum Pathol 1983;14:931–68.

106. Lewis JD, Deren JJ, Lichtenstein GR. Cancer risk in patients with inflammatory bowel disease. Gastroenterol Clin North Am 1999;28:459–77, x.

107. Tytgat GN, Dhir V, Gopinath N. Endoscopic appearance of dysplasia and cancer in inflammatory bowel disease. Eur J Cancer 1995;31A:1174–7.

108. Blackstone MO, Riddell RH, Rogers BH, Levin B. Dysplasia-associated lesion or mass (DALM) detected by colonoscopy in long-standing ulcerative colitis: an indication for colectomy. Gastroenterology 1981;80:366–74.

109. Odze RD. Adenomas and adenoma-like DALMs in chronic ulcerative colitis: a clinical, pathological, and molecular review. Am J Gastroenterol 1999;94:1746–50.

110. Friedman S, Odze RD, Farraye FA. Management of neoplastic polyps in inflammatory bowel disease. Inflamm Bowel Dis 2003;9:260–6.

111. Itzkowitz SH, Harpaz N. Diagnosis and management of dysplasia in patients with inflammatory bowel diseases. Gastroenterology 2004;126:1634–48.

112. Ullman TA, Loftus EV Jr, Kakar S, Burgart LJ, Sandborn WJ, Tremaine WJ. The fate of low grade dysplasia in ulcerative colitis. Am J Gastroenterol 2002;97:922–7.

113. Ullman T, Croog V, Harpaz N, Sachar D, Itzkowitz S. Progression of flat low-grade dysplasia to advanced neoplasia in patients with ulcerative colitis. Gastroenterology 2003;125:1311–9.

114. Bernstein CN, Shanahan F, Weinstein WM. Are we telling patients the truth about surveillance colonoscopy in ulcerative colitis? Lancet 1994;343:71–4.

115. Connell WR, Lennard-Jones JE, Williams CB, Talbot IC, Price AB, Wilkinson KH. Factors affecting the outcome of endoscopic surveillance for cancer in ulcerative colitis. Gastroenterology 1994;107:934–44.

116. Farraye FA, Waye JD, Moscandrew M, Heeren TC, Odze RD. Variability in the diagnosis and management of adenoma-like and non-adenoma-like dysplasia-associated lesions or masses in inflammatory bowel disease: an Internet-based study. Gastrointest Endosc 2007;66:519–29.

117. Rubin PH, Friedman S, Harpaz N, Goldstein E, Weiser J, Schiller J, et al. Colonoscopic polypectomy in chronic colitis: conservative management after endoscopic resection of dysplastic polyps. Gastroenterology 1999;117:1295–300.

118. Odze RD, Farraye FA, Hecht JL, Hornick JL. Long-term follow-up after polypectomy treatment for adenoma-like dysplastic lesions in ulcerative colitis. Clin Gastroenterol Hepatol 2004;2:534–41.

119. Blonski W, Kundu R, Furth EF, Lewis J, Aberra F, Lichtenstein GR. High-grade dysplastic adenoma-like mass lesions are not an indication for colectomy in patients with ulcerative colitis. Scand J Gastroenterol 2008;43:817–20.

120. Rutter MD, Saunders BP, Wilkinson KH, Rumbles S, Schofield G, Kamm MA, et al. Cancer surveillance in long-standing ulcerative colitis: endoscopic appearances help predict cancer risk. Gut 2004;53:1813–6.

121. Rubin CE, Haggitt RC, Burmer GC, Brentnall TA, Stevens AC, Levine DS, et al. DNA aneuploidy in colonic biopsies predicts future development of dysplasia in ulcerative colitis. Gastroenterology 1992;103:1611–20.

122. Kudo S, Tamura S, Nakajima T, Yamano H, Kusaka H, Watanabe H. Diagnosis of colorectal tumorous lesions by magnifying endoscopy. Gastrointest Endosc 1996;44:8–14.

123. Matsumoto T, Iwao Y, Igarashi M, Watanabe K, Otsuka K, Watanabe T, et al. Endoscopic and chromoendoscopic atlas featuring dysplastic lesions in surveillance colonoscopy for patients with long-standing ulcerative colitis. Inflamm Bowel Dis 2008;14:259–64.

124. Rutter MD, Saunders BP, Wilkinson KH, Kamm MA, Williams CB, Forbes A. Most dysplasia in ulcerative colitis is visible at colonoscopy. Gastrointest Endosc 2004;60:334–9.

125. Rubin DT, Rothe JA, Hetzel JT, Cohen RD, Hanauer SB. Are dysplasia and colorectal cancer endoscopically visible in patients with ulcerative colitis? Gastrointest Endosc 2007;65:998–1004.

126. Blonski W, Kundu R, Lewis J, Aberra F, Osterman M, Lichtenstein GR. Is dysplasia visible during surveillance colonoscopy in patients with ulcerative colitis? Scand J Gastroenterol 2008;43:698–703.

127. Rutter M, Bernstein C, Matsumoto T, Kiesslich R, Neurath M. Endoscopic appearance of dysplasia in ulcerative colitis and the role of staining. Endoscopy 2004;36:1109–14.

128. Kiesslich R, Neurath MF. Surveillance colonoscopy in ulcerative colitis: magnifying chromoendoscopy in the spotlight. Gut 2004;53:165–7.

129. Rutter MD, Saunders BP, Schofield G, Forbes A, Price AB, Talbot IC. Pancolonic indigo carmine dye spraying for the detection of dysplasia in ulcerative colitis. Gut 2004;53:256–60.

130. Marion JF, Waye JD, Present DH, Israel Y, Bodian C, Harpaz N, et al. Chromoendoscopy-targeted biopsies are superior to standard colonoscopic surveillance for detecting dysplasia in inflammatory bowel disease patients: a prospective endoscopic trial. Am J Gastroenterol 2008;103:2342–9.

131. Kiesslich R, Fritsch J, Holtmann M, Koehler HH, Stolte M, Kanzler S, et al. Methylene blue-aided chromoendoscopy for the detection of intraepithelial neoplasia and colon cancer in ulcerative colitis. Gastroenterology 2003;124:880–8.

132. Hurlstone DP, Sanders DS, Lobo AJ, McAlindon ME, Cross SS. Indigo carmine–assisted high-magnification chromoscopic colonoscopy for the detection and characterisation of intraepithelial neoplasia in ulcerative colitis: a prospective evaluation. Endoscopy 2005;37:1186–92.

133. Kiesslich R, Goetz M, Lammersdorf K, Schneider C, Burg J, Stolte M, et al. Chromoscopy-guided endomicroscopy increases the diagnostic yield of intraepithelial neoplasia in ulcerative colitis. Gastroenterology 2007;132:874–82.

134. Hurlstone DP, McAlindon ME, Sanders DS, Koegh R, Lobo AJ, Cross SS. Further validation of high-magnification chromoscopic-colonoscopy for the detection of intraepithelial neoplasia and colon cancer in ulcerative colitis. Gastroenterology 2004;126:376–8.

135. Kiesslich R, Galle PR, Neurath MF. Endoscopic surveillance in ulcerative colitis: smart biopsies do it better. Gastroenterology 2007;133:742–5.

136. Machida H, Sano Y, Hamamoto Y, Muto M, Kozu T, Tajiri H, et al. Narrow-band imaging in the diagnosis of colorectal mucosal lesions: a pilot study. Endoscopy 2004;36:1094–8.

137. Gono K, Obi T, Yamaguchi M, Ohyama N, Machida H, Sano Y, et al. Appearance of enhanced tissue features in narrow-band endoscopic imaging. J Biomed Opt 2004;9:568–77.

138. van den Broek FJ, Reitsma JB, Curvers WL, Fockens P, Dekker E. Systematic review of narrow-band imaging for the detection and differentiation of neoplastic and nonneoplastic lesions in the colon (with videos). Gastrointest Endosc 2009;69:124–35.

139. van den Broek FJ, Fockens P, van Eeden S, Reitsma JB, Hardwick JC, Stokkers PC, et al. Endoscopic tri-modal imaging for surveillance in ulcerative colitis: randomised comparison of high-resolution endoscopy and autofluorescence imaging for neoplasia detection; and evaluation of narrow-band imaging for classification of lesions. Gut 2008;57:1083–9.

140. Faigel DO, Fennerty MB. "Cutting the cord" for capsule endoscopy. Gastroenterology 2002;123:1385–8.

141. Cheifetz AS, Lewis BS. Capsule endoscopy retention: is it a complication? J Clin Gastroenterol 2006;40:688–91.

142. Lewis B. Complications and contraindications in capsule endoscopy [abstract]. Gastroenterology 2002;122:A-330.

48

143. Cheifetz AS, Kornbluth AA, Legnani P, Schmelkin I, Brown A, Lichtiger S, et al. The risk of retention of the capsule endoscope in patients with known or suspected Crohn's disease. Am J Gastroenterol 2006;101:2218–22.

144. Buchman AL, Miller FH, Wallin A, Chowdhry AA, Ahn C. Video capsule endoscopy versus barium contrast studies for the diagnosis of Crohn's disease recurrence involving the small intestine. Am J Gastroenterol 2004;99:2171–7.

145. Marmo R, Rotondano G, Piscopo R, Bianco MA, Siani A, Catalano O, et al. Capsule endoscopy versus enteroclysis in the detection of small-bowel involvement in Crohn's disease: a prospective trial. Clin Gastroenterol Hepatol 2005;3:772–6.

146. Voderholzer WA, Beinhoelzl J, Rogalla P, Murrer S, Schachschal G, Lochs H, et al. Small bowel involvement in Crohn's disease: a prospective comparison of wireless capsule endoscopy and computed tomography enteroclysis. Gut 2005;54:369–73.

147. Cave D, Legnani P, de Franchis R, Lewis BS. ICCE consensus for capsule retention. Endoscopy 2005;37:1065–7.

148. Triester SL, Leighton JA, Leontiadis GI, Gurudu SR, Fleischer DE, Hara AK, et al. A meta-analysis of the yield of capsule endoscopy compared to other diagnostic modalities in patients with non-stricturing small bowel Crohn's disease. Am J Gastroenterol 2006;101:954–64.

149. Lorenzo-Zúñiga V, de Vega VM, Domènech E, Cabré E, Mañosa M, Boix J. Impact of capsule endoscopy findings in the management of Crohn's disease. Dig Dis Sci 2009 Mar 3 [Epub ahead of print].

150. Solem CA, Loftus EV Jr, Fletcher JG, Baron TH, Gostout CJ, Petersen BT, et al. Small-bowel imaging in Crohn's disease: a prospective, blinded, 4-way comparison trial. Gastrointest Endosc 2008;68:255–66.

151. Goldstein JL, Eisen GM, Lewis B, Gralnek IM, Zlotnick S, Fort JG. Video capsule endoscopy to prospectively assess small bowel injury with celecoxib, naproxen plus omeprazole, and placebo. Clin Gastroenterol Hepatol 2005;3:133–41.

152. Mehdizadeh S, Chen G, Enayati PJ, Cheng DW, Han NJ, Shaye OA, et al. Diagnostic yield of capsule endoscopy in ulcerative colitis and inflammatory bowel disease of unclassified type (IBDU). Endoscopy 2008;40:30–5.

153. Gal E, Geller A, Fraser G, Levi Z, Niv Y. Assessment and validation of the new capsule endoscopy Crohn's disease activity index (CECDAI). Dig Dis Sci 2008;53:1933–7.

154. Lewis BS, Waye JD. Total small bowel enteroscopy. Gastrointest Endosc 1987;33:435–8.

155. Waye JD. Enteroscopy. Gastrointest Endosc 1997;46:247–56.

156. Landi B, Tkoub M, Gaudric M, Guimbaud R, Cervoni JP, Chaussade S, et al. Diagnostic yield of push-type enteroscopy in relation to indication. Gut 1998;42:421–5.

157. Sidhu R, McAlindon ME, Kapur K, Hurlstone DP, Wheeldon MC, Sanders DS. Push enteroscopy in the era of capsule endoscopy. J Clin Gastroenterol 2008;42:54–8.

158. Yamamoto H, Sekine Y, Sato Y, Higashizawa T, Miyata T, Iino S, et al. Total enteroscopy with a nonsurgical steerable double-balloon method. Gastrointest Endosc 2001;53:216–20.

159. Yamamoto H, Ell C, Binmoeller KF. Double-balloon endoscopy. Endoscopy 2008;40:779–83.

160. Yano T, Yamamoto H. Current state of double balloon endoscopy: the latest approach to small intestinal diseases. J Gastroenterol Hepatol 2009;24:185–92.

161. Pohl J, May A, Nachbar L, Ell C. Diagnostic and therapeutic yield of push-and-pull enteroscopy for symptomatic small bowel Crohn's disease strictures. Eur J Gastroenterol Hepatol 2007;19:529–34.

162. Hotokezaka M, Jimi SI, Hidaka H, Maehara N, Eto TA, Chijiiwa K. Role of intraoperative enteroscopy for surgical decision making with Crohn's disease. Surg Endosc 2007;21:1238–42.

163. Esaki M, Matsumoto T, Hizawa K, Aoyagi K, Mibu R, Iida M, et al. Intraoperative enteroscopy detects more lesions but is not predictive of postoperative recurrence in Crohn's disease. Surg Endosc 2001;15:455–9.

164. Chapman RW, Arborgh BA, Rhodes JM, Summerfield JA, Dick R, Scheuer PJ, et al. Primary sclerosing cholangitis: a review of its clinical features, cholangiography, and hepatic histology. Gut 1980;21:870–7.

165. Thorpe ME, Scheuer PJ, Sherlock S. Primary sclerosing cholangitis, the biliary tree, and ulcerative colitis. Gut 1967;8:435–48.

166. Fausa O, Schrumpf E, Elgjo K. Relationship of inflammatory bowel disease and primary sclerosing cholangitis. Semin Liver Dis 1991;11:31–9.

167. MacCarty RL, LaRusso NF, Wiesner RH, Ludwig J. Primary sclerosing cholangitis: findings on cholangiography and pancreatography. Radiology 1983;149:39–44.

168. Wiesner RH, LaRusso NF. Clinicopathologic features of the syndrome of primary sclerosing cholangitis. Gastroenterology 1980;79:200–6.

169. Adler DG, Baron TH, Davila RE, Egan J, Hirota WK, Leighton JA, et al. ASGE guideline: the role of ERCP in diseases of the biliary tract and the pancreas. Gastrointest Endosc 2005;62:1–8.

170. Ponsioen CY, Vrouenraets SM, van Milligen de Wit AW, Sturm P, Tascilar M, et al. Value of brush cytology for dominant strictures in primary sclerosing cholangitis. Endoscopy 1999;31:305–9.

171. Lindberg B, Arnelo U, Bergquist A, Thorne A, Hjerpe A, Granqvist S, et al. Diagnosis of biliary strictures in conjunction with endoscopic retrograde cholangiopancreaticography, with special reference to patients with primary sclerosing cholangitis. Endoscopy 2002;34:909–16.

172. Athanassiadou P, Grapsa D. Value of endoscopic retrograde cholangiopancreatography-guided brushings in preoperative assessment of pancreaticobiliary strictures: what's new? Acta Cytol 2008;52:24–34.

173. Schwartz DA, Wiersema MJ, Dudiak KM, Fletcher JG, Clain JE, Tremaine WJ, et al. A comparison of endoscopic ultrasound, magnetic resonance imaging, and exam under anesthesia for evaluation of Crohn's perianal fistulas. Gastroenterology 2001;121:1064–72.

174. Schwartz DA, White CM, Wise PE, Herline AJ. Use of endoscopic ultrasound to guide combination medical and surgical therapy for patients with Crohn's perianal fistulas. Inflamm Bowel Dis 2005;11:727–32.

175. Spradlin NM, Wise PE, Herline AJ, Muldoon RL, Rosen M, Schwartz DA. A randomized prospective trial of endoscopic ultrasound to guide combination medical and surgical treatment for Crohn's perianal fistulas. Am J Gastroenterol 2008;103:2527–35.

176. Schwartz DA, Harewood GC, Wiersema MJ. EUS for rectal disease. Gastrointest Endosc 2002;56:100–9.

177. Higaki S, Nohara H, Saitoh Y, Akazawa A, Yanai H, Yoshida T, et al. Increased rectal wall thickness may predict relapse in ulcerative colitis: a pilot follow-up study by ultrasonographic colonoscopy. Endoscopy 2002;34:212–9.

178. Yoshizawa S, Kobayashi K, Katsumata T, Saigenji K, Okayasu I. Clinical usefulness of EUS for active ulcerative colitis. Gastrointest Endosc 2007;65:253–60.

49 Lower Intestinal Bleeding Disorders

Juergen Barnert and Helmut Messmann

Definitions

- *Lower intestinal bleeding* is defined as acute or chronic abnormal blood loss distal to the ligament of Treitz.
- *Acute lower intestinal bleeding* is arbitrarily defined as bleeding of less than 3 days' duration resulting in instability of vital signs, anemia, and/or a need for blood transfusion.
- *Chronic lower intestinal bleeding* is defined as slow blood loss over a period of several days or longer presenting with symptoms of occult fecal blood, intermittent melena, or scant hematochezia.
- *Occult gastrointestinal bleeding* means that the amounts of blood in the feces are too small to be seen but are detectable by chemical tests.
- *Obscure gastrointestinal bleeding* often presents as lower intestinal bleeding and means bleeding from an unclear site that persists or recurs after a negative initial or primary endoscopy.

General Aspects

Epidemiology

The incidence of lower intestinal bleeding is only one-fifth of that in the upper gastrointestinal tract and is estimated at 21–27 cases per 100 000 adults/year [1,2]. Lower intestinal bleeding is usually chronic and self-limiting. Twenty-one of 100 000 adults/year require hospitalization due to severe bleeding. Among these, men and older patients suffer from more severe lower intestinal bleeding [1]. There is a 200-fold increase in the incidence from the third to the ninth decade, due to diverticulosis and angiodysplasia [3]. In a cross-sectional survey, it was found that 15.5% of the population in the United States suffered from rectal bleeding within 1 year, but only 13.9% of those affected sought medical care [4].

Some 20% of all gastrointestinal bleeding disorders occur from colonic and anorectal sources. A small-bowel source is less common. One report found a 1% incidence of recurrent obscure overt bleeding among 2751 patients with gastrointestinal bleeding [5]. Studies of lower gastrointestinal bleeding have noted a 0.5–12% incidence of recurrent bleeding after an initial nondiagnostic colonoscopy result [1,2]. However, some have estimated that a source in the small bowel is the cause of gastrointestinal bleeding in up to 5% of cases [6].

Clinical Course and Prognosis

There is some evidence that upper gastrointestinal bleeding differs in acuteness and severity from lower intestinal bleeding. Patients with lower intestinal bleeding are in shock significantly less often (19% vs. 35%, respectively), require fewer blood transfusions (36% vs. 64%), and have a significantly higher hemoglobin level (84% vs. 61%) [7,8]. Patients with colonic bleeding require fewer blood transfusions in comparison with those who have bleeding from the small intestine [8]. As in upper gastrointestinal bleeding, the majority (80–85%) of cases of bleeding in the lower intestinal tract stop spontaneously. The mortality and morbidity rates increase with age. The overall mortality rate varies between 2.0% and 3.6%. Pa-

tients with bleeding episodes after hospital admission have significantly higher mortality rates (23.1%) in comparison with those who bleed before hospital admission [1].

A study including 252 patients with acute lower intestinal bleeding identified predictive factors that increase the likelihood of a severe course or recurrence of bleeding [9]:
- Heart rate ≥ 100 beats/min
- Systolic blood pressure ≤ 115 mmHg
- Syncope
- Nontender abdominal examination
- Bleeding per rectum during the first 4 h of evaluation
- History of acetylsalicylic acid use
- More than two active comorbid conditions

Velayos et al. [10] identified the following risk factors indicating severe lower intestinal bleeding:
- Hemodynamic instability (blood pressure < 100 mmHg, heart rate > 100 beats/min) 1 h after initial medical evaluation
- Active gross bleeding per rectum
- Initial hematocrit ≤ 35%

Diagnostic Approach

History

A focused history helps differentiate the causes of lower intestinal bleeding. Important points include the duration of bleeding, stool color (melena; massive, intermittent, or scant hematochezia; small quantities of blood in the stool), and frequency. Lower intestinal bleeding is usually suspected when hematochezia is present. This means the passage of maroon or bright red blood or blood clots per rectum. This is different from upper gastrointestinal bleeding, which often presents with hematemesis (vomiting blood) and melena. However, massive upper gastrointestinal bleeding can also present with bright red stool; up to 11% of patients with hematochezia may have upper gastrointestinal bleeding [11]. Clinical symptoms such as pain, weight loss, changes in bowel habits, or fever are helpful in planning the next diagnostic steps. When the patient's medical history is being investigated, note should be made of previous bleeding episodes, abdominal and vascular operations, radiotherapy of the pelvic organs, a history of peptic ulcer disease or inflammatory bowel disease, medication (especially acetylsalicylic acid, nonsteroidal anti-inflammatory drugs, and anticoagulation treatment), a family history of malignant disease, and comorbidity.

Physical Examination

The physical examination helps differentiate acute from chronic bleeding and includes assessment of circulatory stability. Blood loss of less than 250 mL has no influence either on heart rate or blood pressure. Blood loss of more than 800 mL induces a fall in blood pressure of 10 mmHg and a heart rate increase of 10 beats/min. Paleness, weakness, and dizziness are frequent symptoms. Extensive blood loss of more than 1500 mL presents with shock symptoms, tachypnea, and depressed mental status. Digital rectal examination in combination with a test for occult blood helps confirm the patient's description of stool color. A digital rectal examination can also detect 40% of rectal carcinomas; in 2% of patients with massive rectal bleeding, the digital rectal examination detected a rectal cancer [8].

Laboratory Studies

The initial laboratory work-up should include:
- Complete blood count (including hemoglobin, hematocrit, and thrombocytes)
- Coagulation profile
- Serum chemistry (electrolytes and creatinine)
- Sample for type and crossmatch

Endoscopy

Flexible Endoscopy

Flexible endoscopy is now considered the mainstay for evaluation of lower intestinal bleeding. The incidence of serious complications is approximately one in 1000 procedures. Cardiopulmonary problems may account for more than 50% of complications associated with endoscopy; elderly patients and those with cardiovascular or pulmonary diseases are at special risk. Aspiration (in upper endoscopy), oversedation, hypoventilation, and vasovagal events are the major problems. Perforation rarely occurs, even in urgent colonoscopy. Patients should be continuously monitored during urgent endoscopy using electrocardiography and noninvasive measurement of oxygen saturation. If there are unstable vital signs, patients must receive resuscitation before endoscopy.

Esophagogastroduodenoscopy. In patients with hematochezia and hemodynamic instability, esophagogastroduodenoscopy should be undertaken first to exclude an upper gastrointestinal source. Particularly in patients with a history of peptic ulcer and portal hypertension, this should be considered in any case. Although placement of a nasogastric tube is safe and easy, it misses upper gastrointestinal bleeding in 7% of cases. The rate may be even higher in patients with duodenal ulcers, as pylorospasm can prevent reflux of blood into the stomach [12,13].

Colonoscopy. It has been demonstrated in recent years that in experienced hands, colonoscopy plays the same role in acute lower intestinal bleeding as esophagogastroduodenoscopy does in acute upper gastrointestinal bleeding. As in upper gastrointestinal bleeding, there are three main principles underlying urgent colonoscopy:
- Determination of the location and type of the bleeding source
- Identification of patients with ongoing hemorrhage and those who are at high risk for rebleeding
- Assessing the potential for endoscopic intervention

All patients with acute lower intestinal bleeding must be stabilized. Contraindications for colonoscopy are severe active inflammation and also inadequate visibility conditions. The colonoscopy should be aborted if the patient becomes unstable, the bleeding is so severe that identification of a bleeding source is impossible, or the risk of perforation is too high. The diagnostic yield for urgent colonoscopy in acute lower intestinal bleeding reported in the literature is in the range of 48–90% [8,14]. Two publications have reported diagnostic yields of 89–97% [15,16], which is perhaps a reflection of more consistent use of urgent colonoscopy. Two studies demonstrated that early colonoscopy is significantly associated with a shorter hospital stay [9,17]. In most studies, early colonoscopy is defined as examinations conducted within 12–24 h of admission. However, it was shown in a randomized trial addressing this issue that early colonoscopy (after urgent purge preparation) was not superior to a standard care algorithm (including expectant colonoscopy). The rate of finding the source of bleeding and important outcomes (mortality, hospital stay, transfusions requirements, rebleeding, and surgery) did not differ [18,19]. Despite the lack of data, urgent colonoscopy is widely recommended and used. Some physicians perform colonoscopy on an unprepared bowel, as blood is a laxative and the location (height) of blood found in the colon can provide information about the bleeding site. Chaudhry et al. [15] showed that in patients with acute lower intestinal bleeding, a high diagnostic yield (97%) and effective hemostasis was possible even without bowel preparation. They were able to control active bleeding in 17 of 27 patients (63%) by endoscopic intervention. However, current recommendations [20] instead advise cleansing the colon as thoroughly as possible in acute lower gastrointestinal bleeding. This improves evaluation of the mucosa, which in turn enhances recognition of smaller lesions and minimizes the risk of complications resulting from poor visualization. In our institution, bowel cleansing is performed with a polyethylene glycol electrolyte solution. For optimal colon preparation, the patient must consume 3–4 L of the solution. Patients generally tolerate consumption of 1–2 L per hour. It may be helpful to administer a prokinetic antiemetic such as metoclopramide or to administer the solution through a nasogastric tube. The segmental location of fresh blood, or the level above which no blood is present, should be carefully documented by the endoscopist. An attempt should be made to reach the cecum whenever possible. This is important, as a substantial proportion of bleeding sites are located in the right hemicolon. In addition, the endoscopist should try to intubate the terminal ileum. Blood flowing from above is a clear sign of a more proximal bleeding site. Ohyama et al. [16] reported that even in conditions of urgent colonoscopy, it was possible to inspect the cecum in 56% of patients and that advancement as far as the terminal ileum was achieved in 27%. For diagnosing hemorrhoidal bleeding, it is important to inspect the anal transitional zone with a retroflexed instrument and to perform proctoscopy (anoscopy). The second aim in colonoscopy for acute lower intestinal bleeding should be to identify patients with active bleeding or with a risk of rebleeding. By analogy with endoscopic risk stratification in bleeding ulcers, Jensen et al. [21] and Grisolano et al. [22] have shown that evidence of active bleeding, visible vessels, and adherent clot are associated with a severe course or a high rate of rebleeding.

Push enteroscopy. Since colonoscopy visualizes only a small part of the small intestine (the terminal ileum), other investigations need to be carried out when lower intestinal bleeding appears to originate from the small intestine. Push enteroscopy is a procedure similar to traditional upper endoscopy, but with a longer scope in the range of 220–298 cm. However, the diagnostic yield and therapeutic value of push enteroscopy are limited, since only 50–120 cm of the small bowel can be evaluated beyond the ligament of Treitz. Many studies have reported the yield of push enteroscopy in identifying bleeding lesions, with estimates ranging from 3% to 70% [23]. In a meta-analysis of 14 studies on obscure gastrointestinal bleeding, the yield of push enteroscopy for any finding averaged 28% [24]. If a dedicated push enteroscope is not available, a pediatric or standard adult colonoscope can be used instead.

Double-balloon enteroscopy. In 2001, a new enteroscopy technique known as double-balloon enteroscopy or push-and-pull enteroscopy was developed by Yamamoto et al. [25]. The system consists of a 2-m enteroscope and a 145-cm overtube, which both have soft latex balloons at their tips (**Fig. 49.1**). The two balloons can be inflated and deflated using an air-balloon pump controller. The two balloons are operated in combination, and the enteroscope is inserted while simultaneously shortening the intestine. The movement of the double-balloon enteroscope resembles the locomotion of a caterpillar. The double-balloon scope can be inserted through either the mouth or the anus, allowing examination of the entire gastrointestinal tract. It is possible to observe half to two-thirds of the small bowel by each route. The examination is time-consuming and requires sedation or general anesthesia and a high level of technical skill. Currently, enteroscopes with two different diameters are available from Fujinon: the EN-450P5, with an outer diameter of 8.5 mm (the overtube has an external diameter of 12.2 mm) and a working channel diameter of 2.2 mm; and the EN-450T5, with an outer diameter of 9.4 mm (the overtube has an external diameter of 13.2 mm) and a working channel of 2.8 mm. The larger working channel in the EN-450T5 allows a wide range of therapeutic methods to be carried out, including bipolar coagulation and argon plasma coagulation, snare polypectomy, clip placement, injection needle therapy, and balloon dilation. In the clinical setting of obscure gastrointestinal bleeding, the overall diagnostic yield of double-balloon enteroscopy is 43–88% [26–35]. In a Japanese multicenter study including 479 patients with obscure gastrointestinal bleeding, the diagnostic yield was 58% [34]. The highest yield was obtained in patients with overt ongoing bleeding (77%) and in patients with iron-deficiency anemia and continuous positive fecal occult blood testing (71%). In a subgroup of 130 patients at Nagoya University Hospital, the resultant treatments were analyzed. In 28 of 78 patients (36%) in whom small-bowel lesions were identified, endoscopic therapy (electrocoagulation, clipping, and polypectomy) was performed. Bleeding sources were located in the upper gastrointestinal tract in 9% of cases and in the colon in 9%. The complication rate with diagnostic double-balloon enteroscopy is low (0.8%), but it increases in therapeutic double-balloon enteroscopy (5.4%) [36]. Complications include pancreatitis, perforation, and bleeding (after polypectomy).

Single-balloon enteroscopy. Recently, Olympus has presented a single-balloon enteroscope (SIF-Q180) (**Fig. 49.2**). The system consists of a 2-m enteroscope and a flexible overtube with a working length of 132 cm and an outer diameter of 13.2 mm. A latex-free balloon is only attached at the tip of the overtube and is inflated and deflated with air from a pressure-controlled pump. The scope has a working length of 2 m and a wide working channel of 2.8 mm. The tip of the scope is angled and hooked behind a fold to achieve stable positioning of the distal tip, as is achieved with the balloon inflated at the tip of the scope in double-balloon enteroscopy. Preliminary results (from unpublished studies and our own experience) show a similar diagnostic and therapeutic yield in comparison with double-balloon enteroscopy. Single-balloon enteroscopy may be easier to perform than double-balloon enteroscopy.

Intraoperative enteroscopy requires insertion of an endoscope through an enterotomy site or perorally/peranally to examine the small bowel from above or below. The surgeon pleats the bowel over the endoscope, allowing inspection of the entire small bowel in more than 90% of patients. The examination should be performed while the endoscope is being advanced, as surgical manipulation can create artifacts that may be mistaken for potential bleeding lesions. The reported diagnostic yield has been in the range of 60–80%, with rates of recurrent bleeding of 13–60% [37]. However, intraoperative enteroscopy requires considerable amounts of time, staff, and costs. It is associated with a substantial risk of complications and mortality [38]. The mortality associated with the procedure has been up to 11% [39]. Complication rates range from 70% to 100%, and complications include mucosal laceration, intramural hematomas, mesenteric hemorrhage, perforation, prolonged ileus, Ogilvie syndrome, intestinal ischemia, intestinal obstruction, stress ulcer, wound infection, and postoperative pulmonary infection [39].

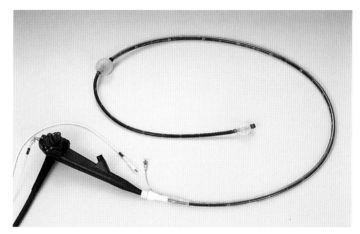

Fig. 49.1 The double-balloon enteroscope, which fits into the overtube (Fujinon). The balloons at the tip of the scope and at the tip of the overtube are both inflated. (Courtesy of Fujinon, Inc.)

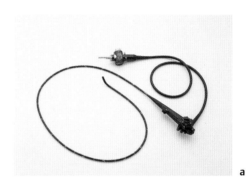

a

49

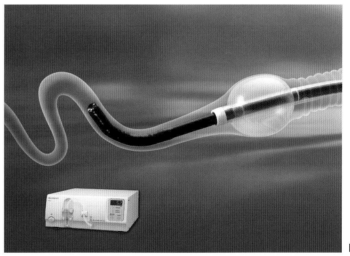

b

Fig. 49.2 The single-balloon enteroscope (Olympus).
a The enteroscope without the overtube (which is similar to that of the double-balloon enteroscope).
b The tip of scope fitted into the overtube; the balloon on the tip of the overtube is inflated. *Lower left:* the balloon pump. (Courtesy of Olympus Corporation.)

Wireless Capsule Endoscopy

In 2000, a paper appeared in the journal *Nature* describing an ingestible miniature camera that was able to send colored images of the small bowel to a portable recording device using radiotelemetry [40]. This wireless capsule endoscope measures 11 × 26 mm, weighs 3.7 g and is produced by Given Imaging, Inc. (**Fig. 49.3a**). Olympus also later presented a similar endoscopic capsule

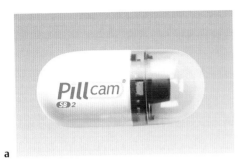

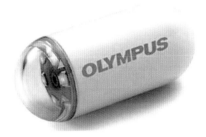

a

b

Fig. 49.3   Video capsule endoscopes.
a   The PillCam SB. (Courtesy of Given Imaging, Inc.)
b   The Endocapsule. (Courtesy of Olympus Corporation.)

Table 49.1   Upper and lower gastrointestinal bleeding sources that may be overlooked

Upper gastrointestinal lesions
Cameron lesions
Fundic varices
Peptic ulcer
Angiectasia
Dieulafoy lesion
Gastric antral vascular ectasia (GAVE)

Lower gastrointestinal lesions
Angiectasia
Neoplasms

(**Fig. 49.3b**). The two devices provide a similar image quality [41]. Examination of the gastrointestinal tract using a disposable endoscopic capsule is noninvasive, well tolerated, and safe, and allows visualization of the mucosa throughout the entire small bowel in approximately 80% of patients [42]. The diagnostic yield of capsule endoscopy in patients with obscure gastrointestinal bleeding is 38–93% [43]. A definitive bleeding source can be identified in approximately half of patients undergoing capsule endoscopy. The most important factors affecting the diagnostic yield are the presence of active bleeding at the time of examination, or a short interval between the last episode of acute bleeding and capsule endoscopy [44,45], and low levels of hemoglobin and high transfusion requirements [46,47]. In a meta-analysis [24] of 14 studies, the yield of capsule endoscopy in obscure gastrointestinal bleeding was found to be twice that of push enteroscopy—63% versus 28% for any finding and 56% versus 26% for clinically significant findings. The diagnostic superiority of capsule endoscopy in this setting was even more marked in comparison with barium radiography [24]. The diagnostic yield for any finding in the three trials analyzed was 67% for capsule endoscopy and 8% for barium radiography. The corresponding figures for clinically significant findings were 42% versus 6%. In the clinical setting of obscure gastrointestinal bleeding, the results of capsule endoscopy and double-balloon enteroscopy appear to be similar. In a meta-analysis by Chen et al. [48], capsule endoscopy was superior if double-balloon enteroscopy was carried out only either via the anal or oral approach (50.3% vs. 45.8%; four fully published trials). This is not surprising, as only performing both approaches in a patient with obscure gastrointestinal bleeding ensures that the whole small intestine is examined with double-balloon enteroscopy. When both approaches are used in obscure gastrointestinal bleeding, double-balloon enteroscopy appears to be superior to capsule endoscopy (87.5% vs. 45.8%). However, only one fully published study including 24 patients is available on this topic [33]. If another study published only in abstract form [31] (with 24 patients evaluated) is also considered, the diagnostic yield of capsule endoscopy and double-balloon enteroscopy (with both ap-

proaches) is equivalent [48]. A recently published study [49] comparing capsule endoscopy and double-balloon enteroscopy did not specifically focus on patients with obscure gastrointestinal bleeding. This study reported a comparable diagnostic yield for the two methods. The global miss rate of capsule endoscopy was reported to be about 11% [50]. This figure can be explained by several factors, such as incompleteness of the examination (occurring in 10–15%), technical limitations (limited battery life and field of view), and suboptimal bowel cleansing (mostly in the distal segments). The risk of retention of the capsule endoscope in patients with occult gastrointestinal bleeding has been reported as between 1% and 5% [44,51–53]. How to prevent capsule retention has yet to be established, as neither the results of radiographic studies nor those with the Given, Inc. patency capsule (Agile) appear to be predictive.

Repeated Endoscopy

In patients with nondiagnostic upper endoscopy and colonoscopy, a repeated endoscopy is helpful in identifying lesions overlooked at the time of the initial endoscopic evaluation (**Table 49.1**). Studies have reported that lesions within the range of a conventional endoscope were detected by small-bowel endoscopy or by a second-look endoscopy in 6–20% of cases [54–58]. In one study, the figure was as high as 64% [59]. Repeated capsule endoscopy is acceptable in patients with obscure gastrointestinal bleeding and negative capsule endoscopy findings. Jones et al. [60] reported a high yield (75%) with repeated capsule endoscopy in patients with obscure gastrointestinal bleeding when the first examination was negative. In addition, these findings led to a change in management in 62.5% of repeated studies. Limited visualization due to blood and debris during the initial capsule endoscopy appears to be a common reason for repeated studies. Recurrent bleeding is another reason.

Nonendoscopic Methods

Nuclear Scintigraphy

Nuclear scintigraphy is a sensitive method of detecting gastrointestinal bleeding at a rate of 0.1 mL/min. It is more sensitive than angiography, but less specific than a positive endoscopic or angiographic examination [61]. The role of nuclear scans, and in particular of ^{99m}Tc-labeled red blood cells, is limited in patients with obscure gastrointestinal bleeding and has substantially declined with the advent of complete endoscopic imaging of the small bowel. A major disadvantage of nuclear imaging is that it localizes bleeding only to an area of the abdomen. For example, bleeding from a redundant sigmoid may appear in the right lower quadrant, suggesting bleeding in the right colon. Another problem is colonic motility, which can move blood in either a peristaltic or antiperistaltic direction. When scans are positive within 2 h, localization is correct in 95–100% of cases, but with positive scans later than 2 h, the accuracy decreases to 57–67% [8]. Scintigraphy may be a useful tool for intermittent gastrointestinal bleeding, when endoscopic methods have failed. It is strongly recommended that every positive radionuclide imaging examination should be confirmed by endoscopy or angiography before definitive therapy is considered—such as surgery, for example.

Radiology

Visceral angiography. It is estimated that visceral angiography can only detect active bleeding of at least 0.5–1.0 mL/min [62,63]. The specificity of this procedure is 100%, but the sensitivity varies with the pattern of bleeding, ranging in one study from 47% with acute to 30% with recurrent bleeding [64]. Data on the clinical utility of angiography in obscure gastrointestinal bleeding are very limited. Advantages of angiography include the lack of a need for bowel preparation, the ability to localize the bleeding source exactly (if identified), and the potential for therapy. Angiography should be reserved for patients who have massive bleeding that precludes colonoscopy or in whom endoscopy has failed to identify the bleeding source. A Hong Kong study compared immediate capsule endoscopy and mesenteric angiography in patients with acute, overt obscure gastrointestinal bleeding. The results showed a higher diagnostic yield with capsule endoscopy [65]. Angiography is not without complications. In a study reviewing 449 consecutive patients with peripheral angiography, the overall complication rate was 9.3% [66]. Hematoma, femoral artery thrombosis, contrast reactions, renal failure, and transient ischemic cerebral attacks were major incidents.

Computed-tomographic angiography (CTA). Studies have shown that CTA is highly sensitive and specific in diagnosing colonic angiodysplasia [67,68]. It appears to be equivalent to visceral angiography in acute gastrointestinal hemorrhage [69]. Bleeding rates < 0.4 mL/min were detectable in an animal experiment [70]. Accuracy rates of 54–79% for localizing colonic bleeding have been reported [71,72]. Potential drawbacks of CTA include the high contrast volume that is administered to the patient if angiography is performed after computed tomography (CT).

Small-bowel radiography. There are two modalities for small-bowel radiography. A small-bowel series (small-bowel follow-through) involves peroral ingestion of a dilute barium solution, followed by serial abdominal imaging. Enteroclysis (the Sellink procedure) is a double-contrast study performed by passing a tube into the proximal small bowel and injecting barium, methylcellulose, and air. The yield of small-bowel barium radiography in obscure gastrointestinal bleeding ranges from 0% to 8% [73–75]. The diagnostic yield of enteroclysis is 4–20% [76–79]. This technique is considered superior to the standard small-bowel follow-through. However, neither of these radiographic studies is capable of diagnosing angiectasias, which are the most common cause of small-intestinal bleeding. Liangpunsakul et al. [80] reported that several ulcers larger than 1 cm found on capsule endoscopy were not detected by enteroclysis, even when the radiologist was unblinded to the capsule endoscopy results. The sensitivity of enteroclysis for diagnosing small-bowel neoplasia approaches 95% [81]. CT enteroclysis is said to have a higher yield in obscure gastrointestinal bleeding. Jain et al. [82] found a source in 47.6% of 21 patients with obscure gastrointestinal bleeding; the yield was higher in patients with overt obscure bleeding in comparison with occult obscure bleeding (64.3% vs. 14.3%). Unless the clinical findings suggest small-bowel obstruction due to neoplasia, Crohn's disease, or prior use of nonsteroidal anti-inflammatory drugs (NSAIDs), there is no role for small-bowel radiography.

Exploratory Laparotomy

Currently, exploratory laparotomy is seldom performed without intraoperative enteroscopy. Lesions have to be identified by simple palpation and transillumination. In two reports, diagnosis was possible at surgery in 64% and 65% of cases, respectively [5,83].

Differential Diagnosis

▣ Colon

The colon accounts for one-third of cases of gastrointestinal bleeding. The frequency of colonic bleeding sources reported varies among publications. One reason for this could be that studies often fail to differentiate between probable and definite sources of bleeding. In addition, the definitions of acute lower intestinal bleeding used are far from uniform. A source of lower intestinal bleeding cannot be definitively identified in up to 25% of patients [84]. **Table 49.2** provides an overview of the frequencies of bleeding sources in patients presenting with hematochezia. Age can provide a clue to the cause of acute lower gastrointestinal bleeding—younger patients tend to bleed from hemorrhoids, vascular malformations, and rectal ulcers, while older patients tend to bleed from diverticula, vascular malformations, and neoplasms.

Diverticula

Diverticula (**Fig. 49.4**) are the reported source of gastrointestinal bleeding in 17–40% of patients (**Table 49.2**). Although most diverticula are located in the left hemicolon, especially in the sigmoid colon, diverticula in the right hemicolon appear to have a greater bleeding tendency. However, the correlation may not always be causal, as diverticula are often cited as the bleeding source in the colon due to lack of evidence of another source. A recent study identified colon diverticula as the bleeding source in 22% of patients with acute lower gastrointestinal bleeding, on the basis either of active bleeding (**Fig. 49.4a**) or of stigmata such as a visible vessel or an adherent clot [21].

Vascular Diseases

Angiodysplasias (**Fig. 49.5**) are cited as the source of lower intestinal bleeding in up to 30% of patients (**Table 49.2**), although a rate of 3–12% is probably more realistic [85]. The majority of angiodysplasias are located in the right hemicolon, and they often occur several at a time. The frequency increases with age. In colonoscopic studies, they are found in 0.83% [86] to 1.4% [87] of the patients examined. Angiodysplasias appear endoscopically as red, circumscribed mu-

Table 49.2 Distribution of sources of hematochezia reported in the literature (based on [85])

Source of bleeding	Frequency (%)
Diverticulum	17–40
Vascular malformation (especially angiectasia)	2–30
Colitis (ischemic, infectious, chronic inflammatory bowel disease, radiation injury)	9–21
Neoplasia, postpolypectomy bleeding	11–14
Anorectal disease (including rectal varices)	4–10
Upper gastrointestinal bleeding	0–11
Small-bowel bleeding	2–9

49

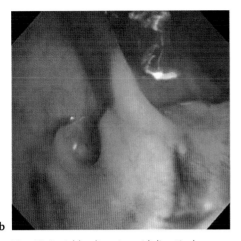

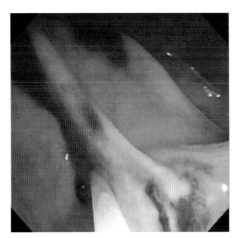

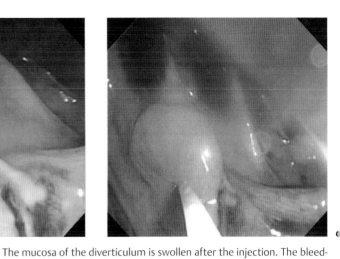

a, b

Fig. 49.4   A bleeding sigmoid diverticulum.
a   A streak of blood from the diverticulum is visible.
b   Needle injection of epinephrine into the wall of the diverticulum.

c   The mucosa of the diverticulum is swollen after the injection. The bleeding has stopped.

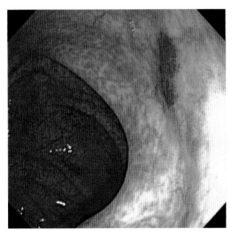

Fig. 49.5   Angiodysplasia in the cecum.

VII

Table 49.3   Criteria for clinical diagnosis of hereditary hemorrhagic telangiectasia (HHT)

Findings
Epistaxis (spontaneous or recurrent)
Telangiectasias on skin and mucosa: multiple, characteristic localizations (face, lips, oral cavity, and fingers)
Visceral arteriovenous malformations (lung, brain, liver, spine) or gastrointestinal telangiectasias (with or without bleeding)
Family history: immediate family member with HHT (according to the above criteria)

Probability of diagnosis
Definitive diagnosis: three or more criteria
Probable diagnosis: two criteria
Improbable: less than two criteria

cosal lesions (**Fig. 49.5**) with a diameter of 1 mm to a few centimeters. The vast majority of affected individuals do not bleed [88,89], and therapy is not always indicated for every angiodysplasia detected on colonoscopy. In consequence, angiodysplasias detected during emergency colonoscopy are not automatically the source of bleeding unless they are bleeding or show stigmata (visible vessel, adherent clot, or submucosal bleeding). It is important to avoid the use of opiates [90,91] and cold-water lavage [92] during colonoscopy as they reduce blood flow in the mucosa, decreasing the diagnostic yield.

Angiodysplasias manifest in the colon in association with numerous syndromes, the most well-known of which is hereditary hemorrhagic telangiectasia (HHT), also known as Osler–Weber–Rendu syndrome. Hereditary hemorrhagic telangiectasia is an autosomal-dominant disease characterized by the formation of abnormal blood vessels. The clinical picture shows attacks involving various organs, primarily the brain, lungs, skin, nose, liver, and gastrointestinal tract. Two clear genetic defects related to hereditary hemorrhagic telangiectasia have been identified. Unlike usual angiectasias, hereditary hemorrhagic telangiectasia affects younger people as well, with involvement of the entire gastrointestinal tract. The diagnosis should be made on the basis of the Curaçao criteria (**Table 49.3**). Gastrointestinal bleeding occurs in one-third of patients with hereditary hemorrhagic telangiectasia [93] and patients over the age of 60 are particularly at risk. The most common localization of hereditary hemorrhagic telangiectasia is the stomach and proximal small bowel (**Fig. 49.6**); the colon is less often affected [94].

Rectal varices. Bleeding, especially from rectal varices (**Fig. 49.7**), is not uncommon in patients with portal hypertension. Rectal varices have a gray-blue color and may be confused with mucosal folds.

Radiation injury. Radiation proctitis (**Fig. 49.8**) due to radiotherapy for pelvic tumors can lead to blood loss, but bleeding generally does not present a problem. A more serious problem is neovascularization resulting from tissue ischemia in radiation-induced endarteritis obliterans. This can lead to considerable morbidity due to recurrent blood loss. Following radiotherapy for prostate carcinoma, 13% of patients report more or less pronounced rectal blood loss over a period of 4–41 months [95]. Another publication has reported a lower rate of 4%; Crook et al. [96] reported that 5% of patients who underwent radiotherapy reported daily blood loss, while 9% reported weekly bleeding. The resulting anemia can become problematic. Chronic radiation injury usually presents endoscopically with multiple telangiectasias, often extending into the anal canal. The mucosa is pale, lacking vessels, and vulnerable. In severe cases, there can also be ulcerations and massive hemorrhage.

Dieulafoy lesion. Bleeding from a Dieulafoy lesion in the stomach is not an unusual finding, but it is an unexpected cause of colonic bleeding. Small mucosal lesions with subsequent erosion of an underlying vessel can lead to spurting hemorrhage.

Colonic ischemia. Hematochezia is not infrequently caused by colonic ischemia. Submucosal hemorrhage, livid-colored mucosa, and

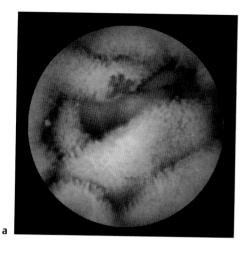

a

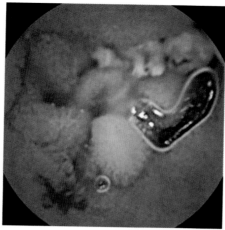

b

Fig. 49.6 Capsule-endoscopic images of angiodysplasias in the small bowel.
a Angiodysplasia in a patient with hereditary hemorrhagic telangiectasia (HHT).
b "Sporadic" angiodysplasia in an older patient.

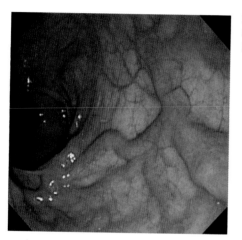

Fig. 49.7 Rectal varices in a patient with portal hypertension.

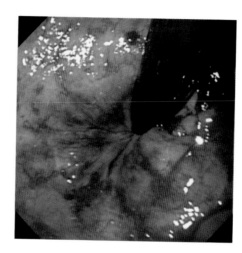

Fig. 49.8 Chronic radiation injury to the rectal mucosa, with multiple angiectasias. (The patient had undergone radiotherapy for prostate carcinoma.) View of the upper margin of the anus and the shaft of the retroflexed scope.

49

mucosal nodularity are typical endoscopic findings in the early stages. The resulting bleeding does not usually cause hemodynamic compromise and is self-limiting in most cases.

Inflammation

Massive hemorrhage leads to hospitalization in 0.1% of patients with ulcerative colitis and 1.2% of patients with Crohn's disease [97]. Among Crohn patients, bleeding locations have been described in one report as being evenly distributed between the small bowel and colon [97]. This is in contrast to the findings of two other studies, one of which describes the colon [98] and the other the ileocolonic junction [99] as the bleeding sites of predilection. In half of all patients with bleeding related to chronic inflammatory bowel disease (IBD), bleeding stops spontaneously. However, the rebleeding rate is 35% [100].

Although infectious colitis and pseudomembranous colitis can present with bloody diarrhea, life-threatening hemorrhage is rare.

NSAIDs can promote bleeding from any number of possible lesions in the gastrointestinal tract. NSAIDs also induce colitis, which may not be visibly discernible from infectious colitis or chronic inflammatory bowel disease. The endoscopic appearance can also include flat and usually irregularly bordered erosions and ulcerations, which are surrounded by an otherwise normal-appearing mucosa.

The causes of lower gastrointestinal bleeding in patients with human immunodeficiency virus (HIV) infection differ from those in other patients. The most common are cytomegalovirus colitis (25%), lymphoma (12%), and idiopathic (unidentifiable) colitis (12%) [101].

The first two causes are especially pronounced in patients with a CD4 lymphocyte count below 200/mm^3. If the cell count is over 200/mm^3, the most common bleeding sources are idiopathic colitis, diverticula, and hemorrhoids. Rebleeding is not uncommon. The 30-day mortality rate related to bleeding is around 14%, and patients with concomitant medical problems, rebleeding, and those requiring surgical intervention are especially at risk. In a study by Chalasani et al. [102], the most common cause of bleeding was also cytomegalovirus infection, followed by hemorrhoids and anal fissures. Thrombocytopenia was a particular risk factor for hemorrhoid bleeding. Colonic histoplasmosis, Kaposi's sarcoma in the colon, and bacterial colitis are further bleeding sources.

Neoplasia

Carcinomas range from 2–9% as the source of hematochezia (**Table 49.2**). Bleeding is the result of erosions on the surface of the tumor.

Colon polyps are reported to be the source of lower intestinal bleeding in 5–11% of patients (**Table 49.2**). Larger polyps with a diameter of more than 1 cm bleed more often. By far the most common cause of lower gastrointestinal bleeding from benign polyps is polypectomy. Bleeding may occur immediately after resection, although the time between polypectomy and bleeding can vary and can occasionally be up to 2 weeks.

Table 49.4 Various causes of obscure gastrointestinal bleeding (in 239 patients) identified by capsule endoscopy and double-balloon enteroscopy [48]

Lesion	Capsule endoscopy	Double-balloon enteroscopy
Angiodysplasia	52%	47%
Ulcer/erosion	21%	18%
Tumor/polyp	16%	19%
Crohn's disease	3%	5%
Diverticulum	<1%	4%
Fresh blood and clot	5%	2%
Others	2%	5%
Overall yield	61%	55%

Table 49.5 Etiology of mid-intestinal bleeding

Younger than 40 years of age
Tumors
Meckel's diverticulum
Dieulafoy lesion
Crohn's disease
Age 40 or older
Angiodysplasia
NSAID enteropathy
Uncommon
Hemobilia
Hemosuccus pancreaticus
Aortoenteric fistula

NSAID, nonsteroidal anti-inflammatory drug.

Anorectal Diseases

Hemorrhoids are the source in 2–9% of patients with acute lower gastrointestinal bleeding (overview in [85]).

Although anal fissures often cause bloodstained stools, acute bleeding is rare. Fissures are relatively easily diagnosed by inspecting the anus. The patient typically has severe pain upon spreading the anus, but the lesion can be carefully and painlessly inspected after injecting a few milliliters of a local anesthetic. Bleeding from fissures usually ceases spontaneously.

Local ischemia appears to play a role in the pathogenesis of solitary rectal ulcers. Internal rectal prolapse or lack of inhibition of the puborectalis muscle during straining are thought to be responsible. Heavy bleeding is rare.

■ Small Bowel

Overt small-bowel bleeding ("mid-intestinal bleeding" or "midgut bleeding") is considered to be a distinct clinical entity, which appears to have a poorer outcome in comparison with colonic and upper gastrointestinal bleeding [103]. The patients require a larger number of diagnostic procedures and blood transfusions and remain in hospital longer. Prakash and Zuckerman reported a mortality rate of 10% in patients with small-bowel bleeding, higher than in those with colonic bleeding and upper gastrointestinal bleeding [103]. However, it must emphasized that this retrospective study was carried out before the advent of capsule endoscopy and double-balloon enteroscopy. The overall incidence and location of specific lesions responsible for small-bowel bleeding are unknown, as there

have been no longitudinal studies addressing this issue. In a meta-analysis comparing the results of capsule endoscopy and double-balloon enteroscopy in patients with obscure gastrointestinal bleeding, angiodysplasias were found to be the most common bleeding source identified by both diagnostic methods, followed by ulcerations/erosions and tumors [48] (**Table 49.4**). A study comparing capsule endoscopy and intraoperative enteroscopy [50,104] and a pooled analysis of capsule endoscopy trials [50] reported similar figures. The causes of obscure gastrointestinal bleeding vary depending on the age of the patient (**Table 49.5**). In a study using push enteroscopy in patients with obscure gastrointestinal bleeding, 40% of patients over the age of 65 had angiodysplasias diagnosed on enteroscopy, in comparison with 12% of patients under 65 [54]. In contrast, the incidence of small-bowel tumors as a cause of obscure gastrointestinal bleeding was noted to be higher in patients under 50 years of age (14%, in comparison with 3% in patients over 50) [105]. This study confirmed that the frequency of arteriovenous malformations increases with age, reaching a maximum in the ninth decade [105].

Angiodysplasia

Sporadic angiectasias (**Figs. 49.5, 49.6**) of the gastrointestinal tract are probably an acquired degenerative lesion associated with the aging process. Factors causing bleeding in angiectasia have not been clearly identified. Increased production of vascular endothelial growth factor (VGEF) and/or quantitative or qualitative defects in von Willebrand factor appear to be involved [106,107]. Angiectasias are the most common source of small-bowel bleeding. Sporadic telangiectasias appear to be a multifocal disease, potentially involving the whole digestive tract. In a recently published study [108], 67% of patients in whom esophagogastroduodenoscopy found telangiectasias also had small-bowel vascular lesions at capsule endoscopy, and 43% had colonic lesions at colonoscopy. Fifty-four percent of patients with positive colonoscopy also had gastroduodenal lesions, and 48% had small-bowel lesions. Patients with associated diseases such as liver cirrhosis, chronic renal failure, or heart valvulopathy presented more severe disease, requiring blood transfusions. The number of blood transfusions correlated with the number of sites affected.

The natural history of vascular lesions in the small bowel has not been well characterized. It is estimated that fewer than 10% of patients with angiodysplasias will eventually bleed. Frequent bleeding episodes and high transfusion requirements are predictive of recurrent bleeding. Angiodysplasia size ≥ 10 mm has been reported to be associated with a more severe clinical impact and a greater likelihood of requiring a therapeutic procedure [109]. These findings support the view that patients with large lesions can benefit from therapeutic interventions with a reduction in the rebleeding rate. In a follow-up study (mean 21 months) [53] including 240 patients with obscure gastrointestinal bleeding, most recurrent bleeding episodes were owing to angiodysplasias. However, the bleeding rate decreased if all angiectasias detected on capsule endoscope were coagulated. This was confirmed by another prospective follow-up study [110], in which nearly all patients with recurrent bleeding showed angiectasias in the small bowel at the initial work-up. All 50 patients had previously been included in a study comparing capsule endoscopy and intraoperative enteroscopy. A retrospective study in Belgium [111] reported follow-up data (with a mean of 635 days) for 92 patients with obscure gastrointestinal bleeding who were examined using capsule endoscopy. Small-bowel angiodysplasias were a clear predictor of a less favorable clinical outcome. The authors hypothesized that the angiectasias may have newly developed or may have been missed at the initial examination.

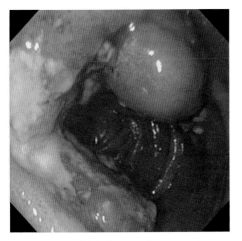

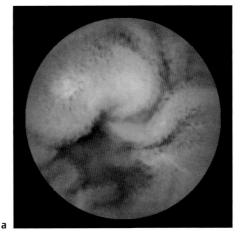

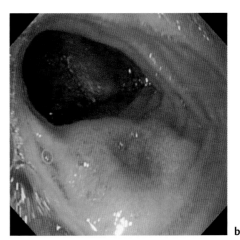

Fig. 49.9 Double-balloon endoscopy: adeno-carcinoma in the jejunum.

Fig. 49.10 Carcinoid tumor in the ileum.
a The capsule-endoscopic appearance.
b The appearance on double-balloon endoscopy.

Tumors

Small-bowel tumors account for 1–3% of all gastrointestinal tumors. In small-bowel tumors, there is a major delay in making the diagnosis after medical help is sought by the patient [112,113]—contributing to the poor prognosis for patients with malignant lesions. In a multicenter European study including 5129 patients who underwent capsule endoscopy, 2.4% of the patients had a small-bowel tumor (112 primary, 12 metastatic). Obscure gastrointestinal bleeding was the indication for capsule endoscopy in 87% of these patients [114]. The lesions were single in 89.5% of cases and multiple in 10.5%. The main type of primary small-bowel lesion was gastrointestinal stromal tumor (GIST; 32%), followed by adenocarcinoma (20%) (**Fig. 49.9**), and carcinoid (15%) (**Fig. 49.10**); 66% of secondary small-bowel tumors were melanomas [114]. In another study [115] including 443 patients examined using capsule endoscopy for obscure gastrointestinal bleeding, 9% of the patients were diagnosed with a small-bowel tumor. In patients under the age of 50, small-bowel tumors were the cause of bleeding even more frequently (13%). Fourteen percent of the tumors were located in the duodenum, 46% in the jejunum, 31% in the ileum, and 10% were multifocal. Of the tumors diagnosed, 48% were malignant. Twenty percent of the tumors were carcinoids, 16% adenocarcinomas, 10% lymphomas, 8% GISTs, and 6% inflammatory polyps. However, a negative capsule endoscopy study does not rule out a small-bowel tumor. A recently published study drew attention to the fact that capsule endoscopy misses a considerable number of small-bowel tumors [116] that are eventually detected on double-balloon enteroscopy.

Diverticula

Meckel's diverticulum (**Fig. 49.11**) is a vestigial remnant of the omphalomesenteric duct and is the most frequent malformation in the gastrointestinal tract. It is present in approximately 2% of the population and is three to four times more common in males. Meckel's diverticulum is located in the distal ileum, usually within 60–100 cm of the ileocecal valve. It is typically 3–5 cm long; giant lesions may be as large as 100 cm in diameter. Heterotopic tissue is present in approximately 50% of all diverticula. The type of tissue most frequently found is gastric mucosa, pancreatic tissue, or a combination of the two. Heterotopic gastric mucosa may lead to bleeding. Approximately 98% of those affected by Meckel's diverticulum are asymptomatic. Symptoms often occur during the first few years of life, but may occur in adults as well. The most common

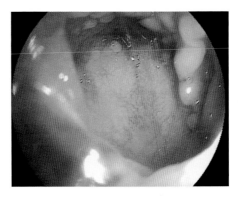

Fig. 49.11 Double-balloon endoscopy, showing a Meckel's diverticulum in the ileum. Fresh blood is visible in the upper part of the diverticulum. The bleeding was stopped by applying clips.

49

presenting symptom is gastrointestinal bleeding, followed by intestinal obstruction, volvulus, and intussusception. The sensitivity of Meckel's scanning using ^{99m}Tc-pertechnate is only 60% in adult patients, but as high as 85–90% in pediatric patients. However, a positive scan only indicates the presence of gastric mucosa in the small bowel, which may or may not represent the bleeding source. Small-bowel follow-through radiography is usually not useful, as the diverticulum may not fill with barium. Enteroclysis examinations show a better yield, because the contrast material, under increased pressure, fills the diverticulum better. The orifice of the diverticulum may be missed on capsule endoscopy or double-balloon enteroscopy, and ileal ulceration may be misdiagnosed as Crohn's disease. However, many case reports in literature show that Meckel's diverticulum can be detected by either of the two methods of small-bowel endoscopy. It has been reported that the capsule endoscope may become trapped in the diverticulum.

Rarely, other types of small-bowel diverticula (apart from Meckel's diverticula) may bleed. They are predominantly located in the duodenum and jejunum.

Erosions and Ulcerations

NSAID enteropathy is a stepwise process involving direct mucosal toxicity, mitochondrial damage, breakdown of intercellular integrity, enterohepatic recirculation, and neutrophil activation by luminal contents, including bacteria. Macroscopic morphologic correlates of this damage include abnormalities ranging from subtle reddening of mucosal folds to discrete erosions (**Fig. 49.12**), ulcers, and occasional bleeding. In a Japanese multicenter study, double-balloon enteroscopy was performed in 1035 patients. Sixty-one of

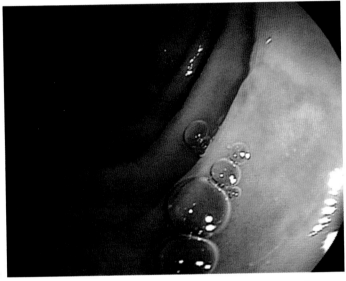

Fig. 49.12 Erosion of the small-bowel mucosa caused by use of nonsteroidal anti-inflammatory drugs (NSAIDs).
a The capsule-endoscopic appearance.
b The appearance on double-balloon endoscopy.

to relate the lesions either to Crohn's disease or NSAID enteropathy on the basis of their endoscopic appearance. The decision should also take the clinical history into account. Other causes of small-bowel ulceration include lymphoma and radiation enteritis.

Therapy

Initial Resuscitation

There are no clear recommendations regarding which patients should be admitted to an intensive-care unit. However, it appears reasonable to monitor patients closely if there is ongoing bleeding and they are at high risk on the basis of the factors mentioned earlier. In addition, patients with a transfusion requirement greater than two units of packed red blood cells and those with significant comorbidity should be admitted to an intensive-care unit. Patients with congestive heart failure or valvular disease may benefit from close monitoring (central venous pressure, pulmonary catheter, pulse contour continuous cardiac output) to minimize the risk of fluid overload. Two large-diameter peripheral catheters or a central venous catheter should be placed for intravenous access. Any coagulopathy (prothrombin time INR > 1.5) should be corrected using fresh frozen plasma or prothrombin complex concentrate and vitamin K. In patients with significant thrombocytopenia (< 50,000/μL), platelet transfusions can be considered. Rapid fluid replacement is indicated in patients with severe hypovolemia or shock. In general, at least 1–2 L of isotonic saline is administered as rapidly as possible in an attempt to restore tissue perfusion. Red blood cells should be used if there is ongoing hemorrhage or severe anemia. The ideal hemoglobin concentration/hematocrit depends on the patient's age, the rate of bleeding, and the presence of comorbid conditions. A young and otherwise healthy person will tolerate a hemoglobin concentration of less than 7–8 g/dL (hematocrit < 20–25%) well, whereas older patients develop symptoms at this level. Maintaining the hemoglobin concentration at around 10 g/dL (hematocrit 30%) in high-risk patients (for instance, an elderly patient with coronary heart disease) is reasonable. However, it must be emphasized that all of these recommendations are given on an empirical basis.

Endoscopy

The efficacy of endoscopic intervention in patients with upper gastrointestinal bleeding is now beyond doubt. Recently, these benefits have also been demonstrated in lower intestinal bleeding [21].

Thermocoagulation

Heat application causes edema, coagulation of tissue protein, and contraction of vessels in the tissue, resulting in hemostasis. In bipolar (BICAP) and monopolar electrocoagulation, electrical current is passed through the tissue and heats it up. In the bipolar modality, the current flows between the two electrodes in the probe tip, and in the monopolar method it is necessary to place a neutral electrode on the patient's body. The coagulation depth is greater with monopolar coagulation than with bipolar [121]. Some monopolar probes have holes in the probe tip for irrigation—e.g., electro-hydrothermal (EHT) probes. A major problem with contact electrocoagulation is the fact that the probe may stick to the tissue; removing the probe entails a risk of tearing off tissue and subsequently inducing bleeding. Perforation occurs in up to 2.5% of patients in whom bipolar coagulation is used in the thin-walled right hemicolon.

the patients were identified as NSAID users and their results were compared with those for 600 control individuals not receiving NSAIDs. Gastrointestinal bleeding was a more frequent indication for double-balloon enteroscopy (79% vs. 44%) in NSAID users. Mucosal breaks were detected in 51% of the NSAID users, in comparison with 5% of the control group. Small-intestinal strictures were seen in 10% of the NSAID users. Acetylsalicylic acid appeared to be less harmful to the small intestine than other NSAIDs [117]. In a postmortem study, Allison et al. [118] found ulcers in the small intestine in 8.4% of 249 NSAID users, in comparison with 0.6% of control individuals; 4.1% of the long-term NSAID users died of perforated small-bowel ulcers. Goldstein et al. [119] compared the effect of a conventional NSAID (naproxen 500 mg twice daily) and a COX-2-specific inhibitor (celecoxib 200 mg twice daily) on the small-bowel mucosa in healthy individuals. Both drugs were given for 2 weeks, and a third group received a placebo. Fifty-five percent of the patients in the naproxen group were found to have mucosal breaks, in comparison with 16% of these receiving celecoxib and 7% of those with the placebo. The COX-2 inhibitor celecoxib thus appears to injure the small-bowel mucosa less than naproxen. A surprising finding was the large number of mucosal breaks in the placebo group.

The question of the specificity of the diagnosis of small-bowel lesions caused by Crohn's disease or NSAIDs was addressed in one capsule endoscopy study [120]. The results suggest that it is difficult

Argon plasma coagulation (APC) transmits energy from ionized argon gas to the tissue without contact between the probe and tissue. The flexible application probe is inserted into the working channel of the endoscope. The penetration depth is 0.8–3.0 mm and it is automatically limited by the desiccation of the tissue. Although valid figures for perforation rates are lacking, they are probably well below 1%.

The heater probe tip consists of a Teflon-coated hollow aluminum cylinder with a heating coil inside. It delivers heat directly to the tissue. The Teflon coating is intended to prevent the probe from adhering to tissue. Data for the complication rate with this method in the colon are lacking.

High-energy laser light causes vaporization of tissue. A flexible optical fiber introduced into the working channel of the scope transmits the laser beam. In the commonly used neodymium: yttrium–aluminum–garnet (Nd:YAG) laser, the optical fiber has to be constantly cooled with carbon dioxide, which can cause considerable bowel distension. The depth of penetration of a single pulse from an Nd:YAG laser is 0.2–6.0 mm and 1–2 mm with an argon beam laser. The deeper necrosis is associated with a higher risk of perforation, especially in the thin-walled right hemicolon.

Injection Therapy

Injection therapy is an inexpensive and easy-to-learn method of achieving hemostasis (**Fig. 49.4**). The injection needles consist of a Teflon sheath with an extendable needle at the tip. For treatment in the colon, a needle extension length of 4 mm should be used in order to limit the depth of penetration. Usually, epinephrine (suprarenin, adrenaline) is used. This causes vasoconstriction and physical compression of the vessel. The individual injection dose should be as low as possible (e.g., 1–2 mL, 1 : 10 000 dilution), as the absorption of catecholamine has systemic effects (tachycardia, arrhythmia, and hypertension). Alternative agents (absolute alcohol, sodium tetradecyl sulfate, ethanolamine, and polidocanol) are not superior to epinephrine and can also cause mucosal injury. Bleeding from rectal varices (**Fig. 49.7**) can often only be stopped by injecting cyanoacrylate glue, as in gastric and esophageal varices. Mucosal injury caused by extravascular injection can result in deep ulcerations and subsequent rebleeding.

Mechanical Methods

Metal clips allow definitive and secure closure of bleeding vessels. The endoscopist can immediately recognize whether a vessel has been occluded. Complications have not been reported so far. Various clips are available, with various jaw angles and lengths. The sheath with the clip is advanced through the working channel of the endoscope. Ligation using rubber bands is used for bleeding hemorrhoids. This is a simple and inexpensive treatment method, but it may be complicated by pain and the risk of rebleeding after the band has fallen off.

▥ Radiologic Angiotherapy

Transcatheter embolization is a more definitive method of controlling hemorrhage than intra-arterial vasopressin infusion. The availability of microcatheters led to the development of microcatheter embolization using microcoils, Gelfoam, and polyvinyl alcohol particles. The success rates reported in the literature range from 70% to 90%, and recurrent hemorrhage occurs in less than 15% of cases [122]. Most interventional radiologists have therefore switched from vasoconstrictive therapy to superselective embolization.

▥ Surgery

Several surgical options are available in the management of lower intestinal bleeding:
- Emergency limited segmental resection for a known bleeding source that cannot be stopped by endoscopic and angiographic intervention
- Emergency segmental resection or subtotal colectomy for an unknown bleeding source
- Elective segmental resection for a known bleeding source such as carcinoma, or for rebleeding from a known lesion

The last resort in the treatment of severe lower intestinal bleeding is surgery, which is said to be necessary in up to 25% of cases. The criteria for emergency surgery are: more than four units of blood per 24 h, or a total of 10 units overall; bleeding continuing for 72 h or more; and significant rebleeding within 1 week of initial cessation [85,123]. Blind segmental colectomy is associated with an unacceptably high morbidity rate (with a rebleeding rate as high as 75%) and mortality (up to 50%). It should be avoided at all costs. Accurate preoperative localization is therefore extremely important. It is worthwhile to inject some methylene blue through the angiographic catheter to stain the affected bowel segment. Directed segmental resection is the treatment of choice because of its low morbidity, mortality (about 4%) and rebleeding rates (about 6%) [123]. The 1-year rebleeding rate has been reduced from 42% without prior angiographic localization to 14% with previous localization.

▥ Pharmacotherapy

Several studies have failed to confirm the efficacy of hormonal therapy for angiodysplasia using estrogen and progestogen. In addition, this treatment approach is hampered by potential side effects. Somatostatin and its analogue, octreotide, have been reported to reduce blood loss from intestinal angiodysplasias. Octreotide at a dosage of 0.05–0.1 mg subcutaneously two to three times a day has been reported to reduce blood loss from intestinal angiodysplasia [124,125]. The response appears to be fast, with disappearance of bleeding within 24 h. Octreotide has also been reported to be effective in patients with bleeding portal hypertensive colopathy [126]. Recent studies have shown that both Osler's disease and nonhereditary intestinal angiodysplasias are characterized by increased production of vascular endothelial growth factor (VGEF). That makes them an attractive target for therapy with direct or indirect VEGF antagonists. The best-known antagonist of angiogenesis is thalidomide. Thalidomide is well-known for its teratogenicity, which correlates with its antiangiogenetic activity. One study has shown that thalidomide prevents rebleeding in patients with angiodysplasias and in patients with severe bleeding related to Crohn's disease [127]. In patients with multiple angiodysplasias of the small bowel, capsule endoscopy showed that thalidomide reduced the number, size, and color intensity of angiodysplasias. This paralleled the clinical efficacy of thalidomide [128]. However, its effectiveness is qualified by its substantial side effects; thalidomide is a potent sedative, causes birth defects, and can induce severe peripheral neuropathy.

49

Differential Endoscopic Therapy

The colon is not as easily accessible for endoscopic therapy as the upper gastrointestinal tract. However, colonoscopic interventions are nowadays widely used to treat bleeding emanating from sources in the colon. Urgent colonoscopy may be difficult due to large amounts of stool and blood, and prior cleansing is therefore advisable. The hemostatic techniques used and the available therapeutic devices are the same in gastroscopy and colonoscopy, apart from the fact that instruments used with colonoscopes have to be longer. In patients with small-bowel bleeding, double-balloon enteroscopy now allows diagnosis and subsequent treatment in most patients. Endoscopic hemostasis was performed in 36% of patients in a Japanese study [34]. Argon plasma coagulation (APC), injection therapy, polypectomy, and clipping can be performed during double-balloon or single-balloon enteroscopy. The endoscopic equipment required for enteroscopy is longer than in colonoscopes. Passage of the accessories through the working channel of a double-balloon or single-balloon enteroscope is more difficult, due to loops and flexion of the scope tip. It can be facilitated by injecting a small amount of silicone oil, for example, into the working channel before the accessories are inserted.

Diverticula

A recent study [21] showed that in acute lower gastrointestinal bleeding emanating from colonic diverticula in which active bleeding (**Fig. 49.4**) or stigmata such as a visible vessel or an adherent clot were identified, patients with endoscopic therapy (epinephrine injection and bipolar coagulation) had no rebleeding, in comparison with 53% of those who did not undergo endoscopic intervention. However, these excellent results are contradicted by another study [129], in which a retrospective analysis of diverticular bleeding was conducted. Using the same endoscopic interventional techniques, this study observed early rebleeding in 38% of cases and late rebleeding in 23%. At first glance, the results of these two studies appear contradictory. A closer look, however, reveals that Jensen et al. [21] consistently advised their patients to discontinue use of NSAIDs or acetylsalicylic acid and to follow a high-fiber diet. It is therefore possible that these additional factors help explain the divergent results and that nonendoscopic factors also play an important role in the treatment outcome. About 80% of the bleeding episodes stop spontaneously. The cumulative risk of rebleeding is 25% after 4 years [1]. A third bleed after a second episode occurs in half of the cases. Surgical resection is therefore recommended after the first rebleeding episode [123]. There is no consensus regarding endoscopic treatment is optimal. In addition to epinephrine injection and coagulation methods, mechanical hemostasis with metal clips is used [130]. Bleeding from Meckel's diverticulum in the ileum is usually treated by surgical resection. In a patient with heavy bleeding from a Meckel's diverticulum, we were able to bridge the period until laparotomy was performed by hemoclipping the bleeding vessel.

Vascular Diseases

Endoscopic thermocoagulation has proved effective in the treatment of angiodysplasias in the colon and rectum. Successful use of heater probes, monopolar and bipolar electrocautery, Nd:YAG laser, and argon plasma coagulation (APC) has been reported. The Wiesbaden group [131] treated angiodysplasias in the small bowel most frequently using argon plasma coagulation, with or without injection of a diluted epinephrine–saline solution (1 : 100,000) during double-balloon enteroscopy. Other groups [132–134] have also used argon plasma coagulation (with a maximum energy output of 20 W) [133] to treat angiodysplasias in the small bowel. Successful injection of fibrin glue has also been reported for bleeding angiodysplasias [132].

Three items should be noted with regard to practical application of thermocoagulation:

- Low power and short application times should be used, especially in the cecum, ascending colon, and small bowel, in order to limit the depth of coagulation. Laser coagulation is not without risk in the right hemicolon and small bowel.
- Larger vascular malformations should first be coagulated around their periphery and then in the center.
- Contact thermocoagulation procedures involve a risk of bleeding, as adherent tissue may be torn off when the probe is withdrawn. Noncontact procedures such as argon plasma coagulation have a distinct advantage.

The treatment of vascular angiectasias in patients with chronic rectal radiation injury is a special problem. Among contact procedures, bipolar probes and heater probes were equally successful [135]. There have been a number of reports on the use of laser treatment for this indication (overview in [136]), with a complication rate in the range of 0–9%. Energy delivery should be kept as low and as short as possible in order to minimize mucosal injury in the damaged tissue. Argon plasma coagulation is a recent and promising treatment option. Its success in the treatment of radiation-induced vascular malformation in the rectum has been repeatedly reported (overview in [136]). As with laser therapy, the power setting should be kept low and the time of application should be short. Several treatment sessions are often necessary.

Treatment of bleeding rectal varices has been reported with methods analogous to the treatment of esophageal and gastric varices, such as band ligation, sclerotherapy, and intravariceal injection of cyanoacrylate glue. In the long run, transjugular intrahepatic portosystemic shunting (TIPS) appears to be a more successful approach [137].

There have been case reports on the successful treatment of bleeding from colonic Dieulafoy lesions using injection of sclerosing agents, thermocoagulation, and hemoclips. Mechanical methods of hemostasis (metal clipping and band ligation) appear to be more effective than injection therapy [138]. May et al. [139] achieved endoscopic hemostasis in Dieulafoy ulcers of the small bowel by using argon plasma coagulation during double-balloon enteroscopy.

Inflammation

In patients with inflammatory bowel disease (IBD), circumscribed colonic bleeding sources can be treated endoscopically. Epinephrine injection and bipolar coagulation [97] have been successful in achieving hemostasis. Injecting a mixture of absolute alcohol and polidocanol [140] and application of metal clips [141] have also stopped bleeding. Schäfer et al. [132] reported successful endoscopic treatment of larger erosions and ulcers in patients with Crohn's disease in the proximal ileum. There are no recommendations for endoscopic therapy of colonic bleeding emanating from NSAID-induced erosions or ulcers. In practice, injection (epinephrine) therapy or clipping devices have been effective in colonic lesions. These methods can also be used during double-balloon enteroscopy.

In a study by Bini et al. [101], colonic bleeding in patients with HIV was controlled endoscopically in nearly all cases using bipolar thermocoagulation probes, with or without epinephrine injection.

Neoplasia

Both laser and argon plasma coagulation allow endoscopic hemostasis in bleeding carcinomas. Contact methods are less suitable, as tearing off tissue after coagulation is completed can cause hemorrhagic oozing. Injection of absolute alcohol into the tumor has also been successful in achieving hemostasis [142]. Metal clips can be tried in circumscribed bleeding sources. Bleeding after polypectomy in the colon may occur immediately, although the time between polypectomy and bleeding can vary and may occasionally be up to 2 weeks. In the event of early postpolypectomy bleeding, hemorrhage can controlled in many cases by resnaring the stalk of the polyp and applying pressure (with or without application of coagulation current). If this fails, a variety of endoscopic techniques have proved to be safe and effective. These include loop or rubber-band ligation of the remaining polyp stalk, thermocoagulation with or without preceding epinephrine injection, and application of metal clips (overview in [85]). Bleeding may also occur after polypectomy during double-balloon enteroscopy. The methods of endoscopic hemostasis here are the same as in the colon.

Anorectal Diseases

Ligation of internal hemorrhoids using rubber bands has proved to be an effective and simple method of treating hemorrhoid bleeding. Jensen et al. [143] compared bipolar coagulation (BICAP) and heater probe treatment for bleeding internal hemorrhoids. Pain was reported more often when the heater probe was used, but in comparison with BICAP the success of the treatment was clearer and followed more quickly. Bleeding is also seen after hemorrhoid surgery and band ligation. Mechanical hemostasis using clip devices as well as epinephrine injection have proved effective. Bleeding from anal fissures usually ceases spontaneously. If necessary, hemostasis can be attempted by injection of an epinephrine solution or with a swab soaked in epinephrine placed in the anus. Heavy bleeding in solitary rectal ulcers is rare. Thermocoagulation, injection therapy, or clipping devices can be used to achieve endoscopic hemostasis in such patients.

Impact of Endoscopy on the Outcome

Endoscopy is now the method of choice for diagnosing and if possible treating acute and chronic lower intestinal bleeding. Patients with chronic bleeding and/or positive occult blood in the feces require colonoscopy, as it has been demonstrated that examining the entire colon results in a significant reduction in the mortality from colon cancer. Colonoscopy is also recommended in the early evaluation of acute lower intestinal bleeding (**Fig. 49.13**). The procedure should be done after the colon has been cleansed using a polyethylene glycol–based solution. The timing of initial colonoscopy after initial presentation varies between 12 and 48 h. Two studies have shown that early colonoscopy is significantly associated with a shorter hospital stay [9,17], but these results are contradicted by another study, which found that early colonoscopy is not superior to a standard care algorithm [18]. In patients with postpolypectomy bleeding, colonoscopy should be carried out without preparation. This also applies to acute ongoing lower intestinal bleeding.

If upper and lower endoscopy are negative, it must be assumed that the small bowel is the source of the bleeding, and capsule endoscopy should be the third test in the evaluation of patients with gastrointestinal bleeding (**Fig. 49.14**) [37]. In patients with active bleeding and anemic patients with chronic bleeding, the diagnostic yield of capsule endoscopy is high. If capsule endoscopy detects the bleeding site, double-balloon or single-balloon enteroscopy can be carried out for endoscopic hemostasis or to take biopsies. In patients with negative capsule endoscopy examinations, the rebleeding rate appears to be low [55,144]. In contrast, patients with positive capsule findings appear to be at high risk (48.4%) for rebleeding [144]. In this study [144], 15 of 31 patients with lesions found on capsule endoscopy underwent further interventions. The highest rebleeding rate was seen in patients with angiodysplasias (58.3%) and active bleeding without identifiable causes on the initial capsule endoscopy (53.8%). Patients with ulcers and erosions seldom re-bled. This may be explained by two factors. Firstly, most of these lesions are related to the use of NSAIDs and resolve on withdrawal of the medication. Secondly, it is known that small-bowel

49

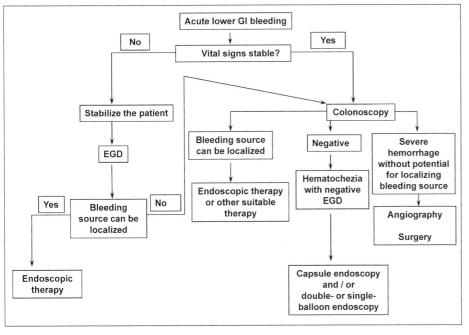

Fig. 49.13 The algorithm for diagnosis and therapy in patients with acute lower gastrointestinal bleeding with hematochezia (adapted from [136]). EGD, esophagogastroduodenoscopy; GI, gastrointestinal.

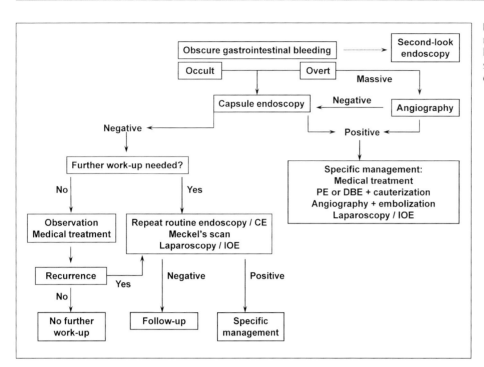

Fig. 49.14 The proposed algorithm for the diagnosis and management of obscure gastrointestinal bleeding (adapted from [136]). CE, capsule endoscopy; DBE, double-balloon enteroscopy; IOE, intraoperative enteroscopy; PE, push enteroscopy.

lesions are found on capsule endoscopy in up to 19% of asymptomatic healthy individuals [119]. A German multicenter study reported a higher rebleeding rate (20%) in patients with negative capsule endoscopy findings [145]. Another large German study included 285 patients with overt or occult obscure gastrointestinal bleeding who underwent capsule endoscopy. Follow-up for a mean of 20 months was possible in 240 of the patients. A bleeding source was detected on capsule endoscopy in 61.4%. The initial capsule endoscopy findings led to treatment in 66.2% of the patients. Rebleeding occurred most often in patients with angiectasias. A lack of anticoagulant medication and negative capsule endoscopy were associated with a low risk of relapse. In a study in Switzerland of patients with suspected small-bowel bleeding, the results of capsule endoscopy only altered the management of the 128 individuals examined in a minority of cases (17%) [146]. Either a "wait-and-see" strategy or supportive medical management alone were the most frequent decisions before and after capsule endoscopy. The indication for surgery was confirmed by capsule endoscopy in seven of 11 patients, and inappropriate surgery was avoided in four patients. An indication for surgery was established in another four patients. Interestingly, four of six cases of small-bowel neoplasia were only diagnosed by capsule endoscopy and not predicted by clinical history or previous examinations. Pennazio et al. [44] showed that the results of capsule endoscopy were able to shorten the time to diagnosis and led to definitive treatment in a relevant proportion of patients.

In most cases, the source of obscure gastrointestinal bleeding is located in the small bowel. Resource utilization is significantly higher in small-bowel bleeding in comparison with colonic bleeding [103]. The main disadvantage of capsule endoscopy is that it does not allow tissue sampling or therapeutic intervention. Double-balloon and single-balloon enteroscopy allow therapeutic approaches, are steerable, and can be carried out even in the presence of small-bowel strictures. The two methods appear to be complementary. Capsule endoscopy is often preferred as the initial diagnostic test because of its noninvasiveness, better tolerance, and the ability to view the entire small bowel. It can also be helpful in determining the initial approach for double-balloon enteroscopy. Double-balloon or single-balloon enteroscopy are indicated as the first procedure in patients with active bleeding, in patients with negative capsule

endoscopy, and in patients with capsule endoscopy findings that require biopsy and therapeutic intervention. The main contraindication to capsule endoscopy is suspected or confirmed gastrointestinal obstruction, stricture, or fistula. In patients with massive lower gastrointestinal bleeding and hemodynamic instability, angiography is the diagnostic and therapeutic procedure of choice.

In younger patients who present with acute or chronic lower gastrointestinal bleeding and negative results on capsule endoscopy, a repeated capsule endoscopy or a (bidirectional) double-balloon enteroscopy should be performed, as small-bowel tumors are the most common cause of obscure gastrointestinal bleeding in this group. Intraoperative enteroscopy should be carried out as a last-resort method in patients with obscure gastrointestinal bleeding.

References

1. Longstreth GF. Epidemiology and outcome of patients hospitalized with acute lower gastrointestinal hemorrhage: a population-based study. Am J Gastroenterol 1997;92:419–24.
2. Bramley PN, Masson JW, McKnight G, Herd K, Fraser A, Park K, et al. The role of an open-access bleeding unit in the management of colonic haemorrhage. A 2-year prospective study. Scand J Gastroenterol 1996;31:764–9.
3. Jensen DM, Machicado GA. Colonoscopy for diagnosis and treatment of severe lower gastrointestinal bleeding. Routine outcomes and cost analysis. Gastrointest Endosc Clin N Am 1997;7:477–98.
4. Talley NJ, Jones M. Self-reported rectal bleeding in a United States community: prevalence, risk factors, and health care seeking. Am J Gastroenterol 1998;93:2179–83.
5. Lau WY, Fan ST, Wong SH, Wong KP, Poon GP, Chu KW, et al. Preoperative and intraoperative localisation of gastrointestinal bleeding of obscure origin. Gut 1987;28:869–77.
6. Lewis BS. Small intestinal bleeding. Gastroenterol Clin North Am 1994;23:67–91.
7. Peura DA, Lanza FL, Gostout CJ, Foutch PG. The American College of Gastroenterology Bleeding Registry: preliminary findings. Am J Gastroenterol 1997;92:924–8.
8. Zuckerman GR, Prakash C. Acute lower intestinal bleeding. Part I: clinical presentation and diagnosis. Gastrointest Endosc 1998;48:606–17.

9. Strate, LL, Syngal S. Timing of colonoscopy: impact on length of hospital stay in patients with acute lower intestinal bleeding. Am J Gastroenterol 2003;98:317–22.

10. Velayos FS, Williamson A, Sousa KH, Lung E, Bostrom A, Weber EJ, et al. Early predictors of severe lower gastrointestinal bleeding and adverse outcomes: a prospective study. Clin Gastroenterol Hepatol 2004;2:485–90.

11. Jensen DM, Machicado GA. Diagnosis and treatment of severe hematochezia. The role of urgent colonoscopy after purge. Gastroenterology 1988;95:1569–74.

12. Luk GD, Bynum TE, Hendrix TR. Gastric aspiration in localization of gastrointestinal hemorrhage. JAMA 1979;241:576–8.

13. Cuellar RE, Gavaler JS, Alexander JA, Brouillette DE, Chien MC, Yoo YK, et al. Gastrointestinal tract hemorrhage. The value of a nasogastric aspirate. Arch Intern Med 1990;150:1381–4.

14. ASGE. The role of endoscopy in the patient with lower gastrointestinal bleeding: Guidelines for clinical application. Gastrointest Endosc 1998;48:685–8.

15. Chaudhry V, Hyser MJ, Gracias VH, Gau FC. Colonoscopy: the initial test for acute lower gastrointestinal bleeding. Am Surg 1998;64:723–8.

16. Ohyama T, Sakurai Y, Ito M, Daito K, Sezai S, Sato Y. Analysis of urgent colonoscopy for lower gastrointestinal tract bleeding. Digestion 2000;61:189–92.

17. Schmulewitz N, Fisher DA, Rockey DC. Early colonoscopy for acute lower GI bleeding predicts shorter hospital stay: a retrospective study of experience in a single center. Gastrointest Endosc 2003;58:841–6.

18. Green BT, Rockey DC, Portwood G, Tarnasky PR, Guarisco S, Branch MS, et al. Urgent colonoscopy for evaluation and management of acute lower gastrointestinal hemorrhage: a randomized controlled trial. Am J Gastroenterol 2005;100:2395–402.

19. Angtuaco TL, Reddy SK, Drapkin S, Harrell LE, Howden CW. The utility of urgent colonoscopy in the evaluation of acute lower gastrointestinal tract bleeding: a 2-year experience from a single center. Am J Gastroenterol 2001;96:1782–5.

20. Davila RE, Rajan E, Adler DG, Egan J, Hirota WK, Leighton JA, et al. ASGE Guideline: the role of endoscopy in the patient with lower-GI bleeding. Gastrointest Endosc 2005;62:656–60.

21. Jensen DM, Machicado GA, Jutabha R, Kovacs TO. Urgent colonoscopy for the diagnosis and treatment of severe diverticular hemorrhage. N Engl J Med 2000;342:78–82.

22. Grisolano SW, Darrell SP, Petersen BT. Stigmata associated with recurrence of lower gastrointestinal hemorrhage [abstract]. Gastrointest Endosc 2003;57:AB117.

23. Raju GS, Gerson L, Das A, Lewis B; American Gastroenterological Association. American Gastroenterological Association (AGA) Institute medical position statement on obscure gastrointestinal bleeding. Gastroenterology 2007;133:1694–6.

24. Triester SL, Leighton JA, Leontiadis GI, Gurudu SR, Fleischer DE, Hara AK, et al. A meta-analysis of the yield of capsule endoscopy compared to other diagnostic modalities in patients with non-stricturing small bowel Crohn's disease. Am J Gastroenterol 2006;101:954–64.

25. Yamamoto H, Sekine Y, Sato Y, Higashizawa T, Miyata T, Iino S, et al. Total enteroscopy with a nonsurgical steerable double-balloon method. Gastrointest Endosc 2001;53:216–20.

26. Nakamura M, Niwa Y, Ohmiya N, Miyahara R, Ohashi A, Itoh A, et al. Preliminary comparison of capsule endoscopy and double-balloon enteroscopy in patients with suspected small-bowel bleeding. Endoscopy 2006;38:59–66.

27. Damian U, Schilling D, Hartmann D. Double-balloon enteroscopy (push and pull enteroscopy) of the small bowel: comparison with video capsule endoscopy and magnetic resonance imaging [abstract]. Gastrointest Endosc 2006;63:AB175.

28. Hadithi M, Heine GD, Jacobs MA, van Bodegraven AA, Mulder CJ. A prospective study comparing video capsule endoscopy with double-balloon enteroscopy in patients with obscure gastrointestinal bleeding. Am J Gastroenterol 2006;101:52–7.

29. Matsumoto T, Esaki M, Moriyama T, Nakamura S, Iida M. Comparison of capsule endoscopy and enteroscopy with the double-balloon method in patients with obscure bleeding and polyposis. Endoscopy 2005;37:827–32.

30. Mehdizadeh S, Roos AS, Leighton J. Double-balloon enteroscopy (DBE) compared to capsule endoscopy (CE) among patients with obscure gastrointestinal bleeding (OGIB): a multicenter U.S. experience [abstract]. Gastrointest Endosc 2006;63:AB90.

31. Kameda N, Higuchi K, Shiba M. A prospective trial comparing wireless capsule endoscopy and double-balloon endoscopy in patients with obscure gastrointestinal bleeding [abstract]. Gastrointest Endosc 2006;63:AB162.

32. Zhong J, Ma T, Zhang C, Sun B, Chen S, Cao Y, Wu Y. A retrospective study of the application on double-balloon enteroscopy in 378 patients with suspected small-bowel diseases. Endoscopy 2007;39:208–15.

33. Zhong J, Zhang CL, Ma TL. Comparative study of double-balloon enteroscopy and capsule endoscopy in etiological diagnosis of small intestine bleeding. Zhonghua Xiaohua Zazhi 2004;24:741–4.

34. Ohmiya N, Yano T, Yamamoto H, Arakawa D, Nakamura M, Honda W, et al. Diagnosis and treatment of obscure GI bleeding at double balloon endoscopy. Gastrointest Endosc 2007;66:S72–7.

35. Manabe N, Tanaka S, Fukumoto A, Nakao M, Kamino D, Chayama K. Double-balloon enteroscopy in patients with GI bleeding of obscure origin. Gastrointest Endosc 2006;64:135–40.

36. Mensink PB, Haringsma J, Kucharzik T, Cellier C, Pérez-Cuadrado E, Mönkemüller K, et al. Complications of double balloon enteroscopy: a multicenter survey. Endoscopy 2007;39:613–5.

37. Raju GS, Gerson L, Das A, Lewis B; American Gastroenterological Association. American Gastroenterological Association (AGA) Institute technical review on obscure gastrointestinal bleeding. Gastroenterology 2007;133:1697–717.

38. Douard R, Wind P, Panis Y, Marteau P, Bouhnik Y, Cellier C, et al. Intraoperative enteroscopy for diagnosis and management of unexplained gastrointestinal bleeding. Am J Surg 2000;180:181–4.

39. Zuckerman GR, Prakash C, Askin MP, Lewis BS. AGA technical review on the evaluation and management of occult and obscure gastrointestinal bleeding. Gastroenterology 2000;118:201–21.

40. Iddan G, Meron G, Glukhovsky A, Swain P. Wireless capsule endoscopy. Nature 2000;405:417.

41. Cave DR, Fleischer DE, Leighton JA, Faigel DO, Heigh RI, Sharma VK, et al. A multicenter randomized comparison of the Endocapsule and the PillCam SB. Gastrointest Endosc 2008;68:487–94.

42. Lewis B, Goldfarb N. Review article: The advent of capsule endoscopy—a not-so-futuristic approach to obscure gastrointestinal bleeding. Aliment Pharmacol Ther 2003;17:1085–96.

43. Pennazio M. Bleeding update. Gastrointest Endosc Clin N Am 2006;16:251–66.

44. Pennazio M, Santucci R, Rondonotti E, Abbiati C, Beccari G, Rossini FP, et al. Outcome of patients with obscure gastrointestinal bleeding after capsule endoscopy: report of 100 consecutive cases. Gastroenterology 2004;126:643–53.

45. Bresci G, Parisi G, Bertoni M, Tumino E, Capria A. The role of video capsule endoscopy for evaluating obscure gastrointestinal bleeding: usefulness of early use. J Gastroenterol 2005;40:256–9.

46. May A, Wardak A, Nachbar L, Remke S, Ell C. Influence of patient selection on the outcome of capsule endoscopy in patients with chronic gastrointestinal bleeding. J Clin Gastroenterol 2005;39:684–8.

47. Estévez E, González-Conde B, Vázquez-Iglesias JL, de Los Angeles Vázquez-Millán M, Pértega S, Alonso PA, et al. Diagnostic yield and clinical outcomes after capsule endoscopy in 100 consecutive patients with obscure gastrointestinal bleeding. Eur J Gastroenterol Hepatol 2006;18:881–8.

48. Chen X, Ran ZH, Tong JL. A meta-analysis of the yield of capsule endoscopy compared to double-balloon enteroscopy in patients with small bowel diseases. World J Gastroenterol 2007;13:4372–8.

49. Pasha SF, Leighton JA, Das A, Harrison ME, Decker GA, Fleischer DE, et al. Double-balloon enteroscopy and capsule endoscopy have comparable diagnostic yield in small-bowel disease: a meta-analysis. Clin Gastroenterol Hepatol 2008;6:671–6.

50. Lewis BS, Eisen GM, Friedman S. A pooled analysis to evaluate results of capsule endoscopy trials. Endoscopy 2005;37:960–5.

51. Sears DM, Avots-Avotins A, Culp K, Gavin MW. Frequency and clinical outcome of capsule retention during capsule endoscopy for GI bleeding of obscure origin. Gastrointest Endosc 2004;60:822–7.

52. Pennazio M, Santucci R, Rondonotti E. Wireless capsule endoscopy in patients with obscure gastrointestinal bleeding: results of the Italian multicentre experience [abstract]. Gastrointest Endosc 2002;55:AB125.

53. Albert JG, Schülbe R, Hahn L, Heinig D, Schoppmeyer K, Porst H, et al. Impact of capsule endoscopy on outcome in mid-intestinal bleeding: a multicentre cohort study in 285 patients. Eur J Gastroenterol Hepatol 2008;20:971–7.

54. Chak A, Koehler MK, Sundaram SN, Cooper GS, Canto MI, Sivak MV Jr. Diagnostic and therapeutic impact of push enteroscopy: analysis of factors associated with positive findings. Gastrointest Endosc 1998;47:18–22.

49

55. Delvaux M, Fassler I, Gay G. Clinical usefulness of the endoscopic video capsule as the initial intestinal investigation in patients with obscure digestive bleeding: validation of a diagnostic strategy based on the patient outcome after 12 months. Endoscopy 2004;36:1067–73.

56. Kitiyakara T, Selby W. Non-small-bowel lesions detected by capsule endoscopy in patients with obscure GI bleeding. Gastrointest Endosc 2005;62:234–8.

57. Tang SJ, Christodoulou D, Zanati S, Dubcenco E, Petroniene R, Cirocco M, et al. Wireless capsule endoscopy for obscure gastrointestinal bleeding: a single-centre, one-year experience. Can J Gastroenterol 2004;18:559–65.

58. Descamps C, Schmit A, Van Gossum A. "Missed" upper gastrointestinal tract lesions may explain "occult" bleeding. Endoscopy 1999;31:452–5.

59. Zaman A, Katon RM. Push enteroscopy for obscure gastrointestinal bleeding yields a high incidence of proximal lesions within reach of a standard endoscope. Gastrointest Endosc 1998;47:372–6.

60. Jones BH, Fleischer DE, Sharma VK, Heigh RI, Shiff AD, Hernandez JL, et al. Yield of repeat wireless video capsule endoscopy in patients with obscure gastrointestinal bleeding. Am J Gastroenterol 2005;100:1058–64.

61. Dusold R, Burke K, Carpentier W, Dyck WP. The accuracy of technetium-99m-labeled red cell scintigraphy in localizing gastrointestinal bleeding. Am J Gastroenterol 1994;89:345–8.

62. Zuckerman DA, Bocchini TP, Birnbaum EH. Massive hemorrhage in the lower gastrointestinal tract in adults: diagnostic imaging and intervention. AJR Am J Roentgenol 1993;161:703–11.

63. Nusbaum M, Baum S. Radiographic demonstration of unknown sites of gastrointestinal bleeding. Surg Forum 1963;14:374–5.

64. Fiorito JJ, Brandt LJ, Kozicky O, Grosman IM, Sprayragen S. The diagnostic yield of superior mesenteric angiography: correlation with the pattern of gastrointestinal bleeding. Am J Gastroenterol 1989;84:878–81.

65. Leung WK, Ho SS, Lau JY. Immediate capsule endoscopy or mesenteric angiogram in patients with acute overt obscure bleeding: interim results of a prospective randomized trial [abstract]. Gastrointest Endosc 2007;65:AB125.

66. Egglin TK, O'Moore PV, Feinstein AR, Waltman AC. Complications of peripheral arteriography: a new system to identify patients at increased risk. J Vasc Surg 1995;22:787–94.

67. Junquera F, Quiroga S, Saperas E, Pérez-Lafuente M, Videla S, Alvarez-Castells A, et al. Accuracy of helical computed tomographic angiography for the diagnosis of colonic angiodysplasia. Gastroenterology 2000;119:293–9.

68. Mindelzun RE, Beaulieu CF. Using biphasic CT to reveal gastrointestinal arteriovenous malformations. AJR Am J Roentgenol 1997;168:437–8.

69. Yoon W, Jeong YY, Shin SS, Lim HS, Song SG, Jang NG, et al. Acute massive gastrointestinal bleeding: detection and localization with arterial phase multi-detector row helical CT. Radiology 2006;239:160–7.

70. Kuhle WG, Sheiman RG. Detection of active colonic hemorrhage with use of helical CT: findings in a swine model. Radiology 2003;228:743–52.

71. Ernst O, Bulois P, Saint-Drenant S, Leroy C, Paris JC, Sergent G. Helical CT in acute lower gastrointestinal bleeding. Eur Radiol 2003;13:114–7.

72. Tew K, Davies RP, Jadun CK, Kew J. MDCT of acute lower gastrointestinal bleeding. AJR Am J Roentgenol 2004;182:427–30.

73. Fried AM, Poulos A, Hatfield DR. The effectiveness of the incidental small-bowel series. Radiology 1981;140:45–6.

74. Rabe FE, Becker GJ, Besozzi MJ, Miller RE. Efficacy study of the small bowel examination. Radiology 1981;140:47–50.

75. Costamagna G, Shah SK, Riccioni ME, Foschia F, Mutignani M, Perri V, et al. A prospective trial comparing small bowel radiographs and video capsule endoscopy for suspected small bowel disease. Gastroenterology 2002;123:999–1005.

76. Rex DK, Lappas JC, Maglinte DD, Malczewski MC, Kopecky KA, Cockerill EM. Enteroclysis in the evaluation of suspected small intestinal bleeding. Gastroenterology 1989;97:58–60.

77. Moch A, Herlinger H, Kochman ML, Levine MS, Rubesin SE, Laufer I. Enteroclysis in the evaluation of obscure gastrointestinal bleeding. AJR Am J Roentgenol 1994;163:1381–4.

78. Dixon PM, Roulston ME, Nolan DJ. The small bowel enema: a ten year review. Clin Radiol 1993;47:46–8.

79. Toth E, Fork FT, Almqvist P. Capsule enteroscopy in obscure gastrointestinal bleeding: a prospective comparative study [abstract]. [Paper presented at the Second International Conference on Capsule Endoscopy, Berlin, 23–25 March 2003.]

80. Liangpunsakul S, Chadalawada V, Rex DK, Maglinte D, Lappas J. Wireless capsule endoscopy detects small bowel ulcers in patients with normal results from state of the art enteroclysis. Am J Gastroenterol 2003;98:1295–8.

81. Bessette JR, Maglinte DD, Kelvin FM, Chernish SM. Primary malignant tumors in the small bowel: a comparison of the small-bowel enema and conventional follow-through examination. AJR Am J Roentgenol 1989;153:741–4.

82. Jain TP, Gulati MS, Makharia GK, Bandhu S, Garg PK. CT enteroclysis in the diagnosis of obscure gastrointestinal bleeding: initial results. Clin Radiol 2007;62:660–7.

83. Brearley S, Hawker PC, Dorricott NJ, Lee JR, Ambrose NS, Silverman SH, et al. The importance of laparotomy in the diagnosis and management of intestinal bleeding of obscure origin. Ann R Coll Surg Engl 1986;68:245–8.

84. Rockey DC. Lower gastrointestinal bleeding. Gastroenterology 2006;130:165–71.

85. Zuckerman GR, Prakash C. Acute lower intestinal bleeding. Part II: etiology, therapy, and outcomes. Gastrointest Endosc 1999;49:228–38.

86. Foutch PG, Rex DK, Lieberman DA. Prevalence and natural history of colonic angiodysplasia among healthy asymptomatic people. Am J Gastroenterol 1995;90:564–7.

87. Richter JM, Hedberg SE, Athanasoulis CA, Schapiro RH. Angiodysplasia. Clinical presentation and colonoscopic diagnosis. Dig Dis Sci 1984;29:481–5.

88. Richter JM, Christensen MR, Colditz GA, Nishioka NS. Angiodysplasia. Natural history and efficacy of therapeutic interventions. Dig Dis Sci 1989;34:1542–6.

89. Foutch PG. Angiodysplasia of the gastrointestinal tract. Am J Gastroenterol 1993;88:807–18.

90. Brandt LJ, Spinnell MK. Ability of naloxone to enhance the colonoscopic appearance of normal colon vasculature and colon vascular ectasias. Gastrointest Endosc 1999;49:79–83.

91. Deal SE, Zfass AM, Duckworth PF. Arteriovenous malformations (AVMs): are they concealed by meperidine? [abstract]. Am J Gastroenterol 1991;86:1552.

92. Brandt LJ, Mukhopadhyay D. Masking of colon vascular ectasias by cold water lavage. Gastrointest Endosc 1999;49:141–2.

93. Kjeldsen AD, Kjeldsen J. Gastrointestinal bleeding in patients with hereditary hemorrhagic telangiectasia. Am J Gastroenterol 2000;95:415–8.

94. Longacre AV, Gross CP, Gallitelli M, Henderson KJ, White RI Jr, Proctor DD. Diagnosis and management of gastrointestinal bleeding in patients with hereditary hemorrhagic telangiectasia. Am J Gastroenterol 2003;98:59–65.

95. Teshima T, Hanks GE, Hanlon AL, Peter RS, Schultheiss TE. Rectal bleeding after conformal 3D treatment of prostate cancer: time to occurrence, response to treatment and duration of morbidity. Int J Radiat Oncol Biol Phys 1997;39:77–83.

96. Crook J, Esche B, Futter N. Effect of pelvic radiotherapy for prostate cancer on bowel, bladder, and sexual function: the patient's perspective. Urology 1996;47:387–94.

97. Pardi DS, Loftus EV Jr, Tremaine WJ, Sandborn WJ, Alexander GL, Balm RK, et al. Acute major gastrointestinal hemorrhage in inflammatory bowel disease. Gastrointest Endosc 1999;49:153–7.

98. Belaiche J, Louis E, D'Haens G, Cabooter M, Naegels S, De Vos M, et al. Acute lower gastrointestinal bleeding in Crohn's disease: characteristics of a unique series of 34 patients. Belgian IBD Research Group. Am J Gastroenterol 1999;94:2177–81.

99. Cirocco WC, Reilly JC, Rusin LC. Life-threatening hemorrhage and exsanguination from Crohn's disease. Report of four cases. Dis Colon Rectum 1995;38:85–95.

100. Robert JR, Sachar DB, Greenstein AJ. Severe gastrointestinal hemorrhage in Crohn's disease. Ann Surg 1991;213:207–11.

101. Bini EJ, Weinshel EH, Falkenstein DB. Risk factors for recurrent bleeding and mortality in human immunodeficiency virus infected patients with acute lower GI hemorrhage. Gastrointest Endosc 1999;49:748–53.

102. Chalasani N, Wilcox CM. Etiology and outcome of lower gastrointestinal bleeding in patients with AIDS. Am J Gastroenterol 1998;93:175–8.

103. Prakash C, Zuckerman GR. Acute small bowel bleeding: a distinct entity with significantly different economic implications compared with GI bleeding from other locations. Gastrointest Endosc 2003;58:330–5.

104. Hartmann D, Schmidt H, Bolz G, Schilling D, Kinzel F, Eickhoff A, et al. A prospective two-center study comparing wireless capsule endoscopy with intraoperative enteroscopy in patients with obscure GI bleeding. Gastrointest Endosc 2005;61:826–32.

105. Lewis BS, Kornbluth A, Waye JD. Small bowel tumours: yield of enteroscopy. Gut 1991;32:763–5.

106. Bauditz J, Lochs H. Angiogenesis and vascular malformations: antiangiogenic drugs for treatment of gastrointestinal bleeding. World J Gastroenterol 2007;13:5979–84.

VII

107. Prochorec-Sobieszek M, Windyga J, Maryniak RK, Misiak A, Szczepanik A. Angiodysplasia as a cause of recurrent bleeding from the small bowel in patients with von Willebrand disease. Report of 4 patients. Pol J Pathol 2004;55:173–6.

108. Polese L, D'Incà R, Angriman I, Scarpa M, Pagano D, Ruffolo C, et al. Gastrointestinal telangiectasia: a study by EGD, colonoscopy, and capsule endoscopy in 75 patients. Endoscopy 2008;40:23–9.

109. Redondo-Cerezo E, Gómez-Ruiz CJ, Sánchez-Manjavacas N, Viñuelas M, Jimeno C, Pérez-Vigara G, et al. Long-term follow-up of patients with small-bowel angiodysplasia on capsule endoscopy. Determinants of a higher clinical impact and rebleeding rate. Rev Esp Enferm Dig 2008;100:202–7.

110. Hartmann D, Schmidt H, Schilling D, Kinze F, Eickhoff A, Weickert U, et al. Follow-up of patients with obscure gastrointestinal bleeding after capsule endoscopy and intraoperative enteroscopy. Hepatogastroenterology 2007;54:780–3.

111. Hindryckx P, Botelberge T, De Vos M, De Looze D. Clinical impact of capsule endoscopy on further strategy and long-term clinical outcome in patients with obscure bleeding. Gastrointest Endosc 2008;68:98–104.

112. Maglinte DD, O'Connor K, Bessette J, Chernish SM, Kelvin FM. The role of the physician in the late diagnosis of primary malignant tumors of the small intestine. Am J Gastroenterol 1991;86:304–8.

113. Gourtsoyiannis NC, Bays D, Papaioannou N, Theotokas J, Barouxis G, Karabelas T. Benign tumors of the small intestine: preoperative evaluation with a barium infusion technique. Eur J Radiol 1993;16:115–25.

114. Rondonotti E, Pennazio M, Toth E, Menchen P, Riccioni ME, De Palma GD. Small-bowel neoplasms in patients undergoing video capsule endoscopy: a multicenter European study. Endoscopy 2008;40:488–95.

115. Cobrin GM, Pittman RH, Lewis BS. Increased diagnostic yield of small bowel tumors with capsule endoscopy. Cancer 2006;107:22–7.

116. Ross A, Mehdizadeh S, Tokar J, Leighton JA, Kamal A, Chen A, et al. Double balloon enteroscopy detects small bowel mass lesions missed by capsule endoscopy. Dig Dis Sci 2008;53:2140–3.

117. Matsumoto T, Kudo T, Esaki M, Yano T, Yamamoto H, Sakamoto C, et al. Prevalence of non-steroidal anti-inflammatory drug-induced enteropathy determined by double-balloon endoscopy: a Japanese multicenter study. Scand J Gastroenterol 2008;43:490–6.

118. Allison MC, Howatson AG, Torrance CJ, Lee FD, Russell RI. Gastrointestinal damage associated with the use of nonsteroidal antiinflammatory drugs. N Engl J Med 1992;327:749–54.

119. Goldstein JL, Eisen GM, Lewis B, Gralnek IM, Zlotnick S, Fort JG, et al. Video capsule endoscopy to prospectively assess small bowel injury with celecoxib, naproxen plus omeprazole, and placebo. Clin Gastroenterol Hepatol 2005;3:133–41.

120. Voderholzer WA, Ortner M, Rogalla P, Beinhölzl J, Lochs H. Diagnostic yield of wireless capsule enteroscopy in comparison with computed tomography enteroclysis. Endoscopy 2003;35:1009–14.

121. Swain CP, Mills TN, Shemesh E, Dark JM, Lewin MR, Clifton JS, et al. Which electrode? A comparison of four endoscopic methods of electrocoagulation in experimental bleeding ulcers. Gut 1984;25:1424–31.

122. Busch OR, van Delden OM, Gouma DJ. Therapeutic options for endoscopic haemostatic failures: the place of the surgeon and radiologist in gastrointestinal tract bleeding. Best Pract Res Clin Gastroenterol 2008;22:341–54.

123. Vernava AM 3rd, Moore BA, Longo WE, Johnson FE. Lower gastrointestinal bleeding. Dis Colon Rectum 1997;40:846–58.

124. Rossini FP, Arrigoni A, Pennazio M. Octreotide in the treatment of bleeding due to angiodysplasia of the small intestine. Am J Gastroenterol 1993;88:1424–7.

125. Torsoli A, Annibale B, Viscardi A. Treatment of bleeding due to diffuse angiodysplasia of the small intestine with somatostatin analogue. Eur J Gastroenterol Hepatol 1991;3:785–7.

126. Yoshie K, Fujita Y, Moriya A, Kawana I, Miyamoto K, Umemura S. Octreotide for severe acute bleeding from portal hypertensive colopathy: a case report. Eur J Gastroenterol Hepatol 2001;13:1111–3.

127. Bauditz J, Schachschal G, Wedel S, Lochs H. Thalidomide for treatment of severe intestinal bleeding. Gut 2004;53:609–12.

128. Bauditz J, Lochs H, Voderholzer W. Macroscopic appearance of intestinal angiodysplasias under antiangiogenic treatment with thalidomide. Endoscopy 2006;38:1036–9.

129. Bloomfeld RS, Rockey DC, Shetzline MA. Endoscopic therapy of acute diverticular hemorrhage. Am J Gastroenterol 2001;96:2367–72.

130. Hokama A, Uehara T, Nakayoshi T, Uezu Y, Tokuyama K, Kinjo F, et al. Utility of endoscopic hemoclipping for colonic diverticular bleeding. Am J Gastroenterol 1997;92:543–6.

131. May A, Nachbar L, Pohl J, Ell C. Endoscopic interventions in the small bowel using double balloon enteroscopy: feasibility and limitations. Am J Gastroenterol 2007;102:527–35.

132. Schäfer C, Rothfuss K, Kreichgauer HP, Stange EF. Efficacy of double-balloon enteroscopy in the evaluation and treatment of bleeding and non-bleeding small bowel disease. Z Gastroenterol 2007;45:237–43.

133. Heine GD, Hadithi M, Groenen MJ, Kuipers EJ, Jacobs MA, Mulder CJ. Double-balloon enteroscopy: indications, diagnostic yield, and complications in a series of 275 patients with suspected small-bowel disease. Endoscopy 2006;38:42–8.

134. Suzuki T, Matsushima M, Okita I, Ito H, Gocho S, Tajima H, et al. Clinical utility of double-balloon enteroscopy for small intestinal bleeding. Dig Dis Sci 2007;52:1914–8.

135. Jensen DM, Machicado GA, Cheng S, Jensen ME, Jutabha R. A randomized prospective study of endoscopic bipolar electrocoagulation and heater probe treatment of chronic rectal bleeding from radiation telangiectasia. Gastrointest Endosc 1997;45:20–5.

136. Barnert J. Acute and chronic lower gastrointestinal bleeding. In: Messmann H, editor. Atlas of colonoscopy: examination techniques and diagnosis. New York: Thieme Medical Publishers; 2006. p. 118–42.

137. Fantin AC, Zala G, Risti B, Debatin JF, Schöpke W, Meyenberger C. Bleeding anorectal varices: successful treatment with transjugular intrahepatic portosystemic shunting (TIPS). Gut 1996;38:932–5.

138. Chung IK, Kim EJ, Lee MS, Kim HS, Park SH, Lee MH, et al. Bleeding Dieulafoy's lesions and the choice of endoscopic method: comparing the hemostatic efficacy of mechanical and injection methods. Gastrointest Endosc 2000;52:721–4.

139. May A, Nachbar L, Ell C. Double-balloon enteroscopy (push-and-pull enteroscopy) of the small bowel: feasibility and diagnostic and therapeutic yield in patients with suspected small bowel disease. Gastrointest Endosc 2005;62:62–70.

140. Hirana H, Atsumi M, Sawai N. A case of ulcerative colitis with local bleeding treated by endoscopic injection of absolute ethanol and 1% polidocanol. Gastroenterol Endosc 1999;4:969–73.

141. Yoshida Y, Kawaguchi A, Mataki N, Matsuzaki K, Hokari R, Iwai A, et al. Endoscopic treatment of massive lower GI hemorrhage in two patients with ulcerative colitis. Gastrointest Endosc 2001;54:779–81.

142. Beejay U, Marcon NE. Endoscopic treatment of lower gastrointestinal bleeding. Curr Opinion Gastroenterol 2002;18:87–93.

143. Jensen DM, Jutabha R, Machicado GA, Jensen ME, Cheng S, Gornbein J, et al. Prospective randomized comparative study of bipolar electrocoagulation versus heater probe for treatment of chronically bleeding internal hemorrhoids. Gastrointest Endosc 1997;46:435–43.

144. Lai LH, Wong GL, Chow DK, Lau JY, Sung JJ, Leung WK. Long-term follow-up of patients with obscure gastrointestinal bleeding after negative capsule endoscopy. Am J Gastroenterol 2006;101:1224–8.

145. Neu B, Ell C, May A, Schmid E, Riemann JF, Hagenmüller F, et al. Capsule endoscopy versus standard tests in influencing management of obscure digestive bleeding: results from a German multicenter trial. Am J Gastroenterol 2005;100:1736–42.

146. Gubler C, Fox M, Hengstler P, Abraham D, Eigenmann F, Bauerfeind P. Capsule endoscopy: impact on clinical decision making in patients with suspected small bowel bleeding. Endoscopy 2007;39:1031–6.

49

50 Anorectal Disease

Joep F.W.M. Bartelsman

Proctitis

Proctitis, or inflammation of the rectum, has several infectious and noninfectious causes (**Table 50.1**). The symptoms and endoscopic appearance of many of these diseases can mimic other conditions and may pose diagnostic difficulties.

Infectious Proctitis

Sexually transmitted proctitis (STP) is common and should be considered when there are rectal symptoms in men who have sex with men. It should also be considered in women if there is a history of anal sex [1,2]. It may be caused by one or several pathogens (**Table 50.2**). The incidence of infectious proctitis and proctocolitis has decreased with the emergence of acquired immune deficiency syndrome (AIDS) and the identification of the human immunodeficiency virus (HIV), leading to a decline in the size of the sexually active subpopulation of homosexual men and the advocation of safer sexual practices. The rates of rectal gonococcal infections decreased dramatically from 1985 to 1995. In Europe and North America, however, the frequency of proctitis caused by lymphogranuloma venereum (LGV) has increased since 2003, particularly in HIV-infected men [3–7].

Gonorrhea

Gonorrhea is often asymptomatic. Symptoms, constipation, pruritus ani, and mucopurulent anal discharge arise about 7 days after exposure [7]. The endoscopic appearance of the rectal mucosa may be normal, but often the mucosa is erythematous and friable, with visible pus. Gram-negative diplococci are visible within the cytoplasm of neutrophilic granulocytes. The sensitivity of a rectal smear is only 60%. Culture for *Neisseria gonorrhoeae* from a swab is still the gold standard for the diagnosis.

Treatment. A single dose of antibiotics—cefixime 400 mg orally, ceftriaxone 250 mg i.m., or spectinomycin 2 g i.m.

Chlamydial Infection

Chlamydia trachomatis (serovars D–K) can cause mild proctitis, comparable with gonorrhea, with mild symptoms of pruritus ani and anal mucopurulent discharge. The rectal mucosa may be normal or erythematous and friable. The diagnosis is made by detecting specific DNA sequences in nucleic acid amplification tests (NAATs) in rectal material. Serologic testing can support the diagnosis [8,9].

Treatment. Azithromycin 1 g orally in a single dose or doxycycline 100 mg twice daily for 7 days.

Lymphogranuloma venereum (LGV) is caused by *Chlamydia trachomatis* serovars L1, L2, and L3. These LGV strains cause a severe proctitis, with severe symptoms of pain, tenesmus, constipation, and bloodstained anal discharge, often accompanied by systemic features—fever, myalgia, arthralgia, malaise, and anorexia. LGV can mimic Crohn's disease, due to the development of perianal fistulas and the endoscopic appearance, with friable rectal mucosa and small erosions or ulcers in the distal 10–15 cm of the rectum [9,10] (**Fig. 50.1**). Biopsies may show granulomatous inflammation, inflammatory cell infiltrates, and crypt abscesses. In contrast to non-LGV chlamydial infections, there are probably no asymptomatic carriers of LGV [11]. A diagnosis of LGV is made by genotyping of positive NAAT material. Polymerase chain reaction (PCR) on rectal biopsy material may detect chlamydial DNA that may not be identified on a swab sample [12]. Positive serology can support the diagnosis.

Treatment. Doxycycline 100 mg orally twice daily for 21 days, tetracycline 500 mg orally four times per day for 21 days, or erythromycin 500 mg orally four times per day for 21 days. It is recommended that a hepatitis C virus RNA test and serological tests for syphilis and HIV should be performed at the time of the LGV diagnosis and 1, 3, and 6 months later [2].

Table 50.1 Causes of proctitis

| Infectious proctitis (see **Table 50.2**) |
| Radiation proctitis |
| Ischemic proctitis |
| Prolapse proctitis |
| • Colitis cystica profunda |
| • Solitary rectal ulcer syndrome (SRUS) |
| Idiopathic hemorrhagic proctitis (ulcerative colitis) |

Table 50.2 Causes of infectious proctitis and proctocolitis

| **Causes of distal proctitis** |
| Neisseria gonorrhoeae |
| Chlamydia trachomatis |
| • Genotype A–K |
| • Genotype L (lymphogranuloma venereum) |
| Treponema pallidum |
| Herpes simplex virus |
| **Causes of proctocolitis** |
| Entamoeba histolytica |
| Campylobacter spp. |
| Salmonella spp. |
| Shigella spp. |
| Cryptosporidium spp. |
| Cytomegalovirus |

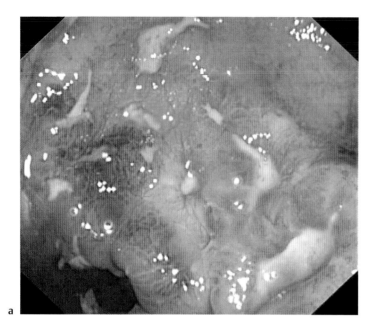

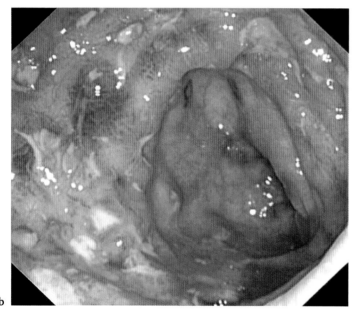

Fig. 50.1a, b Lymphogranuloma venereum (LGV) proctitis: multiple sharply demarcated ulcerations are visible in the rectum.

Syphilis

In active men who have sex with men, syphilis should be considered whenever anorectal lesions are found. In Western countries, the incidence of rectal syphilis is rising in these risk groups [1,2]. Primary rectal syphilis is usually asymptomatic, but it may present as proctitis, rectal ulcer, or pseudotumor [13,14]. Along with tuberculosis and cytomegalovirus infections, syphilis is one of the great masqueraders, which can present as a nonspecific proctitis, not unlike other types of proctitis. The classic anorectal chancre is painless, with well-demarcated indurated edges and a clean base. Generalized rash, fever, and lymphadenopathy may be present. The diagnosis can be made by dark-field microscopy for treponemes, or NAAT for *Treponema pallidum* DNA from biopsies or exudates from an ulcer. Serological tests such as an immunoglobulin G (IgG) anti-treponemal antibody enzyme immunoassay can support the diagnosis. All patients with syphilis should be tested for HIV.

Treatment. Benzathine penicillin 2.4 million units i.m., or in patients allergic to penicillin: doxycycline 100 mg twice daily for 2 weeks.

Herpes Simplex Virus (HSV)

Anorectal HSV infection can be acquired by oral–anal contact or anal intercourse. Most infections are caused by HSV type 2. HSV type 1 accounts for 13% of rectal infections and reflects oro-anal transmission [1,2,9]. A primary infection can involve the perianal skin and extend into the rectum. Patients present with severe proctitis—severe pain, tenesmus, anal discharge, and constipation. In many patients with primary HSV infection, neurological symptoms are present—sacral paresthesia, urinary retention, and impotence. Perianal inspection may reveal vesicles or pustules. Proctoscopy can be painful. The rectal mucosa is friable, with multiple erosions or ulcers in the distal part of the rectum. A large solitary ulcer is sometimes present. The diagnosis can be confirmed by nucleic acid amplification by PCR. Cultures are less sensitive for the diagnosis.

Treatment. Acyclovir 200 mg five times daily for 5 days.

CMV Infection

CMV infection is an important complication in immunocompromised patients, with significant morbidity and mortality. CMV can cause proctocolitis or proctitis. The mucosal lesions in CMV proctitis are due to vasculitis with capillary occlusion, thrombosis, and ischemia: multiple red spots, caused by dilated capillaries in the superficial mucosal layer, and multiple ulcerations [15]. A large solitary ulcer is sometimes present (**Fig. 50.2**). The diagnosis is made by the finding of typical intranuclear inclusion bodies in rectal biopsies taken from the ulcer base.

Treatment. Ganciclovir 10–15 mg/kg daily for 2–3 weeks.

Ischemic Proctitis

Ischemic proctitis is rare. The rectum is spared in most patients with ischemic colitis, because of its abundant collateral vascular supply [16]. Ischemic proctitis accounts for only 5% of cases of ischemic colitis. In most cases, a specific cause is reported, such as vascular surgery or radiotherapy [17,18]. Cocaine can also induce focal rectal ischemia. Vasoconstriction may be the main mechanism in the pathogenesis. In the acute phase, the rectal mucosa is swollen, with large ulcerations. Chronic ischemic proctitis should be suspected whenever ulcer formation is observed endoscopically in the context of atrophic mucosa and multiple whitish scars, with mucosal crypt atrophy and fibrosis evident in biopsy specimens (**Fig. 50.3**).

Treatment of ischemic proctitis depends on the level of ischemia and the underlying cause. Superficial mucosal ischemia can be treated conservatively. In cases of necrosis of the rectal wall and signs of sepsis or perforation, surgery is indicated.

Radiation Proctitis

Chronic radiation proctitis is often seen in patients who have undergone radiotherapy for pelvic malignancies such as carcinoma of the prostate, rectum, and bladder, or gynecologic tumors [19]. Symptoms usually start within the first 2 years after treatment. The

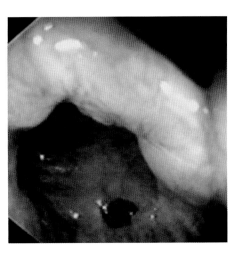
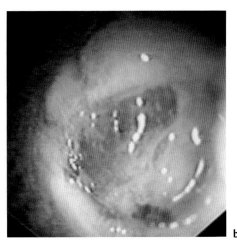

Fig. 50.2a, b A large round solitary ulcer in the distal part of the rectum, caused by cytomegalovirus infection.

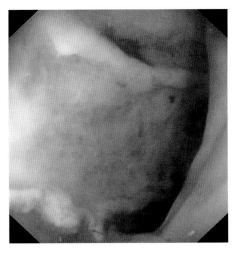
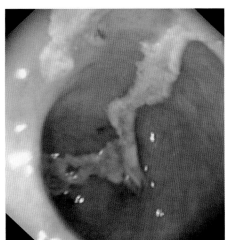

Fig. 50.3a, b Large rectal ulcerations caused by ischemic proctitis after embolization of the hypogastric artery.

50

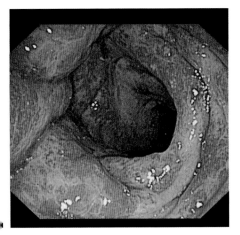
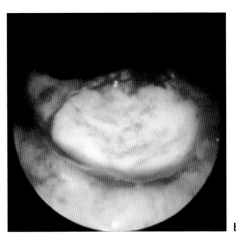

Fig. 50.4
a Radiation proctitis: friable mucosa with multiple telangiectasias.
b Radiation proctitis: a large chronic ischemic ulcer.

etiology of radiation proctitis is chronic mucosal ischemia caused by tissue fibrosis and obliterative endarteritis. The main symptom of radiation proctitis is rectal bleeding due to mucosal friability and neovascular telangiectasias. Rectal pain can be caused by multiple or solitary ulcers. Tenesmus, urgency, increased bowel movements, and occasionally fecal incontinence are caused by decreased rectal compliance. Various endoscopic scoring systems for the endoscopic appearance of radiation proctitis have been used to assess mucosal friability, telangiectasias, and mucosal ulcerations [20], or only for the presence and density of telangiectasias [19] (**Fig. 50.4**).

Treatment. Patients with mild symptoms can be treated conservatively with simple measures such as stool softeners and, in case of anemia, oral iron preparations. However, the majority of patients present with severe hemorrhagic proctitis, which is usually refractory to topical treatment with steroids, 5-aminosalicylic acid, or sucralfate. Other treatment modalities are hyperbaric oxygen therapy and endoscopic therapy with laser or bipolar heater probes.

Currently, the most effective options are topical formalin and argon plasma coagulation (APC) [21,22]. Formalin is administered as a 2% retention enema, prepared by adding 5 mL of commercially available 40% formalin to 100 mL of normal saline. APC is used with an argon flow rate between 1.0 and 1.5 L/min and a voltage of 40–50 W. Single or repeat pulses of less than 1 s are used until the superficial mucosa starts to appear whitish in color and the bleeding stops. Each pulse introduces argon into the bowel, and periodic suctioning is required to deflate the rectum. The aim is to continue APC treatment until there are no more visible bleeding areas or telangiectasis. Often, repeat treatment sessions are necessary after an interval of 2–4 weeks.

Solitary Rectal Ulcer Syndrome

Solitary rectal ulcer syndrome (SRUS) is an uncommon disease of the rectum, characterized by single or multiple ulcerations of the rectal mucosa, associated with symptoms of rectal bleeding, straining on defecation, tenesmus, a sensation of incomplete defecation, and constipation [23–27]. Endoscopically, a single ulcer or sometimes multiple ulcers can be found, mostly located anteriorly 3–10 cm from the anal margin (**Fig. 50.5a, b**). The ulcer is covered by a white, gray, or yellowish slough. The adjacent mucosa can be nodular or granular. SRUS may appear as a polypoid lesion in about 30% of cases (**Fig. 50.5c, d**). In biopsies, SRUS is characterized by erosion of the mucosa, hyperplasia and distortion of the crypt architecture, and fibromuscular obliteration of the lamina propria. The muscularis mucosae is thickened. Misplaced epithelial glandular elements in the submucosa may undergo cystic dilation due to retention of mucin (colitis cystica profunda). It is important to differentiate SRUS from other causes of solitary or multiple ulcers in the rectum (**Table 50.3**).

Table 50.3 Differential diagnosis of solitary rectal ulcer

Inflammatory bowel disease: Crohn's disease, ulcerative colitis

Infection: amebiasis, LGV-type *Chlamydia*, syphilis, CMV, HSV

Malignancy: non-Hodgkin's lymphoma

Ischemia

Radiation

Drug-induced: suppositories, NSAIDs, ergotamine

Stercoral ulcer

Trauma

Colitis cystica profunda

CMV, cytomegalovirus; HSV, herpes simplex virus; LGV, lymphogranuloma venereum; NSAIDs, nonsteroidal anti-inflammatory drugs.

The underlying etiology and pathophysiology are still not completely understood. Rectal prolapse and paradoxical contraction of the puborectal muscle during defecation have been described, resulting in trauma and compression of the anterior rectal wall. This may lead to repeated ischemia of the rectal mucosa, followed by ulceration and fibrosis. However, only a minority of patients with overt rectal prolapse develop SRUS, and mucosal intussusception and rectal prolapse were found in only a minority of patients with SRUS [24]. Most patients with SRUS demonstrate dyssynergia, rectal hypersensitivity, and impaired evacuation in comparison with control individuals.

Treatment. SRUS is difficult to treat and often persists or recurs after treatment. The first step in the treatment is high intake of fluids

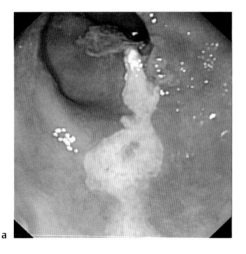
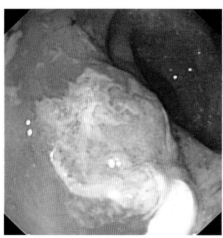

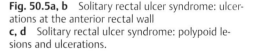
Fig. 50.5a, b Solitary rectal ulcer syndrome: ulcerations at the anterior rectal wall
c, d Solitary rectal ulcer syndrome: polypoid lesions and ulcerations.

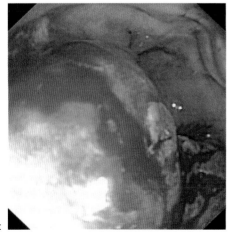
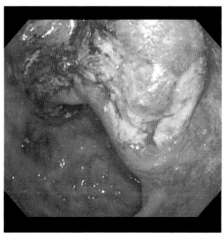

a

b

c

d

and dietary fibers, laxatives, and enemas, and teaching patients to avoid straining on defecation. The second step is biofeedback therapy, which has been shown to lead to improvement of symptoms, anorectal function, and rectal mucosal blood flow and can facilitate healing of ulcerations [12,28,29]. There is a limited place for surgery, with excision of the ulcer, treatment of rectal prolapse by low anterior resection, or rectopexy and colostomy. However, the results of surgical treatment for SRUS are mostly disappointing [23].

Anal Fissure

Anal fissure is a linear tear in the dermal lining of the anal canal, extending from the pectinate line to the anal verge. An acute tear in the mucosa is analogous to a "split lip" of the anus. A fissure is defined as chronic when it remains symptomatic for more than 8 weeks, or when involvement through the submucosa or internal anal sphincter occurs, often accompanied by a sentinel perianal skin tag and a hypertrophic anal papilla [30,31]. Anal fissures are commonly seen in the posterior midline (**Fig. 50.6**). Fissures located off the midline suggest the presence of an underlying disease such as anal cancer, Crohn's disease, syphilis, or tuberculosis.

Constipation is the main predisposing factor for anal fissures. Although the exact mechanism leading to chronic anal fissure is not yet fully understood, current etiological studies are focusing on the tonicity of the internal anal sphincter (IAS) and anal blood flow. Inadequate blood flow in the region of the posterior midline of the anus has been considered to play a major role in the development of anal fissures. Anal sphincter hypertonia may compromise the blood flow even further. This may explain why treatments that improve anal blood flow are associated with better healing rates [32,33].

Anal fissures cause severe pain during and after defecation, with associated fresh red blood on toilet paper or feces. The diagnosis is based on the specific symptoms in combination with physical examination—a visible tear or a sentinel skin tag in combination with a painful rectal examination. Proctoscopy is very painful and not necessary.

Treatment. The treatment of anal fissures is based on the treatment of constipation by diet and laxatives and measures to lower the elevated anal sphincter tone using topical or oral agents, injection therapy, or surgery.
- Initial therapy includes fiber-rich diet (25–30 g of fiber daily) with at least 2 L of fluid daily.
- Topical anesthetics, such as lidocaine 2%, provide variable pain relief and have been shown to be effective in curing anal fissures.
- Glyceryl trinitrate (GTN) and isosorbide dinitrate (ISDN), used in ointments in doses ranging between 0.2% and 0.8%, are able to reduce anal sphincter pressure and show healing rates of about 50%. Problems with topical GTN and ISDN are the short duration of the effect, requiring frequent administration up to six times a day, and the frequent side effects of headache. Topical diltiazem (2%), two to four times daily, has shown equivalent healing rates in comparison with GTN, but with fewer side effects. Diltiazem may also heal 50% of fissures in patients in whom GTN therapy has previously failed.
- Injections with botulinum A toxin are also able to reduce anal sphincter pressure and improve the local blood flow. Healing rates of up to 80%, better than GTN in comparative studies, have been reported, but recurrences are also seen [30]. Botulinum toxin is usually administered at a dosage of 20 U in one to four injections. The ideal location for the injections is not yet clear. The injections are expensive and can be very painful and complicated by temporary fecal incontinence.

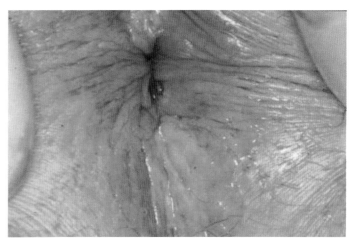

Fig. 50.6 Anal fissure.

Hemorrhoids

Hemorrhoids are enlarged vascular cushions within the anal canal that are fed directly by arteriovenous communications. These cushions are supported by a connective-tissue framework. The combination of weakening of the supporting framework and repeated passage of hard stool and straining can lead to prolapse, bleeding, and thrombosis [34,35]. Hemorrhoids can be classified according to their relation to the pectinate line, which demarcates the transition between the columnar and squamous epithelium within the anal canal. Internal hemorrhoids originate above the pectinate line and external hemorrhoids below it (**Fig. 50.7**). Internal hemorrhoids are classified into four stages, based on the degree of prolapse (**Table 50.4**).

The most common symptom is painless rectal blood loss. Internal hemorrhoids can also cause pruritus, swelling, discharge, and soiling. External hemorrhoids can cause severe anal pain if the hemorrhoid is thrombosed. The diagnosis is easily made on physical examination, followed by rectal examination and proctoscopy. It is important to ask the patient to strain during the examination. Hemorrhoids have to be differentiated from other causes of bleeding from the anal canal such as fissures, tumor, warts, or prolapse. Patients over the age of 40 with rectal blood loss and suspected hemorrhoids as the cause require an additional colonoscopy to exclude colorectal cancer or inflammatory bowel disease.

Treatment. Fiber supplements improve symptoms and bleeding and should be recommended in all stages of hemorrhoidal disease [36,37]. A variety of topical ointments are available and contain a combination of local anesthetics, corticosteroids, and vasoconstrictants. These can sometimes relieve symptoms of pruritus, pain, and discomfort, but no randomized controlled trials are available to support their use. Flavonoids as a dietary supplement have been used as a treatment to reduce congestion and inflammation, but the benefit of this treatment in hemorrhoidal disease is doubtful.

Rubber-band ligation is the most effective outpatient treatment for patients with second- and third-degree internal hemorrhoids. The ligator is introduced into the proctoscope, suction is applied, and the mucosa is drawn into the ligator. Next, a rubber band is pushed over the captured mucosa, the suction is released, and the ligator is removed. Generally, three rubber bands are placed. The bands should be applied above the pectinate line to minimize pain (**Fig. 50.7**). If the patient experiences severe pain directly afterwards, the band can be removed. Mild to moderate complications are seen in about 10% of cases, with discomfort, pain, and slight

50

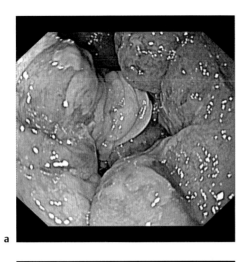

a

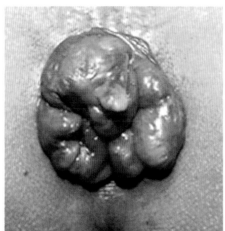

b

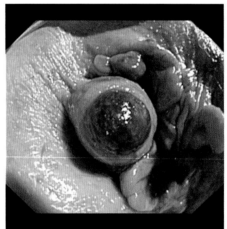

c

d

Fig. 50.7
a Internal hemorrhoids, seen from the rectum (in retroflex visualization).
b Prolapsing hemorrhoids.
c After rubber band ligation.
d External hemorrhoid with thrombus.

Table 50.4 Internal hemorrhoids

Grade 1	Visible in the anal canal, but not prolapsing
Grade 2	Protruding outside the anal canal during straining, but returning spontaneously
Grade 3	Protruding outside the anal canal and requiring manual repositioning
Grade 4	Protruding outside the anal canal and not reducible

bleeding. All patients should be aware of the possibility of severe delayed hemorrhage 5–10 days after the procedure.

Sclerotherapy can be successful in the treatment of first-degree and small second-degree internal hemorrhoids, which are too small to treat with rubber-band ligation. Various solutions are now used, such as 5% oily phenol or 5% sodium morrhuate; 1–2 mL of the sclerosant is injected into the submucosal space. Sclerotherapy is less used nowadays than banding, due to a higher failure rate.

Infrared coagulation involves the application of infrared light to the tissue for 1.5 s, resulting in destruction of the mucosa and submucosa at the application site. It is associated with few complications, but appears to be less effective than banding.

Cryosurgery, bipolar diathermy, and electrotherapy have been used in the past, but are probably less effective than band ligation, sclerotherapy, and infrared coagulation.

Surgical treatment is reserved for grade four hemorrhoids or for lower-grade hemorrhoids that have not responded to conservative treatment. There are several surgical techniques—open and closed hemorrhoidectomy, Doppler ultrasound-guided hemorrhoidal artery ligation, and stapled hemorrhoidopexy.

Thrombosed external hemorrhoids can cause severe debilitating perianal pain. A painful, edematous, bluish and firm mass can be seen during perianal inspection (**Fig. 50.7d**). Sitz baths, ice packs, stool softeners and oral analgesia are usually sufficient, but prompt surgical excision of the thrombus can shorten the recovery period.

External hemorrhoidal skin tags are symptom-free, but may interfere with anal hygiene. If a patient has tags associated with symptoms, another process must be excluded, such as perianal Crohn's disease or carcinoma.

Rectal Prolapse

Rectal prolapse is a distressing condition that most commonly occurs in older women [37]. A complete prolapse is defined as the protrusion of all layers of the rectal wall through the anal canal, with concentric folds evident (**Fig. 50.8**). This appearance is different from the smaller radial folds seen with prolapsing hemorrhoids or distal rectal mucosal prolapse. The protrusion is usually smaller than 15 cm. The protruding mucosa is mostly edematous and vulnerable, with small ulcerations. It is possible to push the prolapse back, unless there is strangulation. Passage of mucus and blood is common. Most patients also have symptoms of fecal incontinence and constipation. In patients in whom overt prolapse is not visible, it can be provoked by a Valsalva maneuver and straining. Often this is only possible if the patient stands, squats, or sits over a toilet while straining. Video defecography can be a useful additional test in evaluating rectal prolapse, to delineate the extent of the prolapse and the presence of associated rectoceles.

Treatment. A complete rectal prolapse can only be treated with surgery. Several operations have been described; the two main approaches are perianal and abdominal, and with each procedure there is a choice for resection or not. Transabdominal rectopexy with or without resection has the lowest recurrence rate. Laparoscopic surgery appears to have similar outcomes to those of open operations. Perianal operations for rectal prolapse are the safest option, but are more often associated with recurrences.

Condylomata Acuminata (Genital Warts)

Condylomata vary from very small lesions to large cauliflower-like lesions on the perianal skin, in the anal canal and transitional epithelium of the distal rectum [37,38] (**Fig. 50.9**). Patients with perianal condyloma may also have such lesions on the penis or vulva, vagina, cervix, and distal urethra. Genital warts are the commonest viral sexually transmitted disease in the Western world. Human papillomavirus (HPV) is the causative agent. HPV types 6 and 11 (with a low oncogenic risk) cause the vast majority of genital warts.

The symptoms of warts vary from no symptoms at all to bleeding and anal wetness. The HPV types that generally cause genital warts do not cause cancer, but some patients are co-infected with high oncogenic risk types. Most of the warts are diagnosed by perianal inspection, but proctoscopy should be performed to assess the anal canal and distal rectum and to rule out associated sexually transmitted diseases of the rectum.

Treatment. Many methods of treating condylomata acuminata have been described—topical methods with caustic or cytotoxic substances, cryotherapy, and more invasive techniques such as electrocautery, laser, and surgical excision. However, recurrences are frequent after all kinds of treatment. The initial treatment of choice is based on the number and location of the lesions. If only a few warts are seen on the perianal skin, and if the lesions are less than 2 mm in size, the initial treatment is local therapy with bi- or trichloroacetic acid every 2–3 weeks. Patients with more extensive lesions or intra-anal lesions and those in whom there is concern regarding anal intraepithelial neoplasia are treated with excision and fulguration. The frequency of follow-up examinations depends on the rapidity with which new warts appear. Appropriate treatment generally clears most warts within 3 months, and it is advisable to see these patients annually for a repeat examination.

Extremely large forms of genital warts are known as giant condylomata acuminata or Buschke–Loewenstein tumors [39]. Most reports favor initial surgical treatment for these giant lesions. Skin grafts may be necessary if a large skin defect is present after excision. Chemotherapy and radiotherapy should only be used in cases of disease recurrence.

Anal Cancer

Histologically, the pectinate line within the anal canal is the border between the proximal columnar epithelium and the external squamous epithelium (**Fig. 50.10**). Lesions distal to the pectinate line typically drain via the inguinal pathway, and lesions proximal to the pectinate line drain abdominally via the mesorectum and pelvic vessels [37]. Squamous cell carcinoma is the most common tumor arising in the anal canal. Variants of squamous cell carcinoma, such as transitional cell carcinoma, basaloid carcinoma, large cell carcinoma, mucoepidermoid carcinoma, and cloacogenic carcinoma have a natural history, patterns of spread, and prognosis similar to those of squamous cell carcinoma [40]. Depending on their location in relation to the pectinate line, tumors arising in the anal canal can

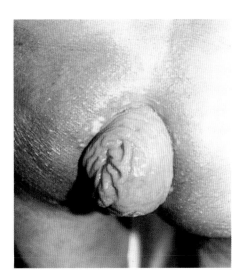

Fig. 50.8 Rectal prolapse.

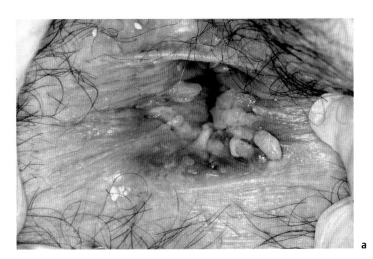

a

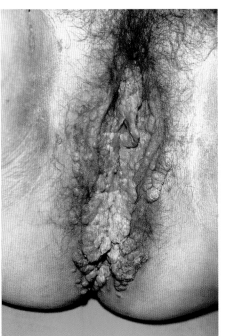

b

Fig. 50.9a, b Condylomata acuminata.

50

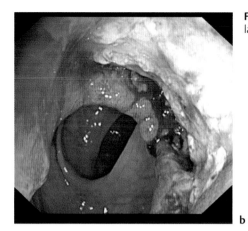

Fig. 50.10a, b   Anal squamous cell carcinoma: a large tumor with central ulceration.

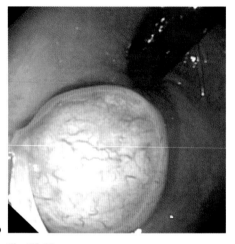
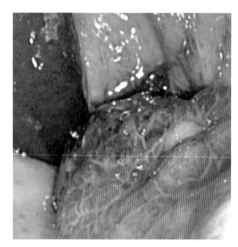
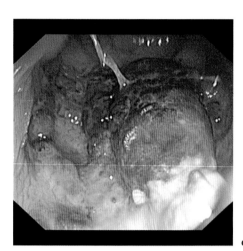

Fig. 50.11
a   A tumor in the distal rectum, covered with normal mucosa: non-Hodgkin's lymphoma.
b, c   A dark red tumor in the distal part of the rectum: Kaposi's sarcoma.

be keratinizing or nonkeratinizing, but both types appear to have similar biology, prognosis, and treatment. However, adenocarcinomas should be treated in the same way as rectal cancers [40,41].

Multiple risk factors, including human papillomavirus (HPV) infection, receptive anal intercourse, cigarette smoking, and immunosuppression have been identified. HIV infection is also associated with anal cancer. There are increasing numbers of HIV-positive patients being diagnosed with the disease. Anal squamous cell carcinoma has to be differentiated from other tumors in the anorectal area: adenocarcinoma, non-Hodgkin's lymphoma, carcinoid, and Kaposi's sarcoma (**Fig. 50.11**).

Most patients with squamous cell carcinoma of the anus present with rectal bleeding. Other symptoms include rectal pain and mass sensation. The diagnosis can be delayed, as blood loss is often ascribed to hemorrhoids. Patients with anal cancer should undergo both physical and radiographic evaluation, including abdominal and pelvic CT scans, and inguinal nodes and any enlarged node should be biopsied to guide further treatment. Recent reports have suggested that FDG-PET scanning can provide better sensitivity in identifying nodal metastases.

Chemoradiotherapy is the standard of care for most patients with squamous cell carcinoma of the anal canal. Intensity-modulated radiotherapy appears to be a promising approach for reducing treatment-related toxicity in anal cancer patients. Intensity-modulated radiotherapy involves the use of computer-aided optimization to design radiation treatment plans that deliver the radiotherapy dose to the target in a highly conformal manner while minimizing the dose to adjacent normal tissues [41]. Abdominoperineal resection is now reserved as salvage therapy for those patients with persistent or recurrent disease after combined chemoradiation.

Anal Intraepithelial Neoplasia

Anal intraepithelial neoplasia is the precursor dysplastic lesion for anal cancer [37,42,43]. Anal intraepithelial neoplasia is classified as grade 1 (low-grade dysplasia) or grades 2 or 3 (high-grade dysplasia). It is believed that the natural progression of dysplasia is from low grade to high grade, with some lesions transforming into invasive squamous cancer. Prolonged microscopic and histological follow-up studies of persistent anal intraepithelial neoplasia grade 3 lesions in the anal canal have shown a sudden change in appearance, with the lesions becoming thickened and palpable and a histological conversion from anal intraepithelial neoplasia grade 3 to carcinoma in situ. The prevalence of anal HPV infection in men who have sex with men of all age groups is high; about 20% have high-risk (oncogenic) HPV in the anal canal.

Taking anal smears using a swab is a well-validated investigation method, with sensitivity and specificity rates comparable to those in cervical cytology. It is advisable for patients with all grades of abnormal lesion to undergo high-resolution anoscopy every 6 months, similar to colposcopy, to identify areas of anal intraepithelial neoplasia.

Successful treatments for small to medium-sized high-grade lesions include trichloroacetic acid, infrared coagulation, and laser. Topical agents for multifocal disease include imiquimod and cidofovir.

References

1. Rompalo AM. Diagnosis and treatment of sexually acquired proctitis and proctocolitis: an update. Clin Infect Dis 1999;28(Suppl 1):S84–90.
2. McMillan A, van Voorst Vader PC, de Vries HJ. Guideline. The 2007 European Guideline (International Union against Sexually Transmitted Infections/World Health Organization) on the management of proctitis, proctocolitis and enteritis caused by sexually transmissible pathogens. Int J STD AIDS 2007;18:514–20.
3. Nieuwenhuis RF, Ossewaarde JM, Götz HM, Dees J, Bing Thio H, Thomeer MGJ, et al. Resurgence of lymphogranuloma venereum in western Europe: an outbreak of Chlamydia trachomatis serovar L2 proctitis in the Netherlands among men who have sex with men. Clin Infect Dis 2004;39:996–1003.
4. Stary G, Stary A. Lymphogranuloma venereum outbreak in Europe. J Dtsch Dermatol Ges 2008;6:935–40.
5. Kapoor S. Re-emergence of lymphogranuloma venereum. J Eur Acad Dermatol Venereal 2008;22:409–16.
6. Jebbari H, Alexander S, Ward H, Evans B, Solomou M, Thornton A, et al. Update on lymphogranuloma venereum in the United Kingdom. Sex Transm Infect 2007;83:324–6.
7. Hamill M, Benn P, Carder C, Copas A, Ward H, Ison C, et al. The clinical manifestation of anorectal infection with lymphogranuloma venereum (LGV) versus non-LGV strains of Chlamydia trachomatis: a case–control study in homosexual men. Int J STD AIDS 2007;18:472–5.
8. McLean CA, Stoner BP, Workowski KA. Treatment of lymphogranuloma venereum. Clin Infect Dis 2007;44:S147–52.
9. Hamlyn E, Taylor C. Sexually transmitted proctitis. Postgrad Med J 2006;82:733–36.
10. Ina K, Kusugami K, Ohta M. Bacterial hemorrhagic enterocolitis. J Gastroenterol 2003;38:111–20.
11. Tinmouth J, Gilmour MW, Kovacs C, Kropp R, Mitterni L, Rachlis A, et al. Is there a reservoir of sub-clinical lymphogranuloma venereum and non-LGV Chlamydia trachomatis infection in men who have sex with men? Int J STD AIDS 2008;19:805–9.
12. Davis BT, Thiim M, Zukerberg LR. Case 2-2006: A 31-year-old, HIV-positive man with rectal pain. N Eng J Med 2006;354:284–9.
13. Furman DL, Patel SK, Arluk GM. Endoscopic and histologic appearance of rectal syphilis. Gastrointest Endosc 2008;67:161–2.
14. Song SH, Jang I, Kim BS, Kim ET, Woo SH, Park MJ, et al. A case of primary syphilis in the rectum. J Korean Med Sci 2005;20:886–7.
15. Alam I, Shanoon D, Alhamdani A, Boyd A, Griffiths AP, Baxter JN. Severe proctitis, perforation and fatal rectal bleeding secondary to cytomegalovirus in an immunocompetent patient: report of a case. Surg Today 2007;37:66–9.
16. Kishiwaka H, Nishida J, Hirano E, Nakano M, Arakawa K, Morishita T, et al. Chronic ischemic proctitis: case report and review. Gastrointest Endosc 2004;60:304–8.
17. Bharucha AE, Tremaine WJ, Johnson CD, Batts KP. Ischemic proctosigmoiditis. Am J Gastroenterol 1996;91:2305–9.
18. Nelson RL, Briley S, Schuler JJ, Abcarian H. Acute ischemic proctitis. Report of six cases. Dis Colon Rectum 1992;35:375–80.
19. Chi KD, Ehrenpreis ED. Accuracy and reliability of the endoscopic classification of chronic radiation-induced proctopathy using a novel grading method. J Clin Gastroenterol 2005;39:42–6.
20. Wachter S, Gerstner N, Goldner G. Endoscopic scoring of late rectal mucosal damage after conformal radiotherapy for prostatic carcinoma. Radiother Oncol 2000;54;11–9.
21. Raman RR. Two percent formalin retention enemas for hemorrhagic radiation proctitis: a preliminary report. Dis Colon Rectum 2007;50:1032–9.
22. Postgate A, Saunders B, Tjandra J, Vargo J. Argon plasma coagulation in chronic radiation proctitis. Endoscopy 2007;39:361–5.
23. Felt-Bersma RJ, Cuesta A. Rectal prolapse, rectal intussusception, rectocele, and solitary rectal ulcer syndrome. Gastroenterol Clin North Am 2001;30:199–222.
24. Rao SSC, Ozturk R, De Ocampo S, Stessman M. Pathophysiology and role of biofeedback therapy in solitary rectal ulcer syndrome. Am J Gastroenterol 2006;101:613–8.
25. Keshtgar A. Solitary rectal ulcer syndrome in children. Eur J Gastroenterol Hepatol 2008;20:89–92.
26. Sharara AI, Azar C, Amr SS, Haddad M, Eloubeidi MA. Solitary rectal ulcer syndrome: endoscopic spectrum and review of the literature. Gastrointest Endosc 2005;62:755 –62.
27. Malik AK, Bhaskar KY, Kochhar R, Bhasin DK, Singh K, Mehta SK, et al. Solitary ulcer syndrome of the rectum: a histopathologic characterisation of 33 biopsies. Indian J Pathol Microbiol 1990;33:216–20.
28. Malouf AJ, Vaizey CJ, Kamm MA. Results of behavioral treatment (biofeedback) for solitary ulcer syndrome. Dis Colon Rectum 2001;44:72–6
29. Vaizey CJ, Roy AJ, Kamm MA. Prospective evaluation of the treatment of solitary rectal ulcer syndrome with biofeedback. Gut 2001;46:212–7.
30. Lindsey I, Jones OM, Cunningham C, Mortensen NJ. Chronic anal fissure. Br J Surg 2004;91:270–9.
31. Steele SR, Madoff RD. Systematic review: the treatment of anal fissure. Aliment Pharmacol Ther 2006;24:247–57.
32. Schouten WR, Briel JW, Auwerda JJ, De Graaf EJ. Ischaemic nature of anal fissure. Br J Surg 1996;83:63–5.
33. Schouten WR, Briel JW, Auwerda JJ. Relationship between anal pressure and anal dermal blood flow. The vascular pathogenesis of anal fissures. Dis Colon Rectum 1994;37:664–9.
34. Hulme-Moir M, Bartolo DC. Hemorrhoids. Gastroenterol Clin North Am 2001;30:183–7.
35. Acheson A, Scholefield JH. Management of haemorrhoids. BMJ 2008;336:380–3.
36. Alonso-Coello P, Mills E, Heels-Ansdell D, Lopez-Yarto M, Zhou Q, Johanson JF, et al. Fiber for the treatment of hemorrhoidal complications: a systematic review and meta-analysis. Am J Gastroenterol 2006;101:181–8.
37. Billingham RP, Isler JT, Kimmins MH, Nelson JM, Schweitzer J, Murphy MM. The diagnosis and management of common anorectal disorders. Curr Probl Surg 2004;41:586–645.
38. Goon P, Sonnex C. Frequently asked questions about genital warts in the genitourinary medicine clinic: an update and review of recent literature. Sex Transm Infect 2008;84:3–7.
39. Paraskevas KI, Kyriakos E, Poulios EE, Stathopoulos V, Tzovaras AA, Briana DD. Surgical management of giant condyloma acuminatum (Buschke-Loewenstein tumor) of the perianal region. Dermatol Surg 2007;33:638–44.
40. Uronis HE, Bendell JC. Anal cancer: an overview. Oncologist 2007;12:524–34.
41. Das P, Crane CH, Ajani JA. Current treatment for localized anal carcinoma. Curr Opin Oncol 2007;19:396–400.
42. Fox PA. Human papillomavirus and anal intraepithelial neoplasia. Curr Opin Infect Dis 2006;19:62–6.
43. Nahas CSR, Lin O, Weiser MR, Temple LK, Wong WD, Stier EA. Prevalence of perianal intraepithelial neoplasia in HIV-infected patients referred for high-resolution anoscopy. Dis Colon Rectum 2006;49:1581–6.

50

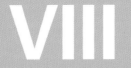

VIII

Biliopancreatic, Hepatic, and Peritoneal Diseases

Section editors:
Charles J. Lightdale, Meinhard Classen, D. Nageshwar Reddy

51 Biliary Tract Diseases

Nathan J. Shores and John Baillie

Introduction

Endoscopic retrograde cholangiopancreatography (ERCP) and endoscopic ultrasonography (EUS) have become major tools in the investigation and treatment of disease of the biliary tract and gallbladder. ERCP evolved rapidly from being a purely diagnostic technique into primarily a therapeutic one with the development of endoscopic sphincterotomy, independently reported in 1974 by Classen and Demling [1], and Kawai et al. [2]. The development of large-channel therapeutic duodenoscopes allowed endoscopists to place endoprostheses of 10 Fr or larger in the biliary tree, starting around 1980. Since that time, diagnostic and therapeutic ERCP have evolved extensively, allowing us to treat a wide spectrum of biliary and pancreatic disorders. Such sophistication requires well-trained and experienced endoscopists to ensure that the procedures are applied appropriately and with the minimum morbidity. Assessed in relation to the complication rate, ERCP is the most dangerous procedure routinely performed by endoscopists. Although ERCP remains the "gold standard" for investigating the biliary tree and pancreatic ductal system, it is just one of a growing number of imaging modalities available to us. These range from relatively non-invasive ones, such as abdominal ultrasound, computed tomography (CT), and magnetic resonance cholangiopancreatography (MRCP) to percutaneous transhepatic cholangiography (PTC), which is the most invasive of all. EUS has rapidly emerged as a technique of great value in the management of hepatobiliary and pancreatic disorders. Using specially modified endoscopes with ultrasound probes attached to the tip, high-resolution ultrasound images can be obtained of the wall of the bowel, as well as adjacent organs and tissues. Using linear-array technology, directed fine-needle aspiration (FNA) can be carried out using EUS for target guidance. This has greatly increased our ability to target and diagnose lesions in the extrahepatic bile duct and pancreas. As with ERCP, EUS requires procedure-specific, supervised training. Given the need to learn EUS anatomy, there is a long learning curve. Until recently, there were limited opportunities in the United States for training in this technique; the procedure was largely confined to teaching hospitals and large regional centers of excellence. There are considerable benefits to parallel training in ERCP and EUS.

Procedures

General Indications for ERCP and EUS (Tables 51.1, 51.2)

Patient Preparation

Informed consent, preferably in writing, should be obtained from patients before all endoscopic procedures. The discussion has to be particularly detailed in the case of ERCP, given the complexity of the procedure and its potentially life-threatening complications (e. g., pancreatitis, bleeding, perforation, infection). EUS-guided fine-needle aspiration and celiac neurolysis are also invasive procedures, albeit with small—but not minimal—risks that the patient must understand and agree to accept. There is a great deal of variation in the reported rates of morbidity and mortality of ERCP. Many of the

data are based on older surveys and require updating in the light of improved technology and procedural skills. The morbidity of ERCP is generally quoted to be in the range of 3–10 %, with mortality ranging from 0.1 % to 1.0 % [3–5]. A recent prospective study of complications of biliary sphincterotomy at the time of ERCP found an overall complication rate of 9.8 %, with a procedure-related mortality of 0.4 % [6]. Particular risk factors for complications included suspected sphincter of Oddi dysfunction (SOD), the presence of liver cirrhosis, and performance of precut papillotomy. As patients are sedated for ERCP and EUS, particular attention must be paid to medical problems that may affect the type of sedation given. Those patients who have previously shown intolerance of ERCP under conscious ("moderate") sedation should have monitored anesthesia care or general anesthesia. Children and mentally impaired adults should undergo ERCP and EUS examinations under general anesthesia.

Antibiotic Coverage

There are no data to support the routine use of prophylactic antibiotics in patients undergoing ERCP. Although the data supporting antibiotic prophylaxis against cholangitis in patients with known biliary obstruction, suspected choledocholithiasis, biliary leaks, etc., are scant, most endoscopists give antibiotics in these situations, and recent specialty guidelines endorse the practice [7]. The antibiotics used must penetrate into bile as well. In the past, we used to use a combination of ampicillin and gentamicin, substituting vancomycin in penicillin-sensitive patients. This prophylaxis is not suitable for

Table 51.1 Diagnostic indications (biliary) for endoscopic retrograde cholangiopancreatography

| Choledocholithiasis* |
| Biliary strictures* |
| Malignancy of the biliary tree (cholangiocarcinoma) (including brushing)* |
| Presurgical and postsurgical evaluation of the biliary tree (selected cases)* |
| Detection of congenital abnormalities (e. g., choledochal cysts)* |
| Detection of cystic duct and gallbladder pathology* |
| Evaluation of space-occupying lesions in the liver |
| Evaluation of unexplained liver function test abnormalities |
| Manometry of the sphincter of Oddi |

*Also an indication for endoscopic ultrasonography.

Table 51.2 Therapeutic indications (biliary) for endoscopic retrograde cholangiopancreatography

| Choledocholithiasis |
| Extraction of cystic duct and (rarely) gallbladder stones |
| Dilation and stenting of benign and malignant strictures |
| Stenting of ampullary tumors |
| Decompression in sphincter of Oddi dysfunction/papillary stenosis |
| Removal of intrabiliary foreign bodies (e. g., parasites) |
| Treatment of bile leaks |

patients with renal impairment, and is expensive. We now tend to substitute a fluoroquinolone, such as ciprofloxacin, or a broad-spectrum cephalosporin. If a complication such as a contained or free perforation of the biliary tree is suspected during or after ERCP or EUS with FNA, antibiotic coverage should be broadened to include an agent that is active against anaerobic bacteria (e. g., metronidazole or piperacillin–tazobactam). The effect of antibiotics depends on the tissue concentration; simply injecting antibiotics into the biliary tree has no useful effect against the organisms that cause cholangitis. Although most endoscopists use parenteral antibiotics, there are data to suggest that oral ciprofloxacin may be equally effective [8]. The culture of bile has rather fallen out of favor. We recommend the collection blood for culture and sensitivity determination when sepsis is suspected or known to be present.

Contrast Allergy

It has been the practice of endoscopists for many years to administer antihistamines and steroids as prophylaxis against contrast allergy in patients undergoing ERCP. This is controversial, and there are scant data supporting this practice [9]. Although the routine use of low-osmolality, nonionic contrast media (LOCM) has been advocated, there are insufficient data to support this approach. Nonionic contrast media are expensive and should therefore be reserved for patients with a documented history of major allergic reactions to iodinated contrast agents. Combining steroid pretreatment with intravenous LOCM has been shown to result in fewer adverse reactions than placebo with LOCM [10]. The amount of ERCP contrast that is absorbed into the circulation is probably minimal in comparison with the intravenous boluses given for CT scans, intravenous urograms, etc., but as contrast reactions are idiosyncratic and not dose-related, those performing ERCP are held to the same safety standards as radiologists. It is not clear whether severe contrast reactions can be prevented by steroid prophylaxis. However, it can be assumed that an effort to provide prophylaxis is better than none at all. In our unit, we give five divided doses of prednisone 20 mg orally at 6-h intervals, starting 30 h before the procedure.

Difficult Anatomy

In experienced hands, cannulation of the bile duct and pancreatic duct can be achieved in the vast majority of ERCP procedures attempted. An expert ERCP endoscopist will usually have a biliary cannulation success rate exceeding 90%. However, the endoscopic approach to the biliary tree (and pancreas) can be rendered difficult or impossible by surgical rearrangement (e. g., Billroth II gastrectomy reconstruction) or strictures (e. g., postbulbar stricture in the duodenum) (**Fig. 51.1**). For experts, the ERCP success rate in patients with prior Billroth II gastrectomy is in the range of 80–90%, with some modification of the therapeutic technique (e. g., needle-knife papillotomy over a stent). The increasingly widespread use of bariatric surgery is a further challenge for the ERCP endoscopist. Double-balloon endoscopy (DBE) has been reported to allow cannulation of the duodenal papilla via a long Roux-en-Y limb in up to 80% of cases requiring therapeutic intervention [11]. However, endoscopic therapy was only successful in 30% of attempts [11]. Similarly, EUS can be made difficult or impossible by anatomic problems. Perforations related to EUS are very rare, but those that have been reported are typically in the setting of "blind dilation" of an esophageal stricture. The use of miniprobes to evaluate tight strictures should reduce the risk of EUS-related perforations using larger instruments.

Failed ERCP has significant financial implications for the healthcare system. Varadarajulu et al. have shown that in comparison with

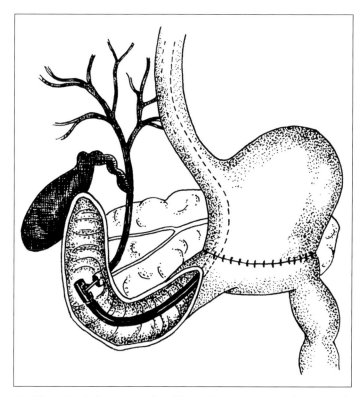

Fig. 51.1 Surgical anatomy after Billroth II gastrectomy, with retrograde access to the duodenal papilla for endoscopic retrograde cholangiopancreatography.

51

controls, the cost of failure to complete an ERCP was not insignificant ($ 1458 vs. $ 5668). In 1814 ERCPs performed during their study, 216 of the patients (11.9%) had previously undergone failed ERCPs at outside hospitals [12]. The authors succeeded in completing ERCP in 95% of the patients. For expert endoscopists in referral centers, failure to complete an ERCP is uncommon, but not unknown. Appropriate radiologic and surgical back-up ensure that these cases are managed without significant excess of morbidity or mortality.

The Normal Cholangiogram

Injection of radiographic contrast medium into the biliary tree through the main papilla (**Fig. 51.2**) provides excellent anatomic detail. In the majority of cases, the following structures can be identified: the common bile duct (CBD), the common hepatic duct, the cystic duct leading to the gallbladder, the gallbladder itself, the liver hilum with the confluence of the right and left main intrahepatic ducts, and secondary and tertiary ducts draining into these. In the standard prone position used for ERCP, the left intrahepatic ducts are usually filled preferentially. Adequate visualization of the right system may require repositioning or the use of an occlusion (balloon) technique. Care must be taken not to overinterpret radiologic findings when the gallbladder is opacified during ERCP; it is easy to miss small stones or polyps, especially when using dense contrast. When assessing biliary anatomy, endoscopists need to be aware of the normal structures and their common variants, including high and low "take-off" of the cystic duct. The upper limit of the normal diameter for the common bile duct (measured by convention in the mid-duct) is 7 mm, and the diameter can be roughly estimated fluoroscopically by comparison with the duodenoscope (10 mm). However, it is not uncommon for elderly patients to have gross dilation of the bile duct without clear pathology. The release of

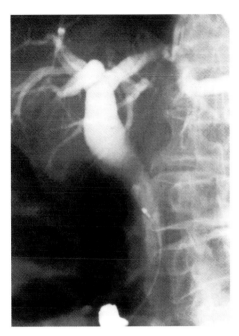

Fig. 51.2 Cholangiography (during endoscopic retrograde cholangiopancreatography) in a patient with post-Billroth II anatomy.

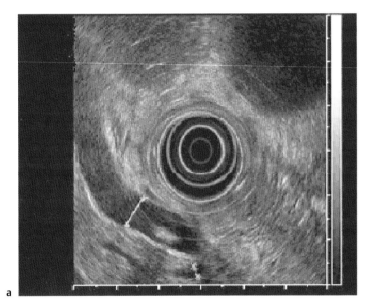

a

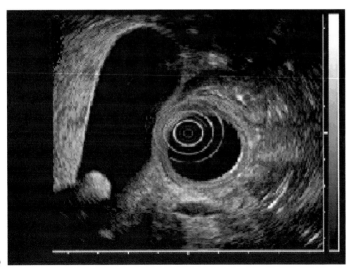

b

Fig. 51.3 a Choledocholithiasis. **b** Cholelithiasis. There is a hyperechoic focus (arrow) with postacoustic shadowing within the gallbladder, consistent with cholelithiasis, as imaged by endoscopic ultrasonography. (Images courtesy of Dr. Jason Conway.)

bile into the duodenum is not continuous, but regulated by the activity of the sphincter of Oddi, a ring of smooth muscle at the level of the ampulla of Vater. Sphincter of Oddi dysfunction (SOD) is a syndrome of recurrent biliary pain, with or without abnormal liver function tests (LFTs) and/or dilation of the bile duct. In most individuals, the CBD is joined by the main pancreatic duct (the Wirsung duct) at the ampulla, where they share a final common channel into the duodenum. In patients with pancreas divisum, however, the main (dorsal) pancreatic duct empties into the duodenum through the minor duodenal papilla.

Cholelithiasis

A gallbladder packed with small stones may be identified easily when the organ fills with contrast during ERCP. However, as previously noted, ERCP is not a particularly sensitive way to detect cholelithiasis. EUS is a much more sensitive tool in the hunt for gallbladder stones. The management of stones in the biliary tree has been one of the success stories of ERCP. Approximately 20 million Americans have gallstones, and some half a million cholecystectomies are performed annually in the United States. Symptoms relating to gallstones are a common cause of hospital admission in the U.S., with estimated direct health costs exceeding $2 billion annually. There are two basic types of gallstone: cholesterol stones and pigment stones (the latter divided between black stones and brown pigment stones). Cholesterol gallstones account for 75–80% of gallstones in the United States. They are most commonly found in middle-aged women, overweight individuals, and patients with ileal disease or those who have undergone small-bowel resection. Pigment stones are composed principally of calcium bilirubinate and phosphate and carbonate salts. They are associated with chronic bacterial or parasitic infections (brown stones) and chronic hemolysis (black pigment stones). Gallstones usually form within the gallbladder. The majority of individuals with gallstones are asymptomatic. However, acute cholecystitis can develop when a stone lodges in the neck of the gallbladder or in the cystic duct. Patients who have had a previous episode of biliary colic have a 60–70% chance of developing recurrent gallstone-related problems. Removal of the gallbladder (typically carried out using the laparoscopic route) is now recommended for this group of patients.

Transabdominal ultrasonography reportedly has a sensitivity of more than 95% for diagnosing gallbladder stones [13]. Given the high prevalence of disease and the excellent sensitivity of conventional transabdominal US, it is unlikely that EUS will ever play a major role in diagnosing cholelithiasis. However, the number of symptomatic patients with normal transabdominal US examinations is still significant. The clinical dilemma is whether or not their symptoms are really biliary in origin and, if so, whether they are related to microlithiasis that is missed by standard transabdominal US. The EUS findings of cholelithiasis are based on at least one of three criteria:

- Stones > 2 mm have associated acoustic shadowing (**Fig. 51.3**)
- Sludge, identified as mobile, low-amplitude echoes that layer in the most dependent part of the gallbladder lumen without acoustic shadowing
- Microlithiasis (or "minilithiasis"), defined as mobile hyperechoic foci 1–2 mm in size, without acoustic shadowing

It has been suggested that detecting cholesterol or bilirubinate crystals in bile aspirates may be helpful in identifying patients with cholelithiasis who have negative ultrasound findings. However, the sensitivity of microscopic examination of bile for detecting cholesterol crystals is very variable and probably no greater than 70% [13,14]. There is a very small body of literature suggesting that combining EUS and stimulated drainage of bile is accurate in predicting the presence of sludge or microlithiasis, or both [15,16]. The finding of biliary sludge or microlithiasis is more sensitive than microscopic bile examination in detecting cholelithiasis. In addition, EUS is more sensitive than transabdominal US for detecting sludge and small stones. These small studies also demonstrated symptom relief or resolution after cholecystectomy in patients with positive tests. However, flawed scientific design and methodology in the studies makes it difficult to draw solid conclusions [17,18].

Currently, there are three clinical situations in which EUS is recommended for diagnosing cholelithiasis. The first scenario is idiopathic acute pancreatitis with negative transabdominal US examinations. Amouyal et al. [19] studied 44 nonalcoholic patients with idiopathic acute pancreatitis. In 29 patients, biliary lithiasis was confirmed by surgery, ERCP, or microscopic examination. In 28 of these 29 patients, EUS demonstrated the presence of microlithiasis in the gallbladder. The second indication for EUS involves the evaluation of obese subjects with biliary colic and a negative transabdominal US examination. The sensitivity of conventional transabdominal US is low in this population. Pieken et al. [20] reported a small experience of identifying cholelithiasis by EUS in obese patients who had negative transabdominal US examinations. The third clinical situation concerns patients with successive negative transabdominal US examinations who have typical biliary colic or cholangitis. The sensitivity and specificity rates for EUS in the diagnosis of microlithiasis not detected by transabdominal US were 96 % and 86 %, respectively, in the study by Amouyal et al. [19]. Needless to say, positive EUS findings usually lead to cholecystectomy.

Some investigators have been successful in placing drains in the gallbladder through the cystic duct in poor surgical candidates [21]. These nasocystic drains have been used to wash out sludge and infected bile. There have also been reports of the removal of small gallstones endoscopically through patent cystic ducts after balloon dilation. Endoscopic stenting of the cystic duct in patients with advanced cirrhosis with symptomatic cholelithiasis appears relatively safe and effective in expert hands, in comparison with the high morbidity and mortality of cholecystectomy reported in Child–Pugh–Turcotte class B and C patients [22–24]. These procedures are technical *tours de force;* in everyday ERCP practice, however, there is rarely an indication to perform transcystic intervention.

Choledocholithiasis

▓ Background

Most CBD stones form within the gallbladder and migrate into the bile duct. However, de novo formation of stones within the biliary tree can occur both before and after cholecystectomy. Patients with periampullary diverticula are at increased risk of developing common bile duct stones (**Fig. 51.4**). This may be due to SOD caused by the presence of the diverticulum, bacterial overgrowth within the diverticulum (encouraging colonization of the adjacent bile duct), or a combination of the two. In countries in which biliary parasites (e. g. , *Fasciola, Ascaris,* and *Clonorchis)* are common, the eggs and dead organisms can form a nidus for stone formation. As previously stated, chronic hemolysis predisposes to biliary pigment stone formation. Bile duct stones predispose to infection (cholangitis), obstruction (jaundice with or without cholangitis), and gallstone (biliary) pancreatitis. Acute cholangitis is a medical emergency that has a high mortality rate if left untreated [25]. The classic Charcot triad consists of pain, jaundice, and fever [26]. When hypotension and confusion are added (evidence of systemic infection), the condition is known as the pentad of Reynolds [26]. One of the most important roles of the ERCP endoscopist is to relieve biliary obstruction caused by stones (choledocholithiasis). If the stone or stones cannot be

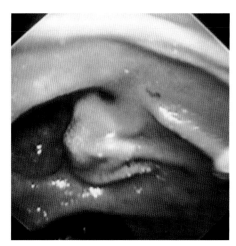

Fig. 51.4 Periampullary diverticulum. This type of diverticulum predisposes to choledocholithiasis, and can make endoscopic retrograde cholangiopancreatography quite difficult by altering the position of the duodenal papilla relative to the duodenoscope.

removed, effective biliary drainage must be established by endoscopic, radiographic, or (if necessary) surgical means. As any ERCP may lead to a therapeutic procedure, ERCP endoscopists must be trained and skilled in techniques for biliary decompression.

▓ ERCP, EUS, or MRCP to Diagnose Choledocholithiasis?

Bile duct stones (choledocholithiasis) complicate gallstone disease in up to 20 % of patients [27]. These stones can cause cholangitis and pancreatitis. ERCP and intraoperative cholangiography are considered to be the gold standards in the diagnosis of choledocholithiasis. However, the accuracy of the diagnosis depends on the operator's expertise. Technical problems, such as air bubbles injected into the biliary tree, may cause erroneous diagnosis of choledocholithiasis, and small stones can be missed. The sensitivity of ERCP for diagnosing choledocholithiasis is reported to be in the range of 79–95 %, with a specificity in the range of 92–98 %. Overall, the accuracy of ERCP for diagnosing choledocholithiasis may be as high as 97 % [28,29]. The incidence of pancreatitis associated with diagnostic ERCP (i. e., without sphincterotomy) is 3–6 % [30,31]. If sphincterotomy is performed, the complication rate increases to 9.8 % [6]. Abnormal LFTs correlate poorly with the actual presence of a common bile duct stone. Nomograms are available that can help predict the presence or absence of choledocholithiasis based on the pattern of the LFTs and the bile duct diameter [32].

Transabdominal US is the least expensive and invasive imaging test available to look for choledocholithiasis, and should therefore be performed first. Despite high specificity (95 %), the sensitivity of transabdominal US is low, ranging from 20 % to 80 % in the literature [33–39]. The presence of small stones or a nondilated bile duct lowers the sensitivity of transabdominal US. In addition, most calculi settle in the intrapancreatic portion of the distal CBD, a location that is particularly troublesome to image using transabdominal US. Computed tomography also has limitations in the diagnosis of choledocholithiasis, especially when the diameter of the stones is less than the thickness of the CT slices. Although the specificity of CT for detecting choledocholithiasis is more than 95 %, the sensitivity is poor, ranging from 23 % to 85 % [34–40]. The overall accuracy rate for CT in identifying choledocholithiasis appears to be around 70 % [28,33,38,41].

Recently, EUS has emerged as a highly accurate way to evaluate the extrahepatic bile duct. The distal intrapancreatic CBD can be visualized reproducibly from the second portion of the duodenum, whereas the proximal CBD and common hepatic duct are viewed from the duodenal bulb. The CBD can be completely inspected in 96–100 % of cases [33,38,41]. However, limitations such as post-

51

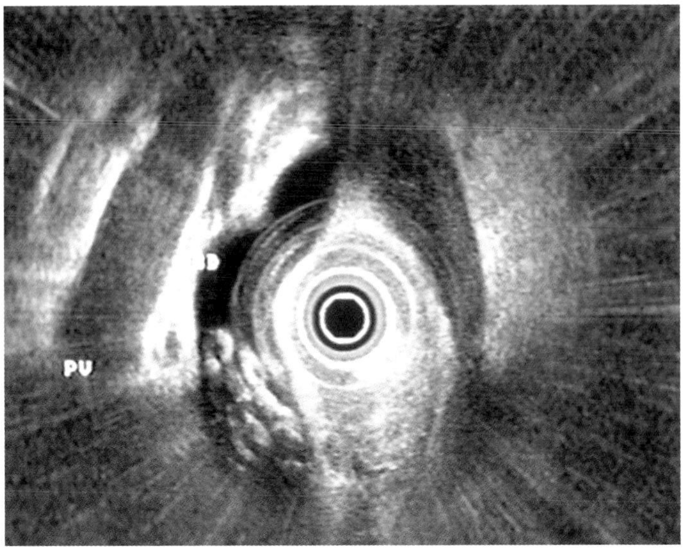

Fig. 51.5 Choledocholithiasis. Multiple hyperechoic foci with postacoustic shadowing are seen within the distal common bile duct. CBD, common bile duct; PV, portal vein.

Billroth II gastrectomy anatomy and significant stenoses may preclude the use of EUS for examining the extrahepatic bile duct. The sensitivity and specificity of EUS for diagnosing choledocholithiasis are reported to be 88–96 % and 96–100 %, respectively (**Fig. 51.5**). Unlike transabdominal US and CT, EUS is able to detect calculi regardless of stone size or bile duct diameter [38]. This has been confirmed in numerous studies in which the diagnostic accuracy of EUS for choledocholithiasis was approximately 95 % [28]. In direct comparisons, EUS was more sensitive (96 %) and specific (100 %) than ultrasonography (63 % and 95 %) and CT (71 % and 97 %), respectively. EUS compares favorably with ERCP in detecting choledocholithiasis, without statistically significant differences in the sensitivity and specificity. The overall accuracy is also similar—94 % for EUS and 97 % for ERCP [42–45].

Magnetic resonance cholangiopancreatography (MRCP) has rapidly evolved as a valuable tool for investigating pancreatic and biliary disorders. Its sensitivity ranges from 71 % to 100 % [46]. In a comparative study, the overall accuracy of EUS in comparison with MRCP for the diagnosis of choledocholithiasis was 97 % vs. 82 % [47]. However, MRCP can fail to detect small stones, especially in an undilated bile duct. One study reported a sensitivity of only 40 % in this particular subgroup [48]. It can be expected that the sensitivity of MRCP for detecting small bile duct stones will increase with operator experience and technological developments. At present, many are limiting their use of MRCP to those patients in whom sedation for EUS or ERCP is contraindicated, or those with altered or distorted anatomy.

What is the role of EUS in identifying choledocholithiasis? It is as accurate as ERCP, with a high negative predictive value, which means that ERCP is unnecessary if stones cannot be seen at EUS. The impressive safety profile of EUS (with a complication rate of less than one in 2000 cases) and its extremely low failure rate compare favorably with ERCP, which has a 5–10 % morbidity and a significant failure rate in inexperienced hands [49,50]. There is increasing interest in "risk stratification" when deciding on preoperative investigations in gallstone patients (**Table 51.3**).

Transabdominal US should be the first-line study, in view of its low cost, safety, and high degree of specificity. The algorithm for investigating and managing choledocholithiasis depends on whether or not intraoperative cholangiography will be performed. In patients with a predicted high risk of having choledocholithiasis, preoperative ERCP is appropriate for stone identification and recovery. In patients whose risk of choledocholithiasis is considered moderate, indeterminate, or low, it is more cost-effective to use preoperative EUS, with ERCP being reserved for patients positively identified as having stones. "Low-risk" patients are expected to have choledocholithiasis in only 2–3 % of cases, and it is therefore acceptable to proceed to surgery without a preoperative study and manage the patient expectantly afterwards [51]. EUS may be the test of choice for choledocholithiasis evaluation in pregnant women and patients with contrast allergy, as this imaging modality avoids exposure to ionizing radiation and iodinated contrast media.

A group in Montreal recently devised a decision-tree simulation to model the cost effectiveness of ERCP, MRCP then ERCP, EUS then ERCP (on separate days), or EUS then ERCP (on the same day) for diagnosing and managing suspected bile duct stones [52]. Their data indicate that ERCP alone, MRCP then ERCP, and EUS then ERCP (on the same day) all appear to be cost-effective. MRCP should be used when the probability of choledocholithiasis is low. Conversely, ERCP appears to be most cost-effective when the pretest probability of a retained duct stone is high.

Endoscopic Management

Sphincterotomy. Endoscopic sphincterotomy (EST) revolutionized the management of CBD stones. Before its introduction in 1974, CBD stones had to be removed surgically using an open surgical procedure that was associated with a not inconsiderable morbidity rate. The current endoscopic approach to CBD stones is successful in at least 90 % of cases in skilled hands, with morbidity and mortality rates that compare favorably with surgery in similarly expert hands. EST can be performed with a mortality of less than 0.5 % and a procedure-related morbidity of less than 10 % [6]. However, it must be remembered that EST is the most invasive procedure routinely performed by gastrointestinal endoscopists.

A sphincterotome (or papillotome) is a modified cannula with an exposed wire at the distal end, through which electric current is transmitted. The sphincterotome is inserted into the bile duct, and

Table 51.3 Determination of risk groups for choledocholithiasis

Positive bile duct stone on US or CT	History of gallstones			
	Negative bile duct stone on US or CT			
	Dilated CBD (>7 mm)		Nondilated CBD	
	T bilirubin > 2 mg/dL (> 35 µmol/L)	Any T bilirubin	T bilirubin < 2 mg/dL (< 35 µmol/L)	Normal bilirubin
	Elevated AP	Elevated AP	Elevated AP	Normal AP
	ALT > 2 × normal	ALT > 2 × normal	ALT > 2 × normal	ALT normal
	Fever	No fever	No fever	No fever
High risk	**High risk**	**Moderate risk**	**Indeterminate risk**	**Low risk**

CBD, common bile duct; CT, computed tomography; ALT, alanine aminotransferase; AP, alkaline phosphatase; US, ultrasonography. Adapted from Canto et al. 1998 [28].

short bursts of current are applied to incise the roof of the ampulla (including the sphincter of Oddi). A variety of less controlled techniques, collectively known as precut papillotomy, have been developed to access the biliary tree in cases of anatomic difficulty (**Fig. 51.6**). Precut techniques carry increased morbidity in comparison with standard sphincterotomy, and should only be used by experts for therapeutic access to the biliary tree.

In the study by Freeman et al. [6], 9.8% of patients undergoing EST had complications, including pancreatitis (5.4%), bleeding (2%), cholangitis (1%), and perforation (<0.5%). The incidence of late complications of biliary sphincterotomy in studies with extended follow-up (5–10 years or more) ranges from 10% to 24% [53]. These late complications include stenosis of the sphincterotomy site, recurrent choledocholithiasis, and cholangitis. This rate of complications compares favorably with the results of surgical exploration and drainage of the CBD. Most of the late complications of ERCP can be managed by endoscopic therapy.

Stone extraction after sphincterotomy. Following successful EST, removal of common bile duct stones can be achieved in 80–95% of patients. Although small stones may pass spontaneously after sphincterotomy, it is unwise to assume that this will occur. A variety of endoscopic balloons and basket catheters are available to retrieve stones. Forceful extraction against resistance should be avoided, as this risks traumatic extension of the sphincterotomy incision. Occasionally, a stone is trapped within a basket catheter in the bile duct in such a way that it cannot be removed or disengaged. In the past, this was a very serious problem that sometimes required surgery. Nowadays, an over-the-catheter lithotripsy system is available that uses a cranking device to pull the wires of the basket against a metal oversleeve. Either the stone or the basket breaks, resolving the problem.

Stone extraction through the intact papilla. Although sphincterotomy is frequently used to enlarge the opening to the CBD for stone extraction, it has been demonstrated that small stones can be removed safely through the intact papilla using balloon or basket catheters. This avoids the immediate and late complications of sphincterotomy, which are particularly likely in the presence of a nondilated bile duct. It is desirable to preserve the biliary sphincter, especially in young patients. MacMathuna et al. [54] demonstrated the use of balloon dilation of the papilla to allow large stones (up to and exceeding 20 mm) to be removed from the CBD without sphincterotomy. They termed this procedure "balloon sphincteroplasty."

Stone extraction without sphincterotomy can cause significant edema of the papilla and make it difficult to remove all the stone fragments and debris. When the papilla is already swollen, as in gallstone pancreatitis with an obstructing calculus, endoscopic sphincterotomy may be necessary to improve biliary drainage—so balloon dilation has its limitations [55]. A multicenter, prospective, randomized trial of endoscopic sphincterotomy versus balloon sphincteroplasty revealed a three times higher incidence of pancreatitis in the balloon sphincteroplasty group, and two of the patients in that group died of severe pancreatitis complicating the procedure. Although subsequent data from the same group suggest that complications from the two techniques may be more similar than originally indicated, this sobering study considerably reduced the initial enthusiasm for the use of balloon sphincteroplasty as a first-line technique for stone recovery [56].

Difficult bile duct stones. Common bile duct stones that are larger than 15 mm in diameter are difficult to retrieve, as they do not pass easily through a standard sphincterotomy site. Smaller stones may present difficulty when they are located proximal to a bile duct stricture or in a tortuous, dilated bile duct (where they may be difficult to capture in a basket). Intrahepatic stones are particularly

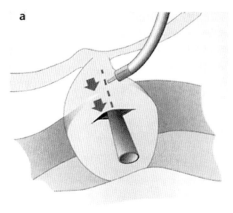

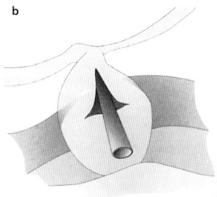

Fig. 51.6 Precut papillotomy over a stent.
a Using a needle-knife papillotome, the bile duct is deroofed over a prepositioned endoprosthesis (stent). This is a useful technique when there are technical difficulties in achieving a standard biliary sphincterotomy.
b After an opening has been created, the stent is removed.

difficult, due to their inaccessibility. A variety of techniques are available to facilitate the removal of biliary stones, including mechanical lithotripsy [57], contact lithotripsy—electrohydraulic [58], laser [59], or extracorporeal shock-wave lithotripsy [60]—and chemical dissolution. Almost all biliary calculi can be removed using one or more of these techniques.

Mechanical lithotripsy. Mechanical lithotriptors consist of a reinforced basket with a mechanical cranking device (**Fig. 51.7**). After the stone has been captured, the wires of the basket are tightened around it using a cranking mechanism. The closed basket is pulled tight against a spiral meal sheath, breaking it by mechanical force. Modern mechanical lithotriptors are highly effective, with success rates of 75–100% being reported [61].

Electrohydraulic lithotripsy (EHL). EHL has been used by urologists for many years to fragment stones in the urinary bladder, renal pelvis, and ureters. This technology has been adapted for use through percutaneous tracts into the liver, and in a retrograde direction into the bile duct through a choledochoscope. In EHL, rapid conversion of a liquid into its gaseous form results in sudden volume expansion, creating a shock wave that fractures the stone. Once suitably small fragments have been created (this is usually a rapid process), conventional stone retrieval techniques are used to complete the duct clearance. Overall, EHL is safe and effective, with success rates reported to be around 80%. However, equipment costs and the need for a second well-trained endoscopist to handle the choledochoscope limit this technique to a small number of specialist centers. The new SpyGlass endoscopic platform, a miniscope system (Boston Scientific, Natick, Massachusetts, USA), requires only one operator and may broaden the practice of therapeutic and diagnostic choledochoscopy.

51

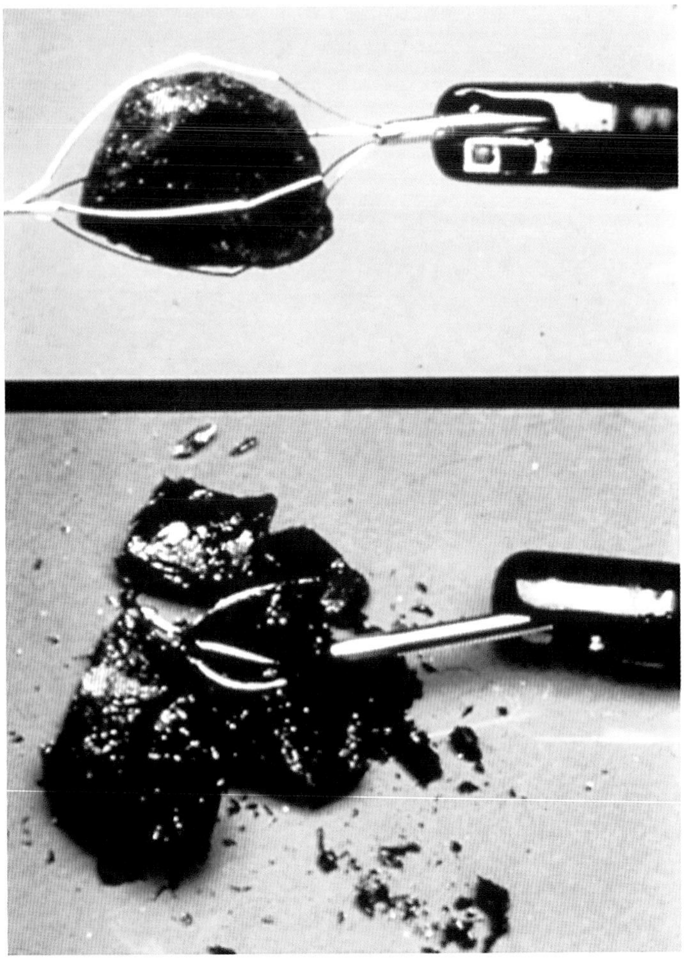

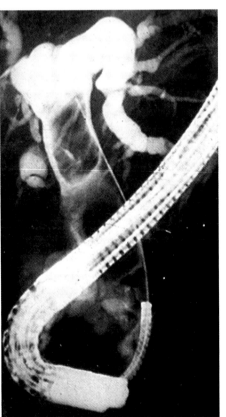

Laser lithotripsy Laser energy can be used to fragment bile duct stones, with a mechanism similar to that of EHL (i. e., the creation of a shock wave from a burst of energy at the stone's surface). A pulsed laser that emits discrete bursts of energy, usually at a frequency of around 10 Hz, is required. For this purpose, a tunable dye laser is ideal. The laser light guide (fiber) is brought into contact with the stone after passing through the instrument channel of a choledochoscope (**Fig. 51.8**). To reduce the risk of collateral damage to the bile duct wall, "smart" lasers have been developed that incorporate automated stone detection (i. e., they do not fire unless they are in contact with a stone). Although laser lithotripsy of bile duct stones can be very effective, it is also very expensive. The equipment is costly and delicate, and requires frequent maintenance. As with EHL, several operators are needed. For these reasons, laser lithotripsy is not widely available.

Extracorporeal shock-wave lithotripsy (ESWL) of common bile duct stones is another adaptation of technology that was first developed by urologists. ESWL was pioneered in Europe for the treatment of gallbladder stones. However, it is also useful for managing difficult bile duct stones, especially when contact methods of fragmentation are unavailable or have failed. ESWL procedures for CBD stones are usually carried out under fluoroscopic guidance, with contrast being injected through a nasobiliary drain placed at the time of ERCP (**Fig. 51.9**) or via a percutaneous catheter. Some ESWL machines use ultrasound rather than fluoroscopy for targeting. Although ESWL is no longer in widespread use for the treatment of gallbladder stones (having been superseded by laparoscopic cholecystectomy), many centers still have ESWL available for urological procedures. The gastroenterologist can usually obtain time on the ESWL machine to treat the occasional patient with difficult biliary calculi.

Chemical dissolution. Dissolving bile duct stones by infusing chemical agents through a nasobiliary drain or percutaneous catheter is an attractive concept, but in practice the results have been disappointing. The earliest dissolution agent used was monoctanoin, a fatty-acid derivative that was infused over a period of 5–8 days [62]. The dissolution rates for pure cholesterol stones were in the range of 40–60%, but the treatment often had to be discontinued due to patient intolerance of the agent (e. g., due to nausea, abdominal cramps, diarrhea) or the nasobiliary tube. Monoctanoin is not suitable for mixed stones, which make up a significant proportion of CBD stones. When methyl *tert*-butyl ether (MTBE) was being evaluated for treating cholesterol stones in the gallbladder, there was interest in modifying it to deal with CBD stones. Unfortunately, it proved impossible to contain this volatile and toxic agent reliably within the bile duct. MTBE leaking from the bile duct into the duodenum can cause severe duodenitis, and if enough ether is absorbed, it causes profound sedation and a variety of unpleasant systemic effects (e. g., hemolysis). For this reason, MTBE is not recommended for use in the biliary tree to dissolve stones. The search is continuing for an agent capable of reliably disaggregating mixed bile duct stones, but none has been identified so far.

Stents for stones. When endoscopic techniques fail to clear the bile duct of stones completely, good biliary drainage must be established before the procedure is completed. An endoscopic prosthesis (stent) should be placed in the bile duct to prevent biliary obstruction and its sequel, cholangitis (**Fig. 51.10**). Thereafter, the patient can be brought back for a further procedure when local edema or bleeding has settled, or the patient can be referred to an expert at another hospital. Ursodeoxycholic acid therapy may be a useful adjunctive treatment, but the research results have been contradictory and have included small numbers of patients [63]. As many elderly, frail patients are poor candidates for repeated endoscopy, biliary stents have been used for long-term management of some bile duct stones.

Fig. 51.7 a, b Mechanical lithotripsy (using a crushing basket) for bile duct stones. The stones are crushed by the wires of a specially hardened basket catheter. (Images courtesy of Dr. Peter Cotton.)

Fig. 51.8 Laser lithotripsy for bile duct stones. A laser light guide is advanced into the bile duct using a thin-caliber choledochoscope, advanced through a large-channel duodenoscope. (Image courtesy of Dr. Richard Kozarek.)

On the whole, this is a successful strategy; however, a large prospective study from Amsterdam suggested that long-term stenting is not without risk (e.g., cholangitis) [64].

ERCP in relation to laparoscopic cholecystectomy. Laparoscopic cholecystectomy is now widely available as the first-line treatment for symptomatic choledocholithiasis. This has affected biliary endoscopists' practice in a number of ways. When laparoscopic cholecystectomy was first introduced, endoscopists saw many patients with iatrogenic bile duct injuries and cystic duct leaks. This early rush of complications reflected the learning curve of the surgeons performing this laparoscopic procedure. Although biliary problems related to laparoscopic cholecystectomy have greatly diminished, endoscopists still see them from time to time.

Common bile duct stones. It has been necessary to develop an algorithm for the management of suspected or proven bile duct stones in patients undergoing laparoscopic cholecystectomy (**Fig. 51.11**). There are ample data in the surgical literature to allow stratification of patients with cholelithiasis into those at low risk (<5%) and those at medium or high risk (>20%) for having choledocholithiasis. The risk factors include cholestatic LFTs, jaundice, dilated bile duct on transabdominal US (with or without stones seen), and cholangitis. Interestingly, recent pancreatitis is not a reliable predictor of choledocholithiasis, as small stones that cause pancreatitis tend to pass spontaneously. Some surgeons request ERCP before laparoscopic cholecystectomy in order to assess the bile duct for stones and, if necessary, remove them. This strategy allows the surgeon to plan a single procedure—i.e., if the endoscopist fails to cannulate the bile duct or remove stones that have been seen, the surgeon can perform an intraoperative cholangiogram or, where appropriate, convert a laparoscopic procedure to an open one to deal with bile duct stones. In our opinion, routine ERCP before laparoscopic cholecystectomy cannot be justified [65]. The yield of bile duct stones is low in the absence of risk factors, and ERCP exposes patients to the risk of complications, some of which can be severe. ERCP should not be used solely to define biliary anatomy, as there is no evidence that this prior knowledge reduces the risk of operative complications. As we know from existing published studies [66–68], patients who have biliary (gallstone) pancreatitis with biliary obstruction (jaundice, cholangitis) may benefit from early ERCP and sphincterotomy (or stenting) to decompress the biliary tree. This is a select subgroup of patients in whom ERCP is justified before laparoscopic cholecystectomy. Also, in patients in whom there is genuine doubt about the likely success of ERCP (e.g., after Billroth II gastrectomy), a preoperative study may be justified to plan subsequent management. The preferred management for suspected choledocholithiasis in the absence of progressive jaundice or cholangitis is to proceed with laparoscopic cholecystectomy and have intraoperative cholangiography performed. The few patients in whom bile duct stones are identified by intraoperative cholangiography can have ERCP and duct clearance before leaving the hospital, usually the day after surgery. There is increasing evidence suggesting that even the presence of a confirmed stone in the setting of acute pancreatitis is not an absolute indication for therapeutic ERCP [69]. A meta-analysis of 450 patients randomly assigned to ERCP for acute biliary pancreatitis concluded that only those patients with evidence of cholangitis benefited from the intervention statistically [70]. Clearly, the current use of ERCP in relation to laparoscopic cholecystectomy is greatly influenced by the skill of the individual endoscopist and by the willingness and ability of the surgeon to perform intraoperative cholangiography.

Bile duct leaks. Bile leaks most commonly follow gallbladder surgery, but can result from ductal injury related to blunt or sharp trauma or iatrogenic injury (e.g., liver biopsy). A patient who develops abdominal pain and low-grade fever soon after laparoscopic cholecystectomy requires investigation for a possible bile leak or

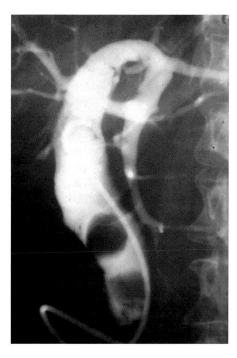

Fig. 51.9 Nasobiliary cholangiogram. Contrast injection via an endoscopically-placed nasobiliary tube reveals several large filling defects (stones) in the common bile duct.

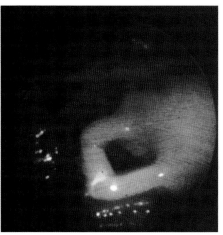

Fig. 51.10 A biliary stent placed to palliate stone obstruction. In this case, pus is seen coming out of the stent. This patient had cholangitis and septicemia, causing a severe coagulopathy—a contraindication for biliary sphincterotomy.

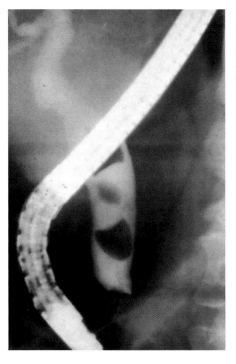

Fig. 51.11 Choledocholithiasis (common bile duct stones). Endoscopic retrograde cholangiopancreatography shows bile duct stones.

51

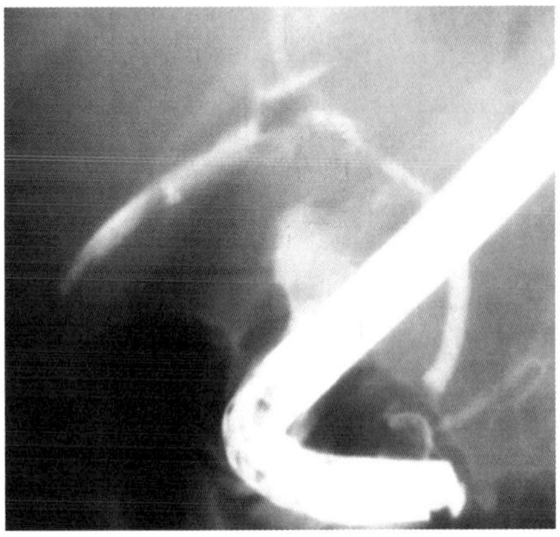

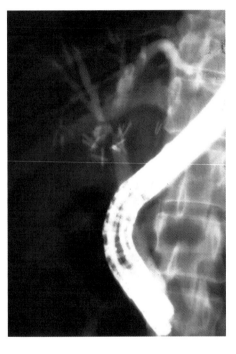

Fig. 51.12 Cystic duct stump leak. The small white cloud at the center of the image is contrast medium leaking from the cystic duct stump on endoscopic retrograde cholangio-pancreatography.

Fig. 51.13 Postsurgical hilar bile duct stricture. Note the surgical clips (linear densities) at the level of the obstruction. This type of injury often requires surgical repair.

other complication of the surgery [71]. Cross-sectional imaging (e. g., CT or transabdominal US) may detect a localized collection of bile (biloma) or sometimes bile lying free in the peritoneal cavity. Any significant collection of bile needs to be drained, either percutaneously or (when peritonitis is present) surgically. Although radionuclide scanning—e. g., a hepato-iminodiacetic acid (HIDA) scan—may suggest or confirm the presence of a bile leak, cholangiography is necessary to define the leak site. ERCP is the preferred approach in most centers, with percutaneous transhepatic cholangiography (PTC) being reserved for patients in whom endoscopic access has failed, or who have leaks from inaccessible areas of the liver (e. g., sequestered segments). The vast majority of bile duct leaks seen by biliary endoscopists arise from the cystic duct stump (**Fig. 51.12**). Injuries to the common hepatic duct, hilum, or intrahepatic ducts can cause leaks that are less straightforward to define. Particularly if a segment or even a lobe of the liver has been sequestered, a combination of PTC and CT scanning may be necessary to identify the lesion. As the bile ducts are usually not dilated when a leak has occurred, PTC in this setting is technically quite challenging, and requires the services of a skilled vascular radiologist.

When a cystic duct leak is identified at ERCP, placing a stent across the duodenal papilla is usually adequate therapy. Routinely performing endoscopic sphincterotomy is unnecessary; although effective, it exposes the patient to some additional risk. Sphincter-

otomy should be reserved for patients with mechanical obstruction at the papilla (e. g., obstructing stone, true papillary stenosis). The length of the stent probably has little to do with whether or not the bile fistula closes. It is probably sufficient to place a stent that is just long enough to bridge the duodenal papilla, thereby reducing transpapillary pressure. Several studies have shown resolution of leaks in post surgical and noniatrogenic biliary injury without stents traversing the level of the leak [72,73]. We tend to leave these stents in place for 2–4 weeks, by which time most bile leaks have resolved.

Persistent bile leaks are often an indication for PTC to look for unexpected accessory or aberrant bile ducts [74]. It is rare for any patient with a bile duct leak to require surgery, although sometimes the leak site is so large that it will not close spontaneously (e. g., avulsed cystic duct stump). An interim analysis of a pilot study using removable covered self-expanding metal stents (SEMS) to treat biliary leaks yielded a 93 % success rate with one migration event—a successful but expensive approach that is unlikely to become the norm [75]. In a different approach, Seewald et al. reported successful closure of seven of nine biliary fistulas that were refractory to standard drainage with N-butyl-2-cyanoacrylate, avoiding the need for a repeat procedure [76]. The published results for endoscopic management of bile duct leaks suggest that this is a largely successful and cost-effective management strategy with standard plastic stents [77,78]. This may not be true if covered SEMS are used. Drastic injuries to the bile duct, such as transection, result in leaks that cannot be managed effectively by endoscopic or percutaneous means and require surgery for bile duct repair. Bile leaks are not uncommon after liver transplantation, especially when the biliary anastomosis is fashioned over a T-tube. When the T-tubes are removed, there may be leakage from the fistulous tract. Endoscopic therapy is usually successful, although our experience has been that stents or drains have to be left in place much longer than in patients who are not immunocompromised, to guarantee healing of the leak. Breakdown of the biliary anastomosis after liver transplantation is usually ischemic and requires surgery.

Postsurgical biliary strictures. A detailed discussion of postsurgical bile duct strictures and their potential endoscopic management is beyond the scope of this review. However, iatrogenic injury at the time of cholecystectomy is probably the commonest cause of benign bile duct stricture [79] (**Fig. 51.13**). Postsurgical strictures are not uncommon after orthotopic liver transplantation, particularly at the site of the biliary anastomosis. Complete transection of a bile duct is a catastrophic injury that declares itself within days. Lesser degrees of ductal injury (short of transection) may result in early or late strictures. Many of these injuries result from trauma to the local vasculature, causing ischemic injury. Other causes of bile duct stricture, such as chronic pancreatitis, pancreatic pseudocysts, or stones in the gallbladder neck or cystic duct (Mirizzi syndrome, **Fig. 51.14**) need to be considered (**Table 51.4**).

The first step in evaluating a benign biliary stricture is to make sure that it is truly benign. If there is any doubt about this, endoscopic brush cytology should be performed, and CT scanning should be carried out to look for an adjacent mass that might indicate malignancy. New technology designed to facilitate single-operator cholangioscopy has shown some success aiding accurate diagnosis of biliary strictures. It has been reported that intraductal use of a miniscope during ERCP resulted in a modified diagnosis in 20 of 29 cases and confirmed the existing diagnosis in 10 of 13 cases. This approach is costly, but there may be a useful diagnostic niche for it given the poor sensitivity of ductal brush cytology. If the stricture is in the extrahepatic bile duct or at the biliary confluence (hilum) (**Fig. 51.13**), it is justifiable to attempt endoscopic or percutaneous radiological dilation, with or without stenting. Strictures (especially when multiple) that involve the smaller intrahepatic bile ducts are not amenable to these interventions. Once accessible benign biliary strictures have been dilated, we like to stent them and leave the stent in place for 3 months. Previously, a clinically significant biliary stricture that persisted beyond two or three dilations and stent exchanges was thought unlikely to resolve spontaneously, and surgical intervention (e. g., a diversion procedure) was recommended. However, the long-term patency data on surgical repair of benign biliary strictures show new stricturing at the surgical anastomosis in 12–22 % of cases [80,81].

Larghi et al. report success in treating postoperative hilar strictures with serial dilations, placing 10-Fr plastic stents every 3–5 months until the stricture resolves. This approach has begun to supplant the traditional early reconstructive surgical approach [82]. Patients with persistent or progressive "benign" strictures should be carefully monitored for the development of malignancy, especially in primary sclerosing cholangitis (see below). In the current state of their development, metal mesh stents should not be used for benign biliary strictures [83], as they have a tendency to epithelialize and occlude. Increasingly, published studies of coated stents are showing promising patency rates, without epithelial hypertrophy and embedding, in patients with benign disease [84].

Gallbladder Lesions

Retrograde cholangiography can identify certain gallbladder lesions, provided that the cystic duct is patent. While large gallbladder stones (> 1 cm) are easily seen, small ones are not infrequently missed, particularly if the gallbladder is underfilled. It is difficult to tell whether a large mass in the gallbladder is a tumor or a matted collection of stones. Standard retrograde cholangiography is rarely sensitive enough to detect small gallbladder polyps. Therapeutic ERCP involving the gallbladder (e. g., placing stents or nasocystic drains, and occasional stone extraction) is technically difficult and rarely indicated clinically. As mentioned above, patients who are at high risk for surgical mortality, such as those with advanced cirrhosis, might be considered for this approach. In all cases, care must be taken when instrumenting the cystic duct and gallbladder to avoid trauma that might cause perforation.

Conventional transabdominal US is commonly performed when cholelithiasis is suspected. With the increasing use of transabdominal ultrasound, polypoid lesions of the gallbladder are frequently discovered. It can be quite difficult to differentiate stones from small polypoid lesions (< 20 mm) using standard low-frequency ultrasound. In addition, overlying bowel gas and body habitus can interfere with ultrasound imaging. With high-frequency probes in close proximity to the gallbladder, EUS has proved useful for investigating suspected gallbladder polyps seen on transabdominal US. The gallbladder can generally be imaged from either the gastric antrum or the duodenal bulb. Cholesterol polyps are the most common polypoid lesions occurring in the gallbladder; they are generally < 10 mm in diameter and appear as echogenic pedunculated masses without associated acoustic shadowing [85–87]. Larger cholesterol polyps may appear heterogeneous or hypoechoic on transabdominal US, making differentiation from adenocarcinoma challenging. Accurate imaging is required, as some small polypoid carcinomas of the gallbladder can be resected for cure.

The normal thickness of the gallbladder wall is 3 mm or less in patients without calculous disease. In chronic cholecystitis, the thickened gallbladder wall retains its normal multilayered appearance as viewed with EUS. Indeed, EUS adds little to the investigation of a thickened gallbladder wall, unless gallbladder cancer is considered a possible diagnosis. However, the integrity of the gallbladder wall is a key factor in the diagnosis of depth of invasion of gallblad-

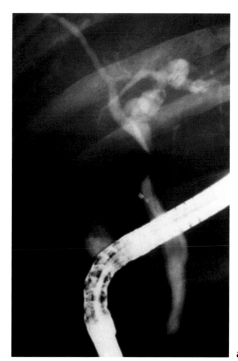

Fig. 51.14 Mirizzi syndrome.
a A smooth stricture at the level of the common hepatic duct, caused by extrinsic pressure from a stone lodged in the cystic duct or neck of the gallbladder.
b Faint calcification reveals the presence of a stone adjacent to the common hepatic duct (arrow).

a

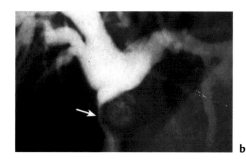

b

Table 51.4 Causes of benign bile duct strictures

Congenital
Acquired
Trauma (surgical or nonsurgical)
Sclerosing cholangitis
Liver transplantation
Chronic pancreatitis
Pancreatic pseudocysts
Mirizzi syndrome
Vascular indentation
Congenital hepatic cysts

der cancer. EUS can detect gallbladder tumors with a sensitivity of more than 90 % [88]. However, accurate staging by depth of invasion proves difficult. As the majority of patients with gallbladder cancer present with advanced disease, EUS evaluation is likely to add little to surgical exploration and management. However, successful EUS-guided cholecystostomy through the duodenal wall for acute cholecystitis in elderly patients who are poor surgical candidates, as reported by a group in Korea, might be feasible for palliation in malignancy as well [89]. Work in this area is ongoing.

51

Biliary Malignancy

■ Malignancy Affecting the Biliary Tree (Table 51.5)

Malignancies resulting in bile duct strictures can be divided into primary and secondary types. Primary malignancies are those arising from the biliary epithelium or closely adjacent tissues, and include cholangiocarcinoma, hepatoma, and gallbladder cancer. Secondary malignancies cause biliary strictures by extrinsic compression of the bile ducts; they include pancreatic tumors (e.g., adenocarcinoma, lymphoma) and metastatic malignancy (e.g., from the colon, breast, or bronchus). As the management of each type of these malignancies is unique, a vigorous effort must be made to identify the tissue of origin. A minority of tumors causing biliary strictures are amenable to surgical resection, but it is important to identify these cases, since removal of the tumor may be the patient's only hope for cure or prolonged survival. Staging of such tumors includes CT scanning, with or without portography and hepatic arteriography. Vascular encasement or invasion is often (but not always) evidence of unresectability. Portal vein invasion does not necessarily exclude surgery, but arterial involvement usually does. While curative resection may be impossible, surgery for biliary and sometimes gastric bypass provides useful palliation in carefully

Table 51.5 Malignant tumors of the biliary tree

Primary
Cholangiocarcinoma
Hepatoma
Gallbladder carcinoma
Secondary
Pancreatic tumors, including adenocarcinoma and lymphoma
Metastatic malignancy

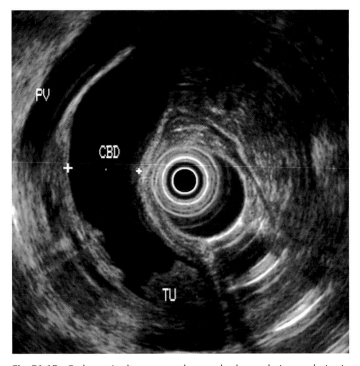

Fig. 51.15 Endoscopic ultrasonography reveals a hypoechoic mass lesion in the distal common bile duct, consistent with cholangiocarcinoma rather than an intra-ampullary carcinoma. CBD, common bile duct (diameter 18 mm); PV, portal vein; TU, tumor.

selected cases. In patients with distal bile duct strictures, laparoscopic biliary and gastric bypass may be an option. The gallbladder should not be used for biliary bypass if the tumor is within 2 cm of the cystic duct take-off, as tumor ingrowth will quickly lead to occlusion and the patient will become jaundiced again [90]. Endoscopic and percutaneous stenting procedures remain the mainstay of palliation for malignant biliary obstruction.

■ A Potpourri of Imaging Techniques

Many imaging techniques are available for studying the biliary tree, including transabdominal US, CT, magnetic resonance imaging (MRI), arteriography, and, most recently, EUS and positron-emission tomography (PET). ERCP and PTC are direct techniques for accessing and imaging the bile ducts, and offer the potential for cytological diagnosis and palliative treatment (e.g., biliary drainage using stents or drains). A detailed discussion of the relative merits of all these imaging modalities is beyond the scope of this review. However, a combination of techniques (e.g., CT plus ERCP, or MRI plus PTC) will provide a higher diagnostic yield in most cases than a single technique used alone. Patients with complex hilar strictures may be best served by PTC and external biliary drainage (usually bilateral); using this method of access, self-expanding metallic stents can be placed for palliation of unresectable tumors [91]. Local irradiation (brachytherapy) can be applied to suitable bile duct tumors using a ^{192}Ir source advanced over a percutaneously placed guide wire [92].

■ EUS or ERCP in the Diagnosis of Biliary Malignancy

Bile duct cancer (cholangiocarcinoma) is rare, with an estimated 2000–3000 new cases annually in the United States. The lesions can be intrahepatic, perihilar (bifurcation to cystic duct origin), or distal extrahepatic (common bile duct) [93]. These cancers are challenging to detect, with small tumors (< 20 mm) being especially problematic for transabdominal US and CT imaging. The detection rate for small carcinomas approaches 100% with EUS and ERCP [94]. ERCP with biopsy and cytological brushing is the most sensitive and specific way to diagnose and localize malignancy in the biliary tree; however, it cannot offer staging information, such as the extent of tumor invasion [95]. Given the proximity of the extrahepatic bile duct to the duodenum, EUS can visualize bile duct tumors and provide useful staging information that can help determine the appropriate treatment (**Fig. 51.15**).

The distal CBD is best viewed by EUS from the descending duodenum at the level of the ampulla. The more proximal CBD and common hepatic duct can be viewed from the duodenal bulb. In general, EUS cannot reliably image the bifurcation of the right and left main intrahepatic ducts. However, one author reported very accurate staging of Klatskin tumors using EUS [96].

Staging of bile duct cancer is done according to the TNM (tumor, node, metastasis) classification (see below). EUS is highly accurate for assessing the T stage of extrahepatic bile duct tumors, with accuracy rates of 81–85% in comparison with surgery [94,95,97]. Given the extremely thin wall layers of the bile duct, and the fact that they can frequently be obscured in the setting of inflammation, it can be quite difficult to distinguish between T1 and T2 lesions. Fortunately, the differentiation between these tumor stages usually does not influence therapeutic management. In contrast, vascular invasion or gross invasion into adjacent organs will likely alter treatment. EUS is capable of distinguishing T3 from T1–2 lesions with an 88% level of accuracy [67]. The nodal staging of cholangiocarcinoma with EUS has an accuracy of 53–81% [94,95,97]. Studies using cytologic sampling via fine-needle aspiration may detect an additional 17–20 % of involved lymph nodes not previously identified with other imaging methods, affecting surgical decision-making, especially with regard to liver transplantation [98,99].

Intraductal ultrasonography (IDUS) uses selective cannulation of the bile duct with a 6-Fr high-frequency (20-MHz) miniprobe. This technique requires fluoroscopy, but allows examination of the entire extrahepatic bile duct and the right and left hepatic ducts. The main advantage of this technique is that staging can be performed during the initial diagnostic and/or therapeutic ERCP. In addition, IDUS can assess portal vein invasion at the liver hilum and invasion of the right hepatic artery. It is difficult to image the liver hilum with EUS; in one study, bile duct tumors were inadequately visualized at this site [100]. IDUS may be more accurate in assessing pancreatic parenchymal invasion by bile duct cancer than EUS [101]. IDUS cannot be performed if the miniprobe cannot cross the malignant bile duct stricture. It also cannot reliably distinguish between tumor stages T1 and T2. As stated previously, differentiation between T3 and T1–2 tumors is most important, as this affects management. When the accuracy of EUS (88 %) is compared with that of IDUS (80 %), there does not appear to be a significant difference in the ability of these techniques to identify the T stage [102].

Tissue Sampling

Brush cytology. Using an endoscopic brush, malignant cells can be scraped from the surface of biliary tumors for cytological examination (**Fig. 51.16**). Foutch [103] reviewed the literature on this subject and reported an overall sensitivity for brush cytology of 59 %, with higher sensitivity in cholangiocarcinoma than in pancreatic head adenocarcinoma. Repeated brushing may increase the cytological yield. Lee et al. [104] evaluated endoscopic bile duct brush cytology, stratifying samples into benign, low-grade dysplasia, and high-grade dysplasia. Overall, the finding of dysplasia had a 37 % sensitivity and a 100 % specificity for bile duct cancer. The combination of brush cytology, FNA, and forceps biopsy has a greater sensitivity (around 80 %) than any single modality alone [105].

Fine-needle aspiration (FNA) and forceps biopsy. Howell et al. [106] reported a 61 % sensitivity (16 of 26 patients) for endoscopic FNA of malignant bile duct strictures. Kubota et al. [107] found a sensitivity of 81 % for transpapillary stricture biopsy in 43 patients with pancreatic and bile duct cancer (**Fig. 51.17**). Nimura et al. [108] reported a high diagnostic yield (> 85 %) for cholangiocarcinoma using forceps biopsy by the percutaneous route. Percutaneous FNA with radiographic guidance has very variable results, but an acceptably low complication rate. Sherman et al. [109] carried out "triple sampling" in 127 patients using Geenen cytology brushes, Howell aspiration needles (Cook Medical Inc., Winston-Salem, North Carolina, USA; two thrusts) and endobiliary forceps biopsy (three or four bites). The overall sensitivity was 71 %. EUS-FNA cytology has emerged as a sensitive test for cholangiocarcinoma, even in patients with negative brush cytology or conventional imaging negative for a mass. Sensitivity ranges from 77 % to 91 %, but negative predictive values (37–67 %) for EUS-FNA are not adequate to rule out malignancy in a negative examination [99,110].

Molecular markers. "Ploidy" refers to the DNA content of cells. The association between aneuploidy and malignant transformation makes evaluation of the ploidy status of biopsy samples potentially useful. Two techniques that can evaluate the DNA content of cells are flow cytometry and absorptive cytometry; the latter requires a much smaller tissue sample, and appears to be superior for diagnosing cancer. Patients with aneuploidy appear to have a shorter survival than those whose cells have diploid DNA content [111]. Mutations in the K-*ras* oncogene have been reported in 75–100 %

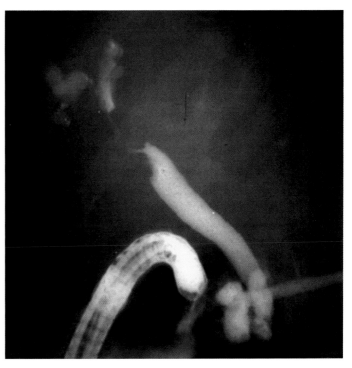

Fig. 51.16 A suitable case for cytological brushing. This cholangiogram shows that a tight hilar stricture is the cause of obstructive jaundice.

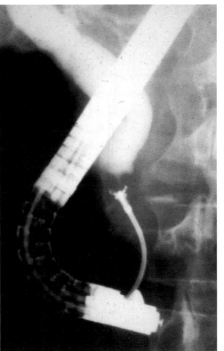

Fig. 51.17
Transpapillary forceps biopsy of a malignant mid-common bile duct stricture.

of pancreatic cancers [112]. Tada et al. [113] noted a high incidence of *ras* gene mutations in bile duct cancers. The mutation occurs at the codon 12 position. The role of this mutation in the genesis of cholangiocarcinoma is uncertain. Other mutations that have been described in pancreatic and biliary cancers include the p53 mutation and loss of integrity of chromosomes 5 and 17 [114,115]. There has been considerable interest in telomerase as a marker of malignant transformation in pancreatic and bile duct cancer [116]. CA-19–9, a Lewis antigen expressed in 95 % of the population, may be elevated

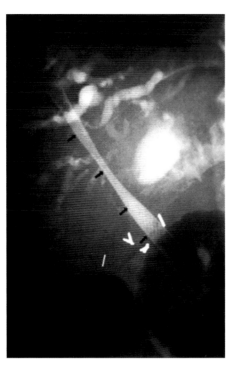

Fig. 51.18 A biliary metal mesh stent (Wallstent) occluded by tumor ingrowth (arrows). It has deployed incompletely, as evidenced by the "waist."

Table 51.6 Classification of sclerosing cholangitis

Primary
Unknown/associated with other diseases (e. g., ulcerative colitis)
Secondary (known or suspected causes)
Surgical trauma
Bile duct stones
Cholangiocarcinoma
Toxic chemicals (e. g., formaldehyde)
Intrahepatic arterial infusion of floxuridine and its derivatives
Liver transplant rejection
Histiocytosis X
AIDS (*Cryptosporidium* infection)

Adapted from Lu and Kaplowitz [124].

in those able to express the protein. The sensitivity of CA-19–9 depends on the cut-off level established for abnormality. Certainly, a CA-19–9 level > 1000 IU/L warrants a search for occult malignancy; and a decline in CA-19–9 after pancreatic cancer therapy is encouraging [117]. However, CA 19–9 is not specific for the pancreas, as it is elevated in some patients with bile duct cancers (cholangiocarcinomas), hepatomas, and even nongastroenterologic solid tumors (e. g., pulmonary tumors).

Staging of Bile Duct Tumors

As noted previously, the TNM classification is being used increasingly to categorize cholangiocarcinoma into four stages: stage I is limited to the mucosa, stage II has periductal invasion but without nodal disease or metastases, stage III has regional lymph nodes involved, and stage IV involves adjacent structures and/or distant metastases. Malignancies of the bile duct are also classified according to their location. Tumors in the upper third involve the common hepatic duct and confluence; those in the middle third arise from the common bile duct between the cystic duct and the upper border

of the duodenum; and tumors in the lower third arise from the common bile duct between the upper border of the duodenum and the ampulla of Vater. For endoscopists, the Bismuth classification [118] is helpful: type I tumors are located within the common hepatic duct, type II involve the right and left main hepatic ducts, and type III involve the secondary intrahepatic bile ducts (IIIa, the right duct; IIIb, the left ones). A more advanced stage, in which both right and left ducts are involved, is sometimes referred to as type IV. The following findings on imaging studies commonly indicate a lack of resectability [119]: bilateral intrahepatic bile duct spread or multifocal disease; involvement of the main trunk of the portal vein; involvement of both branches of the portal vein or bilateral involvement of the hepatic artery and portal vein; and vascular involvement on one side of the liver with extensive bile duct involvement on the other.

Biliary Stenting

Endoscopic stenting is a well-established form of palliative treatment for malignant biliary obstruction. Hilar strictures are much more difficult to bridge than more distal ones. Two prospective, randomized trials have compared plastic and metal endoprostheses for distal biliary obstruction [120,121]. In one study, the overall survival was the same; however, the medium time to stent occlusion was longer for metal stents (33 % after 273 days) than for plastic ones (54 % after 123 days). The second study showed occlusion rates for metal stents of 22 % and 43 % for plastic ones during the lifetime of the patient. Patients stented for hilar obstruction suffer recurrent jaundice and cholangitis more frequently than those with other sites of obstruction. A distinct advantage of the percutaneous approach in hilar malignancy is the ability to place two stents simultaneously through the right and left biliary systems. This can also be done endoscopically, but it is technically difficult to deploy multiple endoscopic stents simultaneously. Bilateral placement of metal mesh stents has become common for palliating unresectable hilar bile duct tumors. Unfortunately, these metal mesh stents have a tendency to occlude due to tumor ingrowth (**Fig. 51.18**). When these stents block, it is sometimes possible to relieve the obstruction by advancing a plastic stent endoscopically through the metal stent lumen. The use of coated metal stents attempts to address the problem of tumor ingrowth. The duration of patency may be improved with coated stents, but an additional risk of acute cholecystitis (3.8 %) is incurred if the cystic duct is incidentally obstructed [122]. The choice of palliation used for patients with unresectable cholangiocarcinoma depends on the overall condition of the patient and his or her expected survival time. Comparison of surgical, endoscopic, and radiological palliation of distal common bile duct strictures shows comparable survival and quality of life.

Miscellaneous Conditions in the Biliary Tree

Primary Sclerosing Cholangitis

Primary sclerosing cholangitis (PSC) is a chronic cholestatic disorder characterized by diffuse inflammatory fibrosis of the intrahepatic and extrahepatic bile ducts [123]. Although the pathogenesis of PSC remains unclear, it is one of several conditions commonly associated with inflammatory bowel disease, especially ulcerative colitis (**Table 51.6**) [124].

The cholangiographic appearances of PSC are almost (but not quite) unique [125]; ERCP increased the number of patients being diagnosed with PSC at an asymptomatic stage. Thinning of the intrahepatic bile ducts, with multifocal strictures and areas of dilation are characteristic in PSC (**Fig. 51.19**). In the extrahepatic biliary tree, PSC may be manifest as a solitary stricture (**Fig. 51.20**), which may be dominant in terms of symptoms and biochemical abnormalities. ERCP helps determine the severity and extent of intrahepatic and extrahepatic involvement in PSC. As the disease progresses, patients can develop worsening cholestasis and intermittent cholangitis. In the absence of effective medical therapy, perhaps a third of PSC patients will eventually require liver transplantation [126]. PSC is a good indication for liver transplantation, as the operative morbidity and mortality are low, with excellent survival. The intrahepatic strictures of PSC are generally diffuse and multifocal and therefore rarely amenable to endoscopic therapy. If a dominant extrahepatic stricture is the cause of recurrent cholangitis, endoscopic therapy with stricture dilation should be considered, as this is likely to reduce the risk of cholestasis and infectious complications.

For the endoscopist considering ERCP as a way to diagnose and treat PSC, the following questions are appropriate. First, what is the indication for the procedure? For initial screening, MRCP followed by ERCP (in patients with negative MRCP) appears to be cost-effective and is our preferred approach [127]. Therapeutic indications for ERCP include stricture dilation and stenting (after cytological brushing), as well as stone removal. These therapeutic interventions may offer the patient symptomatic improvement, but there is no evidence that they reverse the underlying pathological process. Patients with progressive liver disease in PSC who are destined for liver transplantation can be kept well by endoscopic and/or interventional radiological procedures until they are ready to receive their new liver.

The second consideration for the endoscopist in the PSC patient is whether or not the intended intervention may make the surgeon's job more difficult, either for biliary bypass or liver transplantation. For this reason, most endoscopists believe that expandable metal mesh stents should not be placed in the bile duct in benign disease. Practice patterns may shift, however, as removable covered self-expanding metal stents (CSEMS) are starting to be used to manage benign biliary strictures, with encouraging results [84]. Before any endoscopic intervention in PSC, it is important to provide antibiotic prophylaxis against Gram-negative sepsis.

The third question for endoscopists performing ERCP in patients with PSC is to determine whether a new stricture is malignant. There is a strong association between sclerosing cholangitis and the development of cholangiocarcinoma (risk 7–9%) [128]. Often, these tumors cannot be visualized on CT scanning (at least in their early stages), and endoscopic brushing and other tissue sampling methods are therefore very important. Overall, the sensitivity of endoscopic brush cytology is in the range of 40–60% [129]. The yield of malignant diagnoses can be increased by adjunctive techniques such as flow cytometry [111], ploidy studies, determining K-*ras* oncogene status [130], and fluorescent in-situ hybridization (FISH), etc. Direct biopsy of accessible biliary tumors and core biopsies or aspiration specimens are also excellent tools for diagnosing malignancy. CA-19-9, as a serological maker for certain malignancies, is helpful in the diagnosis of cholangiocarcinoma and is useful in scant cellular material when combined with other modalities [131]. Dilation of the bile ducts proximal to an extrahepatic biliary stricture may suggest the development of malignancy. As sclerosing cholangitis is a chronic fibrosing condition, it is difficult for the bile ducts to dilate unless there is a significant pressure gradient generated by obstruction. In our experience, bile duct dilation proximal to dominant stricture is often the first clue that malignancy has developed. In patients who have progressive cholestasis, with liver injury due to extensive PSC, liver transplantation may be the definitive treatment. In such patients, endoscopic maneuvers such as dilation and stenting of strictures are temporizing. In other patients whose PSC is not associated with chronic liver disease but who have problems with recurrent cholangitis, biliary bypass surgery remains

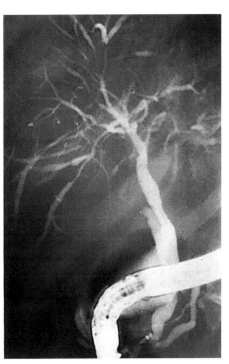

Fig. 51.19 Multiple stenoses in the intrahepatic biliary tree. The confluence with the pancreatic duct system is unremarkable.

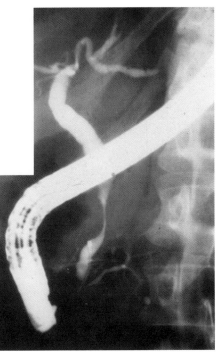

Fig. 51.20 A solitary extrahepatic biliary stricture in primary sclerosing cholangitis.

an option [132]. In view of the potential for PSC patients to need some form of biliary surgery (up to and including transplantation), it is important for the endoscopist, the interventional radiologist, and the surgeon to work together as an interdisciplinary team. The Amsterdam group [133] reported favorable experience with short-term stenting of strictures in PSC. However, in an accompanying editorial, Al-Kawas [134] argued that when it comes to the endoscopic management of PSC, "less is better." There is considerable interest in magnetic resonance cholangiography (MRC) as a noninvasive method of imaging the biliary tree in PSC (**Fig. 51.21**) [135,136]. MRC is preferable to ERCP for periodic surveillance of the progression of PSC in asymptomatic patients.

51

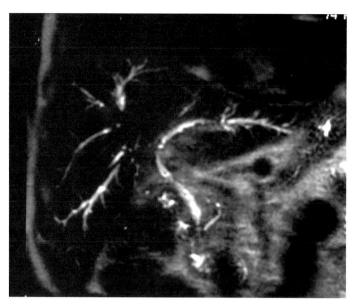

Fig. 51.21 Intrahepatic ducts in primary sclerosing cholangitis, as imaged on magnetic resonance cholangiopancreatography.

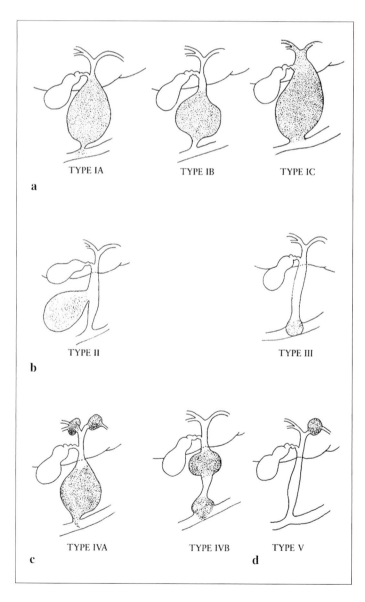

Choledochal Cysts

Bile duct cysts can occur at any level in the biliary tree, from the common bile duct to the intrahepatic ducts. Since the original description of choledochal cysts in the early 1700s, there have been over 1000 case reports in the medical literature. Choledochal cysts are uncommon in Western countries, with an estimated incidence of one in 150,000 [137]. More than one-third of reported cases have occurred in Japanese patients [138]. While the etiology of choledochal cysts has not been fully clarified, they are generally considered to be congenital in origin. However, many choledochal cysts are asymptomatic during childhood and early adulthood, sometimes presenting as late as the sixth or seventh decade. This suggests that environmental factors may be involved in addition to a genetic predisposition. The original classification included just three types of extrahepatic cyst. As some patients with extrahepatic involvement also have intrahepatic cysts, a modified classification was introduced by Todani et al. [139]. Their scheme distinguished five types and two subtypes of choledochal cyst (**Fig. 51.22**). Type I lesions consist of cystic dilations of the common bile duct or cystic duct; these are the most common choledochal cysts, making up 80–90 % of the total. Type II lesions are diverticulum-like, eccentric lesions of the common bile duct, representing less than 3 % of cases. The type III lesion, or choledochocele, is an intramural cystic dilation of the distal common bile duct that appears endoscopically as a compressible, smooth-surfaced bulge in the duodenum. The type IV lesion is divided into types IVA and IVB; in type IVA, there are multiple cysts involving the intrahepatic and extrahepatic bile ducts, whereas in type IVB there are multiple cysts confined to the extrahepatic bile ducts. Type V has single or multiple cysts involving the intrahepatic ducts, and is known as Caroli disease.

The clinical presentation of choledochal cysts varies according to the age of the patient. In infants, there is frequently painless, intermittent jaundice. Nausea, vomiting, and failure to thrive may also occur. The majority of affected children have a palpable mass in the right upper abdomen. Many adults with choledochal cysts are asymptomatic. When symptoms do occur, they are usually related to obstruction, such as pain or jaundice, or both, due to cholangitis. Due to the frequent presence of an anomalous pancreaticobiliary ductal union and choledocholithiasis (**Fig. 51.23**), recurrent pancreatitis may be another presenting complaint in patients with choledochal cysts. Long-standing (especially low-grade) biliary obstruction may result in secondary biliary cirrhosis. Malignant transformation is also a recognized late complication of choledochal cysts. Transabdominal US is often the first imaging test obtained during the work-up in these patients. Although cystic dilations of the bile duct are easily seen on transabdominal US, it lacks sensitivity for changes in the distal CBD when it is obscured by overlying gas. Transabdominal US rarely identifies an anomalous pancreaticobiliary ductal union. There are similar problems with abdominal CT and biliary scintigraphy (e. g., HIDA scanning). MRCP has greatly improved noninvasive imaging of the biliary tree [140] (**Fig. 51.21**)

Fig. 51.22 Todani's classification of choledochal cysts.
a Type IA, localized extrahepatic; type IB, segmental dilation; type IC, diffuse or cylindrical dilation.
b Type II, extrahepatic diverticulum; type III, choledochocele.
c Type IVA, multiple intrahepatic and extrahepatic cysts; type IVB, multiple extrahepatic cysts only.
d Type V, solitary intrahepatic cyst.

VIII

and is the first-line option for diagnosis in asymptomatic patients. PTC may occasionally be needed to define complete biliary anatomy, especially when the biliary tree cannot be cannulated at ERCP. The association of choledochal cysts with cholangiocarcinoma was first described by Irwin and Morison in 1944, and has been well documented since that time [141]. The overall incidence of cholangio-carcinoma in untreated patients with choledochal cysts is reported to be between 3% and 20% [142,143], representing a 5–40-fold increased risk in comparison with the normal population. For patients with type III choledochal cysts, the risk is thought to be at the lower end of the range. The incidence of cholangiocarcinoma appears to increase with age. In patients under 10 years of age, the cancer risk in less than 1%, but it increases to more than 14% after 20 years of age [144]. Other complications of choledochal cysts include cyst rupture, formation of stones within the cysts, cholangitis, and secondary biliary cirrhosis.

Once the diagnosis of a choledochal cyst has been made, the treatment of choice is usually surgical, except in the elderly and those with major comorbidities. Choledochoceles may be an exception, given their low risk of malignant transformation. Type I cysts are usually managed by complete resection of the affected area, with Roux-en-Y hepaticojejunostomy for biliary drainage. The major risks of cyst excision are vascular injury (hepatic artery, portal vein) and damage to the pancreatic duct in the head of the pancreas. Bypass procedures without cyst resection are sometimes performed, but the risk of malignant transformation will then persist. Type II cysts can usually be treated by surgical resection, with or without a drainage procedure. Traditionally, type III choledochal cysts (choledochoceles) have been treated by transduodenal cyst excision and surgical sphincteroplasty. Endoscopic opening of small choledochoceles (either with standard or needle-knife papillotomy) is frequently undertaken; this procedure does not seem to be associated with an increased risk of complications. We are not aware of cholangiocarcinoma having developed in any patient after endoscopic drainage of a choledochocele. We believe that the available data from patients treated endoscopically are insufficient to be able to state with confidence that endoscopic drainage prevents the development of malignant transformation. The risks and benefits always have to be weighed between surgery and endoscopic decompression. After about the age of 60, the risk–benefit ratio is increasingly weighted in favor of endoscopic (i.e., nonsurgical) management alone. Type IV and V choledochal cysts offer some difficult management issues. Complete cyst excision with wide hepaticojejunostomy is an acceptable approach in patients with type IVA cysts. In other cases, isolated resection of the extrahepatic disease, leaving the intrahepatic cysts in place, is performed. Although the intrahepatic cysts sometimes regress, malignancy has been reported to arise from these intrahepatic lesions [145]. Defining the biliary tree by cholangiography is an important first step in planning surgical strategy in these patients. Treatment of patients with Caroli disease (type V) can be difficult, and depends on the extent of liver involvement. For limited forms not complicated by malignancy, partial liver resection may be feasible. Patients with extensive intrahepatic cyst formation may suffer recurrent cholangitis: hepaticojejunostomy may afford significant relief. Endoscopic therapy in combination with extracorporeal shock-wave lithotripsy has been reported as helpful in Caroli disease [146] when surgery is not an option. Finally, orthotopic liver transplantation may be possible in highly selected patients with Caroli disease without cholangiocarcinoma. Caroli disease should not be confused with Oriental cholangiohepatitis, another disease in which stricturing and focal dilation of the intrahepatic bile ducts in prominent (**Fig. 51.24**).

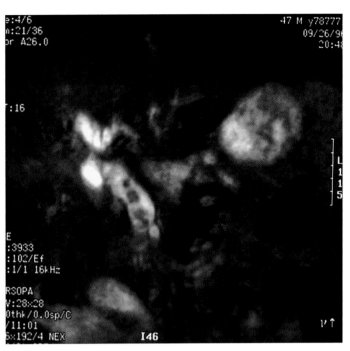

Fig. 51.23 The magnetic resonance cholangiogram shows choledocholithiasis (a string of stones is clearly seen in the bile duct).

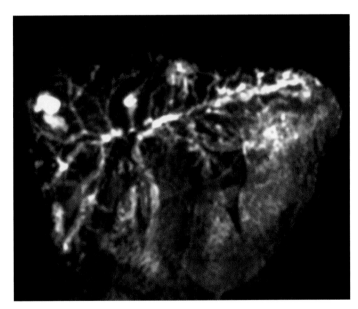

Fig. 51.24 The magnetic resonance cholangiogram shows Oriental cholangiohepatitis.

Sphincter of Oddi Dysfunction

The flow of bile into the duodenum is regulated by the sphincter of Oddi, a ring of smooth muscle that encircles the distal common bile duct at the level of the ampulla. The papilla of Vater and its muscular sphincter represent the junction of the biliary and pancreatic ducts. The physiology of the sphincter of Oddi is complex and incompletely understood, but probably involves a combination of neural, paracrine, and endocrine inputs. When the gallbladder contracts, the sphincter of Oddi relaxes to allow a bolus of bile to be expelled into the duodenum to aid digestion. Manometric measurement of the sphincter of Oddi can be performed during ERCP using a specialized triple-lumen perfusion catheter, first developed by Arndorfer. The catheter is introduced into the common bile duct orifice, sometimes

Table 51.7 The Geenen–Hogan classification of sphincter of Oddi dysfunction [147]

Type	Pain	Abnormal LFTs on two or more occasions	Dilated bile duct ≥ 12 mm
I	Yes	Yes	Yes
II	Yes	Yes	No
	Yes	No	Yes
III	Yes	No	No

LFTs, liver function tests.

over a guide wire with a diameter of 0.018 inches, and advanced until it is deep in the duct. The catheter is then withdrawn in increments, stopping at each port along the length of the catheter tip (marked in 2-mm increments). Sphincter pressures are recorded several times at each of five or six pressure ports; the pressure data are determined using preset calibrations on the manometry recording strip. Modern solid-state pressure transducers with automated recording devices can simplify the work of the endoscopist. The normal resting pressure of the sphincter of Oddi is 5–15 mmHg. Phasic contractions occur three to seven times each minute; these raise the pressure to 30–150 mmHg. Reading the manometric strip is as much an art as a science. Unfortunately, the interpretation of manometric data is inconsistent between major centers, and often within them, too. For this reason, it is important that sphincter of Oddi manometry should be performed by experienced personnel in centers with a sufficient volume of cases to maintain proficiency.

Sphincter of Oddi dysfunction (SOD) is a relatively uncommon clinical syndrome that should be suspected in patients with episodic biliary-type pain after cholecystectomy [147]. This syndrome clearly represents a spectrum of diverse and poorly defined disorders. Papillary stenosis is a structural abnormality that describes fibrosis and subsequent narrowing of the sphincteric portion of the distal common bile duct. The pathophysiological events involved are poorly understood. Papillary stenosis may result from repeated trauma from passage of small biliary stones. Papillitis, an inflammation of the duodenal papilla, occurs mainly in immunosuppressed patients and is sometimes associated with viral infection (e. g., cytomegalovirus, human immunodeficiency virus) [148]. Patients with papillary stenosis typically have typical biliary-type pain, abnormal liver function tests, and radiographic evidence of bile duct dilation. The symptoms usually persist or worsen after cholecystectomy, which removes a distensible reservoir (gallbladder) and exacerbates the effects of the impaired bile flow. This is one form of the condition known as the postcholecystectomy syndrome. The histories of patients presenting with papillary stenosis often show that they have undergone cholecystectomy for presumed gallstones. However, when examined by a pathologist, the gallbladder may appear entirely normal. The fibrotic nature of papillary stenosis makes endoscopic cannulation of the bile duct technically difficult in many cases. When the endoscopic approach fails, percutaneous access (alone, or as a combined procedure) may be considered. Recurrent stenosis develops at papillotomy sites in a few patients, who may require formal surgical procedures such as sphincteroplasty. Endoscopic sphincterotomy for papillary stenosis carries an increased risk of complications, including pancreatitis, perforation, and bleeding. However, when undertaken successfully in the right circumstances, sphincterotomy usually provides permanent relief of the symptoms. Endoscopic stenting or balloon dilation of the papilla rarely improve matters in papillary stenosis, and carry a significant risk of causing pancreatitis in this particular patient population.

In their classic 1989 paper in the *New England Journal of Medicine*, Geenen et al. [147] (**Table 51.7**) suggested that sphincter stenosis and dysmotility should be considered together as part of an SOD syndrome. Type I patients present with typical biliary pain, elevated liver tests (transaminases and/or alkaline phosphatase) documented on two or more occasions with normalization between attacks, a dilated common bile duct (> 12 mm in diameter), or delayed drainage of contrast (> 45 min) from the common bile duct. (Most modern ERCP endoscopists have dropped the bile duct drainage time from the classification, due to its variability related to patient positioning.) Using sphincter of Oddi manometry, motor dysfunction has been recorded in approximately 70 % of these patients. Sphincter stenosis appears to predominate in this patient group. Endoscopic sphincterotomy is almost always successful in abolishing symptoms in type I patients. For this reason, most experts consider sphincter of Oddi manometry to be unnecessary; the endoscopist can proceed directly to perform biliary sphincterotomy. Type II patients have biliary-type pain, but only one of the other two criteria listed for type I; manometry can be helpful in assessing type II patients. In a randomized double-blind prospective study of type II patients, those with manometric abnormalities were significantly more likely to benefit from sphincterotomy (pain response > 90 %) than those with normal sphincter of Oddi manometry (pain response about 25 %). Type III patients present clinically with a pain syndrome only. Although the pain may be caused by SOD, it is more often a manifestation of irritable bowel syndrome or some other chronic, functional abdominal, or chest wall pain. In type III, less than 20 % of patients have abnormal manometry. Even in this subgroup, only 50 % of patients will improve after sphincterotomy. Biliary (sphincter of Oddi) manometry and sphincterotomy should only be performed in type III patients after detailed clinical evaluation and a careful explanation of the risks and benefits. (There is a similar classification for pancreatic sphincter dysfunction, which is discussed in Chapter 52).

SOD is recognized manometrically by a high resting sphincter pressure (> 40 mmHg), sustained elevation in pressures during contraction, and an abnormal response to cholecystokinin or a fatty meal. Dysfunction of the sphincter of Oddi consists of two distinct entities: papillary stenosis (a structural abnormality) and sphincter of Oddi (biliary) dyskinesia (a motility disorder). In type I SOD patients, 70–80 % or more will have sustained symptomatic relief after endoscopic sphincterotomy. The risk of post-ERCP pancreatitis in patients with suspected SOD is quite high—21.7 % in the study by Freeman et al. [6]. Careful selection of patients for ERCP and sphincterotomy is very important, and rewards attention to stratification using radiological and biochemical criteria and symptoms.

Clostridium botulinum toxin (Botox), which destroys postganglionic acetylcholine receptors in certain nerve cells, has been used locally in an effort to treat gastrointestinal motility disorders (such as achalasia and anal sphincter spasm). When injected endoscopically though the duodenal wall into the fibers of the sphincter of Oddi, botulinum A toxin may reduce sphincter of Oddi pressure by 50 % [149]. Wehrmann et al. [150] investigated the potential role of endoscopic injection of botulinum toxin into the duodenal papilla to relieve symptoms of suspected SOD, as a way of predicting the outcome of endoscopic sphincterotomy. Twenty-two postcholecystectomy patients with manometrically confirmed type III SOD received a single dose of 100 mouse units of botulinum toxin injected directly into the duodenal papilla. One patient developed postprocedural pancreatitis. Twelve patients (55 %) were symptom-free 6 weeks after botulinum toxin injection. Sphincter of Oddi pressures returned to normal in five of the ten patients without symptomatic benefit, but none had symptomatic relief after subsequent endoscopic sphincterotomy. Two of five patients had persistently high sphincter of Oddi pressures and benefited from endoscopic sphincterotomy. Eleven of the 12 patients who initially responded to botulinum toxin had recurrent symptoms at 6 months; all had elevated sphincter of Oddi pressures, and all benefited from endoscopic sphincterotomy. The authors suggest that botulinum toxin injection may predict whether SOD type III patients will benefit from endoscopic sphincterotomy.

A similar attempt to treat SOD without the risk of sphincterotomy has been made with sildenafil, a drug better known for its use in erectile dysfunction via selective smooth muscle relaxation [151]. The authors studied seven patients (six women, one man; age range 31–57 years) with an intact sphincter of Oddi and suspected SOD. They excluded patients younger than 18 years and older than 65 years; those who had a difficult cannulation; patients with previous post-ERCP pancreatitis; those with American Society of Anesthesiologists (ASA) grade ≥ 3; those who had used sildenafil within the previous 7 days; patients with creatinine clearance < 30 mL/min; and pregnant women. The results showed that administration of sildenafil markedly reduced basal sphincter of Oddi pressure in patients with suspected SOD. Pretreatment and posttreatment pressures were 82 ± 52 mmHg and 29 ± 27 mmHg, respectively. The mean reduction in pressure was an impressive 53 ± 40 mmHg. These findings are intriguing, and further studies using this agent are certainly warranted. Regrettably, the authors did not provide data on the patients' symptomatic response to sildenafil [151].

Referrals for possible biliary pain are common in specialist biliary clinics. Often, these patients have undergone extensive clinical, radiological, and laboratory testing without a diagnosis having been made. It must be remembered that right upper quadrant pain may come from a variety of sources. Desautels et al. [152] confirmed the suspicions of many of those who treat SOD patients that the pain may not originate solely from the biliary tree. Using duodenal and rectal barostat studies, the authors found that SOD type III patients exhibit duodenal but not rectal hyperalgesia in comparison with matched control individuals. These patients also showed high levels of somatization, depression, obsessive-compulsive behavior, and anxiety. ERCP with biliary (sphincter of Oddi) manometry must be reserved for patients who appear to have a true biliary pain syndrome, as otherwise many patients who have no hope of benefiting from diagnostic and therapeutic ERCP may be put at unnecessary risk of complications, especially post-ERCP pancreatitis.

The whole subject of SOD and its diagnosis has become more complex with recent observations, such as persistent high pressure despite sphincterotomy, asymmetry of the sphincter muscle [153], and concurrent pancreatic hypertension in perhaps the majority of patients with biliary sphincter hypertension [154]. Sphincter of Oddi manometry should probably be confined to large regional centers at which a sufficiently large number of patients can be treated each year to build up and maintain experience. Endoscopists performing ERCP on patients with SOD should be skilled at placing prophylactic pancreatic stents, which have been shown to significantly reduce the incidence and severity of post-sphincter of Oddi manometry pancreatitis [155,156]. Given the concern about procedure-related pancreatitis, less invasive radiological techniques such as quantitative cholescintigraphy [157] and secretin-stimulated MRCP may supersede sphincter of Oddi manometry. However, more data are required before a radionuclide or MRI scan can be considered equivalent to direct pressure measurement. Recent data from the United Kingdom correlated a 1-mm increase in pancreatic duct diameter on MRCP in response to secretin infusion with a durable response to endoscopic biliary sphincterotomy in patients with manometrically proven SOD type II [158]. In this small study, no patients with a negative secretin stimulation MRCP (ss-MRCP) responded to endoscopic therapy.

Biliary Parasites

A variety of parasites inhabit the biliary tree. *Echinococcus* causes hydatid disease. Dumas et al. [159] reported on 28 patients with diffuse hepatic hydatid disease who underwent ERCP preoperatively (n = 19) or in the postoperative period (n = 9). Preoperative ERCP with biliary sphincterotomy was effective in treating all seven patients who presented with acute cholangitis (due to cyst rupture into the bile ducts). It was also helpful in two of three patients with acute pain presumed to be secondary to papillary stenosis in this condition. These encouraging data are supported by those of Rodriguez et al. [160].

A variety of liver flukes, including *Fasciola hepatica* and *Clonorchis sinensis*, as well as the roundworm *Ascaris lumbricoides*, may colonize the biliary tree, where they lay their eggs. In affected patients, fluke or worm eggs are often found to provide the nidus for biliary stone formation. Live or dead worms may occlude the intrahepatic and extrahepatic bile ducts, causing obstruction and sometimes infection (cholangitis). *Fasciola* infects humans through ingestion of contaminated vegetables, especially watercress. It may be quite resistant to standard drug therapy for parasitosis. Dowidar et al. [161] described their treatment of nine patients with fluke infections resistant to oral agents. They flushed the bile ducts with a 2.5 % solution of povidone–iodine during ERCP. Apparently the treatment was effective; all of the patients were found to be negative for *Fasciola* ova when their stools were examined during the follow-up.

Some Recent Developments

Antibiotics and ERCP. Several authors have recently addressed the issue of antibiotic therapy in ERCP. Harris et al. [162] performed a meta-analysis of the published data on the subject. After a review of 49 abstracts, seven randomized, placebo-controlled trials of antibiotic prophylaxis prior to ERCP were identified. Two studies were excluded, because the patients had received antibiotics before and after ERCP. Four studies investigated bacteremia, and five studies looked at the clinical outcome in cholangitis/septicemia. The summary relative risk of the association between antibiotic prophylaxis and bacteremia was 0.39 (95 % CI, 0.12 to 1.29). For cholangitis/septicemia, the summary relative risk was 0.91 (95 % CI, 0.39 to 2.15). The authors concluded that antibiotic prophylaxis prior to ERCP may reduce the incidence of bacteremia, but that this has little clinical relevance. Prophylaxis does not substantially reduce the incidence of cholangitis/septicemia, and in the authors' view routine antibiotic prophylaxis can therefore not be recommended. Lorenz et al. [163] studied 99 consecutive patients with biliary obstruction who underwent ERCP or PTC with biliary drainage, using sequential blood cultures before and up to 60 min after endoscopic intervention, and bile cultures obtained using a drain. The incidence of bacteremia was surprisingly low (11 %), as 73.2 % of 56 bile cultures were positive for organisms (25 species). A pathogen was found in only 19 %, while mixed growth (two to six species) was found in the majority (81 %). Notably, the use of proton-pump inhibitors was found to be a risk factor for developing postprocedural bacteremia (26 % vs. 7.5 %; *P* = 0.02). The most effective antibiotics, as judged by in vitro testing, were imipenem, followed by trimethoprim and sulfamethoxazole, amoxicillin with clavulanic acid (Augmentin), vancomycin, and ofloxacin.

Stenting of malignant biliary strictures. The search for the perfect biliary stent continues. The in vitro advantages of the Teflon stent do not appear to hold up in direct clinical comparisons with polyethylene stents [164]. It has been suggested that stents placed entirely

51

within the bile duct may be less likely to occlude than those placed across the papilla (due to lack of colonization of bile in the former). A Danish group [165] studied this in a prospective, randomized trial, and found no difference in stent survival between the groups (89 versus 82 days), although there was a significantly higher rate of stent migration with the "internal" stents (nine versus two cases). Metal stents are many times more expensive than their plastic counterparts, making it difficult to choose the "right" stent for individual patients. Yeoh et al. [166] from the Medical University of South Carolina compared three different stenting strategies in malignant biliary obstruction using a decision analysis: plastic stent, with exchange for another plastic stent on occlusion; metal stent, with placement of a coaxial plastic stent on occlusion; and plastic stent, with replacement by metal mesh stent on occlusion. The authors found that initial placement of a plastic stent, followed by metal stent placement at first occlusion in survivors, was the most cost-effective approach. Kaassis et al. found that primary metal mesh stent placement for pancreatobiliary malignancy without liver metastasis is cost-effective if the patient's life expectancy is greater than 3 months [167].

Endoscopic papillary balloon dilation versus endoscopic sphincterotomy. Endoscopic papillary balloon dilation (EPBD) is an alternative to endoscopic sphincterotomy for retrieving stones from the bile duct. Huibregtse [168] considered that EPBD should be reserved for patients with uncorrectable coagulopathy who are at high risk for bleeding from endoscopic sphincterotomy. Ohashi et al. [55] carried out a univariate and multivariate analysis of the factors predicting success or failure of EPBD for stones. The overall success rate (complete clearance) was 94% after one to six sessions (mean 1.6). However, when the bile duct was over 15 mm in diameter, the mean number of sessions needed to clear the duct was significantly higher. Stone size and number, and the need for mechanical lithotripsy, were independent variables influencing the success of EPBD.

Pharmacological relaxation of the papilla has been proposed as a method of accessing and removing bile duct stones since the 1980s [169]. Minami et al. [170] were able to extract 33 of 35 multiple and large CBD stones using a combination of EPBD, mechanical lithotripsy, and an intravenous infusion of isosorbide dinitrate at a rate of 5 mg/h. There has been a recent vogue for sphincterotomy followed by balloon dilation to enlarge the opening for the removal of large ductal stones (> 1.5 cm). The technique appears to be effective, but bleeding complications have reportedly been as high as 8–32% [171–173].

References

1. Classen M, Demling L. [Endoscopic sphincterotomy of the papilla of Vater and extraction of stones from the choledochal duct (author's transl)]. Dtsch Med Wochenschr 1974;99:496–7. German.
2. Kawai K, Akasaka Y, Murakami K, Tada M, Koli Y. Endoscopic sphincterotomy of the ampulla of Vater. Gastrointest Endosc 1974;20:148–51.
3. Aliperti G. Complications related to diagnostic and therapeutic endoscopic retrograde cholangiopancreatography. Gastrointest Endosc Clin N Am 1996;6:379–407.
4. Baillie J. Complications of endoscopy. Endoscopy 1994;26:185–203.
5. Ostroff J. Complications of endoscopic sphincterotomy. In: Jacobsen I, editor. Diagnostic and therapeutic applications. New York: Elsevier; 1989. p.61–73.
6. Freeman ML, Nelson DB, Sherman S, Haber GB, Herman ME, Dorsher PJ, et al. Complications of endoscopic biliary sphincterotomy. N Engl J Med 1996;335:909–18.
7. ASGE Standards of Practice Committee; Banerjee S, Shen B, Baron TH, Nelson DB, Anderson MA, et al. Antibiotic prophylaxis for GI endoscopy. Gastrointest Endosc 2008;67:791–8.
8. Leung JW, Libby ED, Morck DW, McKay SG, Liu Y, Lam K, et al. Is prophylactic ciprofloxacin effective in delaying biliary stent blockage? Gastro-

intest Endosc 2000;52:175–82.
9. Draganov P, Cotton PB. Iodinated contrast sensitivity in ERCP. Am J Gastroenterol 2000;95:1398–401.
10. Lasser EC, Berry CC, Mishkin MM, Williamson B, Zheutlin N, Silverman JM. Pretreatment with corticosteroids to prevent adverse reactions to nonionic contrast media. AJR Am J Roentgenol 1994;162:523–6.
11. Emmett DS, Mallat DB. Double-balloon ERCP in patients who have undergone Roux-en-Y surgery: a case series. Gastrointest Endosc 2007;66:1038–41.
12. Varadarajulu S, Trevino J, Wilcox C. The financial and clinical implications of failure at ERCP [abstract]. Gastrointest Endosc 2008;67(5):1.
13. Amouyal G, Amouyal P. Endoscopic ultrasonography in gallbladder stones. Gastrointest Endosc Clin N Am 1995;5:825–30.
14. Marks JW, Bonorris G. Intermittency of cholesterol crystals in duodenal bile from gallstone patients. Gastroenterology 1984;87:622–7.
15. Dill JE, Hill S, Callis J, Berkhouse L, Evans P, Martin D, et al. Combined endoscopic ultrasound and stimulated biliary drainage in cholecystitis and microlithiasis—diagnoses and outcomes. Endoscopy 1995;27:424–7.
16. Dill JE. Symptom resolution or relief after cholecystectomy correlates strongly with positive combined endoscopic ultrasound and stimulated biliary drainage. Endoscopy 1997;29:646–8.
17. Mirbagheri SA, Mohamadnejad M, Nasiri J, Vahid AA, Ghadimi R, Malekzadeh R. Prospective evaluation of endoscopic ultrasonography in the diagnosis of biliary microlithiasis in patients with normal transabdominal ultrasonography. J Gastrointest Surg 2005;9:961–4.
18. Coyle WJ, Lawson JM. Combined endoscopic ultrasound and stimulated biliary drainage in cholecystitis and microlithiasis: diagnosis and outcomes. Gastrointest Endosc 1996;44:102–3.
19. Amouyal P, Amouyal G, Lévy P, Tuzet S, Palazzo L, Vilgrain V, et al. Diagnosis of choledocholithiasis by endoscopic ultrasonography. Gastroenterology 1994;106:1062–7.
20. Pieken S. Role of endosonography in the diagnosis of gallstone disease in obese subjects [abstract]. Gastroenterology 1992;104:A328.
21. Toyota N, Takada T, Amano H, Yoshida M, Miura F, Wada K. Endoscopic naso-gallbladder drainage in the treatment of acute cholecystitis: alleviates inflammation and fixes operator's aim during early laparoscopic cholecystectomy. J Hepatobiliary Pancreat Surg 2006;13:80–5.
22. Conway JD, Russo MW, Shrestha R. Endoscopic stent insertion into the gallbladder for symptomatic gallbladder disease in patients with end-stage liver disease. Gastrointest Endosc 2005;61:32–6.
23. Schlenker C, Trotter JF, Shah RJ, Everson G, Chen YK, Antillon D, et al. Endoscopic gallbladder stent placement for treatment of symptomatic cholelithiasis in patients with end-stage liver disease. Am J Gastroenterol 2006;101:278–83.
24. Shrestha R, Trouillot TE, Everson GT. Endoscopic stenting of the gallbladder for symptomatic gallbladder disease in patients with end-stage liver disease awaiting orthotopic liver transplantation. Liver Transpl Surg 1999;5:275–81.
25. Leung JW, Chung SC, Sung JJ, Banez VP, Li AK. Urgent endoscopic drainage for acute suppurative cholangitis. Lancet 1989;1(8650):1307–9.
26. Browning JD, Sreenarasimhaiah J. Gallstone disease. In: Feldman M, Friedman LS, Brandt LJ, editors. Sleisinger and Fordtran's gastrointestinal and liver disease: pathophysiology, diagnosis, management. 8th ed. Philadelphia: Saunders Elsevier; 2006. p.1387–418.
27. Hermann RE. The spectrum of biliary stone disease. Am J Surg 1989;158:171–3.
28. Canto MI, Chak A, Stellato T, Sivak MV Jr. Endoscopic ultrasonography versus cholangiography for the diagnosis of choledocholithiasis. Gastrointest Endosc 1998;47:439–48.
29. Norton SA, Alderson D. Prospective comparison of endoscopic ultrasonography and endoscopic retrograde cholangiopancreatography in the detection of bile duct stones. Br J Surg 1997;84:1366–9.
30. Cotton PB. ERCP. Gut 1977;18:316–41.
31. Shimizu S, Tada M, Kawai K. Diagnostic ERCP. Endoscopy 1994;26:88–92.
32. Onken J. Accurate prediction of choledocholithiasis [abstract]. Gastroenterology 1994;106:A20.
33. Chak A, Hawes RH, Cooper GS, Hoffman B, Catalano MF, Wong RC, et al. Prospective assessment of the utility of EUS in the evaluation of gallstone pancreatitis. Gastrointest Endosc 1999;49:599–604.
34. Cronan JJ. US diagnosis of choledocholithiasis: a reappraisal. Radiology 1986;161:133–4.
35. Dong B, Chen M. Improved sonographic visualization of choledocholithiasis. J Clin Ultrasound 1987;15:185–90.
36. Pasanen P, Partanen K, Pikkarainen P, Alhava E, Pirinen A, Janatuinen E. Ultrasonography, CT, and ERCP in the diagnosis of choledochal stones. Acta Radiol 1992;33:53–6.

37. Stott MA, Farrands PA, Guyer PB, Dewbury KC, Browning JJ, Sutton R. Ultrasound of the common bile duct in patients undergoing cholecystectomy. J Clin Ultrasound 1991;19:73–6.

38. Sugiyama M, Atomi Y. Endoscopic ultrasonography for diagnosing choledocholithiasis: a prospective comparative study with ultrasonography and computed tomography. Gastrointest Endosc 1997;45:143–6.

39. Wermke W. Sonographic diagnosis of bile duct calculi: results of a prospective study of 222 cases of choledocholithiasis. Ultraschall Med 1987;8:116–20.

40. Baron RL. Common bile duct stones: reassessment of criteria for CT diagnosis. Radiology 1987;162:419–24.

41. Aubertin JM, Levoir D, Bouillot JL, Becheur H, Bloch F, Aouad K, et al. Endoscopic ultrasonography immediately prior to laparoscopic cholecystectomy: a prospective evaluation. Endoscopy 1996;28:667–73.

42. Denis B. Accuracy of endoscopic ultrasonography for diagnosis of common bile duct stones [abstract]. Gastroenterology 1993;104:A358.

43. Napoleon B. Prospective study of the accuracy of echoendoscopy for the diagnosis of bile duct stones [abstract]. Endoscopy 1994;26:422.

44. Salmeron M, Simon JF, Houart R, Lémann M, Johannet H. Endoscopic ultrasonography versus invasive methods for the diagnosis of common bile duct stones [abstract]. Gastroenterology 1994;106:A357.

45. Shim CS, Joo JH, Park CW, Kim YS, Lee JS, Lee MS, et al. Effectiveness of endoscopic ultrasonography in the diagnosis of choledocholithiasis prior to laparoscopic cholecystectomy. Endoscopy 1995;27:428–32.

46. Barish MA, Yucel EK, Ferrucci JT. Magnetic resonance cholangiopancreatography. N Engl J Med 1999;341:258–64.

47. de Lédinghen V, Lecesne R, Raymond JM, Gense V, Amouretti M, Drouillard J, et al. Diagnosis of choledocholithiasis: EUS or magnetic resonance cholangiography? A prospective controlled study. Gastrointest Endosc 1999;49:26–31.

48. Guibaud L, Bret PM, Reinhold C, Atri M, Barkun AN. Bile duct obstruction and choledocholithiasis: diagnosis with MR cholangiography. Radiology 1995;197:109–15.

49. Cotton PB. Endoscopic retrograde cholangiopancreatography and laparoscopic cholecystectomy. Am J Surg 1993;165:474–8.

50. Rösch T. Major complications of endoscopic ultrasonography: results of a survey of 42 105 cases [abstract]. Gastrointest Endosc 1993;39:1.

51. Palazzo L. Which test for common bile duct stones? Endoscopic and intraductal ultrasonography. Endoscopy 1997;29:655–65.

52. EB da Silveira AB. Cost-effectiveness analysis of MRCP, EUS and ERCP in patients with suspected choledocholithiasis. [Paper presented at Digestive Disease Week, San Diego, California, May 17–22, 2008.]

53. Bergman JJ, van der Mey S, Rauws EA, Tijssen JG, Gouma DJ, Tytgat GN, et al. Long-term follow-up after endoscopic sphincterotomy for bile duct stones in patients younger than 60 years of age. Gastrointest Endosc 1996; 44:643–9.

54. MacMathuna P, White P, Clarke E, Lennon J, Crowe J. Endoscopic sphincteroplasty: a novel and safe alternative to papillotomy in the management of bile duct stones. Gut 1994;35:127–9.

55. Ohashi A, Tamada K, Tomiyama T, Aizawa T, Wada S, Miyata T, et al. Influence of bile duct diameter on the therapeutic quality of endoscopic balloon sphincteroplasty. Endoscopy 1999;31:137–41.

56. DiSario JA, Ogara MM, Price S, Hilden K, EDES group. Long-term follow-up on endoscopic papillary balloon dilation compared to endoscopic sphincterotomy for the extraction of bile duct stones [abstract]. Am J Gastroenterol 2007;102:S 188.

57. Siegel JH, Ben-Zvi JS, Pullano WE. Mechanical lithotripsy of common duct stones. Gastrointest Endosc 1990;36:351–6.

58. Hixson LJ, Fennerty MB, Jaffee PE, Pulju JH, Palley SL. Peroral cholangioscopy with intracorporeal electrohydraulic lithotripsy for choledocholithiasis. Am J Gastroenterol 1992;87:296–9.

59. Cotton PB, Kozarek RA, Schapiro RH, Nishioka NS, Kelsey PB, Ball TJ, et al. Endoscopic laser lithotripsy of large bile duct stones. Gastroenterology 1990;99:1128–33.

60. Sauerbruch T, Stern M. Fragmentation of bile duct stones by extracorporeal shock waves. A new approach to biliary calculi after failure of routine endoscopic measures. Gastroenterology 1989;96:146–52.

61. Shaw MJ, Mackie RD, Moore JP, Dorsher PJ, Freeman ML, Meier PB, et al. Results of a multicenter trial using a mechanical lithotripter for the treatment of large bile duct stones. Am J Gastroenterol 1993;88:730–3.

62. Palmer KR, Hofmann AF. Intraductal mono-octanoin for the direct dissolution of bile duct stones: experience in 343 patients. Gut 1986;27: 196–202.

63. Venneman NG, Besselink MG, Keulemans YC, Vanberge-Henegouwen GP, Boermeester MA, Broeders IA, et al. Ursodeoxycholic acid exerts no beneficial effect in patients with symptomatic gallstones awaiting cholecystectomy. Hepatology 2006;43:1276–83.

64. Bergman JJ, Rauws EA, Tijssen JG, Tytgat GN, Huibregtse K. Biliary endoprostheses in elderly patients with endoscopically irretrievable common bile duct stones: report on 117 patients. Gastrointest Endosc 1995;42: 195–201.

65. Baillie J. Treatment of acute biliary pancreatitis. N Engl J Med 1997;336: 286–7.

66. Fan ST, Lai EC, Mok FP, Lo CM, Zheng SS, Wong J. Early treatment of acute biliary pancreatitis by endoscopic papillotomy. N Engl J Med 1993;328: 228–32.

67. Folsch UR, Nitsche R, Ludtke R, Hilgers RA, Creutzfeldt W. Early ERCP and papillotomy compared with conservative treatment for acute biliary pancreatitis. The German Study Group on Acute Biliary Pancreatitis. N Engl J Med 1997;336:237–42.

68. Neoptolemos JP, Carr-Locke DL, London NJ, Bailey IA, James D, Fossard DP. Controlled trial of urgent endoscopic retrograde cholangiopancreatography and endoscopic sphincterotomy versus conservative treatment for acute pancreatitis due to gallstones. Lancet 1988;2(8618):979–83.

69. Baillie J. Should urgent ERCP be performed in patients with acute biliary pancreatitis without acute cholangitis? Nat Clin Pract Gastroenterol Hepatol 2008;5:484–5.

70. Petrov MS, Uchugina AF, Kukosh MV. Does endoscopic retrograde cholangiopancreatography reduce the risk of local pancreatic complications in acute pancreatitis? A systematic review and metaanalysis. Surg Endosc 2008;22:2338–43.

71. Doctor N, Dooley JS, Dick R, Watkinson A, Rolles K, Davidson BR. Multidisciplinary approach to biliary complications of laparoscopic cholecystectomy. Br J Surg 1998;85:627–32.

72. Bridges A, Wilcox CM, Varadarajulu S. Endoscopic management of traumatic bile leaks. Gastrointest Endosc 2007;65:1081–5.

73. Bhattacharjya S, Puleston J, Davidson BR, Dooley JS. Outcome of early endoscopic biliary drainage in the management of bile leaks after hepatic resection. Gastrointest Endosc 2003;57:526–30.

74. Mergener K, Strobel JC, Suhocki P, Jowell PS, Enns RA, Branch MS, et al. The role of ERCP in diagnosis and management of accessory bile duct leaks after cholecystectomy. Gastrointest Endosc 1999;50:527–31.

75. Kahaleh M, Sundaram V, Condron SL, De La Rue SA, Hall JD, Tokar J, et al. Temporary placement of covered self-expandable metallic stents in patients with biliary leak: midterm evaluation of a pilot study. Gastrointest Endosc 2007;66:52–9.

76. Seewald S, Groth S, Sriram PV, Xikun H, Akaraviputh T, Mendoza G, et al. Endoscopic treatment of biliary leakage with N-butyl-2-cyanoacrylate. Gastrointest Endosc 2002;56:916–9.

77. Barkun AN, Rezieg M, Mehta SN, Pavone E, Landry S, Barkun JS, et al. Postcholecystectomy biliary leaks in the laparoscopic era: risk factors, presentation, and management. McGill Gallstone Treatment Group. Gastrointest Endosc 1997;45:277–82.

78. Chow S, Bosco JJ, Heiss FW, Shea JA, Qaseem T, Howell D. Successful treatment of post-cholecystectomy bile leaks using nasobiliary tube drainage and sphincterotomy. Am J Gastroenterol 1997;92:1839–43.

79. Kozarek RA. Endoscopic techniques in management of biliary tract injuries. Surg Clin North Am 1994;74:883–93; discussion 895–6.

80. Kaman L, Behera A, Singh R, Katariya RN. Management of major bile duct injuries after laparoscopic cholecystectomy. Surg Endosc 2004;18: 1196–9.

81. Nuzzo G, Giuliante F, Giovannini I, Murazio M, D'Acapito F, Ardito F, et al. Advantages of multidisciplinary management of bile duct injuries occurring during cholecystectomy. Am J Surg 2008;195:763–9.

82. Larghi A, Tringali A, Lecca PG, Giordano M, Costamagna G. Management of hilar biliary strictures. Am J Gastroenterol 2008;103:458–73.

83. Dumonceau JM, Devière J, Delhaye M, Baize M, Cremer M. Plastic and metal stents for postoperative benign bile duct strictures: the best and the worst. Gastrointest Endosc 1998;47:8–17.

84. Kahaleh M, Behm B, Clarke BW, Brock A, Shami VM, De La Rue SA, et al. Temporary placement of covered self-expandable metal stents in benign biliary strictures: a new paradigm? (with video). Gastrointest Endosc 2008;67:446–54.

85. Jeffrey RB RP. Sonography of the abdomen New York: Raven Press; 1995.

86. Price RJ, Stewart ET, Foley WD, Dodds WJ. Sonography of polypoid cholesterolosis. AJR Am J Roentgenol 1982;139:1197–8.

87. Sugiyama M, Atomi Y, Kuroda A, Muto T, Wada N. Large cholesterol polyps of the gallbladder: diagnosis by means of US and endoscopic US. Radiology 1995;196:493–7.

88. Inui K, Nakazawa S. [Diagnosis of depth of invasion of gallbladder carcinoma with endosonography]. Nippon Geka Gakkai Zasshi 1998;99(10): 696–9. Japanese.

51

89. Lee SS, Park do H, Hwang CY, Ahn CS, Lee TY, Seo DW, et al. EUS-guided transmural cholecystostomy as rescue management for acute cholecystitis in elderly or high-risk patients: a prospective feasibility study. Gastrointest Endosc 2007;66:1008–12.

90. Tarnasky PR, England RE, Lail LM, Pappas TN, Cotton PB. Cystic duct patency in malignant obstructive jaundice. An ERCP-based study relevant to the role of laparoscopic cholecystojejunostomy. Ann Surg 1995;221:265–71.

91. Stoker J, Lameris JS, van Blankenstein M. Percutaneous metallic self-expandable endoprostheses in malignant hilar biliary obstruction. Gastrointest Endosc 1993;39:43–9.

92. Lai EC, Tompkins RK, Mann LL, Roslyn JJ. Proximal bile duct cancer. Quality of survival. Ann Surg 1987;205:111–8.

93. de Groen PC, Gores GJ, LaRusso NF, Gunderson LL, Nagorney DM. Biliary tract cancers. N Engl J Med 1999;341:1368–78.

94. Mukai H, Yasuda K, Nakajima M. Tumors of the papilla and distal common bile duct. Diagnosis and staging by endoscopic ultrasonography. Gastrointest Endosc Clin N Am 1995;5:763–72.

95. Mukai H, Nakajima M, Yasuda K, Mizuno S, Kawai K. Evaluation of endoscopic ultrasonography in the pre-operative staging of carcinoma of the ampulla of Vater and common bile duct. Gastrointest Endosc 1992;38:676–83.

96. Tio TL. Proximal bile duct tumors. Gastrointest Endosc Clin N Am 1995;5:773–80.

97. Tamada K, Kanai N, Ueno N, Ichiyama M, Tomiyama T, Wada S, et al. Limitations of intraductal ultrasonography in differentiating between bile duct cancer in stage T1 and stage T2: in-vitro and in-vivo studies. Endoscopy 1997;29:721–5.

98. Gleeson FC, Rajan E, Levy MJ, Clain JE, Topazian MD, Harewood GC, et al. EUS-guided FNA of regional lymph nodes in patients with unresectable hilar cholangiocarcinoma. Gastrointest Endosc 2008;67:438–43.

99. Rauws EA, Kloek JJ, Gouma DJ, Van Gulik TM. Staging of cholangiocarcinoma: the role of endoscopy. HPB (Oxford) 2008;10(2):110–2.

100. Tio TL, Cheng J, Wijers OB, Sars PR, Tytgat GN. Endosonographic TNM staging of extrahepatic bile duct cancer: comparison with pathological staging. Gastroenterology 1991;100:1351–61.

101. Tamada K, Ido K, Ueno N, Kimura K, Ichiyama M, Tomiyama T. Preoperative staging of extrahepatic bile duct cancer with intraductal ultrasonography. Am J Gastroenterol 1995;90:239–46.

102. Tamada K, Ueno N, Ichiyama M, Tomiyama T, Nishizono T, Wada S, et al. Assessment of pancreatic parenchymal invasion by bile duct cancer using intraductal ultrasonography. Endoscopy 1996;28:492–6.

103. Foutch PG. Diagnosis of cancer by cytologic methods performed during ERCP. Gastrointest Endosc 1994;40:249–52.

104. Lee JG, Leung JW, Baillie J, Layfield LJ, Cotton PB. Benign, dysplastic, or malignant—making sense of endoscopic bile duct brush cytology: results in 149 consecutive patients. Am J Gastroenterol 1995;90:722–6.

105. Fogel EL, Sherman S. How to improve the accuracy of diagnosis of malignant biliary strictures. Endoscopy 1999;31:758–60.

106. Howell DA, Beveridge RP, Bosco J, Jones M. Endoscopic needle aspiration biopsy at ERCP in the diagnosis of biliary strictures. Gastrointest Endosc 1992;38:531–5.

107. Kubota Y, Takaoka M, Tani K, Ogura M, Kin H, Fujimura K, et al. Endoscopic transpapillary biopsy for diagnosis of patients with pancreaticobiliary ductal strictures. Am J Gastroenterol 1993;88:1700–4.

108. Nimura Y, Shionoya S, Hayakawa N, Kamiya J, Kondo S, Yasui A. Value of percutaneous transhepatic cholangioscopy (PTCS). Surg Endosc 1988;2:213–9.

109. Sherman S, Esher EJE, Pezzi JS. Yield of ERCP tissue sampling of biliary strictures by brush, forceps, and needle aspiration methods [abstract]. Gastrointest Endosc 1995;41:478.

110. DeWitt J, Misra VL, Leblanc JK, McHenry L, Sherman S. EUS-guided FNA of proximal biliary strictures after negative ERCP brush cytology results. Gastrointest Endosc 2006;64:325–33.

111. Ryan ME, Baldauf MC. Comparison of flow cytometry for DNA content and brush cytology for detection of malignancy in pancreaticobiliary strictures. Gastrointest Endosc 1994;40:133–9.

112. Almoguera C, Shibata D, Forrester K, Martin J, Arnheim N, Perucho M. Most human carcinomas of the exocrine pancreas contain mutant c-K-*ras* genes. Cell 1988;53:549–54.

113. Tada M, Omata M, Ohto M. High incidence of *ras* gene mutation in intrahepatic cholangiocarcinoma. Cancer 1992;69:1115–8.

114. Ding SF, Delhanty JD, Bowles L, Dooley JS, Wood CB, Habib NA. Loss of constitutional heterozygosity on chromosomes 5 and 17 in cholangiocarcinoma. Br J Cancer 1993;67:1007–10.

115. Hurwitz M, Sawicki M, Samara G, Passaro E Jr. Diagnostic and prognostic molecular markers in cancer. Am J Surg 1992;164:299–306.

116. Itoi T, Shinohara Y, Takeda K, Takei K, Ohno H, Ohyashiki K, et al. Detection of telomerase activity in biopsy specimens for diagnosis of biliary tract cancers. Gastrointest Endosc 2000;52:380–6.

117. Boeck S, Stieber P, Holdenrieder S, Wilkowski R, Heinemann V. Prognostic and therapeutic significance of carbohydrate antigen 19–9 as tumor marker in patients with pancreatic cancer. Oncology 2006;70:255–64.

118. Bismuth H, Nakache R, Diamond T. Management strategies in resection for hilar cholangiocarcinoma. Ann Surg 1992;215:31–8.

119. Looser C, Stain SC, Baer HU, Triller J, Blumgart LH. Staging of hilar cholangiocarcinoma by ultrasound and duplex sonography: a comparison with angiography and operative findings. Br J Radiol 1992;65:871–7.

120. Knyrim K, Wagner HJ, Pausch J, Vakil N. A prospective, randomized, controlled trial of metal stents for malignant obstruction of the common bile duct. Endoscopy 1993;25:207–12.

121. Wagner HJ, Knyrim K, Vakil N, Klose KJ. Plastic endoprostheses versus metal stents in the palliative treatment of malignant hilar biliary obstruction. A prospective and randomized trial. Endoscopy 1993;25:213–8.

122. Fanelli F, Orgera G, Bezzi M, Rossi P, Allegritti M, Passariello R. Management of malignant biliary obstruction: technical and clinical results using an expanded polytetrafluoroethylene fluorinated ethylene propylene (ePTFE/FEP)-covered metallic stent after 6-year experience. Eur Radiol 2008;18:911–9.

123. Lee YM, Kaplan MM. Primary sclerosing cholangitis. N Engl J Med 1995;332:924–33.

124. Lu S, Kaplowitz N. Diseases of the biliary tree. In: Yamada T, editor. Textbook of gastroenterology. Philadelphia: Lippincott; 1991. p.1990–2021.

125. Chen LY, Goldberg HI. Sclerosing cholangitis: broad spectrum of radiographic features. Gastrointest Radiol 1984;9:39–47.

126. Broomé U, Olsson R, Lööf L, Bodemar G, Hultcrantz R, Danielsson A, et al. Natural history and prognostic factors in 305 Swedish patients with primary sclerosing cholangitis. Gut 1996;38:610–5.

127. Meagher S, Yusoff I, Kennedy W, Martel M, Adam V, Barkun A. The roles of magnetic resonance and endoscopic retrograde cholangiopancreatography (MRCP and ERCP) in the diagnosis of patients with suspected sclerosing cholangitis: a cost-effectiveness analysis. Endoscopy 2007;39:222–8.

128. Rosen CB, Nagorney DM. Cholangiocarcinoma complicating primary sclerosing cholangitis. Semin Liver Dis 1991;11:26–30.

129. McGuire DE, Venu RP, Brown RD, Etzkorn KP, Glaws WR, Abu-Hammour A. Brush cytology for pancreatic carcinoma: an analysis of factors influencing results. Gastrointest Endosc 1996;44:300–4.

130. Van Laethem JL, Vertongen P, Devière J, Van Rampelbergh J, Rickaert F, Cremer M, et al. Detection of c-Ki-*ras* gene codon 12 mutations from pancreatic duct brushings in the diagnosis of pancreatic tumours. Gut 1995;36:781–7.

131. Charatcharoenwitthaya P, Enders FB, Halling KC, Lindor KD. Utility of serum tumor markers, imaging, and biliary cytology for detecting cholangiocarcinoma in primary sclerosing cholangitis. Hepatology 2008;48:1106–11.

132. Pitt HA, Thompson HH, Tompkins RK, Longmire WP Jr. Primary sclerosing cholangitis: results of an aggressive surgical approach. Ann Surg 1982;196:259–68.

133. Ponsioen CY, Lam K, van Milligen de Wit AW, Huibregtse K, Tytgat GN. Four years experience with short term stenting in primary sclerosing cholangitis. Am J Gastroenterol 1999;94:2403–7.

134. Al-Kawas FH. Endoscopic management of primary sclerosing cholangitis: less is better! Am J Gastroenterol 1999;94:2235–6.

135. Vitellas KM, Keogan MT, Freed KS, Enns RA, Spritzer CE, Baillie JM, et al. Radiologic manifestations of sclerosing cholangitis with emphasis on MR cholangiopancreatography. Radiographics 2000;20:959–75.

136. Vitellas KM, Keogan MT, Spritzer CE, Nelson RC. MR cholangiopancreatography of bile and pancreatic duct abnormalities with emphasis on the single-shot fast spin-echo technique. Radiographics 2000;20:939–57.

137. Deeg HJ, Rominger JM, Shah AN. Choledochal cyst and pancreatic carcinoma demonstrated simultaneously by endoscopic retrograde cholangiopancreatography. South Med J 1980;73:1678–9.

138. Vanderpool D, Lane BW, Winter JW, Ettinger J. Choledochal cysts. Surg Gynecol Obstet 1988;167:447–51.

139. Todani T, Watanabe Y, Narusue M, Tabuchi K, Okajima K. Congenital bile duct cysts: Classification, operative procedures, and review of thirty-seven cases including cancer arising from choledochal cyst. Am J Surg 1977;134:263–9.

140. Irie H, Honda H, Jimi M, Yokohata K, Chijiiwa K, Kuroiwa T, et al. Value of MR cholangiopancreatography in evaluating choledochal cysts. AJR Am J Roentgenol 1998;171:1381–5.

VIII

141. Bismuth H, Krissat J. Choledochal cystic malignancies. Ann Oncol 1999;10 Suppl 4:94–8.

142. Rossi RL, Silverman ML, Braasch JW, Munson JL, ReMine SG. Carcinomas arising in cystic conditions of the bile ducts. A clinical and pathologic study. Ann Surg 1987;205:377–84.

143. Yamaguchi M. Congenital choledochal cyst. Analysis of 1,433 patients in the Japanese literature. Am J Surg 1980;140:653–7.

144. Voyles CR, Smadja C, Shands WC, Blumgart LH. Carcinoma in choledochal cysts. Age-related incidence. Arch Surg 1983;118:986–8.

145. Tajiri K, Takenawa H, Yamaoka K, Yamane M, Marumo F, Sato C. Choledochal cyst with adenocarcinoma in the cystically dilated intrahepatic bile duct. Abdom Imaging 1997;22:190–3.

146. Caroli-Bosc FX, Demarquay JF, Conio M, Peten EP, Buckley MJ, Paolini O, et al. The role of therapeutic endoscopy associated with extracorporeal shock-wave lithotripsy and bile acid treatment in the management of Caroli's disease. Endoscopy 1998;30:559–63.

147. Geenen JE, Hogan WJ, Dodds WJ, Toouli J, Venu RP. The efficacy of endoscopic sphincterotomy after cholecystectomy in patients with sphincter-of-Oddi dysfunction. N Engl J Med 1989;320:82–7.

148. Kumar M, Murthy A, Duggal L, Sud R. AIDS associated cholangiopathy. Trop Gastroenterol 1998;19:155–6.

149. Sand J, Nordback I, Arvola P, Porsti I, Kalloo A, Pasricha P. Effects of botulinum toxin A on the sphincter of Oddi: an in vivo and in vitro study. Gut 1998;42:507–10.

150. Wehrmann T, Seifert H, Seipp M, Lembcke B, Caspary WF. Endoscopic injection of botulinum toxin for biliary sphincter of Oddi dysfunction. Endoscopy 1998;30:702–7.

151. Ruff KC, Triester S, Crowell MD, Harrison ME. The effect of sildenafil on sphincter of Oddi pressure in patients undergoing ERCP for suspected sphincter of Oddi dysfunction. [Paper presented at Digestive Disease Week, May 17–22, 2008, San Diego, California.]

152. Desautels SG, Slivka A, Hutson WR, Chun A, Mitrani C, DiLorenzo C, et al. Postcholecystectomy pain syndrome: pathophysiology of abdominal pain in sphincter of Oddi type III. Gastroenterology 1999;116:900–5.

153. Takeda T, Tohma H, Yoshida J, Naritomi G, Konomi H, Deng ZL, et al. Vector manometric study of the sphincter of Oddi in the dog: functional and morphological correlation. J Gastroenterol 1998;33:860–3.

154. Eversman D, Fogel EL, Rusche M, Sherman S, Lehman GA. Frequency of abnormal pancreatic and biliary sphincter manometry compared with clinical suspicion of sphincter of Oddi dysfunction. Gastrointest Endosc 1999;50:637–41.

155. Das A, Singh P, Sivak MV Jr, Chak A. Pancreatic-stent placement for prevention of post-ERCP pancreatitis: a cost-effectiveness analysis. Gastrointest Endosc 2007;65:960–8.

156. Fazel A, Quadri A, Catalano MF, Meyerson SM, Geenen JE. Does a pancreatic duct stent prevent post-ERCP pancreatitis? A prospective randomized study. Gastrointest Endosc 2003;57:291–4.

157. Peng NJ, Lai KH, Tsay DG, Liu RS, Su KL, Yeh SH. Efficacy of quantitative cholescintigraphy in the diagnosis of sphincter of Oddi dysfunction. Nucl Med Commun 1994;15:899–904.

158. Pereira SP, Gillams A, Sgouros SN, Webster GJ, Hatfield AR. Prospective comparison of secretin-stimulated magnetic resonance cholangiopancreatography with manometry in the diagnosis of sphincter of Oddi dysfunction types II and III. Gut 2007;56:809–13.

159. Dumas R, Le Gall P, Hastier P, Buckley MJ, Conio M, Delmont JP. The role of endoscopic retrograde cholangiopancreatography in the management of hepatic hydatid disease. Endoscopy 1999;31:242–7.

160. Rodriguez AN, Sanchez del Rio AL, Alguacil LV, De Dios Vega JF, Fugarolas GM. Effectiveness of endoscopic sphincterotomy in complicated hepatic hydatid disease. Gastrointest Endosc 1998;48:593–7.

161. Dowidar N, El Sayad M, Osman M, Salem A. Endoscopic therapy of fascioliasis resistant to oral therapy. Gastrointest Endosc 1999;50:345–51.

162. Harris A, Chan AC, Torres-Viera C, Hammett R, Carr-Locke D. Meta-analysis of antibiotic prophylaxis in endoscopic retrograde cholangiopancreatography (ERCP). Endoscopy 1999;31:718–24.

163. Lorenz R, Herrmann M, Kassem AM, Lehn N, Neuhaus H, Classen M. Microbiological examinations and in-vitro testing of different antibiotics in therapeutic endoscopy of the biliary system. Endoscopy 1998;30:708–12.

164. van Berkel AM, Boland C, Redekop WK, Bergman JJ, Groen AK, Tytgat GN, et al. A prospective randomized trial of Teflon versus polyethylene stents for distal malignant biliary obstruction. Endoscopy 1998;30:681–6.

165. Pedersen FM, Lassen AT, Schaffalitzky de Muckadell OB. Randomized trial of stent placed above and across the sphincter of Oddi in malignant bile duct obstruction. Gastrointest Endosc 1998;48:574–9.

166. Yeoh KG, Zimmerman MJ, Cunningham JT, Cotton PB. Comparative costs of metal versus plastic biliary stent strategies for malignant obstructive jaundice by decision analysis. Gastrointest Endosc 1999;49:466–71.

167. Kaassis M, Boyer J, Dumas R, Ponchon T, Coumaros D, Delcenserie R, et al. Plastic or metal stents for malignant stricture of the common bile duct? Results of a randomized prospective study. Gastrointest Endosc 2003;57:178–82.

168. Huibregtse K. Biliary sphincter balloon dilation; who, when and how? Can J Gastroenterol 1999;13:499–500.

169. Staritz M, Poralla T, Dormeyer HH, Meyer zum Buschenfelde KH. Endoscopic removal of common bile duct stones through the intact papilla after medical sphincter dilation. Gastroenterology 1985;88:1807–11.

170. Minami A, Maeta T, Kohi F, Nakatsu T, Morshed SA, Nishioka M. Endoscopic papillary dilation by balloon and isosorbide dinitrate drip infusion for removing bile duct stone. Scand J Gastroenterol 1998;33:765–8.

171. Attasaranya S, Sherman S. Balloon dilation of the papilla after sphincterotomy: rescue therapy for difficult bile duct stones. Endoscopy 2007;39:1023–5.

172. Kim GH, Kang DH, Song GA, Heo J, Park CH, Ha TI, et al. Endoscopic removal of bile-duct stones by using a rotatable papillotome and a large-balloon dilator in patients with a Billroth II gastrectomy (with video). Gastrointest Endosc 2008;67:1134–8.

173. Misra SP, Dwivedi M. Large-diameter balloon dilation after endoscopic sphincterotomy for removal of difficult bile duct stones. Endoscopy 2008;40:209–13.

51

52 Pancreatic Disease

Evan L. Fogel, Furqaan Ahmed, and Stuart Sherman

Introduction

The management of pancreatic disease has changed significantly during the last 30 years. This has resulted from a variety of factors, including improved medications (such as enteric-coated pancreatic enzyme supplements and octreotide); improved surgical techniques (including postoperative intensive-care management of very ill patients); better noninvasive imaging tests (including ultrasound, computed tomography scanning—especially the spiral type—and magnetic resonance cholangiopancreatography); greater understanding of the genetics of some pancreatic diseases (hereditary pancreatitis); and improved endoscopic diagnostic and therapeutic techniques (including endoscopic ultrasonography). This chapter mostly addresses the latter issues, but refers to other aspects to the extent that they relate to endoscopic techniques. The general aspects of endoscopic retrograde cholangiopancreatography (ERCP), sphincterotomy, and stenting in pancreatic disease are covered in Chapters 15, 34, and 36.

Developmental Anomalies of the Pancreas

Pancreas Divisum: Diagnosis and Therapy

Approximately 10% of the general population have congenital anomalies and variants of the pancreas (**Table 52.1**), and these conditions are therefore encountered periodically at ERCP. The term "congenital anomaly" indicates that atypical development has occurred during embryological maturation, resulting in an abnormality that may cause some form of disability, limitation, or disease. Developmental alterations that are generally of limited clinical importance might be best termed congenital variants. While many congenital anomalies and variants of the pancreas are found coincidentally at endoscopy, surgery, or autopsy, some of them are clinically significant and cause symptoms in childhood or adulthood. Approximately 7% of autopsy series (range 1–14%) report pancreas divisum, the most common pancreatic anatomic variant. The frequency of finding this condition varies greatly among ERCP series, depending on the population studied (frequency of pancreatitis patients) and the vigor with which complete pancreatography is pursued. While the antemortem diagnosis of pancreas divisum was previously limited to ERCP series, the diagnosis can now be suggested by magnetic resonance cholangiopancreatography (MRCP), particularly when secretin is used to enhance the image quality. In expert hands, endoscopic ultrasonography (EUS) may also be helpful in suggesting this diagnosis [1].

Prenatal development. The pancreas is derived from dorsal and ventral buds that develop from the embryological foregut. The ventral system also gives rise to the hepatobiliary system. At approximately the eighth intrauterine week of life, the ventral pancreas rotates posterior to the duodenum and comes to rest posterior and inferior to the head portion of the dorsal pancreas. Parenchymal fusion nearly always occurs, although a tissue plane may be evident histologically, surgically, or radiographically between the dorsal and the ventral pancreas.

Table 52.1 Anatomic categorization of congenital pancreatic anomalies and variants

1	Ventral/dorsal ductal malfusion
	a Pancreas divisum
	b Incomplete pancreas divisum
	c Isolated dorsal segment
2	Rotation/migration problems
	a Annular pancreas
	b Ectopic pancreas
	c Ectopic papillae
3	Agenesis/hypoplasia
4	Ductal duplication
5	Atypical ductal configuration
6	Anomalous pancreaticobiliary junction
7	Cystic malformations

Pancreatic parenchymal textural or contour differences may be evident between the dorsal and ventral pancreas in up to 75% of normal individuals examined using endoscopic ultrasound [2]. Pancreatitis may obscure this plane. The ventral pancreas represents 2–20% of the pancreatic parenchymal mass. Fusion of the ductal system occurs in just over 90% of individuals, although variations in patency of the accessory duct (Santorini duct) occur. **Figure 52.1** shows the variations in anatomy that are grouped under the heading of pancreas divisum. **Figures 52.1 c** and **52.1 d** show the classic pancreas divisum anatomy, with a small ventral duct that drains through the larger, major papilla and the larger dorsal duct that drains through the smaller, minor papilla. **Figure 52.1 f** shows a pancreas in which the entire pancreatic ductal system drains through the minor papilla via the dorsal duct. The branch to the uncinate process represents the ventral pancreas. **Figure 52.1 e** shows incomplete pancreas divisum, in which a small branch of the ventral duct communicates with the dorsal duct. Fifteen percent of pancreas divisum cases are of the incomplete type. The clinical implications of incomplete pancreas divisum are the same as those in complete pancreas divisum, except that modest to full visualization of the dorsal duct may occur using vigorous major papilla contrast injection. **Figure 52.1 i** shows a "reverse" divisum, in which there is an isolated small segment of dorsal pancreas. This occurs when the duct of Santorini does not connect with the genu of the main pancreatic duct. This is of no physiological significance, but can be frustrating for the endoscopist attempting to cannulate the minor papilla in order to visualize the entire pancreas. The rare case of pancreatic cancer that does not involve the main duct may mimic reverse divisum, as the tumor may obstruct the duct of Santorini.

Clinical relevance. Pancreas divisum has clinical significance in three major respects:
- The small ventral duct has to be differentiated from various forms of main pancreatic duct cut-off, such as that seen in pancreatic cancer (**Fig. 52.2**).

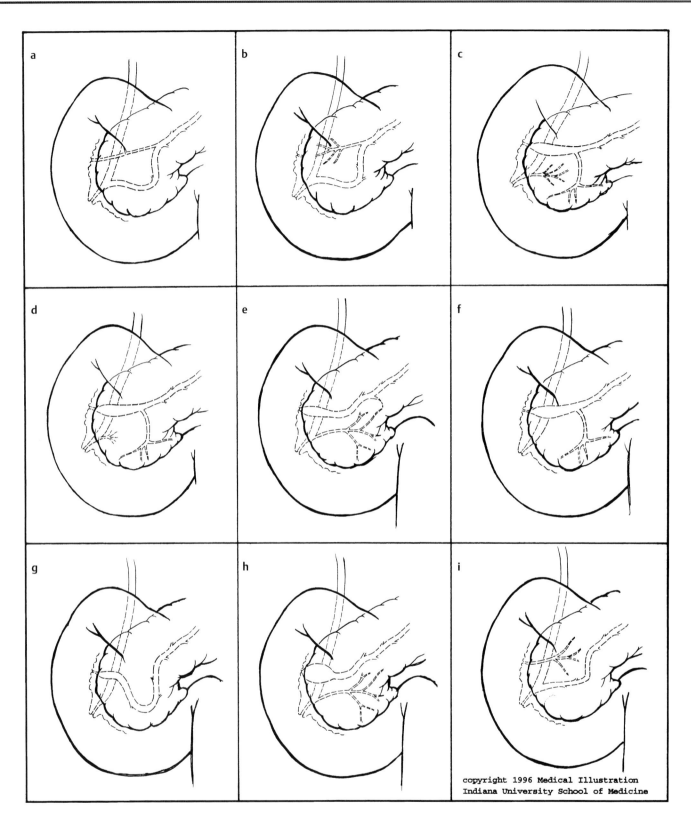

copyright 1996 Medical Illustration
Indiana University School of Medicine

Fig. 52.1 Diagrams of variant forms of pancreatic ductal anatomy (courtesy of the Department of Medical Illustration, Indiana University School of Medicine).

a The main pancreatic duct drains through the major papilla. The accessory duct is patent and drains through the minor papilla.

b Same as **a**, except that the minor papilla is not patent and the accessory duct and branches terminate near the duodenal wall.

c Typical pancreas divisum, with a small ventral duct draining through the major papilla. There is a large dorsal duct draining through the minor papilla.

d A tiny ventral duct that can easily be overlooked on endoscopic retrograde cholangiopancreatography.

e Incomplete pancreas divisum. Same as **c**, except that a small branch of the ventral duct communicates with the dorsal duct.

f A variant of pancreas divisum in which the entire pancreatic ductal system drains through the minor papilla. There is no pancreatic duct connecting to the major papilla.

g Variant of **f**, except that the dorsal duct initially extends caudally in an ansa contour.

h The terminal dorsal duct shows saccular dilation (this is also termed Santorinicele).

i Reversed pancreas divisum, with the accessory ductal system draining a small portion of the pancreatic parenchyma through the minor papilla. The major part of the pancreas drains through the main pancreatic duct, through the major papilla.

- At ERCP, only the ventral part of the pancreas can be viewed using standard major papilla cannulation. This results in incomplete ductography, and the dorsal pancreas remains unevaluated unless minor papilla cannulation is performed.
- In a small proportion of pancreas divisum patients, the minor papilla orifice is so small that excessively high intrapancreatic dorsal duct pressure occurs during active secretion, which may result in inadequate drainage, ductal distension, pain, or pancreatitis. The acute pancreatitis tends to be mild, but pseudocysts, calculi, and other more severe complications are occasionally seen. Pancreas divisum is found in an unexpectedly high proportion of patients with idiopathic pancreatitis [3]. If ductal obstruction occurs, the problem is relative stenosis of the minor papilla rather than pancreas divisum per se. As a consequence, some authors prefer to call this condition the "dominant dorsal duct syndrome" [4].

The majority of pancreas divisum patients have no pancreatic symptoms throughout their lifetime; this type of anatomy therefore appears to be merely a condition that predisposes the individual to the above events. Such a low frequency of symptom manifestation has led to considerable controversy as to whether pancreas divisum and its associated small minor papilla orifice are ever a cause of obstructive pancreatitis. Since it is estimated that less than 5 % of pancreas divisum patients ever develop pancreatic symptoms, the silent majority may statistically obscure any cause-and-effect relationships that may be involved.

Ventral pancreas. **Figure 52.2** illustrates typical small ventral ductal systems. Characteristically, the main ventral duct is 1–4 cm long and tapers terminally into multiple small side branches. This ductal system does not cross over the midline of the spine, and acinarization quickly occurs if contrast injection is continued. Pain usually occurs during acinarization, which can be seen fluoroscopically as a focal, fluffy collection of contrast with generally sharp peripheral margins. This type of event has to be differentiated from a submucosal injection, which has fuzzy peripheral margins; acinarization of a side branch due to excessively deep cannulation; and filling of another cavity, such as a pseudocyst, diverticulum, or necrotic tumor. After acinarization of the ventral pancreas, the contrast will drain promptly within one or two minutes, and films taken during this drainage interval will identify the underlying ductal system. Alternatively, the duct can be reinjected with lesser amounts of contrast to visualize the ductal system. The relatively small ventral duct usually shows additional pathology, but will occasionally show chronic pancreatitis changes (generally associated with similar changes on dorsal ductography) or tumor (**Fig. 52.2 c**). Very rarely, the ventral pancreas will be abnormal while the dorsal duct remains normal [5,6]. In up to one-third of patients with pancreas divisum, no pancreatic duct can be identified connecting to the major papilla (**Fig. 52.1 f**). In such cases, the entire ventral portion of the pancreas generally drains cephalad through a branch of the dorsal duct. Since the ductal systems described by Wirsung, Santorini, and others generally refer to ductal systems in individuals without pancreas divisum, these eponyms are not readily applicable to pancreas divisum and are not used here.

Until complete dorsal ductography is obtained, it may be quite difficult at ERCP to differentiate between a ventral duct in pancreas divisum and pancreatic cancer or a benign stricture. Pathological processes that separate the dorsal and ventral portions of the gland result in acquired pancreas divisum. Complementary information from endoscopic ultrasound, computed tomography (CT), or histological sampling may be required.

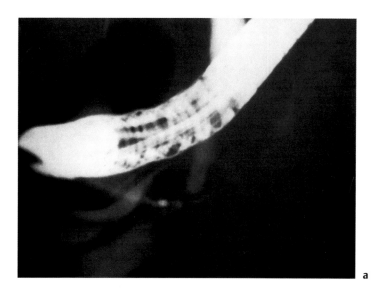

a

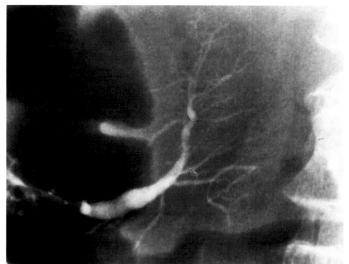

b

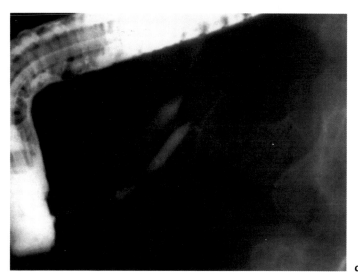

c

Fig. 52.2
a Ductography showing a very tiny ventral duct. This may be missed fluoroscopically unless magnification views are used.
b A typical normal ventral ductogram.
c Pancreatic cancer with main duct cut-off. This has to be differentiated from a ventral pancreas in pancreas divisum. The common bile duct is also narrowed here.

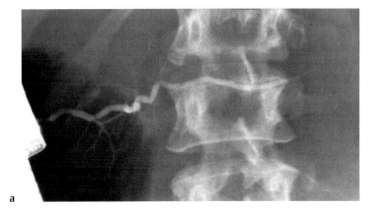

a

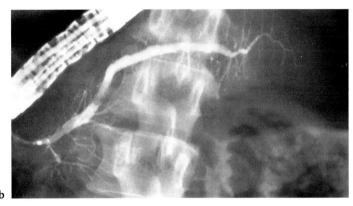

b

VIII

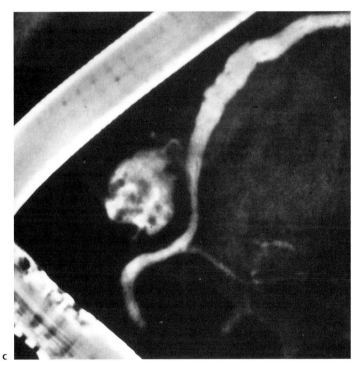

c

Fig. 52.3
a   A normal dorsal ductogram.
b   Mild chronic pancreatitis seen on dorsal ductography. The patient had a clinical history of idiopathic recurrent pancreatitis on two occasions.
c   A dorsal ductogram, showing a small pseudocyst and beading of the dorsal duct.

Dorsal ductography via minor papilla cannulation. Minor papilla cannulation and dorsal ductography are essential to evaluate the pancreatic ductal system in pancreas divisum fully. Minor papilla cannulation should generally be attempted in cases in which a ventral duct is viewed via the major papilla. The minor papilla is nearly always located in the right upper quadrant portion of the visual field when facing the major papilla. It may be as close as 10 mm from the major papilla orifice, and may be located at the cephalad rim of the longitudinal fold to the major papilla, but generally it is 2–3 cm more cephalad and anterior to the major papilla. Cannulation is generally best achieved with the endoscope in the long position, along the greater curve of the stomach. Duodenal motility should be stopped with glucagon or other smooth-muscle relaxants. A variety of devices are potentially useful in achieving cannulation of the minor papilla. Rarely, a standard 5-Fr catheter with a tapered tip will suffice. The highly tapered 5-Fr catheter, with a 23-gauge or 24-gauge blunt needle tip protruding 1–2 mm beyond the catheter tip, is the one that is most helpful in achieving cannulation. The needle tip should be gently inserted into the minor papilla orifice to avoid tissue trauma and blurring of the landmarks. The contrast media used, patient positioning, and fluoroscopic techniques are the same as in conventional ERCP. Deep cannulation is generally best accomplished with a guide wire 0.018 inches in diameter (this may require grooming so that the wire tip curves upward) inside a 3-Fr catheter, highly tapered 5-Fr catheter, or 23-gauge needle-tipped catheter. Once deep cannulation is achieved, it is often advantageous to withdraw the endoscope into the short position (along the lesser curvature of the stomach) to provide a better film quality and to apply dilation forces if needed.

In approximately one-third of cases, the orifice to the minor papilla will not be evident initially. Secretin can be administered intravenously to facilitate identification of the orifice. New genetically engineered human and porcine secretins are now available [7], which generally result in vigorous pancreatic exocrine juice flow and obvious dilation of the orifice. During vigorous juice flow, it is difficult to force contrast medium retrograde to the pancreatic tail, and using such force may precipitate postductography pancreatitis. The use of secretin should therefore be reserved for cases of difficult cannulation. At times, pancreatic juice flow after secretin stimulation may still be inconspicuous. In such cases, spraying a dilute (1 : 10) methylene blue solution over the face of the minor papilla will often help identify the orifice, which is evident when clear juice washes away the background blue dye.

In experienced centers, minor papilla cannulation can be achieved in approximately 95 % of pancreas divisum patients. Patients in whom the procedure fails will generally be those with minor papilla distortion due to inflammation (e. g., in pancreatitis or peptic ulcer disease), diverticula, tumor, or altered gastroduodenal anatomy, such as Billroth I or II operations. The findings at dorsal ductography correlate with the indication for the examination (**Fig. 52.3**). Patients with documented pancreatitis or mass lesions on CT are much more likely to have abnormal dorsal ductography. Patients with biliary tract disease or pain without other objective findings have a low probability of abnormal dorsal ductography. Dorsal ductograms are generally identical to standard major papilla pancreatograms (without divisum), except that the duct–duodenal junction is more perpendicular. An exception to this rule is saccular terminal dorsal duct dilation (**Fig. 52.1 h**). In approximately 2 % of patients, dorsal ductography will only reveal an isolated small ductal system (isolated dorsal segment) (**Fig. 52.1 i**) that simulates a typical ventral pancreas. This type of ductal anatomy is generally of no pathological significance. Once it has been detected, the endoscopist must return to the major papilla to cannulate and view the main pancreatic duct.

Clinical management of pancreas divisum patients. *Coincidental finding.* If pancreas divisum is detected in the setting of biliary pathology, and the patient has no CT abnormalities in the pancreas and no clinical history of pancreatitis, the pancreas divisum ductal anatomy is clinically irrelevant and can be ignored. Indeed, in the setting of a common duct stone, pancreas divisum is probably an asset. Serious gallstone pancreatitis is probably not possible, as gallstone obstruction at the major papilla will only block the small ventral duct, and major papilla sphincterotomy can be carried out more aggressively, because again only a small portion of the pancreas may be disturbed. In the rare cases in which the minor papilla is on the cephalad rim of the longitudinal fold to the major papilla, this anatomy needs to be recognized in order to avoid injury during standard biliary sphincterotomy. A new treatment for pancreas divisum has been described by Wehrmann et al. [8], who found that botulinum toxin injection into the minor papilla led to resolution of recurrent pancreatitis for a period of 8–10 months, followed by relapse. Such patients then responded to minor papilla sphincterotomy. This suggests that there is a muscular sphincter at the minor papilla. Whether this can be used as a method of predicting the outcome of sphincterotomy remains to be assessed in a study including a larger group of patients.

Minimal symptoms. Patients with pancreas divisum and mild or infrequent bouts of pain or pancreatitis can generally be managed with a trial of medical therapy, which may include a low-fat diet, analgesics, anticholinergics, and pancreatic enzyme supplements. This type of treatment may offer some symptomatic benefit, although it does not directly address the underlying ductal anatomy. It is controversial whether persons with mild symptoms should undergo aggressive therapy with the aim of preventing progression to more advanced disease. In patients with mild symptoms who nevertheless have dorsal duct calcifications, pseudocysts, or ductal dilation, a more aggressive approach is warranted.

Moderate/severe pain or pancreatitis. Patients with recurrent pancreaticobiliary-type pain, or pancreatitis associated with clinically significant disability, warrant thorough evaluation of the dorsal pancreas and minor papilla. We generally evaluate the dorsal pancreas and perform minor papilla therapy in patients who have had two or more bouts of pancreatitis requiring less than 10 days of hospitalization, or one bout of more severe pancreatitis.

Methods of evaluating pathological narrowing of the minor papilla. **Table 52.2** lists methods of evaluating narrowing of the minor papilla and factors suggesting that minor papilla stenosis is present. Some of these factors are valuable as clinically diagnostic tools, but others are only suggestive retrospectively, such as in the resected pancreas specimen.

Noninvasive methods. Simple noninvasive methods capable of identifying patients with pathological minor papilla narrowing are needed. Such tools would ideally selectively identify candidates for invasive therapy. A standard CT scan of the pancreas may identify dilation of the dorsal duct and changes associated with chronic pancreatitis that are confined to the dorsal portion of the pancreas. More commonly, the CT scan merely shows nonspecific prominence of the pancreatic head. Visualization of a fat plane [9] between the dorsal and ventral portions can diagnose pancreas divisum, but does not generally separate symptomatic from coincidental states. The normal pancreas shows dilation of the main pancreatic duct for a period of 5–10 min after intravenous secretin stimulation [10]. Using transcutaneous ultrasonography to monitor dorsal duct diameter, Warshaw et al. [11] and Tulassay et al. [10] observed that patients with pancreatic outlet obstruction may have dorsal duct dilation that persists for more than 15 min. The precise criteria for a positive test have not yet been established. Warshaw et al. [11] found a correlation between the ultrasound findings and the outcome of therapy. Patients with positive findings (an abnormal test) had a 90 % chance of obtaining clinical relief with minor papilla

Table 52.2 Methods and observations that can evaluate for pathological minor papilla narrowing and its effects on the dorsal pancreas

Histology
Observation of parenchymal chronic pancreatitis changes limited to the dorsal pancreas
Noninvasive
Dorsal duct dilation or chronic pancreatitis changes confined to the dorsal pancreas as seen on CT scan
Prolonged dilation of the dorsal duct diameter after intravenous secretin stimulation, as monitored by transcutaneous ultrasound (or CT or EUS)
Diagnostic ERCP
Abnormal dorsal ductography (dilation and/or chronic pancreatitis changes) in combination with a normal ventral ductogram
Cystic dilation of the terminal dorsal duct (Santorinicele)
Slow drainage of contrast from the dorsal duct (> 12 min)
Pain provocation during dorsal ductography
Special/therapeutic ERCP
Collection of pure pancreatic juice after deep dorsal duct cannulation and intravenous secretin stimulation. (Abnormal bicarbonate level < 105 mEq/L or volume < 3 mL/min)
Manometry of the minor papilla. (Abnormal ? > 40 mmHg)
Observation of the degree of resistance to passage of a 0.035-inch diameter guide wire and/or 3, 4, or 5 Fr dilation catheter over a guide wire passed into the dorsal duct
Diagnostic/therapeutic trial of minor papilla dilation, stenting, and/or sphincterotomy
Intraoperative
Resistance to passage of a 0.75-mm diameter lacrimal probe into the minor papilla (after laparotomy and duodenostomy)
Observation of parenchymal chronic pancreatitis changes limited to the dorsal pancreas

CT, computed tomography; ERCP, endoscopic retrograde cholangiography; EUS, endoscopic ultrasonography.

therapy, whereas patients with normal tests (no abnormal dilation) had a 60 % chance of not obtaining relief if minor papilla therapy was still performed. Confirmation of these results is needed from other centers. In addition, patients with chronic pancreatitis are problematic, as they may have hyposecretory exocrine function and the dorsal duct may not dilate in spite of significant minor papilla narrowing. If obesity or overlying gas precludes standard transcutaneous ultrasonography, the test can be performed under endoscopic ultrasonography observation even with CT observation. MRCP has been able to detect pancreas divisum in at least three-quarters of patients with pancreas divisum. To date, MRCP techniques for differentiating between symptomatic and asymptomatic pancreas divisum have not been successful.

Diagnostic ERCP. Ventral and dorsal ductography may provide additional clues. An abnormal dorsal duct ductogram (dilation and/or chronic pancreatitis changes) in combination with a normal ventral duct suggests pathological minor papilla narrowing. Dorsal duct dilation is a relatively uncommon finding. Eisen et al. [12] observed cystic dilation of the very terminal portion of the dorsal duct in four of 44 patients, and coined the term "Santorinicele" for this (**Fig. 52.1 h**). In such cases, the minor papilla is commonly only a pinpoint size, with a web-like surface. This may occur particularly when the minor papilla is located in a diverticulum. Pain is occasionally provoked during dorsal ductography, but the significance of this is uncertain.

Special/therapeutic ERCP techniques. Even in the setting of normal ventral and dorsal ductography, evidence of chronic pancreatitis can be obtained by collecting pure pancreatic juice, especially from the dorsal duct. A bicarbonate concentration of less than 105 mEq/L and secretion of pancreatic juice at a volume less than 3 mL/min support a diagnosis of chronic pancreatitis.

Manometry of the minor papilla has been performed infrequently. Normal minor papilla basal pressures have not been defined. Nevertheless, it is interesting to speculate that if a basal pressure of >40 mmHg is abnormal for the major papilla, it may be appropriate to use the same figure for the minor papilla, as the pancreas presumably does not want to secrete against an excessively high barrier at either orifice. Manometry observations have largely been limited to patients in whom the pancreas has very large orifices that can be cannulated with a 5-Fr catheter, or in the post-therapy setting in which cannulation can be achieved with a 5-Fr manometric catheter. Staritz and Meyer zum Buschenfelde [13] studied pancreas divisum patients and showed that the group had high intraductal basal pressures in the dorsal duct in comparison with minor papilla cannulation and accessory duct pressures in nondivisum patients (with patent major papilla orifices). They did not report whether the patients were symptomatic or not. These studies need to be repeated with small-caliber (possibly 3-Fr) catheters that measure both intraductal and intrapapillary (intrasphincteric) pressure. Once a guide wire has been passed into the dorsal duct, observation of the degree of resistance to passage of a 3-Fr, 4-Fr, or 5-Fr catheter might be a gauge of the degree of minor papilla narrowing. This is unstandardized, but it might be possible to extrapolate the findings to the intraoperative observations used by surgeons to evaluate sphincter patency (see below).

Lastly, trial therapy of enlarging the orifice of the minor papilla may provide clinically helpful observations. The therapeutic response in patients with daily, or at least weekly, symptoms can be observed after minor papilla dilation, stenting, or sphincterotomy. A response to such therapy strongly implies that the minor papilla orifice was previously too narrow. Short-term observations are difficult, since a placebo effect may be present. Patients with bouts of pancreatitis occurring infrequently (perhaps one to two times per year) may require several years of observation before the benefits of trial therapy can be determined.

Intraoperative observations. Historically, the surgeon determined patency of the minor papilla by assessing the resistance to passage of a 0.75-mm diameter lacrimal probe into the minor papilla. This requires laparotomy and duodenotomy. Endoscopic cannulation of most minor papillae with guide wires more than 0.021 inches in diameter is usually difficult (the standard 0.035-inch diameter guide wire is equivalent to 0.89 mm). It is understandable how surgeons reached this criterion for minor papilla evaluation. Warshaw et al. [11] found that patients with minor papilla narrowing as assessed by lacrimal probe patency had a high probability of responding to therapy, whereas patients with a patent minor papilla orifice as assessed by lacrimal probe patency had a low probability of responding to minor papilla sphincteroplasty. Also, the surgeon may find chronic pancreatitis changes restricted to the dorsal pancreas, again suggesting minor papilla disease.

Surgical minor papilla sphincterotomy and sphincteroplasty. Endoscopic management must be evaluated against the background of available surgical management methods for adults and children [14]. The results of adult minor papilla therapy show that approximately 80% of patients with acute recurrent pancreatitis report improved clinical status. Patients with pain syndromes alone, or with chronic pancreatitis, have a lesser response [3].

Most surgeons also include cholecystectomy and major papilla sphincteroplasty in the treatment, making the pathophysiological interpretation less precise. In wedge resections of the minor papilla, fibrosis or inflammation have been found in one-third of specimens [15]. Where patient categorization is detailed, it is evident that

patients with attacks of acute recurrent pancreatitis or epigastric pain generally experience improvement with this type of minor papilla therapy. By contrast, patients with established chronic pancreatitis and those with chronic continuous pain have a lower response to such therapy. The largest series, published by Warshaw et al. [11], indicates that the response to ultrasound-monitored secretin stimulation tests and the clinical history help identify responders—for example, 19 of 21 patients (90%) with recurrent attacks of pain and positive ultrasound-monitored secretin tests had symptomatic improvement, whereas three of 14 patients (21%) with continuous pain and a negative secretin response benefited from sphincteroplasty. Similarly, if the minor papilla was stenotic, as evidenced by difficult passage of a 0.75-mm lacrimal probe, the patient was more likely to benefit from surgery. In another published series including 32 patients with symptomatic pancreas divisum, 24 (75%) were symptom-free at the last follow-up (mean 31 months) [16]. Surgical sphincterotomy series and sphincteroplasty series appear to have similar outcomes. Generally, if appropriate patients are selected, the surgical response rates appear to be excellent. Reporting of complications from surgery has not been standardized, but the morbidity rate is approximately 10%, and postoperative deaths have occurred.

Patients with obviously dilated dorsal ducts may be candidates for the Puestow procedure, but this is a distinct minority. One study has suggested that patients with a normal-caliber dorsal duct can become good candidates for lateral pancreaticojejunostomy by metal stent placement and duct expansion (**Fig. 52.4**). Madura and colleagues [17] evaluated 35 patients with chronic pancreatitis and a small-caliber main pancreatic duct; 31 had pancreas divisum. After a period of transpapillary dilation and stenting of the duct, a 10-mm expandable metal stent was placed, and the stent was removed approximately 14 days later at laparotomy when the lateral pancreaticojejunostomy was performed. Seventy-one percent of the patients noted improved pain scores, and a quarter of the patients were able to come off narcotics entirely.

Severely symptomatic patients who do not respond to duct decompression may be candidates for pancreatic denervation or resection, but the results of both procedures are variable. Total pancreatectomy has controlled incapacitating pain in a limited number of patients, and severe malabsorption and brittle diabetes are inevitable. Salvaging and reinfusion of the islet cells, or auto-transplantation, is now an available alternative, with promising results. More than 40% of adult patients [18–20] and 56% of children [21] have achieved insulin independence at least 1 year after total pancreatectomy with islet cell autotransplantation (TP-IAT). When the procedure is performed for chronic pancreatitis, 50–80% of patients become independent of narcotics postoperatively [18,20,22]. However, many patients cannot be weaned off narcotics, particularly those who have used narcotics on a daily basis for at least 3 months preoperatively [23].

Minor papilla endoscopic dilation and stenting. The minor papilla orifice may be opened endoscopically by dilation, stenting, or sphincterotomy. Dilation may be achieved by passing a tapered-tip dilating catheter (5–10 Fr) over a guide wire or by passing a small-diameter balloon (4–5 mm). Dilation alone without associated stenting may provoke serious pancreatitis; these techniques are therefore generally not recommended.

Stenting has been applied to the minor papilla in a therapeutic trial (short-term and long-term basis). In patients who are having daily pain, placement of a transpapillary decompressing stent can serve as a therapeutic trial (i.e., regarding whether ductal decompression resolves the pain). In patients who only have episodic pain or pancreatitis, perhaps one or two times a year, trials of short-term stenting (1–2 months) are of no benefit. Lans et al. [24] have reported a prospective randomized stenting trial in idiopathic recurrent pancreatitis. The patients were prospectively randomized to receive sham therapy versus placement of a stent 3–7 cm long with multiple side holes in the dorsal duct. The stents were exchanged every 3–4 months, and were left in place for 1 year. Control patients received no therapy. The control patients had significantly more frequent hospitalizations, emergency room visits, and pancreatitis episodes than the treated patients. Overall, 90% of the stented patients experienced improvement in comparison with 11% of the controls. The benefit generally persisted over a mean 24-month follow-up period after stent removal. Ertan reported an uncontrolled series in which similar benefits were seen with stenting of the minor papilla [25].

The potential adverse effects of prolonged pancreatic stenting are numerous and include stent occlusion or migration, pancreatitis, pancreatic duct perforation, and pseudocyst formation. A major concern in treating minor papilla stenosis with long-term stenting is that it may induce ductal changes indicating or stimulating chronic pancreatitis [26]. Smith et al. reported that a proportion of such changes may not be reversible [27]. Placement of 5-Fr polyethylene stents in the normal dog pancreas over a 2–4-month interval has shown very worrisome induction of ductal and periductal changes of chronic fibrosis, inflammation, and atrophy [28]. Because of these observations, prolonged stent therapy is not recommended in patients with a relatively normal dorsal duct. When advanced chronic pancreatitis has become established in the dorsal duct system, short-term dorsal duct stenting (for approximately 3 months) or long-term dorsal duct stenting (for several years) was thought to be beneficial in approximately two-thirds of 16 such patients [29].

Endoscopic minor papilla sphincterotomy. Endoscopic sphincterotomy has become the method of choice for opening the minor papilla. The term "papillotomy" may be preferred, as a true sphincter may not be present. Cotton [30] reported the first sphincter ablation of this type, and subsequently several small series with brief follow-up periods have been reported (**Table 52.3**) [31–37]. Two techniques have generally been used: a) using a minipapillotome or standard papillotome (generally wire-guided) to make a 4–6-mm incision in approximately the 10–12-o'clock position, after initial dilation of the orifice with a 5-Fr catheter; or b) placement of a 3–5-Fr plastic unflanged stent, followed by a needle-knife cut, generally in the 10–12-o'clock position, to a depth of 3–4 mm and a height of 4–5 mm, using the stent as a guide (**Fig. 52.5**). The cut is extended 1–2 mm into the duodenal wall beyond the papillary mound. In the Santorinicele patient, unroofing of the bulbous segment and visualization of the dilated duct is the goal. Our experience in more than 600 cases of this type of endoscopic therapy has shown that the two techniques are similarly effective. Data from other centers also suggest similar efficacy and safety with the two techniques [38]. Placement of a stent without an internal flange usually results in spontaneous passage [39]. In patients with a Santorinicele or a very dilated dorsal duct, sphincterotomy without stenting may be adequate. **Table 52.3** shows that using global pain score methods, approximately 75% of idiopathic acute recurrent pancreatitis patients experience improvement after endoscopic therapy. Recent

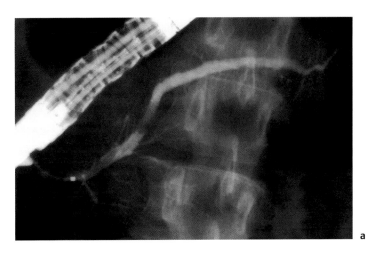

a

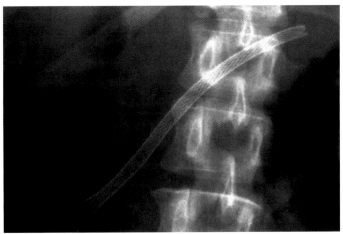

b

Fig. 52.4
a A dorsal ductogram showing chronic pancreatitis. Minor papilla sphincterotomy resolved the symptoms, but recurrent stenosis followed.
b A 68-mm expandable metal stent has been placed (photo on the day of placement). After 12 days had been allowed for duct expansion, the stent was surgically removed during a lateral pancreatojejunostomy, with an anastomosis being formed from the duct mucosa to the jejunal mucosa.

52

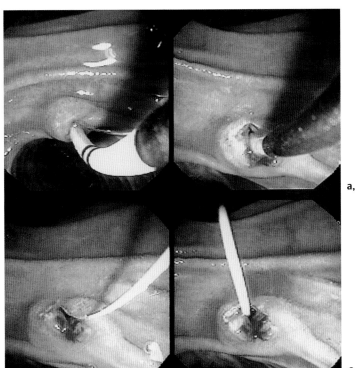

a, b

c, d

Fig. 52.5
a The minor papilla before treatment.
b After pull sphincterotomy. The sphincterotome has been advanced into the duct and bowed and is being pulled back to evaluate the size of the orifice.
c After sphincterotomy, the guide wire is in place.
d A 4-Fr stent without an intraductal barb has been left in the dorsal duct to ensure that the minor papilla remains patent during the immediate post-sphincterotomy period.

Table 52.3 Pancreas divisum: endoscopic sphincterotomy therapy in the minor papilla

First author, ref.	Year	Patients (n)	Improvement1		Recurrent acute pancreatitis*			Pain alone*			Chronic pancreatitis*			Recurrent stenosis		Major complications (n)	Deaths (n)	Mean follow-up (months)
			n	%	n	Σ	%	n	Σ	%	n	Σ	%	n	Σ			
Soehendra [35]	1986	6	6	100	2	2	100				4	4	100			0	0	ca. 3
Russell [36]	1984	5†	1	20												0	(1)‡	ca. 8
Coleman [31]	1993	13	7	54	3	4	75	0			4	9	44			0	0	14
Lehman [32]	1993	51	22	43	13	17	77	6	23	26	3	11	27	10	51	2	1§	20
Liguory [33]	1986	8	5	63	5	8	63							3	8	0	0	ca. 24
Kozarek [34]	1995	39	18	46	11	15	73	1	5	20	6	19	32					20
Toth [37]	2001	83	53	64	35	48	73	18	35	51				15	83	0	0	48
Total		205	112	55	69	94	73	25	63	40	17	43	40	28	142	2	1	ca. 30

* Global symptom assessment.
† Five sphincterotomies achieved in 12 patients attempted.
‡ Death after Whipple's procedure (after failed endoscopic therapy).
§ Minor papilla cannulation and therapy failed.

reports show that patients with improvement have significantly fewer pancreatitis attacks and hospitalization periods after therapy in comparison with the pretherapy period [40]. In patients with chronic pancreatitis and those with pain suggestive of pancreatic origin but no other documented evidence of pancreatic disease, approximately half experienced some pain reduction, but only a quarter of the group had at least a 50 % pain improvement. Chacko and colleagues recently evaluated the outcome of minor papilla endotherapy in 57 patients with pancreas divisum [41]. Patients were classified according to their symptoms as follows: recurrent pancreatitis with pain-free intervals and no radiographic evidence of chronic pancreatitis, chronic abdominal pain without evidence of chronic pancreatitis, or chronic abdominal pain with radiologic evidence of chronic pancreatitis. Clinical improvement was defined as a 50 % reduction in pain scores, narcotic use, or number of emergency room visits or hospitalizations. With a median follow-up of 20 months (range 12–39), clinical improvement was noted in 76 % of patients with recurrent pancreatitis, 33 % with chronic abdominal pain alone, and 42 % with chronic pancreatitis. While these results are consistent with the findings of previous studies, they should be interpreted with caution. Recall bias was likely in this retrospective study. Furthermore, six of the 57 patients (11 %) had undergone prior minor papilla therapy. Perhaps most importantly, recurrent pancreatitis is an episodic illness, and patients might be asymptomatic for long periods between acute attacks. In the absence of long-term follow-up, considering a patient "improved" might be premature. In an ongoing prospective randomized study of 33 patients with pancreas divisum with pain but no documented pancreatitis [42], a 50 % pain improvement (global pain score) was seen in 44 % of the treated patients and 24 % of the control patients (P=0.2). A trend toward benefit from treatment was observed, but a larger series of patients is needed to confirm this. These controlled observations, as well as other uncontrolled studies, indicate that less than half of such pain syndrome patients benefit from intervention. In truly disabled patients, this 40–50 % chance of pain improvement may justify trial therapy.

The overall reported response rate to minor papilla endoscopic therapy (stenting with or without sphincterotomy) is similar to that with surgical sphincteroplasty in similar patient categories (acute recurrent pancreatitis, chronic pancreatitis, chronic abdominal pain). Endoscopic techniques seem preferable, as they avoid the need for laparotomy. The clinically significant short-term complication rate for endoscopic minor papilla sphincterotomy appears to be similar to that in endoscopic major papilla biliary sphincterotomy, although the patient numbers are still limited and reports have

come only from experienced centers. The re-stenosis rate for any therapy of the minor papilla is estimated to be 20 %, although methods of calibrating re-stenosis are uncertain. High-grade strictures of the terminal 10 mm of the dorsal duct are estimated to occur in 2–3 % of patients. These are particularly problematic, as the narrowing extends beyond the duodenal wall and a pancreatic head resection or Puestow drainage procedure may be required. Lifelong follow-up will be needed for both surgical and endoscopic treatments. Since similar techniques are now being used in children [14,43], long-term outcomes are especially important in this group.

Associated abnormalities. Pancreas divisum is associated with other pancreaticobiliary abnormalities. Approximately one-third to one-half of patients with annular pancreas also have pancreas divisum [44,45], with simultaneous rotational and fusional abnormalities. There is evidence that up to half of patients with pancreas divisum have elevated sphincter of Oddi biliary basal pressures [15,46]. These data are based on studies of sphincter manometry and common duct flow and pressure. The frequency of pain relief from major papilla sphincterotomy alone in such pancreas divisum patients has not been reported. In addition, patients with pancreas divisum and partial agenesis of the dorsal pancreas have been reported [47,48]. It has been suggested that pancreas divisum might predispose to biliary tract malignancies. In our review of 875 pancreas divisum patients, 2.06 % were found to have cholangiocarcinoma or ampullary carcinoma [49]. However, this was not statistically different (P=0.86) from 101 such cancer patients identified among 4695 patients (2.15 %) without pancreas divisum who were seen during the same interval. Furthermore, the frequencies of known risk factors for biliary malignancies (primary sclerosing cholangitis, anomalous pancreaticobiliary junction, choledochal cyst, intrahepatic stones) were equally distributed amongst cases and controls, eliminating any confounders.

Annular Pancreas

Annular pancreas arises from failed rotation of a portion of the ventral pancreas during embryological development (**Fig. 52.6**). It is seen in approximately one in 500–1000 ERCPs. Typically, a branch of the ventral pancreas passes posteriorly to the descending duodenum and circles approximately three-quarters of the descending duodenum. This typically produces a ring-like narrowing of the descending duodenum. The major papilla is located distal to the ring, while the minor papilla may be found just proximal, distal or

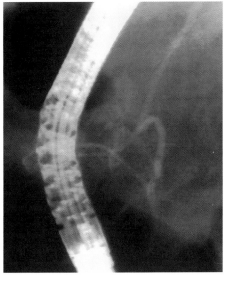

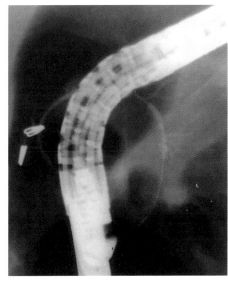

b

Fig. 52.6
a Annular pancreas without pancreas divisum; this is the most common type.
b Annular pancreas with pancreas divisum. The ventral duct encircles the duodenum.
c Annular pancreas with the entire main duct of the pancreatic head encircling the duodenum. No upstream ductal dilation is seen.
d Same patient as **c**. The endoscope has been pulled back, showing the narrowed duodenal lumen in relation to the annular duct. This is a rare variant.

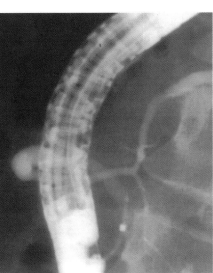

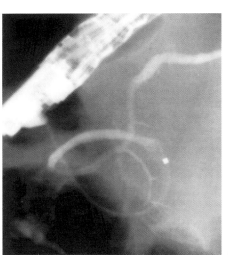

d

52

on the ring itself. The narrowing may be subtle enough to be missed initially if the endoscopic examination is not conducted carefully. While children with annular pancreas tend to present with symptoms of gastric outlet obstruction, adults do so less frequently, although typically the duodenal bulb is enlarged. More commonly, adult patients present with abdominal pain or pancreatitis, perhaps due to the association with pancreas divisum. In children, annular pancreas is often associated with other congenital anomalies, while in adults there is an increased incidence of pancreaticobiliary neoplasia [50]. **Figure 52.6 a** shows a typical annular branch from the ventral pancreas. **Figure 52.6 c** shows the entire ventral portion of the main duct encircling the duodenum and connecting with the dorsal duct. The relationship between annular pancreas and duodenal obstruction is well known; the relationship between pancreatitis and annular pancreas is less certain, particularly in patients without pancreas divisum. Pancreatitis occurring in the annulus for any reason might well produce duodenal obstruction. Most annular branches do not show evidence of chronic pancreatitis.

Pancreatic Agenesis

Complete agenesis of the pancreas is incompatible with life. Approximately one in 1000 ERCPs shows agenesis of part of the pancreas, usually the dorsal system. This can only be definitively diag-

nosed when the major and minor papillae are seen with their associated ducts, but a CT scan shows no duct extending to the left of the spine. This must be differentiated from necrosis of that portion of the pancreas after a bout of serious pancreatitis (**Fig. 52.7**).

Anomalous Pancreaticobiliary Ductal Junction

By definition, this anomaly is present when there is an anomalously long common channel between the biliary tree and the pancreatic ductal system (**Fig. 52.8**). The long channel extends cephalad to the sphincter mechanisms. There is therefore free reflux of pancreatic juice into the bile duct and of bile into the pancreas. The common channel may be quite long, up to 25 mm. This condition is easy to recognize at ERCP, as initial contrast infusion shows a long common channel with free filling of both ductal systems. There is an increased frequency of gallbladder and bile duct cancers, choledochal cysts, and pancreatitis in this setting. Two series showed that common channel sphincterotomy and improved flow of both bile and pancreatic juice to the duodenum resolved the pancreatitis in the majority of the patients treated [51,52].

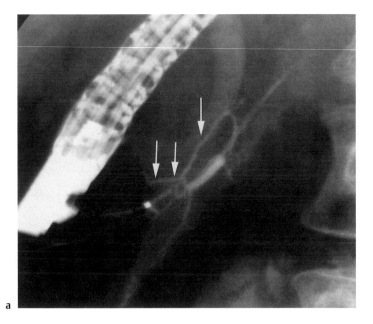

a

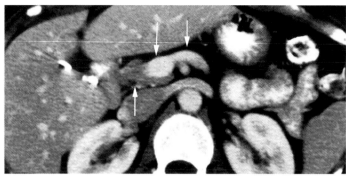

Fig. 52.7
a Partial agenesis of the dorsal pancreas. A rudimentary accessory duct (arrows) extends back toward the minor papilla.
b Computed tomography showed no body or tail of the pancreas. There is no pancreas ventral to the portal vein and no pancreatic tissue adjacent to the splenic vein (arrows: portal and splenic veins).

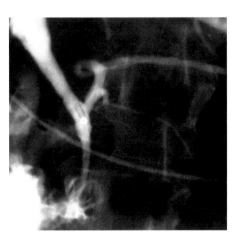

Fig. 52.8 An anomalous pancreaticobiliary ductal junction. The sphincter of Oddi lies entirely distal to the pancreaticobiliary union.

Acute Pancreatitis

Acute Gallstone Pancreatitis

In Western countries, gallstone disease is the leading cause of acute pancreatitis, accounting for nearly half of all cases. Most patients with acute gallstone pancreatitis (AGP) have a mild attack and can be treated conservatively. However, the case fatality rate in severe pancreatitis remains unacceptably high, approaching 10 %.

The passage of one or more stones from the common duct through the papilla of Vater into the duodenum appears to be the necessary event in the development of gallstone pancreatitis (**Fig. 52.9**). This theory is supported by the finding that virtually all patients with gallstone pancreatitis have stones present in their feces, compared with a 10 % recovery in hospitalized patients with biliary colic but no pancreatitis [53]. Although the mechanism by which passage of a stone triggers the acute pancreatitis is still a matter of debate, the evidence in favor of Opie's common-channel reflux hypothesis is now substantial [54].

The diagnosis of gallstone pancreatitis requires that three criteria be met: confirmation of acute pancreatitis, detection of gallstones, and exclusion of other causes of acute pancreatitis. The diagnosis of pancreatitis is dependent on the finding of an elevated serum pan-

creatic enzyme level (amylase and/or lipase usually more than three times the upper limit of normal) or radiographic changes of pancreatitis in the presence of a compatible clinical picture. Transcutaneous abdominal ultrasound is the most common technique used to assess patients for gallbladder stones, as it has an accuracy of > 95 %. However, in the setting of acute pancreatitis, the accuracy decreases to 60–80 %—partly due to the large amount of intestinal gas, which makes visualization of the gallbladder more difficult, and partly because of the small stone size (microlithiasis, with stones < 3 mm in diameter) frequently seen in many of these patients [55]. Endoscopic ultrasound may help identify small gallbladder stones in patients with acute pancreatitis previously labeled as idiopathic [56]. The sensitivity of abdominal ultrasound and CT for detecting common duct stones is at best 50–60 %. ERCP has traditionally been considered to be the most accurate of all imaging techniques, with a sensitivity of more than 95 % for detecting bile duct stones. Because of its risks, ERCP should be restricted to patients who are likely to require endoscopic therapy. MRCP and spiral CT cholangiography are less invasive techniques, with reported sensitivity rates for detecting bile duct stones in the range of 80–95 %. Recently, endoscopic ultrasound has been advocated as a first-line test for the evaluation of subtle common bile duct stones that are not detected using standard techniques, with sensitivity rates at least as high as ERCP. However, these tests are operator-dependent and are not universally available. The role of these techniques in relation to the small ductal stones typical of gallstone pancreatitis is currently under being investigated.

The most useful biochemical predictor for a biliary cause of pancreatitis appears to be elevated serum alanine aminotransferase (ALT). The results of a meta-analysis conducted by Tenner et al. [57] suggested that an ALT level elevated at least threefold had a positive predictive value of 95 % in diagnosing gallstone pancreatitis.

The first line of management in AGP is the same as in any form of acute pancreatitis. Specifically, supportive measures should be immediately instituted (intravenous fluids, parenteral analgesia, nil by mouth diet, etc.), and an assessment of the severity of the pancreatitis should be undertaken. The role and timing of ERCP are fairly unique in this form of pancreatitis.

In the open cholecystectomy era, urgent surgical intervention for severe AGP did not gain general acceptance, due to the increased morbidity and mortality associated with this approach. These surgical reports coincided with uncontrolled endoscopic series report-

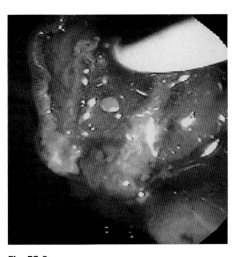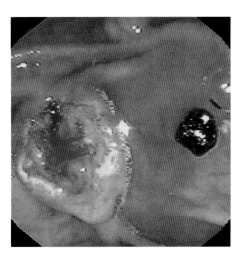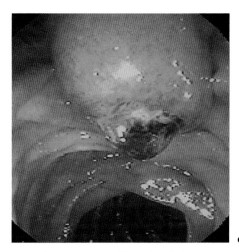

c

Fig. 52.9
a   A stone less than 2 mm in diameter that was removed from the common bile duct in gallstone pancreatitis.
b   A typical small pigment stone that was removed from the distal common bile duct in gallstone pancreatitis.
c   An impacted stone in the major papilla, causing gallstone pancreatitis.

Table 52.4 Results of a prospective randomized trial of conventional treatment in comparison with endoscopic retrograde cholangiopancreatography (ERCP), with or without endoscopic sphincterotomy (EST), in patients with suspected acute gallstone pancreatitis [60]

Group, treatment	n	Complications			Total	
		Pseudo-cysts	Systemic	Deaths	n	%
Mild						
Conventional	34	4	0	0	4	11.8
ERCP ± EST	34	3	1	0	4	11.8
Severe						
Conventional	28	8	12	5	17	60.7
ERCP ± EST	25	3	3	1	6	24.0*

* $P = 0.007$ (vs. conventional).

52

ing the efficacy and safety of ERCP and endoscopic sphincterotomy in the setting of AGP [58,59]. Although the results were encouraging, the studies varied in the criteria used for patient selection and in the timing of endoscopic sphincterotomy in relation to the acute attack (many procedures were performed in the recovery phase, when surgery is also safe). These early series prompted the four randomized controlled trials [60–63] that now serve as the basis for the endoscopic treatment of AGP. The therapeutic principle for endoscopic sphincterotomy in AGP is simply removal of the obstructing calculus and reestablishment of bile and pancreatic juice flow.

In a randomized prospective controlled trial in the United Kingdom, 121 AGP patients received either conventional therapy (i.e., gut rest, analgesics, intravenous fluids, and antibiotics) or underwent urgent ERCP (within 72 h of admission) with endoscopic sphincterotomy and stone extraction (if stones were present in the common bile duct at the time of ERCP) [60]. Patients were stratified according to the predicted severity of their attacks, using the modified Glasgow system. Choledocholithiasis was found in 25% of patients with predicted mild attacks and in 63% of those with predicted severe attacks. The results are shown in **Table 52.4**. The four important findings were: a) ERCP can be safely performed in the setting of gallstone pancreatitis; b) there was a significant reduction in the major complications of patients who underwent urgent ERCP and endoscopic sphincterotomy ($P = 0.03$); c) reduced morbidity was only evident in patients with predicted severe attacks ($P = 0.007$); and d) there was a significant reduction in the hospital stay for those with severe attacks treated with urgent ERCP and endoscopic sphincterotomy (median 9.5 days vs. 17 days, $P = 0.03$). The mortality rate improved numerically, but not to a

statistically significant degree. This trial was criticized because it was believed that the benefits observed were due to the relief of concomitant acute cholangitis (six patients in the urgent ERCP group and five in the conservatively treated group) rather than of pancreatitis. However, excluding patients with acute cholangitis still resulted in an overall benefit for the urgent ERCP group (complication rate 11% vs. 33%, $P = 0.02$), which was more pronounced in severe cases alone (complication rate 15% vs. 60%, $P = 0.003$) [64].

A second randomized controlled study was carried out in the Department of Surgery at the University of Hong Kong [61]. A total of 195 patients with acute pancreatitis were randomly assigned to undergo early ERCP (within 24 h of admission) or conservative therapy. Although the methodology, patient selection, and assessment of severity of acute pancreatitis used in this study differed from those in the British study, the results in the subgroup of patients with gallstone pancreatitis (n = 127) were quite similar (**Table 52.5**). Patients with mild pancreatitis had similar morbidity and mortality rates, regardless of the therapy. In contrast, patients with predicted severe attacks who underwent endoscopic therapy had a lower complication rate (54% vs. 13%, $P = 0.003$) and a lower mortality rate (18% vs. 3%, $P = 0.07$) than patients treated conservatively.

The third study [62] was a prospective multicenter, randomized, controlled study conducted in Germany in which 238 patients with AGP and no evidence of severe biliary obstruction (defined as a bilirubin level > 5 mg/dL) were randomly assigned to ERCP with endoscopic sphincterotomy and stone extraction or conservative therapy within 72 h of symptom onset. This study attempted to address the major criticism of the British and Hong Kong studies—

Table 52.5 Results of a randomized controlled trial of conventional treatment versus endoscopic retrograde cholangiopancreatography (ERCP) and endoscopic sphincterotomy (EST) in patients with suspected acute gallstone pancreatitis [61]

Group, treatment	n	Complications		Biliary sepsis	Deaths	Total	
		Local	Systemic			n	%
Mild							
Conventional	35	1	1	4	0	6	17
ERCP ± ES	34	4	2	0	0	6	18
Severe							
Conventional	28	8	8	8	5 *	15	54 †
ERCP ± ES	30	3	3	0	1	4	13

* *P = 0.07.*
† *P = 0.003.*

i.e., the need to exclude patients presenting with concomitant cholangitis, as these patients are known to benefit from ERCP. The two treatment groups did not differ with regard to mortality (11% vs. 6% overall mortality, P=0.1; and 8% vs. 4% for AGP mortality, P=0.16, for ERCP vs. conservative therapy) or overall complications (46% vs. 51%, P=0.54 for ERCP vs. conservative therapy), regardless of the predicted severity of the pancreatitis. However, respiratory failure was more frequent in the ERCP group (12% vs. 5%, P=0.03), and jaundice was more frequent in patients who received conservative treatment (11% vs. 1%, P=0.02). Many concerns have been raised about the methodology and the results of this study [54,64]. The first concerns the small number of patients enrolled by many of the centers (19 of the 22 centers enrolled less than two patients per year during the 54-month study period), which could be a reflection of inadequate levels of ERCP expertise. The second concern relates to the unexplained increased incidence of respiratory failure in the ERCP group, which was not found in the Hong Kong or United Kingdom studies. Finally, it is unclear why 12% of the patients in the ERCP group developed cholangitis, especially since patients with cholangitis were excluded from the study.

The final study was conducted in Poland and has been published only as an abstract [63]. In this study, 280 consecutive patients with AGP underwent duodenoscopy within 24 h of admission. Seventy-five patients were found to have a stone impacted in the ampulla and underwent immediate sphincterotomy and stone removal. The remaining 205 patients with a normal papilla were randomly assigned to receive immediate ERCP and endoscopic sphincterotomy or conventional therapy. There were significantly fewer complications (36.3% vs. 16.9%, P<0.001) and lower mortality rate (12.8% vs. 2.3%, P<0.001) in patients undergoing ERCP and endoscopic sphincterotomy. This significant reduction in morbidity and mortality was found for patients with predicted mild and severe pancreatitis. Among patients treated with ERCP and endoscopic sphincterotomy, the best results were obtained when the interval between the onset of AGP and endoscopic sphincterotomy was less than 24 h (7% complications and 0% mortality). The poorest outcome occurred when this interval exceeded 72 h (22% complications and 8% mortality).

These studies have produced some conflicting results. A meta-analysis was performed to estimate the overall efficacy and safety of endoscopic intervention [65]. The pooled data revealed a statistically significant reduction in the rate of complications in the endoscopic group (25% vs. 38.2%, P<0.001). Approximately eight patients with AGP would need to be treated with ERCP and endoscopic sphincterotomy to prevent one complication. The pooled data also revealed a statistically significant reduction in mortality in the ERCP and endoscopic sphincterotomy group in comparison with the conventional therapy group (5.2% vs. 9.1%, P<0.05). Approximately 26 patients would need to be treated with ERCP and endoscopic sphincterotomy to prevent one death. The authors of this meta-analysis recommended ERCP and endoscopic sphincterotomy for all patients, regardless of the severity of the pancreatitis.

It should be appreciated that these four studies differed in terms of the timing of patient enrollment and intervention, ethnic and environmental factors, presence of cholangitis or biliary obstruction, methods of assessing the severity of pancreatitis, incidence of gallstones, and perhaps also the level of endoscopic expertise. As a result, the data may not be readily pooled and applied to the general population of patients with AGP. Despite this uncertainty, it has generally been our practice to proceed with early ERCP in the setting of severe, nonobstructive AGP. More recently, a randomized controlled trial by Oría and colleagues [66] evaluated 103 patients with AGP, all with a serum bilirubin level ≥ 1.2 mg/dL and a dilated bile duct (≥ 8 mm). In the 51 patients undergoing ERCP, the procedure was performed within 48 h after the onset of the attack in 46 patients, and within 48–72 h in the remaining five patients. Patients with cholangitis were excluded. While 72% of the patients randomly assigned to ERCP did have bile duct stones removed, there were no differences in the incidence of organ failure, CT severity index, local complications, morbidity, or mortality. The data show that ERCP is clearly indicated in patients with AGP complicated by cholangitis or biliary obstruction. However, these studies taken as a whole suggest that its role in the setting of severe, nonobstructive AGP warrants further investigation. Moreover, the applicability of the results of such studies to community practice will need to be assessed.

The natural history of AGP is that further attacks are likely to occur unless the gallbladder is removed (assuming that a sphincterotomy or other biliary drainage procedure has not been performed). A cholecystectomy is therefore indicated, and if a preoperative cholangiogram has not been done, an intraoperative cholangiogram is highly recommended. Since repeat attacks may occur within weeks of the first attack, most authorities advocate cholecystectomy towards the end of the index hospitalization. In patients who have a high surgical risk or refuse surgery, endoscopic sphincterotomy appears to be an effective method of preventing recurrent pancreatitis.

Acute Recurrent Pancreatitis of Known or Unknown Cause

The etiology of an episode of pancreatitis may be obvious from the clinical history or laboratory data. A heavy alcohol ingestion history, recent significant abdominal trauma, ingestion of pancreatotoxic drugs, or a serum triglyceride level of more than 1000 in the acute setting, all suggest an obvious etiology. The use of ERCP in such cases is generally reserved for diagnosis and management of suspected or noninvasively viewed complications, such as strictures, stones or pseudocysts. It is our practice to perform ERCP with manometry in such cases after three or four bouts of pancreatitis, in hope of finding an endoscopically treatable component of the disease.

Idiopathic pancreatitis is defined as clinical pancreatitis occurring in the absence of any identifiable causes based on the patient history, laboratory testing (including serum triglycerides, calcium, liver function tests) and radiological evaluation (usually an abdominal ultrasound and CT scan). A few series [67] have reported a high frequency of gallstone pancreatitis in this setting, but if patients with any liver test abnormalities are excluded, then the finding of subtle gallstones is less than 10%. The findings of an ERCP examination correlate significantly with the age of the patients being studied (i.e., neoplasms are uncommon in patients under 40 years of age) and with the detail with which manometry is performed on both the bile duct and pancreas. **Table 52.6** shows a series of 1241 patients with idiopathic pancreatitis studied in our institution. The high frequency of sphincter of Oddi dysfunction should be noted (pancreatic and biliary manometry were carried out routinely). Sphincter of Oddi manometry has been used increasingly during the last decade. As can be seen from **Table 52.6**, if manometry had not been performed, nearly half of the patients with idiopathic pancreatitis would not have had a cause detected. A study by Eversman et al. [68] emphasized the importance of studying both sphincters lest a portion of the sphincter disease go undetected. Studies vary in their reported success rates in preventing relapses of idiopathic pancreatitis with just biliary therapy alone. The most pessimistic was by Guelrud et al. [69], who found that only 28% of idiopathic pancreatitis patients with pancreatic sphincter hypertension responded to biliary sphincterotomy alone. Generally, two clinical approaches are practical: a) evaluating and treating the biliary sphincter if abnormal, and then awaiting the clinical response; or b) evaluating and treating both biliary and pancreatic sphincters at the initial session. Jacob and colleagues [70] postulated that sphincter of Oddi dysfunction might cause recurrent pancreatitis even though the sphincter of Oddi manometry was normal and pancreatic stenting may prevent further attacks. In a randomized trial, 34 patients with idiopathic recurrent pancreatitis, normal pancreatic duct sphincter manometry, ERCP, and secretin testing were treated with pancreatic stents (n = 19; 5–7 Fr, with stents exchanged three times over a 1-year period) or conservative therapy (n = 15). During a 3-year follow-up period, pancreatitis occurred in 53% of patients in the control group and 11% of those in the stent group ($P < 0.02$). This study suggests that sphincter of Oddi manometry may be an imperfect test, as patients may have sphincter of Oddi dysfunction but not be detected at the time of manometry. However, long-term studies are needed to evaluate the outcome after removal of stents, and concern remains regarding stent-induced ductal and parenchymal changes. Idiopathic pancreatitis unfortunately has a high complication rate with standard diagnostic ERCP and biliary sphincterotomy alone. Prospective randomized trials evaluating stent placement to protect the pancreas during the treatment session have shown a reduction in the frequency and severity of pancreatitis after the procedure by more than 50% [71].

Overall, ERCP with manometry is recommended in idiopathic pancreatitis after two bouts of mild pancreatitis, especially in young persons, or after a single bout of more severe pancreatitis of uncertain etiology, especially if the CT scan shows ductal dilation or raises any concern about a structural lesion.

It should be appreciated that endoscopic ultrasound has assumed a central role in the evaluation of patients with unexplained pancreatitis. The findings on EUS may direct an alternative therapy (e.g., cholecystectomy for microlithiasis) and obviate a more invasive ERCP, or may be helpful in triage for ERCP (e.g., a finding of bile duct stones). Clearly, EUS can identify small tumors of the pancreas not seen on other imaging tests, which may also be missed at ERCP. Magnetic resonance imaging (MRI) and MRCP have also assumed a

Table 52.6 Endoscopic retrograde cholangiopancreatography findings in 1241 patients with "idiopathic" pancreatitis

Postprocedural diagnosis	Patients	
	n	%
Sphincter of Oddi dysfunction	501	40.4
Pancreas divisum	233	18.8
Periampullary diverticulum	75	6.0
Intraductal mucinous tumors	52	4.2
Choledocholithiasis, ductal sludge	19	1.5
Cholelithiasis, gallbladder sludge	19	1.5
Choledochal cysts	10	0.8
Anomalous pancreaticobiliary junction	7	0.6
Papilla of Vater adenoma/cancer	4	0.3
Annular pancreas	4	0.3
Primary sclerosing cholangitis	3	0.2

Some patients had more than one diagnosis.

vital role in the evaluation of these patients, as they provide high-quality imaging of parenchymal and ductal structures. Secretin stimulation can add to the diagnostic accuracy of this test. Both EUS and MRI/MRCP are operator-dependent, and their sensitivity and specificity in identifying a cause for the pancreatitis will depend on local expertise and availability.

■ Unresolving Acute Pancreatitis

The role of ERCP in the active acute pancreatitis setting appears limited, except when there is a clinical suspicion of gallstone pancreatitis. Few data are available regarding the evaluation of ERCP in nongallstone acute pancreatitis, but concerns over aggravating pancreatic injury or infecting pancreatic necrosis early in the course make most endoscopists cautious.

For patients with diffuse inflammatory changes of the pancreas or slowly resolving peripancreatic fluid collections, most experts recommend 4–8 weeks of total gut rest and parenteral or enteral nutrition to aid in resolving, localizing, or encapsulating inflammatory processes. At this point, management choices have to be made in patients in whom the condition has not resolved—between a) surgical exploration, debridement and drainage; b) application of diagnostic and if possible therapeutic ERCP; or c) a further interval of gut rest and nutritional support. The Seattle group reported a series of such patients (see below in the section on pseudocysts) and noted that the majority had treatable ductal leaks that healed with endoscopic therapy.

Rerknimitr et al. [72] published a preliminary report on 153 patients with ductal leaks (**Table 52.7**). The leaks were categorized according to the leak site (**Fig. 52.10**). This series showed that patients with small duct disruption and partial main duct disruption had a high frequency of resolution of ductal leak with endoscopic sphincterotomy and stenting (**Fig. 52.10**). In 32 patients with complete duct disruption, the fluid collections resolved in 20, who were therefore able to avoid surgery at least initially. Further data are needed to determine whether complete disruptions can be distinguished from partial disruptions by noninvasive imaging methods such as MRCP.

Patients with extensive necrosis and suspected duct disruption need a team approach, as some fluid collections can be managed percutaneously. Some of these patients need surgery, particularly those with disconnected tail syndrome—i.e., necrosis of the neck or body of the pancreas with the residual tail secreting juice into the retroperitoneum. This needs to be identified and surgically cor-

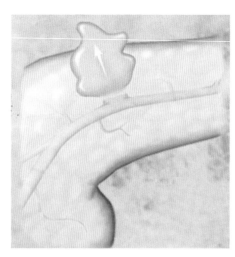

Fig. 52.10 Diagrams of the various types of pancreatic ductal disruption, categorized by the site and degree of main duct injury (courtesy of the Department of Medical Illustration, Indiana University School of Medicine).

a A small ductal leak, caused by a side branch disruption.

b A partial (lateral) main duct disruption. The main pancreatic duct is visualized upstream from the pancreatic duct leak.

c Optimally, the stent tip is placed upstream from the leak site. Alternatively, the stent or drainage tube may be positioned in the fluid collection.

d Complete main pancreatic duct disruption (transected duct). Endoscopically, it is usually not possible to pass a guide wire into the upstream duct.

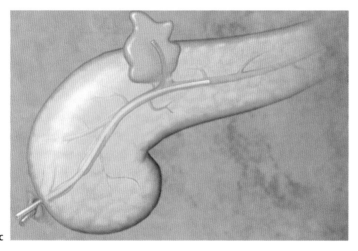

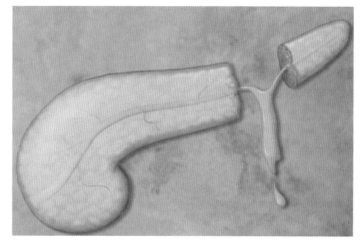

Table 52.7 Pancreatogram findings and results of endoscopic therapy in patients with ductal leaks [72]

Leak type	CPDD	PPDD	SDL	Total
Patients (n)	37	89	27	153
Direct to surgery	5	1	0	6
Endoscopic therapy success/attempt	20/32	79/81	8/8	107/121
Mean duration of therapy (in months)	2.9	2.8	2.6	2.8
Mean number of procedures	2.8	3.0	2.1	2.9
Surgery for failed endoscopic therapy	12/32	2/81	0/8	14/21
Mean follow-up (months)	30	27	26	27

CPDD, complete pancreatic main duct disruption; PPDD, partial pancreatic main duct disruption; SDL, small duct leak.

rected, as percutaneous or endoscopic approaches typically have not led to ultimate success (**Fig. 52.11**). If surgery does not take place and endoscopic therapy is undertaken with transgastric stenting of fluid collections, some experts advocate chronic stenting, as the collection will recur following stent removal. Long-term outcome data are needed in this setting.

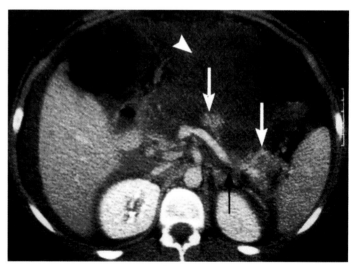

Fig. 52.11 Extensive necrosis, with small areas of residual surviving parenchyma in the pancreatic body and tail (white arrows). Arrowhead: fluid collection; black arrow: splenic vein.

Chronic Pancreatitis

Chronic pancreatitis is an inflammatory process characterized by irreversible destruction of pancreatic parenchyma and ductal structures, with formation of fibrosis. Abdominal pain, steatorrhea, and diabetes are common sequelae. Analgesics, nerve blocks, oral enzyme supplements, and octreotide are variably effective in relieving pain. Pancreatic duct pressure is generally increased in patients with chronic pancreatitis, regardless of the etiology and whether or not the main pancreatic duct is dilated. Ductal and interstitial hypertension and possibly pancreatic ischemia play an important role in the etiology of pain.

The aim of endoscopic therapy (and decompressive surgical therapy) for patients with chronic pancreatitis presenting with pain or clinical episodes of acute pancreatitis, or both, is to alleviate the obstruction of exocrine juice outflow. Certain pathological alterations of the pancreatic duct, bile duct, and/or sphincter lend themselves to endoscopic therapy. Techniques such as sphincterotomy, dilation, and stenting have been adapted for use in the pancreatic duct. Although there are limited data comparing the endoscopic approach to surgery, endoscopic drainage is appealing in that it may offer an alternative to surgical drainage procedures, with generally less morbidity and mortality. In addition, endoscopic procedures do not preclude subsequent surgery if it becomes necessary, and the outcome after reducing the intraductal pressure by endoscopic methods may be a predictor for the success of surgical drainage [73].

Outcome data following endoscopic therapy in chronic pancreatitis are often difficult to interpret due to heterogeneous study populations, with one or more pathological processes being treated (e. g., pancreatic duct stones, strictures, pseudocysts) and multiple therapies being performed in each patient (e. g., stricture dilation, stone extraction, bile duct and/or pancreatic duct endoscopic sphincterotomy). Controlled studies have not been reported to date.

▦ Pancreatic Strictures

Benign strictures of the main pancreatic duct may be a complication of a previous embedded stone, or a consequence of acute inflammatory changes around the main pancreatic duct. Given the putative role of ductal hypertension in the genesis of symptoms in a subpopulation of patients, the value of pancreatic duct stenting to treat pancreatic duct strictures has been evaluated [74–82]. The best candidates for stenting are patients with a stricture of the pancreatic head main duct and upstream dilation (type IV pancreatitis) [75]. For optimal results, the therapy must address both the pancreatic duct stricture and any associated ductal stones (see below).

Pancreatic stent placement technique. The technique for placing a stent in the pancreatic duct is similar to that used for inserting a biliary stent (Chapter 36). A guide wire needs to be maneuvered upstream to the narrowing. Hydrophilic flexible-tipped wires are especially helpful for this, and wires that can be torqued are occasionally necessary. Most pancreatic stents are simply standard polyethylene biliary stents with extra side holes at approximately 1-cm intervals to allow better juice flow from the side branches. In general, the size of stent should not exceed the size of the normal downstream duct. Stents of 4–7 Fr are therefore commonly used in small ducts, whereas stents of 10–11.5 Fr can be used in advanced chronic pancreatitis and grossly dilated ducts. Alternatively, multiple smaller-diameter, softer stents can be placed in these dilated ducts so as to potentially cause less ductal irritation. Most stents for diagnostic trial or short-term therapy are left in place for 2–4 weeks. By contrast, stents for long-term therapy have been left in place for 3–116 months [75]. The need for stent exchange or removal depends on whether the disease being treated has resolved. Although luminal occlusion occurs in most pancreatic stents within the first few weeks [83], clinical improvement may persist much longer than this, perhaps as a result of pancreatic juice siphoning along the stent.

A pancreatic sphincterotomy (major and/or minor papilla) is often performed before (or after) placing a pancreatic stent. There are two methods of cutting the major papilla pancreatic sphincter. A standard pull-type sphincterotome (with or without a wire guide) is inserted into the pancreatic duct and oriented along the axis of the pancreatic duct (usually in the 12-o'clock to 2-o'clock positions). Although the landmarks for determining the length of the incision are imprecise, most authors recommend cutting 6–10 mm. The cutting wire should not extend more than 6–7 mm up the duct when electrocautery is applied, in order to prevent deep ductal injury. Alternatively, a needle-knife can be used to perform the sphincterotomy over a previously placed pancreatic stent. However, performing a biliary sphincterotomy first can expose the pancreaticobiliary septum and allow the length of the cut to be gauged more accurately.

Efficacy of stenting. Evaluation of pancreatic stenting has been difficult, as this technique is frequently combined with pancreatic sphincterotomy, stricture dilation and/or stone removal (**Fig. 52.12**). Wilcox recently summarized the results of pancreatic duct stent placement, usually with ancillary procedures [75,77,80–82,84,85]. Among the 1500 patients treated in 15 series, benefit was seen in 31 %–100 % of patients during a follow-up interval of 8–72 months. The greatest benefit is seen in patients with dominant strictures and dilated ducts [86]. Like surgical decompressive procedures, it appears that the response attenuates over time. However, quantification of the degree of improvement is often poorly defined. Partial or complete symptom improvement after stenting suggests that intraductal hypertension was an etiologic factor. Continued symptom relief after stent removal indicates adequate dilation of the narrowing. Differentiation of these two types of improvement is, unfortunately, not clarified in some reports. In the largest published study, 1018 patients with chronic pancreatitis were followed prospectively for a mean of 4.9 years after endoscopic intervention [87]. At follow-up, 60 % of the patients had completed endotherapy, 16 % were still undergoing endoscopic treatments, and 24 % had undergone surgery. Complete (69 %) or partial (19 %) technical success of endoscopic therapy was achieved in 88 %. All patients had pain initially, but only 34 % had pain at follow-up ($P < 0.0001$); significant reduction in pain (no or weak pain) was achieved in 85 %. Rates of pain relief were similar in patients with dominant strictures in the head and/or body, pancreatic stones in the head and/or body, combination of stones and strictures, and complex pathology.

The appropriate duration of pancreatic stent placement is unknown. Available options include leaving the stent in place either until symptoms or complications occur, or for a predetermined interval (e. g., 3 months). If the patient fails to respond, then the stent should be removed, as ductal hypertension is unlikely to be the cause of the pain. If stenting is clearly beneficial, then one can remove the stent and follow the patient clinically, continue stenting for a more extended period, or carry out a surgical drainage procedure. The latter option assumes that the results of endoscopic therapy will predict the surgical outcome. Two preliminary studies have supported this concept [88,89], but longer-term results are awaited.

Symptomatic improvement may continue after stent removal, in spite of partial persistence of the stricture [75,80–82] (**Table 52.8**), as several other factors may account for the outcome. Firstly, other treatments performed at the time of stenting (e. g., pancreatic stone removal or pancreatic sphincterotomy) may contribute to the benefit. Secondly, many of the strictures that did not resolve showed improved luminal patency (but without the lumen returning to normal). Thirdly, the pain caused by chronic pancreatitis tends to

52

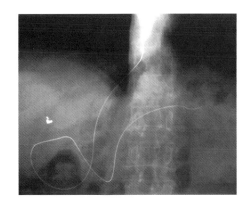

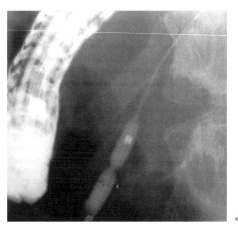

a, b

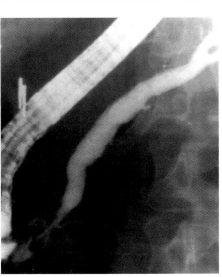

d

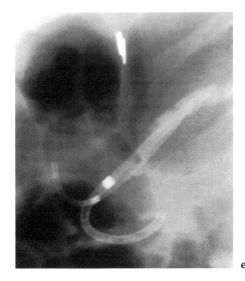

e

Fig. 52.12 Stricture management.
a A stricture of the terminal dorsal duct in a patient with prior surgical sphincteroplasty of the minor papilla.
b The stricture was so tight that only a 0.035-inch guide wire would pass it. The guide wire was left in overnight. The next day, it was possible to pass a balloon catheter.
c Balloon dilation (diameter 4 mm). There is a significant waistline, which resolved when the balloon was inflated to 12 atmospheres. A 7-Fr stent was placed.
d When the stent was removed 3 months later, there was improved patency in the terminal duct.
e Two additional stents were placed, neither of which had an intraductal barb, to allow spontaneous passage. Three years later, the stricture and pancreatitis recurred, and the sequence was repeated.

Table 52.8 Clinical outcome and main pancreatic duct stricture resolution after endoscopic stent removal

First author, year (ref.)	Persistent symptom improvement after endoscopic stent removal			Median follow-up after stent removal (months)	Stricture resolution by ductographic appearance		
	n	Σ	%		n	Σ	%
Ponchon (1995) [81]	12	21	57	14	8	21	38
Smits (1995) [82]	23	33	70	29	10	33	30
Total	35	54	65	23	18	54	33

decrease with time, and it may resolve when marked deterioration of pancreatic function occurs [90].

As noted above, a single large-caliber (10–11.5Fr) pancreatic stent has typically been placed in patients with advanced chronic pancreatitis with pancreatic strictures and grossly dilated ducts. Costamagna and colleagues recently investigated the feasibility, efficacy and long-term results of multiple pancreatic stents in this patient population [91]. Nineteen patients (16 men, three women; mean age 45 years) with severe chronic pancreatitis and a dominant stricture in the pancreatic head had as many stents (8.5–11.5 Fr) placed as possible, limited only by stricture "tightness" and duct diameter. Stents were removed after 6–12 months. The median number of stents placed was three. Only one patient (out of 19; 5.5%) had a persistent stricture after the stenting interval. During the mean follow-up of 38 months after final stent removal, 16 patients (84%) remained asymptomatic and two patients (10.5%) had symptomatic stricture recurrence. No major complications were noted. The authors concluded that multiple stenting of dominant pancreatic duct strictures is a feasible and safe technique, with promising results.

With appropriate patient selection, surgical intervention relieves pain in the majority of patients, and this response is reasonably durable, lasting for years. It is now clear, however, that endoscopic therapy may be an alternative to surgery in select patients. Endotherapy has been compared with surgical therapy in two randomized trials. Díte and colleagues [92] reported the results of a randomized study comparing surgical therapy to endoscopic treatment in 72 patients with a dilated pancreatic duct with stones, strictures, or both. An additional 68 patients who declined randomization and opted for endoscopic therapy (n = 28) or surgery (n = 40) were included in the total results. Of note, extracorporeal shock-wave lithotripsy (ESWL; see below) was not available for stone fragmentation in this trial. At 1 year after the intervention, 92% of the patients in each group had complete or partial pain relief. After

VIII

5 years, the rates were 65 % of the endotherapy patients and 86 % of the surgical patients (complete resolution, 14 % vs. 37 %, respectively; $P = 0.002$; and partial relief, 51 % vs. 49 %; not significant). Weight gain was similarly common in the two groups at 1 year (66 % vs. 60 % respectively), but significantly more patients had gained weight in the surgical group (52 %) than in the endotherapy group (27 %) by 5 years. Outcomes in the randomized group were similar to those for the total group. Despite the many methodologic problems associated with this study, the data suggest that surgical outcomes are more durable.

Cahen et al. recently published results from a randomized trial of 39 patients with chronic pancreatitis and distal pancreatic duct obstruction who were randomly assigned to endoscopic transpapillary drainage with or without ESWL, or surgical pancreaticojejunostomy [93]. At the end of the 24-month follow-up period, higher rates of pain relief were reported in the patients assigned to surgical drainage (75 vs. 32 %). Interestingly, four patients who were initially in the endotherapy group subsequently underwent surgery, with only one of these patients achieving relief postoperatively. Criticisms of this study include the small sample size, a less than aggressive endoscopic approach with short-term stenting, and the use of stents without side holes. Additional long-term trials comparing endoscopic, surgical, and medical management of patients with pancreatic strictures would be of great interest.

A subset of patients may have impassable pancreatic duct strictures, perhaps due to duct angulation, a loop in the pancreatic duct (i.e., ansa pancreatica), or altered surgical anatomy. The Belgian group recently described EUS-guided pancreatogastrostomy and pancreatobulbostomy as alternatives to surgery in this difficult patient population [94]. In their series of 36 patients, technical success with duct access was achieved in 33. With a median follow-up of 14.5 months, pain relief was complete or partial in 25 patients (69 %). Major complications occurred in two patients (one hematoma, one case of severe pancreatitis). The Mayo Clinic group recently described their experience with percutaneous pancreatography, where the pancreatic duct was accessed percutaneously and a pancreatic duct stent was placed, allowing successful endoscopic management of pancreatic duct obstruction [95]. Continued experience is necessary with these new, exciting techniques.

Complications associated with pancreatic stents. True complication rates are difficult to determine due to the simultaneous performance of other procedures (e. g., pancreatic sphincterotomy and stricture dilation), the heterogeneous patient populations treated (i. e., patients with acute or chronic pancreatitis), and the lack of a uniform definition of a complication and absence of a standard system for grading the severity of complications. Complications related directly to stent therapy are listed in **Table 52.9** [27,96]. The rate of pancreatic stent occlusion appears to be similar to that for biliary stents. Fifty percent of pancreatic stents (primarily 5–7 Fr) were found to be occluded within 8 weeks of placement when carefully evaluated using water flow methods [83]. More than 80 % of these early occlusions were not associated with adverse clinical events. In such circumstances, the stent is perhaps serving as a dilator or a wick. Similarly, stents reported to be clinically patent for as long as 38 months have been found to be clearly occluded when water flow testing was carried out [75].

Stent migration may be upstream (i. e., into the duct) or downstream (i. e., into the duodenum). Migration in either direction may be heralded by a return of pain and pancreatitis. Proximal stent migration into the duct is especially problematic and may require surgical, percutaneous, or tedious endoscopic removal. Modifications in pancreatic stent design may reduce the frequency of such occurrences. We have found that a three-quarter or single duodenal pigtail design has eliminated inward migration (unpublished data).

Table 52.9 Complications directly related to pancreatic duct stents or guide wires used to place stents [27,96]

Stent occlusion or foreign body-induced pain and/or pancreatitis
Duodenal erosions
Ductal perforation
Stone formation
Migration into or out of duct
Pancreatic infection
Ductal and parenchymal changes
Pseudocysts

Although therapeutic benefit has been reported for polyethylene pancreatic stenting, it has become evident that morphological changes in the pancreatic duct directly related to this form of treatment occur in the majority of patients. In eight published series [26,27,32,39,97–100], new ductal changes were seen in 36 % (range 24–83 %) of 776 patients. It appears that these stent-induced changes are less likely to occur with smaller-diameter (3-Fr) stents [39]. If one excludes the study in which 3-Fr stents were used most commonly [39] from the above series, new ductal changes were seen in 54 % of 297 patients. Limited observations to date indicate a tendency of these ductal changes to improve with time after stent exchange or removal [26,27,39,97,99,100]. It remains uncertain what the long-term consequences of these stent-induced ductal changes are in the majority of patients; however, permanent strictures have been seen in a small number of patients. Moreover, the long-term parenchymal effects have not been studied in humans. Parenchymal changes (hypoechoic areas around the stent, heterogeneity, and cystic changes) were seen on endoscopic ultrasound in 17 of 25 patients who underwent short-term pancreatic duct stenting [101]. Four patients who had parenchymal changes at stent removal were included in a follow-up study after a mean of 16 months. Two patients had new changes suggestive of chronic pancreatitis (heterogeneous echo texture, echogenic foci in the parenchyma, and a thickened, hyperechoic, irregular pancreatic duct) in the stented region. While such damage might have significant long-term consequences in a normal pancreas, the outcome in patients with advanced chronic pancreatitis may be inconsequential. Further studies addressing issues of stent diameter, as well as the composition and duration of therapy in relation to safety and efficacy, are needed. These potentially serious stent-induced ductal changes should discourage the endoscopist from placing long-term plastic stents in patients with a normal downstream duct.

Pancreatic Ductal Stones

Alcohol-induced, tropical, and idiopathic pancreatitis are the main categories of chronic calcific pancreatitis. Alcohol appears to be directly toxic to the pancreas and produces a dysregulation of secretion of pancreatic enzymes (including zymogens), citrate (a potent calcium chelator), lithostathine (pancreatic stone protein) and calcium. These changes favor the formation of a protein plug as a nidus for stone formation, followed by precipitation of calcium carbonate to form a stone.

There is debate as to whether pancreatic calculi aggravate the clinical course of chronic pancreatitis (manifested as increased abdominal pain or recurrent attacks of acute pancreatitis, or both), or are simply the inevitable sequelae of ongoing gland destruction. It has been postulated that increased intraductal pressure proximal (upstream) to an obstructed focus within the pancreatic duct, as with pancreatic duct stones, is one of the potential mechanisms responsible for attacks of acute pancreatitis or exacerbations of

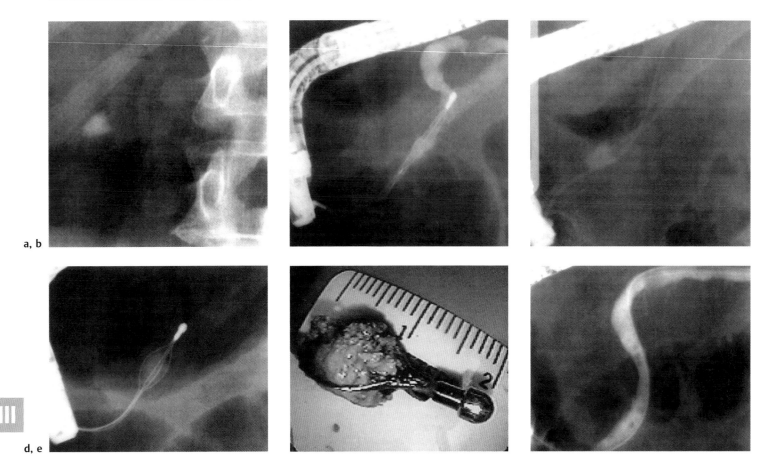

a, b

VIII

d, e

Fig. 52.13 Pancreatic stone.
a There is a bullet-shaped stone in the main duct in the pancreatic head.
b Ductogram. The contrast medium makes it difficult to see the calcified stone.

c A temporary stent was placed for palliation.
d Basketing of the stone.
e View of the removed stone.
f The final patent pancreatogram.

chronic abdominal pain in patients with chronic pancreatitis [78]. This notion is supported by reports indicating that endoscopic removal of pancreatic calculi (with or without extracorporeal shockwave lithotripsy) or surgical removal of calculi results in symptomatic improvement [102–112]. Moreover, stone impaction may cause further trauma to the pancreatic duct, with epithelial destruction and stricture formation. Identification of main pancreatic ductal stones in a symptomatic patient therefore warrants consideration of removal.

Endoscopic techniques. Pancreatic sphincterotomy is usually required to facilitate access to the duct before attempts at stone removal. Whether it is possible to remove a stone by endoscopic methods alone depends on the size and number of the stones, the duct location, the presence of a downstream stricture, and the degree of impaction [109]. Downstream strictures usually require dilation, either with catheters or hydrostatic balloons. Standard stone retrieval balloons and baskets are the most common accessories used (**Fig. 52.13**). Passage of these instruments around a tortuous duct can be difficult, but use of over-the-wire accessories is usually helpful. Stone removal is then performed in the same way as bile duct stone extraction.

Endoscopic results. Sherman et al. [109] attempted to identify patients with predominately main pancreatic duct stones that were most amenable to endoscopic removal, and to determine the effects on the patients' clinical courses of this type of removal. Thirty-two patients with ductographic evidence of chronic pancreatitis and pancreatic duct stones underwent attempted endoscopic removal,

using various techniques including bile duct and/or pancreatic duct sphincterotomy, stricture dilation, pancreatic duct stenting, stone basketing, and balloon extraction and/or flushing. Of these patients, 72% had complete or partial stone removal, and 68% experienced improvement after endoscopic therapy. Symptomatic improvement was most evident in the group of patients with chronic relapsing pain episodes (compared with those presenting with chronic continuous pain alone: 83% vs. 46%). Factors favoring complete stone removal included: three or less stones; stones confined to the head and/or body of the pancreas; absence of a downstream stricture; stone diameter < 10 mm; and absence of impacted stones. After successful stone removal, 25% of the patients had regression of the ductographic changes of chronic pancreatitis, and 42% had a decrease in the main pancreatic duct diameter. The only complication of the treatment was mild pancreatitis in 8%. These data suggest that removal of pancreatic duct stones may result in symptomatic improvement. Longer follow-up periods will be necessary to determine the stone recurrence rate and whether endoscopic success results in persistent clinical improvement or permanent regression of the morphologic changes, or both.

Smits et al. [111] reported their results in 53 patients with pancreatic duct stones that were treated primarily by endoscopic methods alone (eight of the patients underwent extracorporeal shockwave lithotripsy). Stone removal was successful in 42 patients (79%; complete in 39 and partial in three), with initial relief of symptoms in 38 (90%). As with the results reported by Sherman et al. [109], three of 11 patients (27%) in this series with failed stone removal had improvement in symptoms, suggesting that some of the clinical response may be related to other therapies performed at the time of

Table 52.10 Endoscopic therapy for pancreatic ductal stones using adjunctive extracorporeal shock-wave lithotripsy (ESWL). None of the series reported any mortalities

First author, year (ref.)	Patients (n)	Mean ESWL sessions (n)	Complete stone clearance (%)	Major complications (%)	Mean follow-up (months)	Patients with symptom improvement * (%)
Delhaye (1992) [113]	123	1.8	59	36	14	63
Neuhaus (1991) [110]	12	1.6	67	0	8	91
Sauerbruch (1992) [106]	24	1.5	42	9	24	83
Schneider (1994) [115]	50	2.4	60	0	20	90
Sherman (1995) [116]	26	1.2	61	12	26	81
Soehendra (1989) [117]	8	n/a	100	0	6	75
van der Hul (1994) [118]	17	1.9	41	6	30	65
Costamagna (1997) [119]	35	1.9/1.3	74	0	27	72
Total	295	1.8	60	17	19[†]	72

N/a, not available/no data.
* Global symptom assessment.
† Estimate.

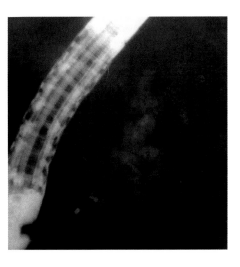

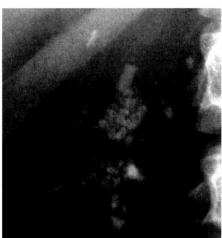

Fig. 52.14
a Multiple stones in the pancreatic head (before treatment).
b After extracorporeal shock-wave lithotripsy. The stone has a more granular appearance. Multiple fragments were removed during subsequent endoscopic retrograde cholangiopancreatography.

52

attempted stone removal (e.g., pancreatic sphincterotomy). During a median follow-up period of 33 months, 13 patients had recurrent symptoms due to stone recurrence. The stones were successfully removed in 10 patients (77 %). None of the factors evaluated (etiology of pancreatitis, presentation with pain or pancreatitis, presence of single or multiple stones, location of stones, presence or absence of a stricture) was shown to predict successful stone treatment (defined as complete or partial removal of stones resulting in relief of symptoms).

Lithotripsy. As noted above, endoscopic methods alone are likely to fail in the presence of large or impacted stones and stones proximal to a stricture. ESWL can be used to fragment stones and facilitate their removal [106,110,113,114] (**Fig. 52.14**). This procedure is therefore complementary to endoscopic techniques, and improves the success of nonsurgical ductal decompression. Patients with obstructing prepapillary concretions and upstream ductal dilation appear to be the best candidates for ESWL. **Table 52.10** summarizes the results of eight series reporting the efficacy and safety of adjunctive ESWL [106,110,113,115–119].

In the largest reported series [113], 123 patients with main pancreatic duct stones and proximal dilation were treated with the electromagnetic lithotriptor, usually before pancreatic duct sphincterotomy. Stones were successfully fragmented in 99 % of cases, resulting in a reduction in ductal dilation in 90 %. The main pancreatic duct was completely cleared of all stones in 59 %. Eighty-five

percent of patients reported pain improvement during a mean follow-up period of 14 months. However, 41 % of patients had a clinical relapse due to stone migration into the main pancreatic duct, progressive structure, or stent occlusion. The same group compared the results of pancreatic stone removal before the availability of ESWL and after the introduction of adjunctive ESWL therapy [112]. Stones were successfully cleared in 18 of 40 patients (45 %) by endoscopic methods alone, compared to 22 of 28 (78.6 %) with ESWL.

A meta-analysis of 16 studies published studies between 1989 and 2002 including 588 patients showed that ESWL had a significant impact on reducing pancreatic stone burden and improvement in pain [120]. Brand and colleagues [121] showed that the global quality of life was improved in 68 % of patients undergoing ESWL. These data suggest that removal of pancreatic duct stones may result in symptomatic benefit. Longer follow-up periods will be necessary to determine the stone recurrence rate and whether endoscopic success results in persistent clinical improvement or permanent regression of the morphological changes. Overall, the endoscopist is encouraged to remove pancreatic duct stones, in symptomatic patients, when they are located in the main duct (in the head and/or body) and are thus readily accessible. The currently available data suggest that the clinical outcome after successful endoscopic removal is similar to the surgical outcome, with lower morbidity and mortality. Long-term follow-up studies have shown that ESWL combined with ERCP may avoid the need for surgery in approximately two-thirds of patients on an intention-to-treat basis [122]. However, to date, no comparative trials have been done in patients with pancreatic stones alone.

There are limited data on the influence of ESWL on the metabolic consequences of chronic pancreatitis. Adamek et al. [114] studied 80 patients with unretrievable obstructive pancreatic duct stones who underwent ESWL with a piezoelectric lithotriptor. While complete duct clearance was achieved in only 43 patients (54%), 61 patients experienced considerable or complete relief of pain. Frequent and fatty stools were observed in 19 patients before treatment. At the end of a mean follow-up period of 40 months (range 24–92 months), bowel symptoms improved in nine patients, whereas eight patients experienced no change. In two patients, stools worsened after ESWL. Of the 40 patients who had lost weight before ESWL, 31 reported an increase in weight irrespective of the success of the treatment. Preexisting diabetes mellitus (n = 21) was unchanged or impaired after ESWL, while six patients developed diabetes after treatment. These results confirm earlier findings that the metabolic function of the pancreas is not notably improved after endoscopic therapy for chronic pancreatitis, although weight gain is often observed [123].

Intraductal laser lithotripsy historically has been used very rarely for the management of pancreatic duct stones. Pancreatoscopy (traditionally via a mother–baby scope system) can be used to visualize laser fiber contact with the stone directly, and to aid fragmentation. Craigie et al. [124] reported their experience in 10 patients with pancreatic stones who underwent intraoperative endoscopy with electrohydraulic lithotripsy (EHL). Attempts at endoscopic therapy alone had previously failed in all of them, with an average EHL time of 65 min. The authors concluded that EHL represents a valuable adjunct in the management of patients with chronic pancreatitis and unretrievable ductal stones in the pancreatic head region. However, intraductal maneuverability remains very limited. Preliminary experience with SpyGlass pancreatoscopy (Boston Scientific, Natick, Massachusetts, USA) and EHL, on the other hand, has shown promising results [125]. Using this single-operator system, Chen and colleagues evaluated 17 patients with pancreatic duct stones (16 in the pancreatic head, one in the tail). The mean diameter of the largest stone in each case was 9.4 mm. EHL was attempted in 10 patients and stone clearance was achieved in eight (80%) after a mean of 1.2 sessions. No serious adverse events related to pancreatoscopy were reported.

Stone dissolution via ductal irrigation (contact dissolution) or an oral agent is an attractive endoscopic adjunct for stone removal. Berger et al. [126] carried out nasopancreatic drainage in six patients with main pancreatic duct stones. The pancreatic duct was perfused with a mixture of isotonic citrate and saline at 3 mL/min for 4 days. A stone-free state was achieved in all cases. Pancreatic pain disappeared during the perfusion, and four patients remained free of pain during the follow-up period (1–12 months). The remaining two patients had repeat therapy, which resulted in pain resolution. Pancreatic exocrine function was improved in three of five evaluated patients. Our experience with a similar number of patients is that infusion rates greater than 0.5 mL/min are poorly tolerated. Trimethadione, an epileptic agent and a weak organic acid, has been shown in vitro to induce a concentration-dependent increase in calcium solubility. Noda et al. [127] reported promising results for trimethadione in a dog model of pancreatic stones. Unfortunately, the doses used in dogs could potentially be toxic if extrapolated to humans. At present, no rapidly effective solvent for human use is available to treat pancreatic stones. Further trials are needed to establish a role for medical therapy (either alone or as an aid to endoscopic measures) in treating patients with symptomatic pancreatic duct stones.

Pancreatic Pseudocysts and Fistulas

Pancreatic pseudocysts are defined as encapsulated collections (without an epithelial lining) of pancreatic juice—which may be pure or may contain necrotic debris, or blood, or both—which are situated either outside or within the limits of the pancreas from which they arise. Conventional therapy for symptomatic pancreatic pseudocysts has been primarily surgical. More recently, percutaneous and endoscopic techniques have been used. Patients with pseudocysts who are the best candidates for endoscopic drainage have a single mature cyst (without pancreatic necrosis, residual adjacent inflammation, or portal hypertension) that abuts the stomach or duodenum or remains in continuity with the ductal system. Patients with more complex conditions are generally best managed using a multidisciplinary approach, with input from surgery, medicine, and interventional radiology.

The aim of endoscopic therapy is to create a communication between the pseudocyst and the bowel lumen (**Fig. 52.15**). Two approaches can be applied, depending on whether the cyst communicates with the pancreatic duct [78,128–135]. Cysts communicating with the ductal system can be drained by a transpapillary approach [129,130,133–136]. The proximal tip of the endoprosthesis has generally been placed in the cystic cavity [128]. A pancreatic sphincterotomy may be required. As with all indications for pancreatic duct stenting, the size, length, and shape of the endoprosthesis should be adapted to the anatomy and the diameter of the duct.

Noncommunicating pseudocysts can be treated by direct endoscopic cystoenterostomy via the stomach (cystogastrostomy) or duodenum (cystoduodenostomy), creating a communication between the cystic cavity and the gastric or duodenal lumen. Two prerequisites should be fulfilled before this treatment is attempted: bulging due to the cyst should be obvious during upper endoscopy, and the distance between the cyst and lumen should not exceed 1 cm. This distance can usually be assessed by CT scanning, ultrasound, or endosonography; however, when the compression is visible, the distance between the cyst and the lumen is usually less than 1 cm. The cyst wall should be mature. A double-lumen or triple-lumen beveled-tip needle-knife is used to burrow a hole (usually using blended current) into the cyst cavity. A cystoenterostome is now commercially available [134]. A guide wire is advanced into the cyst and looped 360° to secure positioning. Puncture should be performed perpendicularly to the cyst wall, and a duodenoscope is therefore preferred. The newly created tract is then balloon-dilated to 8–10 mm. Vigorous flow of pseudocyst fluid into the gut lumen generally occurs, and this must be aspirated to maintain the endoscopic view. Two or more double-pigtail plastic stents are then placed, bridging the cyst and intestinal lumen (using pigtail stents prevents inward migration). When significant debris or necrotic tissue is present, a nasocystic drain should be considered to allow for lavage of the cyst cavity. It is appropriate to keep the patient on a nil-by-mouth diet with intravenous broad-spectrum antibiotics for 24–48 h if the cyst is > 6 cm. Diabetics, patients with debris in the cyst, and immunosuppressed patients may need a longer nil-by-mouth interval, as oral intake allows food and a greater concentration of bacteria to enter the residual cyst. The pseudocyst size is followed using ultrasound or CT examinations at intervals of 4–6 weeks. After resolution (usually in 1–2 months), the stents are removed endoscopically and follow-up pancreatography is carried out.

Table 52.11 shows the results with endoscopic management reported by large centers [78,128–131,133,135,136]. Technical success rates are around 90%. Pseudocysts recur in 10–20% of endoscopically managed cases, especially in patients with ductal cut-off on the pancreatogram. These results certainly support the use of

VIII

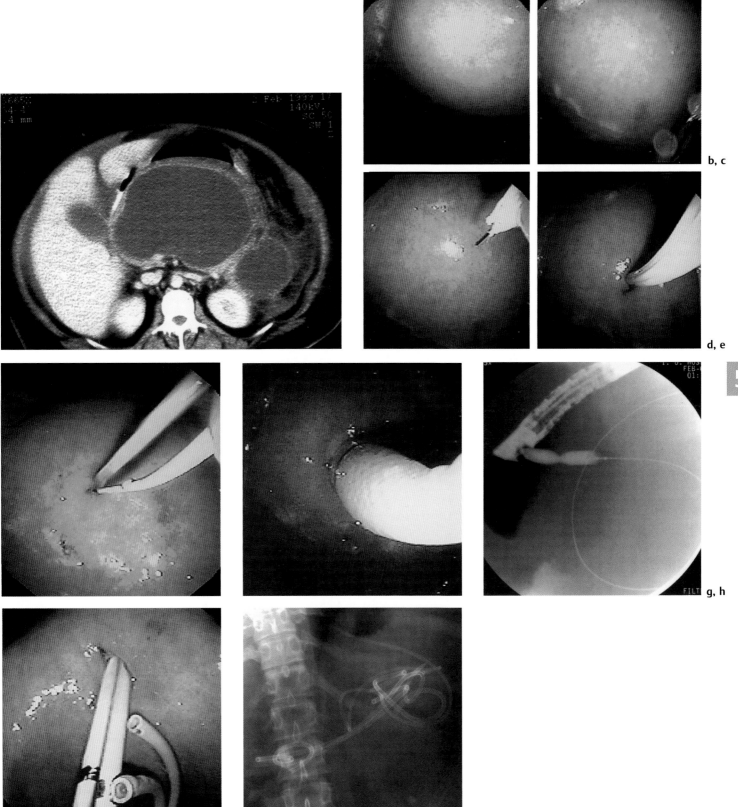

52

Fig. 52.15

a   A large retrogastric pseudocyst causing pressure on the duodenum and stomach.

b, c   The view from the gastric antrum, showing bulging caused by the pseudocyst.

d   The needle-knife is positioned for perpendicular puncture.

e   The 5-Fr catheter of the needle knife has entered the cyst, and a 0.035-inch guide wire has been passed and looped into the cyst.

f   Pancreatic juice is seen exiting from the cyst adjacent to the wire.

g, h   The hydrostatic balloon, with a diameter of 8 mm, is being expanded. The waistline fully resolved with further inflation.

i   Two 7-Fr double-pigtail stents are in place.

j   The final radiograph, with an additional nasocystic drain in place. Despite the presence of some debris in the cyst (not seen on computed tomography), all inflammatory changes and fluid collections resolved during the subsequent 3 months. The nasocystic tube was removed after 10 days, and the stents were removed after 4 months.

Table 52.11 Results of endoscopic therapy for pseudocysts

First author, year (ref.)	Technical success	Transpapillary (n)	Cystogastrostomy (n)	Cystoduode- nostomy (n)	Complications (n)	Deaths (n)
Grimm (1989) [78]	14/16	5	1	8	5	1
Cremer (1989) [131]	32/33	0	11	21	3	0
Kozarek (1991) [133]	12/14	12	0	0	5	0
Sahel (1991) [128]	58/67*	26	1	31	9	1
Catalano (1995) [130]	17/21	17	0	9	1	0
Smits (1995) [135]	31/37*	16	8	7	6	0
Binmoeller (1995) [129]	47/53*	31	6	10	6	0
Howell (1995) [136]	100/108	37	38	25	25	0
Total	311/349 (89%)	144	65	102	66 (17%)	2 (1%)

Combination therapy in several.

endoscopic therapy in appropriate candidates. When compared to other endoscopic techniques, this procedure has a relatively high bleeding and perforation rate. Bleeding complications can be reduced by avoiding cyst puncture high along the lesser curvature (the left gastric artery area) and by using a hydrostatic balloon (not a sphincterotome) to enlarge the tract orifice, or by initial puncture with a needle catheter instead of the needle-knife. Nevertheless, the overall complication rate probably compares favorably with that of surgical series. Coordination with the surgeon is necessary when performing this procedure.

Recently, the Virginia group evaluated covered self-expanding metal stents for endoscopic drainage of pseudocysts [137]. In 18 patients, 17 responded successfully, with 14 (78%) achieving complete resolution of the pseudocyst and three (17%) with a decrease in the size of the collection. A prospective randomized study with a cost-effective analysis comparing these metal stents with conventional plastic stents needs to be performed before this technique can be advocated for routine use.

Endoscopic ultrasound has become increasingly used in the evaluation and therapy of pancreatic fluid collections. This endoscopic procedure can: 1, determine whether there is significant solid debris within a collection; 2, differentiate between a pseudocyst and other noninflammatory cystic lesions; 3, guide transmural drainage; and 4, be used to perform the pseudocyst drainage. Because a visible luminal bulge is not required for direct EUS pseudocyst drainage, the number of potential patients available for endoscopic therapy has increased.

Pancreatic duct disruptions or leaks occur as a result of acute or chronic pancreatitis, trauma, or surgical injury and can produce pancreatic ascites, pseudocyst formation, pleural effusions, and cutaneous fistulas. Pancreatic leaks and fistulas can be successfully treated with transpapillary stents. Telford and colleagues [138] reported that 25 of 43 (58%) disruptions resolved with pancreatic stenting, with no recurrences during a 2-year follow-up interval. Bridging the disruption was found on multivariate analysis to be predictive of a successful outcome [138,139]. Endoscopic injection of tissue glue has also been used to close pancreatic fistulas [140].

Disconnected pancreatic duct syndrome is a recognized complication of severe acute pancreatitis. Here, there is viable pancreatic tissue upstream from the site of duct disruption, typically corresponding to a site of pancreatic necrosis. Secretion of pancreatic juice into the retroperitoneal space may therefore serve as a source of ongoing inflammation and pain. While surgery remains the gold standard for management of these patients, the role of endoscopy is being investigated, as noted above. In one study of 31 patients with a disconnected pancreatic duct, 26 underwent initial endoscopic drainage of pancreatic fluid collections and five went directly to surgery [141]. Of the patients treated endoscopically, 19 had long-

term improvement, while endoscopic treatment failed in seven patients, who required surgery. These results suggest that endoscopic therapy may be an option for a selected group of patients. Further study is needed to better define this group and to determine long-term success. Endoscopic therapy has also been used to treat sterile organized necrosis for symptomatic patients [142]. The procedure is more technically difficult, has a higher rate of complications and a lower "cure rate," and tends to occur in more severely ill patients than those with pseudocysts.

Biliary Obstruction in Chronic Pancreatitis

Intrapancreatic common bile duct strictures have been reported to occur in 2.7–45.6% of patients which chronic pancreatitis. Such strictures are the result of a fibrotic inflammatory restriction, or sometimes compression by a pseudocyst. Since long-standing biliary obstruction can lead to secondary biliary cirrhosis or recurrent cholangitis, or both, biliary decompression has been recommended. Surgical therapy has been the traditional approach. However, in view of the excellent outcome (with low morbidity) of endoscopic biliary stenting in postoperative strictures, several studies have evaluated similar techniques for bile duct strictures complicating chronic pancreatitis. In the absence of cholangitis or jaundice, most experts advocate biliary decompression when the alkaline phosphatase is found to be consistently more than twice the upper limit of normal during a 6-month period of observation.

Polyethylene stents. Results of early studies using plastic biliary stents in patients with chronic pancreatitis and distal bile duct strictures were disappointing [143–145]. While cholestasis, jaundice and cholangitis responded to stent placement, only 20–30% of patients had complete clinical recovery (resolution of symptoms), biological recovery (normalization of cholestatic liver tests), and radiological recovery (resolution of biliary stricture and upstream dilation), allowing for removal of the stent with long-term follow-up.

Vitale et al. [146] evaluated 25 patients with distal biliary strictures secondary to chronic pancreatitis. The indications for biliary decompression were jaundice, persistent cholestasis, or cholangitis. Eight patients had concomitant bile duct stones. Four patients (16%) had chronic calcific pancreatitis and four patients had a pancreatic pseudocyst. Endoscopic therapy consisted of biliary sphincterotomy, stricture dilation, and polyethylene stent placement (7–11.5 Fr) in all patients. When necessary, pancreatic sphincterotomy, biliary or pancreatic stone removal, pancreatic stenting, and pseudocyst drainage were also performed. Whenever possible, two biliary stents were placed side by side at follow-up sessions. Stents were exchanged electively at intervals of 3–4 months, with a mean stenting period of 13.3 months (range 3–28 months). All patients achieved prompt relief of jaundice and cholestasis. Mean serum alkaline phosphatase and bilirubin levels decreased from 484 to 161 U/L and from 4.8 to 1.4 mg/dL, respectively, after endoscopic drainage. After a mean follow-up period of 32 months, 20 of the 25 patients remained stent-free, without stricture recurrence. Complications consisted of six episodes of cholangitis and nine episodes of pancreatitis. The authors concluded that endoscopic stenting provides definitive treatment in most of these patients and that it can be regarded as a viable alternative to standard surgical bypass treatment. This study contradicts the findings of the other large series [143–145] noted earlier. The shorter follow-up period, use of double biliary stents, and infrequent calcific pancreatitis in this study (16 % vs. 60–70 % in other series) may account for the discrepancy. The Milwaukee group has also reported better outcomes with multiple stents than with a single stent [147]. In addition, Kiehne et al. [148] found that 12 of 14 patients did not comply with the arranged dates for stent exchange, and were repeatedly admitted on an emergency basis with cholangitis or biliary sepsis.

Self-expanding metal stents. Because of the largely disappointing long-term results with plastic stents, and concern regarding the high morbidity associated with surgically performed biliary drainage procedures in alcoholic patients, the group in Brussels evaluated the use of uncoated expandable metal stents for this indication [149]. Twenty patients were treated using a metal stent 34 mm long that expands to a full diameter of 10 mm. The short length of the stent was chosen so that surgical bypass treatment would still be possible if necessary. Cholestasis (n = 20), jaundice (n = 7), and cholangitis (n = 3) resolved in all patients. Eighteen patients had no further biliary problems during a follow-up period of 33 months (range 24–42 months). Two patients (10 %) developed epithelial hyperplasia within the stent, resulting in recurrent cholestasis in one and jaundice in the other. These patients were treated endoscopically with standard plastic stents, and one of the patients ultimately required surgical drainage. The authors concluded that this therapy could be an effective alternative to surgical biliary diversion, but longer follow-up periods and controlled trials will be necessary to confirm these results. Trials of membrane-coated metal stents and removable coil-spring stents are underway.

▪ Autoimmune Pancreatitis

Autoimmune pancreatitis (AIP) is a unique form of chronic pancreatitis characterized by swelling of the gland, irregular narrowing of the pancreatic duct, and lymphoplasmacytic infiltration of the pancreas. Much of the early experience with this disease was in Asia, with prevalence estimates of AIP in patients with chronic pancreatitis reaching 5 %. It is now recognized as a worldwide disease, however, and the Mayo Clinic group recently identified AIP in 27 of 254 patients (11.0 %) with chronic pancreatitis [150]. While AIP is characterized by a dramatic response to steroid therapy, endoscopists need to be aware of the condition, as up to 70 % of patients present with obstructive jaundice leading to evaluation with ERCP. Computed tomography scans may demonstrate a diffusely enlarged pancreas ("sausage-shaped") or a pancreatic mass (**Fig. 52.16 c, d**). When ERCP is performed, a diffusely narrowed pancreatic duct is often seen, and a distal biliary stricture may reflect pancreatic involvement (**Fig. 52.16 a**). The challenge is to differentiate AIP from pancreatic cancer preoperatively. **Figure 52.16 b** represents a case of AIP with resolution of pancreatic and biliary strictures following steroid therapy. Occasionally, proximal biliary strictures may be seen superior to the pancreas, illustrating the point that AIP is not only confined to the pancreas but may reflect a more widespread,

systemic disease process. The bile duct, kidneys, lungs, thyroid, prostate, retroperitoneum, liver, and gallbladder may also be involved.

Histologically, AIP is characterized by an immunoglobulin G4 (IgG4)-positive lymphoplasmacytic infiltration of the pancreas or other affected organs. Chari and colleagues [151] recently evaluated the role of EUS core biopsy in AIP in 16 patients. While seven of the 16 patients (44 %) had diagnostic histology, 15 (96 %) had diagnostic IgG4 immunostaining. This technique shows promise; however, EUS core biopsy is not widely available and experience to date has been limited to expert centers. Serum IgG4 has been suggested as a reasonable marker of AIP, with a sensitivity approaching 75 % [152]. However, our experience in Indiana [153] has demonstrated a sensitivity of only 13 % (two of 15), suggesting that the IgG4 prevalence may differ among patient populations. Ampullary biopsy at ERCP, on the other hand, does appear to show promise as a simple screening tool for AIP. Using a cut-off of > 10 IgG4 immunostain-positive cells per high-powered field, Kamisawa et al. [154] found a sensitivity of 80 % (eight of 10) in AIP patients, and 0 % (none of 10) in pancreas cancer patients. Endoscopists need to have a heightened awareness to establish an accurate diagnosis of AIP, in an effort to preserve pancreatic function and possibly avoid resective surgery.

▪ Sphincter of Oddi Dysfunction

Although sphincter of Oddi dysfunction (SOD) is a known cause of acute recurrent pancreatitis, its role in the pathogenesis of chronic pancreatitis is much less certain. Studies using modern manometric techniques have shown a high frequency of basal sphincter pressure abnormalities, especially in the pancreatic sphincter, in patients with established chronic pancreatitis [155,156]. A review of pancreatic basal sphincter pressure in 106 patients with ductographic abnormalities showed an elevated basal pressure ≥ 40 mmHg in 61 % of cases. Tarnasky and colleagues [157] carried out sphincter of Oddi manometry in 104 consecutive patients with unexplained upper abdominal pain. All of the patients also underwent evaluation for chronic pancreatitis using pancreatic ductography, endoscopic ultrasonography, and assessment of the pancreatic fluid bicarbonate concentration. Patients with SOD were four times more likely (odds ratio 4.6; P = 0.01) to meet the criteria for chronic pancreatitis than those patients with normal sphincter of Oddi manometry. Of the 68 patients with SOD, 20 (29 %) had evidence of chronic pancreatitis. Twenty of 23 patients (87 %) with chronic pancreatitis had abnormal sphincter of Oddi manometry. However, it is not known whether the sphincter at times becomes dysfunctional as part of the overall general scarring process, or whether it has a role in the pathogenesis of chronic pancreatitis. Longitudinal follow-up is required.

The surgical literature, although limited, suggests that in chronic pancreatitis patients with documented or suspected sphincter of Oddi dysfunction, ablation alone of both the biliary and pancreatic sphincters benefits 30–60 % of those affected [158,159]. Bagley et al. [159] reported a surgical series of 67 patients with mild to moderate chronic pancreatitis who underwent empirical biliary and pancreatic sphincterotomy (n = 33) or sphincteroplasty (n = 34). During a 5-year follow-up period, 44 % of the patients had pain relief. The outcome for patients with idiopathic chronic pancreatitis was similar to that in patients with alcohol-induced chronic pancreatitis. However, 11 of 12 patients (92 %) who stopped alcohol consumption showed clinical improvement, in comparison with two of 16 patients (12.5 %) who continued to drink. Since endoscopic pancreatic sphincterotomy has only recently been performed with increasing frequency, its role in the management of pancreatic sphincter stenosis has not been clearly defined. The value of endoscopic sphincter ablation as the only therapy in patients with chronic pancreatitis awaits further study, preferably in randomized controlled trials.

52

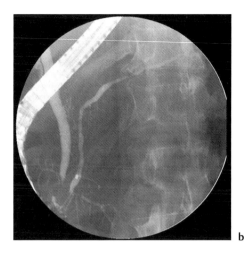

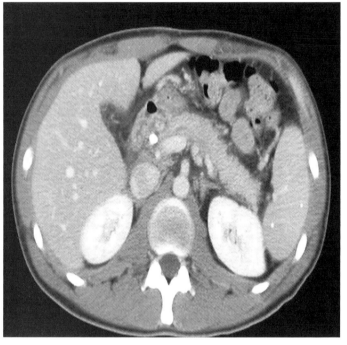

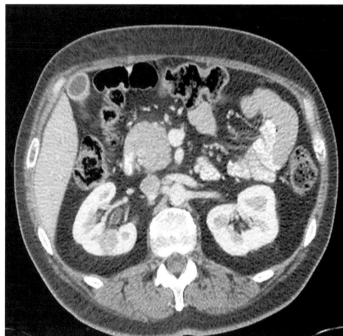

Fig. 52.16
a Biliary and pancreatic duct strictures in a patient with autoimmune pancreatitis.
b Virtual resolution of the strictures in the same patient following a course of steroid therapy.

c Computed tomography demonstrating the classic "sausage" pancreas seen in autoimmune pancreatitis.
d Computed tomography showing a mass in the head of the pancreas, worrisome for tumor, which turned out to be autoimmune pancreatitis.

Pancreatic Neoplasms

Routine ductal origin carcinomas account for more than 90% of pancreatic neoplasms. These lesions are discussed elsewhere in this volume in the sections on ERCP, stenting, endoscopic ultrasound, and tissue sampling (Chapters 15, 20, 22, and 35). This section therefore focuses on less frequent pancreatic neoplasms, with the emphasis on mucin-producing neoplasms, as these are the ones that are most clinically relevant.

Mucin-producing and cystic pancreatic neoplasms (**Fig. 52.17**) have been increasingly recognized in the last decade. Such lesions are more common among Asians, but are seen worldwide. **Table 52.12** shows the categorization of these lesions. Recent classifications [160,161] of cystic neoplasms have made mucinous cyst adenoma/carcinoma into a category separate from intraductal papillary mucin-producing tumors, previously known as mucinous duct ectasia. Current evidence supports the view that mucin-producing neoplasms that cause ductal dilation belong to the same family of lesions that cause frankly cystic lesions. The latter appear to involve occlusion of smaller ducts and perhaps thicker mucus, which therefore form cystic lesions. Combinations of dilated ducts and cysts are common. The management of such lesions is largely dependent on the clinical probability of associated invasive cancer. The majority of patients affected present with pancreatitis and pancreatic-type pain. Steatorrhea, diabetes, and weight loss are predominant in a minority of patients. A few asymptomatic lesions are found in studies such as chest CT scanning (with upper abdominal views included).

Noninvasive imaging is essential in such lesions, as nearly all patients will have a dilated pancreatic ductal system or cystic lesions. The cysts may be small (a few millimeters) or large (10–15 cm). The presence of septa within a cyst, or the absence of a history of pancreatitis or pancreatic trauma, increases the concern regarding neoplasm (versus pseudocyst). The clinician should remember that approximately 10% of cystic lesions are cystic neoplasms.

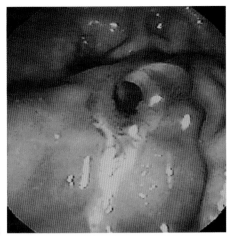

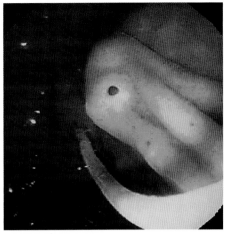

b

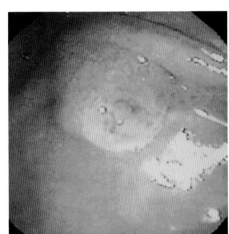

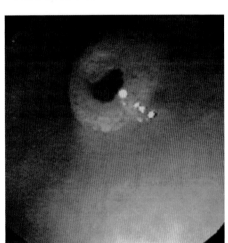

d

Fig. 52.17 Endoscopic views of mucus-secreting pancreatic tumors.
a Mucus exiting a patulous major papilla pancreatic orifice.
b Mucus exiting the minor papilla; there is a catheter in the major papilla.
c A normal major papilla (with closed orifice).
d The same patient and major papilla as in **c**, with a patulous orifice during mucus flow. Approximately one-third of mucus tumors have an intermittently open orifice.

ERCP recognition of cystic neoplasms is critical for appropriate management of the lesions (**Fig. 52.18**). Mucin-producing neoplasms of the pancreas are benign in their early phases, but must be regarded as similar to villous adenomas of the colon–i.e., as having a high malignant potential with increasing age and size. ERCP diagnosis starts with recognition of a patulous pancreatic orifice with mucus exiting. This is seen as gross dilation of the ampullary orifice in about half of such cases. This type of dilation may be intermittent, and observation of the papilla for a few minutes is recommended in questionable cases. Ductography should be performed slowly, and multiple early films should be taken to look for filling defects within the partially contrast-filled duct. Excessively rapid injection will flush mucus in the head of the gland back to the tail, causing mucus to be diluted in the contrast so that it disappears radiologically. Attention should be paid to small filling defects, and juice aspirated from the duct should be analyzed for mucus, goblet cells, cellular atypia, and tumor markers. The role of ERCP is to identify the mucus in the duct, to allow juice to be aspirated for neoplastic evaluation, and to assess the region of the lesion in relation to the area of the pancreas that will likely require resection. Usually, a combination of CT and ductography will show the area of maximal ductal dilation and cyst formation. Lesions in the pancreatic head will commonly leave the tail normal, and a Whipple's resection will be adequate. Lesions in the tail will commonly have less dilation of the main duct of the head, and an upstream hemipancreatectomy will be adequate. Intraoperative evaluation of frozen sections from the surgical margin is recommended. Preoperative or intraoperative pancreatoscopy may be of value. Despite their premalignant potential, not all mucin-producing cystic neoplasms need to be resected. Such lesions grow quite

Table 52.12 Cystic neoplasms of the pancreas, in approximate order of frequency

Mucin-producing cystic tumor	Intraductal papillary mucinous tumor Cystadenocarcinoma
Adenocarcinoma of ductal origin	With necrosis that appears cyst-like
Serous cystadenoma	Microcystic and macrocystic
Lymphoma/sarcoma	With necrosis that appears cyst-like
Islet-cell tumors	Cystic variant
Solid pseudopapillary tumor	
Miscellaneous	Cystic teratoma Acinar-cell cystadenocarcinoma Lymphangioma Hemangioendothelioma Numerous other very rare lesions

slowly, and elderly patients with a significant surgical risk can receive observation alone; many such lesions go 5–15 years before frankly invasive pancreatic carcinoma develops.

A variety of other cystic lesions of the pancreas may be encountered initially on CT or ERCP (**Fig. 52.19**). Most other cystic lesions of the pancreas do not communicate with the ductal system and are identified by displacement or obstruction of the pancreatic ductal system. Many other lesions have a low malignant potential and can generally be observed unless the overall clinical suspicion for neoplasm remains high. Lesions with mixed solid and cystic components have a high malignant potential (mucinous cystadenocarcinoma, cystic islet cell tumors, necrotic pancreatic ductal origin

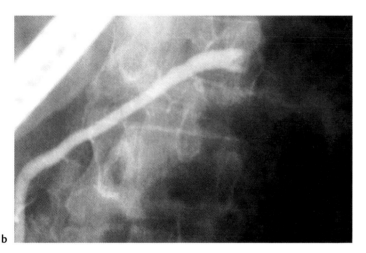

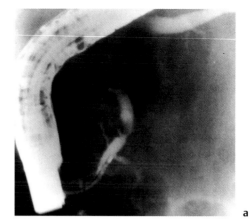

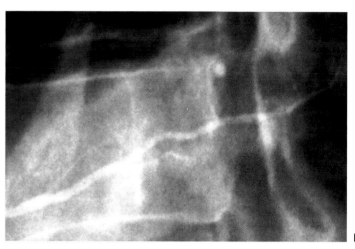

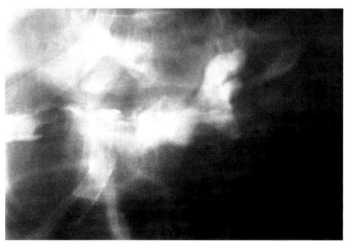

Fig. 52.18

a A cystic lesion in the tail of the pancreas in a 52-year-old man who had had two episodes of acute pancreatitis. The cyst is connected with the downstream duct; this represents mucus entering the duct.

b The endoscopic retrograde cholangiopancreatogram (ERCP) shows a dilated main duct in the pancreatic tail, with a cut-off caused by a mucus plug.

c After the catheter has been advanced into the cyst (to aspirate mucus for cytology), a further contrast injection shows puddling of dye in the cyst. The resected specimen was found to be a mucinous cystadenocarcinoma, with no spread outside the pancreas. There was no evidence of recurrence on follow-up computed tomography and ERCP examinations after 4 years.

Fig. 52.19

a A focal collection of mucus in the main duct in the pancreatic head. Care must be taken during pancreatography to look for mucus filling defects in the early filling phase of films, to ensure that the mucus is not "washed away" to the tail and missed. The resected specimen was found to be an intraductal papillary mucin-producing tumor, with focal adenocarcinoma.

b A 47-year-old woman with recurrent pancreatitis. Endoscopic retrograde cholangiopancreatography was normal, and a trace of linear filling defect was evident on the main duct of the pancreatic body only in retrospect.

c Six years later, there is obvious cast-like mucus present in the main duct of the pancreatic body and tail.

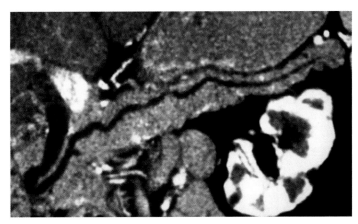

Fig. 52.20 Computed tomography of a normal pancreas and terminal common bile duct. The reconstruction is curvilinear, allowing a single-slice view of the entire pancreas.

carcinomas). A detailed discussion of each of the other cystic lesions of the pancreas is beyond the scope of this chapter.

Conclusions

There has been substantial progress in endoscopic techniques in the field of pancreatic disease during the last 20 years, but many pancreatic diseases remain poorly controlled and treated. Continued improvements in endoscopes and endoscopic accessories can be expected. Scientific studies will further define the precise roles of endoscopic, surgical, medical, and other forms of treatment. We are optimistic that patient management will continue to improve and that noninvasive imaging techniques—particularly MRCP and CT (**Fig. 52.20**)—will continue to make further advances.

References

1. Lai R, Freeman ML, Cass OW, Mallery S. Accurate diagnosis of pancreas divisum by linear-array endoscopic ultrasonography. Endoscopy 2004;36:705–9.
2. Savides TJ, Gress FG, Zaidi SA, Ikenberry SO, Hawes RH. Detection of embryologic ventral pancreatic parenchyma with endoscopic ultrasound. Gastrointest Endosc 1996;43:14–9.
3. Fogel EL, Toth TG, Lehman GA, DiMagno MJ, DiMagno EP. Does endoscopic therapy favorably affect the outcome of patients who have recurrent acute pancreatitis and pancreas divisum? Pancreas 2007;34:21–45.
4. Warshaw AL, Simeone JF, Schapiro RH, Flavin-Warshaw B. Evaluation and treatment of dominant dorsal duct syndrome: pancreas divisum redefined. Am J Surg 1990;159:59–66.
5. Grech P, Jowell P, Cotton PB. Isolated ventral chronic calcific pancreatitis in pancreas divisum. Gastrointest Endosc 1992;38:715–8.
6. Saltzberg DM, Schreiber JB, Smith K, Cameron JL. Isolated ventral pancreatitis in a patient with pancreas divisum. Am J Gastroenterol 1990;85:1407–10.
7. Devereaux BM, Lehman GA, Fein S, Phillips S, Fogel EL, Sherman S. Facilitation of pancreatic duct cannulation using a new synthetic porcine secretin. Am J Gastroenterol 2002;97:2279–81.
8. Wehrmann T, Schmitt T, Seifert H. Endoscopic botulinum toxin injection into the minor papilla for treatment of idiopathic recurrent pancreatitis in patients with pancreas divisum. Gastrointest Endosc 1999;50:545–7.
9. Zeman RK, McVay LV, Silverman PM, Cattau EL, Benjamin SB, Fleischer DF, et al. Pancreas divisum: thin-section CT. Radiology 1988;169:395–8.
10. Tulassay Z, Jakab Z, Vadsz A, Keleman E, Gupta R. Secretin provocation ultrasonography in the diagnosis of papillary obstruction in pancreas divisum. Gastroenterol J 1991;51:47–50.
11. Warshaw AL, Compton CC, Lewandrowski K, Cardenosa G, Mueller PR. Cystic tumors of the pancreas: new clinical, radiologic, and pathologic observations in 67 patients. Ann Surg 1990;212:432–5.
12. Eisen G, Schutz S, Metzler D, Baillie J, Cotton PB. Santorinicele: new evidence for obstruction in pancreas divisum. Gastrointest Endosc 1994;40:73–6.
13. Staritz M, Meyer zum Buschenfelde KH. Elevated pressure in the dorsal part of pancreas divisum: the cause of chronic pancreatitis? Pancreas 1988;3:108–10.
14. Wagner CW, Golladay ES. Pancreas divisum and pancreatitis in children. Am Surg 1988;54:22–6.
15. Madura JA, Fiore AC, O'Connor KW, Lehman GA, McCammon RL. Pancreas divisum: detection and management. Am Surg 1985;51:353–7.
16. Madura JA. Pancreas divisum: stenosis of the dorsally dominant pancreatic duct. Am J Surg 1986:151:742–5.
17. Madura JA, Canal DF, Lehman GA. Wall stent-enhanced lateral pancreaticojejunostomy for small-duct pancreatitis. Arch Surg 2003;138:644–9.
18. Ahmad SA, Lowy AM, Wray CJ, D'Alessio D, Choe KA, James LE, et al. Factors associated with insulin and narcotic independence after islet autotransplantation in patients with severe chronic pancreatitis. J Am Coll Surg 2005;201:680–7.
19. Clayton HA, Davies JE, Pollard CA, White SA, Musto PP, Dennison AR. Pancreatectomy with islet autotransplantation for the treatment of severe chronic pancreatitis: the first 40 patients at the Leicester General Hospital. Transplantation 2003;76:92–8.
20. Rodriguez Rilo HL, Ahmad SA, D'Alessio D, Iwanaga Y, Kim J, Choe KA, et al. Total pancreatectomy and autologous islet cell transplantation as a means to treat severe chronic pancreatitis. J Gastrointest Surg 2003;7:978–89.
21. Bellin MD, Carlson AM, Kobayashi T, Gruessner AC, Hering BJ, Moran A, et al. Outcome after pancreatectomy and islet autotransplantation in a pediatric population. J Pediatr Gastroenterol Nutr 2008:47:37–44.
22. Sutherland DER, Gruessner RWG, Jie T. Pancreatic islet autotransplantation for chronic pancreatitis. Clin Transplant 2004;18(Suppl 13):17.
23. Alexakis N, Connor S, Ghaneh P, Raraty M, Lombard M, Smart H, et al. Influence of opioid use on surgical and long-term outcome after resection for chronic pancreatitis. Surgery 2004;136:600–8.
24. Lans JI, Geenen JE, Johanson JF, Hogan WJ. Endoscopic therapy in patients with pancreas divisum and acute pancreatitis: a prospective, randomized, controlled clinical trial. Gastrointest Endosc 1992;38:430–4.
25. Ertan A. Long term results after endoscopic pancreatic stent placement without pancreatic papillotomy in acute recurrent pancreatitis due to pancreas divisum. Gastrointest Endosc 2000;52:9–14.
26. Kozarek RA. Pancreatic stents can induce ductal changes consistent with chronic pancreatitis. Gastrointest Endosc 1990;36:93–5.
27. Smith MT, Sherman S, Ikenberry SO, Hawes RH, Lehman GA. Alterations in pancreatic ductal morphology following polyethylene pancreatic duct stenting. Gastrointest Endosc 1996;44:268–75.
28. Sherman S, Alvarez C, Robert M, Ashley SW, Reber HA, Lehman GA. Polyethylene pancreatic duct stent-induced changes in the normal dog pancreas. Gastrointest Endosc 1993;39:658–64.
29. Boerma D, Huibregtse K, Gulik TM, Rauws EA, Obertop H, Gouma DJ. Long-term outcome of endoscopic stent placement for chronic pancreatitis associated with pancreas divisum. Endoscopy 2000;32:452–6.
30. Cotton PB. Duodenoscopic papillotomy at the minor papilla for recurrent dorsal pancreatitis. Endosc Dig 1978;3:27–8.
31. Coleman SD, Cotton PB. Endoscopic accessory sphincterotomy and stenting in pancreas divisum. Gastrointest Endosc 1993;39:312.
32. Lehman GA, Sherman S, Nisi R, Hawes RH. Pancreas divisum: results of minor papilla sphincterotomy. Gastrointest Endosc 1993;39:108.
33. Liguory C, Lefebvre JF, Canard JM, Bonnel D, Fritsch J, Etienne JP. [Pancreas divisum: clinical and therapeutic study in man, apropos of 87 cases.] Gastroenterol Clin Biol 1986;10:820–5. French.
34. Kozarek RS, Ball TJ, Brandabur JJ, Raltz SL. Endoscopic approach to pancreas. Dig Dis Sci 1995;40:1974–81.
35. Soehendra N, Kempeneers I, Nam VC, Grimm H. Endoscopic dilatation and papillotomy of the accessory papilla and internal drainage in pancreas divisum. Endoscopy 1986;18:129–32.
36. Russell RCG, Wong NW, Cotton PB. Accessory sphincterotomy (endoscopic and surgical) in patients with pancreas divisum. Br J Surg 1984;71;954–7.
37. Toth TG, Sherman S, Fogel E, Fukushima T, Phillips SD, Lehman GA. Pancreas divisum: efficacy of endoscopic minor papilla therapy of primarily and secondarily treated patients [abstract]. Gastrointest Endosc 2001;53:AB135.
38. Attwell A, Borak G, Hawes R, Cotton P, Romagnuolo J. Endoscopic pancreatic sphincterotomy for pancreas divisum by using needle-knife or standard pull-type technique: safety and reintervention rates. Gastrointest Endosc 2006;64:705–11.

52

39. Rashdan A, Fogel EL, McHenry L, Sherman S, Temkit M, Lehman GA. Improved stent characteristics for prophylaxis of post-ERCP pancreatitis. Clin Gastro Hep 2004;2:322–9.

40. Kwan V, Loh SM, Walsh PR, Williams SJ, Bourke MJ. Minor papilla sphincterotomy for pancreatitis due to pancreas divisum. ANZ J Surg 2008;78:257–61.

41. Chacko LN, Chen YK, Shah RJ. Clinical outcomes and nonendoscopic interventions after minor papilla endotherapy in patients with symptomatic pancreas divisum. Gastrointest Endosc 2008;68:667–73.

42. Sherman S, Hawes R, Nisi R, Bucksot L, Earle D, Lehman GA. Randomized controlled trial of minor papilla sphincterotomy (MiES) in pancreas divisum (Pdiv) patients with pain only. Gastrointest Endosc 1994;40:125P.

43. Lemmel T, Hawes R, Sherman S, Earle D, Lehman GA. Endoscopic evaluation and therapy or recurrent pancreatitis (RP) and pancreatobiliary pain (PBP) in the pediatric population [abstract]. Gastrointest Endosc 1993;39:317A.

44. Lehman GA, O'Connor KW. Coexistence of annular pancreas and pancreas divisum: ERCP diagnosis. Gastrointest Endosc 1985;31:25–8.

45. Fogel EL, Zyromski N, McHenry L, Watkins JL, Schmidt S, Lazzell-Pannell L, et al. Annular pancreas (AP) in the adult: experience at a large pancreatobiliary endoscopy center [abstract]. Gastrointest Endosc 2006;63:308A.

46. Gregg JA. Function and dysfunction of the sphincter of Oddi. In: Jacobson IM, editor. ERCP: diagnosis and therapeutic applications. New York: Elsevier Science; 1989. p.138–70.

47. Lehman GA, Kopecky KK, Rogge JD. Partial pancreatic agenesis combined with pancreas divisum and duodenum reflex. Gastrointest Endosc 1987;33:445–8.

48. Wildling R, Schnedl WJ, Reisinger EC, Schreiber F, Lipp RW, Lederer A, et al. Agenesis of the dorsal pancreas in a woman with diabetes mellitus and in both of her sons. Gastroenterology 1993;104:1182–6.

49. Fatima H, Malcolm M, Sherman S, Fogel EL, McHenry L, Watkins JL, et al. Pancreas divisum: a retrospective review to evaluate the risk of biliary tract neoplasms. Pract Gastroenterol 2007;31:24–34.

50. Zyromski NJ, Sandoval JA, Pitt HA, Ladd AP, Fogel EL, Mattar WE, et al. Annular pancreas: dramatic differences between children an adults. J Am Coll Surg 2008;206:1019–27.

51. Samavedy R, Sherman S, Lehman GA. Endoscopic therapy in anomalous pancreatobiliary duct junction. Gastrointest Endosc 2000;50:623–7.

52. Guelrud M, Morera C, Rodriguez M, Prados JG, Jaen D. Normal and anomalous pancreatobiliary union in children and adolescents. Gastrointest Endosc 1999;50:189–93.

53. Acosta J, Ledesma C. Gallstone migration as a cause of acute pancreatitis. N Engl J Med 1974;290:484–7.

54. Soetikno RM, Carr-Locke DL. Endoscopic management of acute gallstone pancreatitis. Gastrointest Endosc Clin N Am 1998;8:1–12.

55. Neoptolemos JP, Hall AW, Finlay DF, Berry JM, Carr-Locke DL, Fossard DP. The urgent diagnosis of gallstones in acute pancreatitis: a prospective study of three methods. Br J Surg 1984;71:230–3.

56. Chi-Leung L, Lo CM, Chan JKF, Poon RTP, Fan ST. EUS for detection of occult cholelithiasis in patients with idiopathic pancreatitis. Gastrointest Endosc 2000;51:28–32.

57. Tenner S, Dubner H, Steinberg W. Predicting gallstone pancreatitis with laboratory parameters: a meta-analysis. Am J Gastroenterol 1994;89:1863–6.

58. Safrany L, Cotton PB. A preliminary report: urgent duodenoscopic sphincterotomy for acute gallstone pancreatitis. Surgery 1981;89:424–8.

59. Van der Spuy A. Endoscopic sphincterotomy in the management of gallstone pancreatitis. Endoscopy 1981;13:25–6.

60. Neoptolemos JP, London NJ, Carr-Locke DL, London NJ, Bailey IA, James D, et al. Controlled trial of urgent endoscopic retrograde cholangiopancreatography and endoscopic sphincterotomy versus conservative treatment for acute pancreatitis due to gallstones. Lancet 1988;2:979–83.

61. Fan ST, Lai EC, Mok FP, Lo CM, Zheng SS, Wong J. Early treatment of acute biliary pancreatitis by endoscopic papillotomy. N Engl J Med 1993;328:228–32.

62. Folsch U, Nitsche R, Ludtke R, Hilgers RA, Creutzfeld W. Early ERCP and papillotomy versus conventional management in acute biliary pancreatitis. N Engl J Med 1997;336:237–42.

63. Nowak A, Nowakowska-Dulawa E, Marek T, Rybicka J. Final results of the prospective, randomized, controlled study on endoscopic sphincterotomy versus conventional management in acute biliary pancreatitis [abstract]. Gastroenterology 1995;108:380A.

64. Baillie J. Treatment of acute biliary pancreatitis. N Engl J Med 1997;336:286–7.

65. Sharma VK, Howden CW. Meta-analysis of randomized controlled trials of endoscopic retrograde cholangiography and endoscopic sphincterotomy for the treatment of acute biliary pancreatitis. Am J Gastroenterol 1999;94:3211–4.

66. Oría A, Cimmino D, Ocampo C, Silva W, Kohan G, Zandalazini H, et al. Early endoscopic intervention versus early conservative management in patients with acute gallstone pancreatitis and biliopancreatic obstruction: a randomized clinical trial. Ann Surg 2007;245:10–7.

67. Ros E, Navarro S, Bru C, Garcia-Pugés A, Valderrama R. Occult microlithiasis in "idiopathic" acute pancreatitis: prevention of relapse by cholecystectomy or ursodeoxycholic acid therapy. Gastroenterology 1991;101:1701–9.

68. Eversman D, Fogel E, Rusche M, Sherman S, Lehman G. Frequency of abnormal pancreatic and biliary sphincter manometry compared with clinical suspicion of sphincter of Oddi dysfunction. Gastrointest Endosc 1999;50:637–41.

69. Guelrud M, Plaz J, Mendoza S, Beker B, Rojas A, Rossiter G. Endoscopic treatment in type II pancreatic sphincter dysfunction [abstract]. Gastrointest Endosc 1995;41:A398.

70. Jacob L, Geenen JE, Catalano MF, Geenen DJ. Prevention of pancreatitis in patients with idiopathic recurrent pancreatitis: a prospective nonblinded randomized study using endoscopic stents. Endoscopy 2001;33:559–62.

71. Singh P, Das A, Isenberg G, Wong RC, Sivak MV Jr, Agrawal D, et al. Does prophylactic pancreatic stent placement reduce the risk of post-ERCP acute pancreatitis? A meta-analysis of controlled trials. Gastrointest Endosc 2004;60:544–50.

72. Rerknimitr R, Sherman S, Fogel EL, Bucksot L, Fay P, Shelly LA, et al. Pancreatic duct leaks: results of endoscopic management [abstract]. Gastrointest Endosc 2000;51:AB139.

73. Huibregtse K, Smits ME. Endoscopic management of diseases of the pancreas. Am J Gastroenterol 1994;89(Suppl):566–77.

74. McCarthy J, Geenen JE, Hogan WJ. Preliminary experience with endoscopic stent placement in benign pancreatic disease. Gastrointest Endosc 1988;34:16–8.

75. Cremer M, Devière J, Delhaye M, Baize M, Vandermeeren A. Stenting in severe chronic pancreatitis: results of medium-term follow-up in 76 patients. Endoscopy 1991;23:171–6.

76. Huibregtse K, Schneider B, Vrij AA, Tytgat GN. Endoscopic pancreatic drainage in chronic pancreatitis. Gastrointest Endosc 1988;34:9–15.

77. Kozarek RA, Patterson DJ, Ball TJ, Traverso LW. Endoscopic placement of pancreatic stents and drains in the management of pancreatitis. Ann Surg 1989;209:261–6.

78. Grimm H, Meyer WH, Nam VC, Soehendra N. New modalities for treating chronic pancreatitis. Endoscopy 1994;21:70–4.

79. Kozarek RA, Ball TJ, Patterson DJ, Traverso LW, Raltz S. Endoscopic pancreatic duct sphincterotomy: indications, technique, and analysis of results. Gastrointest Endosc 1994;40:592–8.

80. Binmoeller KF, Jue P, Seifert H, Nam WC, Izbicki J, Soehendra N. Endoscopic pancreatic stent drainage in chronic pancreatitis and a dominant stricture: long-term results. Endoscopy 1995;27:638–44.

81. Ponchon T, Bory RM, Hedelius F, Roubein LD, Paliard P, Napoleon B, et al. Endoscopic stenting for pain relief in chronic pancreatitis: results of a standardized protocol. Gastrointest Endosc 1995;42:452–6.

82. Smits ME, Badiga SM, Rauws EAJ, Tytgat GN, Huibregtse K. Long-term results of pancreatic stents in chronic pancreatitis. Gastrointest Endosc 1995;42:461–7.

83. Ikenberry SO, Sherman S, Hawes RH, Smith M, Lehman GA. The occlusion rate of pancreatic stents. Gastrointest Endosc 1994;40:611–3.

84. Wilcox CM. Endoscopic therapy for pain in chronic pancreatitis: is it time for the naysayers to throw in the towel? [Editorial]. Gastrointest Endosc 2005;61:582–6.

85. Binmoeller KF, Rathod VD, Soehendra N. Endoscopic therapy of pancreatic strictures. Gastrointest Endosc Clin N Am 1998;8:125–42.

86. Gabbrielli A, Pandolfi M, Mutignani M, Spada C, Perri V, Petruzziello L, et al. Efficacy of main pancreatic duct endoscopic drainage in patients with chronic pancreatitis, continuous pain, and dilated duct. Gastrointest Endosc 2005;61:576–81.

87. Rösch T, Daniel S, Scholz M, Huibregtse K, Smits M, Schneider T, et al. Endoscopic treatment of chronic pancreatitis: a multicenter study of 1000 patients with long-term follow-up. Endoscopy 2002;34:765–71.

88. McHenry L, Gore DC, DeMaria EJ, Zfass AM. Endoscopic treatment of dilated-duct chronic pancreatitis with pancreatic stents: preliminary results of a sham-controlled, blinded, crossover trial to predict surgical outcome [abstract]. Am J Gastroenterol 1993;88:1536A.

89. Duvall GA, Schneider DM, Kortan P, Haber GB. Is the outcome of endoscopic therapy of chronic pancreatitis predictive of surgical success? [abstract] Gastrointest Endosc 1996;43:405A.

VIII

90. Ammann RW, Akovbiantz A, Larglader F, Scheuler G. Course and outcome of chronic pancreatitis: longitudinal study of a mixed medical–surgical series of 245 patients. Gastroenterology 1984:86:820–8.

91. Costamagna G, Bulajic M, Tringali A, Pandolfi M, Gabbrielli A, Spada C, et al. Multiple stenting of refractory pancreatic duct strictures in severe chronic pancreatitis: long-term results. Endoscopy 2006;38:254–9.

92. Díte P, Ruzicka M, Zboril V, Novotný I. A prospective, randomized trial comparing endoscopic and surgical therapy for chronic pancreatitis. Endoscopy 2003;35:553–8.

93. Cahen DL, Gouma DJ, Nio Y, Rauws EA, Boermeester MA, Busch OR, et al. Endoscopic versus surgical drainage of the pancreatic duct in chronic pancreatitis. N Engl J Med 2007;356:676–84.

94. Tessier G, Bories E, Arvanitakis M, Hittelet A, Pesenti C, Le Moine O, et al. EUS-guided pancreatogastrostomy and pancreatobulbostomy for the treatment of pain in patients with pancreatic ductal dilatation inaccessible for transpapillary endoscopic therapy. Gastrointest Endosc 2007;65: 233–41.

95. Simmons DT, Baron TH, LeRoy A, Petersen BT. Percutaneous pancreatography for treatment of complicated pancreatic duct strictures. Pancreatology 2008;8:194–8.

96. Siegel J, Veerappan A. Endoscopic management of pancreatic disorders: potential risks of pancreatic prosthesis. Endoscopy 1991;23:177–80.

97. Derfus GA, Geenen JE, Hogan WJ. Effect of endoscopic pancreatic duct stent placement on pancreatic ductal morphology [abstract]. Gastrointest Endosc 1990;36:206A.

98. Rossos PG, Kortan P, Haber GB. Complications associated with pancreatic duct stenting [abstract]. Gastrointest Endosc 1992;38:252A.

99. Burdick JS, Geenen JE, Venu RP, Schmalz MJ, Johnson GK, Shakoor T, et al. Ductal morphological changes due to pancreatic stent therapy: a randomized controlled study [abstract]. Am J Gastroenterol 1992;87:155A.

100. Eisen G, Coleman S, Troughton A, Cotton PB. Morphological changes of the pancreatic duct after stent placement for benign disease [abstract]. Gastrointest Endosc 1994;40:107A.

101. Sherman S, Hawes RH, Savides TJ, Gress FJ, Ikenberry SO, Smith MT, et al. Stent-induced pancreatic ductal and parenchymal changes: correlation of endoscopic ultrasound with ERCP. Gastrointest Endosc 1996;44:276–82.

102. Schneider MU, Lux G. Floating pancreatic duct concrements in chronic pancreatitis. Endoscopy 1987;17:8–10.

103. Delhaye M, Vandermeeren A, Baize M, Cremer M. Extracorporeal shockwave lithotripsy of pancreatic calculi. Gastroenterology 1992;102: 610–20.

104. Ponsky JL, Duppler DW. Endoscopic sphincterotomy and removal of pancreatic duct stones. Am Surg 1987;53:613–6.

105. Fuji T, Amano H, Harima K, Aibe T, Asagami F, Kinukawa K, et al. Pancreatic sphincterotomy and pancreatic endoprosthesis. Endoscopy 1985;17: 69–72.

106. Sauerbruch T, Holl J, Sackman M, Paumgartner G. Extracorporeal lithotripsy of pancreatic stones in patients with chronic pancreatitis and pain: a prospective follow-up study. Gut 1992;33:613–6.

107. Hansell DT, Gillespie G, Imrie CW. Operative transpapillary extraction of pancreatic calculi. Surg Gynecol Obstet 1986;163:17–20.

108. Kozarek RA, Ball TJ, Patterson DJ. Endoscopic approach to pancreatic duct calculi and obstructive pancreatitis. Am J Gastroenterol 1992;87:600–3.

109. Sherman S, Lehman GA, Hawes RA, Ponich T, Miller LS, Cohen LB, et al. Pancreatic ductal stones: frequency of successful endoscopic removal and improvement of symptoms. Gastrointest Endosc 1991;37:511–7.

110. Neuhaus H. Fragmentation of pancreatic stones by ESWL. Endoscopy 1991;23:161–5.

111. Smits ME, Rauws EA, Tytgat GNJ, Huibregtse K. Endoscopic treatment of pancreatic stones in patients with chronic pancreatitis. Gastrointest Endosc 1996;23:161–5.

112. Cremer M, Devière J, Delhaye M, Vandermeeren A, Baize M. Endoscopic management of chronic pancreatitis. Acta Gastroenterol Belg 1993;56: 192–200.

113. Delhaye M, Cremer M. Clinical significance of pancreas divisum. Acta Gastroenterol Belg 1992;55:59–66.

114. Adamek HE, Jakobs R, Buttman A, Adamek MU, Schneider ARJ, Riemann JF. Long term follow-up of patients with chronic pancreatitis and pancreatic stones treated with extracorporeal shock-wave lithotripsy. Gut 1999;45:402–5.

115. Schneider HT, May A, Benninger J, Rabenstein T, Hahn EG, Katalinic A, et al. Piezoelectric shock wave lithotripsy of pancreatic duct stones. Am J Gastroenterol 1994;89:2042–8.

116. Sherman S, Rahaman S, Gottlieb K, Hawes R, Smith M, Kopecky K, et al. Lithotripsy in the management of pancreatic duct (PD) stones [abstract]. Gastrointest Endosc 1995;41:429A.

117. Soehendra N, Grimm H, Meyer HW, Schreiber HW. [Extracorporeal shock-wave lithotripsy in chronic pancreatitis]. Dtsch Med Wochenschr 1989;114:1402–6. German.

118. Van der Hul R, Plaiser P, Jeekel J, Terpstra O, den Toom R, Bruining H. Extracorporeal shock-wave lithotripsy of pancreatic duct stones: immediate and long-term results. Endoscopy 1994;26:573–8.

119. Costamagna G, Gabbrielli A, Mutignani M, Perri V, Pandolfi M, Boscaini M, et al. Extracorporeal shock-wave lithotripsy of pancreatic stones in chronic pancreatitis: immediate and medium-term results. Gastrointest Endosc 1997;46:231–6.

120. Guda NM, Partington S, Freeman ML. Extracorporeal shockwave lithotripsy in the management of chronic calcific pancreatitis: a meta-analysis. J Pancreas 1005;6:6–12.

121. Brand B, Kahl M, Sidhu S, Nam VC, Sriram PV, Jaeckle S, et al. Prospective evaluation of morphology, function, and quality of life after extracorporeal shockwave lithotripsy and endoscopic treatment of chronic calcific pancreatitis. Am J Gastroenterol 2000;95:3428–38.

122. Delhaye M, Arvanitakis M, Verset G, Cremer M, Devière J. Long-term clinical outcome after endoscopic pancreatic ductal drainage for patients with painful chronic pancreatitis. Clin Gastroenterol Hepatol 2004;2: 1096–106.

123. Von Tirpitz C, Glasbrenner B, Mayer D, Malfertheiner P, Adler G. Comparison of different endocrine stimulation tests in nondiabetic patients with chronic pancreatitis. Hepatogastroenterology 1998;45:1111–6.

124. Craigie JE, Adams DB, Byme TK, Tagge EP, Tarnasky PR, Cunningham JT, et al. Endoscopic electrohydraulic lithotripsy in the management of pancreatobiliary lithiasis. Surg Endosc 1998;12:405–8.

125. Chen YK, Tarnasky PR, Raijman I. Peroral pancreatoscopy (PP) for pancreatic stone therapy and investigation of suspected pancreatic lesions—first human experience using the SpyGlass direct visualization system (SDVS) [abstract]. Gastrointest Endosc 2008;67:AB108.

126. Berger Z, Topa L, Takacs T, Pap A. Nasopancreatic drainage for chronic calcifying pancreatitis (CCP) [abstract]. Digestion 1992;52:70A.

127. Noda A, Shibata T, Ogawa Y, Hayakawa T, Kameya S, Hiramatsu E, et al. Dissolution of pancreatic stones by oral trimethadione in a dog experimental model. Gastroenterology 1996;43:1002–8.

128. Sahel J. Endoscopic drainage of pancreatic cysts. Endoscopy 1991;23: 181–4.

129. Binmoeller KF, Seifert H, Walter A, Soehendra N. Transpapillary and transmural drainage of pancreatic pseudocysts. Gastrointest Endosc 1995;42:219–24.

130. Catalano MF, Geenen JE, Schmalz MJ, Johnson GK, Dean RS, Hogan WJ. Treatment of pancreatic pseudocysts with ductal communication by transpapillary pancreatic duct endoprosthesis. Gastrointest Endosc 1995;42:219–24.

131. Cremer M, Devière J, Engelholm L. Endoscopic management of cysts and pseudocysts in chronic pancreatitis: long-term follow-up after 7 years of experience. Gastrointest Endosc 1989;35:1–9.

132. Elton E, Howell DA, Lehman GA, Baron TH, Sherman S, Qaseem T, et al. Acute vs. chronic pancreatitis: implications for endoscopic pseudocyst drainage [abstract]. Gastrointest Endosc 1997;45:157A.

133. Kozarek RA, Ball TJ, Patterson DJ, Freemy PC, Ryan JA, Traverso LW. Endoscopic transpapillary therapy for disrupted pancreatic duct and peripancreatic fluid collections. Gastroenterology 1991;100:1362–70.

134. Barthet M, Sahel J, Bodiou B, Bernard JP. Endoscopic transpapillary drainage of pancreatic pseudocysts. Gastrointest Endosc 1995;42:208–13.

135. Smits ME, Rauws EAJ, Tytgat GNJ, Huibregtse K. The efficacy of endoscopic treatment of pancreatic pseudocysts. Gastrointest Endosc 1995;42: 202–7.

136. Howell DA, Baron TH, Lehman GA, Sherman S, Parsons WG, Thaggard EG, et al. Endoscopic drainage of pancreatic pseudocysts in the setting of necrotizing pancreatitis: a multicenter analysis [abstract]. Gastrointest Endosc 1995;41:423A.

137. Talreja JP, Shami VM, Ku J. Endoscopic drainage of pancreatic fluid collections with fully covered metallic stents (CSEMS). How does it compare to conventional drainage with plastic stents? [abstract]. Gastrointest Endosc 2008;67:AB108.

138. Telford JJ, Farrell JJ, Saltzman JR, Shields SJ, Banks PA, Lichtenstein DR, et al. Pancreatic stent placement for duct disruption. Gastrointest Endosc 2002;56:18–24.

139. Varadarajulu S, Noone TC, Tutuian R, Hawes RH, Cotton PB. Predictors of outcome in pancreatic duct disruption managed by endoscopic transpapillary stent placement. Gastrointest Endosc 2005;61:568–75.

140. Seewald S, Brand B, Groth S, Omar S, Mendoza G, Seitz U, et al. Endoscopic sealing of pancreatic fistula by using N-butyl-2-cyanoacrylate. Gastrointest Endosc 2004;59:463–70.

52

141. Pelaez-Luna M, Vege SS, Petersen BT, Chari ST, Clain JE, Levy MJ, et al. Disconnected pancreatic duct syndrome in severe acute pancreatitis: clinical imaging characteristics and outcomes in a cohort of 31 cases. Gastrointest Endosc 2008;68:91–7.

142. Baron TH, Harewood GC, Morgan DE, Yates MR. Outcome differences after endoscopic drainage of pancreatic necrosis, acute pancreatic pseudocysts, and chronic pancreatic pseudocysts. Gastrointest Endosc 2002; 56:7–17.

143. Devière J, Devaere S, Baize M, Cremer M. Endoscopic biliary drainage in chronic pancreatitis. Gastrointest Endosc 1990;36:96–100.

144. Barthet M, Bernard JP, Duval JL, Affiat C, Sahel J. Biliary stenting in benign biliary stenosis complicating chronic calcifying pancreatitis. Endoscopy 1994;26:569–72.

145. Smits ME, Rauws EAJ, van Gulik TM, Gouma DJ, Tytgat GN, Huibregtse K. Long-term results of endoscopic stenting and surgical drainage for biliary stricture due to chronic pancreatitis. Br J Surg 1996;8:764–8.

146. Vitale GC, Reed DN Jr, Nguyen CT. Endoscopic treatment of distal bile duct stricture from chronic pancreatitis. Surg Endosc 2000;14:227–31.

147. Catalano MF, Linder JD, George S, Alcocer E, Geenen JE. Treatment of symptomatic distal common bile duct stenosis secondary to chronic pancreatitis: comparison of single vs. multiple simultaneous stents. Gastrointest Endosc 2004;60:945–52.

148. Kiehne K, Folsch UR, Nitsche R. High complication rate of bile duct stents in patients with chronic alcoholic pancreatitis due to noncompliance. Endoscopy 2000;32:377–80.

149. Devière J, Cremer M, Love J, Sugai B. Management of common bile duct strictures caused by chronic pancreatitis with metal mesh self-expandable stents. Gut 1994;35:122–6.

150. Pearson RK, Longnecker DS, Chari ST, Smyrk TC, Okazaki K, Frulloni L, et al. Controversies in clinical pancreatology: autoimmune pancreatitis: does it exist? Pancreas 2003;27:1–13.

151. Chari ST, Smyrk TC, Levy MJ, Topazian MD, Takahashi N, Zhang L, et al. Diagnosis of autoimmune pancreatitis: the Mayo Clinic experience. Clin Gastroenterol Hepatol 2006;4:1010–6.

152. Ghazale A, Chari ST, Smyrk TC, Levy MJ, Topazian MD, Takahashi N, et al. Value of serum IgG4 in the diagnosis of autoimmune pancreatitis and in distinguishing it from pancreatic cancer. Am J Gastroenterol 2007;102: 1646–53.

153. Moore S, Cummings O, Sandrasegaran K, Al-Haddad M, Dewitt J, Sherman S et al. Autoimmune pancreatitis in the midwest U.S. population: should we rely on elevated IgG4 for establishing the diagnosis? Am J Gastroenterol 2008:103:S 83.

154. Kamisawa T, Tu Y, Egawa N, Tsuruta K, Okamoto A. A new diagnostic tool for autoimmune pancreatitis. Gastrointest Endosc 2008;68:358–61.

155. Vestergaard H, Krause A, Rokkjaer M, Frombert O, Thommesen P, Funch-Jensen P. Endoscopic manometry of the sphincter of Oddi and the pancreatic and biliary ducts in patients with chronic pancreatitis. Scand J Gastroenterol 1994;29:188–92.

156. Ugljesic M, Bulajic M, Milosavljevic T, Stimec B. Endoscopic manometry of the sphincter of Oddi and pancreatic and biliary ducts in patients with chronic pancreatitis. Int J Pancreatol 1996;19:191–5.

157. Tarnasky PR, Hoffman B, Aabakken L, Knapple WL, Coyle W, Pineau B, et al. Sphincter of Oddi dysfunction is associated with chronic pancreatitis. Am J Gastroenterol 1997;92:1125–9.

158. Sherman S, Hawes RH, Madura JA, Lehman GA. Comparison of intraoperative and endoscopic manometry of the sphincter of Oddi. Surg Gynecol Obstet 1992;175:410–8.

159. Bagley FH, Fraasch JW, Taylor RH, Warren RW. Sphincterotomy or sphincteroplasty in the treatment of pathologically mild chronic pancreatitis. Am J Surg 1981;141:418–22.

160. Kloppel G, Solcia E, Longnecker DS, Capella C, Sobin LH. World Health Organization international histological classification of tumours: histological typing of tumors of the endocrine pancreas. 2nd ed. Berlin: Springer, 1996. p.1–6.

161. Solcia E, Capella C, Kloppel G. Tumors of the pancreas. Washington, DC: Armed Forces Institute of Pathology; 1997. p.1–262. (Atlas of tumor pathology, fascicle 20, 3 rd series.)

53 Diseases of the Liver and Peritoneum

H. Juergen Nord

Introduction

Unlike other parts of the intestinal tract, in which the mucosal linings are amenable to direct endoscopic inspection and biopsy through natural body orifices, the abdominal cavity and its organs, such as the liver, spleen, and intestines, are all covered by peritoneum and do not offer themselves readily to endoscopy. Evaluation of the abdominal cavity has therefore primarily relied on serological and imaging studies such as transcutaneous ultrasonography, computed tomography (CT), magnetic resonance imaging (MRI), and imaging-guided biopsy. Direct inspection of the abdominal cavity (laparoscopy) requires a small incision, creation of a pneumoperitoneum to form a space above the viscera, and insertion of a laparoscope. Diagnostic laparoscopy is one of the oldest endoscopic procedures, dating back to the turn of the 20th century. Throughout the decades it has been practiced, primarily by gastroenterologists, as one of the most accurate diagnostic tools, especially when combined with direct-vision biopsy in the evaluation of diffuse and focal liver diseases, as well as peritoneal disorders. However, in recent years there has been an unfortunate decline in diagnostic laparoscopy. Most procedures are now performed by gynecologists and abdominal surgeons for other indications, and very few if any by gastroenterologists and hepatologists.

With the advent of laparoscopic cholecystectomy, surgeons have embraced, expanded, and rediscovered this well-established procedure in a way unparalleled by any other surgical procedure, past and present. While therapeutic applications dominated initially, more and more surgeons are now performing diagnostic laparoscopy either by necessity or by default. However, the main indications for laparoscopy by surgeons are still therapeutic rather than diagnostic.

Possible reasons for the decline in the use of laparoscopy by gastroenterologists include the increasing popularity of noninvasive imaging studies, the popularity of imaging-guided biopsies, and misconceptions about its diagnostic accuracy, safety, and complications of the procedure. With the emergence of natural orifice transluminal endoscopic surgery (NOTES) as a new field of endoscopic surgery and the excitement about its potential, rapidly evolving techniques, and its ultimate position among minimally invasive procedures (see Chapter 23), it is surprising that gastroenterologists rushing to embrace NOTES do not to appear to have shown any interest in diagnostic laparoscopy. Diagnostic laparoscopy is easily performed in the endoscopy suite, and without excessive costs. It is an ideal introduction to peritoneal anatomy and an ideal preparation for NOTES.

The role of laparoscopy in the rapid and accurate evaluation of disorders of the liver, gastrointestinal tract, peritoneum, and pelvic organs is well established, and many well-designed studies have shown that it is superior to other noninvasive imaging studies—especially in focal liver disease, the staging of intra-abdominal malignancies, ascites of unknown cause, and other conditions. Laparoscopy has an excellent safety record and can be performed at low cost, especially when it is conducted in the endoscopy suite using only sedation and analgesia. Unfortunately, advantage is not taken of these significant cost savings by surgeons who perform even simple diagnostic procedures in the operating room, often using general anesthesia. The technical aspects of the procedure are described in Chapter 23.

Diseases of the Liver and Biliary System

▥ Normal Findings

The first view through the endoscope from the classic laparoscopy insertion site, approximately two fingerbreadths to the left of and above the umbilicus, shows the left liver lobe, the falciform ligament, and the right hepatic lobe with the gallbladder (**Fig. 53.1**). The edge of the liver does not extend beyond the right costal margin, which is easily identified. Any caudal extension beyond this suggests hepatomegaly. The hepatic surface is smooth, with a clear and undistorted light reflection. A liver surface with multiple small highlights suggests an irregular, often nodular surface, with possible cirrhosis. The normal liver color is a dark red-brown, and the edge is sharp, frequently with an increased grayish-white thickening of the capsule (**Fig. 53.2**). Increased capsule thickening at the edge of the liver may be confused with fibrosis or cirrhosis. Biopsies should be placed more centrally, and surgical wedge biopsies should be supplemented by a central core needle biopsy.

While the hepatic surface is smooth, a lobular pattern may be identified with close-up inspection, as well as transparent lymphatic vessels (**Fig. 53.3**). A rounded edge always suggests an infiltrative process such as fatty liver or cirrhosis (**Fig. 53.4**), as does spontaneous presentation of the undersurface, which is usually not directly visible. The falciform ligament separating the right and left lobe is stretched in a sail-like fashion, due to the pneumoperitoneum (**Fig. 53.5**). It has a finely reticulated vascular pattern. The round ligament is at its free edge, often with various degrees of fat infiltration. The vessels in the falciform ligament become easily engorged early in portal hypertension, long before esophageal varices and ascites develop.

There are many variants of normal findings. The falciform ligament may have an asymmetrical insertion—e.g., to the left of the

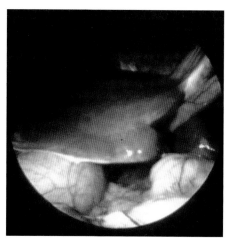

Fig. 53.1 Normal liver and right upper quadrant.

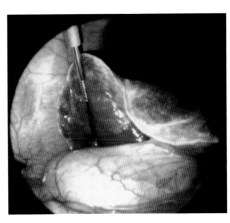

Fig. 53.2 Right upper quadrant with palpating probe, lifting the right lateral lobe. Capsule thickening at the edge of the liver.

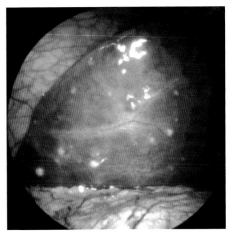

Fig. 53.3 Increased lobular pattern in a patient with mild cholestasis. There is a transparent lymphatic vessel in the foreground. The white nodules represent noncaseating granulomas, in a patient with tuberculous hepatitis.

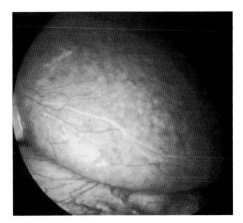

Fig. 53.4 The rounded edge of the left hepatic lobe, with fatty infiltration. There is an increased vascular pattern and a transparent lymphatic vessel in the foreground. The hepatic color is a golden bronze color due to the increased fat content.

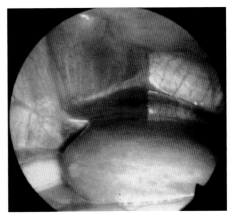

Fig. 53.5 View of the upper mid-abdomen, showing the falciform ligament with a delicate vascular pattern, a smooth left lobe, and the tendineus portion of the diaphragm. There is a small hepatic cyst on the anterior medial aspect of the left liver lobe.

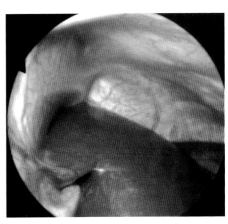

Fig. 53.6 Asymmetrical insertion of the round ligament into the left lobe.

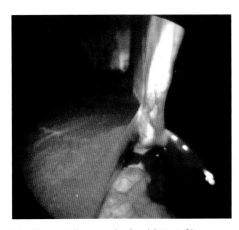

Fig. 53.7 Yellow patch—focal fatty infiltration on the right of the falciform ligament. This has no clinical significance.

midline in the left lobe (**Fig. 53.6**). Focal fatty infiltration, such as a yellow patch either to the right or left of the falciform ligament (**Fig. 53.7**), is observed in 5–10 % of patients. This may be a source of confusion due to the striking difference in color, but it has no pathologic significance and is found in otherwise normal livers. A sagittal groove in the right lobe, caused by an impression of a diaphragmatic fold, is also known as the anomaly of Zahn (**Fig. 53.8**). In older scintigraphic studies, it was often confused with a hepatic filling defect.

The gallbladder has a robin's-egg bluish color, with prominent vascular markings (**Fig. 53.1**). Its insertion at the undersurface of the right hepatic lobe is highly variable and may create a notch at the edge of the liver, of various degrees (**Fig. 53.9**). The normal gallbladder is easily indented with the palpating probe, as is the large atonic gallbladder often found in cirrhosis (**Fig. 53.10**). It has to be differentiated from the distended gallbladder seen in obstructive jaundice (Courvoisier sign), which feels tight and cannot be indented.

▮ Fatty Liver

Fatty infiltration of the liver is a common finding and is frequently the cause of isolated aminotransferase elevations without other abnormalities. Ultrasonography and CT are often strongly suggestive or diagnostic. Since hepatic steatosis is a diffuse process, it can easily be diagnosed by percutaneous liver biopsy and is not an indication for laparoscopy. Fatty liver may have many causes, such as obesity, metabolic syndrome, hyperlipidemia, diabetes mellitus, alcohol (with and without alcoholic hepatitis), drugs, etc. The liver has a golden-yellow color (**Fig. 53.4**). The hepatic architecture is preserved, and the lobular pattern is readily apparent on close-up inspection. The liver is usually enlarged, clearly extending beyond the right costal margin. The edge is no longer sharp, but rounded, and often the hepatic undersurface is spontaneously visible. The yellow color of the liver can easily be demonstrated through a technique called xanthography ("yellow writing") (**Fig. 53.11**). Stroking the palpating probe over the liver surface will temporarily displace blood, leaving the yellow color of the fat-infiltrated paren-

VIII

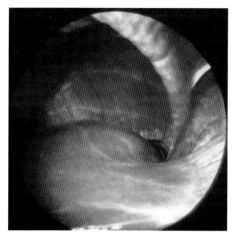

Fig. 53.8 There is a sagittal groove in the dome of the right lobe due, to a longitudinal fold in the diaphragm (Zahn anomaly).

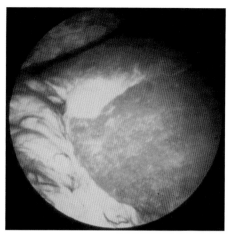

Fig. 53.9 A notch is seen in the anterior edge of the right lobe, due to insertion of the gallbladder.

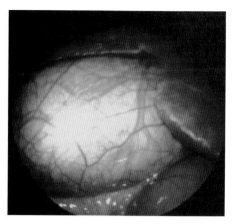

Fig. 53.10 Distended gallbladder in cirrhosis. The gallbladder has the appearance of a robin's egg, with a blue color and vascular markings.

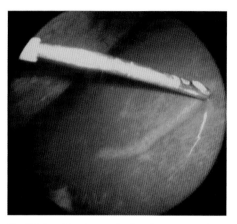

Fig. 53.11 Xanthography ("yellow writing") on a fatty liver, using a palpating probe.

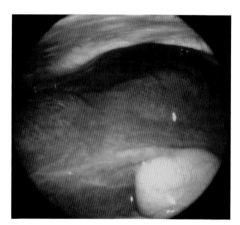

Fig. 53.12 Focal fatty infiltration in a patient with alcohol abuse. This condition may be confused with liver tumor on imaging studies. The undersurface of the liver is spontaneously visible, suggesting infiltration. The former edge is visible in the form of a grayish-white capsule thickening, extending from the gallbladder to the left of the image.

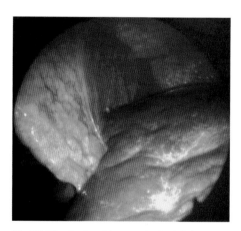

Fig. 53.13 Dystrophic scars in the left hepatic lobe after acute viral hepatitis. Although they are morphologically dramatic, these changes are not usually associated with impaired hepatic function.

chyma behind. The yellow streak will slowly fill in again and blend in with the rest of the liver surface.

In some cases, fat may be focal, similar to the physiologic yellow patch described above. Focal fatty metamorphosis is usually diagnosed with imaging studies and gives rise to confusion, even when an imaging-guided biopsy shows fatty liver—e. g., in a patient with alcohol abuse (**Fig. 53.12**). The question still remains of whether the finding represents a primary or secondary malignancy. Laparoscopy can quickly settle the issue. The different yellow color is characteristic, as is the normal lobular pattern, lack of distorted architecture, and neovascularity. Guided needle biopsies confirm the diagnosis.

Acute and Chronic Hepatitis

With the advent of newer, vastly improved serological facilities in the diagnosis of viral hepatitis, there is no indication for laparoscopy or biopsy in this condition, since patient management would not be affected by the biopsy findings. However, the way in which acute viral hepatitis progresses to chronic hepatitis and cirrhosis was demonstrated by Heinz Kalk, the father of modern laparoscopy,

through systematic and serial laparoscopic examinations and by correlating the clinical, endoscopic, and histologic findings [1,2].

Acute viral hepatitis is rarely if ever an indication for laparoscopy. In the unusual cases in which a biopsy is needed for the differential diagnosis, a percutaneous biopsy is sufficient, or a transjugular biopsy when there are coagulation abnormalities. Since the inflammatory process is diffuse and homogeneous, these methods usually yield a representative morphologic picture. Classic textbooks and atlases of laparoscopy describe hepatomegaly, usually with a rounded edge, marked erythema, and a lobular pattern that is no longer distinguishable [3]. On close inspection, increased lymphatic vessels are seen. The hepatic surface is smooth. The spleen is frequently enlarged, with rounded edges. After resolution of the acute process, there is usually full restitution, with normalization of aminotransferase levels and the laparoscopic picture. An increased lobular pattern suggestive of intralobular fibrosis may be observed. In some patients, significant dystrophic scarring or areas of atrophy may result (**Figs. 53.13, 53.14**) [4]. This may lead to deep, irregular scars, with dramatic-appearing laparoscopic images in which the findings may be confused with cirrhosis. Significant atrophy can result, and a multilobular pattern that can be described as "potato

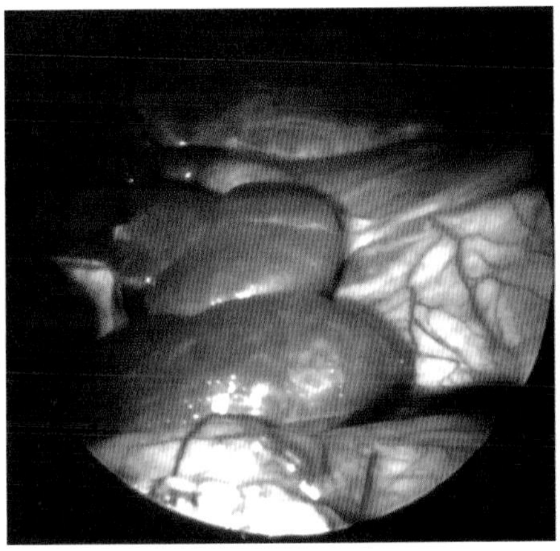

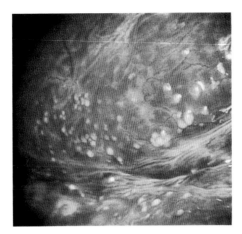

Fig. 53.14 Partial dystrophy resulting in deep scars and pseudolobular formation, known as "potato liver." This finding is not associated with portal hypertension and should not be confused with cirrhosis.

Fig. 53.15 Chronic hepatitis with marked activity, fibrosis, and an increased vascular pattern.

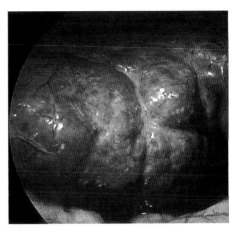

Fig. 53.16 Primary biliary cirrhosis. Map-like darker areas separated by lighter fields are characteristic. There is an increased vascular pattern on the surface.

liver" is seen. Imaging studies can be quite confusing in this setting, and a percutaneous biopsy may be hazardous, since these livers are frequently smaller and irregular, with small pseudolobules. Laparoscopy is the ideal method of evaluating these patients. Hepatic function is usually within normal limits, and these changes do not result in portal hypertension.

Chronic hepatitis. The availability of newer treatments for chronic inflammatory conditions such as chronic hepatitis B and C, autoimmune hepatitis, as well as Wilson disease, hemochromatosis, and primary biliary cirrhosis, makes increased diagnostic accuracy mandatory. It is often assumed that chronic inflammatory changes are diffuse parenchymal processes for which a percutaneous biopsy will be representative. However, blind percutaneous liver biopsies have been shown to be unreliable, since chronic hepatitis can be patchy. The same applies to fibrosis and cirrhosis, often the end stage of chronic hepatitis, which has long been recognized by laparoscopists to be difficult to exclude using a blind needle biopsy [5].

The laparoscopic findings in chronic hepatitis are varied and nonspecific. The surface is frequently irregular and undulating, with a break-up of the light reflex. The color varies from pink to patchy red, reflecting the inflammatory process. On close-up, an increased vascular pattern may be noticeable. White markings represent fibrous changes, and fibrotic bands may be noticeable in more advanced cases (**Figs. 53.15, 53.16**). It is impossible to distinguish endoscopically chronic hepatitis B and C or autoimmune hepatitis. Laparoscopy is only one of various parameters that need to be taken into account, including serology and histology. In alcoholic hepatitis, the above findings are often combined with fatty infiltration, frequently with a transition to fibrosis and ultimately the cobblestone pattern of cirrhosis.

Since chronic hepatitis without cirrhosis is a more diffuse and presumably homogeneous process, one would expect a single biopsy to be representative. However, in 20 of 85 patients (23.5%), Jeffers et al. noted different histological findings in imaging-guided biopsies taken from the right and left lobe [6]. In 35% of these, a different diagnosis was made. In 65%, a different degree of inflammation between the two lobes was noted. In more than half of the cases, the disease was more advanced in one lobe than in the other. The findings were similar in the two lobes in only 5%. The implications of this for the evaluation of new therapeutic agents for chronic hepatitis using a simple follow-up biopsy are significant. These data suggest that conclusions from therapeutic trails using only a single

pretherapy and post-therapy biopsy from a single lobe are unreliable.

It is difficult to identify fibrosis without cirrhosis laparoscopically. Increased firmness to palpation with the palpating probe is not always reliable. There is a subtle transition in the microscopic picture from milder forms of chronic hepatitis to progressive moderate chronic disease ("active" hepatitis), with an increasingly mottled surface appearance due to whitish bands (fibrous bands and inflammatory infiltrates) interspersed with more reddish areas (increased blood vessels, regenerative tissue). With increasing fibrosis, the liver develops an irregular surface with a variegated appearance. This is the result of regenerating tissue and new vessel proliferation, with deposition of whitish fibrous tissue in between. The fibrosis may be so diffuse on the surface as to cause a "sugar coating," giving the appearance of a white liver.

Detection of fibrosis laparoscopically can be improved using intravenous indocyanine green (ICG) [7]. ICG is taken up by the hepatocytes and produces a greenish hue that contrasts with the white to yellow appearance of connective tissue. In a study of 19 patients with histologically confirmed fibrosis, the diagnostic yield was doubled using ICG. ICG staining correlated with the amount of hepatic ligandin in the subcapsular tissue—a binding protein that prevents reflux of ICG into plasma [8].

The superiority of laparoscopy over other imaging studies such as ultrasonography in diffuse liver disease (fatty liver, chronic hepatitis, cirrhosis) was confirmed in a 1997 study by Cardi et al. [9]. The false-negative rates with ultrasound for fatty liver, chronic hepatitis, and cirrhosis were 79%, 33%, and 31%. The specificity was 89% for cirrhosis, but only 72% for chronic hepatitis. Laparoscopy found eight small hepatocellular carcinomas incidentally in 114 cirrhotic patients, while ultrasound detected only one [9]. Unfortunately, the laparoscopic findings in chronic hepatitis C do not allow reliable assessment of the response to interferon therapy [10]. Neither the topographic appearance of the hepatic surface (smooth, granular, or nodular) nor the histology (presence or absence of bridging fibrosis) were found to correlate with the response to therapy. Bridging fibrosis did not correlate well with hepatic surface changes. Sixty-one percent of patients with a smooth liver surface had fibrosis, and 43% of patients without bridging fibrosis had a granular liver.

Cirrhosis and its complications. Chronic liver disease and its end stage, cirrhosis, are still among the main indications for laparoscopy and imaging-guided liver biopsy. The endoscopic findings of cirrhosis are classic and specific, so that a diagnosis can often be made on

VIII

inspection alone—an advantage if marked clotting abnormalities prevent a biopsy. Laparoscopy therefore has a higher sensitivity than a blind biopsy, which can miss cirrhosis in one in four patients [5].

Laparoscopic characteristics are based on surface changes, size, induration, color, and associated findings such as lymphatic cysts, distension of the gallbladder, signs of portal hypertension, ascites and associated hepatocellular carcinoma (**Table 53.1**).

Cirrhosis is characterized by regenerating nodules on the hepatic surface, with circumferential whitish, fibrotic retractions. These nodules can vary in size from less than a millimeter to 1–3 mm and up to several centimeters in size. In purely descriptive terms, cirrhosis is classified into micronodular (≤3 mm nodules) and macronodular cirrhosis (>3 mm to several centimeters) (**Fig. 53.17**). In some forms of micronodular cirrhosis, the nodules are so small that the surface appears smooth; however, multiple highlights reflecting light off the tiny nodules provide a clue. A similar effect can be seen after biopsy, when blood running over the liver surface outlines a fine nodular pattern (**Fig. 53.18**).

The color varies from pink to red-brown. Fibrous tissue creates a more grayish-white color, and fatty infiltration in alcoholic cirrhosis—especially with superimposed alcoholic hepatitis—gives a more golden hue.

The size of the liver is highly variable in cirrhosis. The insertion of the round ligament usually coincides with the edge of the costal margin. Both are easily identified as classic landmarks. Due to proliferation of connective tissue, the liver increases in size and extends well beyond the right costal margin (**Figs. 53.19, 53.20**). Infiltration will also increase liver size in the anterior–posterior direction, allowing spontaneous inspection of the undersurface of the organ (**Fig. 53.12**). The usually sharp edge of the liver becomes more rounded and is often totally obliterated. Only increased fibrous tissue, in the form of capsule thickening, indicates the former edge. The change in size may involve both lobes or may be more pronounced in one lobe than in the other.

The consistency of the liver becomes denser in cirrhosis and is best appreciated using the palpating probe, which gives excellent tactile sensation. The normal liver is soft, easily indented, and drapes itself over the probe when lifted up (**Fig. 53.2**). In cirrhosis, the organ is stiff, has no pliability, and lifts in toto rather than showing a draping effect.

Table 53.1 Laparoscopic classification of cirrhosis

Surface changes

Regenerating nodules
    Micronodular, ≤3 mm nodules
    Macronodular, >3 mm nodules
    Mixed nodularity

Fibrosis
    Circumferential fibrotic retractions
    Deep dystrophic scars
    Capsule thickening

Vasculature
    Increased, often congested surface vessels
    Prominent congested lymphatics
    Lymph cysts

Size—hepatomegaly
Extension of one or both lobes beyond the right costal margin
Spontaneous presentation of the undersurface (increase in anterior–posterior diameter)

Associated conditions, complications
Portal hypertension
Increased collaterals—falciform ligament, phrenicocolic ligament, in adhesions
Recanalized umbilical vein
Ascites—clear, chylous (rare)
Hepatocellular carcinoma

53

Laparoscopy and percutaneous liver biopsy are invasive tests associated with certain risks, and noninvasive tests have therefore been developed for staging of fibrosis and cirrhosis. Transient elastography (FibroScan) is a novel noninvasive method of assessing hepatic fibrosis. It is simple, rapid, and can be used at the bedside. Magnetic resonance elastography is another method of assessing the mechanical properties of soft tissues. A recent meta-analysis of nine studies reported estimated sensitivity and specificity rates of 87% and 91%, respectively, for stage 4 fibrosis (cirrhosis). The estimates for stage 2–4 fibrosis were lower (sensitivity 70%, specificity

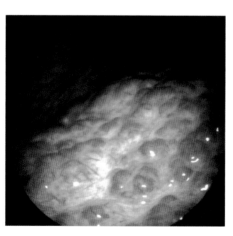

Fig. 53.17 Cirrhosis hepatis, with regenerating nodules of a few millimeters to 1 cm in size. The nodules are surrounded by broad whitish fibrous bands. There are irregular highlights of varying size reflecting light off the regenerating nodules.

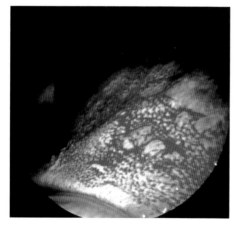

Fig. 53.18 Micronodular cirrhosis due to alcohol. The nodular pattern is accentuated after biopsy, due to blood surrounding more prominent nodules.

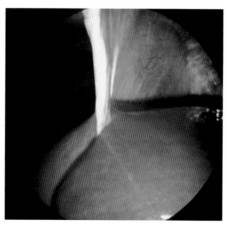

Fig. 53.19 Marked hepatomegaly. Extension of the right and left lobe well beyond the insertion of the round ligament. Fatty liver with fibrosis.

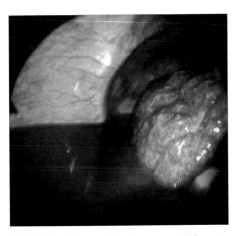

Fig. 53.20   Micronodular cirrhosis, with hepatomegaly and ascites. The liver has a grossly irregular surface, due to dystrophy. The small highlights are characteristic of a micronodular pattern. The liver extends well beyond the right costal margin.

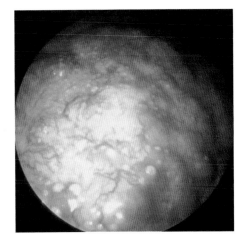

Fig. 53.21   Small lymphatic cysts on the surface of the liver.

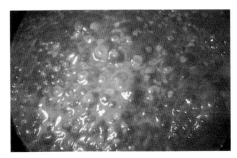

Fig. 53.22   Idiopathic hemochromatosis with complete cirrhotic transformation. The area of small to moderate nodular transformation is slightly concealed by dense lymphoceles. The regenerating areas are dark brown to gray in color. There is no sign of inflammatory activity.

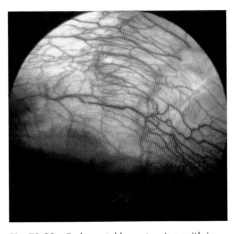

Fig. 53.23   Early portal hypertension, with increased collaterals in the falciform ligament extending to the anterior abdominal wall.

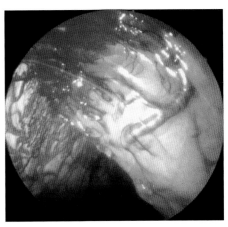

Fig. 53.24   Portosystemic collaterals in postoperative adhesions after cholecystectomy.

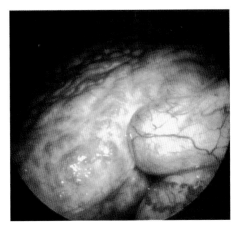

Fig. 53.25   Micronodular cirrhosis, with a recanalized umbilical vein (Cruveilhier–Baumgarten syndrome). These collaterals can develop to finger-sized structures.

84%) [11]. In 101 patients, staging with FibroScan had a sensitivity of 88.2% and a specificity of 85.4% for stage 4 fibrosis/cirrhosis when histology and/or gross nodularity on laparoscopy with guided biopsies from both liver lobes were used as the gold standard [12]. Markers of serum fibrosis (hyaluronic acid, type IV collagen, type IV collagen 7S domain, and type III procollagen N-peptide) are not as accurate in staging fibrosis and cirrhosis as the FibroScan and are best when used in conjunction with transient elastography [13].

Surface vessels are often increased and congested, including prominent lymphatic vessels. Small, glass-clear cysts, often less than 1 mm in size, may cover the hepatic surface (**Figs. 53.21, 53.22**). These are lymph cysts and form as a result of the blockage of lymphatic flow. Pathognomonic of cirrhosis, they are often overlooked and present at a pre-ascitic stage.

The gallbladder can be markedly distended due to poor emptying. It may be confused with a Courvoisier gallbladder, tensely distended in obstructive jaundice, especially if cirrhosis is associated with cholestasis and a dark greenish liver color (**Fig. 53.10**). However, the gallbladder in cirrhosis is soft and easily indented with the probe, while it is tense like a tight balloon in obstructive jaundice.

Portal hypertension. Signs of portal hypertension through passive venous congestion and the development of collateral vessels are easily noted at laparoscopy and develop long before esophageal varices and ascites are clinically apparent. Portosystemic collaterals can form wherever the portal circulation is able to find access to the systemic venous system in the form of collaterals. One of the earliest signs of portosystemic collaterals is vessels in the region of the phrenicocolic ligament in the left upper quadrant. The falciform ligament is another site of early collateral formation (**Fig. 53.23**). The collaterals here may range from a delicate, increased network to large, congested vessels. Postoperative adhesions are a convenient bridge to the systemic circulation, and often a network of extensive collaterals is noted, especially after operations in the upper abdomen such as open cholecystectomy (**Fig. 53.24**). Some of the vessels may be pencil-thick, presenting a risk of significant hemorrhage—e.g., during blind percutaneous liver biopsy—if they are accidentally punctured. This is an additional argument for using imaging-guided biopsies in patients with cirrhosis and portal hypertension. The umbilical vein can recanalize to an impressive size, usually with prominent vasa vasorum [11] (**Fig. 53.25**). Large veins may extend through the ligamentum teres to the umbilicus and ulti-

VIII

mately give rise to a caput medusae. A recanalized umbilical vein has been reported in 20 of 224 cases of cirrhosis (9%). Although one might expect decompression of the portal bed as a result of these large collaterals, they did not prevent the development of esophageal varices in 50% of patients with the syndrome [14].

Ascites as a complication of cirrhosis and portal hypertension is closely associated with alterations in lymphatic flow in the liver [15] (**Fig. 53.20**). Lymphatic vessels on the liver surface are congested as the result of hepatic fibrous transformation and restriction of flow (**Fig. 53.26**). Ultimately, they lose their ability to drain into the thoracic duct via the porta hepatis. The lymphocysts mentioned above form and then rupture, draining into the abdominal cavity, with resulting ascites. Chylous ascites as a complication of cirrhosis without retroperitoneal tumor obstruction of the lymphatic system has been described, but is rare.

There is little correlation between laparoscopic characteristics and etiology of cirrhosis. In patients with chronic alcohol abuse, a micronodular cirrhotic pattern is found more often, while macronodular cirrhosis is more common after chronic viral and autoimmune hepatitis, with necrosis leading to large regenerating nodules. However, there is wide overlap between the multiple causes of cirrhosis and the endoscopic presentation.

However, laparoscopic findings do appear to correlate with the prognosis of cirrhosis. In an attempt to correlate laparoscopy with the prognosis, a Japanese study compared cumulative survival data in 372 patients. When the nodularity was classified into grade I (mild nodularity), grade II (distinctly elevated nodules), and grade III (hemispheric nodules over the entire surface), the 5-year survival rates for patients in each of these groups were 81.9%, 64.4%, and 50.6%, respectively. The differences between grades I and II, and between grades II and III, were significant. An absence of small lymphatic cysts (the pre-ascitic stage) suggested a much better prognosis (73% vs. 52.6%), even if only a small number of cysts were present. The size of the right lobe, but not of the left lobe, was also significant. The 5-year survival rate in patients with an enlarged right lobe was 78%, in comparison with 61.4% in those with an atrophic right lobe.

Liver biopsy in cirrhosis. The high false-negative rate of percutaneous liver biopsy in patients with cirrhosis is well established in the literature. A review of 6242 cases of cirrhosis evaluated by blind percutaneous liver biopsy reported a false-negative rate of 1–61%, with an average of 24%, or one in four patients [5]. Due to the characteristic surface changes, laparoscopy has a high diagnostic yield, especially if the findings are confirmed with direct-vision biopsy, and more so if a cutting-type needle is used. Aspiration needles and the use of a Menghini technique yield an often fragmented specimen that is inadequate for correct diagnosis, which requires the presence of regenerating nodules, perinodular fibrosis, and distortion of the normal hepatic architecture [16,17]. In a review of 1251 cases in which laparoscopy and direct-vision biopsies were compared, the false-negative biopsy rate varied from 7% to 57%, with an average of 29%—similar to the percutaneous biopsy rate. The false-negative rate for laparoscopy varied from 4% to 18%, with an average of 9% [5]. In a randomized prospective study, percutaneous biopsy gave a correct diagnosis in 82% of 64 patients, laparoscopy with biopsy gave a correct diagnosis in 100% [18]. The value of combining the macroscopic picture of laparoscopy with the microscopic histological picture of direct-vision biopsy was demonstrated by Orlando et al. Laparoscopy and guided biopsy yielded almost identical rates of correct diagnosis in 78.4% and 78.8%, respectively. Combining the two procedures increased the accuracy to 97.7% [19]. Further support for this argument was provided by a large retrospective study conducted at the University of Miami. Of 434 patients with suspected liver diseases, 169 were diagnosed with cirrhosis at laparoscopy. Only 115 of these diagnoses were confirmed histologically, resulting in a false-negative rate of 32%. Of the 54 false-

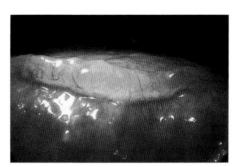

Fig. 53.26 Occlusion of the lymphatic vessels. A lymphatic vessel occluded and dilated to the thickness of a pencil, on the right caudal margin of the liver. Incomplete cirrhotic transformation.

negative patients identified by histology, 91% were in Child–Pugh grades A and B, while 9% of Child–Pugh grade C cirrhotic patients were missed by biopsy. Of the 263 patients without cirrhosis at laparoscopy, only two had cirrhosis on biopsy, resulting in a false-negative rate of 0.8% for laparoscopy [20]. Of 142 patients evaluated laparoscopically for various liver diseases such as fatty liver, chronic hepatitis. and fibrosis, as well as cirrhosis, laparoscopy had a sensitivity of 100% for cirrhosis, with a specificity of 97%. Histology missed 6% of patients with cirrhosis [21].

The evidence is overwhelming that laparoscopy and direct-vision biopsy should be the preferred method of evaluation for patients with suspected cirrhosis. Valuable prognostic information can be obtained, such as evidence of portal hypertension, hypertensive collateral circulation, lymphatic cysts, lobe atrophy, and possible associated hepatocellular carcinoma. A proper biopsy site can be selected, both lobes can be biopsied, large collaterals can be avoided—especially if adhesions are present—and postbiopsy bleeding can be controlled. In addition, laparoscopy can be combined with laparoscopic ultrasound for better evaluation of deeper organ sites.

Hepatocellular carcinoma. This complication of cirrhosis is discussed under focal liver disease and staging of malignancies, below.

Metastatic tumors in cirrhosis. Hepatocellular carcinoma is the dominant tumor complicating cirrhosis, but metastatic tumors have also been observed—although with a much lower frequency than in the noncirrhotic liver. An Italian study found only 19 cases of metastasis in 2538 patients with cirrhosis who underwent laparoscopy. Primary liver tumors were seen in 140 patients—an almost tenfold increase [22]. In an autopsy series of 1073 cases of cirrhosis, 190 primary liver tumors were found in 22 cases of metastasis in 98 extrahepatic neoplasms. Another autopsy series of 498 cases of cirrhosis demonstrated 71 hepatocellular carcinomas and 18 metastases in 58 extrahepatic neoplasms. In the laparoscopy series, there was a predominance of esophageal carcinomas (31.8%), which led to liver metastases in only 3.7% of cases. The autopsy series found predominantly intra-abdominal tumors, draining through the portal system, with liver metastases in 35.2% of cases. The altered hepatic architecture and blood flow may play a role in this phenomenon. Tumors are frequently overlooked with imaging studies, which may be misleading due to the distorted liver architecture.

Focal Liver Lesions

Benign Focal Lesions

Hepatic cysts. Benign hepatic cysts are a common finding on imaging studies and are usually of no pathologic consequence. Their sharply demarcated contours, round or oval shape, and water-density measurement on CT rarely give rise to consideration of other types of focal lesion. Cysts are therefore an incidental finding at laparoscopy. Laparoscopy is rarely indicated to differentiate a suspected cyst from any other type of focal lesion. Cyst puncture is usually not indicated.. We have seen only one cyst in 30 years that

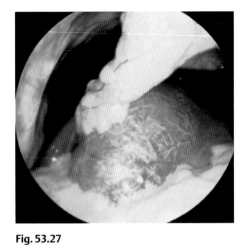

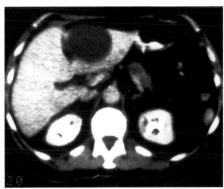

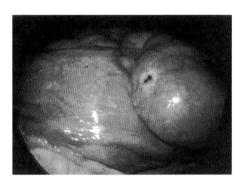

Fig. 53.27
a A large, benign hepatic cyst several centimeters in size in the left lobe. There is a bluish-gray color, with a normal vascular network in the normal liver capsule.
b The corresponding computed-tomography scan shows the large cyst in the anterior left lobe.

Fig. 53.28 A small hemangioma in an otherwise normal liver. The hemangioma was not detected on imaging studies.

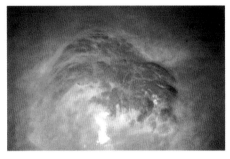

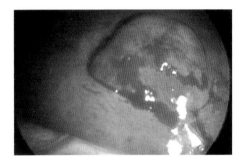

Fig. 53.29 Hemangioma. A large, flat, and prominent hemangioma, ca. 3 × 2 cm in size, with a spongy structure and livid red coloring. On palpation, it had a firmly elastic consistency. The preliminary ultrasound diagnosis was a tumor of unclear malignancy.

Fig. 53.30 Hepatocellular adenoma. Two fingerbreadths above the left margin of the liver, a pink-red tumor ca. 2 × 3 cm in size and with smooth contours is seen, clearly distinct from the normal parenchyma. It had an increased consistency on palpation. There are traces of blood after two biopsies.

Fig. 53.31 Focal nodular hyperplasia. Nodular deformation of the entire right lobe of the liver. The maximum diameter of the nodes was 9 cm. Marked vascularization is seen, with varix-like venous distension, and there was a solid consistency on palpation. There is a coagulated biopsy scar after pulsating hemorrhage following a biopsy.

caused compression of the common bile duct and obstructive jaundice due to its size and location. Liver cysts present at various sizes, from 1 mm to several centimeters in diameter; rarely, they may be quite large (**Fig. 53.27**). Their color is bluish-gray, depending on the thickness of the overlying hepatic parenchyma and capsule.

Polycystic disease of the liver, which may accompany polycystic renal disease, is a rare disorder with multiple cystic lesions, leading to cystic transformation of the organ [23]. Liver function is usually normal in these patients, but the size and number of cysts may give rise to mechanical compression of the common bile duct or may compromise portal blood flow, leading to portal hypertension and esophageal varices. Cyst drainage and surgical unroofing of the larger cysts may be beneficial in selected cases [24].

Hemangioma. Hepatic hemangiomas are the most common benign hepatic tumors, usually identified on imaging studies or incidentally during exploratory laparoscopy. A hemangioma may be suspected and confirmed by a dynamic CT scan with a rapid bolus injection of intravenous contrast medium, or using MRI or angiography. Hemangiomas can vary in size from a few millimeters to centimeters (**Fig. 53.28**). In some cases, they can be large enough to occupy a major portion of a liver lobe. Their color is purplish-blue, resembling that of blood vessels. Larger lesions have an irregular nodular surface and can extend prominently beyond the hepatic surface (**Fig. 53.29**). The bleeding risk even from large lesions is low [25]. The need for surgical intervention is dictated by the overall size of

the lesion and its relationship to, and effect on, other intra-abdominal structures. Laparoscopy can assist in the proper staging for resectability.

Hepatic adenoma, focal nodular hyperplasia, and peliosis hepatis.
Hepatic adenomas are rare tumors. They present as focal defects on imaging studies and are not associated with abnormal liver function tests. They vary in size and may extend to several centimeters in diameter. Adenomas present endoscopically as reddish-pink, sharply demarcated tumors that usually extend beyond the hepatic surface. The diagnosis is made by needle biopsy (**Fig. 53.30**). Spontaneous rupture with catastrophic intra-abdominal hemorrhage may occur in large tumors. Hepatic adenomas have been linked to estrogen therapy; they were more frequently observed during the 1970s and 1980s. The recent decrease in their frequency may be related to different formulations of supplementary estrogen drugs and birth-control pills.

Focal nodular hyperphasia is characterized by small, benign, regenerating nodules of normal liver tissue. Macronodular regeneration occurs rarely. The picture may be confused with cirrhosis, and a large-core biopsy is usually required for correct diagnosis (**Fig. 53.31**). Focal nodular hyperplasia has been associated with various medical conditions—mainly hematological disorders and after immunosuppressive therapy [26]. In some patients with immunosuppressive therapy after renal transplantation, micronodular

VIII

transformation was associated with peliosis hepatis and was thought to be due to azathioprine and possibly cyclosporine [27].

Peliosis hepatis is characterized by bluish-black irregular markings on the hepatic surface, usually only a few millimeters in size, but often becoming confluent to form a large network covering the liver surface. This is an incidental finding of no pathological consequence and has been associated with androgens as well as various medications [27].

Sarcoidosis. The hepatic surface is almost always involved in sarcoidosis of the liver. Since the lesions are focal, they may be missed by a blind percutaneous liver biopsy. Sarcoidosis is characterized by small, whitish nodules on the hepatic surface, which measure no more than 1–2 mm in size [28]. They are therefore not identified on imaging studies. In patients in the proper clinical setting and with isolated elevations of the hepatocanalicular enzymes, laparoscopy with guided liver biopsy is the ideal investigation. In some patients, these lesions are larger, probably due to confluence of smaller nodules, and they may be confused macroscopically with metastatic tumor (**Fig. 53.32**). The lack of neovascularity in this setting argues against malignancy.

Focal Malignant Lesions

With advances in medical and surgical therapy for malignancies, accurate tumor staging has a major impact on the proper selection of treatment and on the prognosis. The prospective pretreatment patient evaluation usually requires histologic biopsy assessment. Staging must have an impact on the appropriate selection of therapy. If a patient requires a laparotomy because of an obstructing colon carcinoma, staging for local spread is not appropriate. However, staging for distant metastases may have implications for subsequent treatment, such as chemotherapy.

It is appropriate to start the staging work-up with serologic and noninvasive imaging studies before advancing to other tests. There may be different clinical scenarios—the patient may have a known primary carcinoma, with liver metastases being suspected on the basis of the clinical evaluation and laboratory tests. The true nature of the hepatic lesion will have a major impact on the patient's future treatment course and outlook. In another case, imaging studies carried out for other reasons may reveal a focal liver lesion; the differential diagnosis lies between a benign and malignant lesion. Finally, imaging tests may be negative in a patient with a known primary tumor. However, absence or presence of metastases will have a major impact on the subsequent patient management, with a choice between palliative measures and resection with curative intent. Laparoscopy is ideally suited to settle these questions.

In patients with squamous cell carcinoma of the esophagus or pancreatic carcinoma associated with alcohol use, imaging studies may not be able to differentiate between chronic liver disease due to alcohol or tumor.

In tumors that do not require a laparotomy for therapy—e. g., carcinomas of the lung, breast, or in some cases esophagus—laparoscopy can identify hepatic and peritoneal metastases in a significant number of patients and should be seriously considered [29–31]. Many studies have shown that laparoscopy and direct-vision biopsy can provide an accurate diagnosis of malignancies involving the liver and peritoneum in 80–90 % of cases and that the false-negative rate with CT is unacceptably high [32–34].

Brush cytology combined with direct-vision biopsy further increases the histological yield and can be used when postbiopsy bleeding is a concern [35]. Fine-needle aspiration of the tumor is safe and effective if there is concern regarding tumor spread that might jeopardize a future curative resection, as in the case of hepatocellular carcinoma [36].

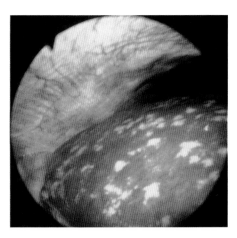

Fig. 53.32 Sarcoidosis. The larger irregular whitish plaques are due to the confluence of smaller miliary nodules. Marked hepatomegaly, with extension of the right hepatic lobe beyond the costal margin.

Laparoscopic ultrasound has been used to help assess resectability in both primary and limited metastatic disease [37]. In 19 of 24 patients, 18 of whom had metastatic lesions and six of whom had hepatocellular carcinoma, laparoscopic ultrasonography identified six of eight unresectable patients who had been considered resectable on the basis of prelaparoscopy tests.

Diagnostic accuracy. Surgical and autopsy series have demonstrated that the hepatic surface is involved in 90 % of patients if liver metastases are present. Two-thirds of the hepatic surface can be inspected at laparoscopy when the proper techniques are used [38]. Lesions as small as 1–2 mm can be identified and biopsied, a size that is clearly below the resolution of the most modern scanners [34,39]. Prospective controlled trials have shown that CT-directed and direct-vision biopsies yield similar results in patients with focal lesions on imaging studies (80 % vs. 93 %) [32]. The high false-negative rate for CT has been confirmed in three prospective studies. Cancer was found at laparoscopy in 21 % of 19 patients with negative scans in whom intra-abdominal malignancies were suspected. The negative predictive value for CT was only 50 %, in comparison with 89 % for laparoscopy. The same authors found liver and peritoneal metastases in 48 % of patients with a negative CT scan but with malignancy suspected on clinical grounds [31,33]. In 40 patients with pancreatic carcinomas considered resectable on the basis of the preoperative work-up, laparoscopy detected lesions in 35 %. In 26 patients who underwent laparotomy, three had false-negative laparoscopy findings. In two of the three, the examination had to be considered incomplete, since a palpating probe was not used to assist in the inspection of the liver undersurfaces. Most lesions were small implants of only a few millimeters in diameter (**Fig. 53.33**). The authors considered that many of these lesions would have been overlooked at open laparotomy. In an update of this experience in 114 patients with pancreatic cancer, which included angiography as part of the work-up, laparoscopy was found to have a sensitivity of 93 % and a specificity of 100 % [40].

In addition to inspection and biopsy peritoneal washing cytology can add to the diagnostic accuracy [41]. Positive cytology of peritoneal lavage was especially helpful in patients in whom laparoscopy failed to detect any lesions. The survival rates in this group were similar to those in patients with confirmed metastases, in comparison with the survival with patients with negative cytology. Peritoneal washing cytology is a simple and inexpensive technique and should be added at the time of staging laparotomy.

Esophageal carcinoma. Esophageal carcinoma—particularly squamous cell carcinoma—usually presents late in the course, since dysphagia is a late warning sign. The overall 5-year survival is only 7 %, worse than for any other form of cancer. Most patients

53

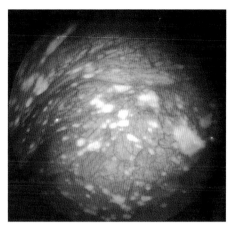

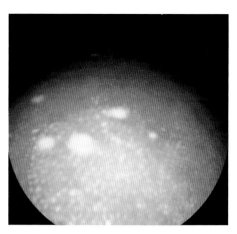

Fig. 53.33 Metastatic pancreatic carcinoma. There a small, 1-mm peritoneal implant between the left liver lobe and the stomach. The engorged mesenteric veins should be noted.

Fig 53.34 Metastatic gastric carcinoma. There are small implants on the parietal peritoneum that were not visible on other imaging studies.

Fig. 53.35 Metastatic pancreatic carcinoma. These lesions, only a few millimeters in diameter, were not detected with other imaging studies.

are therefore unresectable at the time of diagnosis, and palliation with radiotherapy, stent placement, and/or laser therapy has to be considered. Surgical palliation is not acceptable due to its high morbidity and mortality, and accurate staging is mandatory. Surgical therapy should only be considered if a curative resection seems feasible. In patients with advanced cirrhosis due to alcohol abuse, one of the risk factors for esophageal carcinoma, surgery is contraindicated even if the tumor is at a resectable stage. These patients are also best identified at laparoscopy.

In a large series of 369 patients with esophageal cancer and carcinoma of the cardia, preoperative laparoscopy detected liver and peritoneal metastases in 24% of cases. The false-negative rate for laparoscopy was only 4%. Cirrhosis was noted in 14% of the patients [31].

Another large study used laparoscopic ultrasound and peritoneal lavage cytology as additional measures in patients with carcinoma of the esophagus and cardia. In 127 patients, metastases were found in 19%, a positive cytology in 10%, and cirrhosis in 6% [42]. Similar results have been reported by other investigators. In 90 patients with similar tumors, laparoscopy was superior to CT in detecting liver lesions (88% vs. 56%) and peritoneal metastases (89% vs. 0%) and was only slightly better in detecting malignant lymph nodes (51% vs. 31%) [43]. The addition of laparoscopic ultrasound actually down-staged some patients who had successful resections [44]. Similar results were found in two additional studies [45,46]. The sensitivity for detecting metastases was 82% with laparoscopic ultrasound, 67% with laparoscopy, and 55% with CT. The accuracy rates for detecting resectability were 96%, 88%, and 68%, respectively. Laparoscopy has also been combined with thoracoscopy in the staging of esophageal cancer [47]. Thoracoscopy assessed 28 of 30 patients as N0 and two as N1; 26 of the N0 cases were confirmed after resection, and the surgical findings showed that two patients with stage N1 had been missed. Endoscopic ultrasonography (EUS) has been compared with laparoscopy and thoracoscopy [48]. Laparoscopy prevented only 6% of unnecessary operations, but the combination of laparoscopy and thoracoscopy was superior to EUS in staging lymph-node metastases.

Gastric carcinoma. In spite of the use of EUS, ultrasonography, and CT, the staging of gastric carcinoma is often inadequate, particularly in the case of small peritoneal implants and liver metastases, as well as invasion of adjacent organs. Especially when it is combined with laparoscopic ultrasound and cytology, laparoscopy can change the staging significantly, avoiding unnecessary laparotomies in a significant number of patients (**Fig. 53.34**). In a study of 40 patients

considered resectable using all other criteria, 40% were judged unresectable on the basis of the laparoscopic findings alone, due to locally advanced disease in 27.5% of cases and distant metastases in 12.5% [49]. Resectability was confirmed in 87% of the operated patients, with an overall diagnostic accuracy for laparoscopy of 91.6%. Similar results were obtained in four studies including 350 patients [50–53]. When the TNM system was used to compare laparoscopy with ultrasonography and CT, laparoscopy showed a staging accuracy of 68.6%, in comparison with 32.8% for ultrasound and CT. As the T stage increased, the differences became more pronounced—T3 69.7% vs. 12.1%, and T4 84.2% vs. 42.1%. Laparoscopy staged all metastases correctly, but ultrasound and CT falsely assessed 18 of 70 patients as having stage M0 [53]. The overall TNM accuracy for laparoscopy was 72%, compared with 38% for CT and ultrasonography. In a prospective multicenter study, laparoscopy was found to have a diagnostic accuracy of 98.6% (70 of 71 patients). However, CT was not used in all patients [54]. The yield of laparoscopy can be increased by including laparoscopic exploration of the lesser sac and using laparoscopic ultrasound and cytology [55,56]. In 111 patients with advanced gastric cancer—T3 and T4 on CT and EUS—extended laparoscopy using the above techniques resulted in up-staging in 25.2% of cases and down-staging in 15.3%, more than half of which were from T4 to T2 [56]. Extended diagnostic laparoscopy appears to be the technique with the greatest accuracy and the highest yield in tumor staging.

Cytology of peritoneal washings during laparoscopy may increase the diagnostic yield. In a prospective study of 40 patients with esophageal and gastric carcinoma, laparoscopy up-staged 21 patients (52.5%). Cytology alone failed to identify 45% of patients with positive findings at laparoscopy. The addition of cytology added no additional stage IV patients to the laparoscopy-negative group [57] (see Chapter 23).

Pancreatic carcinoma. Since the early reports by Meyer-Burg et al. reporting direct inspection of the pancreas, initially through a supragastric approach, further publications have described various techniques for the diagnosis and biopsy of pancreatic carcinoma [58–60]. These techniques allow inspection and biopsy of the body and tail, but not of the pancreatic head. Since tumors in these parts are diagnosed late, with a very poor outlook, laparoscopy rarely contributes to patient management, and fine-needle aspiration biopsy can be accomplished using an imaging-guided approach.

The main value of laparoscopy lies in its ability to assist in staging and detecting liver and peritoneal metastases—particularly very small lesions, as mentioned earlier [34] (**Figs. 53.33–53.35**). The yield is significantly enhanced by use of laparoscopic ultrasonography and cytology. When CT, MRI, angiography, and laparoscopy were compared in an extension of a previous study [34], Warshaw et al. were able to identify 90% of unresectable lesions correctly [61]. In 27 of 88 patients, small liver and peritoneal metastases were confirmed. CT missed all but two of these lesions, but laparoscopy with biopsy detected 96% of metastases. In 73 patients with pre-operative laparoscopy, 42 were correctly staged. However, five of nine patients judged to be resectable at laparoscopy were found to be unresectable at laparotomy [62]. Shortcomings of laparoscopy were demonstrated when CT was compared with laparoscopy. In patients considered unresectable on CT, laparoscopy confirmed this in only 75% of cases. However, of the 25% (n = 9) considered potentially resectable, eight underwent laparotomy and all eight were unresectable [63]. If CT suggested resectability, laparoscopy prevented futile surgery in 38% of cases; however, it predicted resectability correctly in only 50%. In a study of 109 patients, surgery was prevented in 29% of those with metastases [64]. There is little question that laparoscopic ultrasonography increases the diagnostic yield. The unresectability rate can be increased from 35% to 60% [65]. Laparoscopic ultrasound is especially useful in evaluating pancreatic vascular encasement and invasion [66]. Peritoneal washing for cytology should also be used in an attempt to reduce the number of unresectable tumors found at laparotomy [34,67,68]. This technique is especially helpful if the laparoscopic exploration is negative for metastases, and it should be used routinely.

Hepatocellular carcinoma (HCC). In the United States and western Europe, HCC is diagnosed in one to five patients per 100,000 population. It is often associated with chronic hepatitis B and C and other chronic liver diseases, and it usually develops against a background of cirrhosis. At the time of diagnosis, HCC is usually far advanced, with a poor prognosis and short survival time. This limited survival time, coupled with a short duration of symptoms, has led to the misconception that HCC is a rapidly growing tumor. However, HCC develops as a slow-growing malignancy [69]. The recognition of high-risk groups makes it mandatory to carry out surveillance for small asymptomatic tumors that may be potentially curable with surgery. Patients with more advanced and symptomatic tumors require accurate diagnosis and tumor staging to avoid unnecessary surgery.

Initial screening is usually carried out using alpha-fetoprotein and ultrasonography. In comparison with CT, ultrasonography has the highest detection rate for small lesions <3 cm in diameter (92.2% vs. 73.2%) and is the initial imaging study of choice [70]. In most cases, HCC occurs in a multinodular fashion and often involves both lobes. In rare cases, it may be diffusely infiltrating.

Laparoscopy is best suited for confirming the diagnosis using direct-vision biopsy and/or cytology, for detecting peritoneal spread, and for assessing the extent and severity of associated cirrhosis, which frequently determines the prognosis and resectability of otherwise localized disease. In patients in whom curative resection seems possible, forceps or core needle biopsies should be avoided, in order to prevent possible tumor spread. The same applies to the risk of bleeding in patients with coagulopathy or vascular tumors, especially with large surface vessels. Fine-needle aspiration and brush cytology are safe and have an accuracy of 100% [71–73].

HCC is characterized by one or multiple nodules, often multichromatic, often due to bleeding or bile production. It is characterized by marked neovascularity and is extremely firm to palpation and easily differentiated in cirrhosis (**Fig. 53.36**). Smaller lesions may be difficult to detect. The typical umbilication and crater like appearance of metastatic adenocarcinoma is frequently absent.

Small intrahepatic tumors without involvement of the hepatic surface occur in 10% of cases, and vascular invasion of either the

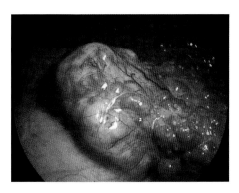

Fig. 53.36 Hepatocellular carcinoma.

hepatic or portal vein can be detected using ultrasonography, illustrating the complementary nature of the two procedures [74]. The superiority of laparoscopy over other imaging studies has repeatedly been demonstrated, as well as its ability to diagnose small peritoneal metastases [73,75,76]. In 115 cases of HCC, cytology and biopsy gave a combined accuracy of 95.6% [77]. Early diagnosis of HCC remains elusive. Yellow hepatic surface nodules are an indicator of early HCC. Histological alterations such as fatty changes, "nodule-within-nodule" formation, increased nuclear-to-cytoplasmic ratio, and hypercellularity have been found to correlate with HCC. The greater the number of these histological findings, the greater the chance of concomitant HCC [78]. HCC may present as minute nodules. The lesions are small, yellow, and often larger than 5 mm. Histologically, small cells with severe fatty metamorphosis are found, compatible with a well-differentiated HCC [79]. Routine biopsy of all nodules and suspicious lesions should be carried out, since HCC is not always macroscopically apparent. In a study of the selective preoperative use of laparoscopy in 60 patients with potentially resectable HCC, 14 of 19 inoperable patients (74%) were identified by means of laparoscopy, which increased the resectability rate from 68% to 89%. These patients had less blood loss and shorter operating-room times and hospital stays. Clinically apparent cirrhosis and radiographic evidence of major vascular tumor invasion, as well as bilobular tumors, were (not unexpectedly) predictive of inoperable disease at laparoscopy [80].

Cirrhosis will frequently render HCC unresectable, especially if the tumor is advanced or associated with extensive collaterals, even if it is otherwise localized. Cirrhosis may not always be suspected on clinical grounds or from the laboratory data and can be missed on imaging studies. In a retrospective analysis of 54 patients with HCC who underwent ultrasonography and laparoscopy, ultrasound diagnosed cirrhosis in only 35 patients while laparoscopy identified it in 42 [74].

With the recent introduction of laparoscopic partial hepatectomy for HCC, the role of preoperative laparoscopic staging has been expanded, especially in combination with laparoscopic ultrasonography. In a group of 119 patients with HCC, 34% were found to be unresectable after laparoscopy and laparoscopic ultrasonography. Sixty-one percent underwent curative resection (laparoscopic and open). The median hospital stay for the laparoscopic liver resection group (22 patients) was significantly shorter than that for the open resection group (51 patients): 8 vs. 13 days [81].

There have been initial attempts to develop endoscopic treatments for smaller lesions using microwave techniques. It is too early to say whether curative coagulation of small lesions or effective palliation of larger lesions can reasonably be expected [82,83].

Liver transplantation is increasingly being used to treat small, limited HCC lesions. Accurate preoperative staging is paramount for long-term success. Laparoscopy, preferably combined with laparoscopic ultrasonography, would thus be ideally suited for accurate pretransplantation staging.

53

Carcinoma of the gallbladder. Carcinoma of the gallbladder rarely presents with signs or symptoms that might lead the clinician to suspect the diagnosis. It is usually diagnosed late, and metastases— either hepatic or peritoneal—are almost always present. Dense adhesions in response to the neoplastic process often make direct inspection and biopsy of the tumor difficult. In one of the largest laparoscopic evaluations of gallbladder cancer, the gallbladder could only be examined in 48 of 98 patients; 78 had hepatic spread, and 22 had peritoneal spread. A malignancy was confirmed in 89 patients, suggesting that adhesions were not a major limiting factor [84]. When ultrasound was compared with laparoscopy, laparoscopy was found to exclude malignancy correctly when ultrasound suggested tumor. Laparoscopy was correct in 95.8 % of cases, while ultrasound detected only 62.5 %. Distant metastases were correctly diagnosed by laparoscopy in 95 % and by ultrasound in 51.2 %. A combination of the two methods gave a diagnostic accuracy of 100 %. Laparoscopy again avoided unnecessary surgery in 83.3 % of patients [85].

Lymphoma. Laparoscopy is especially useful in the evaluation and staging of lymphomas, especially Hodgkin's disease. It is well known that liver function tests and scans may have false-negative rates as high as 20 % [86]. Since Hodgkin's involvement of the liver is characterized by small whitish nodules, often less than a centimeter in size, it is not surprising that scanning and blind biopsies have a high miss rate. Liver or splenic involvement indicates stage IV disease. Staging must have an impact on therapy, and it is therefore important to be familiar with the latest treatment protocol, which may already include chemotherapy for stage III disease. In these cases, staging laparoscopy may add little to the management. The diagnostic accuracy of laparoscopy approaches that of staging laparotomy [87]. It is imperative that multiple biopsies are taken from both liver lobes, since surface changes may be absent. When staging laparotomy was compared with laparoscopy, Hodgkin's disease of the liver was diagnosed in four of 34 patients. In the remaining 30, who underwent laparotomy, only one additional case was diagnosed [88]. In one large series, laparoscopy resulted in up-staging from stages I or II to stages III or IV in 35 % of cases [89]. When laparoscopy was compared with CT in 112 patients with Hodgkin's and non-Hodgkin's lymphoma, hepatic involvement was found in 8.5 % of the Hodgkin's patients and in 24.5 % of those with non-Hodgkin's lymphoma. Laparoscopy up-staged 50 % of patients to stage IV [90]. Splenic biopsy can be carried out safely, but it has a low accuracy rate in the absence of surface involvement [91]. Complete laparoscopic staging, including splenectomy in six cases, has been reported [92]. Laparoscopy can be extremely helpful in the follow-up of these patients. Therapy may leave scars in the hepatic parenchyma that may be confusing on imaging studies. Laparoscopy with guided biopsy can rule out or confirm recurrences.

Other malignancies. Carcinoma of the lung and breast are tumors in which hepatic and peritoneal spread are usually not considered at the initial staging evaluation. However, tumor involvement in the abdominal cavity will radically change prognosis and treatment.

A total of 131 patients with small cell carcinoma of the lung were found to have hepatic metastases in 25 % of cases, diagnosed at laparoscopy and ultrasonography with fine-needle aspiration biopsy [93]. Seven percent of them had false-negative laparoscopies and 14 % had false-negative findings on ultrasonography.

Laparoscopy can be complimentary in the staging of carcinoma of the breast. One study reported liver metastases smaller than 1 cm in 8.5 % of patients, in whom the lesions had not been detected by previous imaging studies [94].

Laparoscopy and laparoscopic ultrasound can be an alternative to a second-look laparotomy in patients in whom recurrent colorectal carcinoma is suspected. Laparoscopic ultrasound increased the detection of nodal metastases over laparoscopy and CT, but overestimated the nodal involvement in some cases [95].

Peritoneal Disorders

Primary Peritoneal Disease

Most of the visceral and parietal peritoneum can be inspected at laparoscopy. This includes the ligaments, such as the falciform, hepatophrenic, phrenicocolic, splenophrenic, and others, which may be confused with adhesions by novices. Using the palpating probe and lifting the undersurfaces of the liver, or moving the greater omentum, allows exploration of most of the viscera covered by peritoneum, including the small and large intestine, as well as female pelvic structures. (**Figs. 53.37–53.39**) Laparoscopy is therefore ideally suited for abdominal exploration and for the evaluation of peritoneal disorders, especially if the lesions are small. These abnormalities are usually not detected with other imaging studies, and blind peritoneal biopsies are unreliable.

Mesothelioma is the primary peritoneal malignancy. In many patients, the pleura is involved as well, and it may often be the only organ system afflicted. Exposure to the carcinogen asbestos, especially among shipbuilding workers, is a well-established cause.

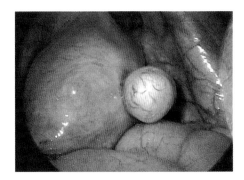

Fig. 53.37 Uterine myoma. Intramural myoma formation causing a slightly enlarged uterus in dextroposition. There is a cherry-sized, broad-based subserous myoma located on the dorso-cranial circumference.

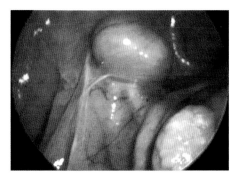

Fig. 53.38 Parovarian cyst. On the lower right, the left fallopian tube can be seen, with a grayish-white left ovary. At a distance of 3 cm from it there is a thick-walled ovarian cyst, located on the common iliac artery. There had been no change in the findings during the previous 6 years.

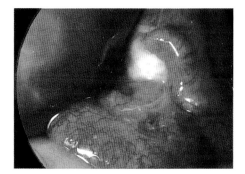

Fig. 53.39 Acute adnexitis. There is an extremely sinuous and thickened right fallopian tube, with acute vascular congestion and some inflammatory adhesion to the ovary, visible in white.

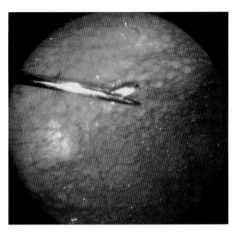

Fig. 53.40 Mesothelioma. Nodular unifocal involvement of the parietal and visceral peritoneum.

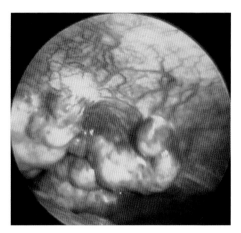

Fig. 53.41 An undifferentiated carcinoma of the tongue with metastasis to the peritoneum. The anterior abdominal wall shows marked neovascularity and ascites.

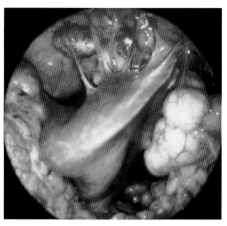

Fig. 53.42 Metastatic leiomyosarcoma from the small bowel, with grape-like nodules involving only the peritoneum, seen here in the region of the left liver lobe.

The clinical presentation is nonspecific. Patients report abdominal pain, weakness, weight loss, and abdominal distension in the case of ascites. Ascites studies reveal an exudate, but ascites cytology is usually negative for malignant cells. Laparoscopy with biopsy is the procedure of choice for a definitive diagnosis [96,97]. The laparoscopic picture is characterized by multiple small miliary lesions, which stud the visceral and parietal peritoneum in a homogeneous pattern. While the uniform small nodular pattern is characteristic, it is not diagnostic (**Fig. 53.40**). Biopsy, usually with cup forceps, is required for a definitive diagnosis. Most patients with peritoneal mesothelioma present with ascites. It is not possible to differentiate the condition with certainty from metastatic peritoneal spread from other primary tumors by visual inspection alone, and even tuberculous peritonitis should be included in the differential diagnosis. In metastatic peritoneal diseases, the nodularity is usually more irregular and varied. Neovascularity and inflammatory adhesions are common. In a series of 36 patients with pulmonary mesothelioma, with 12 equivocal CT findings for diaphragmatic extension and peritoneal disease, laparoscopy was used as a preoperative staging procedure. In six patients, definitive diaphragmatic and peritoneal involvement was diagnosed [97].

Metastatic Disease

Next to the liver, the peritoneum is one of the most common sites of metastatic carcinoma, especially adenocarcinoma. As mentioned earlier, carcinomas with hepatic and peritoneal metastases originate in organs drained by the portal system, such as the stomach, pancreas, and colon, but may also originate in the ovaries or uterus, or outside the abdominal cavity in sites such as the esophagus, breast, or other more distant sites. Peritoneal seeding occurs in lymphoma, especially in non-Hodgkin's lymphoma in patients with acquired immune deficiency syndrome (AIDS), multiple myeloma, malignant carcinoid, and others. Ascites is again one of the dominating features, together with abdominal pain, distension, weight loss, and malaise. Imaging studies will reveal ascites in cases where it is present. They are otherwise even less sensitive than in metastatic liver disease. Since ascites may be due to benign or malignant liver disease, laparoscopy is the only method of achieving quick differentiation. The laparoscopic image is variable and less homogeneous than in mesothelioma. Lesions may be miliary, whitish and flat, or more confluent and of varying sizes, with marked

nodularity. Neovascularity is a prominent feature, as are inflammatory adhesions (**Figs. 53.33, 53.34, 53.41, 53.42**). Metastases may sometimes be only few in number, measuring 1–2 mm in size, and they may be easily overlooked if a careful total abdominal exploration is not carried out, including the use of a palpating probe. Small lesions of the omentum are particularly easily overlooked because of its yellow color.

In patients with AIDS, the peritoneum may be involved with lymphoma. In 54 patients with human immunodeficiency virus (HIV) infection, 44 of whom had AIDS, 13 had peritoneal disease. Eight of these had non-Hodgkin's lymphoma. In half of the patients, the laparoscopic diagnosis led to a change in management. In these patients, a diagnosis had not been previously established on clinical grounds or by CT scan [98]. Biopsy of all lesions is required in order to establish a correct diagnosis and to differentiate between a malignant lesion and granuloma in tuberculous peritonitis.

Pseudomyxoma peritonei is a rare and unusual tumor, with gelatinous, transparent peritoneal aggregates. Most of these lesions are associated with carcinoma. Half of the lesions originate from cystadenocarcinoma of the ovaries, and a quarter from appendiceal carcinoma. However, they may also be caused by a ruptured appendiceal mucocele or ovarian cystadenoma [99]. Patients require careful abdominal exploration, with biopsies and special attention to the ovaries and appendix.

Technical advances may further aid in the diagnosis of peritoneal metastatic disease, with the use of a minilaparoscope with a diameter of 1.9 mm and only a single incision (with the Veress needle being exchanged for the minilaparoscope). Peritoneal metastases were confirmed in 23 of 36 patients and definitely ruled out in 13. CT missed the tumor spread in 12 of these 23 patients, with one false-positive diagnosis. The sensitivity and specificity of minilaparoscopy were 100% and 85%, respectively, in comparison with 48% and 97% for CT. This study further demonstrates that even modern CT imaging can diagnose peritoneal metastases in only about half of the cases [100].

Fluorescence, achieved by photosensitizing tumors, may lead to better tumor staging, as it allows small lesions that are not visible in white light to be detected. Thirteen patients with ovarian carcinoma underwent intraperitoneal instillation of 5-aminolevulinic acid 5 h before a second-look staging laparoscopy. In 12 of the 13 patients, laparoscopy revealed metastases, identified by their strong red fluorescence. In four of the patients, the lesions had not been detected with white light, probably due to their small size. Peritoneal

53

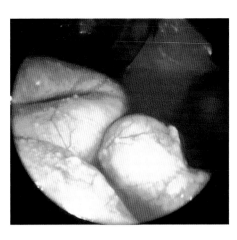

Fig. 53.43 Tuberculous peritonitis with ascites.

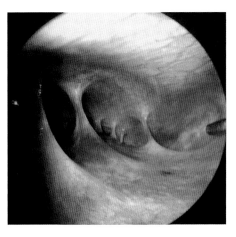

Fig. 53.44 Curtis–Fitz-Hugh syndrome. Perihepatitis is usually due to gonococcal infection, with "violin-string" adhesions between the right liver lobe and the anterior abdominal wall.

lavage cytology was positive in only four patients. Fluorescence for detecting metastases had a sensitivity and specificity of 92% and 95%, respectively [101].

Infectious Diseases

Tuberculous peritonitis. Tuberculous peritonitis is the most common and clinically most significant peritoneal infection. Although it is more prevalent in developing countries rather than developed ones, tuberculous peritonitis has become more frequent in recent years because of different patterns of migration and an increased number of patients with immunosuppression, especially those with AIDS.

In one of the largest series, including 135 patients, the clinical presentation was as follows: abdominal distension in 96%; weight loss in 80%; abdominal pain in 82%; weakness in 76%; anorexia in 73%; and fever in 69% [102]. The abdominal distension is usually due to ascites. Ascites studies reveal an exudate and an ascitic fluid cell count of more than 300/mL, with a predominance of lymphocytes. The ascites fluid is yellowish and cloudy. Smears and cultures for acid-fast bacilli are usually negative. The majority of patients do not have pulmonary or other organ tuberculosis. The study found that only two of the 135 had pulmonary lesions, while 10 had liver involvement [102]. The value of laparoscopy with peritoneal biopsy for achieving a rapid and correct diagnosis has repeatedly been demonstrated [102–107]. Laparoscopy reveals whitish-yellowish nodules, uniformly located over most if not all of the peritoneum. The nodules are miliary and 1–5 mm in diameter. Some may be confluent. The neovascularity does not allow differentiation between neoplastic and tuberculous lesions (**Fig. 53.43**). Biopsy material should be sent not only for histology, but also for tissue culture.

In the proliferative phase, the peritoneum will be thickened, dull, and irregular, with dense adhesions, especially between bowel loops. Laparoscopy at this stage may be hazardous, with a risk of intestinal perforation. In HIV-positive patients, atypical tuberculous peritonitis due to *Mycobacterium avium-intracellulare* may be found [98].

The liver may be involved in extrapulmonary tuberculosis (**Fig. 53.3**). Miliary lesions, which are often noncaseating in the liver, involve the entire parenchyma, including the hepatic surface, and may be indistinguishable from sarcoidosis. Biopsy for histology and culture is mandatory for a correct diagnosis.

Ascites of Unknown Cause

In most patients, the correct diagnosis of the cause of ascites can be made by routine laboratory screening tests, bacterial cultures, ascites amylase testing, and cytology studies of a cell block after centrifugation of the ascites fluid. Imaging studies with guided biopsy are useful as well. Laparoscopy is unsurpassed as the ideal test for evaluating patients with ascites of unknown cause. In a large study from Taiwan including 129 patients, carcinomatosis was found to be the most common cause, in 61% of the patients. Most of the patients were suffering from adenocarcinoma, with one mesothelioma; 20% had tuberculous peritonitis; and 5.4% had unsuspected cirrhosis [108]. Ovarian carcinoma is one of the most common causes of peritoneal spread in ascites. The undersurfaces of the diaphragm are a common site for seeding and should be carefully explored in all cases of ascites of unknown cause [109]. Other studies confirm that laparoscopy is the procedure of choice in this clinical setting.

Trujillo established a correct diagnosis in 89% of 43 patients with ascites of unknown cause [110]. Thirty-three percent were suffering from unsuspected cirrhosis, 26% from metastatic carcinoma, 21% had ovarian carcinoma, and 19% had tuberculous peritonitis. The different percentages for the same disease entities in these studies are of less importance, since disease patterns vary from one part of the world to another.

Perihepatitis

Right upper quadrant abdominal pain secondary to perihepatitis and adhesions from the anterior liver capsule to the anterior abdominal wall and diaphragm is known as Curtis–Fitz-Hugh syndrome. It is related to pelvic inflammation, most commonly gonococcal salpingitis and resulting peritonitis and perihepatitis [111,112]. Laparoscopy reveals adhesions with a "violin-string" appearance (**Fig. 53.44**). Laparoscopy must be carried out with the patient under mild sedation and not general anesthesia. Manipulation of the adhesions will reproduce the pain and may then allow lysis and pain relief.

Chronic and Acute Pain Syndromes

Postoperative adhesions are common, but usually asymptomatic. However, adhesions may become symptomatic short of intestinal obstruction, with sharp and circumscribed abdominal pain. If the pain is sharp, persistent, located in one region of the abdomen, remaining in the same location, more radiating, and is aggravated by activities that produce stretching between the pelvic organs, other abdominal structures, and the parietal peritoneum, it is often caused by adhesions. Gynecologists are more ready to accept this concept than surgeons or internists. Laparoscopy under sedation and analgesia is preferable over general anesthesia in this setting.

In a study spanning almost 20 years, the role of laparoscopy was explored in patients with acute and chronic abdominal pain [113]. In 265 well-selected patients with chronic pain, the laparoscopic findings were normal in 24%. A definitive diagnosis was made in 128 of the remaining 201 patients (64%), in whom laparoscopic operations were carried out—e. g., for adhesiolysis. In the remaining 73 patients (36%), multiple diagnoses were made.

In acute abdominal pain, a definitive diagnosis was made in 119 of 121 patients. Fifty-three had laparoscopic operations, 45 were treated medically, and 21 underwent laparotomy [113]. Similar results were obtained in 70 patients with chronic abdominal pain. With adhesiolysis, appendectomy, cholecystectomy, or hernia repair, more than 70% of patients experienced long-term pain relief [114].

There has been an explosive increase during the last 20 years in surgical applications extending beyond laparoscopic cholecystectomy. The diagnosis and management of patients with an acute abdomen remains a clinical challenge. If properly used, laparoscopy can reduce the incidence of unnecessary surgical procedures, such as appendectomy. This is especially important in women of childbearing age. In 65 patients with a generalized acute abdomen, laparoscopy led to a change in the surgical approach in 58% of cases, or to avoidance of unnecessary surgery [115]. In a retrospective study of 1220 patients, those undergoing a classic McBurney appendectomy had a normal appendix in 25%. For those in the laparoscopy group, the figure was only 8.2% [116]. In a multicenter study evaluating the role of laparoscopy in 1043 patients with a clinical diagnosis of appendicitis, appendectomy was performed in only 79%, with an appendicitis rate of 75%. Sixty-one percent of the appendectomies were carried out laparoscopically. A gynecological disorder was diagnosed in 15% of the women [117].

Intestinal obstruction with failure of medical management may best be managed laparoscopically rather than with an open laparotomy. In 167 patients who underwent diagnostic laparoscopy for intestinal obstruction, the most common etiologies were adhesions, hernias, and adenocarcinoma of the colon. Almost all patients were successfully treated laparoscopically [118].

Acute Abdomen, Blunt Abdominal Trauma

Laparoscopy is ideally suited for the evaluation and management of patients with an acute abdomen and blunt abdominal trauma after conventional evaluation, if they are hemodynamically stabile. Small-caliber laparoscopes (minilaparoscopy) can simplify the procedure without compromising visibility [119].

In a study of 100 patients with acute abdominal findings, a diagnosis was established laparoscopically in 92% of cases, followed by operative laparoscopy for appendectomy, cholecystectomy, and operations for ovarian cysts. Only 11% of the procedures had to be converted to open laparotomy. Eight percent were managed with primary laparotomy [120]. In 99 hemodynamically stable patients with abdominal trauma, which was blunt in 28 patients and penetrating in 71, laparoscopy was negative in 61% of those with blunt trauma and 60% of those with penetrating trauma. None of the laparoscopy-negative patients required a subsequent laparotomy. Laparoscopy shortened the hospital stay and was more cost-effective than laparotomy [121].

Minilaparoscopy can be safely carried out at the bedside in the intensive-care unit in critically ill patients in whom an abdominal cause of illness is suspected. In many cases, intestinal ischemia is identified [122].

The role of laparoscopy in patients with disorders of the liver and peritoneum is well established and is continuing to expand. Gastroenterologists should continue to foster this effective tool, which has stood the test of time.

References

1. Kalk H. Die chronischen Verlaufsformen der Hepatitis epidemica in Beziehung zu ihren anatomischen Grundlagen. Dtsch Med Wochenschr 1947;72:308–13.
2. Kalk H, Brühl W, Sieke E. Die gezielte Leberpunktion. Dtsch Med Wochenschr 1943;69:693.
3. Henning H, Lightdale CJ, Look D. Color atlas of laparoscopy. New York: Thieme; 1994.
4. Nakajima Y. Laparoscopic study of the scarred liver. Gastroenterol Endosc 1986;28:25–38.
5. Nord HJ. Biopsy diagnosis of cirrhosis: blind percutaneous versus guided direct vision techniques: a review. Gastrointest Endosc 1982;28:102–4.
6. Jeffers LJ, Findor A, Thung SN, Reddy R, Silva M, Schiff ER. Minimizing sampling error with laparoscopic guided liver biopsy of right and left lobes [abstract]. Gastrointest Endosc 1991;37:A266.
7. Abei M, Tanaka N, Matsumoto H, Chiba T, Matsuzaki Y, Nishi M, et al. Laparoscopic observation of liver colored with indocyanine green in chronic hepatitis, 1: improved sensitivity for diagnosis of fibrosis. Gastrointest Endosc 1993;39:406–9.
8. Abei M, Tanaka N, Matsumoto H, Matsuzaki Y, Osuga T. Laparoscopic observation of liver colored with indocyanine green in chronic hepatitis, 2: correlation with subcapsular ligandin. Gastrointest Endosc 1993;39:410–2.
9. Cardi M, Muttillo IA, Amadori L, Petroni R, Mingazzini P, Barillari P, et al. Superiority of laparoscopy compared to ultrasonography in diagnosis of widespread liver diseases. Dig Dis Sci 1997;42:546–8.
10. Ohkawa K, Hayashi N, Yuki N, Kasahara A, Oshita M, Mochizuki K, et al. Disease stage of chronic hepatitis C assessed by both peritoneoscopic and histologic findings and its relationship with response to interferon therapy. Gastrointest Endosc 1997;45:168–75.
11. Talwalkar JA, Kurtz DM, Schoenleber SJ, West CP, Montori VM. Ultrasound-based elastography for the detection of hepatic fibrosis: systematic review and meta-analysis. Clin Gastroenterol Hepatol 2007; 5: 1214–20.
12. Nudo CG, Jeffers LJ, Bejararo PA, Servin-Abad LA, Leibovici Z, De Medina M, et al. Correlation of laparoscopic liver biopsy to elasticity measurements (FibroScan) in patients with chronic liver disease. Gastroenterol Hepatol 2008;4:862–70.
13. Tatsumi C, Kudo M, Ueshima K, Kitai S, Takahashi S, Inoue T, et al. Noninvasive evaluation of hepatic fibrosis using serum fibrotic markers, transient elastography (FibroScan) and real-time tissue elastography. Intervirology 2008;51(Suppl 1):27–33.
14. Henning H, Look D. Das Cruveilhier-von Baumgarten Syndrom aus laparoskopischer Sicht. Z Gastroenterol 1970;8:133.
15. Meyer-Burg J. The lymphatic system of the liver, 2: direct laparoscopic observation of the lymphatic drainage with patent blue [98]Au and Lipiodol. Endoscopy 1973;5:32.
16. Tameda Y, Yoshizawa N, Takase K, Nakano T, Kosaka Y. Prognostic value of peritoneoscopic findings in cirrhosis of the liver. Gastrointest Endosc 1990;36:34–8.
17. Zotti S, Papaleo E, Marin G. Laparoscopy and liver biopsy in the morphological diagnosis of cirrhosis: concordance and diagnostic validity. Ital J Gastroenterol 1981;13:14–7.
18. Pagliaro L, Rinaldi F, Craxi A, Di Piazza S, Filippazzo G, Gatto G, et al. Percutaneous blind biopsy versus laparoscopy with guided biopsy in diagnosis of cirrhosis: a prospective randomized trial. Dig Dis Sci 1983;28:39–43.
19. Orlando R, Lirussi F, Okolicsangl L. Laparoscopy and liver biopsy—further evidence that the two procedures improve the diagnosis of cirrhosis: a retrospective study of 1,003 consecutive examinations. J Clin Gastroenterol 1990;12:47–52.
20. Poniachik J, Bernstein DE, Reddy KR, Jeffers LJ, Coelho-Little ME, Civantos F, et al. The role of laparoscopy in the diagnosis of cirrhosis. Gastrointest Endosc 1996;43:568–71.
21. Jalan R, Harrison DJ, Dillon JF, Elton RA, Finlayson ND, Hayes PC. Laparoscopy and histology in the diagnosis of chronic liver disease. QJM 1995;88:559–64.
22. Zotti S, Piccigallo E, Rumpinelli L, Romagnoli G, Tufano A, Dagnini G. Primary and metastatic tumors of the liver associated with cirrhosis: a study based on laparoscopy and autopsy. Gastrointest Endosc 1986;32:91–5.
23. Van Erpecum KJ, Janssens AR, Terpstra JL, Tjon A, Tham RT. Highly symptomatic adult polycystic disease of the liver. J Hepatol 1987;5:109–17.

53

24. Jeng KS, Yang FS, Kao CR, Huang SH. Management of symptomatic polycystic liver diseases: laparoscopy adjuvant with alcohol sclerotherapy. J Gastroenterol Hepatol 1995;10:359–62.

25. Eckardt V, Beck K. Benigne Hämiangiome der Leber. Leber Magen Darm 1974;4:337–42.

26. Wanless IR, Godwin TA, Allen F, Feder R. Nodular regenerative hyperplasias of the liver in hematologic disorders: a possible response to obliterative portal venography. Medicine 1980;59:367–79.

27. Izumi S, Nishiuchi M, Kameda Y, Nagano S, Fukunishi T, Kohro T, et al. Laparoscopic study of peliosis hepatis and nodular transformation of the liver before and after renal transplantation: natural history and aetiology in follow-up cases. J Hepatol 1994;20:129–37.

28. Ursin E, Spech HJ, Liehr H. Laparoskopie und Lebersarkoidose. Med Klin 1974;69:681–6.

29. Mulshine JL, Makuch RW, Johnston-Early A, Matthews MJ, Carney DN, Ihde DC, et al. Diagnosis and significance of liver metastases in small cell carcinoma of the lung. J Clin Oncol 1984;2:733–41.

30. DeSouza LJ, Shinde SR. The value of laparoscopic liver examination in the management of breast cancer. J Surg Oncol 1980;14:97–103.

31. Dagnini G, Caldironi MW, Marin G, Buzzaccarini O, Tremolada C, Ruol A. Laparoscopy in abdominal staging of esophageal carcinoma: report of 369 cases. Gastrointest Endosc 1986;32:400–2.

32. Brady PG, Goldschmid S, Chappel G, Slone FL, Boyd WP. A comparison of biopsy techniques in suspected focal liver disease. Gastrointest Endosc 1987;33:289–92.

33. Brady PG, Peebles M, Goldschmid S. Role of laparoscopy in the evaluation of patients with suspected hepatic or peritoneal malignancy. Gastrointest Endosc 1991;37:27–30.

34. Warshaw AL, Tepper JE, Shipley WV. Laparoscopy in staging and planning of therapy for pancreatic cancer. Am J Surg 1986;151:76–80.

35. Lightdale CJ, Hajdu SI, Luisi CB. Cytology of liver, spleen and peritoneum obtained by sheathed brush during laparoscopy. Am J Gastroenterol 1980;74:21–4.

36. Jeffers L, Spieglman G, Reddy R, Dubow R, Nadji M, Ganjei P, et al. Laparoscopically directed fine needle aspiration for the diagnosis of hepatocellular carcinoma: a safe and accurate technique. Gastrointest Endosc 1988;34:235–7.

37. Barbot DJ, Marks JH, Feld RI, Liu JB, Rosato FE. Improved staging of liver tumors using laparoscopic intraoperative ultrasound. J Surg Oncol 1997; 64:63–7.

38. Boyce HW, Nord HJ, Berci G. Laparoscopy. In: Yamada T, Alpers DH, Owyange C, Powell DW, Silverstein FE, editors. Textbook of gastroenterology. 2nd ed. Philadelphia: Lippincott; 1995. p. 2818–36.

39. Nord HJ. Technique of laparoscopy. In: Sivak MV, editor. Gastroenterologic endoscopy. 2nd ed. Philadelphia: Saunders; 2000. p. 1476–503.

40. Rivera JA, Fernandez del Castillo C, Warshaw AL. The preoperative staging of pancreatic adenocarcinoma. Adv Surg 1996;30:97–122.

41. Makary MA, Warshaw AL, Centeno BA, Willet CG, Rattner DW, Fernandez-del Castillo C. Implications of peritoneal cytology for pancreatic cancer management. Arch Surg 1998;133:361–5.

42. Stein HJ, Kraemer SJM, Feussner H, Fink U, Siewert JR. Clinical value of diagnostic laparoscopy with laparoscopic ultrasound in patients with cancer of the esophagus or cardia. J Gastrointest Surg 1997;1:167–73.

43. Watt I, Stewart I, Anderson D. Laparoscopy, ultrasound and computed tomography in cancer of the esophagus and gastric cardia: a prospective comparison for detecting intra-abdominal metastases. Br J Surg 1989;76:1038–9.

44. Hünerbein M, Rau B, Schlag PM. Laparoscopy and laparoscopic ultrasound for staging of upper gastrointestinal tumors. Eur J Surg Oncol 1995;21: 50–5.

45. Rau B, Hünerbein M, Reingruber B, Hohenberger P, Schlag PM. Laparoscopic lymph node assessment in pretherapeutic staging of gastric and esophageal cancer. Recent Results Cancer Res 1996;142:209–15.

46. Finch MD, John TG, Garden OJ, Allan PL, Paterson-Brown S. Laparoscopic ultrasonography for staging gastroesophageal cancer. Surgery 1997;121: 10–7.

47. Krasna MJ, Flowers JL, Attars S, McLaughlin J. Combined thoracoscopic/laparoscopic staging of esophageal cancer. J Thorac Cardiovasc Surg 1996;111:800–7.

48. Luketich JD, Schauer P, Landreneau R, Nguyen N, Urso K, Ferson P, et al. Minimally invasive surgical staging is superior to endoscopic ultrasound in detecting lymph node metastases in esophageal cancer. J Thorac Cardiovasc Surg 1997;114:817–21.

49. Kriplani AK, Kapur BML. Laparoscopy for pre-operative staging and assessment of operability of gastric carcinomas. Gastrointest Endosc 1991;37:441–3.

50. Burke EC, Karpeh MS, Conlon KC, Brennan ME. Laparoscopy in the management of gastric adenocarcinoma. Ann Surg 1997;225:262–7.

51. Lowy AM, Mansfield PF, Leach SD, Ajani J. Laparoscopic staging for gastric cancer. Surgery 1996;119:611–4.

52. Stell DA, Carter CR, Stewart I, Anderson JR. Prospective comparison of laparoscopy, ultrasonography and computed tomography in the staging of gastric cancer. Br J Surg 1996;83:1260–2.

53. D'Ugo DM, Coppola R, Persiani R, Ronconi P, Caracciolo F, Picciocchi A. Immediately preoperative laparoscopic staging for gastric cancer. Surg Endosc 1996;10:996–9.

54. Asencio F, Aguilo J, Salvador JL, Villar A, De la Morena E, Ahamad M, et al. Video-laparoscopic staging of gastric cancer: a prospective multicenter comparison with noninvasive techniques. Surg Endosc 1997;11:1153–8.

55. Charukhehyan SA. Lesser sac endoscopy in gastric carcinoma: operability assessment. Surg Laparosc Endosc 1998;8:9–13.

56. Feussner H, Omote K, Fink U, Walker SJ, Siewert JR. Pretherapeutic laparoscopic staging in advanced gastric carcinoma. Endoscopy 1999;31: 342–7.

57. Wilkiemeyer MB, Bieligk SC, Ashfaq R, Jones DB, Rege RV, Fleming JB. Laparoscopy alone is superior to peritoneal cytology in staging gastric and esophageal carcinomas. Surg Endosc 2004;18:852–6.

58. Meyer-Burg J. The inspection, palpation and biopsy for the pancreas. Endoscopy 1972;4:99–101.

59. Meyer-Burg J, Ziegler U, Kirstaedter HJ, Palmer G. Peritoneoscopy in carcinoma of the pancreas: report of 20 cases. Endoscopy 1973;5:86–90.

60. Ishida H. Peritoneoscopy and pancreas biopsy in the diagnosis of pancreatic diseases. 1983;29:211–8.

61. Warshaw AL, Gu ZY, Wittenberg J, Waltman AC. Preoperative staging and assessment of resectability of pancreatic cancer. Arch Surg 1990;125: 230–3.

62. Cuschieri A. Laparoscopy for pancreatic cancer: does it benefit the patient? Eur J Surg Oncol 1988;14:41–4.

63. Andrén-Sandberg A, Lindberg CG, Lundstedt C, Ihse I. Computed tomography and laparoscopy in the assessment of the patient with pancreatic cancer. J Am Coll Surg 1998;186:35–40.

64. Reddy KR, Levi J, Livingstone A, Jeffers L, Molina E, Kligerman S, et al. Experience with staging laparoscopy in pancreatic malignancy. Gastrointest Endosc 1999;49:498–503.

65. John TG, Greig JD, Carter DC, Garden OJ. Carcinoma of the pancreatic head and periampullary region: tumor staging with laparoscopy and laparoscopic ultrasonography. Ann Surg 1995;221:156–64.

66. Hann LE, Conlon KC, Dougherty EC, Hilton S, Bach AM, Brennan ME Laparoscopic sonography of peripancreatic tumors: preliminary experience. AJR Am J Roentgenol 1997;169:1257–62.

67. Fernandez-del Castillo C, Warshaw AL. Laparoscopy for staging in pancreatic carcinoma. Surg Oncol 1993;2:25–9.

68. Meduri F, Diana F, Merenda R, Caldironi MW, Zuin A, Losacco L, et al. Implication of laparoscopy and peritoneal cytology in the staging of early pancreatic cancer. Zentralbl Pathol 1994;140:243–6.

69. Nord HJ, Brady PG. Endoscopic diagnosis and therapy of hepatocellular carcinoma. Endoscopy 1993;25:126–30.

70. Shinagawa T, Ohio M, Kimura K, Tsunetomi S, Morita M, Saisho H, et al. Diagnosis and clinical features of small hepatocellular carcinoma with emphasis on the utility of real-time ultrasonography: a study in 51 patients. Gastroenterology 1984;86:495–502.

71. Lightdale CJ, Hajdu SI, Luisi CB. Cytology of the liver, spleen and peritoneum obtained by sheathed brush during laparoscopy. Am J Gastroenterol 1980;74:21–4.

72. Hajidu S, D'Ambrosio BA, Fields V. Aspiration and brush cytology of the liver. Semin Diagn Pathol 1986;3:238–77.

73. Jeffers L, Spieglman G, Reddy R, Dubow R, Nadji M, Ganjei P, et al. Laparoscopically directed fine needle aspiration for the diagnosis of hepatocellular carcinoma: a safe and accurate technique. Gastrointest Endosc 1988;34:235–7.

74. Gandolfi L, Muratori R, Solmi L, Rossi A, Leo P. Laparoscopy compared with ultrasonography in the diagnosis of hepatocellular carcinoma. Gastrointest Endosc 1989;35:508–11.

75. Fornari F, Rapaccini GL, Cavanna L, Civardi G, Anti M, Fedeli G, et al. Diagnosis of hepatic lesions: ultrasonically guided fine needle biopsy or laparoscopy? Gastrointest Endosc 1988;34:231–4.

76. Lightdale CJ. Laparoscopy and biopsy in malignant liver disease. Cancer 1982;50:2672–5.

77. Cusso X, Marti-Vicente A, Mones-Xiol J, Vilardell E. Laparoscopic cytology: an evaluation. Endoscopy 1988;20:102–3.

VIII

78. Kameda Y, Shinji Y. Early detection of hepatocellular carcinoma by laparoscopy: yellow nodules as diagnostic indications. Gastrointest Endosc 1992;38:554–9.

79. Kameda Y, Shinji T, Nishiuchi M. Detection of minute hepatocellular carcinoma with fatty metamorphosis by laparoscopy [abstract]. Endoscopy 1988;20 (Suppl):A29.

80. Weitz J, D'Angelica M, Jarnagin W, Gonen M, Fong Y, Blumgart L, et al. Selective use of diagnostic laparoscopy prior to planned hepatectomy for patients with hepatocellular carcinoma. Surgery 2004;135:273–81.

81. Lai EC, Tang CN, Ha JP, Tsui DK, Li MK. The evolving influence of laparoscopy and laparoscopic ultrasonography on patients with hepatocellular carcinoma. Am J Surg 2008;196:736–40.

82. Yamanaka N, Okamoto E, Tanaka T, Oriyama T, Fujimoto J, Furukawa K, et al. Laparoscopic microwave coagulonecrotic therapy for hepatocellular carcinoma. Surg Laparosc Endosc 1995;5:444–9.

83. Ido K, Isoda N, Kawamoto C, Hozumi M, Suzuki T, Nagamine N, et al. Laparoscopic microwave coagulation therapy for solitary hepatocellular carcinoma performed under laparoscopic ultrasonography. Gastrointest Endosc 1997;45:415–20.

84. Dagnini G, Marin G, Patella M, Zotti S. Laparoscopy in the diagnosis of primary carcinoma of the gallbladder. Gastrointest Endosc 1984;30:289–91.

85. Kriplani AK, Jagant S, Kapur BML. Laparoscopy in primary carcinoma of the gallbladder. Gastrointest Endosc 1992;38:326–9.

86. Givler RL, Brunk SF, Haas CA, Gulesserian HP. Problems of interpretation of liver biopsy in Hodgkin's disease. Cancer 1971;28:1335–42.

87. DeVita VT Jr, Bagley CM Jr, Goodell B, O'Kieffe DA, Trujillo NP. Peritoneoscopy in the staging of Hodgkin's disease. Cancer Res 1971; 31:1746–50.

88. Coleman M, Lightdale CJ, Vinciguerra VP, Degnan TJ, Goldstein M. Horwitz T, et al. Peritoneoscopy in Hodgkin's disease: confirmation of results by laparotomy. JAMA 1976;236:2634–6.

89. Dagnini G. Laparoscopy and imaging techniques. Berlin: Springer; 1990.

90. Sans M, Andreu V, Bordas JM, Llach J, Lopez-Guillermo A, Cervantes F, et al. Usefulness of laparoscopy with liver biopsy in the assessment of liver involvement at diagnosis of Hodgkin's and non-Hodgkin's lymphomas. Gastrointest Endosc 1998;47:391–5.

91. Beretta G, Spinelli P, Rilke F, Tancini G, Canetta R, Gennari L, et al. Sequential laparoscopy and laparotomy combined with bone marrow biopsy in staging Hodgkin's disease. Cancer Treat Rep 1976;60:1231–7.

92. Ferzli G, Fiorillo MA, Solis R, Sayad P, Riina L, Hallak A, et al. Laparoscopic staging of Hodgkin's disease. J Laparoendosc Adv Surg Tech A 1997;7:353–5.

93. Hansen SW, Jensen F, Pedersen NT, Pedersen AG, Hansen HH. Detection of liver metastases in small-cell lung cancer: a comparison of peritoneoscopy with liver biopsy and ultrasonography with fine-needle aspiration. J Clin Oncol 1987;5:255–9.

94. DeSouza LJ, Shinde SR. The value of laparoscopic liver examination in the management of breast cancer. J Surg Oncol 1980;14:97–103.

95. Goletti O, Celona G, Galatioto C, Viaggi B, Lippolis PV, Pieri L, et al. Is laparoscopic sonography a reliable and sensitive procedure for staging colorectal cancer? A comparative study. Surg Endosc 1998;12:1236–41.

96. Salky BA. Laparoscopic diagnosis of peritoneal mesothelioma. Gastrointest Endosc 1983;29:65–6.

97. Conion KC, Rusch VW, Gillerns S. Laparoscopy: an important tool in the staging of malignant pleural mesothelioma. Ann Surg Oncol 1996;3:489–94.

98. Jeffers LJ, Alzate I, Aguilar H, Reddy KR, Idrovo V, Cheinquer H, et al. Laparoscopic and histologic finding in patients with the human immunodeficiency virus. Gastrointest Endosc 1994;40:160–4.

99. Fernandez RN, Daly JM. Pseudomyxoma peritonei. Arch Surg 1980;115:409–14.

100. Denzer U, Hoffmann S, Helmreich-Becker I, Kauczor HU, Thelen M, Kanzler S, et al. Minilaparoscopy in the diagnosis of peritoneal tumor spread: prospective controlled comparison with computed tomography. Surg Endosc 2004;18:1067–70.

101. Löning M, Diddens H, Küpker W, Diedrich K, Hüttmann G. Laparoscopic fluorescence detection of ovarian carcinoma metastases using 5-aminolevulinic acid–induced protoporphyrin IX. Cancer 2004;100:1650–6.

102. Sandikci MU, Colakoglu S, Ergun Y, Unal S, Akkiz H, Sandikci S, et al. Presentation and role of peritoneoscopy in the diagnosis of tuberculosis peritonitis. J Gastroenterol Hepatol 1992;7:298–301.

103. Mimica M. Usefulness and limitations of laparoscopy in the diagnosis of tuberculosis peritonitis. Endoscopy 1992;24:588–91.

104. Bhargava DK, Shriniwas MD, Chopra P. Peritoneal tuberculosis: laparoscopic patterns and its diagnostic accuracy. Am J Gastroenterol 1992;87:109–12.

105. Nafeh MA, Medhat A, Abdul-Hameed AG, Ahmad YA, Rashwan NM, Strickland GT. Tuberculous peritonitis in Egypt: the value of laparoscopy in diagnosis. Am J Trop Med Hyg 1992;47:470–7.

106. Hossain J, Al-Aska AK, Mofleh IA. Laparoscopy in tuberculous peritonitis. J R Soc Med 1992;85:89–91.

107. Al Quorain AA, Satti MB, al Gindan YM, al Ghassab GA, al Freihi HM. Tuberculous peritonitis: the value of laparoscopy. Hepatogastroenterology 1991;38(Suppl 1):37–40.

108. Chu CM, Lin SM, Peng SM, Wu CS, Liaw YE. The role of laparoscopy in the evaluation of ascites of unknown origin. Gastrointest Endosc 1994;40: 285–9.

109. Bagley CM Jr, Young RC, Schein PS, Chabner BA, DeVita VT. Ovarian carcinoma metastatic to the diaphragm—frequently undiagnosed at laparotomy: a preliminary report. Am J Obstet Gynecol 1973;116:397–400.

110. Trujillo NP. Peritoneoscopy and guided biopsy in the diagnosis of intraabdominal disease. Gastroenterology 1976;71:1083–5.

111. Curtis AH. A cause of adhesions in the right upper quadrant. JAMA 1930;94:1221–2.

112. Fitz-Hugh T Jr. Acute gonococcic peritonitis of the right upper quadrant in women. JAMA 1934;102:2094–6.

113. Salky BA, Edye MB. The role of laparoscopy in the diagnosis and treatment of abdominal pain syndromes. Surg Endosc 1998;12:911–4.

114. Onders RP, Mittendorf EA. Utility of laparoscopy in chronic abdominal pain. Surgery 2003;134:549–52.

115. Cuesta MA, Eijsbouts QA, Gordijn RV, Borgstein PJ, de Jong D. Diagnostic laparoscopy in patients with an acute abdomen of uncertain etiology. Surg Endosc 1998;12:915–7.

116. Barrat C, Catheline JM, Rizk N, Champault GG. Does laparoscopy reduce the incidence of unnecessary appendicectomies? Surg Laparosc Endosc 1999;9:27–31.

117. Moberg AC, Ahlberg G, Leijonmarck CE, Montgomery A, Reiertsen O, Rosseland AR, et al. Diagnostic laparoscopy in 1043 patients with suspected acute appendicitis. Eur J Surg 1998;164:833–40.

118. Franklin ME Jr, Gonzalez JJ Jr, Miter DB, Glass JL, Paulson D. Laparoscopic diagnosis and treatment of intestinal obstruction. Surg Endosc 2004;18:26–30.

119. Helmreich-Becker I, Meyer zum Büschenfelde KH, Louse AW. Safety and feasibility of a new minimally invasive diagnostic laparoscopy technique. Endoscopy 1998;30:756–62.

120. Ahmad TA, Shelbaya E, Razek SA, Mohamed RA, Tajima Y, Ali SM, et al. Experience of laparoscopic management in 100 patients with acute abdomen. Hepatogastroenterology 2001;48:733–6.

121. Taner AS, Topgul K, Kucukel F, Demir A, Sari S. Diagnostic laparoscopy decreases the rate of unnecessary laparotomies and reduces hospital costs in trauma patients. J Laparoendosc Adv Surg Tech 2001;11:207–11.

122. Pecoraro AP, Cacchione RN, Sayad P, Williams ME, Ferzli GS. The routine use of diagnostic laparoscopy in the intensive care unit. Surg Endosc 2001;15:638–41.

53

IX

Infectious Diseases of the Gastrointestinal Tract

Section editors:
Guido N.J. Tytgat, Charles J. Lightdale, Michael B. Wallace

54 Infectious Diseases of the Intestines

Paul Feuerstadt and Lawrence J. Brandt

Introduction

Patients usually consider diarrhea to be an increased frequency or liquidity of their stool. By contrast, physicians' definitions are more quantitative—e. g., an increase in the frequency of stool to three or more episodes per day, or a weight greater than 200 g in 24 h, without mention of stool consistency [1]. Diarrhea can be classified on the basis of its causative mechanisms—i. e., osmotic or secretory—and the duration of disease, with acute diarrhea lasting less than 2 weeks, persistent diarrhea being more than 2 weeks, and chronic diarrhea lasting longer than 4 weeks [2]. Acute diarrhea is a frequently encountered problem, with an estimated 1.0–1.4 cases per person per year [3]. Although the most common etiology of acute diarrhea is infection, and physicians are consulted for over 8 million cases yearly, a specific etiology is identified in only a minority of such cases [4,5]. In cases for which history, physical examination, stool microbiology, and serologic studies do not clarify the diagnosis, endoscopy may be useful, offering direct visualization of the affected bowel surfaces and the ability to obtain tissue specimens.

Clinical Features

History

The differential diagnosis of acute infectious diarrhea is very broad, but a comprehensive clinical history is useful to help the clinician guide evaluation and diagnosis. This history should include risk factors for human immunodeficiency virus and acquired immune deficiency syndrome (HIV/AIDS) and other co-morbid medical conditions resulting in chronic immunosuppression (e. g., diabetes, malignancy, liver disease, or organ transplantation), as these factors will broaden the list of infectious etiologies that should be considered. The presence of immunosuppression, however, only expands the number of possible infections to which the affected patient is prone, and so the traditional medical history, including exposure to potentially infectious persons, new medications, recently ingested food, travel, etc., is still clinically important.

Characteristics of the stool, such as its volume, consistency, and the presence of blood also are useful in determining the cause of diarrhea. Large-volume, watery bowel movements with diffuse, cramping abdominal pain are most consistent with a small-bowel etiology. Alternatively, colonic disease presents with a smaller volume of more formed stool accompanied by blood and mucus, as well as lower abdominal cramping and rectal symptoms, including tenesmus and urgency. Given the fluid-absorptive properties of the colon, disease of this organ can sometimes be localized on the basis of the consistency of the stool, with looser stool associated with causes in the proximal colon and more formed stool resulting from disease in the distal colon.

When an infectious etiology of diarrhea is being considered, obtaining a history of recent travel, hospitalization, contact with other ill individuals, and food intake is useful. Individuals who have recently been to mountainous areas should be tested for *Giardia lamblia*. Alternatively, if the patient has been hospitalized or has had a course of antibiotics, *Clostridium difficile* should be considered.

Giardia, Cryptosporidium, and *Shigella* are likely etiologies in patients who have spent time in day-care facilities for children. If a food-borne or water-borne pathogen is likely, the time since ingestion is important. Symptoms presenting within 6 h of ingestion are consistent with preformed bacterial toxins (e. g., *Staphylococcus aureus* or *Bacillus cereus*). Alternatively, if symptoms occur within 8–14 hours of ingestion, *Clostridium perfringens* is likely. Finally, a viral etiology is most likely when the lapse between ingestion and the onset of diarrhea is greater than 14 h.

It is important to consider noninfectious causes of diarrhea as well. Any recent changes in medication or diet are essential for a complete history. The addition of nutritional supplements (e. g., magnesium) or illicit drugs (e. g., cocaine) should be considered. Sugar-free products (possibly containing sorbitol and other poorly absorbed sugars, resulting in osmotic diarrhea), increased alcohol intake, or caffeine can alter bowel habits as well. Finally, one must consider index presentations of inflammatory bowel disease, irritable bowel syndrome, ischemic disorders, and fecal impaction as possible etiologies; it is rare, however, for Crohn's disease and ulcerative colitis to have their onset in a person with immunocompromise due to advanced HIV infection.

Physical Examination

In assessing a patient with acute infectious diarrhea, the physical examination is useful for establishing the severity of disease. Signs of severe infection include fever, hypovolemia (tachycardia, hypotension, dry mucous membranes, and low urine output), severe abdominal pain, distension, and decreased bowel sounds. These and other "alarm symptoms"—such as an inability to tolerate oral fluids, stools that contain blood and mucus, dysentery (passage of six or more stools, often with blood and mucus, per 24-h period or duration of illness ≥ 48 h), diarrhea with severe abdominal pain in immunocompromised patients (AIDS, transplant patients, patients whom have received chemotherapy) or persons ≥ 50 years of age—should indicate to the clinician the need for prompt medical evaluation [6]. Using this information, one can decide whether hospitalization or immediate intervention is necessary. Patients with dysentery may benefit from antimicrobial therapy [7]. The most common pathogens to cause diarrhea are *Campylobacter, Shigella, Salmonella,* and invasive *Escherichia coli* [6]. Patients who are immunocompromised or over 50 years of age are at higher risk for complications and fatality related to diarrhea [8–10].

Diagnostic Testing

As most acute diarrheal illness is self-limited (lasting < 24 h), patients presenting within 1 day of symptomatic onset do not usually require further investigation and management unless they are dehydrated, febrile, or have blood or pus in their stool [3]. These patients should have their blood drawn for a complete blood count, electrolytes, blood urea nitrogen, creatinine, and culture.

Stool cultures should *not* be obtained routinely, as the diagnostic yield of routine stool culture is estimated to be only 2–12 % [11–13].

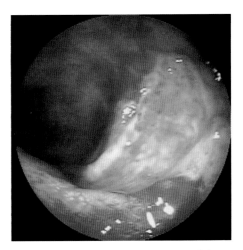

Fig. 54.1 The endoscopic appearance of this large rectal ulcer is consistent with cytomegalovirus (CMV), but biopsy indicated both CMV and *Cryptosporidium.*

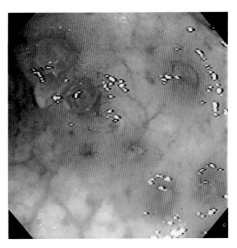

Fig. 54.2 The endoscopic appearance is consistent with cytomegalovirus (CMV), but the biopsy results showed acid-fast bacilli and no CMV inclusion bodies.

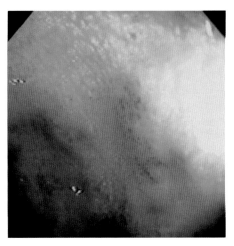

Fig. 54.3 Endoscopic appearance of infectious colitis: patchy erythema and ulceration is characteristic, but not pathognomonic, of this usually self-limited disease.

The diagnostic yield of a stool culture, however, increases in patients with high fever (temperature > 38.5 °C, 101.5 °F), bloody diarrhea, or if the stool contains leukocytes, lactoferrin, or occult blood [6]; these factors are predictive for identifying bacterial pathogens [11–14]. Tests of colonic inflammation such as fecal leukocytes, lactoferrin, or fecal occult blood are useful, as elevations in any of these are commonly caused by *E. coli* O157:H7, *Shigella, Salmonella, Campylobacter,* and less often *Aeromonas, Yersinia,* and noncholera vibrios [14–16]. All of these pathogens can be found on routine stool culture, and although some states require screening for *E. coli* O157:H7 in all patients with bloody diarrhea, only 68 % of hospitals screen for this pathogen [17–19]. In patients presenting with bloody diarrhea and with a low fecal leukocyte count, the clinician should consider *Entamoeba histolytica* amebiasis [20,21] .

Routine evaluation of stool for ova and parasites—e. g., for *Giardia lamblia, Trichuris trichiura, Entamoeba histolytica, Ascaris lumbricoides,* and *Strongyloides stercoralis*—should not be conducted in all patients with acute diarrhea, as it is not a cost-effective test [22–24]. The utility of a stool ova and parasite examination increases if patients have traveled to an endemic area, are recent immigrants from an endemic area, or have children in day care. In such individuals, one to two stool specimens should be sent for ova and parasite analysis [25,26]. In the past decade, the use of alternative stool tests for rapid results has increased. The enzyme immunoassay and fluorescent antibody assay tests for both *Giardia* and *Cryptosporidium* have shown excellent sensitivity and specificity when indicated [27–29].

In patients with acute infectious diarrhea, the American College of Gastroenterology recommends that colonoscopy be performed only in those with persistent diarrhea that has not responded to a course of therapy or in homosexual men with diarrhea. In immunocompromised patients, flexible sigmoidoscopy is recommended for tenesmus, increased fecal leukocytes and blood, dysentery, or stools with low bulk [6]. Colonoscopy is indicated in patients with chronic or nonspecific diarrhea with stool studies and barium enema that are unrevealing [30,31]. In order to maximize the diagnostic yield of colonoscopy in patients with diarrhea, random mucosal biopsies and ileoscopy should be performed [32–34]. Direct endoscopic inspection sometimes can be characteristic of a certain infection, while the mucosal biopsy specimen may reveal another organism (**Fig. 54.1**) or even a different diagnosis (**Fig. 54.2**). Culturing fluid obtained during the colonoscopy and biopsy specimens

also increases the information obtained during the procedure, but one should be aware of the potential contamination with *Pseudomonas* or *Serratia* found in tap water used to rinse endoscopes after disinfection [35,36].

■ Differentiating Infectious Colitis from Inflammatory Bowel Disease

Infectious etiologies and inflammatory bowel disease (IBD) must be considered in the differential diagnosis for an acute diarrheal illness. The history a patient provides can help differentiate the two entities. Infectious colitis usually has an acute onset, fever early in the course of disease, and more than 10 bowel movements in 24 h; IBD typically has an insidious onset, fewer than six stools a day, and fever that is delayed unless the patient is severely ill [37]. Physical examination can also provide some insight into the location of the disease, although it usually does not help differentiate infectious diarrhea from IBD. Although an elevated white blood cell count does not favor either diagnosis, anemia, thrombocytosis, and a decrease in albumin all support IBD.

Direct mucosal visualization can be helpful during prolonged illness, acute illness when steroids are being considered, or when a specific diagnosis is needed. Infectious colitis and Crohn's disease are typically patchy (**Fig. 54.3**) in comparison with the continuous disease seen in ulcerative colitis (**Fig. 54.4 a**) and occasionally in bypass colitis (**Fig. 54.4 b**). Random biopsies taken from both affected and unaffected mucosa can help yield a diagnosis, although it is rare that a specific infection—e. g., amebiasis, schistosomiasis, tuberculosis, and some others—can be diagnosed. In infectious colitis, the crypt architecture usually is preserved, the inflammatory infiltrate typically includes neutrophils without an increase in lymphocytes or plasma cells between the crypt base and the muscularis mucosa, and there is sparse basilar infiltration (**Fig. 54.5**) [38]. Conversely, crypt atrophy and crypt distortion (branching of glands), mixed acute and chronic cell–induced inflammation of the lamina propria, and basilar plasma cells with or without lymphocytes are typical of IBD (**Fig. 54.6**) [38–40].

54

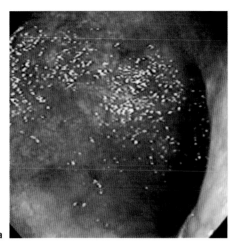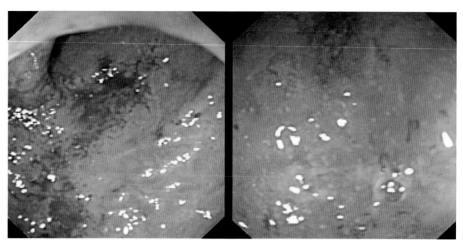

a

b

Fig. 54.4 Endoscopic appearance of ulcerative colitis and bypass colitis. **a** Ulcerative colitis is characterized by diffuse mucosal edema, granularity, microerosions, and friability.

b Bypass colitis may mimick infectious colitis when inflammatory abnormalities are patchy or diffuse (b).

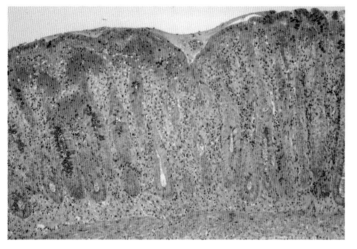

Fig. 54.5 Histology of infectious colitis (acute *Salmonella* colitis). Note the preservation of the normal crypt architecture, with straight glands, and the predominantly acute inflammation with polymorphonuclear leukocytes throughout the lamina propria.

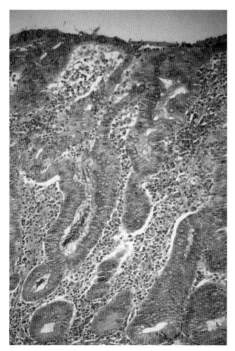

Fig. 54.6 Histology of ulcerative colitis. Note the distorted crypts and basal lamina propria inflammation, with lymphocytes and plasma cells.

Treatment

Assessing the volume status is of primary concern in the initial management of a patient with acute diarrhea. Patients with volume depletion should be evaluated and rehydrated quickly. The method used to rehydrate the patient depends on the clinical scenario. Most patients will respond to a standard formulation of oral rehydration therapy using a glucose-based electrolyte solution; patients with profuse watery diarrhea, however, may have extensive small-intestinal injury that can impair absorption of oral solutions and cause a subsequent secondary osmotic diarrhea. Intravenous fluids are most appropriate both in this circumstance and when the patients are severely hypovolemic or lack sufficient mental status to take oral solutions [1]. Alternatively, a diet of bananas, rice, apple sauce and toast (the "BRAT" diet) while avoiding milk products can be recommended, despite limited evidence to support its efficacy [41].

Antimotility agents should not be used in patients with bloody or suspected inflammatory diarrhea if the patients are severely ill. These agents have been implicated in the development of toxic megacolon in patients with *C. difficile* infection and hemolytic–uremic syndrome in children infected with Shiga toxin–producing *E. coli* [42]. Loperamide is the antimotility drug of choice in adults, given its ability to produce symptomatic relief without penetration of the nervous system and minimal risk of addiction [43]. Despite decreased efficacy in comparison with loperamide, bismuth subsalicylate has also been shown to diminish diarrhea, nausea, and abdominal pain in patients with traveler's diarrhea [44,45].

Patients should be carefully assessed before antibiotic treatment is considered. If the etiology of suspected infectious diarrhea is not known, it may not be wise to use antibiotics, as they are believed to prolong the shedding of certain bacteria (salmonella or *C. difficile*) and to increase the complication rate in patients with Shiga toxin–producing *E. coli* infection [46,47]. In patients who are severely ill, or in those who are believed to have a bacterial pathogen, empiric fluoroquinolones are the agent of choice [48]. The second-line empiric therapy for those allergic to fluoroquinolones is trimethoprim-sulfamethoxazole, although there is growing bacterial resistance to this drug in the community. When the cause of the diarrhea is known, there are specific guidelines for each etiology.

Specific Organisms

Viruses

Endoscopy plays a role in the diagnosis of viral infections mainly for evaluating colitis in immunosuppressed individuals. The endoscopic appearance of viral colitis ranges from normal-appearing mucosa, characteristic features (e. g., amphophilic or eosinophilic nuclear inclusions, predominantly affecting the surface epithelium and characteristically involving goblet cells in adenovirus colitis), to severe ulcerations (CMV colitis). Biopsies taken in children with viral gastroenteritis can show flattening of the small-intestinal villi.

Cytomegalovirus (CMV) is the most common viral cause of diarrhea in AIDS patients and may affect any part of the gastrointestinal tract. It also causes invasive disease in patients with solid organ transplants [49,50] and can cause severe infection in immunocompetent individuals [51,52]. Latent CMV is believed to reactivate in immunocompromised individuals, leading to viremia, deposition of viral particles in the vascular endothelium, vasculitis, and resultant submucosal ischemia and ulceration [49].

Endoscopy plays an important role in the diagnosis of CMV colitis [53]. As some reports have shown that more than one-third of the affected individuals have gross disease only proximal to the sigmoid colon, colonoscopy rather than flexible sigmoidoscopy may be needed to locate evidence of infection [54]. The appearance of the mucosa on endoscopy may resemble that of ulcerative colitis, with granularity and mucosal friability, and patients may occasionally have mass lesions that may be mistaken for colonic neoplasms. More typical of CMV infection, however, is the presence of colitis alone (defined by edema and subepithelial hemorrhage, **Fig. 54.7**), colitis with ulceration, or discrete, variably sized ulcers ranging from 5 mm to < 2 cm in areas of otherwise normal mucosa [55,56].

A definitive diagnosis of CMV colitis is made by identifying typical inclusion bodies in biopsy specimens, and not by serologic studies or culture of biopsy material [57]. CMV can be confirmed as the cause of inclusions using immunoperoxidase staining, in situ hybridization, or PCR. Multiple biopsies from the centers of ulcerations are recommended, as viral inclusions are found most frequently in the endothelial cells of the deeper layers of the gut wall. Treatment with intravenous ganciclovir, foscarnet, or cidofovir has improved symptoms, but not mortality [58,59].

Herpes simplex virus (HSV) is a common cause of proctitis, along with *Neisseria gonorrhoeae*, *Chlamdyia trachomatis*, and *Treponema pallidum* in men who have sex with men [60]. Typically, transmission is via direct inoculation during anoreceptive intercourse. Symptoms of HSV proctitis include anorectal burning, pruritus ani, tenesmus, diarrhea, constipation, and mucoid or bloody bowel movements, often with bilateral tender inguinal lymphadenopathy. Some patients also develop symptoms suggestive of lumbosacral radiculopathy, including impotence, pain localized to the thigh, buttocks, and lower abdomen, and inability to urinate [61].

Approximately 1–3 weeks following infection, the perianal skin, anal canal, and rectum will be affected with multiple vesicles, which soon evolve into aphthous ulcers. Endoscopically, involvement tends to be localized to the distal 5–10 cm of the rectum, where the initial lesions are seen as small single or grouped vesicles surrounded by erythema. These lesions subsequently coalesce to form aphthous ulcers. Biopsy of the rectum or anal canal may reveal typical intranuclear inclusion bodies or multinucleated giant cells. Viral culture is usually not necessary. Symptomatic treatment includes sitz baths, topical anesthetics, and oral pain medication; acyclovir (first-line treatment), valacyclovir, and famciclovir are potential antiviral treatments [61].

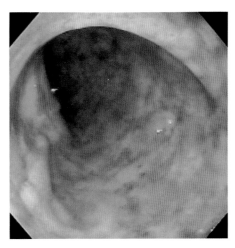

Fig. 54.7 Cytomegalovirus colitis. The endoscopic image shows the sigmoid colon, with edema and diffuse subepithelial hemorrhage. While the appearance is not pathognomonic of cytomegalovirus, these features are characteristic.

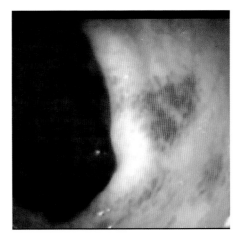

Fig. 54.8 *Shigella* colitis. Note the nonspecific inflammation, edema, and submucosal hemorrhage with punctate lesions.

54

Bacteria

Shigella. Humans and other primates are the only reservoir of *Shigella,* and all infection is therefore the result of person-to-person spread, either directly or through contaminated food or water. Approximately 6.3 cases of shigellosis per 100 000 people, most of which are caused by *S. sonnei*, occur in the United States each year [62]. Shigellosis, also known as acute bacillary dysentery, tends to occur in members of confined groups where there is crowding, poor sanitation, or a large number of children (typically aged 1–4 years) [63].

Shigella is extremely infectious, and ingestion of small numbers of organisms may produce disease in healthy individuals, in part because the bacterium is resistant to gastric acid [64,65]. Those infected with *Shigella* may experience fever, signs and symptoms of systemic toxicity, nausea, cramps and watery followed by bloody diarrhea with tenesmus, the sequence of symptoms paralleling the descent of the organisms down through the gastrointestinal tract [66]. The typical incubation period is 1–7 days. Initially, organisms multiply in the small bowel, causing secretion of fluid and electrolytes. Later, *Shigella* bacteria penetrate colonic mucosal epithelial cells, multiply, and spread, producing inflammation and superficial ulcerations [67]. Colonoscopy can reveal continuous, diffuse, nonspecific inflammation, edema (**Fig. 54.8**), and occasionally ulcerations with overlying exudates, friability, and punctate lesions, depending on the timing of the procedure from the onset of infection [68]. The colonic manifestations of *Shigella* are usually seen in the rectosigmoid region, with decreased findings proximally [69]. Given these macroscopic findings, occasionally a subacute presentation of

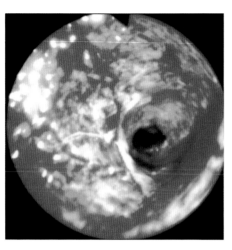

Fig. 54.9 *Campylobacter* colitis. Note the diffuse colitis and bleeding.

shigellosis can be confused with ulcerative colitis. Biopsies of affected areas reveal an intense acute inflammatory reaction with polymorphonuclear leukocytes, hemorrhage, and ulcer. Typically there is also edema, crypt abscess formation, crypt architecture distortion, loss of goblet cells, and organisms in the colonic mucosa [67]. The diagnosis is typically clinical, although stool culture and PCR may be helpful. Currently, there are no useful serological tests. Although shigellosis is usually a self-limited disease, treatment with antibiotics such as fluoroquinolones, azithromycin, and ceftriaxone shortens the duration of symptoms and stool carriage of the organism [70].

Salmonella infection produces a variety of overlapping clinical syndromes, including acute gastroenteritis or enterocolitis with diarrhea, enteric fever with diarrhea that may be complicated by intestinal hemorrhage, and a carrier state. The estimated incidence in the United States is 14.92 cases per 100 000, the vast majority of which are caused by the various serotypes of *S. enteritidis* [62]. *Salmonella* is a major cause of food-borne outbreaks of diarrheal disease from poultry, meat, eggs, and dairy products.

Ingestion of *S. typhi* may result in systemic manifestations, as well as abdominal pain, bloating, and constipation, followed by diarrhea. Colonoscopy is of little use in establishing *S. typhi* as the cause of symptoms, since focal hemorrhage, friability, and ulcerations are nonspecific findings that may resemble those in other infectious diarrheas or in IBD [71]. Toxic megacolon and perforation may complicate typhoid fever, and caution is therefore needed when considering colonoscopy in these patients [72]. The diagnosis of typhoid fever is confirmed by blood and stool cultures and serologic tests.

Nontyphoidal salmonellae also are transmitted via ingestion and may produce many of the clinical symptoms of *S. typhi*, although acute gastroenteritis and enterocolitis are the most common. *Salmonella* gastroenteritis and enterocolitis are characterized by a sudden onset of vomiting, colicky abdominal pain, and diarrhea that is the color and consistency of pea soup. Diarrheal stools may contain occult or gross blood, and affected individuals have systemic signs and symptoms of bacterial infection. Colonoscopy reveals only nonspecific changes, and the diagnosis is made on the basis of a history of potential exposure, the clinical presentation, the presence of leukocytes in the stool, and a positive stool culture. Transient carriers of *Salmonella* and most patients with enterocolitis do not require antibiotic therapy, which actually may prolong excretion of organisms in stool and increase the relapse rate, although patients who are very sick, the elderly, and those with AIDS should be treated [73].

Campylobacter jejuni is responsible for more than 98 % of enteric infections from *Campylobacter* species, and is the second most common cause of infectious colitis in the United States after *Salmo-*nella [62]. Person-to-person spread through fecal–oral transmission is the most common route of infection, although campylobacteriosis is also caused by ingestion of contaminated milk, exposure to sick pets, and ingestion of tainted poultry, eggs, or contaminated water supplies.

Individuals infected with *Campylobacter* usually develop nausea, anorexia, cramping abdominal pain, and either profuse watery or grossly bloody diarrhea 1–6 days after ingesting the organism [74]. Abdominal pain and tenderness in patients with campylobacteriosis (as in yersiniosis) may mimic appendicitis [75]. *C. jejuni* probably invades and injures the colonic epithelium in a manner similar to *Shigella,* involving multiple bacterial virulence factors and epithelial cell invasion [76].

As in salmonellosis and shigellosis, the inflammatory changes seen on biopsy specimens from patients with chronic disease are nonspecific and resemble those of IBD, especially ulcerative colitis. Definitive diagnosis only can be made via stool culture, although thorough clinical assessment and microscopic examination of the stool showing sheets of motile, comma-shaped rods may support the diagnosis. Colonoscopy may show patchy areas of erythema and erosion (**Fig. 54.9**), and biopsy specimens show findings ranging from minor nonspecific colitis to more severe colitis with goblet cell depletion and crypt abscess formation. Although the infection is usually self-limited, studies have shown that treatment with antibiotics such as macrolides and fluoroquinolones (with growing resistance) within the first 3 days of symptom onset can shorten the duration of disease [77].

Yersinia enterocolitica is seen infrequently in the United States, with an estimated annual incidence of 0.36 per 100 000 people [62]. Yersiniosis is most common in children under 5 years of age and is usually less severe in adults. It is transmitted via ingestion of products from streams and lake water, animals either as food sources or pets, as well as contaminated food such as milk and ice cream [78].

Patients can present with several syndromes when infected with *Yersinia,* enterocolitis being the most common. Fever, abdominal cramping, and diarrhea for 1–3 weeks are characteristic of this infection, and profuse watery diarrhea is sometimes observed [79]. *Y. enterocolitica* usually targets and invades the epithelium overlying Peyer patches in the terminal ileum. Following invasion of the epithelium, it proliferates in the lymphoid follicles and then spreads to the lamina propria. Given the resultant adenitis and ileal inflammation, disease presentations can be confused with appendicitis and possibly IBD [80]. Stool culture is the only way to diagnose Y. enterocolitica definitively. Given the nature of the infection, colonoscopy is unlikely to aid in the diagnosis. Antibiotic treatment is not usually indicated, as the diagnosis is usually made after the patient has started to improve and there is no evidence showing that treatment alters the clinical course [81].

Escherichia coli belongs to the normal flora found in the bowel in humans and animals. Although most species are not pathogenic, three classes of *E. coli* (enterotoxigenic, enteropathogenic, and enteroadherent) affect the small bowel, producing secretory diarrhea, and two other classes—enteroinvasive *E. coli* (EIEC) and enterohemorrhagic *E. coli* (EHEC)—cause proctocolitis with bloody diarrhea.

E. coli O157:H7, the principal EHEC responsible for hemorrhagic colitis, is seen relatively infrequently in the population, but occurs in outbreaks from infected undercooked beef, produce, and many other vectors [82]. A common timeline of E. coli O157:H7 infection begins with an incubation period of 3–8 days, followed by 1–2 days of nonbloody diarrhea progressing to bloody diarrhea [83]. Hemorrhagic colitis may be complicated by the hemolytic uremic syndrome (HUS) in 10–30 % of patients, resulting from the effects of two shiga-like toxins [84]. Pathologically, bacterial adherence factors aid in attaching the organism to the intestinal epithelium and allow direct delivery of cytotoxic substances (e. g., Stx2 toxin) to the gut mucosa and endothelial cells.

Endoscopic examination of patients with hemorrhagic colitis due to E. coli O157:H7 demonstrates focal, segmental, submucosal hemorrhage and edema, erythema, superficial ulcerations and pseudomembranes, and changes that may resemble those of ischemic colitis. *E. coli* O157:H7 toxins induce vascular thrombi and may produce colonic ischemia. The most severe changes typically occur in the ascending and transverse colon, as segmental colitis [85,86]. Barium enema radiography may reveal thumbprinting (**Fig. 54.10**), and biopsy specimens show superficial inflammation, an ischemic appearance, and early pseudomembrane formation. As in all forms of infectious colitis, diagnosis depends on a thorough clinical evaluation, followed by microscopic examination and culture of stool to establish the specific etiology. Although many clinical microbiology laboratories are now routinely checking stool culture specimens for E. coli O157:H7, some centers require specific requests for culture on McConkey sorbitol agar, since E. coli O157:H7 colonies are characteristically sorbitol-negative [87]. Uncomplicated *E. coli* O157:H7 infection usually lasts 5–10 days and resolves spontaneously, although in some outbreaks more than 40% of patients have needed hospitalization. Management of patients with mild to moderate infection is controversial, but most recommendations favor avoidance of antibiotics and antidiarrheal agents; use of these agents may foster the release and binding of toxins from dying organisms. Treatment of severe disease and HUS is beyond the scope of this chapter [83].

Tuberculosis. Both *Mycobacterium tuberculosis* and *Mycobacterium avium complex* (MAC) infections can occur in immunocompetent hosts, as well as in AIDS patients. The clinical presentation of gastrointestinal tuberculosis is variable. The most common features, in descending order of frequency, include abdominal pain, distension, weight loss, diarrhea, nausea, vomiting, and a palpable right lower quadrant mass [88]. The gastrointestinal virulence is believed to be caused by ingested bacilli passing through Peyer patches and then being transported to mesenteric lymph nodes via macrophages. The resulting mucosal inflammatory cell infiltration, lymph-node enlargement, and edema are believed to cause symptomatic disease [89].

Patients with MAC typically have diarrheal disease in the setting of systemic infection. Endoscopic evaluation may be entirely normal or may reveal erythema, edema, erosions, ulcers, or whitish nodules (**Fig. 54.11**). The changes may resemble those in Crohn's disease when the ileocecal area is affected. Colonic biopsies are diagnostically reliable, but peripheral blood culture is a more sensitive test for disseminated MAC [90]. Stool culture is the best way to differentiate MAC from tuberculosis.

Gastrointestinal tuberculosis most often involves the terminal ileum and cecum (**Fig. 54.12**), and can therefore occasionally be confused with Crohn's disease. The ascending and transverse colon and anorectum may also be affected, even in the absence of ileocecal disease (**Fig. 54.13**) [91]. Three patterns of disease are recognized: ulcerative, hypertrophic, and a mixed form. The ulcerative form appears as multiple superficial lesions of the epithelial surface, whereas the hypertrophic variety is characterized by scarring, fibrotic changes, and mass lesions that resemble carcinoma. The mixed type has combined features of the other two [92].

Colonoscopic examination shows segmental disease (usually with two or more segments involved), the mucosal surface being erythematous, edematous, and ulcerated, often with cobblestoning (**Fig. 54.14**) [93]. In contrast to the ulcers in Crohn's disease, which tend to parallel the longitudinal axis of the bowel, tuberculous ulcers tend to be circumferential, with their long axis perpendicular to the bowel lumen. When these ulcers heal, they produce strictures that narrow the lumen. Radiologic imaging may show these lesions, along with bowel wall thickening. Diagnosis is made by identifying the organisms in the tissues and by culture. Colonic biopsy may

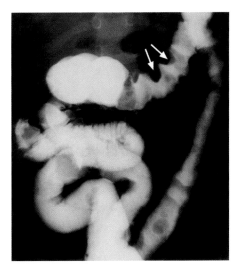

Fig. 54.10 Barium enema, demonstrating thumbprinting pattern (arrows) in the transverse colon of a child with *E. coli* O157:H7 hemorrhagic colitis. (Photograph provided by Phillip Tarr, MD and Dennis Shaw MD, Seattle; reprinted courtesy of the *New England Journal of Medicine*.)

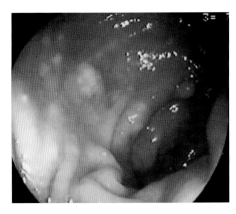

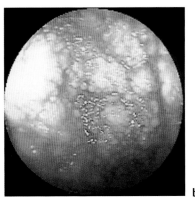

Fig. 54.11 *Mycobacterium avium* complex colitis.
a Erythema and edema.
b Whitish nodules.

54

show granulomas, sometimes without caseation, in the mucosa and submucosa. Although evidence is limited, a three-drug treatment with isoniazid, pyrazinamide, and rifampin (with addition of ethambutol or streptomycin in AIDS patients) are the standard of care [94].

Clostridium difficile-induced pseudomembranous colitis (PMC) has an estimated incidence in the United States of 6.9 cases per 100 000 people and is rapidly increasing [95]. While *C. difficile* is not considered to be part of the normal bowel flora, it is found in the stools of up to 3% of healthy adults, in many infants [96,97], and in up to 30% of hospitalized patients [98]. Pseudomembranous colitis (PMC) most commonly occurs after antibiotic therapy has disturbed the ecology of the colon, allowing *C. difficile* to proliferate. In addition, PMC may occur spontaneously in critically ill individuals, is believed by some to occur almost twice as often in patients treated with proton-pump inhibitors, and is found with increased frequency in the elderly and those with immunocompromise, including patients with HIV/AIDS [99].

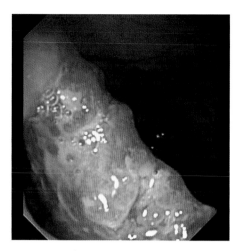

Fig. 54.12 Characteristic tuberculous ulceration of the ileocecal valve.

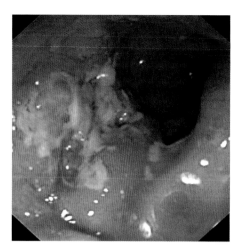

Fig. 54.13 Confluent tuberculous ulceration. Note the absence of longitudinal alignment of the ulcers.

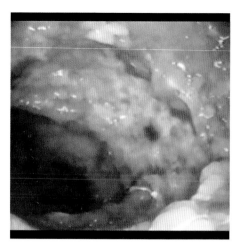

Fig. 54.14 *Mycobacterium tuberculosis* colitis, showing mucosal erythema, edema, and a large ulcer with an irregular nodular base.

PMC is caused by toxins formed by *C. difficile*. The organism itself is not invasive and its pathogenicity is toxin-based. The two most common toxins, A and B, are known to cause cytoskeletal damage, loss of tight junctions, mucosal injury, inflammation, fluid secretion, and electrophysiologic changes in colonocytes [100]. Symptoms of PMC may develop within 48 h of the start of treatment with an antibiotic, or as long as 10 weeks after therapy has been completed. Most affected individuals will have fever, leukocytosis, and abdominal pain, accompanied by watery diarrhea that contains occult blood. Gross bleeding occurs in less than 10% of patients. Severely affected patients will have fever, abdominal distension, and ileus and may even develop toxic megacolon.

Endoscopic evaluation of patients suspected of having PMC may reveal characteristic cream-colored plaques 2–8 mm in diameter, although such plaques are not always present and may spare the rectum; similar plaques, although usually not quite as distinct, may be seen in patients with other forms of infectious colitis or with colonic ischemia (**Fig. 54.15**) [101]. Thus, colonoscopy in PMC is neither absolutely sensitive nor specific, and stool-toxin assays should be used to confirm the diagnosis. The diagnosis is based on a history of exposure to an antibiotic and the presence of toxin in the stool [102]. Cholestyramine and colestipol bind *C. difficile* toxins and may provide symptomatic relief in mild cases. Metronidazole or oral vancomycin are used to treat the infection [103].

Parasitic Diseases

Giardiasis, caused by *Giardia lamblia,* is a common cause of diarrhea in the United States [104]. Although *Giardia* is most commonly spread via contaminated water, it can also be transmitted through food by fecal–oral transmission [105]. Patients with giardiasis typically have watery diarrhea with malabsorption, cramping upper abdominal pain, and flatulence [106].

On ingestion of the infectious cysts, gastric acid and intestinal proteases cause release of trophozoites, which then multiply by binary fission and become adherent to enterocytes in the upper small intestine. It is currently unclear how *Giardia* trophozoites induce the malabsorptive diarrhea that is frequently seen, but they do not directly invade the mucosa. Endoscopically, the duodenum usually appears normal, and biopsies may reveal trophozoites near the epithelium between villi. Diagnosis is most commonly made via stool ova and parasite assessment, although the sensitivity of multiple samples is only around 50%. Enzyme immunoassay studies have recently been developed for diagnosis, although these are not frequently used [29,107]. Metronidazole is the most commonly studied treatment for giardiasis, with tinidazole and nitazoxanide as alternative treatments. In one head-to-head trial of alternative treatments, tinidazole was found to be more effective than nitazoxanide [108].

Amebiasis. It is estimated that over 500 million individuals worldwide are infected with *Entamoeba*, although only 1–11% are infected with the pathogenic strain, *Entamoeba histolytica*. *E. histolytica* is the third leading parasitic cause of death in the world after malaria and schistosomiasis [109]. In Western countries, persons who are especially susceptible to amebiasis include previous residents of endemic areas, immunosuppressed individuals, and male homosexuals. Humans are the principal natural reservoir for *E. histolytica*, and disease is spread from person to person by fecal–oral contamination. *E. histolytica* exists in two principal forms: ineffective cysts responsible for transmission of parasites from one individual to another, and trophozoites with the capacity to invade the bowel mucosa and cause disease. Ingested cysts pass intact into the distal small intestine, where the cyst walls disintegrate, liberating metacystic amebae that divide into trophozoites. Trophozoites are swept by the fecal stream into the colon, where they may multiply and invade the intestinal wall [21].

E. histolytica infection may produce noninvasive colonization, acute or chronic colitis, and diarrhea, which may be mild or severe, and bland or hemorrhagic [110]. Endoscopically, the initial colonic

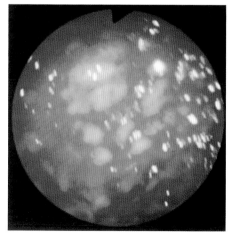

Fig. 54.15 Colonoscopy revealing typical yellow plaques in a patient with pseudomembranous colitis.

lesions are small areas of necrosis and superficial ulceration (**Fig. 54.16**). Early on, the ulcers are separated from each other by normal mucosa and may mimic Crohn's disease [111]. Later, as the ameba invade through the mucosa into the submucosa and then laterally within the submucosa, they form the classic flask-shaped ulcers, seen best on barium enema examination (**Fig. 54.17**) [109]. There may be lateral and downward extension of the macroscopic ulceration, producing irregular ulcers with overhanging edges (collar-button ulcers) and necrotic, gelatinous bases covered by a thick, purulent membrane. Healing may cause fibrosis and thickening of the bowel wall, but strictures occur in less than 1 % of patients with amebic dysentery. A similar percentage of patients will develop a mass of granulation tissue (ameboma) in the cecum or rectosigmoid that may resemble a neoplasm. Diagnostically, organisms are better detected on smears prepared from the surface mucus overlying the ulcers than they are by microscopic examination of biopsy specimens. *E. histolytica* is most commonly diagnosed with microscopic stool examination, with multiple (usually three) samples providing the greatest sensitivity [112]. Noninvasive colitis, defined by asymptomatic luminal infection, is frequently treated with paromomycin. Symptomatic invasive disease and extraintestinal disease is treated with tinidazole or metronidazole, with another broad-spectrum antibiotic for 10 days, followed by 7 days of paromomycin [21,110].

Schistosomiasis. Intestinal schistosomiasis is caused by *Schistosoma mansoni* (Africa, South and Central America, and the Caribbean), *S. japonicum* (Far East) and *S. haematobium*. Although schistosomiasis is uncommonly seen in the United States, 200 million people worldwide are infected and approximately 20 million have severe illness [113].

The life cycle of these blood flukes begins with developmental stages in snails living in fresh water. The fluke enters the human body through cercarial penetration of the skin. They then migrate through the venous circulation to the lungs, followed by the heart, and then the liver, where the larvae mature. Following maturation, the worms migrate to the mesenteric vessels of the bowel or bladder, from where they are disseminated in the feces or urine [114].

Symptoms found in acute disease include fever, malaise, urticaria, abdominal discomfort, diarrhea, and weight loss with blood tests showing eosinophilia. Persons with chronic disease, which typically develops 2–5 years after initial infection, may also have abdominal pain, diarrhea, and weight loss [115]. Colitis develops only when the eggs are deposited in the viscera, evoking an intense inflammatory response. S. japonicum infects the ascending colon, S. mansoni the descending colon, and S. haematobium the rectum (and bladder). Endoscopically, in acute disease, affected portions of the mucosa are congested, granular, and ulcerated [116]. Mucosal abnormalities are seen most frequently in the proximal colon, and colonoscopy is therefore preferable to flexible sigmoidoscopy for assessing schistosomiasis. If the disease progresses, pseudopolyps (often with surface exudate) and strictures may develop. Ulcers may develop into fistulas opening on the perineum or buttocks, or into sinus tracks extending into the ischiorectal fossa, where they may form abscesses. Occasionally, large masses of inflammatory tissue (pseudopolyps) resembling tumors obstruct the bowel or prolapse from the rectum [117]. The most sensitive diagnostic technique involves a crush preparation made from a fresh mucosal biopsy, with microscopic visualization of the larvae, although examination of the stool for ova and parasites is easier and is the more commonly used method of diagnosis [114]. Praziquantel is the mainstay of treatment for schistosomiasis [118].

Cryptosporidia are protozoan parasites that are commonly found in cattle and many other animals. *C. hominis* is the species that most frequently infects human gastrointestinal epithelia [119]. Patients with advanced AIDS are most often affected, but infected immunocompetent individuals who have persistent diarrhea are increas-

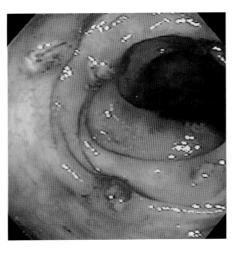

Fig. 54.16 Amebic colitis, showing shallow ulcers in the colonic mucosa.

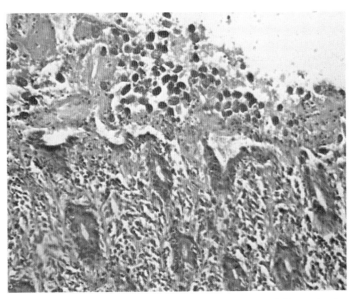

Fig. 54.17 Histology of amebic colitis (periodic acid–Schiff stain). The exudate overlying the surface epithelium, with trophozoites and inflammatory cells, should be noted. (Image reprinted with permission from Forbes A, Misiewicz JJ, Compton CC, et al, editors. *Atlas of Clinical Gastroenterology.* 3 rd ed. Edinburgh: Elsevier Mosby, 2005.)

ingly being recognized [120]. Outbreaks are usually water-borne, given the resistance of the parasite to chlorine and low infectious dose.

The life cycle of cryptosporidia is characterized by cysts, which after ingestion release sporozoites into the lumen of the small intestine. The sporozoite then attaches to the microvilli, a process that triggers the epithelial cell to surround the infectious agent with an extracytoplasmic vacuole. The sporozoite subsequently divides by binary fission, releasing merozoites into the intestinal lumen, where they can attach onto another epithelial cell, reproduce sexually, or be shed into the feces.

In immunocompromised individuals, cryptosporidial diarrhea is usually large-volume, watery, and clinically does not improve without treatment. It may be accompanied by nausea, vomiting, and abdominal pain. In immunocompetent individuals, after a 7-day incubation period, a self-limited watery diarrheal illness lasting 2 weeks is common [121]. *Cryptosporidium* testing is not routine in stool studies and has to be specifically requested. A modified acid-fast stain of the stool is usually used for detection; more recently, enzyme-linked immunosorbent assay (ELISA) tests have been developed. Endoscopy is usually unrevealing, but biopsy specimens of the intestine may aid in the diagnosis, especially if electron micro-

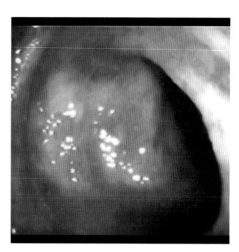

Fig. 54.18 *Strongyloides stercoralis*. There is a nonspecific appearance of erythema, loss of vascular markings, and ulceration that can be seen in self-limited colitis or in specific entities such as ulcerative colitis.

scopy is done [121]. Currently, treatment is limited and immunocompetent patients usually need only supportive measures. Patients with advanced HIV/AIDS respond best when their immune status has been reconstituted with highly active antiretroviral therapy (HAART). If HAART therapy is not possible or the patient is not responsive, treatment with either paromomycin, azithromycin, or nitazoxanide with an antidiarrheal agent is recommended [122].

Isospora belli is most commonly a cause of disease in immunocompromised people, especially residents of tropical areas. In the United States, outbreaks have been reported in mental health institutions and day-care centers. The life cycle of *Isospora* has not been extensively studied, but is believed to be similar to that of *Cryptosporidium*. Infected immunocompetent individuals experience a self-limited watery diarrhea with abdominal pain for 2–4 weeks, in contrast to immunocompromised patients, who commonly have a protracted diarrheal illness with malabsorption and weight loss [123]. Diagnosis is most frequently made with modified acid-fast staining of the stool. *Isospora* infection is sometimes associated with a peripheral eosinophilia, unlike other protozoan infections. Endoscopy is normal, with biopsies sometimes aiding in diagnosis. Treatment with trimethoprim-sulfamethoxazole is usually helpful; immunocompromised patients require 4 weeks of treatment, in contrast to immunocompetent patients, who only require 10 days of therapy [123].

Strongyloides stercoralis has a worldwide distribution, but is much more common in tropical climates. Its life cycle is relatively complicated, with both parasitic and free-living cycles. The rhabditiform larvae, which hatch from eggs during intestinal transit, are passed in the stool, transform to infective filariform larvae in the soil, penetrate the intact skin of the host, and complete a typical lung–intestine cycle [124]. The parasite usually inhabits the upper small intestine and causes epigastric pain, nausea, vomiting, recurrent diarrhea, weight loss, and urticaria [125].

Hyperinfection can occur when the rhabditiform larvae develop into filariform larvae in the host's body, usually in conditions of immunologic compromise, as in patients receiving glucocorticoids, immunosuppressive drugs, or in those with AIDS. It is with hyperinfection that the colon is involved and with hyperinfection, marked eosinophilia (e. g., 10–40 %) suggests the diagnosis and examination of the stool reveals filariform larvae. Colon involvement may produce a picture similar to that of chronic ulcerative colitis (**Fig. 54.18**). Current treatment for uncomplicated disease includes thiabendazole, ivermectin, and albendazole. For hyperinfection or disseminated disease, ivermectin is the most useful medication, with albendazole as a potential alternative [125].

References

1. Thielman NM, Guerrant RL. Clinical practice. Acute infectious diarrhea. N Engl J Med 2004;350:38–47.
2. Guerrant RL, Van Gilder T, Steiner TS, Thielman NM, Slutsker L, Tauxe RV, et al. Practice guidelines for the management of infectious diarrhea. Clin Infect Dis 2001;32:331–51.
3. Herikstad H, Yang S, Van Gilder TJ, Vugia D, Hadler J, Blake P, et al. A population-based estimate of the burden of diarrhoeal illness in the United States: FoodNet, 1996-7. Epidemiol Infect 2002;129:9–17.
4. Selby W. Diarrhoea—differential diagnosis. Aust Fam Physician 1990;19: 1683–6, 1688–9.
5. Garthright WE, Archer DL, Kvenberg JE. Estimates of incidence and costs of intestinal infectious diseases in the United States. Public Health Rep 1988;103:107–15.
6. DuPont HL. Guidelines on acute infectious diarrhea in adults. The Practice Parameters Committee of the American College of Gastroenterology. Am J Gastroenterol 1997;92:1962–75.
7. Oldfield EC 3 rd, Bourgeois AL, Omar AK, Pazzaglia GL. Empirical treatment of *Shigella* dysentery with trimethoprim: five-day course vs. single dose. Am J Trop Med Hyg 1987;37:616–23.
8. Gangarosa RE, Glass RI, Lew JF, Boring JR. Hospitalizations involving gastroenteritis in the United States, 1985: the special burden of the disease among the elderly. Am J Epidemiol 1992;135:281–90.
9. Slotwiner-Nie PK, Brandt LJ. Infectious diarrhea in the elderly. Gastroenterol Clin North Am 2001;30:625–35.
10. DuPont HL, Marshall GD. HIV-associated diarrhoea and wasting. Lancet 1995;346:352–6.
11. Guerrant RL, Shields DS, Thorson SM, Schorling JB, Gröschel DH. Evaluation and diagnosis of acute infectious diarrhea. Am J Med 1985;78:91–8.
12. Koplan JP, Fineberg HV, Ferraro MJ, Rosenberg ML. Value of stool cultures. Lancet 1980;2(8191):413–6.
13. Ethelberg S, Olsen KE, Gerner-Smidt P, Mølbak K. The significance of the number of submitted samples and patient-related factors for faecal bacterial diagnostics. Clin Microbiol Infect 2007;13:1095–9.
14. Bardhan PK, Beltinger J, Beltinger RW, Hossain A, Mahalanabis D, Gyr K. Screening of patients with acute infectious diarrhoea: evaluation of clinical features, faecal microscopy, and faecal occult blood testing. Scand J Gastroenterol 2000;35:54–60.
15. McNeely WS, Dupont HL, Mathewson JJ, Oberhelman RA, Ericsson CD. Occult blood versus fecal leukocytes in the diagnosis of bacterial diarrhea: a study of U.S. travelers to Mexico and Mexican children. Am J Trop Med Hyg 1996;55:430–3.
16. Harris JC, Dupont HL, Hornick RB. Fecal leukocytes in diarrheal illness. Ann Intern Med 1972;76:697–703.
17. Voetsch AC, Angulo FJ, Rabatsky-Ehr T, Shallow S, Cassidy M, Thomas SM, et al. Laboratory practices for stool-specimen culture for bacterial pathogens, including *Escherichia coli* O157:H7, in the FoodNet sites, 1995–2000. Clin Infect Dis 2004;38(Suppl 3):S 190–7.
18. Morris JG Jr, Black RE. Cholera and other vibrioses in the United States. N Engl J Med 1985 Feb 7;312(6):343–50.
19. Metchock B, Lonsway DR, Carter GP, Lee LA, McGowan JE Jr. *Yersinia enterocolitica:* a frequent seasonal stool isolate from children at an urban hospital in the southeast United States. J Clin Microbiol 1991;29:2868–9.
20. Ravdin JI. Amebiasis. Clin Infect Dis 1995;20:1453–64; quiz 1465–6.
21. Haque R, Huston CD, Hughes M, Houpt E, Petri WA Jr. Amebiasis. N Engl J Med 2003;348:1565–73.
22. Siegel DL, Edelstein PH, Nachamkin I. Inappropriate testing for diarrheal diseases in the hospital. JAMA 1990;263:979–82.
23. Morris AJ, Wilson ML, Reller LB. Application of rejection criteria for stool ovum and parasite examinations. J Clin Microbiol 1992;30:3213–6.
24. Meropol SB, Luberti AA, De Jong AR. Yield from stool testing of pediatric inpatients. Arch Pediatr Adolesc Med 1997;151:142–5.
25. Branda JA, Lin TY, Rosenberg ES, Halpern EF, Ferraro MJ. A rational approach to the stool ova and parasite examination. Clin Infect Dis 2006;42:972–8.
26. Cartwright CP. Utility of multiple-stool-specimen ova and parasite examinations in a high-prevalence setting. J Clin Microbiol 1999;37:2408–11.
27. Mayer CL, Palmer CJ. Evaluation of PCR, nested PCR, and fluorescent antibodies for detection of *Giardia* and *Cryptosporidium* species in wastewater. Appl Environ Microbiol 1996;62:2081–5.
28. Garcia LS, Shimizu RY. Evaluation of nine immunoassay kits (enzyme immunoassay and direct fluorescence) for detection of *Giardia lamblia* and *Cryptosporidium parvum* in human fecal specimens. J Clin Microbiol 1997;35:1526–9.

IX

29. Garcia LS, Shimizu RY, Novak S, Carroll M, Chan F. Commercial assay for detection of *Giardia lamblia* and *Cryptosporidium parvum* antigens in human fecal specimens by rapid solid-phase qualitative immunochromatography. J Clin Microbiol 2003;41:209–12.

30. Gonvers JJ, Bochud M, Burnand B, Froehlich F, Dubois RW, Vader JP. 10. Appropriateness of colonoscopy: diarrhea. Endoscopy 1999;31:641–6.

31. Lipsky MS, Adelman M. Chronic diarrhea: evaluation and treatment. Am Fam Physician 1993;48:1461–6.

32. Yusoff IF, Ormonde DG, Hoffman NE. Routine colonic mucosal biopsy and ileoscopy increases diagnostic yield in patients undergoing colonoscopy for diarrhea. J Gastroenterol Hepatol 2002;17:276–80.

33. Harewood GC, Olson JS, Mattek NC, Holub JL, Lieberman DA. Colonic biopsy practice for evaluation of diarrhea in patients with normal endoscopic findings: results from a national endoscopic database. Gastrointest Endosc 2005;61:371–5.

34. Schiller LR. Chronic diarrhea: To biopsy or not to biopsy. Gastrointest Endosc 2005;61:376–7.

35. Barbut F, Beaugerie L, Delas N, Fossati-Marchal S, Aygalenq P, Petit JC. Comparative value of colonic biopsy and intraluminal fluid culture for diagnosis of bacterial acute colitis in immunocompetent patients. Infectious Colitis Study Group. Clin Infect Dis 1999;29:356–60.

36. Matsumoto T, Iida M, Kimura Y, Fujishima M. Culture of colonoscopically obtained biopsy specimens in acute infectious colitis. Gastrointest Endosc 1994;40:184–7.

37. Schumacher G, Kollberg B, Sandstedt B. A prospective study of first attacks of inflammatory bowel disease and infectious colitis. Histologic course during the 1st year after presentation. Scand J Gastroenterol 1994;29:318–32.

38. Abreu MT, Harpaz N. Diagnosis of colitis: making the initial diagnosis. Clin Gastroenterol Hepatol 2007;5:295–301.

39. Tanaka M, Saito H, Fukuda S, Sasaki Y, Munakata A, Kudo H. Simple mucosal biopsy criteria differentiating among Crohn's disease, ulcerative colitis, and other forms of colitis: measurement of validity. Scand J Gastroenterol 2000;35:281–6.

40. Tanaka M, Masuda T, Yao T, Saito H, Kusumi T, Nagura H, et al. Observer variation of diagnoses based on simple biopsy criteria differentiating among Crohn's disease, ulcerative colitis, and other forms of colitis. J Gastroenterol Hepatol 2001;16:1368–72.

41. King CK, Glass R, Bresee JS, Duggan C; Centers for Disease Control and Prevention. Managing acute gastroenteritis among children: oral rehydration, maintenance, and nutritional therapy. MMWR Recomm Rep 2003;52:1–16.

42. Cimolai N, Basalyga S, Mah DG, Morrison BJ, Carter JE. A continuing assessment of risk factors for the development of Escherichia coli O157:H7-associated hemolytic uremic syndrome. Clin Nephrol 1994;42:85–9.

43. DuPont HL, Flores Sanchez J, Ericsson CD, Mendiola Gomez J, DuPont MW, Cruz Luna A, et al. Comparative efficacy of loperamide hydrochloride and bismuth subsalicylate in the management of acute diarrhea. Am J Med 1990;88:15S–19S.

44. Johnson PC, Ericsson CD, DuPont HL, Morgan DR, Bitsura JA, Wood LV. Comparison of loperamide with bismuth subsalicylate for the treatment of acute travelers' diarrhea. JAMA 1986;255:757–60.

45. DuPont HL, Sullivan P, Pickering LK, Haynes G, Ackerman PB. Symptomatic treatment of diarrhea with bismuth subsalicylate among students attending a Mexican university. Gastroenterology 1977;73:715–8.

46. Johnson S, Homann SR, Bettin KM, Quick JN, Clabots CR, Peterson LR, Gerding DN. Treatment of asymptomatic *Clostridium difficile* carriers (fecal excretors) with vancomycin or metronidazole. A randomized, placebo-controlled trial. Ann Intern Med 1992;117:297–302.

47. Wong CS, Jelacic S, Habeeb RL, Watkins SL, Tarr PI. The risk of the hemolytic-uremic syndrome after antibiotic treatment of *Escherichia coli* O157:H7 infections. N Engl J Med 2000;342:1930–6.

48. Wiström J, Jertborn M, Ekwall E, Norlin K, Söderquist B, Strömberg A, et al. Empiric treatment of acute diarrheal disease with norfloxacin. A randomized, placebo-controlled study. Swedish Study Group. Ann Intern Med 1992;117:202–8.

49. Emery VC. Investigation of CMV disease in immunocompromised patients. J Clin Pathol 2001;54:84–8.

50. Fishman JA, Emery V, Freeman R, Pascual M, Rostaing L, Schlitt HJ, et al. Cytomegalovirus in transplantation—challenging the status quo. Clin Transplant 2007;21:149–58.

51. Carter D, Olchovsky D, Pokroy R, Ezra D. Cytomegalovirus-associated colitis causing diarrhea in an immunocompetent patient. World J Gastroenterol 2006;12:6898–9.

52. Rafailidis PI, Mourtzoukou EG, Varbobitis IC, Falagas ME. Severe cytomegalovirus infection in apparently immunocompetent patients: a systematic review. Virol J 2008;5:47.

53. Smith PD, Quinn TC, Strober W, Janoff EN, Masur H. NIH conference. Gastrointestinal infections in AIDS. Ann Intern Med 1992;116:63–77.

54. Dieterich DT, Rahmin M. Cytomegalovirus colitis in AIDS: presentation in 44 patients and a review of the literature. J Acquir Immune Defic Syndr 1991;4(Suppl 1):S29–35.

55. Marques O Jr, Averbach M, Zanoni EC, Corrêa PA, Paccos JL, Cutait R. Cytomegaloviral colitis in HIV positive patients: endoscopic findings. Arq Gastroenterol 2007;44:315–9.

56. Wilcox CM, Chalasani N, Lazenby A, Schwartz DA. Cytomegalovirus colitis in acquired immunodeficiency syndrome: a clinical and endoscopic study. Gastrointest Endosc 1998;48:39–43.

57. Mönkemüller KE, Bussian AH, Lazenby AJ, Wilcox CM. Special histologic stains are rarely beneficial for the evaluation of HIV-related gastrointestinal infections. Am J Clin Pathol 2000;114:387–94.

58. Blanshard C, Benhamou Y, Dohin E, Lernestedt JO, Gazzard BG, Katlama C. Treatment of AIDS-associated gastrointestinal cytomegalovirus infection with foscarnet and ganciclovir: a randomized comparison. J Infect Dis 1995;172:622–8.

59. Bobak DA. Gastrointestinal infections caused by cytomegalovirus. Curr Infect Dis Rep 2003;5:101–7.

60. Klausner JD, Kohn R, Kent C. Etiology of clinical proctitis among men who have sex with men. Clin Infect Dis 2004;38:300–2.

61. Hamlyn E, Taylor C. Sexually transmitted proctitis. Postgrad Med J 2006;82:733–6.

62. Centers for Disease Control and Prevention (CDC). Preliminary FoodNet data on the incidence of infection with pathogens transmitted commonly through food—10 states, 2007. MMWR Morb Mortal Wkly Rep 2008;57:366–70.

63. Sur D, Ramamurthy T, Deen J, Bhattacharya SK. Shigellosis: challenges & management issues. Indian J Med Res 2004;120:454–62.

64. Gorden J, Small PL. Acid resistance in enteric bacteria. Infect Immun 1993;61:364–7.

65. DuPont HL, Levine MM, Hornick RB, Formal SB. Inoculum size in shigellosis and implications for expected mode of transmission. J Infect Dis 1989;159:1126–8.

66. von Seidlein L, Kim DR, Ali M, Lee H, Wang X, Thiem VD, et al. A multicentre study of *Shigella* diarrhoea in six Asian countries: disease burden, clinical manifestations, and microbiology. PLoS Med 2006;3:e353.

67. Niyogi SK. Shigellosis. J Microbiol 2005;43:133–43.

68. Khuroo MS, Mahajan R, Zargar SA, Panhotra BR, Bhat RL, Javid G, Mahajan B. The colon in shigellosis: serial colonoscopic appearances in *Shigella dysenteriae* I. Endoscopy 1990;22:35–8.

69. Speelman P, Kabir I, Islam M. Distribution and spread of colonic lesions in shigellosis: a colonoscopic study. J Infect Dis 1984;150:899–903.

70. Bhattacharya SK, Sur D. An evaluation of current shigellosis treatment. Expert Opin Pharmacother 2003;4:1315–20.

71. Saffouri B, Bartolomeo RS, Fuchs B. Colonic involvement in salmonellosis. Dig Dis Sci 1979;24:203–8.

72. Schofield PF, Mandal BK, Ironside AG. Toxic dilatation of the colon in salmonella colitis and inflammatory bowel disease. Br J Surg 1979;66:5–8.

73. Sirinavin S, Garner P. Antibiotics for treating salmonella gut infections. Cochrane Database Syst Rev 2000;(2):CD001167.

74. Allos BM. *Campylobacter jejuni* infections: update on emerging issues and trends. Clin Infect Dis 2001;32:1201–6.

75. Blakelock RT, Beasley SW. Infection and the gut. Semin Pediatr Surg 2003;12:265–74.

76. Zilbauer M, Dorrell N, Wren BW, Bajaj-Elliott M. *Campylobacter jejuni*-mediated disease pathogenesis: an update. Trans R Soc Trop Med Hyg 2008;102:123–9.

77. Pichler HE, Diridl G, Stickler K, Wolf D. Clinical efficacy of ciprofloxacin compared with placebo in bacterial diarrhea. Am J Med 1987;82:329–32.

78. Ackers ML, Schoenfeld S, Markman J, Smith MG, Nicholson MA, DeWitt W, et al. An outbreak of *Yersinia enterocolitica* O:8 infections associated with pasteurized milk. J Infect Dis 2000;181:1834–7.

79. Vantrappen G, Geboes K, Ponette E. *Yersinia* enteritis. Med Clin North Am 1982;66:639–53.

80. Naktin J, Beavis KG. *Yersinia enterocolitica* and *Yersinia pseudotuberculosis*. Clin Lab Med 1999;19:523–36, vi.

81. Pai CH, Gillis F, Tuomanen E, Marks MI. Placebo-controlled double-blind evaluation of trimethoprim-sulfamethoxazole treatment of *Yersinia enterocolitica* gastroenteritis. J Pediatr 1984;104:308–11.

54

82. Rangel JM, Sparling PH, Crowe C, Griffin PM, Swerdlow DL. Epidemiology of *Escherichia coli* O157:H7 outbreaks, United States, 1982–2002. Emerg Infect Dis 2005;11:603–9.

83. Lawson JM. Update on *Escherichia coli* O157:H7. Curr Gastroenterol Rep 2004;6:297–301.

84. Moake JL. Thrombotic microangiopathies. N Engl J Med 2002;347:589–600.

85. Shigeno T, Akamatsu T, Fujimori K, Nakatsuji Y, Nagata A. The clinical significance of colonoscopy in hemorrhagic colitis due to enterohemorrhagic *Escherichia coli* O157:H7 infection. Endoscopy 2002;34:311–4.

86. Su C, Brandt LJ. *Escherichia coli* O157:H7 infection in humans. Ann Intern Med 1995 Nov 1;123(9):698–714.

87. Ina K, Kusugami K, Ohta M. Bacterial hemorrhagic enterocolitis. J Gastroenterol 2003;38:111–20.

88. Underwood MJ, Thompson MM, Sayers RD, Hall AW. Presentation of abdominal tuberculosis to general surgeons. Br J Surg 1992;79:1077–9.

89. Rasheed S, Zinicola R, Watson D, Bajwa A, McDonald PJ. Intra-abdominal and gastrointestinal tuberculosis. Colorectal Dis 2007;9:773–83.

90. Poorman JC, Katon RM. Small bowel involvement by *Mycobacterium avium* complex in a patient with AIDS: endoscopic, histologic, and radiographic similarities to Whipple's disease. Gastrointest Endosc 1994;40:753–9.

91. Addison NV. Abdominal tuberculosis—a disease revived. Ann R Coll Surg Engl 1983;65:105–11.

92. Horvath KD, Whelan RL. Intestinal tuberculosis: return of an old disease. Am J Gastroenterol 1998;93:692–6.

93. Shah S, Thomas V, Mathan M, Chacko A, Chandy G, Ramakrishna BS, et al. Colonoscopic study of 50 patients with colonic tuberculosis. Gut 1992;33:347–51.

94. Leung VK, Law ST, Lam CW, Luk IS, Chau TN, Loke TK, et al. Intestinal tuberculosis in a regional hospital in Hong Kong: a 10-year experience. Hong Kong Med J 2006;12:264–71.

95. Centers for Disease Control and Prevention (CDC). Surveillance for community-associated *Clostridium difficile*—Connecticut, 2006. MMWR Morb Mortal Wkly Rep 2008;57:340–3.

96. Stark PL, Lee A, Parsonage BD. Colonization of the large bowel by *Clostridium difficile* in healthy infants: quantitative study. Infect Immun 1982;35:895–9.

97. Viscidi R, Willey S, Bartlett JG. Isolation rates and toxigenic potential of *Clostridium difficile* isolates from various patient populations. Gastroenterology 1981;81:5–9.

98. Riggs MM, Sethi AK, Zabarsky TF, Eckstein EC, Jump RL, Donskey CJ. Asymptomatic carriers are a potential source for transmission of epidemic and nonepidemic *Clostridium difficile* strains among long-term care facility residents. Clin Infect Dis 2007;45:992–8.

99. Cloud J, Kelly CP. Update on *Clostridium difficile* associated disease. Curr Opin Gastroenterol 2007;23:4–9.

100. Riegler M, Sedivy R, Pothoulakis C, Hamilton G, Zacherl J, Bischof G, et al. *Clostridium difficile* toxin B is more potent than toxin A in damaging human colonic epithelium in vitro. J Clin Invest 1995;95:2004–11.

101. Goldman WM, Avicolli AS, Lutwick S. *Clostridium difficile* colitis. N Engl J Med 1994;330:1755.

102. Lyerly DM, Neville LM, Evans DT, Fill J, Allen S, Greene W, et al. Multicenter evaluation of the Clostridium difficile TOX A/B TEST. J Clin Microbiol 1998;36:184–90.

103. Pépin J, Valiquette L, Gagnon S, Routhier S, Brazeau I. Outcomes of *Clostridium difficile*–associated disease treated with metronidazole or vancomycin before and after the emergence of NAP1/027. Am J Gastroenterol 2007;102:2781–8.

104. Yoder JS, Beach MJ; Centers for Disease Control and Prevention (CDC). Giardiasis surveillance—United States, 2003–2005. MMWR Surveill Summ 2007;56:11–8.

105. White KE, Hedberg CW, Edmonson LM, Jones DB, Osterholm MT, MacDonald KL. An outbreak of giardiasis in a nursing home with evidence for multiple modes of transmission. J Infect Dis 1989;160:298–304.

106. Osterholm MT, Forfang JC, Ristinen TL, Dean AG, Washburn JW, Godes JR, et al. An outbreak of foodborne giardiasis. N Engl J Med 1981;304:24–8.

107. Garcia LS, Shimizu RY. Evaluation of nine immunoassay kits (enzyme immunoassay and direct fluorescence) for detection of *Giardia lamblia* and *Cryptosporidium parvum* in human fecal specimens. J Clin Microbiol 1997;35:1526–9.

108. Escobedo AA, Alvarez G, González ME, Almirall P, Cañete R, Cimerman S, et al. The treatment of giardiasis in children: single-dose tinidazole compared with 3 days of nitazoxanide. Ann Trop Med Parasitol 2008;102:199–207.

109. Stanley SL Jr. Amoebiasis. Lancet 2003;361:1025–34.

110. Bercu TE, Petri WA, Behm JW. Amebic colitis: new insights into pathogenesis and treatment. Curr Gastroenterol Rep 2007;9:429–33.

111. Tucker PC, Webster PD, Kilpatrick ZM. Amebic colitis mistaken for inflammatory bowel disease. Arch Intern Med 1975;135:681–5.

112. González-Ruiz A, Haque R, Aguirre A, Castañón G, Hall A, Guhl F, et al. Value of microscopy in the diagnosis of dysentery associated with invasive *Entamoeba histolytica*. J Clin Pathol 1994;47:236–9.

113. Chitsulo L, Engels D, Montresor A, Savioli L. The global status of schistosomiasis and its control. Acta Trop 2000;77:41–51.

114. Ross AG, Bartley PB, Sleigh AC, Olds GR, Li Y, Williams GM, et al. Schistosomiasis. N Engl J Med 2002;346:1212–20.

115. Zhou H, Ross AG, Hartel GF, Sleigh AC, Williams GM, McManus DP, et al. Diagnosis of schistosomiasis japonica in Chinese schoolchildren by administration of a questionnaire. Trans R Soc Trop Med Hyg 1998;92:245–50.

116. Nebel OT, el-Masry NA, Castell DO, Farid Z, Fornes MF, Sparks HA. Schistosomal colonic polyposis: endoscopic and histologic characteristics. Gastrointest Endosc 1974;20:99–101.

117. Chen MC, Wang SC, Chang PY, Chuang CY, Chen YJ, Tang YC, et al. Granulomatous disease of the large intestine secondary to schistosome infestation. A study of 229 cases. Chin Med J (Engl) 1978;4:371–8.

118. Thomas H, Gönnert R. The efficacy of praziquantel against cestodes in animals. Z Parasitenkd 1977;52:117–27.

119. Xiao L, Fayer R, Ryan U, Upton SJ. *Cryptosporidium* taxonomy: recent advances and implications for public health. Clin Microbiol Rev 2004;17:72–97.

120. Navin TR, Weber R, Vugia DJ, Rimland D, Roberts JM, Addiss DG, et al. Declining CD 4 + T-lymphocyte counts are associated with increased risk of enteric parasitosis and chronic diarrhea: results of a 3-year longitudinal study. J Acquir Immune Defic Syndr Hum Retrovirol 1999;20:154–9.

121. Chen XM, Keithly JS, Paya CV, LaRusso NF. Cryptosporidiosis. N Engl J Med 2002;346:1723–31.

122. Rossignol JF, Ayoub A, Ayers MS. Treatment of diarrhea caused by *Cryptosporidium parvum:* a prospective randomized, double-blind, placebo-controlled study of Nitazoxanide. J Infect Dis 2001;184:103–6.

123. Lewthwaite P, Gill GV, Hart CA, Beeching NJ. Gastrointestinal parasites in the immunocompromised. Curr Opin Infect Dis 2005;18:427–35.

124. Concha R, Harrington W Jr, Rogers AI. Intestinal strongyloidiasis: recognition, management, and determinants of outcome. J Clin Gastroenterol 2005;39:203–11.

125. Segarra-Newnham M. Manifestations, diagnosis, and treatment of *Strongyloides stercoralis* infection. Ann Pharmacother 2007;41:1992–2001.

IX

55 Intestinal Abnormalities in AIDS

Andrew T. Pellecchia and Lawrence J. Brandt

Introduction

The increasingly beneficial effects of the newer antiretroviral regimens and the continuing increase in knowledge concerning the prevention and treatment of human immunodeficiency virus (HIV) infection have resulted in a progressive change in the face of the acquired immune deficiency syndrome (AIDS) epidemic in the United States. The number of new cases of HIV/AIDS acquired in the United States per year is continuing to decline, with 40,608 cases diagnosed in 2005 compared with 58 254 cases diagnosed just 8 years earlier in 1997 [1]. Similarly, the age-adjusted death rate from HIV infection in the United States, 4.5 per 100 000 in 2004, has been in a continuous decline since 1995, and AIDS has not been in the list of the top 15 causes of death in the United States since 1997 [2]. Moreover, there has been a sharp decline in hospital use for HIV-infected patients. AIDS patients had 12,000 fewer hospitalizations in 2005 than in 2000, and the length of stay in the hospital was down to an average of 7.5 days—1.9 days less than in 2005 [3].

Despite this good news, however, the slopes of the downward trends in mortality and incidence appear to be leveling off and there continues to be a disproportionate impact of the epidemic on certain ethnic and minority populations. Men who have sex with men (MSM) continue to remain a population at high risk for HIV infection, representing 71 % of all men diagnosed with HIV in 2005 [4]. In addition, a recent study examining HIV in five major cities found that the prevalence of HIV in black MSM (46 %) was more than twice that in white MSM (21 %). By the end of 2005, an estimated 217 323 MSM in the United States were living with HIV. Looking at minority populations as a whole, blacks accounted for 49 % of those newly-diagnosed with HIV/AIDS in 2006, while Hispanics/Latinos accounted for 17 % in 2005 [5,6]. Clearly, these are the populations most in need of assistance if the successes of the past decade are to be built upon in the years to come.

Outside of the United States and other developed nations, the HIV/AIDS epidemic continues virtually unchecked. The total number of people living with HIV/AIDS is continuing to increase every year. It is estimated that in 2005, 38.6 million individuals worldwide were infected with HIV and that over 95 % of those were living in the developing world. The majority of these individuals—approximately 24.5 million men, women, and children—were living in sub-Saharan Africa [7]. Most will die during the next 10 years, joining the 25 million lives claimed worldwide by the AIDS epidemic so far. AIDS continues to be the leading cause of death in Africa, as well as the fourth leading cause of death worldwide [8]. It is little wonder that the 2004 World Health Report from the World Health Organization identified HIV as the world's most urgent public health challenge, as AIDS is perhaps the greatest lethal epidemic in the history of the civilized world.

The gastrointestinal tract remains a major target for pathogens and diseases in patients infected with HIV. The entire gastrointestinal tract from mouth to anus can be affected. Approximately 50 % of patients with HIV present with gastrointestinal diseases, and virtually all patients will develop gastrointestinal complications during the course of their disease [9].

Endoscopy has come to play a very important role in both the diagnosis and therapy of a variety of AIDS-related gastrointestinal diseases. Despite the persistence of a sometimes negative approach by some physicians to the evaluation of HIV-afflicted patients, endoscopy remains the gold standard for diagnosis in most cases. Demonstration of a tissue pathogen or disease can be critical in a patient with nonspecific symptoms or a life-threatening presentation or exacerbation of disease.

Using a symptom-based approach, this chapter reviews the application of endoscopy to the diagnosis and therapy of AIDS-related gastroenterologic disease. We do not discuss specific treatment strategies, as these are reviewed in depth elsewhere. We also briefly discuss safety issues for the clinician performing endoscopic examinations in patients with HIV disease.

Dysphagia and Odynophagia

Both dysphagia (difficulty in swallowing) and odynophagia (painful swallowing) are manifestations of esophageal disease. In AIDS, disorders of the esophagus are found in as many as 30–40 % of patients at some point in the course of the disease [10]. Endoscopy is the definitive diagnostic test for esophageal disease in the AIDS patient. The timing and necessity of routine endoscopy in patients with AIDS and esophageal symptoms have changed in the last decade. In the past, endoscopy was performed in virtually all patients with AIDS and dysphagia. Given the fact that candidal esophagitis is the most common etiology of dysphagia in this patient population, there has been a trend towards treating patients empirically with antifungal agents and only performing endoscopy in the subset of patients who have persistent symptoms [11,12].

▦ Etiology (Table 55.1)

Candida albicans, cytomegalovirus (CMV), herpes simplex virus (HSV), idiopathic ulceration, and Kaposi's sarcoma are the most common esophageal lesions in AIDS patients. Candidal infection is the most common, and in the era before highly active antiretroviral therapy (HAART) it affected 40–70 % of patients with AIDS. With the

Table 55.1 Most common esophageal pathology involved in HIV-associated dysphagia/odynophagia

Candida species
Cytomegalovirus
Idiopathic esophageal ulcer
Herpes simplex
Peptic
Kaposi's sarcoma
Mycobacterium avium-intracellulare
Mycobacterium tuberculosis (rare)
Histoplasma capsulatum (rare)
Cryptosporidium parvum (rare)
Pneumocystis carinii (rare)

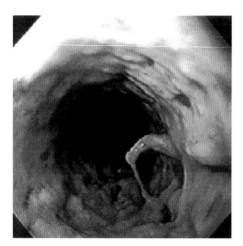

Fig. 55.1   Severe candidal esophagitis.

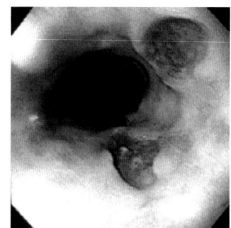

Fig. 55.2   Cytomegalovirus-induced esophageal ulceration.

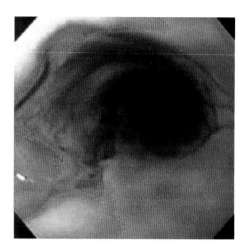

Fig. 55.3   Idiopathic esophageal ulceration.

widespread institution of HAART, however, the incidence of all HIV-related opportunistic infections has decreased dramatically [13]. In a study by Mocroft et al., there was a 32% decline in the incidence of esophageal candidiasis from 1995 to 2004 [14]. Despite this decrease, the overall incidence of gastrointestinal opportunistic infections in patients on HAART is still almost 10%, with much higher incidences for patients not receiving antiretroviral treatment [15].

Candida Esophagitis

Most patients (66%) with *Candida* esophagitis also have thrush. On endoscopy, creamy white or yellow plaques with surrounding erythematous mucosa are typical (**Fig. 55.1**). The plaques are usually isolated, but can become circumferential and completely involve the entire esophagus. Ulcers may also be present, but should raise the suspicion of a concomitant viral pathogen (e.g., HSV, CMV).

On biopsy, a neutrophilic infiltrate at the squamous epithelial surface and a pseudomembrane are usually found. The *Candida albicans* fungus, identified by its budding yeast forms and pseudohyphae, can be invasive. Brushing is almost always more sensitive than biopsy alone, and both should probably be performed.

Cytomegalovirus

Endoscopically, the lesions caused by CMV can range from one or more discrete small ulcers to an extremely large (2–10 cm in length) shallow ulceration, or deep ulcers of the esophagus (**Fig. 55.2**). Occasionally, ulceration can be so severe that *no* normal mucosa is seen, only infected granulation tissue. Biopsies should be taken from the ulcer base; CMV inclusions are characteristic. Cytology and viral culture add little to the diagnostic yield as long as at least 10 biopsies are taken from the ulcer [16,17]. In contrast to HSV, inclusions are seen in stromal and endothelial cells rather than squamous cells.

Herpes Simplex Virus

The endoscopic findings in HSV esophagitis vary from vesiculation early in the course of infection to ulceration. Typically, HSV ulcers are round, multiple, well-circumscribed, uniform, and usually smaller than those seen in CMV disease. They may be deep, however, and are associated with severe esophageal spasm and odynophagia in addition to dysphagia.

In contrast to the recommendation to biopsy the ulcer base in suspected CMV, biopsies are more often diagnostic of HSV infection if taken from the ulcer edge. Necrotic squamous epithelium is seen, with both acute and chronic inflammation; diagnostic nuclear changes are also present, and consist of a homogeneous ground-glass appearance and multinucleate squamous cells. Cowdry type A inclusions are rarely found [18]. Obviously, if the cause of the ulcer is not known, numerous biopsies should be obtained from both the ulcer base and edge.

Idiopathic (Aphthous) Ulcers

Idiopathic esophageal ulceration (**Fig. 55.3**) is diagnosed when large, irregular mid-esophageal and distal esophageal ulcers are seen endoscopically and no specific etiological agent can be identified. Idiopathic esophageal ulcers resemble CMV-induced ulcers, but are more often solitary and deep [19,20]. Severe odynophagia and associated weight loss are typical.

The pathogenesis of idiopathic esophageal ulcers is poorly understood, but it is probably related to dysfunctional immunoregulation. On biopsy, there is a nonspecific mixed inflammatory infiltrate, with numerous eosinophils and granulation tissue [18]. These patients often have a dramatic response to oral prednisone, but relapse is common [21]. Thalidomide, which has been shown both to stimulate T-lymphocyte proliferation and to inhibit tumor necrosis factor-α (TNF-α) activity, has also been found to be effective [22,23], with perhaps a lower relapse rate than that seen with corticosteroid treatment [24].

Other

In AIDS patients, as in immunocompetent patients, gastroesophageal reflux with esophagitis or peptic stricturing, pill-induced esophagitis, and carcinoma can also be found, although they are uncommon. Esophageal tuberculosis [25], histoplasmosis [26], cryptosporidiosis [27], Kaposi's sarcoma (**Figs. 55.4, 55.5**), and *Pneumocystis* infection [28] have all been reported, albeit rarely.

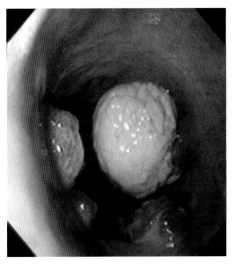

Fig. 55.4 Extensive multifocal Kaposi's sarcoma of the esophagus.

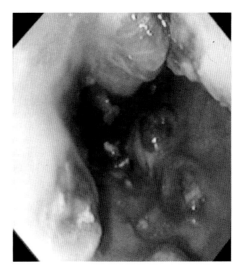

Fig. 55.5 Kaposi's sarcoma.

Table 55.2 Differential diagnosis of abdominal pain in the AIDS patient

Location of pain	Source	Etiology
Mid-epigastric	Stomach	Peptic, CMV, Kaposi's sarcoma, lymphoma, acalculous cholecystitis
Diffuse	Mesentery, pancreas, small or large bowel	*Mycobacterium avium-intracellulare*, acute or chronic pancreatitis, CMV, lymphoma, mesenteric ischemia
Right upper quadrant	Gallbladder, biliary tree, liver	Acalculous cholecystitis, AIDS cholangiopathy, gallstone disease, liver disease (hepatitis, tumor)
Left lower quadrant	Sigmoid colon	CMV, lymphoma, ameba
Right lower quadrant	Cecum, right hemicolon, terminal ileum, appendix	CMV, lymphoma, ameba, appendicitis and periappendicitis

CMV: cytomegalovirus.

Abdominal Pain

The approach to the AIDS patient with abdominal pain should follow the same algorithm as in immunocompetent patients. Certain infections and conditions, however, are limited to this patient population and should be kept in mind during evaluations (**Table 55.2**).

Gastric Diseases

Whereas upper gastrointestinal symptoms are quite common in the AIDS patient and are often cited as a reason for discontinuing HAART, gastric diseases are relatively uncommon in this patient population; presentations include epigastric pain, nausea, or vomiting [29]. Peptic ulcers occur infrequently, as *Helicobacter pylori* infection is found less often in the AIDS patient than in control populations [29,30], and hypochlorhydria is present in up to 25% of patients with advanced AIDS [31]. There are now several studies, however, that show that the prevalence of H. pylori–associated disease, as well as its severity, is directly related to the severity of immune deterioration [31,32]. It must be noted that positive serologic testing for *H. pylori* infection appears to be directly related to higher CD4 counts [33], and thus negative serologic testing for *H. pylori* does not rule out this infection in patients who have low CD4 counts.

Cytomegalovirus

CMV is the most frequent opportunistic gastric infection in AIDS and may be the most commonly identified cause of peptic ulcer disease in symptomatic AIDS patients [34,35]. Endoscopically, the appearance of CMV is variable, but it usually presents as a patchy gastritis (**Fig. 55.6**) or as multiple small ulcers. On biopsy of the stomach, CMV inclusions often are seen in epithelial cells, whereas such inclusions are rare in intestinal epithelial cells [18].

Kaposi's Sarcoma

Kaposi's sarcoma, the most common AIDS-related malignancy, frequently affects the stomach. Most often, it affects the skin, but in one study of 50 patients with cutaneous Kaposi's sarcoma, 40% had gastrointestinal lesions [36,37]. Intestinal and gastric Kaposi's sarcoma is frequently asymptomatic, but gastric involvement can result in pyloric obstruction, pain, or upper gastrointestinal bleeding. It typically appears endoscopically as submucosal violet-red nodules, plaques, or polyps (**Figs. 55.7, 55.8**). Given its submucosal location, it is not surprising that false-negative rates for endoscopic biopsy are as high as 77% [36]. Biopsies characteristically reveal spindle cells and irregular, jagged, slit-like spaces lined by atypical endothelial cells. Extravasated red cells, hemosiderin, and eosinophilic round cytoplasmic globules are often seen [18]. Human herpesvirus 8 has been implicated as the agent inciting the development of Kaposi's sarcoma [38].

55

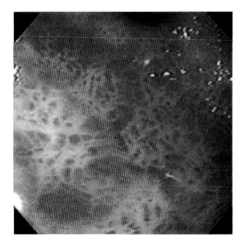

Fig. 55.6 Cytomegalovirus-induced gastritis.

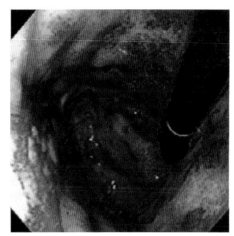

Fig. 55.7 Gastric Kaposi's sarcoma.

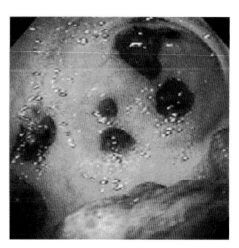

Fig. 55.8 Bulky purplish antral plaques and polyps in gastric Kaposi's sarcoma.

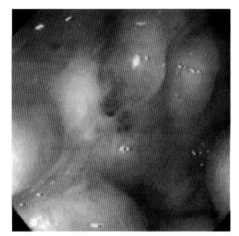

Fig. 55.9 Ulcerated gastric lymphoma.

Lymphoma

Gastric lymphoma, by contrast, almost always results in epigastric pain or symptoms of gastric outlet obstruction. AIDS-related gastric lymphomas are commonly multifocal and extensive at initial presentation (stage IV). Extranodal non-Hodgkin's lymphomas occur in approximately 10 % of HIV-infected patients [39,40]. They present in the gastrointestinal tract in approximately 30 % of patients, and are often fatal. At least 95 % are B cell lymphomas, and they are typically immunoblastic or large cell types [39]. On endoscopy, lymphomas can be difficult to distinguish from adenocarcinoma (**Fig. 55.9**), as both usually present as ulcerated mass lesions. Biopsy, however, is conclusive.

Mycobacterium avium complex (MAC)

Cramping periumbilical abdominal pain, associated with weight loss, fever, or diarrhea, as discussed above, is a frequent symptom in patients with HIV disease. One of the more common etiological agents for these symptoms is MAC, the most common mycobacterial infection in AIDS. Most often, MAC is disseminated, and mesenteric lymphadenitis with diffuse abdominal pain is often found. In a recent review of the endoscopic findings in patients with disseminated MAC [41], the most common finding was multiple raised nodules (38%), followed by normal mucosa (36%); other less frequently seen findings were ulcerations, erythema, edema, friability,

reduced mucosal vascular pattern, stricture, and aphthous erosions. The diagnosis is established by biopsy, with acid-fast staining of bone marrow, liver, or gastrointestinal tract specimens. The diagnosis can also be made with blood or stool cultures. Treatment with multiple antimycobacterial antibiotics is prolonged and difficult, but effective.

Pancreaticobiliary Diseases

Pancreatitis

Asymptomatic hyperamylasemia is seen in up to 46 % of HIV patients [42,43], but pancreatitis was rare until the use of didanosine and pentamidine became more widespread. Didanosine has been reported to cause pancreatitis in up to 23 % of patients treated with this agent [44]. The clinical course is most often mild, but severe and even fatal cases of pancreatitis have been reported.

Infectious etiologies of pancreatitis are multiple, but the diagnosis is rarely confirmed except at autopsy, as pancreatic biopsy is not done routinely. CMV, HSV, *Cryptosporidium*, MAC, and *Toxoplasma* have all been reported to cause pancreatitis [45]. The incidence of pancreatic ductal changes suggestive of chronic pancreatitis in patients with AIDS is between 37 % and 54 %. Some studies have shown a strong correlation between pancreatic ductal changes and AIDS-related sclerosing cholangitis, while others have cast doubt on this association [46,47].

The presentation and treatment in the AIDS patient with pancreatitis are no different from those in pancreatitis in nonimmunocompromised patients. Treatment includes close observation, nothing by mouth, supportive care, and analgesia.

Acalculous Cholecystitis

Acute cholecystitis is the most common indication for urgent abdominal surgery in patients with AIDS, and over one-third of these patients will have acalculous cholecystitis. Despite this frequency, acalculous cholecystitis is still a relatively rare entity, albeit one with significant morbidity and mortality for the patient with AIDS [48,49]. Infections of the gallbladder with CMV, *Cryptosporidium,* and MAC have all been reported [50], but most cases are idiopathic. Patients present with clinical symptoms and signs similar to those of calculous cholecystitis, with right upper quadrant abdominal pain seen in 90 % and nausea in 83 % [50]. Hepatobiliary scintigraphy with diisopropyl iminodiacetic acid (DISIDA) and hepatoiminodiacetic acid (HIDA) scanning usually reveals cystic duct obstruction. The alkaline phosphatase level is elevated in most patients. The definitive diagnosis and treatment is with cholecystectomy. The mortality can be even more significant if the diagnosis is missed and gallbladder gangrene, perforation, or both develop—a situation that occurs especially with CMV infection.

AIDS Cholangiopathy (Fig. 55.10)

AIDS cholangiopathy is a spectrum of disorders seen in severely immunosuppressed patients with AIDS (CD 4 count < 50/mm^3). The disorder consists of four distinct entities: papillary stenosis with common bile duct dilation; sclerosing cholangitis; papillary stenosis and sclerosing cholangitis; and long extrahepatic bile duct strictures. The most common variant is having both papillary stenosis and sclerosing cholangitis.

Etiologically, infection of the biliary tree by *Cryptosporidium*, microsporidia, or CMV is most frequent. Up to 85 % of patients present with right upper quadrant or epigastric abdominal pain with or without fever (fever is seen in 60 % of patients). Diarrhea and weight loss also are common. Most patients have elevated alkaline phosphatase levels, and elevated bilirubin is seen in only 15 % [51,52].

The diagnosis is established at endoscopic retrograde cholangiopancreatography (ERCP) with characteristic cholangiographic findings (e.g., a dilated common bile duct in papillary stenosis and intrahepatic ducts that are alternately strictured and dilated). Biopsy and culture of bile and tissue can yield a definitive pathogen in approximately 50 % of cases [52,53]. It has been suggested that microsporidia may be missed in a large proportion of the remainder, as this pathogen is hard to detect [53].

Management consists of treating the underlying infection and also relieving the biliary obstruction. This is achieved by endoscopic sphincterotomy for papillary stenosis, often in combination with stenting to provide drainage of strictured segments of the biliary system. Most series have shown that pain is relieved in 60–80 % of cases after endoscopic therapy. Unfortunately, endoscopic intervention has not been associated with improvement in mortality for these patients, and their long-term survival remains poor [54]. This is not unexpected, given the advanced stage of AIDS at the time of presentation. It also should be noted that alkaline phosphatase levels may continue to rise despite pain relief, because of continued disease progression.

Diarrhea

Chronic diarrhea remains the most common AIDS-related gastrointestinal complaint in patients with HIV-related disease. Diarrhea occurs at some time during the course of the disease in up to 60 % of patients in developed nations, while in developing countries persistent diarrhea has been reported to affect up to 95 % of patients [55,56]. The incidence of diarrhea has been reported to be 14.2 per 100 person-years, and the probability of developing diarrhea within 2 years with a CD 4 lymphocyte count < 500/mm^3 is 74.3 % [56].

Chronic diarrhea has an obvious adverse effect on quality of life, and it is an independent predictor of poor survival among patients with HIV infection [55]. There is a reported 10-month mortality rate of 72 % in patients with AIDS and chronic diarrhea. Without doubt, it is also responsible for continued high health-care costs [57].

The pathophysiology of AIDS-related diarrhea is multifactorial. Both opportunistic infections (with an identifiable enteric pathogen) and ongoing intestinal immunological dysregulation result in diarrhea in these patients by several pathogenic mechanisms (**Table**

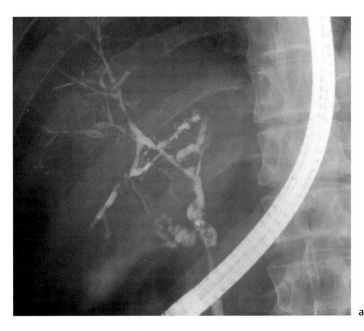
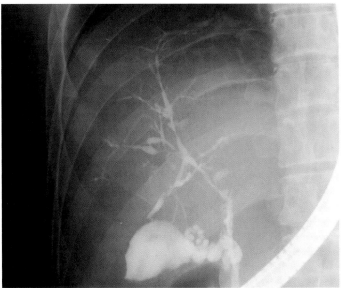

Fig. 55.10 a, b Sclerosing cholangitis variant of AIDS cholangiopathy. The alternately strictured and dilated ("chain of lakes") appearance of the intrahepatic biliary system should be noted.

55.3) [58]. Gastrointestinal endoscopy has proved useful for evaluating patients with HIV-related diarrhea, but its optimal use remains poorly studied, particularly with regard to the timing and type of endoscopy performed.

Pathogens

An etiology can be established in 44–80 % of patients with HIV-associated diarrhea, depending on the thoroughness of diagnostic testing [57]. In a study of 1933 patients [56], the most common pathogens (**Table 55.4**) were *Cryptosporidium* (12–15 %); nontubercular mycobacteria (8–14 %); microsporidia (5–11 %); and bacteria (*Salmonella, Shigella, Campylobacter,* and *Escherichia coli*; 10 %). Cytomegalovirus is found in 5–15 %. Enteric pathogen-caused diarrhea in patients with AIDS is strongly associated with severe immunodeficiency, and a total of 90 % of all such pathogens are found in patients with CD 4 lymphocyte counts < 200/mm^3.

Table 55.3 Pathophysiological factors involved in AIDS-related diarrhea [58]

Pathogenic mechanism	Etiological agent
Decreased mucosal surface area	*Cryptosporidium*, microsporidia, *Isospora*
Altered secretion of inflammatory mediators (e. g., interleukin-1)	Mycobacterium avium-intracellulare, Clostridium difficile
Ileal dysfunction	HIV enteropathy
Exudative enteropathy	Mycobacterium avium-intracellulare
Altered motility	HIV enteropathy
Bacterial overgrowth	HIV enteropathy
Chronic mucosal inflammation, infection of enterochromaffin cells, interaction of gp120 with VIP receptor, antiproliferative effects, direct effects on enterocyte function	Direct HIV infection

HIV, human immunodeficiency virus; VIP, vasoactive intestinal polypeptide.

Table 55.4 Most common pathogens involved in HIV-associated diarrhea [56]

Ova and parasites
- Cryptosporidium
- Microsporidia
- Giardia lamblia

Entamoeba histolytica

Enteropathogenic bacteria
- Salmonella species
- Shigella species
- Campylobacter

Nontuberculous mycobacteria
- Mycobacterium avium-intracellulare

Viruses
- Cytomegalovirus

Isospora belli
- Cyclospora species
- Leishmania
- Strongyloides species

Aeromonas

Verotoxin-producing *Escherichia coli*

Clostridium difficile

The incidence and cause of bacterial diarrhea in a large cohort of patients with HIV infection was reexamined in a retrospective cohort study sponsored by the Centers for Disease Control and Prevention. Data were analyzed from 44,778 persons for the period 1992–2002. During this time, there were 11,320 episodes of diarrheal illness, in which 1091 (9.6%) at least one bacterial organism was listed as a causative agent. The mean incidence of bacterial diarrhea was 7.2 cases per 1000 person-years. The frequencies of bacterial pathogens identified in this study were *Clostridium difficile* 53.6%, *Shigella* 14%, *Campylobacter* 13.8%, and *Salmonella* 7.4% [59].

Intestinal coinfection with two or more pathogens is more unusual than are single infections. Coinfection is diagnosed in approximately 20% of patients [56], and occurs more commonly when *Mycobacterium avium* complex (MAC) or *Cryptosporidium* is present.

Diagnostic Yield

The value of panendoscopy—i. e., esophagogastroduodenoscopy (EGD) and colonoscopy—in patients with HIV-related diarrhea remains controversial. In a prospective study [56], the examination of biopsies obtained at EGD disclosed pathogens that had not been diagnosed by previous stool studies in only 8% of patients, and the addition of colonoscopy after EGD had been performed detected at least one other pathogen in 20% of cases; most frequently, CMV colitis was found.

In another prospective study [57] in which both EGD and colonoscopy were performed in 79 patients with HIV-related diarrhea, an infection not diagnosed by stool culture or ova and parasite examination was found in 28% of patients. Duodenal biopsies, however, yielded no additional pathogens beyond those identified by colonoscopy if the terminal ileum was intubated and sampled. Moreover, 100% of patients with CMV colitis had evidence of the infection on rectosigmoid biopsies, and only a few additional diagnoses were made by examining the colon beyond the rectosigmoid. This is in direct conflict with data from two other studies [60,61], which provided evidence that a significant proportion of pathogens might be limited to the proximal colon. In Bini and Weinshel's series [60], 30% of pathogens (most commonly CMV, *Mycobacterium tuberculosis, Clostridium difficile,* and *Hymenolepis nana*) were identified only on biopsies of the proximal colon, beyond the reach of the sigmoidoscope. In Dieterich and Rahmin's series [61], 24% of patients had CMV disease localized to the right colon or cecum. Despite these data, the American Gastroenterological Association, in a position paper published in 1996 [62], and some respected investigators [63] recommend only a flexible sigmoidoscopy with biopsy if a specific pathogen is not diagnosed on routine stool studies in the AIDS patient with chronic diarrhea.

The value of EGD with duodenal biopsy and/or aspirate is somewhat more controversial. Multiple studies have failed to show a dramatic benefit for these procedures in evaluating chronic HIV-related diarrhea. The diagnostic yield of duodenal biopsy and aspirate is low, ranging from 8% [56] to 13% [64]. If electron microscopy is added to the evaluation, the yield increases to 26% [64], but this is cost-prohibitive and too cumbersome in most clinical situations.

In a study by Bini and Cohen [65], however, an offending organism was found in 29.6% of upper endoscopies. For patients with a CD4 count >100/mm^3, the diagnostic yield was 8.3%, but this increased significantly to 62.8% for patients when the CD4 count was <100/mm^3. When patients with a CD4 count >100/mm^3 were compared with those with a CD4 count <100/mm^3, EGD was associated with a much lower cost of identifying a pathogen by endoscopy for the more severely immunocompromised patients ($21,583 vs. $2943) [65]. The organisms most commonly found on EGD in endoscopy studies are *Cryptosporidium,* microsporidia, CMV, and *Giardia.* Newer evidence [66–70] indicates that microsporidia can be reliably diagnosed using a modified trichrome stain, polymerase chain reaction (PCR) analysis of stool specimens (up to 100% sensitivity compared with electron microscopy in one study), or fluorescent in-situ hybridization.

The preferred algorithm for evaluating AIDS-related diarrhea is shown in **Fig. 55.11** [56]. Specifically, in patients with diarrhea and low CD4 lymphocyte counts (<100/mm^3), when routine stool studies are inconclusive, colonoscopy with terminal ileal intubation and biopsy remains the best overall diagnostic test. In patients with CD4 lymphocyte counts of 100–200/mm^3, flexible sigmoidoscopy with biopsy might prove useful, because the incidence of CMV disease in this group is lower than when CD4 counts are higher. Duodenal biopsy should be performed if the above studies are inconclusive, especially in patients with CD4 lymphocyte counts <100/mm^3.

The importance of obtaining stool studies *first* in patients with AIDS and chronic diarrhea cannot be overemphasized. Routine stool studies identify far more etiologies of chronic diarrhea in AIDS patients than does any endoscopic approach in most series (in one study, up to 47% when six stool specimens from each patient were examined) [71].

IX

A defeatist approach using only antidiarrheal therapy if stool studies are negative (as has been advocated in the past) [72] is no longer appropriate. Specific pathogens and therapies should always be sought in the patient with chronic diarrhea and AIDS.

Specific Pathogens and Endoscopic Appearance

Cytomegalovirus. CMV colitis is notable at endoscopy for its variability: isolated shallow ulcerations, deep circular ulcers, patchy submucosal hemorrhage, mucosal edema, and mucosal friability (**Figs. 55.12, 55.13**); occasionally, CMV appears as an ulcerated mass resembling neoplasia. It can mimic ischemic colitis, Crohn's disease, or ulcerative colitis, all of which rarely arise de novo in patients with severe immunodeficiency. Colonic perforations are well documented with this infection.

Biopsies, most commonly from an ulcer base, reveal stromal and endothelial cells with characteristic CMV inclusions (markedly enlarged cells with amphophilic nuclear inclusions and abundant granular basophilic cytoplasm) [18]. Inflammation and erosions or ulcers usually are present, and parallel the number of inclusions. CMV culture is slow and unreliable, and has little role in clinical practice. Both conventional and real-time PCR can now be used to detect CMV DNA in the blood. Both PCR techniques appear to be equivalent to testing for CMV antigenemia by immunofluorescence. Unlike antigenemia assays, which rely on enumeration of the number of CMV antigen-positive polymorphonucleocytes, the PCR techniques offer an advantage in that they can be used in profoundly neutropenic patients [73].

Mycobacterium avium complex. Gastrointestinal involvement with MAC is often diagnosed more reliably outside of the gastrointestinal tract (e. g., bone marrow biopsy, liver biopsy, or blood culture), because its endoscopic appearance can be subtle, and random tissue sampling can often miss it. Endoscopically, the small-intestinal folds may appear thickened or edematous, with occasional yellow patches, which can become confluent. On small-bowel biopsy specimens, MAC resembles Whipple's disease, as the lamina propria in both diseases contains variable numbers of periodic acid–Schiff (PAS)-positive macrophages; in MAC, macrophages are packed with acid-fast organisms, whereas in Whipple's disease, acid-fast staining is negative. Villous atrophy also is notable [18].

Microsporidia/Cryptosporidium parvum. The endoscopic appearance of the small-bowel mucosa in patients with Cryptosporidium or microsporidia is erythematous and slightly granular, due to irregular, fused, widely-spaced, and shortened villi [18]. On routine biopsy, these organisms can easily be missed. Cryptosporidia are round basophilic bodies 2–5 µm in size, which appear to be on the surface of enterocytes on light microscopy. Electron microscopy, however, shows them to be just below the surface epithelium. The appearance of microsporidia (Enterocytozoon bieneusi and Encephalitozoon intestinalis) is even more subtle than that of cryptosporidia on routine hematoxylin–eosin staining, but they are more easily seen with electron microscopy than with routine light microscopy. The surrounding villi are variably atrophic, with lamina propria neutrophils and crypt abscesses seen infrequently, and more often in cryptosporidial infection. Because infections from the genus Encephalitozoon result in a deeper infection than those with the genus Enterocytozoon, the former may be detected in the urine of some infected patients, whereas urine analysis is not helpful in diagnosing E. bieneusi infection [74,75].

HIV enteropathy. This term is applied to diarrhea in the AIDS patient for which no infectious cause can be found despite extensive investigation. A variety of pathologic findings are seen in biopsies

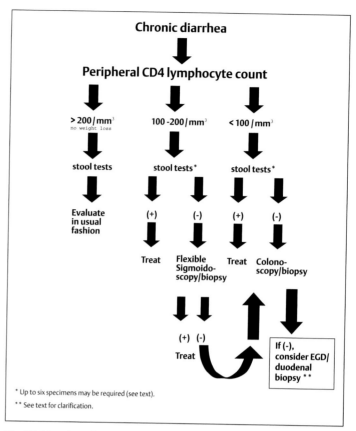

Fig. 55.11 Algorithm for the diagnostic investigation of chronic AIDS-related diarrhea.

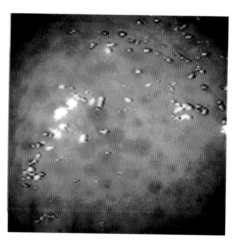

Fig. 55.12 Cytomegalovirus-induced proctocolitis.

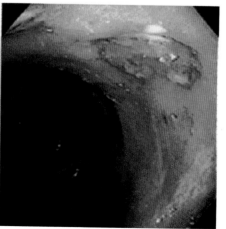

Fig. 55.13 Cytomegalovirus-induced rectal ulceration.

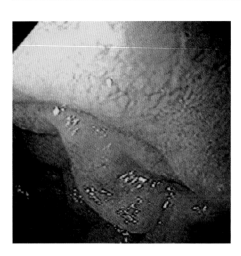

Fig. 55.14 "Frosted" appearance of the duodenal mucosa in a patient with HIV enteropathy.

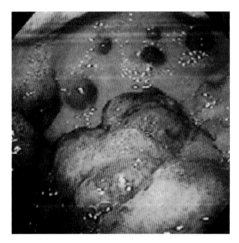

Fig. 55.15 Bulky reddish-purple masses seen in colonic Kaposi's sarcoma.

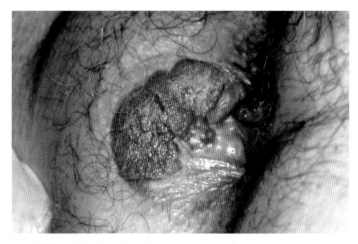

Fig. 55.16 AIDS-related (peri)anal squamous cell carcinoma.

from these patients, ranging from mild villous atrophy to vacuolated enterocytes and mild chronic small-bowel inflammation. Endoscopically, the mucosa may appear "frosted" (**Fig. 55.14**), but this is not a specific finding. Often, there are objective findings of severe malabsorption, including lactose intolerance, vitamin B_{12} and D-xylose malabsorption, and increased intestinal permeability with protein loss. Resolution of not only the clinical symptoms but also the ultrastructural tissue changes has been reported in patients with HIV enteropathy after initiation of HAART therapy [76].

There are two major schools of thought about the pathophysiology of the diarrhea of HIV enteropathy. One hypothesis is that HIV infection of the mucosa results in a change in intestinal permeability through disruption of tight junctions, epithelial cell apoptosis, or both [77]. An alternative, but not mutually exclusive, hypothesis is that the HIV protein gp120 acts through a coreceptor to cause calcium-mediated microtubule loss and thus cellular instability [78].

Gastrointestinal Bleeding

Gastrointestinal bleeding is uncommon in patients with AIDS [79]. When it does occur, however, survival is adversely affected [80–82]. Once again, it is important to remember that the most likely causes of gastrointestinal bleeding in the immunocompetent HIV-positive patient are *not* AIDS-related (e. g., peptic ulcer disease, esophagitis, diverticulosis, and hemorrhoids). As immunosuppression progresses, however, most AIDS patients with gastrointestinal bleeding have unique lesions and conditions directly related to HIV disease that should be investigated and treated endoscopically in all but those with imminently terminal disease.

AIDS-Related Upper Gastrointestinal Bleeding

Kaposi's sarcoma (**Fig. 55.8**) is the most common cause of AIDS-related upper gastrointestinal bleeding in advanced AIDS patients, representing 31% of lesions in one series [79]. Gastroduodenal lymphoma accounted for 30% of bleeding in another series [82]. Neither lesion is very amenable to endoscopic therapy, but attempts to control bleeding temporarily with laser coagulation have been successful. Surgical resection may need to be done as a last resort. Bleeding from portal hypertension, most commonly from esophageal varices, is seen in only approximately 10% of patients—an interesting observation, given the high prevalence of chronic liver disease in this population. A low platelet count is observed in 8–9% of AIDS patients and has been shown to be an independent risk factor for predicting upper gastrointestinal bleeding in this population [82].

AIDS-Related Lower Gastrointestinal Bleeding

CMV disease of the colon is the most common identifiable cause of lower gastrointestinal bleeding in patients with AIDS, seen in 39% of patients in one series [81]; 28% of patients in the same series had idiopathic colonic ulceration. Kaposi's sarcoma of the small bowel was found in 6%, and 8% of patients had bleeding Kaposi's sarcomas of the colon (**Fig. 55.15**) [79]. The in-hospital mortality in patients with AIDS-related lower gastrointestinal bleeding is high, ranging from 28% [81] to 39% [80], but this mortality is most often not related to gastrointestinal bleeding and correlates most with advanced immunodeficiency.

Patients with AIDS can also have bleeding from anorectal sources (**Fig. 55.16**), and these should not be overlooked during the evaluation, especially if the patient is a man who has sex with men. Etiologies of anorectal bleeding can include condylomatous disease (**Fig. 55.17**), herpes simplex infection, idiopathic ulceration, and non-Hodgkin's lymphoma.

IX

AIDS and the Endoscopist

Endoscopic examination has played, and will continue to play, an important role in the evaluation and therapy of the patient with HIV disease. This raises important safety concerns for the practicing endoscopist in avoiding patient-to-patient and patient-to-endoscopist cross-contamination.

Although endoscopic transmission of HIV never has been reported [83], endoscopic instruments have been vectors for mycobacteria, *Salmonella, Pseudomonas* [84], hepatitis B virus [85], and hepatitis C virus in clearly documented cases [86]. In one study, contamination of 20 endoscopes used in patients with AIDS was assessed [87]. Seven of 20 unwashed endoscopes were contaminated with HIV, six were contaminated with *Candida,* and *Pseudomonas* contamination was found in five. Washing alone removed all organisms from 66 of 68 contaminated sites [87]. Furthermore, evidence has been obtained using PCR techniques that mycobacteria, hepatitis B virus, hepatitis C virus, and HIV are readily inactivated by commonly used cleaning methods and germicides [83,88,89].

Thus, if the accepted standards are followed for adequate mechanical cleaning and high-level disinfection of endoscopes (e. g., a 20-min soak at room temperature in 2 % glutaraldehyde solution), patient-to-patient transmission of infectious agents can be kept to a low rate. Special care must be exercised with duodenoscopes and linear echo endoscopes, however, as mechanical cleaning is more difficult, especially around the mobile elevator. Two-tiered systems (e. g., dedicated endoscopes and accessories, or specific procedures for only some patients) are not appropriate.

All endoscopists should practice universal/standard precautions during any endoscopic procedure with any patient (**Table 55.5**). Although this would seem obvious to most, one would be surprised at how many endoscopists "cut corners," even in this day and age [90]. In one large study [91], only 57 % of endoscopists employed barrier precautions for all endoscopic procedures involving possible contact with blood or bodily fluids of patients with *known* blood-borne infections.

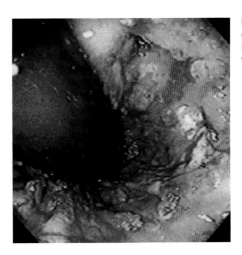

Fig. 55.17 Severe anal condylomatous lesions in a patient with advanced AIDS.

Table 55.5 Standard/universal precautions

Hand washing	Wash hands after touching blood, body fluids, secretions, excretions, and contaminated items, whether or not gloves are worn
Gloves	Wear clean, nonsterile gloves when touching blood, body fluids, secretions, excretions, and contaminated items
Masks, eye protection, face shields	Wear a mask and eye protection or a face shield during procedures that are likely to generate splashes or sprays of blood or body fluids
Gowns	Wear a clean, nonsterile gown to protect skin and to prevent soiling of clothing during procedures and patient care activities that are likely to generate sprays or splashes of blood or body fluids
Patient care equipment	Handle used patient-care equipment soiled with blood or body fluids in a manner that prevents skin and mucous membrane contact or cross-contamination with other patients or the environment. All equipment must be properly cleaned and reprocessed prior to further patient contact

Conclusions

Even though patients with HIV disease in developed countries are far healthier today than they were just a few years ago, the gastrointestinal tract still remains a major target for pathogens and diseases in AIDS. Endoscopic diagnosis will continue to be a mainstay in the evaluation and treatment of this population for the foreseeable future.

References

1. Fastats AIDS/HIV, 2005: www.cdc.gov/nchs/fastats/aids-hiv.htm.
2. Deaths: Final Data for 2004, National Vital Statistics Reports, Volume 55, Number 19, August 21, 2007. http://www.cdc.gov/nchs/data/nvsr/nvsr55/nvsr55_19.pdf.
3. http://www.cdc.gov/nchs/data/hus/hus07.pdf#101.
4. http://www.cdc.gov/hiv/topics/msm/resources/factsheets/msm.htm.
5. http://www.cdc.gov/hiv/topics/aa/resources/factsheets/aa.htm.
6. http://www.cdc.gov/hiv/hispanics/resources/factsheets/hispanic.htm.
7. UNAIDS. 2006 Report on the global AIDS epidemic. Geneva: UNIADS; 2006.
8. http://www.who.int/mediacentre/factsheets/fs314/en/index.html.
9. Knox TA, Spiegelman D, Skinner SC, Gorbach S. Diarrhea and abnormalities of gastrointestinal function in a cohort of men and women with HIV infection. Am J Gastroenterol 2000;95:3482–9.
10. Wilcox CM. Gastrointestinal manifestations of AIDS. In: Brandt LJ, editor. Clinical practice of gastroenterology. Philadelphia: Current Medicine; 1999. p. 1490–9.
11. Lai YP, Wu MS, Chen MY, Chuang CY, Shun CT, Lin JT. Timing and necessity of endoscopy in AIDS patients with dysphagia or odynophagia. Hepatogastroenterology 1998;45:2186–9.
12. Bonacini M. Medical management of benign oesophageal disease in patients with human immunodeficiency virus infection. Dig Liver Dis 2001;33:294–300.
13. Mönkemüller KE, Call SA, Lazenby AJ, Wilcox CM. Declining prevalence of opportunistic gastrointestinal disease in the era of combination antiretroviral therapy. Am J Gastroenterol 2000;95:457–62.
14. Mocroft A, Oancea C, van Lunzen J, Vanhems P, Banhegyi D, Chiesi A, et al. Decline in esophageal candidiasis and use of antimycotics in European patients with HIV. Am J Gastroenterol 2005;100:1446–54.
15. Mönkemüller KE, Lazenby AJ, Lee DH, Loudon R, Wilcox CM. Occurrence of gastrointestinal opportunistic disorders in AIDS despite the use of highly active antiretroviral therapy. Dig Dis Sci 2005;50:230–4.
16. Wilcox CM, Rodgers W, Lazenby A. Prospective comparison of brush cytology, viral culture, and histology for the diagnosis of ulcerative esophagitis in AIDS. Clin Gastroenterol Hepatol 2004;2:564–7.
17. Wilcox CM, Straub RF, Schwartz DA. Prospective evaluation of biopsy number for the diagnosis of viral esophagitis in patients with HIV infection and esophageal ulcer. Gastrointest Endosc 1996;44:587–93.
18. Clayton F, Clayton CH. Gastrointestinal pathology in HIV-infected patients. Gastroenterol Clin North Am 1997;26:191–240.
19. Wilcox CM, Schwartz DA. Endoscopic characterization of idiopathic esophageal ulceration associated with human immunodeficiency virus infection. J Clin Gastroenterol 1993;16:251–6.

55

20. Wilcox CM, Straub RF, Schwartz DA. Prospective endoscopic characterization of cytomegalovirus esophagitis in AIDS. Gastrointest Endosc 1994;40:481–4.

21. Wilcox CM, Schwartz DA. Comparison of two corticosteroid regimens for the treatment of idiopathic esophageal ulcerations associated with HIV infection. Am J Gastroenterol 1994;89:2163–7.

22. Bellomo A, Schorr-Lesnick B. Thalidomide treatment for idiopathic esophageal ulcers in patients with HIV. Gastrointest Endosc 1996;44:729–31.

23. Alexander LN, Wilcox CM. A prospective trial of thalidomide for the treatment of HIV-associated idiopathic esophageal ulcers. AIDS Res Hum Retroviruses 1997;13:301–4.

24. Georghiou PR, Kemp RJ. HIV-associated esophageal ulcers treated with thalidomide. Med J Aus 1990;152:382–3.

25. Mönig SP, Schmidt R, Wolters U, Krug B. [Tuberculosis of the esophagus]. Wien Klin Wochenschr 1995;107:155–7. German.

26. Forsmark CE, Wilcox CM, Darragh TM, Cello JP. Disseminated histoplasmosis in AIDS: an unusual case of esophageal involvement and gastrointestinal bleeding. Gastrointest Endosc 1990;36:604–5.

27. Kazlow PG, Shah K, Benkov KJ, Dische R, LeLeiko NS. Esophageal cryptosporidiosis in a child with acquired immunodeficiency syndrome. Gastroenterology 1986;91:1301–3.

28. Grimes MM, LaPook JD, Bar MH, Wasserman HS, Dwork A. Disseminated *Pneumocystis carinii* infection in a patient with acquired immunodeficiency syndrome. Hum Pathol 1987;18:307–8.

29. Werneck-Silva AL, Prado IB. Dyspepsia in HIV-infected patients under highly active antiretroviral therapy. J Gastroenterol Hepatol 2007;22:1712–6.

30. Vaira D, Miglioli M, Menegatti M, Holton J, Boschini A, Vergura M, et al. *Helicobacter pylori* status, endoscopic findings, and serology in HIV-1 positive patients. Dig Dis Sci 1995;40:1622–6.

31. Welage LS, Carver PL, Revankar S, Pierson C, Kauffman CA. Alterations in gastric acidity in patients infected with human immunodeficiency virus. Clin Infect Dis 1995;21:1431–8.

32. Olmos M, Araya V, Pskorz E, Quesada EC, Concetti H, Perez H, et al. Coinfection: *Helicobacter pylori*/human immunodeficiency virus. Dig Dis Sci 2004;49:1836–9.

33. Fabris P, Bozzola L, Benedetti P, Scagnelli M, Nicolin R, Manfrin V, et al. *H. pylori* infection in HIV-positive patients. A serohistological study. Dig Dis Sci 1997;42:289–92.

34. Chiu HM, Wu MS, Hung CC, Shun CT, Lin JT. Low prevalence of *Helicobacter pylori* but high prevalence of cytomegalovirus-associated peptic ulcer disease in AIDS patients: comparative study of symptomatic subjects evaluated by endoscopy and CD4 counts. J Gastroenterol Hepatol 2004;19:423–8.

35. Varsky CG, Correa MC, Sarmiento N, Bonfanti M, Peluffo G, Dutack A, et al. Prevalence and etiology of gastroduodenal ulcer in HIV-positive patients: a comparative study of 497 symptomatic subjects evaluated by endoscopy. Am J Gastroenterol 1998;93:935–40.

36. Friedman SL, Wright TL, Altman DF. Gastrointestinal Kaposi's sarcoma in patients with acquired immunodeficiency syndrome: endoscopic and autopsy findings. Gastroenterology 1985;89:102–8.

37. Saltz RK, Kurtz RC, Lightdale CJ, Myskowski P, Cunningham-Rundles S, Urmacher C, et al. Kaposi's sarcoma: gastrointestinal involvement correlation with skin findings and immunologic function. Dig Dis Sci 1984;29:817–23.

38. Chang Y, Cesarman E, Pessin MS, Lee F, Culpepper J, Knowles DM, et al. Identification of herpesvirus-like DNA sequences in AIDS-associated Kaposi's sarcoma. Science 1994;266:1865–9.

39. Knowles DM, Chadburn A. Lymphadenopathy and the lymphoid neoplasms associated with the acquired immune deficiency syndrome. In: Knowles DM, editor. Neoplastic hematopathology. 2nd ed. Baltimore: Lippincott Williams and Wilkins; 2000: 987–1090.

40. Krause J. AIDS-related non-Hodgkin's lymphomas. Microsc Res Tech 2005;68:168–75.

41. Sun H, Chen M, Wu M. Endoscopic appearance of GI mycobacteriosis caused by the *Mycobacterium avium* complex in a patient with AIDS: case report and review. Gastrointest Endosc 2005;61:775–9.

42. Zarro JF, Pichon F, Regnier B. HIV and the pancreas. Lancet 1987;ii:1212–3.

43. Schwartz MS, Brandt LJ. Spectrum of pancreatic disorders in patients with the acquired immunodeficiency syndrome. Am J Gastroenterol 1989;84:459–62.

44. Maxson CJ, Green SM, Turner JL. Acute pancreatitis as a common complication of 2,3-dideoxyinosine therapy in the acquired immunodeficiency syndrome. Am J Gastroenterol 1992;87:708–13.

45. Simon D, Brandt LJ. ERCP in patients with AIDS. In: Jacobsen IM, editor. ERCP and its applications. Philadelphia: Lippincott-Raven, 1998: 141–9.

46. Barthet M, Chauveau E, Bonnet E, Petit N, Bernard JP, Gastaut JA, et al. Pancreatic ductal changes in HIV-infected patients. Gastrointest Endosc 1997;45:59–63.

47. Evrard S, Van Laethem JL, Urbain D, Devière J, Cremer M.. Chronic pancreatic alterations in AIDS patients. Pancreas 1999;19:335–8.

48. Ricci M, Puente AO, Rothenberg RE. Open and laparoscopic cholecystectomy in acquired immunodeficiency syndrome: indications and results in fifty-three patients. Surgery 1999;125:172–7.

49. Fiorillo MA, Feuerstadt P, Kuperschmidt D. General surgery indications and outcomes in patients with human immunodeficiency virus (HIV) infection: A 15-year perspective [submitted for publication July 2008].

50. French AL, Beaudet LM, Benator DA, Levy CS, Kass M, Orenstein JM. Cholecystectomy in patients with AIDS: clinical pathologic correlation in 107 cases. Clin Infect Dis 1995;21:852–8.

51. Benhamou Y, Caumes E, Gerosa Y, Cadranel JF, Dohin E, Katlama C, et al. AIDS-related cholangiopathy: critical analysis of a prospective series of 26 patients. Dig Dis Sci 1993;38:1113–8.

52. Cello JP. Acquired immunodeficiency syndrome cholangiopathy: spectrum of disease. Am J Med 1989;86:539–46.

53. Pol S, Romana CA, Richard S, Amouyal P, Desportes-Livage I, Carnot F, et al. Microsporidial infection in patients with the human immunodeficiency virus and unexplained cholangitis. N Engl J Med 1993;328:95–9.

54. Ko WF, Cello JP, Rogers SJ, Lecours A. Prognostic factors for the survival of patients with AIDS cholangiopathy. Am J Gastroenterol 2003;98:2176–81.

55. Thom K, Forrest G. Gastrointestinal infections in immunocompromised hosts. Curr Opin Gastroenterol 2006;22:18–23.

56. Weber R, Ledergerber B, Zbinden R, Altwegg M, Pfyffer GE, Spycher MA, et al. Enteric infections and diarrhea in human immunodeficiency virus-infected persons: prospective community-based cohort study. Swiss HIV Cohort Study. Arch Intern Med 1999;159:1473–80.

57. Kearney DJ, Steuerwald M, Koch J, Cello JP. A prospective study of endoscopy in HIV-associated diarrhea. Am J Gastroenterol 1999;94:596–602.

58. Lu SS. Pathophysiology of HIV-associated diarrhea. Gastroenterol Clin North Am 1987;26:175–89.

59. Sanchez TH, Brooks JT, Sullivan PS, Juhasz M, Mintz E, Dworkin MS, et al. Bacterial diarrhea in persons with HIV infection, United States, 1992–2002. Clin Infect Dis 2005;41:1621–7.

60. Bini E, Weinshel E. Endoscopic evaluation of chronic human immunodeficiency virus-related diarrhea: is colonoscopy superior to flexible sigmoidoscopy? Am J Gastroenterol 1998;93:56–60.

61. Dieterich DT, Rahmin M. Cytomegalovirus colitis in AIDS: presentation in 44 patients and a review of the literature. J Acquir Immune Defic Syndr 1991;4(Suppl 1):S 29–35.

62. [No authors listed.] American Gastroenterological Association medical position statement: guidelines for the management of malnutrition and cachexia, chronic diarrhea, and hepatobiliary disease in patients with human immunodeficiency virus infection. Gastroenterology 1996;111:1722–3.

63. Johanson JF. To scope or not to scope: the role of endoscopy in the evaluation of AIDS-related diarrhea. Am J Gastroenterol 1996;91:2261–2.

64. Bown JW, Savides TJ, Mathews C, Isenberg J, Behling C, Lyche KD. Diagnostic yield of duodenal biopsy and aspirate in AIDS-associated diarrhea. Am J Gastroenterol 1996;91:2289–92.

65. Bini EJ, Cohen J. Diagnostic yield and cost-effectiveness of endoscopy in chronic human immunodeficiency virus-related diarrhea. Gastrointest Endosc 1998;48:354–61.

66. Corcoran GD, Tovey DG, Moody AH, Chiodini PL. Detection and identification of gastrointestinal microsporidia using non-invasive techniques. J Clin Pathol 1995;48:725–27.

67. DeGirolami PC, Ezratty CR, Desai G, McCullough A, Asmuth D, Wanke C, et al. Diagnosis of intestinal microsporidiosis by examination of stool and duodenal aspirate with Weber's modified trichrome and Uvitez 2B stains. J Clin Microbiol 1995;33:805–10.

68. Didier ES, Orenstein JM, Aldras A, Bertucci D, Rogers LB, Janney FA. Comparison of three staining methods for detecting microsporidia in fluids. J Clin Microbiol 1995;33:3138–45.

69. Weber R, Bryan RT, Owen RL, Wilcox CM, Gorelkin L, Visvesvara GS, et al. Improved light-microscopical detection of microsporidia spores in stool and duodenal aspirates. N Engl J Med 1992;326:161–6.

70. Graczyk TK, Johansson MA, Tamang L, Visvesvara GS, Moura LS, DaSilva AJ, et al. Retrospective species identification of microsporidian spores in diarrheic fecal samples from human immunodeficiency virus/AIDS patients by multiplexed fluorescence in situ hybridization. J Clin Microbiol 2007;45:1255–260.

IX

71. Blanshard C, Francis N, Gazzard BG. Investigation of chronic diarrhea in acquired immunodeficiency syndrome: a prospective study of 155 patients. Gut 1996;39:824–32.

72. Johanson JF, Sonnenberg A. Efficient management of diarrhea in the acquired immunodeficiency syndrome (AIDS): a medical decision analysis. Ann Intern Med 1990;112:942–8.

73. Drew WL. Laboratory diagnosis of cytomegalovirus infection and disease in immunocompromised patients. Curr Opin Infect Dis 2007;20:408–11.

74. Notermans DW, Peek R, de Jong MD, Wentink-Bonnema EM, Boom R, van Gool T. Detection and identification of *Enterocytozoon bieneusi* and *Encephalitozoon* species in stool and urine specimens by PCR and differential hybridization. J Clin Microbiol 2005;43:610–4.

75. Molina JM, Chastang C, Goguel J, Michiels JF, Sarfati C, Desportes-Livage I, et al. Albendazole for treatment and prophylaxis of microsporidiosis due to *Encephalitozoon intestinalis* in patients with AIDS: a randomized double-blind controlled trial. J Infect Dis 1998;177:1373–7.

76. Giovanni B, Calabrese C, Manfredi R, Pisi AM, Di Febo G, Hakim R, et al. HIV enteropathy: undescribed ultrastructural changes of duodenal mucosa and their regression after triple antiviral therapy. A case report. Dig Dis Sci 2005;50:617–22.

77. Kotler D. HIV infection and the gastrointestinal tract. AIDS 2005;19: 107–17.

78. Clayton F, Kotler DP, Kuwada SK, Morgan T, Stepan C, Kuang J, et al. Gp 120-induced Bob/GPR15 activation: a possible cause of human immuno-deficiency virus enteropathy. Am J Pathol 2001;159:1933–9.

79. Cello JP, Wilcox CM. Evaluation and treatment of gastrointestinal tract hemorrhage in patients with AIDS. Gastroenterol Clin North Am 1988;17:639–48.

80. Cappell MS, Geller AJ. The high mortality of gastrointestinal bleeding in HIV-seropositive patients: a multivariate analysis of risk factors and warning signs of mortality in 50 consecutive patients. Am J Gastroenterol 1992;87:815–24.

81. Chalasani N, Wilcox CM. Etiology and outcome of lower gastrointestinal bleeding in patients with AIDS. Am J Gastroenterol 1998;93:175–8.

82. Parente F, Cernuschi M, Valsecchi L, Rizzardini G, Musicco M, Lazzarin A, et al. Acute upper gastrointestinal bleeding in patients with AIDS: a relatively uncommon condition associated with reduced survival. Gut 1991;32:987–90.

83. Morris J, Duckworth GJ, Ridgway GL. Gastrointestinal endoscopy decontamination failure and the risk of transmission of blood-borne viruses: a review. J Hosp Infect 2006;63:1–13.

84. Allen JI, Allen MO, Olson MM, Gerding DN, Shanholtzer CJ, Meier PB, Vennes JA, et al. *Pseudomonas* infection of the biliary system resulting from use of a contaminated endoscope. Gastroenterology 1987;92: 759–63.

85. Birnie GG, Quigley EM, Clements GB, Follet EA, Watkinson G. Endoscopic transmission of hepatitis B virus. Gut 1983;24:171–4.

86. Kozarek RA. Transmission of hepatitis C virus during colonoscopy. N Engl J Med 1997;337:1848–9.

87. Hanson PJ, Gor D, Clarke JR, Chadwick MV, Nicholson G, Shah N, et al. Contamination of endoscopes used in AIDS patients. Lancet 1989;ii:86–8.

88. Chanzy B, Duc-Bin DL, Rousset B, Morand P, Morel-Baccard C, Marchetti B, et al. Effectiveness of a manual disinfection procedure in eliminating hepatitis C from experimentally contaminated endoscopes. Gastrointest Endosc 1999;50:147–51.

89. Standards of Practice Committee of the American Society of Gastrointestinal Endoscopy. Infection control during gastrointestinal endoscopy: guidelines for clinical application. Gastrointest Endosc 1999;49:836–41.

90. Shapiro M, Brandt LJ. Endoscopy in the age of HIV: a study of current practices and attitudes. Gastrointest Endosc 1994;40:477–80.

91. Gorse GJ, Messner RL. Infection control practices in gastrointestinal endoscopy in the United States; a national survey. Gastroenterol Nurs 1991;14:72–9.

55

Pediatric Endoscopy

Section editors:
Guido N.J. Tytgat, Charles J. Lightdale, Meinhard Classen

56 Pediatric Endoscopy

Victor L. Fox

Introduction

Gastrointestinal disorders in children include a broad spectrum of acute and chronic conditions similar to those found in adults. A major difference is the relative rarity of malignancies in the pediatric population. Screening and surveillance protocols for tumors or for dysplasia in conditions with malignant potential are therefore only a minor part of pediatric practice. Therapeutic interventions to eradicate early neoplasia or palliate advanced cancers are also rarely needed. On the other hand, pediatricians more often than internists are the first to encounter gastrointestinal manifestations of various genetic syndromes, congenital malformations, metabolic defects, and allergic disease (**Figs. 56.1–56.4**). Endoscopic investigations and therapeutic interventions are commonly carried out in children with unexplained diarrhea, malabsorption, and inflammatory bowel disease, as well as feeding and swallowing disorders, unexplained bleeding, and complications of advanced liver disease.

The production of increasingly smaller-diameter equipment has enabled endoscopists to perform in children nearly all of the diagnostic and therapeutic procedures currently practiced in adults. Despite this, no pediatric endoscopes truly exist, since none have been specifically and optimally designed for use in children. Procedures in small children are therefore difficult to perform, and a potentially higher risk of technical failure or injury must be considered. Furthermore, some advanced techniques such as cholangioscopy and endosonography, which require specialized larger-diameter instruments, are simply not possible in very small children or infants.

Pediatric endoscopists need to apply their specialized knowledge of pediatric anatomy, physiology, and behavior when choosing equipment, procedural technique, and the approach to sedation. Most pediatric endoscopists acquire suitable technical skills and medical knowledge through formal training programs in pediatric gastroenterology. However, pediatric endoscopy is also performed by surgeons who are trained in flexible endoscopy and by adult medicine specialists who have unique expertise in advanced techniques such as endoscopic retrograde cholangiopancreatography [1] and endoscopic ultrasonography. The American Society for Gastrointestinal Endoscopy (ASGE) has modified its practice guidelines to acknowledge differences in the care of adult and pediatric patients [2]. This chapter provides an overview of pediatric endoscopy, including major indications and common findings. Since pediatric endoscopy encompasses most aspects of adult endoscopy, the reader should refer to other chapters in this textbook when greater detail about specific techniques and equipment is desired.

Patient Preparation

▥ Emotional Preparation

Preendoscopy preparation may reduce a child's anxiety about a planned procedure. Reduced anxiety can positively affect various outcome measures of a procedure, such as the amount of medication required for adequate sedation [3], post-traumatic stress symptoms, and the family's level of satisfaction. The preoperative evaluation should include a history about past problems with procedures or sedation, to identify medical and emotional risk factors that might guide subsequent decisions about sedation and postprocedural observation. The procedure should be described in terms that

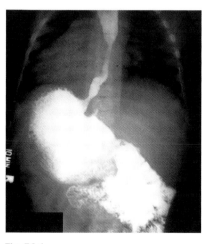 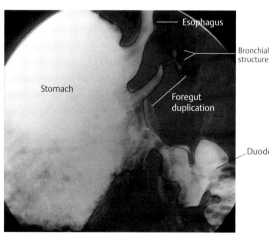 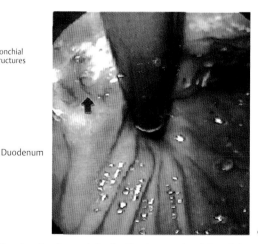

a, b

c

Fig. 56.1
a Barium contrast examination in a 9-year-old boy with Kartagener syndrome (situs inversus totalis and ciliary dyskinesia) and a small foregut duplication arising from the cardia of the stomach. The duplication contained bronchiolar structures (extralobar pulmonary sequestration) and extended into the right chest. There was also a hiatal hernia and severe gastroesophageal reflux, resulting in a long peptic stricture.

b Magnified view showing the foregut duplication just to the right of the gastroesophageal junction. Branching bronchial structures were faintly seen filling with contrast.
c The orifice of the foregut duplication (arrow) arising from the proximal stomach.

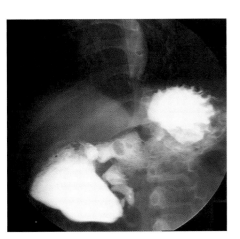

Fig. 56.2 A massively dilated proximal duodenum due to duodenal stenosis in a young boy with trisomy 21.

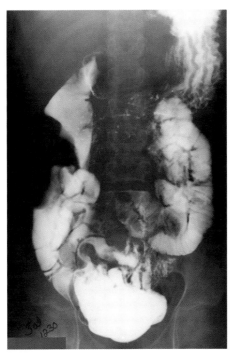

Fig. 56.3 Upper gastrointestinal and small-bowel contrast examination in a 12-year-old girl with mitochondrial neurogastrointestinal encephalomyopathy (MNGIE). Clinical symptoms included abdominal pain, postprandial emesis, intermittent diarrhea, and growth delay. The contrast study shows delayed emptying of barium from the stomach and a dilated duodenum after 3 h due to intestinal pseudo-obstruction. The child developed a rapidly progressive visceral and peripheral neuropathy.

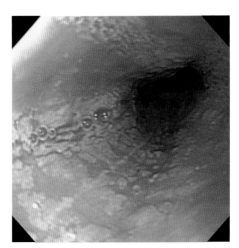

Fig. 56.4 Diffuse exudative esophagitis in 10-year-old boy with allergic eosinophilic esophagitis.

56

match the child's stage of emotional and intellectual development. Children can be given a brief tour of the procedure facility and can even be allowed to handle instruments and devices that they may encounter during their procedure. They should also be encouraged to bring attachment objects, such as a favorite stuffed animal or blanket, to enhance comfort and security.

▪ Dietary Restrictions

Presedation dietary restriction is employed with children, as with adults, to reduce the potential for aspiration of gastric contents. The duration of fasting actually correlates poorly with the volume of retained gastric fluid at the time of endoscopy in children [4]. In one study, no difference was found in gastric volume or pH in children allowed clear liquids 2–3 h before induction of anesthesia in comparison with conventional prolonged overnight fasting [5]. **Table 56.1** presents the presedation dietary guidelines recommended by the Sedation Committee at Children's Hospital Boston.

▪ Sedation

Although gastrointestinal endoscopy has been performed in young children without sedation [6], it is difficult to ethically justify withholding analgesic and hypnotic medications from children who undergo potentially painful or frightening procedures [7]. The emotional trauma suffered during a procedure by an unsedated child is likely to impact negatively on future medical encounters. Most

Table 56.1 Nil per os guidelines for sedation

Patient age	Solids and nonclear liquids*	Clear liquids†
>16 y	Nothing after midnight	Nothing after midnight
36 mo–16 y	6–8 h	2–3 h
6 mo–36 mo	6 h	2–3 h
<6 mo	4–6 h	2 h

Includes nonhuman milk and formula.
† Includes breast milk.

pediatricians and parents support the use of some type of sedation if it can be administered safely during an endoscopic procedure.

Children undergoing sedation require additional skilled personnel for careful monitoring. The sedation practice guidelines issued by the American Academy of Pediatrics in 1992 [8] recommend that one assistant—generally a nurse who is skilled in airway management—should devote exclusive attention to patient monitoring and should not share in other responsibilities of the procedure. A minimum of two assistants is therefore required when sedation is administered for endoscopy in children. One assistant supports the airway and assesses vital signs, while the other prepares or administers additional medication and assists with biopsies or other endoscopic interventions.

Basic monitoring equipment is similar for adults and children and includes pulse oximetry, an electrocardiogram monitor, and a blood-pressure monitor. The endoscopy room must be equipped with a continuous source of pressurized 100% oxygen and suction. Resuscitation equipment should include an anesthesia bag with

Table 56.2 Medications for sedation

Midazolam	Oral presedative: 0.5 mg/kg (maximum dose 20 mg)
	Intravenous: dose 0.05 mg/kg (maximum single dose 2.5 mg), then additional doses every 3 min to maximum dose 0.3 mg/kg or 15 mg
Fentanyl	Intravenous dose 1.0 µg/kg (maximum 50 µg), then additional doses every 5 min to maximum dose of 5 µg/kg or 250 µg
Reversal agents	
Flumazenil (to reverse benzodiazepine effects)	If < 20 kg: i.v. dose 0.01 mg/kg, repeat at 1-min intervals to maximum cumulative dose of 0.05 mg/kg or 1.0 mg, whichever is less
	If ≥ 20 kg: i.v. dose 0.2 mg, repeat at 1-min intervals to maximum cumulative dose of 0.05 mg/kg or 1.0 mg, whichever is less
Naloxone (to reverse opioid effects)	Intravenous initial dose 1 µg/kg; if no response within 90 s, give second dose of 2 µg/kg; if no response within 90 s, give third dose 4 µg/kg. (Maximum dose for all three doses is 400 µg or one ampule)

large and small masks, various-sized laryngoscopes and endotracheal tubes for airway intubation, medications, and a defibrillator.

The optimal approach to sedation is still an unresolved controversy among pediatric endoscopists, due to anecdotal experience and retrospective or inadequately designed studies [9]. Current practice ranges from selective use of intravenous sedation to uniformly applied general anesthesia. Young children and some adolescents are more anxious and less cooperative than adults and therefore require a deeper level of sedation. While the safety and efficacy of intravenous sedation is well documented, many skillful endoscopists are simply unwilling to assume the responsibility of administering sedation to children, deferring this role to an intensive-care specialist or anesthesiologist. Invariably, some children will require general anesthesia due to underlying medical risks or the complexity of the procedure.

Physical differences between adults and young children may contribute to increased risks during sedation for pediatric endoscopy. The soft-walled trachea of an infant may be compressed by a large-diameter endoscope, resulting in acute airway obstruction. The relatively large tongue and prominent adenoid and tonsil tissue in young children may also compromise the airway during sedation. Excessive air distension of the stomach or bowel may impede diaphragm movement and depress ventilation. The use of appropriate equipment and careful technique can minimize these problems.

Elective procedures in children with mild but unresolved upper respiratory tract infection should be deferred until congestion has cleared. Children with neurologic or neuromuscular dysfunction may develop marked upper airway obstruction due to pharyngeal wall hypotonia once sedation has been administered. A history of noisy breathing or night-time snoring should alert the endoscopist to a high-risk airway. The jaw thrust maneuver, an oral airway, or a nasopharyngeal airway may be used to treat this problem acutely. However, children with any airway difficulties should have an anesthesia consultation, with an anticipated need for endotracheal intubation.

Safe, controlled sedation generally requires intravenous access, and establishing intravenous access in a frightened and uncooperative child can be a challenging and frustrating process. The anxiety and pain of inserting an intravenous catheter may be lessened by using oral premedication (e.g., midazolam) [10,11] and dermal anesthesia (e.g., lidocaine 2% plus epinephrine 1 : 100 000). A topical anesthetic—e.g., lidocaine or benzocaine—may be applied to the posterior pharynx to reduce gagging. Sprays work well with most children, and paste can be applied to the pharynx in infants using the tip of a finger or a soft-tipped applicator. Administration of topical pharyngeal anesthesia after partially sedating the child will minimize recall of the unpleasant taste or sensation of the anesthetic. Additional environmental comforts such as dimmed lights, soft music, a warm room temperature, and a steady soothing voice issuing reassuring comments have been recommended in order to enhance successful sedation [12], but their beneficial effect has not been studied. Parents may accompany a child to the procedure room and remain present during the initiation of sedation. However, the continued presence of a parent during a procedure is of no proven benefit to the process and may only serve as an unnecessary distraction.

Few studies have prospectively examined the outcomes of different sedation medications for children undergoing endoscopy [13–17]. At Children's Hospital Boston, the preferred medications for intravenous sedation are midazolam and fentanyl. In children as in adults, these drugs produce rapid-onset anxiolysis, hypnosis, amnesia, and analgesia with a relatively brief duration of action and a comfortable margin of safety against complete loss of consciousness. The reversal agents flumazenil and naloxone are available for midazolam and fentanyl, respectively, but they are not used routinely. Following an initial dose, both midazolam and fentanyl are titrated using incremental doses every 3–5 min until an adequate level of sedation is achieved. **Table 56.2** shows recommended medication dosages in children.

Propofol, a relatively new sedative-hypnotic agent, has generated considerable interest among endoscopists because of its rapid onset, short duration of action, and minimal side effects when administered intravenously. Although typically used to induce a state of anesthesia, propofol can be used to achieve lighter states of sedation when administered in small intermittent doses or continuous infusion. It may be used alone or in combination with short-acting narcotics [18]. Propofol is generally administered to children by an anesthesiologist, since rapid onset of apnea may require skilled control of a compromised airway [19].

The dissociative agent, ketamine, has also attracted attention among pediatric endoscopists because of its capacity to induce potent analgesia, hypnosis, and amnesia without respiratory depression. Ketamine increases oral secretions and enhances protective airway reflexes, leading to an increased risk of laryngospasm. A retrospective series reported an 8.2% incidence of transient laryngospasm among 636 pediatric gastroenterology procedures, 86% of which were upper gastrointestinal endoscopies [20]. Nausea and vomiting after ketamine are not unusual. These properties make this agent less than ideal for use as a sedative for endoscopy.

Intravenous sedation has been shown to be safe and relatively effective in large numbers of children undergoing endoscopy [17]. No deaths, cardiorespiratory arrests, or aspiration events were reported in one study including more than 2500 procedures [21]. Transient oxygen desaturation, easily corrected with supplemental oxygen, has been reported in 3–9% of patients [16,22]. Rates of failure to complete the procedure during intravenous sedation range from 1% to 5% [16,17,23], but will vary with patient selection and individual experience.

General anesthesia is often viewed as a second choice for sedation for routine endoscopy, because of its increased cost [23] and the inconvenience of involving additional skilled personnel and suitable facilities. Although general anesthesia is perceived by some patients and medical personnel as involving higher risk than intravenous sedation, modern anesthetic agents and equipment managed by a pediatric anesthesiologist provide equal, if not superior, sedation with respect to many outcome measures [24]. Major complications such as colonic perforation are rare during general anesthesia [25,26]. Minor complications such as sore throat are common [27]. No randomized prospective studies have compared general anesthesia with intravenous sedation for complication outcomes during pediatric endoscopy.

Antibiotic Prophylaxis

There are few data measuring the rate of endoscopy-related bacteremia and infection in children [28,29]. Recommendations for prophylaxis are generally extrapolated from adult experience and follow the guidelines issued by the American Society for Gastrointestinal Endoscopy and the American Heart Association (AHA). The revised 2007 AHA guidelines have eliminated the recommendation for infective endocarditis prophylaxis for all patients with cardiac disease, including high-risk lesions, regardless of the type of endoscopic procedure. **Table 56.3** lists the recommended doses for prevention of infection during percutaneous endoscopic gastrostomy or high-risk endoscopic retrograde cholangiopancreatography in children.

Contraindications

There are few contraindications to endoscopy in a child. As in adult patients, these include cardiovascular instability, an unstable airway, rapidly deteriorating pulmonary or neurologic status, and bowel perforation. Suspected cervical spine injuries must first be stabilized. Small size is rarely a contraindication for endoscopy, with the exception of extreme prematurity or in neonates weighing less than 1.5–2.0 kg, in whom the indications for endoscopy are exceptional. Mild coagulopathy does not preclude diagnostic endoscopy, although the risk of bleeding and hematoma may be increased.

Equipment

All of the three major endoscopy equipment companies (Olympus, Pentax, and Fujinon) manufacture instruments suitable for use in children. Standard diagnostic endoscopes can be used in school-age children and adolescents. Ultraslim endoscopes (diameter 5–7 mm) are reserved for procedures in small children and infants. Although narrow-diameter endoscopes are commercially available, no instruments have been uniquely designed for use in small children. The length, stiffness, and bending sections are not optimal and result in awkward handling, greater patient discomfort, and frequent mucosal trauma.

Table 56.3 Antibiotic prophylaxis

Percutaneous gastrostomy	Cefazolin 25 mg/kg (maximum 1 g) i.v. or i.m. 30 min before the procedure
ERCP (for biliary obstruction, bile leak, or pancreatic pseudocyst)	Ampicillin/sulbactam 50 mg/kg (maximum 2 g) i.v. 30 min before the procedure or cefazolin 25 mg/kg (maximum 1 g) i.v. or i.m. 30 min before the procedure

Ultraslim endoscopes have operating channels with diameters in the range of 2.0 mm. Commonly used accessories such as biopsy forceps, snares, and some grasping devices are available in sizes that can be advanced through a 2.0-mm operating channel. Other devices, such as multipolar electrocoagulation catheters, hemostatic clips, and detachable snares require a larger operating channel. Small, 5-Fr cannulas and papillotomes barely fit through duodenoscopes with a 2.0-mm operating channel. Devices that attach to the tip of an endoscope, such as the adaptor for elastic band ligation and protective hoods used during foreign-body retrieval, require a minimum tip diameter of 9 mm and can therefore not be used with the smallest-diameter endoscopes. Overtubes are rarely used in children, since their relatively large diameter poses an increased risk of trauma to the esophagus or pharynx.

Upper Gastrointestinal Endoscopy

Esophagogastroduodenoscopy (EGD) is the most frequently performed endoscopic procedure in children. While the basic technique for esophagogastroduodenoscopy is the same for children and adults, a few differences are worth highlighting. Before sedation is administered, orthodontic appliances and any jewelry around the face should be removed to avoid dislodgment and potential injury or aspiration. This applies particularly to adolescents, given the recent popularity of nose and tongue piercing. School-age children may have loose deciduous teeth, which should be noted and sometimes removed as they too pose a risk of aspiration. Infants and young children undergoing conscious sedation may be loosely swaddled for additional restraint.

Direct inspection of the pharynx, arytenoids, and vocal cords is useful to look for potential evidence of acid reflux injury, such as erythema or mucosal thickening (**Fig. 56.5**). Clinically silent incidental findings include heterotopic columnar epithelium in the proximal esophagus ("inlet patch") (**Fig. 56.6**) and heterotopic pancreatic tissue in the gastric antrum (**Fig. 56.7**). Rarely, diverticula

56

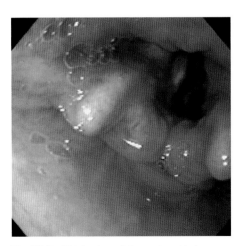

Fig. 56.5 Thickening of the arytenoids in a neurologically impaired adolescent boy with chronic gastroesophageal reflux disease.

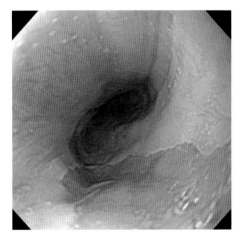

Fig. 56.6 An "inlet patch" of heterotopic columnar epithelium in the proximal esophagus of an adolescent girl with chronic nausea.

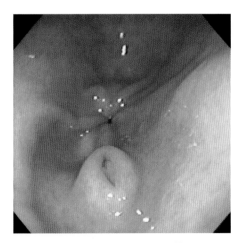

Fig. 56.7 The typical appearance of heterotopic pancreatic tissue in the gastric antrum, consisting of a smooth, round subepithelial mass with central dimple. An incidental finding in an adolescent girl with gastroesophageal reflux disease.

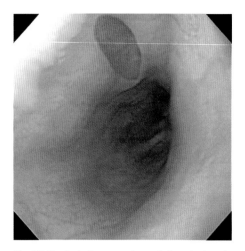

Fig. 56.8 A shallow esophageal diverticulum in an infant boy.

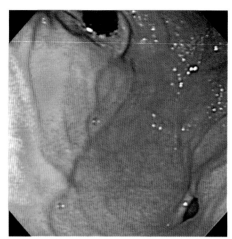

Fig. 56.9 A small diverticulum in the gastric fundus in an adolescent boy.

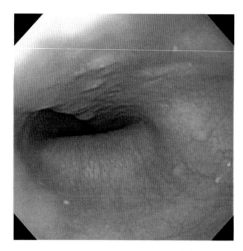

Fig. 56.10 Posterior compression of the proximal esophagus by an aberrant left subclavian artery in an adolescent girl with heartburn symptoms.

Table 56.4 Common indications for esophagogastroduodenoscopy in children

Dysphagia or odynophagia
Unexplained vomiting
Unexplained abdominal or chest pain
Chronic diarrhea or suspected intestinal malabsorption
Chronic infectious or chronic inflammatory disease
Upper gastrointestinal hemorrhage
Chemical or mechanical injury
Removal of foreign body
Placement of enteral feeding tubes

may be found in the esophagus, stomach, or duodenum (**Figs. 56.8, 56.9**). Impingement on the posterior esophagus by an aberrant subclavian artery is generally asymptomatic (**Fig. 56.10**). Other etiologies of swallowing dysfunction should be investigated in children with this finding.

The antrum of the stomach may be difficult to view completely in an infant or small child, due to the relative stiffness and long bending angle of even the smallest-diameter endoscopes. Overstretching of the body of the stomach occurs during deep insertion of the endoscope to bring the pylorus into view. A linear pattern of hemorrhagic mucosal trauma may be seen during withdrawal of the endoscope. Tightly angled portions of the duodenum in young children also limit optimal viewing of all surfaces. Mucosal biopsies from representative segments of the upper gastrointestinal tract are generally recommended in children, even when no gross abnormalities are found, since visual inspection alone may fail to detect significant pathology. This is especially important when searching for evidence of subtle inflammatory or architectural changes seen in such disorders as eosinophilic gastroenteritis, gluten-sensitive enteropathy, or epithelial dysplasia.

Complete upper gastrointestinal endoscopy can also be performed via a gastrostomy. In this case, an endoscope with a diameter of 5–6 mm is usually needed, because of the small-diameter stoma in most children. This approach is particularly useful for children with compromised respiratory function or with unfavorable esophageal anatomy. It can also facilitate wire-guided placement of a small-bowel catheter to be used for feeding or antroduodenal manometry.

Indications and Specific Diagnostic and Therapeutic Applications

Table 56.4 lists common indications for EGD in children.

Dysphagia, odynophagia, and chest pain. Dysphagia, odynophagia, chest pain, or aversive feeding behavior in a child may be signs of esophagitis, stricture, or dysmotility. Oral and esophageal Crohn's disease, herpetic and fungal infection, and pill-induced injury can present with odynophagia (**Fig. 56.11**). Given the inclination of young children to taste the world around them, an impacted foreign body should always be considered (**Fig. 56.12**). Associated respiratory symptoms may indicate recurrent aspiration. Most children with recurrent aspiration have oropharyngeal discoordination accompanying neurologic or neuromuscular disease. Diagnostic endoscopy is of limited value in such cases, although features of coexisting gastroesophageal reflux disease may be revealed. Rarely, a congenital H-type tracheoesophageal fistula will be discovered as the cause of recurrent aspiration and feeding difficulties (**Fig. 56.13**). When the level of suspicion is high and a contrast esophagram fails to identify a fistula, the diagnosis may be established by combining bronchoscopy with EGD. The fistula orifice is more readily found in the trachea than in the esophagus. The opening can be probed, and the fistula tract can be confirmed by injecting dye or contrast through the tract into the esophagus.

Gastroesophageal reflux disease (GERD) is frequently implicated in children with feeding problems, vomiting, chest or abdominal pain, poorly controlled reactive airway disease, and chronic upper respiratory tract symptoms. Endoscopic features of mucosal inflammation can support this diagnosis. Nonerosive changes are the most common finding in children and include a diminished or absent subepithelial vascular pattern and longitudinal furrowing (**Fig. 56.14**). Isolated squamous papillomas are occasionally seen, presumably in response to chronic injury (**Fig. 56.15**). Patterns of erosive esophagitis in children range from focal superficial linear ulceration (**Fig. 56.16**) to extensive circumferential erosion (**Fig. 56.17**). Short and long segments of metaplastic columnar epithelium may be found in the distal esophagus of children with GERD (**Figs. 56.18, 56.19**). Cardia-type histology predominates in young patients, but progression to intestinal-type metaplasia that defines Barrett's esophagus occurs with advancing patient age. A recent multicenter study identified older age and the presence of a hiatal hernia as possible independent risk factors for Barrett's esophagus

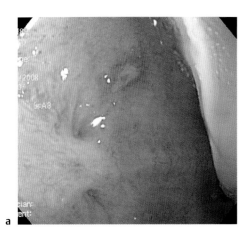

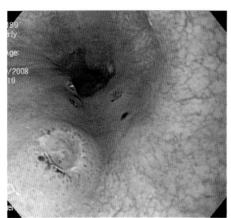

a

b

Fig. 56.11 An adolescent girl with upper gastro-intestinal tract Crohn's disease.
a Aphthous ulcer on the hard palate.
b Multiple shallow ulcers in the esophagus, accentuated by narrow-band imaging.

Fig. 56.12 A disk battery impacted in the proximal esophagus of a 9-month-old infant presenting with 5 days of difficult feeding.

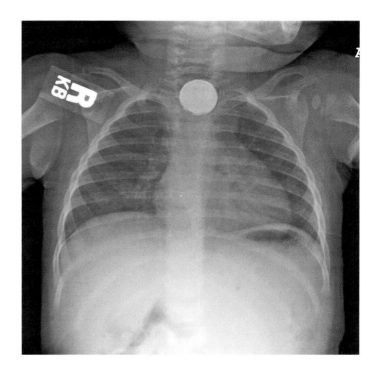

56

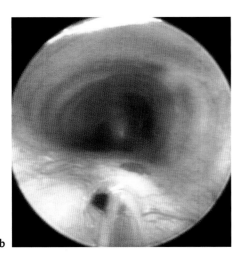

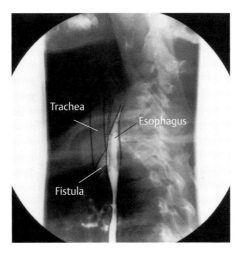

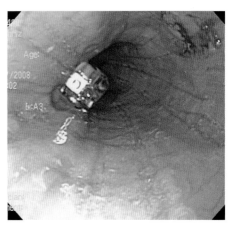

Trachea

Esophagus

Fistula

b

Fig. 56.13
a An H-type fistula in a 3-year-old girl with unexplained recurrent pneumonia. There is a small amount of barium crossing from the proximal esophagus to the trachea, where there is contrast coating the posterior surface.
b The bronchoscopic view, showing a catheter entering a defect in the posterior wall of the trachea. (Images courtesy of Dr. Craig Lillehei.)

Fig. 56.14 A pale, furrowed esophagus with diminished vascular pattern and recently placed Bravo pH capsule in an adolescent girl with symptoms of regurgitation and heartburn.

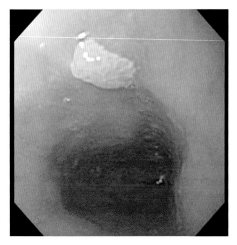

Fig. 56.15   Squamous papilloma in an adolescent boy with gastroesophageal reflux syndrome.

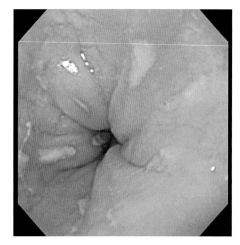

Fig. 56.16   Erosive esophagitis in a 5-year-old boy with chronic vomiting and abdominal pain.

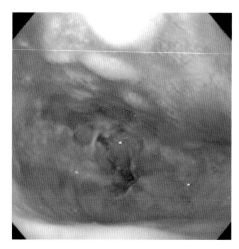

Fig. 56.17   Severe erosive esophagitis in a 5-year-old girl with glutaric acidemia and chronic gastroesophageal reflux disease.

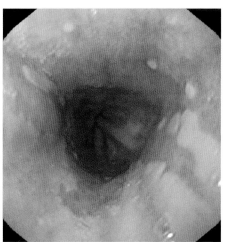

Fig. 56.18   An irregular squamocolumnar junction containing specialized columnar epithelium (Barrett's esophagus) in an adolescent boy with cystic fibrosis and chronic gastroesophageal reflux.

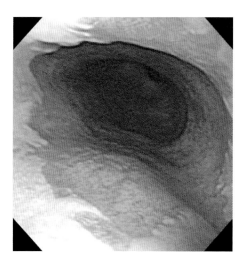

Fig. 56.19   Long-segment Barrett's esophagus in otherwise healthy 9-year-old boy with chronic regurgitation.

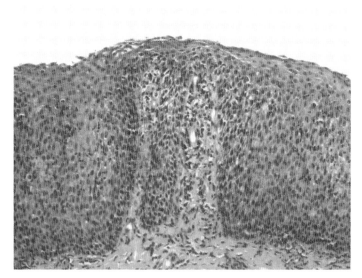

Fig. 56.20   A mucosal biopsy in a case of allergic esophagitis, showing expansion of the basal zone and extensive infiltration of the epithelium with eosinophils (courtesy of Dr. Kamran Badizadegan). The density of eosinophils is typically in the range of 20–40 per high-powered field. Clustering of eosinophils in the superficial epithelium (not shown here) is a unique microscopic feature of this disease.

in children [30]. The natural history of columnar metaplasia in the esophagus of children requires further study before routine childhood surveillance can be recommended for progressive changes of dysplasia or cancer.

Eosinophilic esophagitis is a histopathologic entity that is defined by diffuse high-density infiltration of the epithelium with eosinophils (**Fig. 56.20**) [31]. Although these changes can be induced by excessive acid reflux, they are most often reported in children with a history of atopic disease and detectable sensitivity to food and environmental antigens. Endoscopic features include absent vascular pattern, linear furrowing, and plaques of pinpoint exudate [32] (**Fig. 56.21**). High-resolution endosonography reveals thickening of the esophageal wall, predominantly involving the mucosal and submucosal layers (**Fig. 56.22**) [33]. Dysphagia for solid foods is a common presenting symptom. Impaction may result from the dysmotility associated with active inflammation (**Fig. 56.23**) or from stricture due to subepithelial fibrosis [34,35].

Most esophageal strictures in children are due to a common congenital anomaly, esophageal atresia, at the site of surgical anastomosis (**Figs. 56.24, 56.25**). Congenital esophageal stenosis may also be found in the distal esophagus in children with esophageal atresia (**Fig. 56.26**), or as an isolated malformation. Long-segment strictures, also called narrow or small-caliber esophagus, are increasingly recognized as a childhood complication of chronic eo-

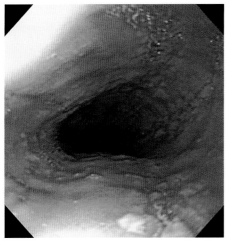
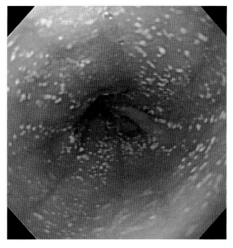
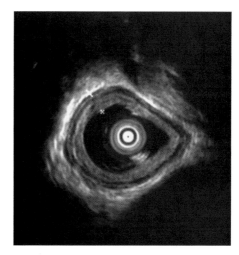

Fig. 56.21 Two children with typical endoscopic features of allergic eosinophilic esophagitis.
a Furrowed pale mucosa with an absent vascular pattern.
b Pinpoint exudate, consisting of eosinophilic microabscesses.

Fig. 56.22 High-resolution endosonography of allergic esophagitis in an adolescent girl, using a 20-MHz catheter probe. The esophageal wall is expanded (3.4 mm), predominantly due to thickening of the mucosal and submucosal layers.

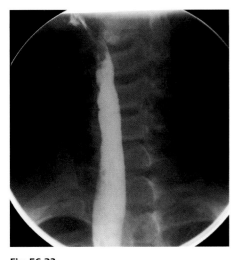
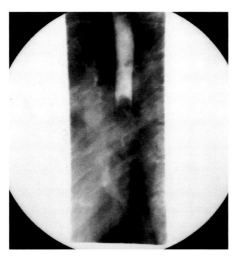
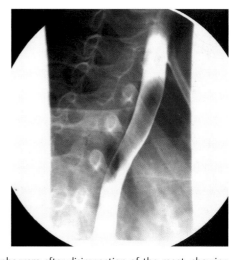

Fig. 56.23
a Ring-like narrowings in the proximal esophagus of an adolescent boy with allergic esophagitis.
b Meat impaction in the proximal esophagus of a patient with allergic esophagitis.

c A repeat barium esophagram after disimpaction of the meat, showing absence of an esophageal stricture.

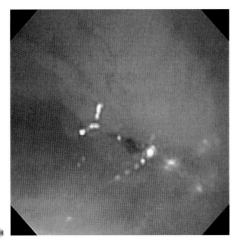
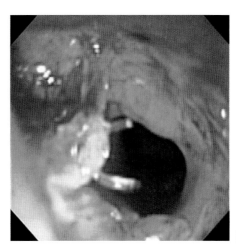

Fig. 56.24 An infant with repaired esophageal atresia.
a The barely patent anastomosis before dilation.
b The widely patent anastomosis, with a visible suture, after balloon dilation.

56

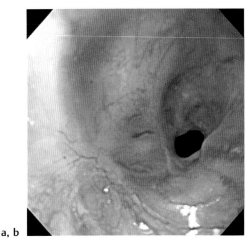
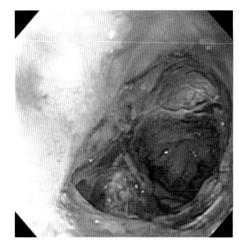
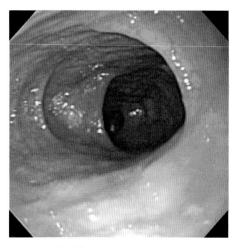

a, b

Fig. 56.25 An infant with repaired esophageal atresia complicated by proximal anastomotic stricture of the colon interposition.
a The anastomotic stricture before dilation.

b The widely patent anastomosis after dilation.
c The neo-esophagus formed by colon interposition.

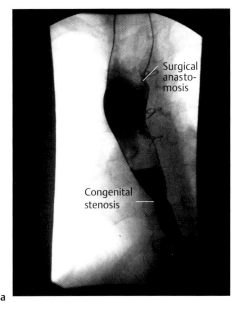
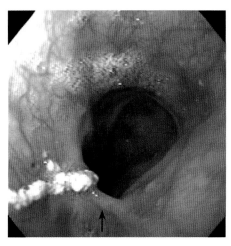
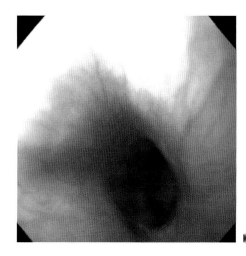

a

Fig. 56.26
a Barium esophagram in a 9-year-old boy with repaired esophageal atresia and tracheoesophageal fistula. The site of the proximal anastomosis is widely patent, but there is a focal congenital stenosis in the distal esophagus. Sternotomy wires following repair of a tetralogy of Fallot cardiac defect are visible.
b The proximal esophagus, showing a shelf-like defect (arrow) adjacent to a widely patent anastomosis. The white material is food debris.
c Distal esophageal narrowing at site of the congenital stenosis. The overlying mucosa is normal.

sinophilic esophagitis (**Fig. 56.27**). This stricturing disease may be overlooked on barium radiography, as no focal narrowing is seen. Effective dilation produces dramatic linear tearing of the mucosa and submucosa (**Fig. 56.28**). Rarely, long-segment strictures are found in children due to chronic peptic injury from GERD (**Fig. 56.29**).

Anastomotic and congenital strictures can be very difficult to dilate, due to transmural fibrosis. High pressures in the range of 100–150 psi (689–1034 kPa) or 10 atmospheres (1013 kPa) may be needed when using balloon dilation catheters. Refractory or recurrent strictures have been successfully treated by combining dilation with intralesional steroid (triamcinolone) injection [36,37] or application of topical mitomycin C [38,39]. Dilation is quite painful and is therefore best performed in a child under general anesthesia. Through-the-scope dilation catheters can be used with standard diagnostic endoscopes in older children, but over-the-wire catheters are needed for dilation in infants when small-caliber endoscopes with a narrow operating channel are being used. Simultaneous fluoroscopy offers the advantage of confirming the position

and reduction of any waist in the balloon during maximal distension. Fluoroscopy also allows immediate recognition or exclusion of a postdilation transmural tear, indicated by extravasation of contrast that has been injected into the esophageal lumen.

Motor disorders of the esophagus and stomach in children require endoscopic evaluation to exclude inflammation, mass lesions, or other structural problems. Significant dysmotility may accompany severe esophagitis, especially eosinophilic esophagitis [40]. Idiopathic achalasia is the most debilitating motor disorder of the esophagus, and although it occurs rarely in childhood, it has been reported in children of all ages (**Fig. 56.30**). The esophagus may appear only minimally dilated during barium contrast radiography, yet primary peristaltic contractions are absent and the lower esophageal sphincter fails to relax normally. Obstructive lesions in the distal esophagus may mimic the signs and symptoms of achalasia and should be excluded endoscopically. Pneumatic balloon dilation of the lower esophageal sphincter results in immediate and dramatic improvement in the majority of children with achalasia. Soft-tipped, wire-guided pneumatic balloons with diameters ranging

X

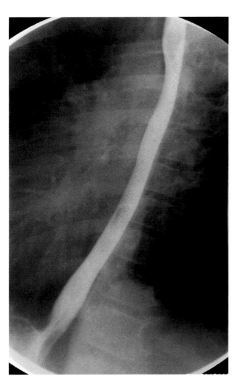

Fig. 56.27 A narrow-caliber esophagus due to stricture from sub-epithelial fibrosis in a 10-year-old boy with allergic eosinophilic esophagitis.

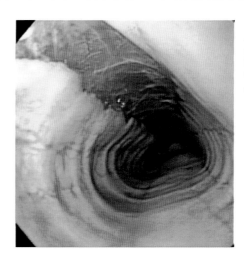

Fig. 56.28 A linear tear after balloon dilation of an esophageal stricture in an adolescent boy with allergic eosinophilic esophagitis.

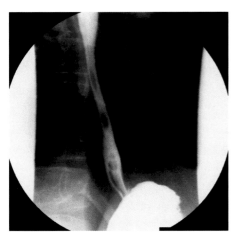

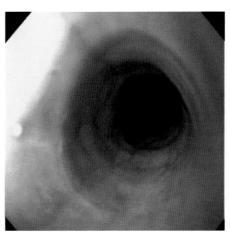

Fig. 56.29
a A long-segment esophageal stricture in a 14-year-old boy with gastroesophageal reflux disease. The patient had minimal heartburn symptoms, but long-standing dysphagia for solid food.
b Endoscopy shows smooth concentric narrowing of the lumen and abnormal mucosa, with an absent vascular pattern.

b

56

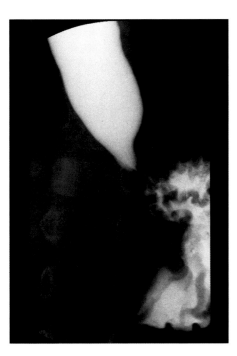

Fig. 56.30 Characteristic radiographic features of achalasia in a 5-year-old boy. The body of the esophagus is dilated, with absent peristaltic contractions and narrowing at the gastroesophageal junction due to a nonrelaxing lower esophageal sphincter.

from 20 mm to 40 mm are chosen roughly in accordance with the size of the child and the diameter of the esophagus. Several dilation sessions are needed to achieve stable long-term improvement. Thoracoscopic and laparoscopic approaches to surgical myotomy are highly effective as a primary treatment or after failed pneumatic dilation [41] (**Fig. 56.31**).

Injection of botulinum toxin (Botox) directly into the lower esophageal sphincter has also proved to be temporarily effective in children with achalasia [42]. Botox is indicated in children when the diagnosis of achalasia is uncertain, when underlying comorbidities warrant the least invasive intervention, or when waxing and waning symptoms persist after pneumatic dilation or surgical myotomy.

Unexplained vomiting and abdominal pain. Unexplained vomiting and abdominal pain in infants and children frequently represents gastroesophageal reflux disease (GERD). Although esophagitis may be found, endoscopy in children with GERD is often negative. However, endoscopic evaluation is warranted to exclude other conditions such as Crohn's disease, allergic gastroenteritis, or peptic ulceration due to exposure to nonsteroidal anti-inflammatory drugs (NSAIDs) or *Helicobacter pylori* infection (**Figs. 56.32, 56.33**). In the

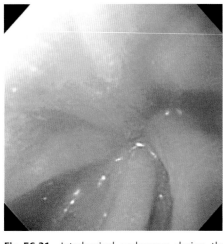
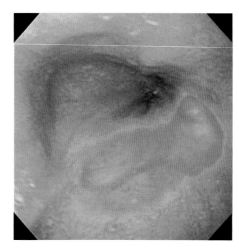
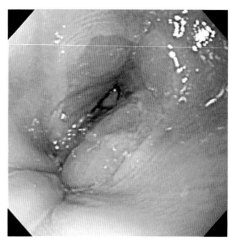

a, b

Fig. 56.31 Intraluminal endoscopy during thoracoscopic myotomy for achalasia in a 14-year-old boy.
a Tight pinch at the gastroesophageal junction before myotomy.

b Transillumination with a thoracoscope during dissection.
c The relaxed gastroesophageal junction after completion of the myotomy.

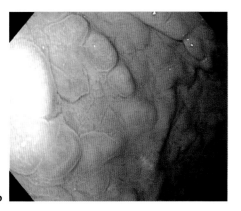
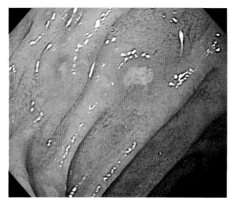
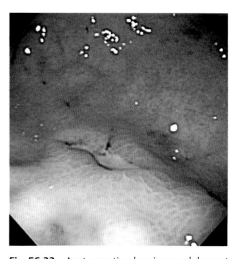

a, b

Fig. 56.32 Two children with upper gastrointestinal tract Crohn's disease.
a Diffuse nodularity in the stomach.
b Multiple aphthous ulcers in the third portion of the duodenum.

Fig. 56.33 Acute peptic ulcer in an adolescent girl taking daily nonsteroidal anti-inflammatory medication.

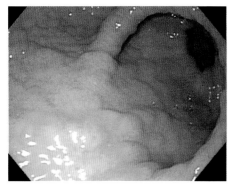

Fig. 56.34 Diffuse nonerosive nodular gastritis associated with chronic *Helicobacter pylori* infection in an 11-year-old boy.

absence of associated peptic ulcer, nodular gastritis induced by *Helicobacter pylori* is an asymptomatic or incidental finding (**Fig. 56.34**). Structural lesions such as hypertrophic pyloric stenosis of infancy, a peptic stricture, a congenital web, and postsurgical changes are important causes of pain and vomiting (**Fig. 56.35**). Foreign bodies must also be considered.

Small-bowel ischemia from vasculitis due to Henoch–Schönlein purpura or polyarteritis nodosa presents with severe cramping abdominal pain. Endoscopy reveals patchy, nonspecific ulceration and mural thickening (**Fig. 56.36**). Nausea or vomiting in the bone-marrow transplant recipient may be a sign of graft-versus-host disease (**Fig. 56.37**). Immunosuppressed patients are also at increased risk for opportunistic infections and Epstein–Barr virus–associated lymphoproliferative disease (**Fig. 56.38**). Motility disorders manifested by pseudoobstruction can also present with pain and vomiting. Diagnosis and treatment may be confounded by prior surgical intervention (**Fig. 56.39**). The diagnostic yield of endoscopy is quite low when performed in children for the sole indication of unexplained abdominal pain. Thakkar and colleagues reported a yield of only 3.6% among 1871 children under 18 years of age reviewed in published series from the English-language literature between 1966 and 2005 [43].

Chronic diarrhea, malabsorption, and small-bowel disease. With the exception of infectious enteritis, celiac disease is the predominant cause of chronic diarrhea and malabsorption in childhood. The diagnosis is often suggested by serologic results, but definitive confirmation relies on endoscopic biopsy of the small bowel. Characteristic endoscopic findings include absence of villi, and notching or scalloping of the circular folds in the duodenum. Nodularity and occasional erosions may also be found. These surface characteristics

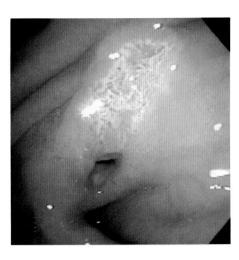

Fig. 56.35 Congenital duodenal web in an adolescent girl presenting with recurrent abdominal pain and vomiting. A tiny opening is seen adjacent to the ampullary orifice.

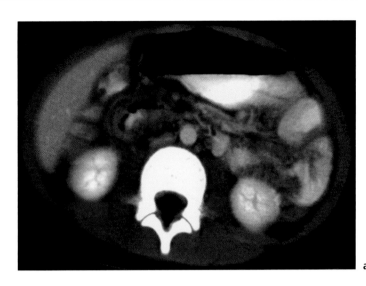

a

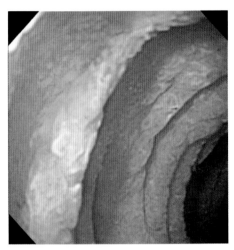

Fig. 56.37 Atrophic mucosa with loss of villi and diffuse superficial erosion in the duodenum of a 7-year-old girl with chronic graft-versus-host disease, after bone-marrow transplantation for acute lymphoblastic leukemia.

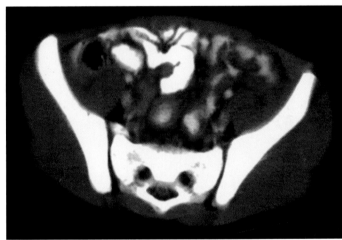

b

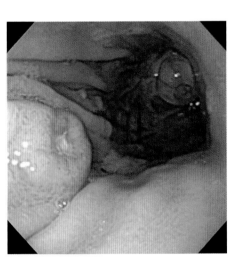

Fig. 56.38 Gastric ulcer due to Epstein–Barr virus–associated lymphoproliferative disease in a 4-year-old child after kidney transplantation.

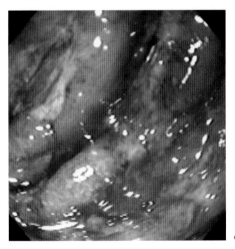

c

Fig. 56.36 a, b Abdominal computed tomography in an 8-year-old boy with Henoch–Schönlein purpura-like vasculitic disease resulting in small-bowel ischemia. There is extensive thickening of the duodenum (**a**) and jejunum (**b**).
c Endoscopy revealed thickened duodenal folds, with superficial ulceration and exudate.

56

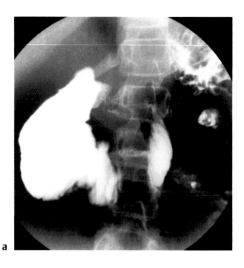

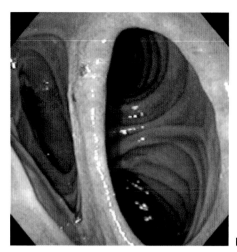

Fig. 56.39
a The dilated proximal duodenum in a 7-year-old girl with recurrent vomiting due to suspected superior mesenteric artery syndrome. A gastrojejunostomy was performed to relieve obstruction.
b The patient continued to vomit intermittently for the next 6 years, due to presumed dysmotility. She improved dramatically after oral erythromycin. Endoscopy confirmed a patent gastrojejunostomy, with native duodenum on the left and afferent and efferent loops of the jejunum on the right.

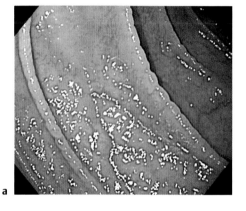

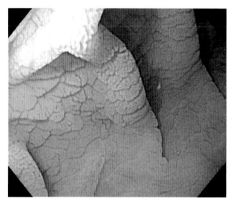

Fig. 56.40 Celiac disease in a 15-year-old girl.
a Notching or scalloping of circular folds.
b Magnified view of the atrophic mucosa, using the fluid immersion technique.

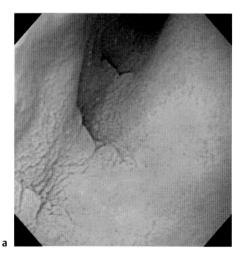

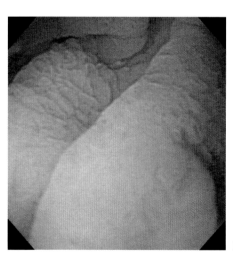

Fig. 56.41 Atrophic mucosa resembling celiac disease.
a A 17-year-old boy with eosinophilic gastroenteritis.
b A 12-year-old boy with epithelial dysplasia (tufted enteropathy).

may be accentuated by imaging the mucosa through a fluid layer or by using a high-definition or magnification endoscope (**Fig. 56.40**). Inspection and tissue sampling from the duodenum is usually sufficient for diagnosis, although patchy involvement may yield equivocal or confusing results. The gross endoscopic features seen with celiac disease are not specific and may be seen in other childhood conditions that induce mucosal and villous atrophy, including allergic enteropathy, autoimmune enteropathy, and rare epithelial dysplasias such as tufting enteropathy (**Fig. 56.41**).

Upper gastrointestinal hemorrhage. Upper gastrointestinal endoscopy is the preferred diagnostic procedure for evaluation of upper gastrointestinal bleeding in children, as with adults. If bleeding is active or severe or endoscopic therapy is likely, general endotracheal anesthesia is warranted in order to facilitate an optimal examination and minimize the risk of aspiration.

Endoscopy is generally recommended for children with acute life-threatening hemorrhage requiring blood transfusion, or with unexplained low-grade recurrent or persistent bleeding (**Fig. 56.42**). Although most pediatric endoscopists apply management algorithms derived from risk of rebleeding in adult studies, this approach has not been validated by outcome data in children.

Several authors have retrospectively analyzed the endoscopic findings in children presenting with upper gastrointestinal bleed-

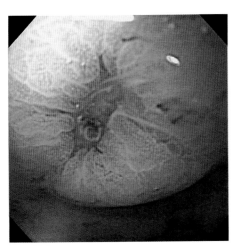
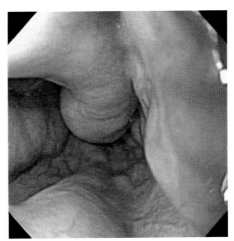
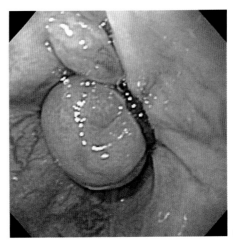

a, b

Fig. 56.42 Gastric ulcer with a visible vessel, in an adolescent girl presenting with massive upper gastrointestinal hemorrhage and syncope.

Fig. 56.43
a Large esophageal varices in a 15-year-old girl with cystic fibrosis–associated cirrhosis and portal hypertension.
b Elastic band ligation of a varix.

ing. Cox and Ament [44] reported the findings in 68 children and adolescents with upper gastrointestinal bleeding. The five most common causes were duodenal ulcer (20%), gastric ulcer (18%), esophagitis (15%), gastritis (13%), and varices (10%). Chang et al. [45] reported the findings in 27 infants. Duodenal ulcer, hemorrhagic gastritis, and gastric erosions were the most common findings. Four of 27 infants (15%) had no identifiable lesion. Bleeding was often preceded by acute viral infection with fever, aspirin ingestion, and diarrhea. Among 29 children reviewed by Quak et al. [46], upper gastrointestinal bleeding was associated with gastric erosion (27.6%), esophagitis (17.2%), esophageal varices (13.8%), duodenal ulcer (10.3%), and Mallory–Weiss tear (3.5%). Eight children (27.6%) had no identified site of bleeding. Factors that alter the relative frequency of reported lesions include patient age, medication exposure, and preexisting disease.

Many of the hemostatic endoscopic techniques used successfully in adult patients—including electrocoagulation, argon plasma coagulation (APC), injection of epinephrine and sclerosants, elastic band ligation, and mechanical clips—have been applied in children. However, with the exception of variceal eradication, published pediatric experience has been limited to case reports [47–50]. Consequently, no conclusions can be made about optimal techniques for treating nonvariceal bleeding in children. Injection techniques are appealing because of simplicity, low cost, portability, and, in the case of epinephrine, lack of tissue destruction. The choices may be limited by the availability of accessories that will fit through a small (2.0–2.2 mm) operating channel. For example, only injection catheters and the 1.5-mm diameter APC catheter can be used with small-diameter operating channels. Endoscopes with an operating channel of 2.8 mm or larger are needed for other hemostatic accessories.

Sclerotherapy for esophageal varices is a well-established hemostatic technique in children. The injection technique and sclerosants used are similar for adults and children, with the exception that relatively smaller volumes of sclerosant are used in children. Most sclerosing agents (sodium morrhuate, ethanolamine oleate, polidocanol, and sodium tetradecyl sulfate, alone or mixed with ethanol) have been used with comparable success. Many pediatric series have been published during the past three decades, representing experience in over 10 countries. Four studies [51–54] involved only children with extrahepatic portal vein obstruction, and only one study [55] dealt exclusively with intrahepatic disease. Clinical outcomes for treatment of these conditions are difficult to interpret, since most reports [56–65] combined patients with both intrahepatic and extrahepatic disease. The reported efficacy for controlling

active bleeding in children exceeds 90%, although active variceal bleeding, witnessed at the time of endoscopy, is infrequently described. Eradication of esophageal varices can be successfully accomplished by sclerotherapy in more than 90% of children. However, bleeding may recur before initial eradication or despite eradication due to another source such as gastric varices, congestive gastritis, and duodenal varices [66,67]. Short-term recurrence of varices and bleeding is more common in children with intrahepatic disease than in children with extrahepatic portal vein obstruction.

Endoscopic management of gastric varices, excluding varices at the gastroesophageal junction, has been infrequently described in children. Conventional sclerosing agents may not adequately control bleeding [68]. Fuster et al. [69] reported using cyanoacrylate (Histoacryl) for gastric varices in children, following reports of successful application in adults.

Elastic band ligation of varices has been performed in children (**Fig. 56.43**), with safety and efficacy comparable to the findings reported in adults [70–76]. In comparison with sclerotherapy, greater endoscopic skill is needed to manipulate the ligation device within the narrow esophagus of a child. Ligation adaptors have an outer diameter in the range of 12–13 mm. They are difficult to use in the esophagus of children under 1 year of age, given their large diameter. Detachable metal clips [77,78] and nylon miniloops [73] have also been used successfully in a small number of children, but these techniques appear to be more cumbersome than multiple-band ligation.

Caustic and foreign-body ingestion. Young children are prone to explore their environment through touch and taste. Injury from chemicals and foreign bodies is an unfortunate outcome of this innocent inquisitiveness. Accidental ingestion of strong alkali or acid is an unfortunately common pediatric problem worldwide. Devastating mucosal injury to the esophagus and stomach can result in severe scarring (**Fig. 56.44**) that may require organ replacement (**Fig. 56.45**). The presence or absence of oropharyngeal lesions does not reliably predict gastroesophageal injury. Endoscopy is therefore often recommended within the first 24–48 h from the time of ingestion, to assess the initial pattern and severity of tissue injury so that early and late complications can be anticipated. Although early endoscopy has been routinely recommended in order to characterize the extent of injury for all witnessed or suspected caustic ingestions, severe injury is rarely identified in completely asymptomatic cases [79,80]. Endoscopy restricted to symptomatic children may therefore be more justifiable. A simple scoring

56

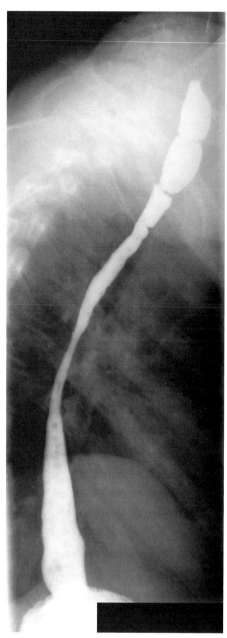

Fig. 56.44
a Multiple ring-like strictures along the length of the esophagus in a 5-year-old boy who had ingested powdered dishwasher detergent, resulting in extensive caustic injury. The mid-esophagus has narrowed to a diameter of 3–4 mm.
b Endoscopic view of the proximal stricture.

a

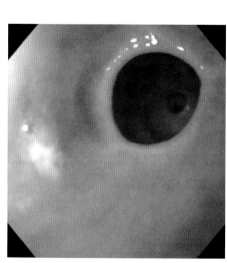

b

system [81] can be used to assess mucosal injury: grade 1, erythema or edema; grade 2, ulceration; grade 3, transmural injury or perforation. Extensive circumferential ulceration or transmural injury of the esophagus increases the risk for stricture formation. Decisions about hospitalization, fluid and nutritional support, prophylactic stenting [82] and dilations, or initiation of medications are based on the extent of injury. Treatment with systemic corticosteroids has not proved to be effective in preventing strictures [83]. Topical application of agents that inhibit fibroblasts, such as mitomycin C, may offer some benefit [38,39,84]. Prevention through public education and altered consumer practices remains the most effective therapy.

Coins are by far the most common foreign body ingested by children, although other small objects within reach of a child must be anticipated [85]. A metallic disk seen on plain radiography may represent a button battery rather than a coin, posing potential serious risk of caustic injury [86]. A complete examination should be performed to look for multiple foreign bodies, to exclude underlying anatomic abnormalities that may have caused retention of the object—e. g., stricture or web—and to assess for injury. Airway protection with endotracheal intubation is recommended during endoscopic foreign-body removal. Although this approach is not universally practiced, it will prevent sudden airway obstruction by an object inadvertently released into the hypopharynx during extraction. Unusual foreign bodies, such as a trichobezoar, may require gastrotomy with operative removal (**Fig. 56.46**).

The general principles and techniques for foreign-body removal are similar for adults and children. Objects lodged in the esophagus should be removed within 24 h, since ulceration begins to occur within this time. Batteries in the esophagus represent a true endoscopic emergency, due to the additional risk of caustic injury. Foreign bodies containing lead, such as lead sinkers, also require urgent attention in order to reduce the risk or severity of lead toxicity [87,88]. Maximal absorption of lead occurs within the acidic environment of the stomach. Urgent evacuation by endoscopic removal or the use of promotility agents and laxatives, along with acid-suppressive medication, are therefore advised, along with careful monitoring for rising lead levels that may require chelation therapy. Although linear sharp objects such as hairpins or needles may pass uneventfully through the intestinal tract, endoscopic removal can prevent potential perforating injury. Long objects that might pass spontaneously in an adult are less likely to pass through the acutely angled duodenum of a small child (**Fig. 56.47**). Nonradiopaque objects such as toothpicks or plastic items are especially problematic, since serial radiographs cannot track their movement; they should therefore be removed endoscopically if there is any risk for delayed perforation or impaction. A plastic cap adaptor, used for band ligation or mucosal resection, is very effective for removing large soft foreign bodies such as impacted meat, as it distributes suction over a large surface area.

Percutaneous endoscopic gastrostomy. Percutaneous endoscopic gastrostomy (PEG), initially devised by Gauderer and Ponsky in 1980 [89], is now among the most frequent therapeutic endoscopic procedures in children. Careful patient selection and meticulous endoscopic technique result in a high rate of technical success, improved nutritional support, parental satisfaction, and few complications [90]. The technique for PEG is the same for children and adults. The pull technique as originally described by Gauderer remains the most popular method. A modification of the original pull technique includes laparoscopy [91,92]. Laparoscopy-assisted PEG may be combined with laparoscopic fundoplication for children undergoing combined procedures. Endoscopy can also be used to facilitate the "push" technique of percutaneous gastrostomy in children [93,94]. In this case, the endoscope is used to insufflate the stomach and visualize the puncture site, followed by a modified

X

56

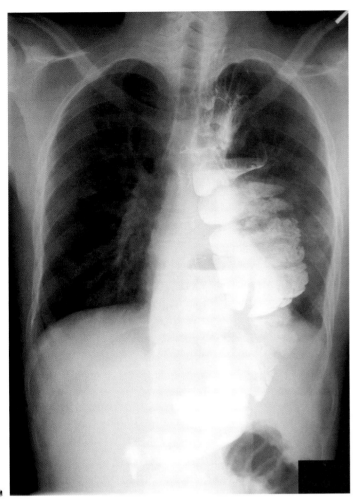
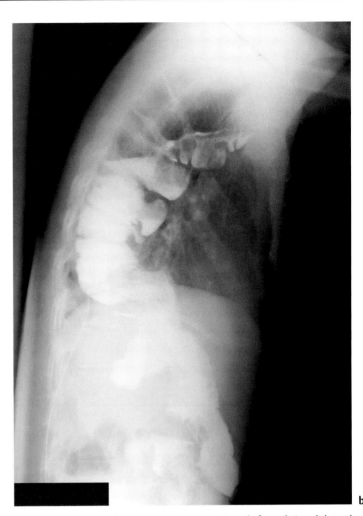

b

Fig. 56.45 a, b   Colon-esophagus in an adolescent boy who had undergone esophageal replacement due to a severe caustic injury (a frontal view, b lateral view).

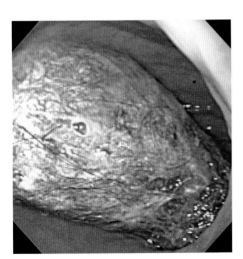

Fig. 56.46   Trichobezoar in a 3-year-old girl with trichotillomania. Surgical removal by gastrotomy was required.

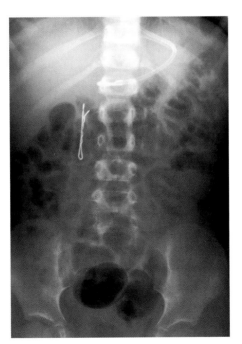
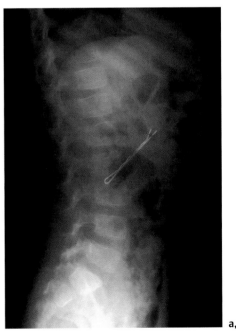

a, b

Fig. 56.47   A straight hairpin lodged in the second or descending portion of the duodenum in a 4-year-old girl.

a   Single anterior-view radiographs of the abdomen were obtained repeatedly over a period of 4 months, during which time the pin was mistakenly assigned to the transverse colon.

b   The pin position in a lateral-view radiograph (right) was inconsistent with the transverse colon. The pin was identified and removed endoscopically without complications.

Seldinger technique for catheter insertion. This technique eliminates bacterial contamination of the gastrostomy tube by oral flora and avoids bumper trauma to the esophagus. The main advantage may be for very small infants (< 2.0 kg) and children with esophageal strictures. One-step skin-level gastrostomy tubes are also available and are often preferred by ambulatory patients [95,96]. PEG catheters may be replaced with gastrojejunal catheters in children with poor gastric motility or excessive esophageal reflux. There is a small published experience with direct percutaneous endoscopic jejunal catheter placement [97].

A moderate number of PEG catheter devices are commercially available for use in children. The catheters are constructed from either silicone or polyurethane materials and have various designs for the internal bumper that provide sufficient pliability for insertion and traction removal yet prevent easy accidental dislodgement. Both silicone and polyurethane materials deteriorate over time, necessitating eventual removal and replacement with a new gastrostomy catheter if necessary. Balloon-type replacement catheters are usually preferred, as nonphysicians are able to replace them with little discomfort or risk to the patient. Several low-profile skin-level devices are available.

The primary indication for gastrostomy in children is severe dysphagia, usually secondary to cerebral palsy or progressive neuropathic disorders but also due to congenital anomalies such as cleft palate or Pierre Robin syndrome. Gastrostomy for enteral access is also indicated for children with normal swallowing function but inadequate calorie intake, due to underlying systemic disease or structural lesions of the esophagus or intestine. Children with congenital heart disease, malignancy, cystic fibrosis, or other chronic lung disease, acquired immunodeficiency syndrome (AIDS), Crohn's disease, severe burns, dystrophic epidermolysis bullosa, esophageal atresia, and short bowel syndrome fall under this category.

Complications. Complications will inevitably occur during endoscopic procedures in children [98]. A single prospective survey published as an abstract provides the only large-scale data in pediatrics [99]. A complication rate of 1.7 % was reported in 2046 upper gastrointestinal endoscopies. This included a single bowel perforation and one incident of postprocedural bleeding.

Duodenal hematoma has been reported in children following routine diagnostic endoscopy [100–105]. The incidence of this serious complication is unknown. Fatal air embolism has also been reported [106]. Most complications in children have been related to percutaneous gastrostomy, esophageal dilation, variceal sclerotherapy, and foreign-body removal.

Complications following PEG in children [107–109] include cellulitis, fasciitis, symptomatic pneumoperitoneum, gastrocolic fistula, and esophageal laceration. Complication rates have ranged from 12 % to 19 % [108,110,111]. PEG catheter removal and replacement with a "button" device has resulted in stoma tract disruption [108,112] and peritonitis in children [113]. Cutting the catheter and allowing the internal bumper to pass spontaneously risks allowing it to become lodged in the distal esophagus or in the small bowel [114,115], resulting in significant morbidity and possible surgical intervention.

Shah and Berman [116] reported a single perforation in 17 children (5.8 %) after 132 balloon dilations (0.8 %) for various esophageal strictures. Most of the serious complications associated with sclerotherapy in adults have also been reported in children. Esophageal stricture is most common, at 5–20 % in most pediatric series. Ischemic spinal cord injury has been reported [117]. Apart from injury due to overtubes [72], which are no longer used since the development of multiligator devices, no major complications have been reported in children after endoscopic band ligation of varices.

Enteroscopy

All forms or techniques of enteroscopy, including peroral push, double-balloon, intraoperative, and capsule endoscopy have been performed in children [118–121]. Limitations are based on the size or age of the child and a history of prior abdominal or intestinal surgery. Total diagnostic enteroscopy can be achieved with the capsule technique in children as young as 1.5–2 years of age [122]. Since young children are less able to cooperate with ingesting a video capsule, endoscopic placement may be necessary (**Fig. 56.48**) [123]. **Table 56.5** indicates the recommended bowel preparation before capsule endoscopy. Therapeutic enteroscopy within the mid- or distal small bowel often requires surgical assistance by laparoscopy or laparotomy, while proximal lesions may be reached with push or balloon enteroscopy techniques.

Gastrointestinal bleeding is the most common indication for enteroscopy in early childhood. The examination may be performed to identify an obscure source of bleeding or to map the extent of a known source such as a vascular malformation (**Fig. 56.49**). Investigation of known or suspected small-bowel Crohn's disease is a

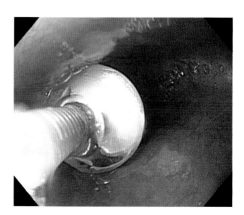

Fig. 56.48 View of a front-loaded video capsule held in the AdvanCE deployment catheter (U.S. Endoscopy, Mentor, Ohio, USA).

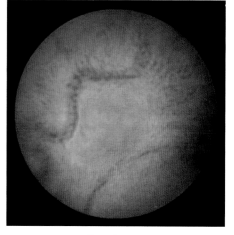
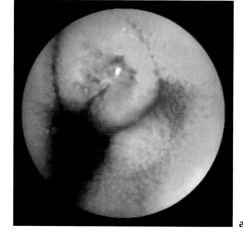

Fig. 56.49 Capsule-endoscopic views of small-bowel vascular anomalies.
a A tortuous vessel in an adolescent boy with multifocal reticular venous malformation involving the small and large intestine.
b One of a multitude of polypoid venous malformations in an 8-year-old boy with blue rubber bleb nevus syndrome.

Table 56.5 Bowel preparation for capsule endoscopy

Day before procedure
Regular diet until 12:00 p.m., then clear liquids only thereafter. No milk or milk products, or juices with pulp
Take polyethylene glycol 3350 (MiraLAX) 17 g in 225 mL clear liquid at 2:00 p.m. and repeat once again in the evening at bedtime

Day of procedure
Continue clear liquids until 2–3 h before the procedure, then nil per os

common indication for enteroscopy in older children and adolescents (**Fig. 56.50**). Crohn's disease of the proximal and distal small bowel is usually detected by upper gastrointestinal endoscopy or colonoscopy during retrograde inspection of the terminal ileum. However, disease is occasionally restricted to less accessible regions of the small bowel. Initial screening by bowel magnetic resonance imaging (MRI) or by capsule endoscopy can identify areas of active disease that may be reached by push enteroscopy or balloon enteroscopy for biopsy confirmation (**Fig. 56.51**).

Other important indications for enteroscopy include intestinal polyposis (**Fig. 56.52**), conditions associated with chronic malabsorption such as autoimmune enteritis (**Fig. 56.53**) or intestinal lymphangiectasia (**Fig. 56.54**), and graft assessment after intestinal transplantation. For bowel transplant recipients, enteroscopy is usually performed via an ileostomy.

Colonoscopy

■ Bowel Preparation

Children can be uncooperative, noncompliant, or intolerant of various regimens used for bowel cleansing or preparation. Failed or suboptimal bowel preparation is therefore a major impediment to successful colonoscopy. Successful strategies use the most palatable agents and diligent supervision by a parent or guardian. For uncooperative or chronically constipated children, supervised administration of cathartics, lavage solutions, and enemas during an inpatient or prolonged outpatient visit may be necessary to ensure success. Extra care must be taken when using reagents capable of inducing large electrolyte or fluid fluxes in infants. Colonic lavage,

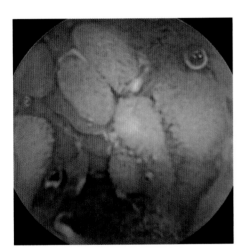

Fig. 56.50 Capsule endoscopy revealing severe multifocal ulceration in the small bowel in a 7-year-old boy with Crohn's disease.

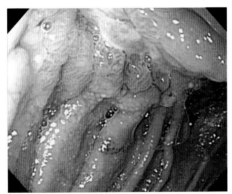

Fig. 56.51 A focal area of nodularity and ulceration found with a single-balloon enteroscope (Olympus) 150 cm beyond the pylorus in a 14-year-old girl with an abnormal bowel magnetic resonance imaging examination but normal findings on upper gastrointestinal endoscopy and ileocolonoscopy.

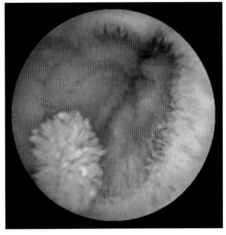

Fig. 56.52 Capsule endoscopy view of a small-bowel hamartomatous polyp in a 9-year-old boy with Peutz–Jeghers syndrome.

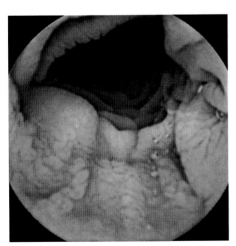

Fig. 56.53 Capsule endoscopy view of diffuse mucosal atrophy in a 10-year-old girl with autoimmune enteritis.

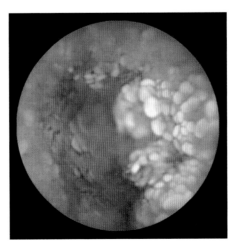

Fig. 56.54 Characteristically thickened white villi in a 2-year-old boy with protein-losing enteropathy due to intestinal lymphangiectasia.

56

Table 56.6 Bowel preparation for children undergoing colonoscopy

Children under 2 years of age
Clear liquid diet with oral cathartic and enema preparation
1   Clear liquids for 2 days before the examination (limit to 12–24 h for young infants exclusively fed breast milk or commercial formula)

2   Senna syrup (nonalcohol) is given for each of 2 days before examination
     1–6 months: 2.5 mL
     6–12 months: 5 mL
     1–2 years: 7.5 mL

3   A saline enema (10 mL/kg to max. of 500 mL) is administered on the evening before and on the morning of the procedure. The saline solution is made by adding half a teaspoon of table salt to 225 mL of water
Children 2–8 years of age
Oral polyethylene glycol 3350 without electrolytes (MiraLAX) with oral cathartic
1   Begin low-residue diet 4 days before the examination and continue this until restricting diet to clear liquids only on the day prior to examination
2   Administer PEG 17 g/225 mL of any liquid for a total of 1.5 g/kg/day (maximum 100 g/day) and divided into two or three doses each day beginning 4 days before the examination. Adjust the amount to produce very soft or pasty liquid stool until 1 day before the examination, when stool should become liquid or diarrheal
3   Beginning 3 days before the examination, administer one dose per day of oral bisacodyl (5 mg) or senna (5 mL or one tab)
Children over 8 years and older
Oral polyethylene glycol 3350 without electrolytes (MiraLAX) with oral cathartic
1   Two days before the examination, begin low-residue diet. One day before the examination, restrict diet to clear liquids only
2   One day before the examination, mix 235 g of PEG (one container of MiraLAX) into 1800 mL clear juice or commercial sports drink. Then ingest the entire mixture by drinking one glass every 20–30 minutes within 6–7 h
3   Beginning 2 days before the examination, administer one dose per day of oral bisacodyl (10 mg) or senna (10 mL or 2 tabs)

PEG, polyethylene glycol.

using commercially available polyethylene glycol–balanced electrolyte solutions ensures safe, effective, and rapid cleansing of the intestine in most patients [124]. However, the unpleasant taste and large volume of this preparation reduce its acceptance and tolerability for outpatients. In one study [125] of 20 children, 40 mL/kg/h resulted in clear stool after a mean of 2.6 hours. Emesis (20%) and nausea (55%) were frequent, and 11 of the 20 patients (55%) either required or requested nasogastric tube administration. Although low-volume oral sodium phosphate preparations may be well tolerated and accepted in adolescents [126], younger children are less tolerant, and there have been increasing reports of severe renal injury in adult patients. Oral sodium phosphate preparations were eliminated from use at Children's Hospital Boston in 2008 and replaced by nearly exclusive use of oral polyethylene glycol 3350 without electrolytes, combined with bisacodyl [127,128]. **Table 56.6** lists recommendations for bowel preparation before colonoscopy.

Equipment

Slim flexible colonoscopes with an insertion tube diameter in the range of 10–11 mm can be used for most school-age children and adolescents. Smaller-diameter and more flexible endoscopes should be used for infants and young children, to avoid wall trauma. Slim-diameter gastroscopes (5–8 mm) or enteroscopes (8–9 mm) can be used, as no suitable colonoscopes are commercially available in this size range.

Basic Technique

The basic principles and technique for colonoscopy in children are the same as in adult patients. Deeply sedated or anesthetized children are easily examined while lying supine with the legs slightly parted or supported in a frog-leg position. The supine position also facilitates easier passage of the endoscope through the ileocecal valve into the distal ileum. Inspection of the distal ileum is frequently performed in children, since diagnosis and reassessment of inflammatory bowel disease, including Crohn's disease, are important indications for the procedure. The advancing tip or light of the endoscope may be palpable or visible through the thin abdominal wall in a young child. Gentle pressure on the abdominal wall can aid in reducing loops that form as the endoscope is advanced through the colon. Forceps biopsies should be obtained from both abnormal and normal-appearing tissue in children so that subtle microscopic disease is not overlooked [129].

Polypectomy

Polypectomy is the most common therapeutic intervention performed during colonoscopy in children. Given the prevalence of polyps in children, it is an essential skill for the pediatric endoscopist. Depending on the nature and size of the polyp, basic or advanced polypectomy techniques must be considered and the endoscopist should be prepared to deal with complications such as hemorrhage immediately. Polyps found beyond the rectum should be removed and retrieved when first encountered, as they may not be found again during the withdrawal phase of the examination. Most polyps in children are of the juvenile inflammatory type, ranging from small sessile to large pedunculated lesions. They are generally excised with an electrocautery snare, but when < 5 mm they can be safely removed using the cold-snare technique. Techniques for hemostasis such as loop ligation or clipping of a stalk are useful to the pediatric endoscopist for prophylactic treatment of large (20–30 mm diameter) juvenile polyps with thick, highly vascularized stalks, and for treatment of unexpected postpolypectomy bleeding (**Figs. 56.55, 56.56**). Large sessile polyps are quite rare in children. Advanced techniques for mucosal resection of sessile polyps are therefore rarely needed.

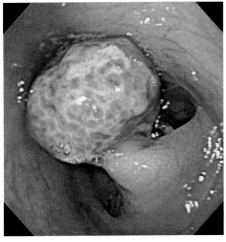
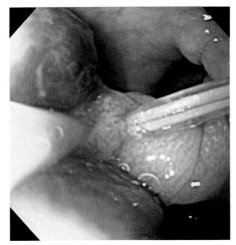
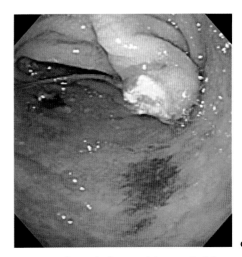

Fig. 56.55 A large (25 mm) juvenile inflammatory polyp presenting with hematochezia and abdominal pain in 4-year-old girl.
a The large polyp, with a slightly lobular and characteristically ulcerated surface, attached to the wall by a thick vascular pedicle.

b Cautery snare resection was performed after applying an Endoloop (Olympus) for hemostasis.
c The polyp stalk with the Endoloop after completion of the polypectomy.

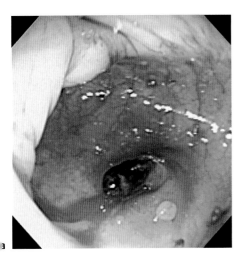
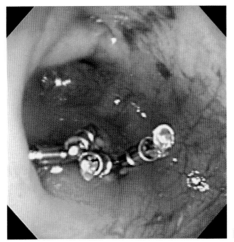

Fig. 56.56 Postpolypectomy bleeding in a 12-year-old boy with familial adenomatous polyposis.
a Active bleeding from the residual polyp stalk.
b The bleeding was arrested after several Quick-Clips (Olympus) had been applied.

56

Indications and Contraindications

The indications for colonoscopy in children are listed in **Table 56.7**. A detailed discussion of specific diagnostic and therapeutic applications for these indications follows. As with adult patients, chronic or recurrent nonspecific abdominal pain in the absence of other findings is not an indication for colonoscopy. Complete colonoscopy should be performed in most children undergoing a large-bowel examination, since the inconvenience and risks of the examination relate primarily to bowel preparation and sedation and more proximal lesions will otherwise be missed. However, a sigmoidoscopic examination may be sufficient to confirm allergic colitis in young infants.

Contraindications for colonoscopy are similar to those for upper gastrointestinal endoscopy. Cardiovascular, respiratory, or neurologic instability usually precludes safe colonoscopy. Coagulopathy should be corrected before proceeding with colonoscopy, particularly when biopsies or more invasive therapeutic interventions are anticipated. Colonoscopy is contraindicated when bowel perfora-

tion is suspected. Neutropenia and bowel ischemia are relative contraindications, due to the increased risk for sepsis and bowel perforation. Inadequate bowel preparation is another relative contraindication, as diagnostic lesions may be overlooked and the endoscope cannot be safely advanced through the lumen with inadequate visualization.

Table 56.7 Common indications for colonoscopy in children

Lower gastrointestinal hemorrhage
Acute or chronic colitis
Chronic diarrhea
Suspected disease of the terminal ileum (Crohn's disease)
Suspected polyposis disorder
Neoplasia or cancer surveillance
Decompression of obstructed colon (sigmoid volvulus)

Specific Diagnostic and Therapeutic Applications

Lower gastrointestinal tract hemorrhage. Colonoscopy is an essential tool in the diagnosis and treatment of lower gastrointestinal bleeding (LGIB) in children. Besides anal fissures, most LGIB in children is due to either colitis or benign juvenile polyps [130]. Colonoscopy is useful in the evaluation of acute colitis when initial stool tests are negative for infectious etiologies. Focal ulceration may occur as a consequence of postoperative ischemic injury, or in the setting of systemic vasculitic disease such as hemolytic–uremic syndrome. Anastomotic ulceration (**Fig. 56.57**) following ileocolonic resection [131,132] and solitary rectal ulcer syndrome (**Fig. 56.58**) [133–135] are other focal ulcerating lesions that present with LGIB in children. Mucosal biopsies are essential for differentiating between infectious, ischemic, allergic, neoplastic, and inflammatory disease.

Juvenile polyps are a common source of rectal bleeding in childhood [136] (**Fig. 56.55**). The characteristic histology of these nonneoplastic polyps reveals dilated cystic spaces, inflammatory cell infiltrate, increased vascularity, and areas of epithelial destruction [137]. Solitary juvenile polyps are found most often in the rectosigmoid colon, but multiple polyps may be found in more than 50 % of cases, with distribution throughout the colon [138]. Polypectomy is indicated to confirm the diagnosis and prevent recurrent bleeding. Children with multiple or recurrent juvenile polyps may have juvenile polyposis syndrome (JPS) (**Fig. 56.59**), a condition associated with germline mutations in either *SMAD4* [139] or *BMPR1A* [140,141] in a total of approximately 40 % of patients and with an autosomal-dominant pattern of inheritance. Adults and older children with JPS are at increased risk for developing adenoma and colon cancer [142]. Bleeding occurs less often in children with other polyposis conditions such as familial adenomatous polyposis or Peutz–Jeghers syndrome.

Vascular anomalies are an uncommon source of LGIB in children and are best characterized by colonoscopy. They may be single or multifocal malformations (**Fig. 56.60**), and may be associated with a multisystem disorder such as the Klippel–Trenaunay syndrome (**Fig. 56.61**) [143], or blue rubber bleb nevus syndrome (**Fig. 56.62**) [144]. Vascular lesions may also represent proliferating tumors such as hemangioma, or diffuse neonatal hemangiomatosis. Hemorrhoids are occasionally seen in children, but in contrast to adult patients, hemorrhoidal bleeding is rare in childhood. Prominent anorectal hemorrhoids or rectal varices should raise a suspicion of elevated portal pressure [67] or isolated venous malformation.

Most endoscopic hemostatic techniques used to treat LGIB in adult patients can be applied in children, including thermocoagulation [145], elastic band ligation, sclerotherapy [67], clipping, and argon plasma coagulation.

Colitis, chronic diarrhea, and idiopathic inflammatory bowel disease. Protein allergy is a common cause of colitis in infants who are fed formula containing cow's milk protein, and less often soy protein [146,147]. Even infants who are exclusively fed breast milk may develop allergic colitis, presumably due to intact proteins

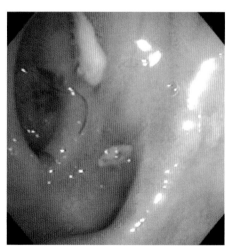

Fig. 56.57 Focal ulceration at the site of an ileocolonic anastomosis after right-sided hemicolectomy in a 12-year-old boy. A residual suture identifies the site of the anastomosis.

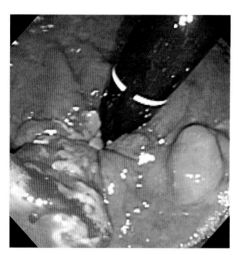

Fig. 56.58 A polypoid form of solitary rectal ulcer in an adolescent boy with an abnormal bowel pattern including frequency, urgency, and pain, as well as chronic hematochezia.

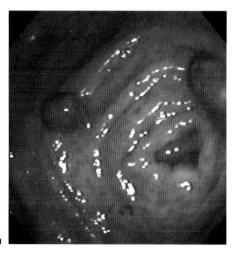

a

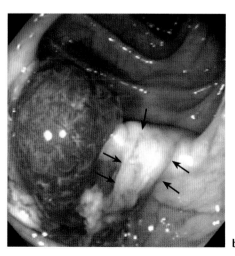

b

Fig. 56.59 Multiple juvenile polyps in a 9-year-old girl with juvenile polyposis syndrome.
a Multiple small uniform polyps with short stalks surrounding the appendiceal orifice.
b A large lobular polyp with a long stalk (arrows) draped over a haustral fold.

X

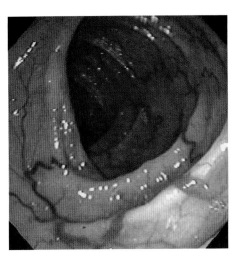

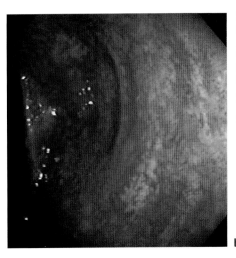

Fig. 56.60 Vascular malformations in the colon.
a Multiple tortuous veins encountered throughout most of the colon in a 15-year-old boy with a venous malformation and intermittent rectal bleeding.
b A transmural lymphaticovenous malformation confined to the sigmoid colon in an 11-year-old boy. The reddish-blue discoloration is due to myriad small vascular channels in the submucosa.

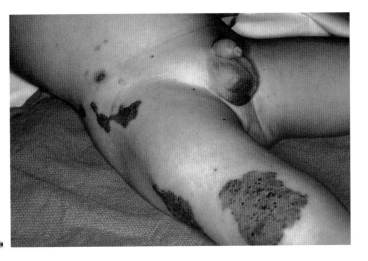

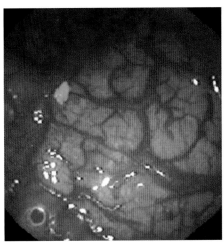

Fig. 56.61
A 22-month-old boy with Klippel–Trenaunay syndrome and rectal bleeding.
a Right leg, hip, and scrotal involvement with capillary lymphaticovenous malformation.
b An abnormal mucosal vascular pattern in the sigmoid colon. (Reproduced with permission from Gastroenterology Clinics of North America [130].)

56

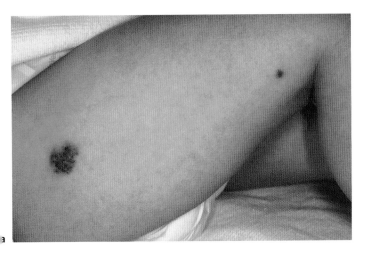

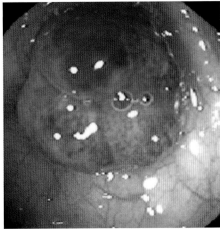

Fig. 56.62 Blue rubber bleb nevus syndrome.
a Typical dark blue nodular lesions of the skin in a 2-year-old boy.
b An oozing polypoid lesion in the colon in a 12-year-old girl.

secreted in human milk [148]. Rarely, the condition may extend into early childhood [149]. Endoscopic features are nonspecific, but include prominent lymphoid nodularity, patchy erythema, and hemorrhage from superficial ulceration (**Fig. 56.63**). Histology shows acute inflammation, characteristically dominated by eosinophilic infiltrate of the epithelium and lamina propria [150,151]. Although the diagnosis is usually established by a clinical response to dietary restriction, endoscopy with biopsies may be useful if signs and symptoms fail to improve.

Colonoscopy is indicated for the evaluation of chronic diarrhea in children when investigation for infection and malabsorption has been unrevealing. The principal diagnosis is idiopathic inflammatory bowel disease (IBD). Total colonoscopy and examination of the terminal ileum should be performed in order to provide the most accurate differentiation between Crohn's disease and ulcerative colitis [152]. The characteristic endoscopic findings for Crohn's disease and ulcerative colitis are the same in children and adults. These include focal aphthous lesions and irregular deeper ulcers in Crohn's

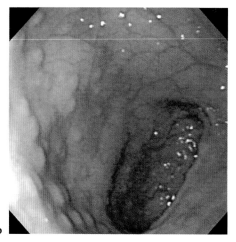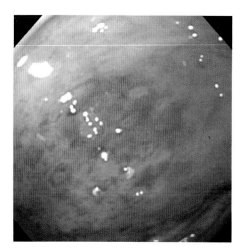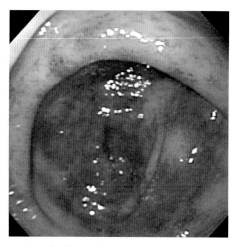

a, b

Fig. 56.63 Allergic colitis induced by cow's milk protein in an infant.
a Prominent lymphoid nodularity.

b Erythematous halo around lymphoid nodules.
c Patchy erythema and hemorrhage.

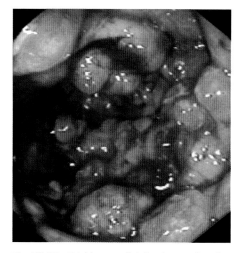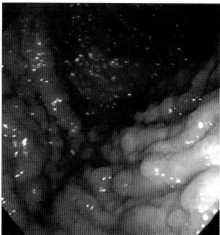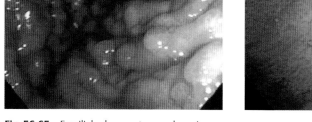

Fig. 56.64 Friable superficially ulcerated nodules in the colon, at times obliterating the lumen, in a 13-year-old girl with non–X-linked hyper-IgM syndrome and lymphoproliferative disease.

Fig. 56.65 Familial adenomatous polyposis.
a Small nodular adenomas in the colon of a 13-year-old girl, who had no symptoms.
b The subtle periampullary rim of an adenoma in an adolescent girl.

disease, and diffuse fine mucosal granularity with continuous superficial ulceration in ulcerative colitis. A discontinuous or patchy pattern of ulceration is not uncommon in early-childhood presentation of ulcerative colitis and does not necessarily imply a diagnosis of Crohn's disease.

Some unusual etiologies of chronic diarrhea include lymphocytic colitis, allergic or eosinophilic gastroenteritis, collagenous colitis, and lymphoproliferative disease associated with congenital immunodeficiencies such as hyper-IgM syndrome (**Fig. 56.64**).

Screening and surveillance for polyposis and neoplasia. Colonoscopy is necessary in the evaluation and management of children and young adults who are at risk for polyposis based on a family history or identified gene mutation. With familial adenomatous polyposis (FAP), flat dysplasia and small nodules can be found in early childhood, and larger polyps usually develop by adolescence (**Fig. 56.65**) [153]. Total colonoscopy should be performed during screening for FAP, since polyps may be sparse and unevenly distributed over the length of the colon. Large polyps should be removed in order to look for areas of high-grade dysplasia or early malignancy, since this will necessitate early or urgent colectomy. In the absence

of high-grade dysplasia, annual colonoscopy is recommended in children with FAP until prophylactic colectomy is performed. Prophylactic colectomy is generally recommended in middle adolescent years, although even earlier may be necessary, since cancers in young children have been reported [154].

Peutz–Jeghers syndrome [155] and juvenile polyposis syndrome [156] are two other important polyposis syndromes encountered during childhood. Both are associated with predominantly hamartomatous polyps, but foci of adenoma may develop in both conditions, which are clearly associated with higher rates of colon cancer [157–159] in comparison with the general population. Although rare, colon cancer has been described in pre-adolescents and adolescents with juvenile polyposis syndrome. The progressive adenoma-to-carcinoma sequence has been recognized in juvenile polyps. Surveillance colonoscopy with prophylactic polypectomy every 1–3 years has been recommended for juvenile polyposis when the number of polyps is not excessive. The endoscopic management of Peutz–Jeghers polyposis in childhood is mostly directed toward removal of large polyps that might result in small-bowel intussusception or otherwise be a source of pain or bleeding (**Fig. 56.66**).

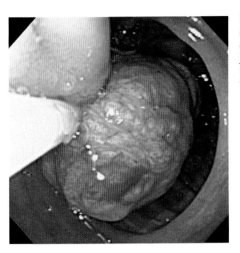

Fig. 56.66 A large duodenal polyp in a 4-year-old boy with Peutz–Jeghers syndrome, presenting with intermittent abdominal pain.

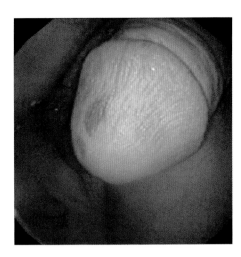

Fig. 56.67 Pigmented macules on penile glans of a child with *PTEN* syndrome. (Image courtesy of Dr. Athos Bousvaros.)

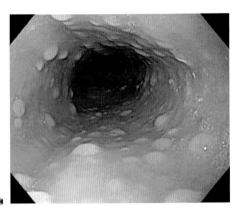

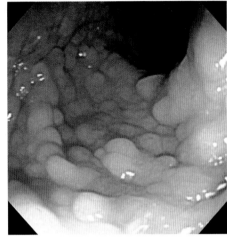

b

Fig. 56.68 *PTEN* syndrome.
a Prominent glycogenic acanthosis in the esophagus.
b Multiple small colonic polyps or nodules consisting of ganglioneuroma.

56

PTEN hamartoma tumor syndrome, a complex and phenotypically heterogeneous disorder that includes Cowden syndrome and Bannayan–Riley–Ruvalcaba syndrome, may present with juvenile inflammatory type polyps in childhood [160]. Penile freckling (**Fig. 56.67**) and macrocephaly are important clues to the diagnosis. Other common endoscopic findings include nodules in the esophagus due to glycogenic acanthosis and small polyps or nodules in the small bowel and colon, consisting of ganglioneuroma (**Figs. 56.68**). An increased risk for intestinal neoplasia has not been proven. In addition to hereditary polyposis, endoscopic surveillance for neoplasia is also indicated in children with chronic colitis for more than 8–10 years [161].

Other therapeutic interventions. Retained foreign bodies in the lower gastrointestinal tract are rare in children. Flexible endoscopes may be used for objects trapped in the colon or terminal ileum [114]. Colonoscopy will occasionally be employed to reduce a sigmoid volvulus or decompress a dilated colon in a child. Colonic strictures may be treated using balloon catheter dilation, as performed in other segments of the gastrointestinal tract. Percutaneous endoscopic cecostomy or sigmoidostomy are alternatives to surgical or percutaneous procedures for colonic irrigation in children with intractable constipation [162,163].

Complications. The major complications of colonoscopy are bowel perforation and hemorrhage. The incidence of perforation during pediatric colonoscopy can only be estimated on the basis of limited reports, but is probably less than 1%. Isolated cases have been reported [25,164–166]. In a review of 1700 pediatric colonoscopies [167], no perforations occurred during diagnostic studies and four perforations occurred following polypectomy. No complications were seen in a study of 42 children who underwent endoscopic polypectomy for a total of 84 polyps [168]. In another polypectomy series [169], there were four complications among 74 children, one of which required surgical intervention. Incomplete or diastatic serosal lacerations have also been described in children [170]. As with perforation, there is no reliable figure for the incidence of hemorrhage following colonoscopy in children. Most significant hemorrhage is related to polypectomy.

Endoscopic Retrograde Cholangio-pancreatography

Introduction

Waye reported the first successful endoscopic retrograde cholangiopancreatography (ERCP) in a child in 1976 [171]. After subsequent improvements in equipment design and extensive experience in adult patients, ERCP is now routinely performed in children with biliary and pancreatic disease at major medical centers throughout the world. Successful cannulation of the bile duct or pancreatic duct is achieved in over 90% of cases in most published series, similar to the experience in adult patients. Recent reports have focused on the efficacy of therapeutic ERCP in children [172–176].

Equipment

Standard diagnostic duodenoscopes with a tip diameter of approximately 11 mm can be used safely in most children over the age of 2–3 years. Therapeutic duodenoscopes with larger operating channels and tip diameters of approximately 13 mm should be reserved for older children. Operating channels with a diameter of at least 3.2 mm will accommodate nearly all types of diagnostic and therapeutic accessories. A duodenoscope with a diameter of 7–8 mm is required for very small children and infants and can be obtained from either Olympus or Pentax. The operating channel of these small-diameter endoscopes is approximately 2.0 mm, which will only accept cannulas and other accessories that have a diameter or 5 Fr or less. The range of tip angulation is similar to that in standard duodenoscopes, but the field of view is narrower. Sphincterotomy and stone extraction are feasible using these ultraslim duodenoscopes.

Patient Preparation and Sedation

Preparation and sedation for children undergoing ERCP are similar to the procedures used in upper gastrointestinal endoscopy. Many endoscopists favor general anesthesia during ERCP in children, for several reasons. Successful duct cannulation and therapeutic interventions require fine control that is difficult to achieve or maintain with a sedated but restless or uncooperative child. Respiratory function may be compromised in a very deeply sedated child, due to limited chest wall and diaphragm movement when the patient is in a prone position. Also, a relatively large-diameter endoscope may compress the soft-walled trachea of an infant or young child. Positive-pressure ventilation via an endotracheal tube can usually overcome the latter two problems.

Basic Technique

The basic techniques for diagnostic and therapeutic ERCP are similar for adults and children. The major and minor papillae, although smaller in infants, are still easily identified. When one is working within a narrow duodenum, only a short length of the cannula can extend out from the endoscope tip before impacting against the opposite wall of the bowel. The operator is forced to work very close to the papilla. A sphincterotome is helpful in this situation, since it adds an extra dimension of cannula tip deflection that is often needed for selective deep cannulation of the bile duct. Tapered-tip sphincterotomes with short cutting wire lengths of 10–15 mm can be obtained commercially or custom-ordered for this purpose.

The mucosal surface and papilla in young infants is easily traumatized by minor mechanical injury. Extra care needs to be taken to avoid forceful cannulation or injection of contrast that might cause tearing, bleeding, or swelling that might obscure the normal anatomic landmarks or obstruct drainage of the ducts. Selective deep cannulation of either the bile duct or the pancreatic duct is often not possible in neonates unless there is abnormal distension of the ducts. Instead, superficial cannulation of the ampulla followed by injection of contrast will often simultaneously fill both ducts. This technique is especially relevant to examinations for suspected biliary atresia. An optimal iodine concentration for children has not been defined, but a range of 150–300 mg iodine/mL appears to work well.

The length and structure of the common channel leading from the biliary and pancreatic ducts to the ampulla must be carefully studied, since congenital variants are associated with important conditions such as choledochal cyst and recurrent pancreatitis in children [177].

Role of the Pediatric Endoscopist

ERCP is the most technically challenging of all endoscopic procedures and carries a significant risk for serious complications. Recently published studies indicate that experience with 200 or more cases is required in order to reliably achieve deep common bile duct (CBD) cannulation [178–180], which is necessary for most therapeutic interventions and many diagnostic studies. The procedure should be not be performed by an endoscopist who lacks sufficient training, experience, or direct supervision to achieve an 80–90% rate of technical success. The relatively small volume of pediatric ERCP cases may not provide sufficient experience for many pediatric endoscopists to acquire or sustain the level of competence needed for this procedure. On the other hand, while adult endoscopists with advanced training in pancreaticobiliary endoscopy have the necessary technical and cognitive skills to manage adult diseases, their understanding of pediatric conditions is usually limited. Pediatric patients are therefore best served when pediatric and adult endoscopists collaborate to achieve optimal patient selection, preparation, and technical outcome [181].

Contraindications

There are few absolute contraindications for ERCP in children. The major contraindications for EGD—cardiovascular, pulmonary, or neurologic instability or bowel perforation—also may be applied to ERCP. An esophageal stricture may preclude safe passage of the side-viewing endoscope until the stricture has been successfully dilated. Acute pancreatitis is a relative contraindication to ERCP, except in the case of gallstone pancreatitis, when relieving obstruction may improve the patient's clinical course. While there is evidence to support this recommendation in adult patients, there are no data to validate the practice in children. Endoscopic cholangiography is rarely feasible in children who have undergone prior biliary reconstruction with a Roux-en-Y choledochojejunostomy. Such a reconstruction is often performed during pediatric liver transplantation. Many biliary complications after liver transplantation therefore require percutaneous or surgical rather than endoscopic intervention. Growing experience with balloon enteroscopy may change this approach [182].

Diagnostic and Therapeutic Indications

The dominant role of ERCP as the primary diagnostic modality for abnormalities of the biliary and pancreatic ducts is now being successfully challenged by magnetic resonance imaging cholangiopancreatography (MRCP) in children as well as adults [183–187]. As the noninvasive technology of MRCP improves, ERCP will be increasingly reserved for therapeutic interventions or for direct sampling of tissue and fluid. Most endoscopic therapies employed in adult patients have been performed in children, with comparable efficacy and safety. However, endoscopists with the necessary skills and experience are not always available, and controlled studies comparing outcomes of medical, endoscopic, radiologic, and surgical therapies have not been conducted in children. The decision to proceed with endoscopic intervention in a child therefore needs to take into consideration local experience and available resources.

The indications for ERCP in children can be separated into two main categories, biliary and pancreatic, each of which has specific diagnostic and therapeutic applications (**Tables 56.8, 56.9**).

▦ Biliary Conditions

Choledocholithiasis is the most common biliary indication for ERCP in children, due primarily to stones that form in the gallbladder. Risk factors include family history, age, gender, ethnicity, hemolytic conditions, metabolic disease, and prior surgery. At times, no predisposing risk factors can be identified, as seen with otherwise healthy infants in whom gallbladder sludge or stones are detected during prenatal ultrasound examinations. This material may never become symptomatic, or it may dissolve or pass spontaneously [188]. Rarely, however, young healthy infants present with obstructive jaundice from stones impacted in the distal common bile duct. Whether these stones were formed prenatally or postnatally is usually unknown in individual cases. The combined effects of prolonged fasting and exposure to parenteral nutrition, diuretics, and repeated blood transfusions contribute to pigment sludge and stones in premature neonates and in infants who have undergone cardiac surgery (**Fig. 56.69**). Chronic hemolytic anemia due to sickling hemoglobinopathies and spherocytosis is a major cause of pigment stone formation in older children and young adults (**Fig. 56.70**). Increasing age, female gender, and obesity are important risk factors for cholesterol stone formation in children (**Fig. 56.71**).

Given the risks of intervention and possibility of spontaneous resolution, a period of waiting with supportive care is appropriate for the infant or child with minimal or easily managed symptoms. Endoscopic intervention is indicated when impacted stones or sludge fail to pass spontaneously. Evidence of superimposed septic cholangitis, with fever or rapidly rising serum transaminases and bilirubin, is an indication for urgent intervention to prevent overwhelming sepsis. Endoscopic sphincterotomy and stone extraction has been performed successfully in children as young as 2 months of age [189]. After sphincterotomy, stones may be removed with either a retrieval balloon catheter or basket. If the stone cannot be re-

Table 56.8 Biliary indications for endoscopic retrograde cholangiopancreatography in children

Diagnostic
Choledocholithiasis
Choledochal cyst
Dilated intrahepatic or extrahepatic bile duct
Biliary stricture
Sclerosing cholangitis
Persistent bile leak
Neonatal cholestasis

Therapeutic
Stone extraction
Stricture dilation
Stent placement
Sphincterotomy

Table 56.9 Pancreatic indications for endoscopic retrograde cholangiopancreatography in children

Diagnostic
Suspected gallstone pancreatitis
Persistent acute, recurrent, or chronic pancreatitis
Suspected developmental pancreatic anomalies
Pancreatic trauma
Pancreatic mass

Therapeutic
Stone extraction
Stricture dilation
Sphincterotomy
Stent placement for pseudocyst drainage (transpapillary or transmural)

56

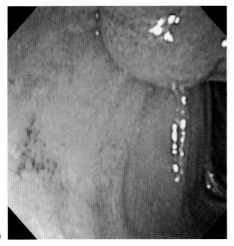
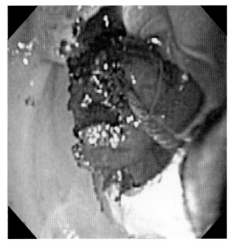
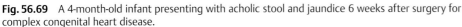
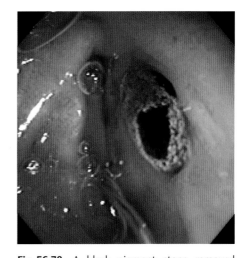

Fig. 56.69 A 4-month-old infant presenting with acholic stool and jaundice 6 weeks after surgery for complex congenital heart disease.
a Bulging papilla darkened by impacted stone.
b A soft pigment stone released after sphincterotomy. (Reproduced with permission from Fox VL. ERCP in children in T.H. Baron et al., editors, *ERCP*. London: Elsevier, 2008.)

Fig. 56.70 A black pigment stone removed from the common bile duct in a 15-year-old girl with sickle-cell disease.

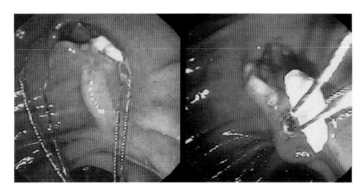

Fig. 56.71   Basket extraction of a white cholesterol-type common bile duct stone in a 15-year-old girl. The patient presented with abdominal pain and a dilated bile duct 7 months after laparoscopic cholecystectomy.

moved at the time of initial endoscopy, a temporary stent can be placed to maintain drainage. Since the long-term risks of sphincterotomy in childhood are unknown, the technique of papillary balloon dilation is, in theory, an attractive alternative. However, there has been little published experience in children [173] and the risk of pancreatitis may be higher than following sphincterotomy. The sequential combination of endoscopic stone removal followed by laparoscopic cholecystectomy is frequently applied in children as in adult patients when stones are present within both the CBD and gallbladder. However, this approach may not be appropriate for all children, especially in the absence of a strong family history or other risk factors for continued stone formation. Prospective outcome data are needed in infants and young children with idiopathic pigment stones before prophylactic cholecystectomy can be routinely recommended after removal of a CBD stone. For the infant with resolved choledocholithiasis and no residual gallbladder stones, the gallbladder may be left in place. Furthermore, once a sphincterotomy has been performed to remove a CBD stone, small residual stones or sludge in the gallbladder may pass spontaneously.

Choledochal cyst.   Suspected choledochal cyst (**Fig. 56.72**) is an important indication for cholangiography in children and adults. **Figure 56.73** shows the different types of congenital bile duct cysts according to the anatomic classification by Todani and colleagues [190]. Cystic changes are very well demonstrated by transabdominal ultrasonography, but finely detailed anatomy of the duct may not be seen, particularly at the distal end of the bile duct. Magnetic resonance cholangiography reveals greater detail of the bile duct, but may also not show the pancreaticobiliary junction as clearly as ERCP. Since a long common channel or anomalous pancreaticobiliary union [177] is found in the majority of patients with a choledochal cyst (**Fig. 56.74**), the absence of an anomalous junction should raise questions about the etiology and proper treatment for a dilated biliary system in a child. For example, biliary obstruction by a stone may in young infants result in marked distension of an otherwise normal extrahepatic bile duct, mimicking a type I choledochal cyst (**Fig. 56.75**). ERCP can also establish most reliably whether or not there is continuity between the bile duct and cystic lesions that may have been identified with other imaging modalities.

Therapeutic ERCP makes it possible to relieve obstruction by stone extraction or temporary stent placement [191]. Once the obstruction has been relieved, definitive surgical excision of a chole-

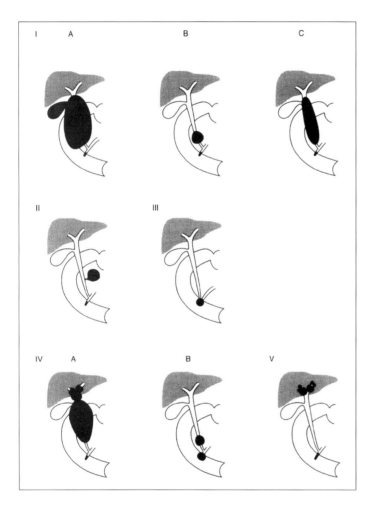

Fig. 56.73   Schematic representation of the anatomic classification of choledochal cysts by Todani. (Reproduced with permission from M. Guelrud et al., *ERCP in pediatric practice: diagnosis and treatment.* Oxford: Isis Medical Media, 1997 with permission.)

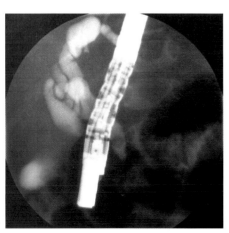
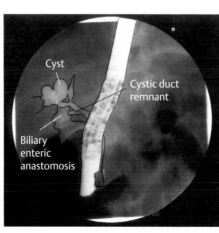

a, b

Fig. 56.72   Choledochal cyst.
a   A residual type V choledochal cyst in a 2-year-old girl. The cyst had originally been detected during prenatal ultrasound at 20 weeks' gestation. The cyst was partially resected and drained via jejunal interposition when the child was 2 months old.
b   A type IV choledochal cyst in a 4-year-old boy presenting with intermittent biliary obstruction due to a stone impacted in the distal common bile duct.

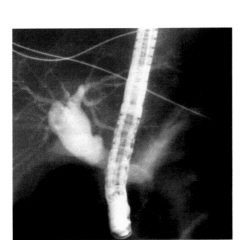

Fig. 56.74 Anomalous pancreaticobiliary union associated with choledochal cyst malformation in an 8-year-old girl.

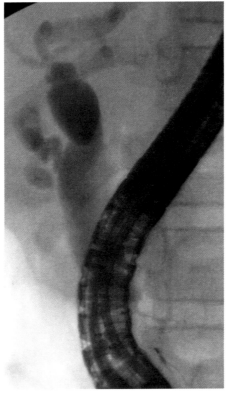

Fig. 56.75 Fusiform dilation of bile duct, resembling a type I choledochal cyst due to a stone impacted in the ampulla in a 3-month-old infant.

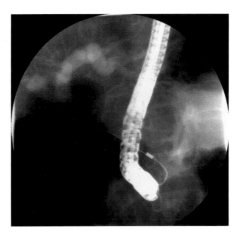

Fig. 56.76 Biliary obstruction at the level of the common hepatic duct in a 2-year-old boy treated for neuroblastoma. The guide wire could not breach the stricture.

56

dochal cyst can proceed on an elective basis. Endoscopic sphincterotomy alone may benefit patients with type III choledochal cysts (choledochoceles) or selected patients with anomalous pancreaticobiliary union and a dilated bile duct [192,193].

Biliary stricture or disruption. Biliary strictures are found in children with primary or autoimmune sclerosing cholangitis; congenital narrowing; bile duct injury from surgery—e. g. biliary anastomotic stricture after liver transplantation; and extrinsic compression from acute or chronic pancreatitis. Tumors are a rare cause of biliary obstruction in children. There is usually extrinsic compression from a tumor mass, or a stricture due to prior radiotherapy or surgery (**Fig. 56.76**).

Sclerosing cholangitis may arise in children with idiopathic inflammatory bowel disease or in association with various immunodeficiency states (**Fig. 56.77**). A nearly normal-appearing cholangiogram may be seen with very early or mild sclerosing cholangitis. In this early stage, the diagnosis is based on suggestive liver histopathology and the biochemical profile. As the disease progresses, the characteristic bile duct changes emerge, with beaded and pruned hepatic branches and irregular common duct contours. Magnetic resonance cholangiography is usually adequate to reveal these gross morphological changes in the ducts. ERCP should be reserved for situations in which MRI is either unavailable or equivocal, or when therapeutic intervention is anticipated. In the author's experience, a common ERCP finding is underfilling of the peripheral hepatic ducts despite deep cannulation. Inject of contrast under pressure using a retrieval balloon to prevent retrograde flow of contrast allows filling of the inflamed and partially occluded hepatic branches.

Focal congenital stricture of the bile duct can be difficult to distinguish from sclerosing cholangitis (**Fig. 56.78**). The liver histology for both shows an active cholangitis with features of chronic

injury. The former should improve with dilation and stenting, or Roux-en-Y jejunal anastomosis [194], while the latter is expected to progress. Strictures associated with congenital and acquired biliary lesions have been successfully treated in children using transendoscopic dilation and placement of stents [172,195] (**Fig. 56.79**). Obstructive jaundice due to pancreatic disease is an ominous sign in an adult, potentially heralding advanced pancreatic cancer. Fortunately, this is rarely the case in children, in whom pancreatic cancer and tumors are quite rare. Acute or chronic pancreatitis is more often the cause, and these conditions are treatable with dilation and temporary stent placement (**Fig. 56.80**). ERCP is also the ideal approach for localization and treatment of bile duct disruption resulting from blunt abdominal trauma (**Fig. 56.81**) or after cholecystectomy (**Fig. 56.82**).

Neonatal cholestasis. Idiopathic neonatal hepatitis and parenteral nutrition are the most common causes of neonatal cholestasis. Cholangiography should be normal in both conditions. Structural causes of neonatal cholestasis include biliary atresia, choledochal cyst, choledocholithiasis and inspissated bile, intrahepatic bile duct paucity or hypoplasia, neonatal sclerosing cholangitis, and congenital bile duct stricture. Cholangiography may confirm or exclude the diagnosis or allow definitive therapy for some of these disorders.

The diagnosis of biliary atresia is excluded by demonstrating free flow of bile into the duodenum. This can be achieved by detecting bile in the duodenum, observing normal excretion of technetium-labeled bile during scintigraphy, or obtaining a normal cholangiogram. Approaches for cholangiography that involve direct injection of contrast include ERCP, percutaneous transhepatic cholangiography, percutaneous transcholecystic cholangiography, and intraoperative cholangiography. The role of ERCP [196,197] remains controversial. Most pediatric gastroenterologists and hepatologists rely on

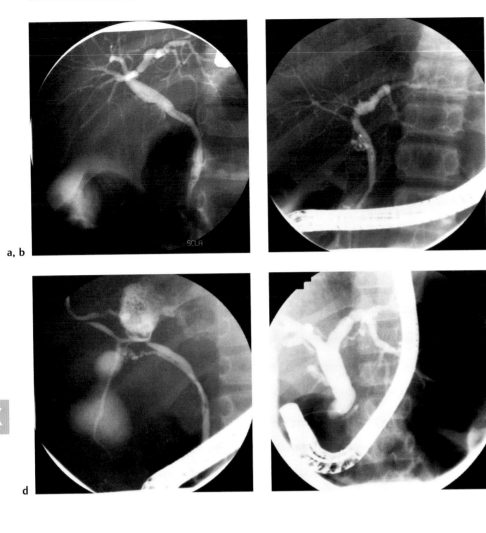

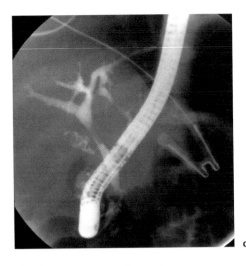

Fig. 56.77 Sclerosing cholangitis.
a Early disease in a 4-year-old boy with recently diagnosed ulcerative colitis. There are subtle irregularities in the common bile duct, but no significant changes in the intrahepatic ducts.
b Advanced disease in a 14-year-old boy with ulcerative colitis.
c Advanced disease in an 8-year-old boy with combined B cell and T cell immunodeficiency disorder.
d An unusual intrahepatic cystic lesion in a 10-year-old boy with Langerhans cell histiocytosis.
e Papillary stenosis in a 13-year-old boy with acquired immune deficiency syndrome.

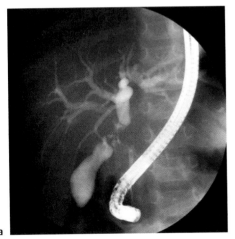

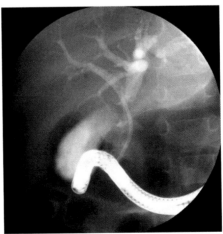

Fig. 56.78
a Presumed congenital stricture of the common hepatic duct in a 20-month-old boy.
b The obstruction was relieved after a 5-Fr stent was placed using the Olympus PJF 7.5 duodenoscope (with a 2.0-mm operating channel).

a combination of clinical presentation, serum chemistries, ultrasonography, biliary scintigraphy, and liver histology rather than ERCP findings when selecting infants for surgical exploration for biliary atresia. ERCP is feasible but technically difficult in young infants. Equipment has not been designed for ERCP in infants, so that the procedure requires an even higher level of skill than is already needed for ERCP in general. Many centers do not have access to a very small-diameter duodenoscope or an endoscopist with the requisite skills who is willing to perform the test. Endoscopic findings [198] that suggest biliary atresia are: an absence of bile in the duodenum; partial filling of the bile duct with abnormal termina-

tion; and failure to fill the bile duct with contrast despite filling of the pancreatic duct. The decision to pursue the diagnosis by surgical exploration therefore often relies on the endoscopist's impression that failure to fill the bile duct is due to atresia and not a technical failure. Endoscopic cholangiography is perhaps most clinically useful when biliary atresia is considered unlikely, but other tests have been equivocal or nondiagnostic. The diagnosis is definitively excluded by demonstrating the presence of a patent duct during retrograde injection of contrast.

Syndromic (Alagille syndrome) and nonsyndromic paucity of intrahepatic bile ducts are important anatomic abnormalities that

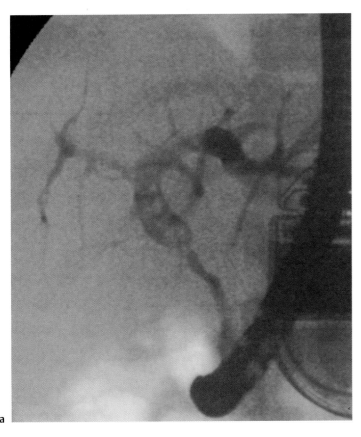

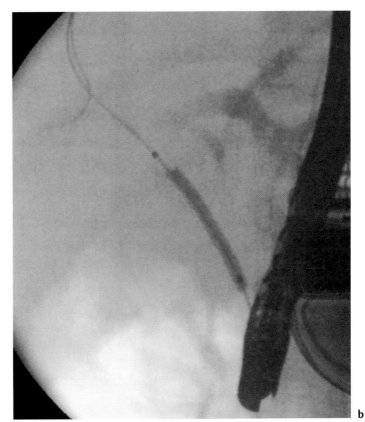

56

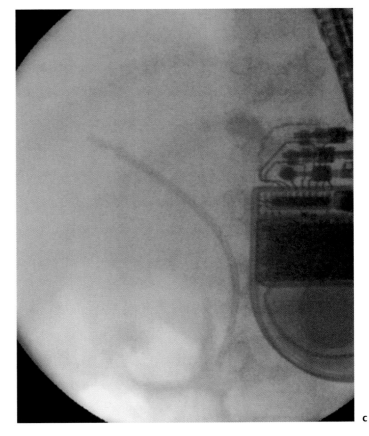

Fig. 56.79 Acquired biliary stricture with a delayed presentation in a 6-year-old boy with hypoplastic left heart syndrome (an implanted defibrillator is seen). The patient had undergone cholecystectomy and common bile duct exploration for cholelithiasis at the age of 2 months.
a Common bile duct stones impacted above the stricture.
b Balloon catheter dilation of the stricture.
c Stent placement.

can mimic biliary atresia in the neonate. Cholangiography may identify findings that suggest Alagille syndrome, although the diagnosis is primarily established by compatible liver histology, genetic testing in some families, and other clinical findings such as the associated facial dysmorphism and cardiovascular abnormalities.

Nonsyndromic paucity of bile ducts is a heterogeneous disorder. Similar cholangiopathic features may be seen in children with sclerosing cholangitis (especially neonatal sclerosing cholangitis), graft-versus-host disease, and liver allograft rejection.

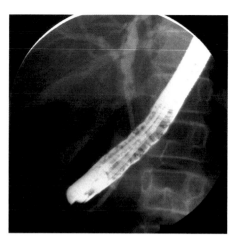
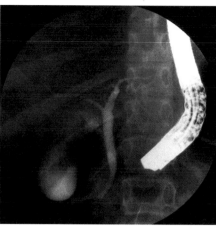

a, b

c

Fig. 56.80
a Biliary stricture due to extrinsic compression of the distal common bile duct by swelling in the head of the pancreas in a 12-year-old with occult pancreatitis.

b A bile duct stent has been advanced across the site of the stricture.
c Persistent irregularity but resolved obstruction after 6 months of stenting.

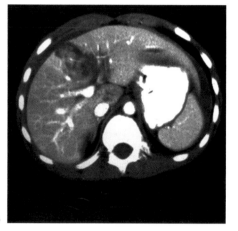
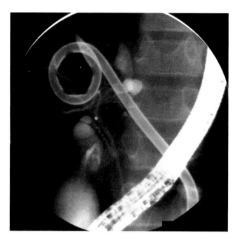
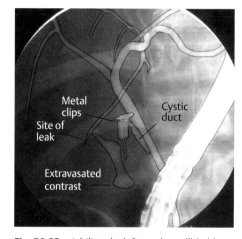

a, b

Fig. 56.81
a Computed tomography showing liver laceration due to blunt abdominal trauma in an 8-year-old boy.
b Contrast injection with the catheter tip in the common hepatic duct shows a leak from the left hepatic duct. The injury healed without further intervention.

Fig. 56.82 A biliary leak from the gallbladder fossa (Luschka duct) following laparoscopic cholecystectomy in a 15-year-old boy.

Pancreatic Conditions

Gallstone pancreatitis. The morbidity in children with gallstone pancreatitis may be less than in adults, and mortality is rarely encountered. There are no controlled data in children to show whether urgent ERCP for stone disimpaction improves the outcome of the pancreatitis, although it may be expected that biliary complications will be reduced.

Persistent acute, recurrent, or chronic pancreatitis. Pancreatography is indicated for children with unexplained persistent acute pancreatitis, recurrent pancreatitis, or chronic pancreatitis. Although transabdominal ultrasonography and computed tomography (CT) will reveal marked distension of the pancreatic duct or major structural abnormalities in the body of the pancreas, these modalities will fail to demonstrate subtle anatomic findings in the pancreatic duct such as strictures, anomalous pancreaticobiliary union, and pancreas divisum. Magnetic resonance pancreatography also lacks sufficient resolution in children to show fine details of the pancreatic duct for an accurate anatomic diagnosis. ERCP is still an essential diagnostic modality for evaluating and managing pancreatitis in children [199].

Developmental anomalies such as anomalous pancreaticobiliary junction (**Fig. 56.83**) [200], annular pancreas [201], dorsal pancreatic agenesis [201], and duodenal duplications [202] have been associated with recurrent attacks of pancreatitis in children and are best demonstrated with endoscopic pancreatography. Pancreas divisum (**Fig. 56.84**) or so-called dominant dorsal duct [203], which is found in 5–10 % of the general population, is the most frequently encountered developmental anomaly. Its role in the pathogenesis of recurrent pancreatitis remains controversial. An improved outcome has been reported after endoscopic therapy in children [204] but the data are limited to case reports and small series.

Chronic progressive pancreatitis in children may result from identified metabolic disease, or from idiopathic biochemical or autoimmune inflammatory conditions. Cystic fibrosis is the prototypic genetic metabolic disorder and most common cause of pancreatic insufficiency in pediatrics. This autosomal-recessive disorder results from mutations in the cystic fibrosis transmembrane conductance regulator (*CFTR*) gene. Children with isolated "idiopathic" chronic or relapsing pancreatitis have also been found to have compound heterozygous genotypes combining severe and variable function mutations, as well as a higher than predicted frequency of single-allele *CFTR* mutations. A greater than predicted

X

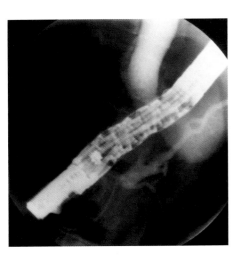

Fig. 56.83 Anomalous pancreaticobiliary union in an 8-year-old girl with recurrent pancreatitis.

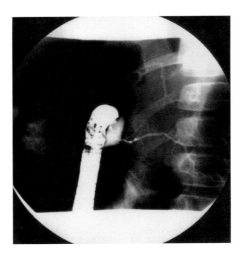

Fig. 56.84 Pancreas divisum or dominant dorsal pancreatic duct in an 8-year-old boy with recurrent pancreatitis. The long scope position was required for injection of the minor papilla.

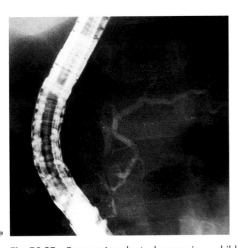

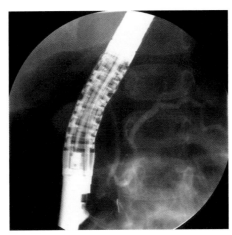

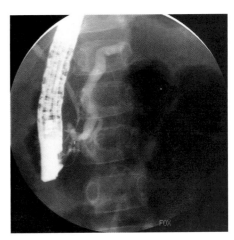

c

Fig. 56.85 Progressive duct changes in a child with chronic idiopathic pancreatitis.
a Mild dilation at 17 months of age. The pancreatic duct is the same diameter or slightly smaller than the bile duct.

b Increasing dilation at 4.5 years of age, showing the pancreatic duct slightly larger than the bile duct.
c Marked dilation of the pancreatic duct at 7.5 years of age.

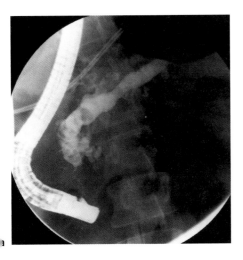

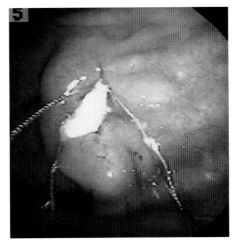

Fig. 56.86
a Marked dilation of the pancreatic duct with stones in an 18-year-old girl with hereditary pancreatitis.
b Basket extraction of a soft white proteinaceous stone.

b

56

frequency of single-allele mutations in the serine peptidase inhibitor, Kazal type 1 (*SPINK1*), alone or in combination with single allele mutations of *CFTR*, is also found in children with chronic pancreatitis. Single-allele mutations in the cationic trypsinogen gene, *PRSS1*, result in autosomal-dominant hereditary pancreatitis. Mutations in genes controlling other metabolic pathways such as the organic acidemias and lipid metabolism are rarer causes of relapsing pancreatitis in children. Although anatomic alterations of the pancreatic duct may be found in children with chronic or relapsing pancreatitis,

the significance of these findings, especially pancreas divisum, in the pathogenesis is changing with the emerging recognition of genetic factors.

Mild dilation of the main pancreatic duct and its side branches may be found in children with early chronic pancreatitis (**Fig. 56.85**). As the disease progresses, the duct may develop marked dilation and tortuosity, and stones or proteinaceous plugs may occlude the lumen (**Figs. 56.86**). The severity of pancreatic disease or duct changes does not necessarily correlate well with the patient's age

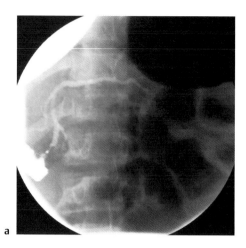

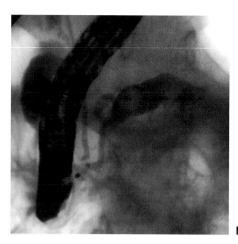

a
b

Fig. 56.87 Siblings of the patient in **Fig. 56.86** with hereditary pancreatitis.
a A 16.-year-old boy with mild dilation of the pancreatic duct.
b A 5-year-old girl with marked dilation of the pancreatic duct and an impacted stone.

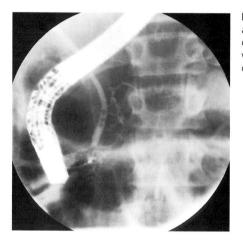

Fig. 56.88 An irregular and atrophic pancreatic duct in a 14-year-old boy with chronic pancreatitis due to cystic fibrosis.

X

or the underlying diagnosis (**Fig. 56.87**). The features of chronic pancreatitis associated with classical cystic fibrosis differ in that the ductal system usually atrophies rather than dilates (**Fig. 56.88**). ERCP with sphincterotomy has been used to relieve potential outflow obstruction of the duct in children [201,204] with recurrent or chronic pain associated with pancreatitis.

Pancreatic pseudocyst. When pseudocysts fail to resolve spontaneously following an attack of pancreatitis, ERCP provides useful diagnostic information for planning a drainage procedure. Endoscopic treatments such as transpapillary stenting, transmural cystoduodenostomy or cystogastrostomy, and combination therapy with transmural and transpapillary drainage are reasonable options for children (see **Fig. 56.96**) [201,204–210].

Pancreatic trauma. ERCP provides important information about the integrity of the pancreatic duct following abdominal trauma [211]. Transection of the duct may be detected early and treated surgically or even endoscopically by placement of a transpapillary stent [204]. The age or size of the child is potentially a limiting factor when attempting pancreatic stent placement, given the very small diameter of the normal pancreatic duct in young children.

Complications. The major complications following ERCP in children include pancreatitis, hemorrhage, infection, and perforation. A single pediatric death has been reported resulting from infection of a pancreatic pseudocyst [212]. This and other severe complications are probably underreported. Pancreatitis is certainly the most com-

mon complication after ERCP. The rate reported in pediatric series ranges from 3% to 8%, which is similar to the experience in adult patients. Hemorrhage and perforation have rarely been reported and are likely to be less than 1%, as reported in adults. The rate of ERCP-related bacteremia in children is not known, and few cases of clinical infection have been reported. Antibiotic prophylaxis during ERCP is recommended for children with an obstructed bile duct or pancreatic pseudocyst (see **Table 56.3**). Finally, the long-term complications of endoscopic sphincterotomy in children are unknown.

Sphincter of Oddi dysmotility. Sphincter of Oddi manometry has been performed in children with biliary-type pain, idiopathic pancreatitis, and malformations of the ductal system, with abnormal results being interpreted on the basis of normal control values from adult patients [206,213–215]. However, the perfusion catheters used in adult patients may fit tightly against the sphincter or within the ducts of a small child and may shift the range of recorded pressures. There are no data to establish the range of pressures or findings in normal children of varied age and size. Sphincter of Oddi dysmotility should therefore be regarded as a provisional diagnosis in children, pending further study.

Gastrointestinal Endosonography

The earliest and still principal clinical indication for gastrointestinal endosonography (EUS) is the investigation and staging of tumors and malignancies. Since these lesions are relatively uncommon in pediatrics, experience with EUS in children remains limited to case reports and small series [216–219]. Low clinical demand, the high cost of the equipment, and limited access to training prevent most pediatric endoscopists from exploring this novel technology. Maximal tip diameters in the range of 13–14 mm and the relatively long nonbending sections in current echoendoscopes impede easy or safe oral passage of these instruments in young children. Catheter-based probes are more adaptable for use in children, as they can be advanced through diagnostic endoscopes with operating channels ≥2.8 mm. Rectal probes are also suitable for use in most children.

The clinical indications for EUS in children include: investigation of subepithelial mass lesions; cancer staging; assessment for pancreatic and biliary disease; and evaluation of anorectal malformations. High-resolution probe endosonography in the esophagus can be used to assess wall layer involvement with inflammatory disease [220] (**Fig. 56.22**) or congenital stenosis [221–223] (**Fig. 56.89**), as well as varices, congenital vascular anomalies (**Fig. 56.90**), and other subepithelial mass lesions (**Fig. 56.91**). Catheter probes can also be used to image subepithelial and vascular lesions in the stomach,

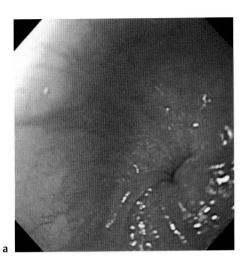

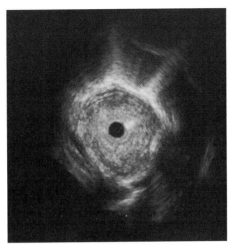

Fig. 56.89 Congenital esophageal stenosis in an 11-month-old boy.
a Severe stenosis in the distal esophagus, covered with normal epithelium.
b High-resolution endoscopic ultrasonography using a 20-MHz probe shows disruption of the normal echo layers, due to replacement of the muscularis propria by fibrous tissue.

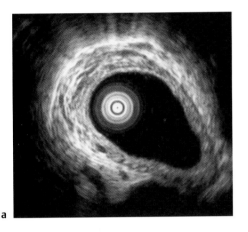

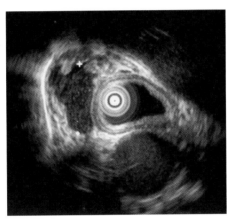

Fig. 56.90 Endosonography of the esophagus using a 20-MHz catheter probe in a 9-year-old girl with lymphaticovenous malformation of the mediastinum and chest.
a The normal echo-layer architecture in the esophageal wall has been replaced by numerous small vascular channels.
b There is a large, irregularly shaped vascular structure (marked by electronic calipers) replacing the azygous vein.

56

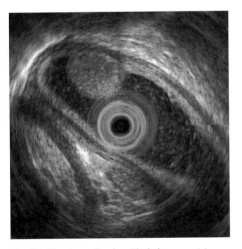

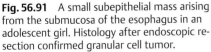

Fig. 56.91 A small subepithelial mass arising from the submucosa of the esophagus in an adolescent girl. Histology after endoscopic resection confirmed granular cell tumor.

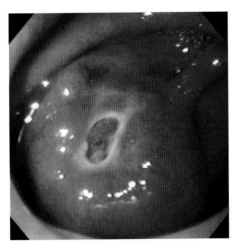

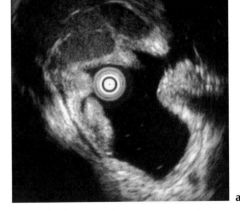

Fig. 56.92 A young adult presenting with recurrent massive bleeding several years after successful liver transplantation.
a Mucosal ulceration over a submucosal mass in the proximal duodenum.
b Endosonography using a 20-MHz catheter probe revealed a hypoechoic vascular structure compatible with duodenal varices. The bleeding subsided after the ulcer had been closed with metal clips.

duodenum, and colon, which in children may include pancreatic heterotopia, lymphoproliferative disease, and varices or vascular anomalies [224] (**Figs. 56.92–56.94**). Echoendoscopes provide a greater depth of imaging and the ability to carry out tissue sampling or interventions, which are generally needed for pancreatic disease, solid tumors, and cystic lesions in children. EUS-guided fine-needle aspiration biopsy (**Fig. 56.95**) and EUS-guided pseudocyst drainage [225] (**Fig. 56.96**) may assist surgical planning or eliminate the need for surgery in some pancreatic conditions in childhood. Endosonography has also been used to assist in the surgical management of anorectal malformations in children [226–229].

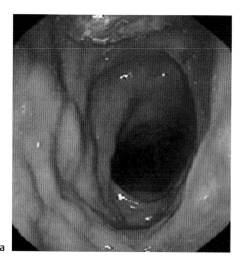

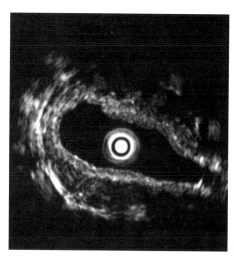

Fig. 56.93
a An irregular mucosal fold pattern in the rectum, due to abnormally expanded submucosal vascular channels.
b Endosonography using a 20-MHz catheter probe in the area corresponding to the rectal wall in **a**. The normal echo layer pattern in the rectal wall is disrupted by the vascular malformation, seen as an expanded hypoechoic zone in the submucosa.

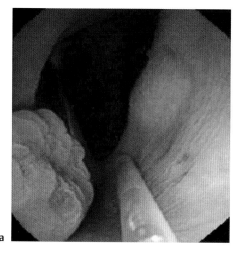

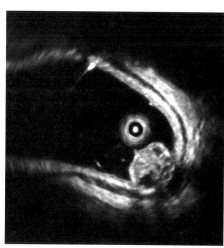

Fig. 56.94 Polypoid venous malformation in blue rubber bleb nevus syndrome.
a An ultrasound catheter probe is positioned next to a colonic lesion in the water-filled lumen.
b Endosonography of the colonic lesion using a 20-MHz catheter probe, demonstrating hypoechoic vascular channels penetrating through the wall into the serosa.

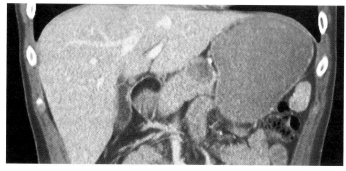

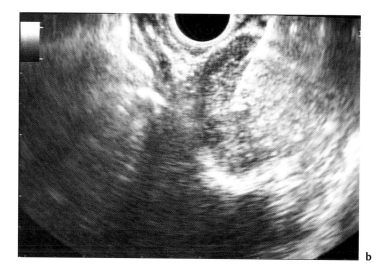

Fig. 56.95 Pseudopapillary tumor of the pancreas in a 14-year-old boy.
a Computed tomography, showing a round, low-density mass in the body of the pancreas.
b Fine-needle aspiration biopsy. The needle is entering the hypoechoic mass lesion.

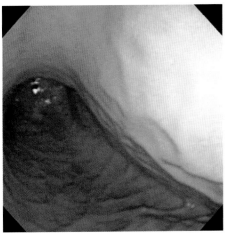
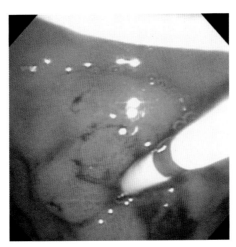
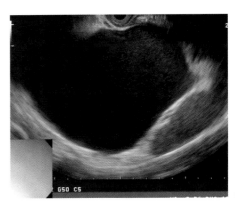

Fig. 56.96 A post-traumatic pancreatic pseudocyst in a 10-year-old boy.
a The bulging posterior wall of stomach is due to the mass effect of the pseudocyst.

b A stent entering the posterior wall of the stomach after endoscopic ultrasound–guided transgastric drainage.
c A large, simple hypoechoic cyst abutting the spleen.

References

1. Green JA, Scheeres DE, Conrad HA, Cloney DL, Schlatter MG. Pediatric ERCP in a multidisciplinary community setting: experience with a fellowship-trained general surgeon. Surg Endosc 2007;21:2187–92.
2. Lee KK, Anderson MA, Baron TH, Banerjee S, Cash BD, Dominitz JA, et al. Modifications in endoscopic practice for pediatric patients. Gastrointest Endosc 2008;67:1–9.
3. Mahajan L, Wyllie R, Steffen R, Kay M, Kitaoka G, Dettorre J, et al. The effects of a psychological preparation program on anxiety in children and adolescents undergoing gastrointestinal endoscopy. J Pediatr Gastroenterol Nutr 1998;27:161–5.
4. Ingebo KR, Rayhorn NJ, Hecht RM, Shelton MT, Silber GH, Shub MD. Sedation in children: adequacy of two-hour fasting. J Pediatr 1997;131:155–8.
5. Schriener MS, Triebwasser A, Keon TP. Ingestion of liquids compared with preoperative fasting in pediatric outpatients. Anesthesiology 1990;72:593–7.
6. Hargrove CB, Ulshen MH, Shub MD. Upper gastrointestinal endoscopy in infants: diagnostic usefulness and safety. Pediatrics 1984;74:828–31.
7. Walco GA, Cassidy RC, Schechter NL. Pain, hurt, and harm. The ethics of pain control in infants and children. N Engl J Med 1994;331:541–4.
8. Committee on Drugs of the American Academy of Pediatrics. Guidelines for monitoring and management of pediatric patients during and after sedation for diagnostic and therapeutic procedures. Pediatrics 1992;89:1110–5.
9. Schwarz SM, Lightdale JR, Liacouras CA. Sedation and anesthesia in pediatric endoscopy: one size does not fit all. J Pediatr Gastroenterol Nutr 2007;44:295–7.
10. Liacouras CA, Mascarenhas M, Poon C, Wenner WJ. Placebo-controlled trial assessing the use of oral midazolam as a premedication to conscious sedation for pediatric endoscopy. Gastrointest Endosc 1998;47:455–60.
11. Fishbein M, Lugo RA, Woodland J, Lininger B, Linscheid T. Evaluation of intranasal midazolam in children undergoing esophagogastroduodenoscopy. J Pediatr Gastroenterol Nutr 1997;25:261–6.
12. Gilger MA. Conscious sedation for endoscopy in the pediatric patient. Gastroenterol Nurs 1993;16:75–9.
13. Figueroa-Colon R, Grunow JE. Randomized study of premedication for esophagogastroduodenoscopy in children and adolescents. J Pediatr Gastroenterol Nutr 1988;7:359–66.
14. Tolia V, Fleming SL, Kauffman RE. Randomized, double-blind trial of midazolam and diazepam for endoscopic sedation in children. Dev Pharmacol Ther 1990;14:141–7.
15. Bahal OMN, Nahata MC, Murray RD, Linscheid TR, Williams T, Heitlinger LA, et al. Efficacy of diazepam and meperidine in ambulatory pediatric patients undergoing endoscopy: a randomized, double-blind trial. J Pediatr Gastroenterol Nutr 1993;16:387–92.
16. Chuang E, Wenner WJ, Piccoli DA, Altschuler SM, Liacouras CA. Intravenous sedation in pediatric upper gastrointestinal endoscopy. Gastrointest Endosc 1995;42:156–60.
17. Mamula P, Markowitz JE, Neiswender K, Zimmerman A, Wood S, Garofolo M, et al. Safety of intravenous midazolam and fentanyl for pediatric GI endoscopy: prospective study of 1578 endoscopies. Gastrointest Endosc 2007;65:203–10.
18. Abu-Shahwan I, Mack D. Propofol and remifentanil for deep sedation in children undergoing gastrointestinal endoscopy. Paediatr Anaesth 2007;17:460–3.
19. Barbi E, Petaros P, Badina L, Pahor T, Giuseppin I, Biasotto E, et al. Deep sedation with propofol for upper gastrointestinal endoscopy in children, administered by specially trained pediatricians: a prospective case series with emphasis on side effects. Endoscopy 2006;38:368–75.
20. Green SM, Klooster M, Harris T, Lynch EL, Rothrock SG. Ketamine sedation for pediatric gastroenterology procedures. J Pediatr Gastroenterol Nutr 2001;32:26–33.
21. Balsells F, Wyllie R, Kay M, Steffen R. Use of conscious sedation for lower and upper gastrointestinal endoscopic examinations in children, adolescents, and young adults: a twelve-year review. Gastrointest Endosc 1997;45:375–80.
22. Gilger MA, Jeiven SJ, Barrish JO, McCarroll LR. Oxygen desaturation and cardiac arrhythmias in children during esophagogastroduodenoscopy using conscious sedation. Gastrointest Endosc 1993;39:392–5.
23. Squires RH, Morriss F, Schluterman S, Drews B, Galyen L, Brown K. Efficacy, safety and cost of intravenous sedation versus general anesthesia in children undergoing endoscopic procedures. Gastrointest Endosc 1995;41:99–104.
24. Lamireau T, Dubreuil M, Daconceicao M. Oxygen saturation during esophagogastroduodenoscopy in children: general anesthesia versus intravenous sedation. J Pediatr Gastroenterol Nutr 1998;27:172–5.
25. Dillon M, Brown S, Casey W, Walsh D, Durnin M, Abubaker K, et al. Colonoscopy under general anesthesia in children. Pediatrics 1998;102:381–3.
26. Stringer MD, Pinfield A, Revell L, McClean P, Puntis JW. A prospective audit of paediatric colonoscopy under general anaesthesia. Acta Paediatr 1999;88:199–202.
27. Steiner SJ, Pfefferkorn MD, Fitzgerald JF. Patient-reported symptoms after pediatric outpatient colonoscopy or flexible sigmoidoscopy under general anesthesia. J Pediatr Gastroenterol Nutr 2006;43:483–6.
28. Byrne WJ, Euler AR, Campbell M, Eisenach KD. Bacteremia in children following upper gastrointestinal endoscopy or colonoscopy. J Pediatr Gastroenterol Nutr 1982;1:551–3.
29. el-Baba M, Tolia V, Lin CH, Dajani A. Absence of bacteremia after gastrointestinal procedures in children. Gastrointest Endosc 1996;44:378–81.
30. El-Serag HB, Gilger MA, Shub MD, Richardson P, Bancroft J. The prevalence of suspected Barrett's esophagus in children and adolescents: a multicenter endoscopic study. Gastrointest Endosc 2006;64:671–5.
31. Collins MH. Histopathologic features of eosinophilic esophagitis. Gastrointest Endosc Clin N Am 2008;18:59–71, viii–ix.
32. Fox VL. Eosinophilic esophagitis: endoscopic findings. Gastrointest Endosc Clin N Am 2008;18:45–57, viii.

56

33. Fox VL, JE Teitelbaum JE, Nurko SN, Furuta GT. High resolution probe endosonography in allergic esophagitis [abstract]. Gastrointest Endosc 2000;51:AB131.

34. Aceves SS, Newbury RO, Dohil R, Bastian JF, Broide DH. Esophageal remodeling in pediatric eosinophilic esophagitis. J Allergy Clin Immunol 2007;119:206–12.

35. Chehade M, Sampson HA, Morotti RA, Magid MS. Esophageal subepithelial fibrosis in children with eosinophilic esophagitis. J Pediatr Gastroenterol Nutr 2007;45:319–28.

36. Berenson GA, Wyllie R, Caulfield M, Steffen R. Intralesional steroids in the treatment of refractory esophageal strictures. J Pediatr Gastroenterol Nutr 1994;18:250–2.

37. Zein NN, Greseth JM, Perrault J. Endoscopic intralesional steroid injections in the management of refractory esophageal strictures. Gastrointest Endosc 1995;41:596–8.

38. Uhlen S, Fayoux P, Vachin F, Guimber D, Gottrand F, Turck D, et al. Mitomycin C: an alternative conservative treatment for refractory esophageal stricture in children? Endoscopy 2006;38:404–7.

39. Rosseneu S, Afzal N, Yerushalmi B, Ibarguen-Secchia E, Lewindon P, Cameron D, et al. Topical application of mitomycin-C in oesophageal strictures. J Pediatr Gastroenterol Nutr 2007;44:336–41.

40. Nurko S, Rosen R. Esophageal dysmotility in patients who have eosinophilic esophagitis. Gastrointest Endosc Clin N Am 2008;18:73–89, ix.

41. Mehra M, Bahar RJ, Ament ME, Waldhausen J, Gershman G, Georgeson K, et al. Laparoscopic and thoracoscopic esophagomyotomy for children with achalasia. J Pediatr Gastroenterol Nutr 2001;33:466–71.

42. Hurwitz M, Vargas J, Ament ME, Tolia V, Molleston J, Reinstein LJ, et al. Evaluation of the use of botulinum toxin in children with achalasia. J Pediatr Gastroenterol Nutr 2000;30:509–14.

43. Thakkar K, Gilger MA, Shulman RJ, El Serag HB. EGD in children with abdominal pain: a systematic review. Am J Gastroenterol 2007;102:654–61.

44. Cox K, Ament ME. Upper gastrointestinal bleeding in children and adolescents. Pediatrics 1979;63:408–13.

45. Chang MH, Wang TH, Hsu JY, Lee TC, Wang CY, Yu JY. Endoscopic examination of the upper gastrointestinal tract in infancy. Gastrointest Endosc 1983;29:15–7.

46. Quak SH, Lam SK, Low PS. Upper gastrointestinal endoscopy in children. Singapore Medical Journal 1990;31:123–6.

47. Noronha PA, Leist MH. Endoscopic laser therapy for gastrointestinal bleeding from congenital vascular lesions. J Pediatr Gastroenterol Nutr 1988;7:375–8.

48. Kato S, Ozawa A, Ebina K, Nakagawa H. Endoscopic ethanol injection for treatment of bleeding peptic ulcer. Eur J Pediatr 1994;153:873–5.

49. Murray KF, Jennings RW, Fox VL. Endoscopic band ligation of a Dieulafoy lesion in the small intestine of a child. Gastrointest Endosc 1996;44:336–9.

50. Ebina K, Kato S, Abukawa D, Nakagawa H. Endoscopic hemostasis of bleeding duodenal ulcer in a child with Henoch–Schönlein purpura. J Pediatr 1997;131:934–6.

51. Kong MS, Wang KL, Wong HF. Endoscopic injection sclerotherapy for esophageal variceal bleeding in children with extrahepatic portal vein obstruction. J Formos Med Assoc 1994;93:885–7.

52. Hassall E, Berquist W, Ament M, Vargas J, Dorney S. Sclerotherapy for extrahepatic portal hypertension in childhood. J Pediatr 1989;115:69–74.

53. Stringer MD, Howard ER. Long term outcome after injection sclerotherapy for oesophageal varices in children with extrahepatic portal hypertension. Gut 1994;35:257–9.

54. Yachha SK, Sharma BC, Kumar M, Khanduri A. Endoscopic sclerotherapy for esophageal varices in children with extrahepatic portal venous obstruction: a follow-up study. J Pediatr Gastroenterol Nutr 1997;24:49–52.

55. Sokal EM, Van Hoorebeeck N, Van Obbergh L, Otte JB, Buts JP. Upper gastrointestinal tract bleeding in cirrhotic children candidates for liver transplantation. Eur J Pediatr 1992;151:326–8.

56. Paquet KJ, Lazar A. Current therapeutic strategy in bleeding esophageal varices in babies and children and long-term results of endoscopic paravariceal sclerotherapy over twenty years. Eur J Pediatr Surg 1994;4:165–72.

57. Hill ID, Bowie MD. Endoscopic sclerotherapy for control of bleeding varices in children. Am J Gastroenterol 1991;86:472–6.

58. Maksoud JG, Goncalves ME. Treatment of portal hypertension in children. World J Surg 1994;18:251–8.

59. Thapa BR, Mehta S. Endoscopic sclerotherapy of esophageal varices in infants and children. J Pediatr Gastroenterol Nutr 1990;10:430–4.

60. Howard E, Stringer M, Mowat A. Assessment of injection sclerotherapy in the management of 152 children with oesophageal varices. Br J Surg 1988;75:404–8.

61. Sarin SK, Misra SP, Singal AK, Thorat V, Broor SL. Endoscopic sclerotherapy for varices in children. J Pediatr Gastroenterol Nutr 1988;7:662–6.

62. Donovan TJ, Ward M, Shepherd RW. Evaluation of endoscopic sclerotherapy of esophageal varices in children. J Pediatr Gastroenterol Nutr 1986;5:696–700.

63. Stellen GP, Lilly JR. Esophageal endosclerosis in children. Surgery 1985;98:970–5.

64. Spence RA, Anderson JR, Johnston GW. Twenty-five years of injection sclerotherapy for bleeding varices. Br J Surg 1985;72:195–8.

65. Vane DW, Boles ET Jr, Clatworthy HW Jr. Esophageal sclerotherapy: an effective modality in children. J Pediatr Surg 1985;20:703–7.

66. Hicsonmez A, Karaguzel G, Tanyel FC. Duodenal varices causing intractable gastrointestinal bleeding in a 12-year-old child. Eur J Pediatr Surg 1994;4:176–7.

67. Heaton ND, Davenport M, Howard ER. Symptomatic hemorrhoids and anorectal varices in children with portal hypertension. J Pediatr Surg 1992;27:833–5.

68. Millar AJ, Brown RA, Hill ID, Rode H, Cywes S. The fundal pile: bleeding gastric varices. J Pediatr Surg 1991;26:707–9.

69. Fuster S, Costaguta A, Tobacco O. Treatment of bleeding gastric varices with tissue adhesive (Histoacryl) in children. Endoscopy 1998;30:S 39–40.

70. Fox VL, Carr-Locke DL, Connors PJ, Leichtner AM. Endoscopic ligation of esophageal varices in children. J Pediatr Gastroenterol Nutr 1995;20:202–8.

71. Cano I, Urruzuno P, Medina E, Vilarino A, Benavent MI, Manzanares J, et al. Treatment of esophageal varices by endoscopic ligation in children. Eur J Pediatr Surg 1995;5:299–302.

72. Price MR, Sartorelli KH, Karrer FM, Narkewicz MR, Sokol RJ, Lilly JR. Management of esophageal varices in children by endoscopic variceal ligation. J Pediatr Surg 1996;31:1056–9.

73. Sasaki T, Hasegawa T, Nakajima K, Tanano H, Wasa M, Fukui Y, et al. Endoscopic variceal ligation in the management of gastroesophageal varices in postoperative biliary atresia. J Pediatr Surg 1998;33:1628–32.

74. McKiernan PJ, Beath SV, Davison SM. A prospective study of endoscopic esophageal variceal ligation using a multiband ligator. J Pediatr Gastroenterol Nutr 2002;34:207–11.

75. Poddar U, Thapa BR, Singh K. Band ligation plus sclerotherapy versus sclerotherapy alone in children with extrahepatic portal venous obstruction. J Clin Gastroenterol 2005;39:626–9.

76. Celinska-Cedro D, Teisseyre M, Woynarowski M, Socha P, Socha J, Ryzko J. Endoscopic ligation of esophageal varices for prophylaxis of first bleeding in children and adolescents with portal hypertension: preliminary results of a prospective study. J Pediatr Surg 2003;38:1008–11.

77. Ohnuma N, Takahashi H, Tanabe M, Yoshida H, Iwai J, Muramatsu T. Endoscopic variceal ligation using a clipping apparatus in children with portal hypertension. Endoscopy 1997;29:86–90.

78. Mitsunaga T, Yoshida H, Kouchi K, Hishiki T, Saito T, Yamada S, et al. Pediatric gastroesophageal varices: treatment strategy and long-term results. J Pediatr Surg 2006;41:1980–3.

79. Gupta SK, Croffie JM, Fitzgerald JF. Is esophagogastroduodenoscopy necessary in all caustic ingestions? J Pediatr Gastroenterol Nutr 2001;32:50–3.

80. Betalli P, Falchetti D, Giuliani S, Pane A, Dall'Oglio L, de Angelis GL, et al. Caustic ingestion in children: is endoscopy always indicated? The results of an Italian multicenter observational study. Gastrointest Endosc 2008;68:434–9.

81. Gaudreault P, Parent M, McGuigan MA, Chicoine L, Lovejoy FH Jr. Predictability of esophageal injury from signs and symptoms: a study of caustic ingestion in 378 children. Pediatrics 1983;71:767–70.

82. De Peppo F, Zaccara A, Dall'Oglio L, Federici di Abriola G, Ponticelli A, Marchetti P, et al. Stenting for caustic strictures: esophageal replacement replaced. J Pediatr Surg 1998;33:54–7.

83. Anderson KD, Rouse TM, Randolph JG. A controlled trial of corticosteroids in children with corrosive injury of the esophagus. N Engl J Med 1990;323:637–40.

84. Olutoye OO, Shulman RJ, Cotton RT. Mitomycin C in the management of pediatric caustic esophageal strictures: a case report. J Pediatr Surg 2006;41:e1–3.

85. Byrne WJ. Foreign bodies, bezoars, and caustic ingestions. Gastrointest Endosc Clin N Am 1994;4:99–119.

86. Litovitz T, Schmitz BF. Ingestion of cylindrical and button batteries: an analysis of 2382 cases. Pediatrics 1992;89(4 Pt 2):747–57.

87. Fergusson JA, Malecky G, Simpson E. Lead foreign body ingestion in children. J Paediatr Child Health 1997;33:542–4.

88. St Clair WS, Benjamin J. Lead intoxication from ingestion of fishing sinkers: a case study and review of the literature. Clin Pediatr (Phila) 2008;47:66–70.

89. Gauderer MW, Ponsky JL, Izant RJ Jr. Gastrostomy without laparotomy: a percutaneous endoscopic technique. J Pediatr Surg 1980;15:872–5.

90. Avitsland TL, Kristensen C, Emblem R, Veenstra M, Mala T, Bjornland K. Percutaneous endoscopic gastrostomy in children: a safe technique with major symptom relief and high parental satisfaction. J Pediatr Gastroenterol Nutr 2006;43:624–8.

91. Croaker GD, Najmaldin AS. Laparoscopically assisted percutaneous endoscopic gastrostomy. Pediatr Surg Int 1997;12:130–1.

92. Kohler H, Razeghi S, Spychalski N, Behrens R, Carbon R. Laparoscopic-assisted percutaneous endoscopic gastrostomy—rendez-vous PEG—in infants, children and adolescents. Endoscopy 2007;39(Suppl 1):E136.

93. Crombleholme TM, Jacir NN. Simplified "push" technique for percutaneous endoscopic gastrostomy in children. J Pediatr Surg 1993;28:1393–5.

94. Robertson FM, Crombleholme TM, Latchaw LA, Jacir NN. Modification of the "push" technique for percutaneous endoscopic gastrostomy in infants and children. J Am Coll Surg 1996;182:215–8.

95. Treem WR, Etienne NL, Hyams JS. Percutaneous endoscopic placement of the "button" gastrostomy tube as the initial procedure in infants and children. J Pediatr Gastroenterol Nutr 1993;17:382–6.

96. Gauderer MW, Abrams RS, Hammond JH. Initial experience with the changeable skin-level port-valve: a new concept for long-term gastrointestinal access. J Pediatr Surg 1998;33:73–5.

97. Virnig DJ, Frech EJ, Delegge MH, Fang JC. Direct percutaneous endoscopic jejunostomy: a case series in pediatric patients. Gastrointest Endosc 2008;67:984–7.

98. Rothbaum RJ. Complications of pediatric endoscopy. Gastrointest Endosc Clin N Am 1996;6:445–59.

99. Ament ME. Prospective study of risks of complication in 6,424 procedures in pediatric gastroenterology [abstract]. Pediatr Res 1981;15:524.

100. Ghishan FK, Werner M, Vieira P, Kuttesch J, DeHaro R. Intramural duodenal hematoma: an unusual complication of endoscopic small bowel biopsy. Am J Gastroenterol 1987;82:368–70.

101. Szajewska H, Albrecht P, Ziolkowski J, Kubica W. Intramural duodenal hematoma: an unusual complication of duodenal biopsy sampling. J Pediatr Gastroenterol Nutr 1993;16:331–3.

102. Karjoo M, Luisiri A, Silberstein M, Kane RE. Duodenal hematoma and acute pancreatitis after upper gastrointestinal endoscopy. Gastrointest Endosc 1994;40:493–5.

103. Lipson SA, Perr HA, Koerper MA, Ostroff JW, Snyder JD, Goldstein RB. Intramural duodenal hematoma after endoscopic biopsy in leukemic patients. Gastrointest Endosc 1996;44:620–3.

104. Ramakrishna J, Treem WR. Duodenal hematoma as a complication of endoscopic biopsy in pediatric bone marrow transplant recipients. J Pediatr Gastroenterol Nutr 1997;25:426–9.

105. Guzman C, Bousvaros A, Buonomo C, Nurko S. Intraduodenal hematoma complicating intestinal biopsy: case reports and review of the literature. Am J Gastroenterol 1998;93:2547–50.

106. Desmond PV, MacMahon RA. Fatal air embolism following endoscopy of a hepatic portoenterostomy. Endoscopy 1990;22:236.

107. Davidson PM, Catto-Smith AG, Beasley SW. Technique and complications of percutaneous endoscopic gastrostomy in children. Aust N Z J Surg 1995;65:194–6.

108. Fox VL, Abel SD, Malas S, Duggan C, Leichtner AM. Complications following percutaneous endoscopic gastrostomy and subsequent catheter replacement in children and young adults. Gastrointest Endosc 1997;45:64–71.

109. Behrens R, Lang T, Muschweck H, Richter T, Hofbeck M. Percutaneous endoscopic gastrostomy in children and adolescents. J Pediatr Gastroenterol Nutr 1997;25:487–91.

110. Marin OE, Glassman MS, Schoen BT, Caplan DB. Safety and efficacy of percutaneous endoscopic gastrostomy in children. Am J Gastroenterol 1994;89:357–61.

111. Khattak IU, Kimber C, Kiely EM, Spitz L. Percutaneous endoscopic gastrostomy in paediatric practice: complications and outcome. J Pediatr Surg 1998;33:67–72.

112. Romero R, Martinez FL, Robinson SYJ, Sullivan K, Hart MH. Complicated PEG-to-skin level gastrostomy conversions: analysis of risk factors for tract disruption. Gastrointest Endosc 1996;44:230–4.

113. Benkov KJ. When "buttoning up" is not sound advice. J Pediatr Gastroenterol Nutr 1993;17:358–60.

114. Berman JH, Radhakrishman J, Kraut JR. Button gastrostomy obstructing the ileocecal valve removed by colonoscopic retrieval. J Pediatr Gastroenterol Nutr 1991;13:426–8.

115. Yaseen M, Steele MI, Grunow JE. Nonendoscopic removal of percutaneous endoscopic gastrostomy tubes: morbidity and mortality in children. Gastrointest Endosc 1996;44:235–8.

116. Shah MD, Berman WF. Endoscopic balloon dilation of esophageal strictures in children. Gastrointest Endosc 1993;39:153–6.

117. Seidman E, Weber A, Morin C, Ethier R, Lamarche J, Guerguerian A, et al. Spinal cord paralysis following sclerotherapy for esophageal varices. Hepatology 1984;4:950–4.

118. Darbari A, Kalloo AN, Cuffari C. Diagnostic yield, safety, and efficacy of push enteroscopy in pediatrics. Gastrointest Endosc 2006;64:224–8.

119. Sidhu R, Sanders DS, McAlindon ME, Thomson M. Capsule endoscopy and enteroscopy: modern modalities to investigate the small bowel in paediatrics. Arch Dis Child 2008;93:154–9.

120. Haruta H, Yamamoto H, Mizuta K, Kita Y, Uno T, Egami S, et al. A case of successful enteroscopic balloon dilation for late anastomotic stricture of choledochojejunostomy after living donor liver transplantation. Liver Transpl 2005;11:1608–10.

121. Leung YK. Double balloon endoscopy in pediatric patients. Gastrointest Endosc 2007;66(3 Suppl):S 54–6.

122. Fox VL. Approach to the pediatric patient. In: Faigel DO, Cave DR, editors. Capsule endoscopy. London: Elsevier; 2008. Chapter 12.

123. Holden JP, Dureja P, Pfau PR, Schwartz DC, Reichelderfer M, Judd RH, et al. Endoscopic placement of the small-bowel video capsule by using a capsule endoscope delivery device. Gastrointest Endosc 2007;65:842–7.

124. Ingebo KB, Heyman MB. Polyethylene glycol–electrolyte solution for intestinal clearance in children with refractory encopresis. A safe and effective therapeutic program. Am J Dis Child 1988;142:340–2.

125. Sondheimer JM, Sokol RJ, Taylor SF, Silverman A. Safety, efficacy, and tolerance of intestinal lavage in pediatric patients undergoing diagnostic colonoscopy. J Pediatr 1991;119:148–52.

126. Sabri M, Di Lorenzo C, Henderson W, Thompson W, Barksdale E Jr, Khan S. Colon cleansing with oral sodium phosphate in adolescents: dose, efficacy, acceptability, and safety. Am J Gastroenterol 2008;103:1533–40.

127. Pashankar DS, Uc A, Bishop WP. Polyethylene glycol 3350 without electrolytes: a new safe, effective, and palatable bowel preparation for colonoscopy in children. J Pediatr 2004;144:358–62.

128. Safder S, Demintieva Y, Rewalt M, Elitsur Y. Stool consistency and stool frequency are excellent clinical markers for adequate colon preparation after polyethylene glycol 3350 cleansing protocol: a prospective clinical study in children. Gastrointest Endosc 2008;68:1131–5.

129. Sanderson IR, Boyle S, Williams CB, Walker-Smith JA. Histologic abnormalities in biopsies from macroscopically normal colonoscopies. Arch Dis Child 1986;61:274–7.

130. Fox VL. Gastrointestinal bleeding in infancy and childhood. Gastroenterol Clin N Am 2000;29:37–66.

131. Sondheimer JM, Sokol RJ, Narkewicz MR, Tyson RW. Anastomotic ulceration: a late complication of ileocolonic anastomosis. J Pediatr 1995;127:225–30.

132. Bhargava SA, Putnam PE, Kocoshis SA. Gastrointestinal bleeding due to delayed perianastomotic ulceration in children. Am J Gastroenterol 1995;90:807–9.

133. Eigenmann PA, Le Coultre C, Cox J, Dederding JP, Belli DC. Solitary rectal ulcer: an unusual cause of rectal bleeding in children. Eur J Pediatr 1992;151:658–60.

134. De la Rubia L, Ruiz Villaespesa A, Cebrero M, Garcia de Frias E. Solitary rectal ulcer syndrome in a child. J Pediatr 1993;122:733–6.

135. Dehghani SM, Haghighat M, Imanieh MH, Geramizadeh B. Solitary rectal ulcer syndrome in children: a prospective study of cases from southern Iran. Eur J Gastroenterol Hepatol 2008;20:93–5.

136. Perisic VN. Colorectal polyps: an important cause of rectal bleeding. Arch Dis Child 1987;62:188–9.

137. Horrilleno EG, Eckert C, Ackerman LV. Polyps of the rectum and colon in children. Cancer 1957;10:131–7.

138. Cynamon HA, Milor DE, Andres JM. Diagnosis and management of colonic polyps in children. J Pediatr 1989;114:593–6.

139. Howe JR, Roth S, Ringold JC, Summers RW, Jarvinen HJ, Sistonen P, et al. Mutations in the SMAD4/DPC4 gene in juvenile polyposis. Science 1998;280:1086–8.

140. Howe JR, Bair JL, Sayed MG, Anderson ME, Mitros FA, Petersen GM, et al. Germline mutations of the gene encoding bone morphogenetic protein receptor 1A in juvenile polyposis. Nat Genet 2001;28:184–7.

141. Zhou XP, Woodford-Richens K, Lehtonen R, Kurose K, Aldred M, Hampel H, et al. Germline mutations in BMPR1A/ALK3 cause a subset of cases of

56

juvenile polyposis syndrome and of Cowden and Bannayan–Riley–Ruval-caba syndromes. Am J Hum Genet 2001;69:704–11.

142. Coburn MC, Pricolo VE, DeLuca FG, Bland KI. Malignant potential in intestinal juvenile polyposis syndromes. Ann Surg Oncol 1995;2:386–91.

143. Azizkhan RG. Life-threatening hematochezia from a rectosigmoid vascular malformation in Klippel–Trenaunay syndrome: long-term palliation using an argon laser. J Pediatr Surg 1991;26:1125–8.

144. Oranje AP. Blue rubber bleb nevus syndrome. Pediatr Dermatol 1986;3:304–10.

145. Tooson JD, Marsano LS, Gates LK Jr. Pediatric rectal Dieulafoy's lesion. Am J Gastroenterol 1995;90:2232–3.

146. Jenkins HR, Pincott JR, Soothill JF, Milla PJ, Harries JT. Food allergy: the major cause of infantile colitis. Arch Dis Child 1984;59:326–9.

147. Odze RD, Wershil BK, Leichtner AM, Antoniolli DA. Allergic colitis in infants. J Pediatr 1995;126:163–70.

148. Lake AM, Whitington PF, Hamilton SR. Dietary protein-induced colitis in breast-fed infants. J Pediatr 1982;101:906–10.

149. Ravelli A, Villanacci V, Chiappa S, Bolognini S, Manenti S, Fuoti M. Dietary protein-induced proctocolitis in childhood. Am J Gastroenterol 2008;103:2605–12.

150. Goldman H, Proujansky R. Allergic proctitis and gastroenteritis in children: clinical and mucosal biopsy features in 53 cases. Am J Surg Pathol 1986;10: 75–86.

151. Odze RD, Bines J, Leichtner AM, Goldman H, Antonioli DA. Allergic proctocolitis in infants: a prospective clinicopathologic biopsy study. Hum Pathol 1993;24:668–74.

152. Holmquist L, Rudic N, Ahren C, Fallstrom SP. The diagnostic value of colonoscopy compared with rectosigmoidoscopy in children and adolescents with symptoms of chronic inflammatory bowel disease of the colon. Scand J Gastroenterol 1988;23:577–84.

153. Cohen M, Thomson M, Taylor C, Donatone J, Quijano G, Drut R. Colonic and duodenal flat adenomas in children with classical familial adenomatous polyposis. Int J Surg Pathol 2006;14:133–40.

154. Jerkic S, Rosewich H, Scharf JG, Perske C, Fuzesi L, Wilichowski E, et al. Colorectal cancer in two pre-teenage siblings with familial adenomatous polyposis. Eur J Pediatr 2005;164:306–10.

155. Tomlinson IP, Houlston RS. Peutz–Jeghers syndrome. J Med Genet 1997;34:1007–11.

156. Giardiello FM, Hamilton SR, Kern SE, Offerhaus GJA, Green PA, Celano P, et al. Colorectal neoplasia in juvenile polyposis or juvenile polyps. Arch Dis Child 1991;66:971–5.

157. Järvinen H, Franssila KO. Familial juvenile polyposis coli: increased risk of colorectal cancer. Gut 1984;25:792–800.

158. Boardman LA, Thibodeau SN, Schaid DJ, Lindor NM, McDonnell SK, Burgart LJ, et al. Increased risk for cancer in patients with the Peutz–Jeghers syndrome. Ann Intern Med 1998;128:896–9.

159. Sharma AK, Sharma SS, Mathur P. Familial juvenile polyposis with adenomatous–carcinomatous change. J Gastroenterol Hepatol 1995;10:131–4.

160. Waite KA, Eng C. Protean PTEN: form and function. Am J Hum Genet 2002;70:829–44.

161. Griffiths AM, Sherman PM. Colonoscopic surveillance for cancer in ulcerative colitis: a critical review. J Pediatr Gastroenterol Nutr 1997;24:202–10.

162. DePeppo F, Iacobelli BD, DeGennaro M, Colajacomo M, Rivosecchi M. Percutaneous endoscopic cecostomy for antegrade colonic irrigation in fecally incontinent children. Endoscopy 1999;31:501–3.

163. Rawat DJ, Haddad M, Geoghegan N, Clarke S, Fell JM. Percutaneous endoscopic colostomy of the left colon: a new technique for management of intractable constipation in children. Gastrointest Endosc 2004;60:39–43.

164. Gans SL, Ament M, Cristie DL. Pediatric endoscopy with flexible fiberscopes. J Pediatr Surg 1975;10:375–80.

165. Holgersen LO, Mossberg SM, Miller RE. Colonoscopy for rectal bleeding in childhood. J Pediatr Surg 1978;13:83–5.

166. Habr-Gama A, Alves PRA, Gama-Rodrigues JJ, Teixeira MG, Barbieri D. Pediatric colonoscopy. Dis Colon Rectum 1979;22:530–5.

167. Howdle PD, Littlewood JM, Firth J, Losowsky MS. Routine colonoscopy service. Arch Dis Child 1984;59:790–3.

168. Bartnik W, Butruk E, Ryzko J, Rondio H, Rasinski A, Orlowska J. Short- and long-term results of colonoscopic polypectomy in children. Gastrointest Endosc 1986;32:389–92.

169. Jalihal A, Misra SP, Arvind AS, Kamath PS. Colonoscopic polypectomy in children. J Pediatr Surg 1992;27:1220–2.

170. Livstone EM, Cohen GM, Troncale FJ, Touloukian RJ. Diastatic serosal lacerations: An unrecognized complication of colonoscopy. Gastroenterology 1974;76:1245–7.

171. Waye JD. Endoscopic retrograde cholangiopancreatography in the infant. Am J Gastroenterol 1976;65:461–3.

172. Brown KO, Goldschmiedt M. Endoscopic therapy of biliary and pancreatic disorders in children. Endoscopy 1994;26:719–23.

173. Tarnasky PR, Tagge EP, Hebra A, Othersen B, Adams DB, Cunningham JT, et al. Minimally invasive therapy for choledocholithiasis in children. Gastrointest Endosc 1998;47:189–92.

174. Guelrud M. Endoscopic therapy of pancreatic disease in children. Gastrointest Endosc Clin N Am 1998;8:195–219.

175. Hsu RK, Draganov P, Leung JW, Tarnasky PR, Yu AS, Hawes RH. Therapeutic ERCP in the management of pancreatitis in children. Gastrointest Endosc 2000;51:396–400.

176. Cheng CL, Fogel EL, Sherman S, McHenry L, Watkins JL, Croffie JM, et al. Diagnostic and therapeutic endoscopic retrograde cholangiopancreatography in children: a large series report. J Pediatr Gastroenterol Nutr 2005;41:445–53.

177. Guelrud M, Morera C, Rodriguez M, Prados JG, Jaen D. Normal and anomalous pancreaticobiliary union in children and adolescents. Gastrointest Endosc 1999;50:189–93.

178. Watkins JL, Etzkorn KP, Wiley TE, DeGuzman L, Harig JM. Assessment of technical competence during ERCP training. Gastrointest Endosc 1996;44:411–5.

179. Jowell PS, Branch S, Affronti J, Bute BP, Browning CL, Baillie J. At least 180 ERCPs are needed to attain competence in diagnostic and therapeutic ERCP [abstract]. Gastrointest Endosc 1996;44:314.

180. Jowell PS, Baillie J, Branch S, Affronti J, Browning CL, Bute BP. Quantitative assessment of procedural competence: a prospective study of training in retrograde cholangiopancreatography. Ann Intern Med 1996;125:983–9.

181. Fox VL, Werlin SL, Heyman MB. ERCP in children: a position statement from the North American Society for Pediatric Gastroenterology and Nutrition. J Pediatr Gastroenterol Nutr 2000;30:335–42.

182. Aabakken L, Bretthauer M, Line PD. Double-balloon enteroscopy for endoscopic retrograde cholangiography in patients with a Roux-en-Y anastomosis. Endoscopy 2007;39:1068–71.

183. Yamataka A, Kuwatsuru R, Shima H, Kobayashi H, Lane G, Segawa O, et al. Initial experience with non-breath-hold magnetic resonance cholangiopancreatography: a new noninvasive technique for the diagnosis of choledochal cyst in children. J Pediatr Surg 1997;32:1560–2.

184. Hirohashi S, Hirohashi R, Uchida H, Akira M, Itoh T, Haku E, et al. Pancreatitis: evaluation with MR cholangiopancreatography in children. Radiology 1997;203:411–5.

185. Ernst O, Gottrand F, Calvo M, Michaud L, Sergent G, Mizrahi D, et al. Congenital hepatic fibrosis: findings at MR cholangiopancreatography. AJR Am J Roentgenol 1998;170:409–12.

186. Miyazaki T, Yamashita Y, Tang Y, Tsuchigame T, Takahashi M, Sera Y. Single-shot MR cholangiopancreatography of neonates, infants, and young children. AJR Am J Roentgenol 1998;170:33–7.

187. Matos C, Nicaise N, Devière J, Cassart M, Metens T, Struyven J, et al. Choledochal cysts: comparison of findings at MR cholangiopancreatography and endoscopic retrograde cholangiopancreatography in eight patients. Radiology 1998;209:443–8.

188. Brown DL, Teele RL, Doubilet PM, DiSalvo DN, Benson CB, Ban Alstyne GA. Echogenic material in the fetal gallbladder: sonographic and clinical observations. Radiology 1992;182:73–6.

189. Wilkinson ML, Clayton PT. Sphincterotomy for jaundice in a neonate. J Pediatr Gastroenterol Nutr 1996;23:507–9.

190. Todani T, Watanabe Y, Narusue M, Tabuchi K, Okajima K. Classification, operative procedures and review of thirty seven cases including cancer arising from choledochal cyst. Am J Surg 1977;134:263–9.

191. Houben CH, Chiu PW, Lau J, Lee KH, Ng EK, Tam YH, et al. Preoperative endoscopic retrograde cholangiopancreatographic treatment of complicated choledochal cysts in children: a retrospective case series. Endoscopy 2007;39:836–9.

192. Venu RP, Geenen JE, Hogan WJ, Dodds WJ, Wilson SW, Stewart ET, et al. Role of endoscopic retrograde cholangiopancreatography in the diagnosis and treatment of choledochocele. Gastroenterology 1984;87:1144–9.

193. Ng WD, Liu K, Wong MK, Kong CK, Lee K, Chan YT, et al. Endoscopic sphincterotomy in young patients with choledochal dilatation and a long common channel: a preliminary report. Br J Surg 1992;79:550–2.

194. Chapoy PR, Kendall RS, Fonkalsrud E, Ament ME. Congenital stricture of the common hepatic duct: an unusual case without jaundice. Gastroenterology 1981;80:380–3.

195. Stoker J, Lameris JS, Robben SG, Dees J, Sinaasappel M. Primary sclerosing cholangitis in a child treated by nonsurgical balloon dilatation and stenting. J Pediatr Gastroenterol Nutr 1993;17:303–6.

X

196. Iinuma Y, Narisawa R, Iwafuchi M, Uchiyama M, Naito M, Yagi M, et al. The role of endoscopic retrograde cholangiopancreatography in infants with cholestasis. J Pediatr Surg 2000;35:545–9.

197. Ohnuma N, Takahashi H, Tanabe M, Yoshida H, Iwai J. The role of ERCP in biliary atresia. Gastrointest Endosc 1997;45:365–70.

198. Guelrud M, Jaen D, Mendoza S, Plaz J, Torres P. ERCP in the diagnosis of extrahepatic biliary atresia. Gastrointest Endosc 1991;37:522–6.

199. Graham KS, Ingram JD, Steinberg SE, Narkewicz MR. ERCP in the management of pediatric pancreatitis. Gastrointest Endosc 1998;47:492–5.

200. Mori K, Nagakawa T, Ohta T, Nakano T, Kayahara M, Akiyama T, et al. Pancreatitis and anomalous union of the pancreaticobiliary ductal system in childhood. J Pediatr Surg 1993;28:67–71.

201. Guelrud M, Mujica C, Jaen D, Plaz J, Arias J. The role of ERCP in the diagnosis and treatment of idiopathic recurrent pancreatitis in children and adolescents. Gastrointest Endosc 1994;40:428–36.

202. Black PR, Welch KJ, Eraklis AJ. Juxtapancreatic intestinal duplication with pancreatic ductal communication: a cause of pancreatitis and recurrent abdominal pain in childhood. J Pediatr Surg 1986;21:257–61.

203. Warshaw A, Simeone J, Schapiro R. Evaluation and treatment of the dominant dorsal duct syndrome (pancreas divisum redefined). Am J Surg 1990;159:59–66.

204. Kozarek R, Christie D, Barklay G. Endoscopic therapy of pancreatitis in the pediatric population. Gastrointest Endosc 1993;39:665–9.

205. Brown CW, Werlin SL, Geenen JE, Schmalz M. The diagnostic and therapeutic role of endoscopic retrograde cholangiopancreatography in children. J Pediatr Gastroenterol Nutr 1993;17:19–23.

206. Lemmel T, Hawes R, Sherman S, Earle D, Lehman G, Smith M, et al. Endoscopic evaluation and therapy of recurrent pancreatitis and pancreatobiliary pain in the pediatric population [abstract]. Gastrointest Endosc 1994;40:54.

207. Kimble RM, Cohen R, Williams S. Successful endoscopic drainage of a posttraumatic pancreatic pseudocyst in a child. J Pediatr Surg 1999;34:1518–20.

208. Patty I, Kalaoui M, Al-Shamali M, Al-Hassan F, Al-Naqeeb B. Endoscopic drainage for pancreatic pseudocyst in children. J Pediatr Surg 2001;36:503–5.

209. Bridoux-Henno L, Dabadie A, Rambeau M, Gall EL, Bretagne JF. Successful endoscopic drainage of a pancreatic pseudocyst in a 17-month-old boy. Eur J Pediatr 2004;163:482–4.

210. Al-Shanafey S, Shun A, Williams S. Endoscopic drainage of pancreatic pseudocysts in children. J Pediatr Surg 2004;39:1062–5.

211. Rescorla FJ, Plumley DA, Sherman S, Scherer LR 3 rd, West KW, Grosfeld JL. The efficacy of early ERCP in pediatric pancreatic trauma. J Pediatr Surg 1995;30:336–40.

212. Reimann JF, Koch H. Endoscopy of the biliary tract and the pancreas in children. Endoscopy 1978;10:166–72.

213. Guelrud M, Morera C, Rodriguez M, Jaen D, Pierre R. Sphincter of Oddi dysfunction in children with recurrent pancreatitis and anomalous pancreatobiliary union: an etiologic concept. Gastrointest Endosc 1999;50:194–9.

214. Varadarajulu S, Wilcox CM. Endoscopic management of sphincter of Oddi dysfunction in children. J Pediatr Gastroenterol Nutr 2006;42:526–30.

215. Misra S, Treanor MR, Vegunta RK, Chen CC. Sphincter of Oddi dysfunction in children with recurrent abdominal pain: 5-year follow-up after endoscopic sphincterotomy. J Gastroenterol Hepatol 2007;22:2246–50.

216. Kato S, Fujita N, Shibuya H, Nakagawa H. Endoscopic ultrasonography in a child with chronic pancreatitis. Acta Paediatr Jpn 1993;35:151–3.

217. Yachha SK, Dhiman RK, Gupta R, Ghoshal UC. Endosonographic evaluation of the rectum in children with extrahepatic portal venous obstruction. J Pediatr Gastroenterol Nutr 1996;23:438–41.

218. Roseau G, Palazzo L, Dumontier I, Mougenot JF, Chaussade S, Navarro J, et al. Endoscopic ultrasonography in the evaluation of pediatric digestive diseases: preliminary results. Endoscopy 1998;30:477–81.

219. Varadarajulu S, Wilcox CM, Eloubeidi MA. Impact of EUS in the evaluation of pancreaticobiliary disorders in children. Gastrointest Endosc 2005;62:239–44.

220. Fox VL, Nurko S, Teitelbaum JE, Badizadegan K, Furuta GT. High-resolution EUS in children with eosinophilic "allergic" esophagitis. Gastrointest Endosc 2003;57:30–6.

221. Takamizawa S, Tsugawa C, Mouri N, Satoh S, Kanegawa K, Nishijima E, et al. Congenital esophageal stenosis: therapeutic strategy based on etiology. J Pediatr Surg 2002;37:197–201.

222. Kouchi K, Yoshida H, Matsunaga T, Ohtsuka Y, Nagatake E, Satoh Y, et al. Endosonographic evaluation in two children with esophageal stenosis. J Pediatr Surg 2002;37:934–6.

223. Usui N, Kamata S, Kawahara H, Sawai T, Nakajima K, Soh H, et al. Usefulness of endoscopic ultrasonography in the diagnosis of congenital esophageal stenosis. J Pediatr Surg 2002;37:1744–6.

224. Fishman SJ, Fox VL. Visceral vascular anomalies. Gastrointest Endosc Clin N Am 2001;11:813–34, viii.

225. Antillon MR, Shah RJ, Stiegmann G, Chen YK. Single-step EUS-guided transmural drainage of simple and complicated pancreatic pseudocysts. Gastrointest Endosc 2006;63:797–803.

226. Emblem R, Diseth T, Morkrid L, Stien R, Bjordal R. Anal endosonography and physiology in adolescents with corrected low anorectal anomalies. J Pediatr Surg 1994;29:447–51.

227. Emblem R, Diseth T, Morkrid L. Anorectal anomalies: anorectal manometric function and anal endosonography in relation to functional outcome. Pediatr Surg Int 1997;12:516–9.

228. Jones NM, Smilgin-Humphreys M, Sullivan PB, Grant HW. Paediatric anal endosonography. Pediatr Surg Int 2003;19:703–6.

229. Keshtgar AS, Ward HC, Richards C, Clayden GS. Outcome of excision of megarectum in children with anorectal malformation. J Pediatr Surg 2007;42:227–33.

56

Index